TEXTBOOK OF
UNCOMMON CANCER

TEXTBOOK OF UNCOMMON CANCER

EDITED BY

C.J. WILLIAMS
CRC Medical Oncology Unit
University of Southampton
Southampton, UK

J.G. KRIKORIAN
Framingham, Massachusetts, USA

M.R. GREEN
Department of Medical Oncology
University of California at San Diego
California, USA

D. RAGHAVAN
Department of Clinical Oncology
Royal Prince Alfred Hospital
Sydney, Australia

A Wiley Medical Publication

JOHN WILEY & SONS
Chichester · New York · Brisbane · Toronto · Singapore

Distributed in the United States of America, Canada and Japan by Alan R. Liss Inc.,
41 East 11th Street, New York, NY 10003, USA.

Library of Congress Cataloging-in-Publication Data

Textbook of uncommon cancer

    (A Wiley medical publication)
    1. Cancer.   I. Williams, C.J. (Christopher John Hacon)   II. Series.
[DNLM: 1. Neoplasms. QZ 200 T3556] RC262. T43 1988   616.99′4   87-23141
ISBN 0 471 90968 8

British Library Cataloguing in Publication Data

Textbook of uncommon cancer
   1. Cancer—Diagnosis
   I. Williams, Chris, *1946–*
   616.99′4075   RC270

ISBN 0 471 90968 8

Printed in Great Britain
at the Alden Press, Osney Mead, Oxford

Contents

Section IX: Ophthalmic Tumours

Section X: Head and Neck Tumours

List of Contributors

B. ADDIS — Consultant Histopathologist, The Brompton Hospital and Institute for Cardiovascular and Chest Medicine, The Brompton Hospital, London, UK

C.R. ANDERSTRÖM — Department of Urology, Kärnsjukhuset, Skövde, Sweden

K.H. ANTMAN — Dana Farber Cancer Institute, Harvard Medical School, Boston, Maryland, USA

J.G. BATSAKIS — Professor of Pathology, MD Anderson Hospital, Houston, Texas, USA

J. BHAWAN — Professor of Dermatology and Pathology, Boston University School of Medicine, Boston, Maryland, USA

J. BILEZIKIAN — Department of Medicine, College of Physicians and Surgeons, Columbia University, New York, New York, USA

J.J. BROOKS — Associate Professor of Pathology, Department of Pathology and Laboratory Medicine, University of Pennsylvania, Philadelphia, Pennsylvania, USA

R.B. BUCHANAN — Department of Radiotherapy, Royal South Hants Hospital, Southampton, UK

M.E. CROWTHER — Gynaecological Oncology Fellow, St Bartholomew's Hospital, London, UK

D.C. DAHLIN — Emeritus Professor of Pathology, Mayo Clinic, Rochester, Minnesota, USA

R.K. DAVIS — Department of Otolaryngology, University of Utah, Salt Lake City, Utah, USA

C.D. DIETZEN — Department of Surgery, Louisiana State University School of Medicine, New Orleans, Louisiana, USA

R. FLORENTIN — Professor, Department of Pathology, Albany Medical Center Hospital, Albany, New York, USA

M. FRIEDLANDER — Department of Clinical Oncology, Royal Prince Alfred Hospital, Camperdown, Australia

H.F. FRIERSON, JR — Assistant Professor of Pathology, University of Virginia Medical Center, Charlottesville, Virginia, USA

S. FUJII	Associate Professor, Department of Gynecology and Obstetrics, Faculty of Medicine, Kyoto University, Kyoto, Japan
T.S. GANESAN	Department of Medical Oncology, St Bartholomew's Hospital, London, UK
W.P.R. GIBSON	University of Sydney, Division of Otolaryngology, Sydney, Australia
H. GOEPFERT	Professor of Surgery, MD Anderson Hospital, Houston, Texas, USA
A. GOLDHIRSCH	Senior Clinical Scientist, Ludwig Institute for Cancer Research, Bern, Switzerland
C.R. HAMILTON	Clinical Academic Unit, The Royal Marsden Hospital, Sutton, Surrey, UK
P. HARNETT	Department of Haematology and Oncology, Westmead Hospital, Westmead, Australia
P.G. HARPER	Medical Oncology Clinic, Guy's Hospital, London, UK
A. HERBERT	Department of Histopathology, Southampton General Hospital, Southampton, UK
A. HIRSCHFIELD	Monteviore Medical Centre, Bronx, New York, USA
L. HOLDEN	Research Assistant, Department of Medical Oncology, Charing Cross Hospital, London, UK
R. HOLLAND	Department of Pathology, University Hospital of Nijmegen, Nijmegen, The Netherlands
W.K. HONG	Professor of Medicine, MD Anderson Hospital, Houston, Texas, USA
A. HORWICH	Professor of Radiotherapy, The Royal Marsden Hospital, Sutton, Surrey, UK
C.N. HUDSON	Consultant Gynaecologist, St Bartholomew's and Homerton Hospitals, London, UK
J. HUNGERFORD	Consultant Ophthalmic Surgeon, St Bartholomew's Hospital, London, UK
M.A. ISRAEL	Molecular Genetics Section, Pediatric Branch, National Cancer Institute, Bethesda, Maryland, USA
M.E. JELBART	Urological Cancer Research Unit, Royal Prince Alfred Hospital, Camperdown, Australia
S.L. JOHANSSON	Professor and Director of Anatomic Pathology, University of Nebraska Medical Center, Omaha, Nebraska, USA
P. KORNBLITH	Monteviore Medical Center, Bronx, New York, USA
M.D. LAGIOS	Senior Surgical Pathologist, Department of Pathology, Children's Hospital of San Francisco, San Francisco, California, USA
P.A. LEVINE	University of Virginia School of Medicine, Charlottesville, Virginia, USA

J. LOEFFLER	Joint Center for Radiation Therapy, Harvard Medical School, Boston, Massachusetts, USA
D. LOWE	Senior Lecturer/Honorary Consultant in Histopathology, St Bartholomew's Hospital Medical College, London, UK
J.S. MACDONALD	Professor of Medicine, Lucille Parker Mackay Cancer Center, University of Kentucky Medical Center, Kentucky, USA
J. MACKINTOSH	Department of Clinical Oncology, Royal Prince Alfred Hospital, Camperdown, Australia
L.T. MALDEN	Royal Prince Alfred Hospital, Sydney, Australia
J.H. MALFETANO	Associate Professor of Obstetrics and Gynecology, Albany Medical College, Albany, New York, USA
G.D. MALKASIAN, JR	Department of Obstetrics and Gynecology, The Mayo Clinic, Rochester, Minnesota, USA
J.C. MANIVEL	Mayo Memorial Building, Minneapolis, Minnesota, USA
D.L. MARCHETTI	Clinician, Department of Gynaecologic Oncology, Roswell Park Memorial Institute, Buffalo, New York, USA
R.J. MARSHALL	Department of Pathology, Royal Cornwall Hospital, Truro, Cornwall, UK
P. MAUCH	Joint Center for Radiation Therapy, Harvard Medical School, Boston, Massachusetts, USA
B.C. McCAUGHAN	Department of Cardiothoracic Surgery, Royal Prince Alfred Hospital, Sydney, Australia
M.S. METCALFE	Assistant Professor of Medicine, University of Kentucky Medical Center, Kentucky, USA
S.E. MILLS	Associate Professor of Pathology, University of Virginia Medical Center, Charlottesville, Virginia, USA
G.H. MILLWARD-SADLER	Consultant Pathologist, University of Southampton Medical School, Southampton, UK
J.M. MONAGHAN	Department of Gynaecological Oncology, Queen Elizabeth Hospital, Tyne and Wear, UK
F.J. MONTZ	Division of Gynecologic Oncology, Women's Hospital, Los Angeles, California, USA
C.P. MORROW	Division of Gynecologic Oncology, Women's Hospital, Los Angeles, California, USA
A.M. NEVILLE	Research Administrator, Ludwig Institute for Cancer Research, Zurich, Switzerland
E.S. NEWLANDS	Senior Lecturer, Department of Medical Oncology, Charing Cross Hospital, London, UK

K. OBERG	Senior Clinical Scientist, Ludwig Institute for Cancer Research, Zurich, Switzerland
C.J. O'BRIEN	Attending Surgeon, Royal Prince Alfred Hospital, Sydney, Australia
F.J. PARADINAS	Senior Lecturer, Department of Histopathology, Charing Cross Hospital, London, UK
B. PEARSON	Urological Cancer Research Unit, Royal Prince Alfred Hospital, Sydney, Australia
M.L. PENSAK	University of Cincinnati Medical Center, Cincinnati, Ohio, USA
G.N. PETERS	Department of Surgery, Baylor University Medical Center, and Sammons Cancer Center, Dallas, Texas, USA
L.J. PETERS	Professor of Radiotherapy, MD Anderson Hospital, Houston, Texas, USA
M.S. PIVER	Chief, Department of Gynaecologic Oncology, Roswell Park Memorial Institute, Buffalo, New York, USA
D. RAGHAVAN	Department of Clinical Oncology, Royal Prince Alfred Hospital, Sydney, Australia
J.C. ROSENBERG	Chief of Surgery, Hutzel Hospital, Wayne State University, Detroit, Michigan, USA
P.J. RUSSELL	Urological Cancer Research Unit, Royal Prince Alfred Hospital, Camperdown, Australia
P. RUSSELL	Department of Anatomical Pathology, Royal Prince Alfred Hospital, Camperdown, Australia
R.W. SHAW	Professor, Academic Department of Obstetrics and Gynaecology, Royal Free Hospital, London, UK
E. SHANE	Department of Medicine, College of Physicians and Surgeons, Columbia University, New York, New York, USA
M. SLEVIN	ICRF Department of Medical Oncology, St Bartholomew's Hospital, London, UK
J.H. SHEPHERD	Consultant Gynaecological Surgeon, St Bartholomew's Hospital, London, UK
P.J. SOUTHALL	CRC Research Fellow in Histopathology, Charing Cross Hospital, London, UK
C.A. SPAULDING	University of Virginia School of Medicine, Charlottesville, Virginia, USA
F.M. STEWART	University of Virginia School of Medicine, Charlottesville, Virginia, USA
R. STUART-HARRIS	Medical Oncology Unit, Department of Medicine, Westmead Hospital, Sydney, Australia

J.A. TALCOTT	Dana Farber Cancer Institute, Harvard Medical School, Boston, Massachusetts, USA
I. TAYLOR	Department of Surgery, University of Southampton, Southampton, UK
D.E. TOWNSEND	Director, Gynecologic and Oncologic Services, University of California, Davis Medical Center, Sacramento, California, USA
U. VAN HOELST	Department of Pathology, University Hospital of Nijmegen, Nijmegen, The Netherlands
G.F. VAWTER	Professor of Pathology, Children's Hospital, Harvard Medical School, Boston, Massachusetts, USA
I.D. VELLACOTT	Academic Department of Obstetrics and Gynaecology, Royal Free Hospital, London, UK
M. WANER	Department of Surgery, University of Sydney, Sydney, Australia
C.C. WANG	Professor of Radiation Therapy, Harvard Medical School, Boston, Massachusetts, USA
N. WEIDNER	Associate Professor of Pathology, Harvard Medical School, Brigham and Women's Hospital, Boston, Massachusetts, USA
M.R. WICK	Mayo Memorial Building, Minneapolis, Minnesota, USA
R.H. WILKINSON	Radiologist and Associate in Medicine, The Children's Hospital, Boston, Massachusetts, USA
C.J. WILLIAMS	CRC Medical Oncology Unit, University of Southampton, Southampton, UK
E.J. WILLS	Department of Anatomical Pathology, Royal Prince Alfred Hospital, Camperdown, Australia
J. WONG	Department of Urology, Royal Prince Alfred Hospital, Sydney, Australia
R. WRIGHT	Professor of Medicine, University of Southampton Medical School, Southampton, UK
M. YOONESSI	State University of New York at Buffalo School of Medicine, Buffalo, New York, USA

Preface

The idea for this book came from the common experience of each of the editors: an excessive expenditure of time and energy, even in this era of computerized searches, needed to collate and evaluate data on uncommon cancers.

We all, surprisingly commonly, look after patients with unusual tumours, and unfortunately major textbooks on general oncology rarely devote more than one or two paragraphs to such cancers. It was for this reason that we set out to collect together comprehensive and critical reviews on many of the rare tumours. Such a goal has called for a truly international effort in order to bring together the enormous range of specialist knowledge necessary to cover the breadth and diversity of the subject. Some ninety contributors from hospitals and research centres throughout the world, led by a team of editors based in the UK, USA and Australia, have contributed their clinical experience to what we believe is a unique and exceptional addition to the current literature on cancer.

Originally we envisaged all chapters following a logical format to ensure that each was as comprehensive and readable as possible. However, uncommon cancers may be divided into two groups: common tumours at rare sites, and uncommon tumours of specific type. Rather than impose an unworkable structure on authors by forcing them to conform to a set of specific rules regarding level of content, style and approach, in a subject which by its very nature varies greatly in the degree of information available, we have elected to abandon the traditional textbook style, and have instead produced a collection of up-to-the-minute reviews, a compendium of the richest source of information that is now available. Since few will read the book from cover to cover, but rather refer to individual chapters as the need arises, we felt the variation in style would not prove problematic. We have tried to ensure that practical information useful in planning management is always included, but some cancers are so rare that little such information is available; the authors of these chapters have, in general, concentrated on reviewing what is known about the biology and pathology of those tumours.

Since cancers may be described as uncommon because of site or specific type there is inevitably some overlap in several sections. This has affected several chapters where a particular tumour has been described more than once, in different detail and from different viewpoints. In such instances we have cross-referenced the alternative description rather than lose information and perspective by deleting one.

Because of the extraordinary diversity of cancer it is inevitable that we have not been able to include all of the rare tumours. It is our intention to update regularly each of the chapters in future editions and we would welcome suggestions for topics which have been neglected. In the first edition we have chosen to omit unusual cancers of the haematopoietic/lymphoid systems and paediatric cancers, apart from those of unusual sites, since these are usually well covered in specific textbooks.

Most practising oncologists have little need to refer to textbooks; they keep up to date on the management of common cancers by reading original papers. However, we are confident that there is a real need for a major textbook on the previously neglected uncommon cancers. Our aim has been to review the available data and to present the clinician with information, when it is available, that will be helpful in planning the optimal management for these challenging patients.

CHRISTOPHER J. WILLIAMS
JOHN G. KRIKORIAN
DEREK RAGHAVAN
MARK R. GREEN

Section 1

Gynaecological Tumours

Textbook of Uncommon Cancer
Edited by C.J. Williams, J.G. Krikorian, M.R. Green and D. Raghavan
Published by John Wiley & Sons Ltd
© 1988 Mayo Foundation

Chapter **1**

Tumors of Granulosa–Theca Cell Derivation

George D. Malkasian, Jr

Chairman, Department of Obstetrics and Gynecology, Mayo Clinic and Mayo Foundation; Professor of Obstetrics and Gynecology, Mayo Medical School, Rochester, Minnesota, USA

INTRODUCTION

In 1973, the World Health Organization published a classification of sex cord stromal tumors that, in 1982, was expanded by Young and Scully (1) (Table 1). Fox (2) further subdivided these tumors. However, even though these subclassifications might be useful to pathologists, they do not provide clinicians with any helpful information regarding care or prognosis, with the exception of sex cord tumors with annular tubules. This chapter presents current information about granulosa cell tumors, thecomas, and sex cord tumors with annular tubules.

Fox (2) summarized current concepts of the histogenesis well, as follows:

> All of these cells are thought to originate ultimately from either the sex cords or the mesenchyme of the embryonic gonad though it has to be admitted that the early stages of gonadal development are still a matter of dispute. Thus some, probably most, embryologists believe that the sex cords are derived as downgrowths from the coelomic epithelium whilst others consider that they originate from gonadal mesenchyme. Argument also exists as to the eventual fate of cells in the sex cords; it is widely believed that these cells differentiate into granulosa cells if the gonad

is destined to become an ovary and into Sertoli cells if development is deflected along a testicular pathway by the presence of H–Y antigen in the germ cells. According to this concept the granulosa and Sertoli cells are homologues of each other, a relationship denied, however, by others who believe that whilst granulosa cells originate from cortical sex cords the Sertoli cells derive from medullary cords of mesonephric origin . . .

> The stromal element of these tumours may be of an indifferent nature or can be differentiated into either thecal or Leydig cells, these latter also being considered as homologous . . .

The cause of any of these tumors remains unknown. Animal models have been established in which granulosa cell tumors can be produced, but application of the derived information to the tumor in humans remains, at best, remote and applicable to only an infinitesimally small number of patients.

GRANULOSA CELL TUMORS

Granulosa cell tumors have been reported to account for 70% of all feminizing ovarian tumors, 28% of all solid malignant ovarian neoplasms, 10% of all solid ovarian tumors, 1.7% of all ovarian tumors, and from 0.6% to

TABLE 1 CLASSIFICATION OF SEX CORD-
STROMAL TUMORS

A. Granulosa–stromal cell tumors
   1. Granulosa cell tumor
      a. Adult type
      b. Juvenile type
   2. Tumors in the thecoma–fibroma group
      a. Thecoma
         i. Typical
        ii. Luteinized
      b. Fibroma–fibrosarcoma
         i. Fibroma
        ii. Cellular fibroma
       iii. Fibrosarcoma
      c. Sclerosing stromal tumor
      d. Unclassified
B. Sertoli-Leydig cell tumors (androblastomas)
   1. Well differentiated
   2. Of intermediate differentiation
   3. Poorly differentiated
   4. With heterologous elements
C. Gynandroblastoma
D. Sex cord tumor with annular tubules
E. Unclassified

4.6% of all malignant ovarian neoplasms (3). Between 32% and 39% occur in women younger than 40 years, and about 5% occur during the prepubertal period (4). Scully (5) described a form of granulosa cell tumor that was clearly different in appearance and nearly always occurred during the first 20 years of life. Therefore, granulosa cell tumors are of the adult type or the juvenile type (Table 1).

Adult Type

The symptoms manifested by granulosa cell tumors relate primarily to menstrual dysfunction, mainly metrorrhagia, menorrhagia, or oligomenorrhea. They may cause prepubertal bleeding, amenorrhea, or postmenopausal bleeding. They are associated with increasing abdominal girth, abdominal or pelvic pain, and, occasionally, virilizing symptoms. They are rarely diagnosed when asymptomatic. Fertility in affected patients is similar to that of the population at large (6, 7).

Young et al. (8) reported that granulosa cell tumors can occur during pregnancy and have been problematic, particularly during the third trimester. Of those reviewed, 76% were of the juvenile type. They noted that when these tumors occur in association with pregnancy they are much less frequently associated with hormonal manifestations and more frequently complicated by rupture. They are all large enough to be palpated or identified as ovarian lesions on ultrasonic examination. No distinctive ultrasonic findings allow discrete diagnosis of the tumor.

The hormonal manifestations of granulosa cell tumors are frequently alluded to, but few studies report serum or urinary estrogen, testosterone, or androstenedione levels. Anikwue et al. (9), in a summary of reports in the literature, found that estrogen levels that were elevated preoperatively returned to normal postoperatively in 10 of 11 patients and remained the same in one. Virilization or hirsutism is reported in up to 7% of patients with granulosa cell tumors (9), but no hormonal studies have been done preoperatively and postoperatively. Nakashima et al. (10) summarized the literature and added 15 more cases; the total number of reported cases of androgen-producing granulosa cell tumors was then 29. Androgenic manifestations were hirsutism in 72%, clitorimegaly in 62%, deepening of the voice in 34%, amenorrhea in 31%, male escutcheon in 28%, and atrophy of the breasts in 10%. All tumors were Stage I at diagnosis. No hormonal studies were reported. Demopoulos and Bell (11) studied the fine structure of a virilizing human granulosa–theca cell tumor in a patient with an elevated serum testosterone value and androstenedione crystalloids of Reinke in the steroidogenic cells; the findings raised the possibility that the functional cells are derived from nonneoplastic preexisting hilus or Leydig cells.

Steroid-binding proteins have been studied in granulosa cell tumors, and androgen- (12–14), progestin- (12, 13, 15, 16), and estrogen- (13, 15, 17) binding sites have been identified. Interestingly, estrogen receptors were not found in most tumors studied; when the receptors were present, the levels were low. This observation may attest to the fact that the

TABLE 2 STUDIES OF GRANULOSA CELL TUMOR

Reference, year	No. of patients	Stage I disease (%)	5-yr survival (%)	Late recurrence (%)	Factors related to survival				
					Stage	Histologic pattern	Cellular atypia	Mitotic activity	Size
Young et al., 1984 (8)	17	100	100	NE[a]	NE	No	No	No	No
Schwartz and Smith, 1976 (18)	51	50.9	68	NE	Yes	NE	NE	NE	NE
Evans et al., 1980 (6)	118	86.1	82.1	5(>13 yr)	Yes	NE	NE	NE	NE
Ohel et al., 1983 (7)	172	44.7	55	NE	Yes	NE	NE	NE	NE
Björkholm and Silfverswärd, 1981 (19)	198	91	85	5(>5 yr)	Yes	No	Yes	Yes	Yes
Anikwue et al., 1978 (9)	32	100	NE	NE	NE	NE	NE	NE	NE
Gee and Russell, 1981 (20)	20	90	95	5(>5 yr)	Yes	No	No	No	No

[a] NE, not evaluated.

receptors are absent or the technique used has not adequately eluted the endogenous estrogens saturating the sites before testing.

In recently reported series (Table 2), the percentage of tumors diagnosed as Stage I disease ranged from 44.7% to 100%, and the 5-year survival rates varied in direct proportion to early diagnosis, from 55% to 100%. Although the course of the disease has repeatedly been shown to be indolent, one consistent factor in prognosis is the stage of the disease at diagnosis (1, 6, 19). Also, tumor rupture during Stage I disease has been shown to lead to decreased survival (19). In the series with long follow-up, 5% of all patients had recurrence 5 or more years after initial diagnosis and treatment. Recurrence has been reported as long as 30 years after initial treatment (21). Once disease recurs, survival is poor, being reported at about 30% (6).

Teyssier et al. (22) summarized the literature regarding chromosome changes in ovarian carcinoma. The most common structural rearrangements associated with ovarian carcinoma were chromosome 6 having a partial deletion or translocation of the long arm. Their study of one granulosa cell tumor showed a similar interstitial deletion of the long arm of chromosome 6; this finding suggested the malignant nature of granulosa cell tumors at the cellular level. The tumor studied was a Stage I lesion, and no clinical follow-up data

were provided to describe the subsequent behaviour of the tumor.

The histologic patterns that have been described for granulosa cell tumors are follicular (macrofollicular and microfollicular), insular, trabecular, moiré silk or watered silk, diffuse or sarcomatoid, and luteinized. Although these types were all carefully described by pathologists, the tumors have a tendency to show more than one pattern when thoroughly studied. The histologic types do not correlate with survival (Table 2).

Fox et al. (23) noted that the size of a tumor at diagnosis had a high correlation with survival. They reported that 10-year survival was 53% if the tumor was larger than 15 cm in diameter, 57% if the tumor was 6 to 15 cm, and 100% if the tumor was 5 cm or less. Björkholm and Silfverswärd (19) showed a significant difference—mortality was 4% in patients with Stage I disease whose tumors were 5 cm or less in diameter and 20% in those whose tumors were more than 5 cm in diameter.

Treatment of granulosa cell tumor is primarily surgical. On the basis of their data, Evans et al. (6) suggested total abdominal hysterectomy and bilateral salpingo-oophorectomy. Of the patients with Stage IA lesions, 9.0% had recurrence of their primary tumor and 7.5% died of their disease. Patients who underwent total abdominal hysterectomy and bilateral salpingo-oophorectomy had a recurrence rate of 6%, and those who had a less extensive operation had a recurrence rate of 25%. Once recurrence was diagnosed, 73% of the patients died of their disease despite radiation or chemotherapy or both. These data are in contrast to Young and Scully's (1) statement that high-grade and recurrent tumors respond favorably to radiation therapy. They also believed that unilateral oophorectomy was adequate for Stage IA disease. We continue to believe that for any stage higher than IA, total abdominal hysterectomy and bilateral salpingo-oophorectomy is indicated, and this opinion was echoed by Slayton (24). Should conservative unilateral oophorectomy be chosen, it should always be preceded by dilatation and curettage because the incidence of associated endometrial cancer has been reported to be 4% (7), 15% (6), 16% (25), and 20% (26). The less worrisome endometrial hyperplasia has been reported to be present in 22% (7), 41% (26), and 55% (6). Anikwue et al. (9), in a cumulative review of the literature, found that the occurrence rate of endometrial hyperplasia was 62% and that of endometrial carcinoma was 13.2%.

Although adjuvant radiation therapy is often suggested and many series report its use, overall data are not available to compare survival by stage of disease with and without it. Retrospective analyses by Ohel et. al. (7) and Evans et al. (6) did not document its efficacy.

Results of chemotherapy for recurrent disease are summarized in Table 3. A few long-term responses were noted with melphalan (Alkeran); cisplatin and doxorubicin (Adriamycin); or actinomycin, 5-fluorouracil, and cyclophosphamide. The better results occurred with multiple drug programs.

Our current treatment of Stage IAii disease or higher is total abdominal hysterectomy and bilateral salpingo-oophorectomy in addition to cyclophosphamide and cisplatin.

Follow-up is for life because of the indolent nature of the disease and the tendency for late recurrence. Our most recent study (6) showed that the average time to recurrence was 6 years and the longest interval to recurrence was 23

TABLE 3 REPORTED RESULTS OF CHEMOTHERAPY FOR RECURRENT GRANULOSA CELL TUMOR

Reference, year	Agent	No. of patients	Response Partial	Response Complete	Duration (months)
Jacobs et al., 1982 (27)	Cisplatin, doxorubicin	2	1	1	18, 24
Malkasian et al., 1974 (28)	Cyclophosphamide	12	3	—	3
	Melphalan	1	—	—	—
	Actinomycin D	1	1	—	3
Young et al., 1984 (8)	Cyclophosphamide, cisplatin, doxorubicin	1	—	1	8
Schwartz and Smith, 1976 (18)	Melphalan	9	1	—	7
	Thiotepa	4	1	—	12
	Actinomycin, fluorouracil, cyclophosphamide	2	—	2	27, 35
Neville et al., 1984 (29)	Cyclophosphamide	1	—	1	12
	Fluorouracil	2	—	—	—
	Melphalan	1	—	1	36
	Cisplatin, hexamethylmelamine	1	—	—	—
	Cyclophosphamide, methrotrexate, fluorouracil,	2	1	—	—
	Vincristine, prednisone	2	1	—	—
Camlibel and Caputo, 1983 (30)	Cytoxan, cisplatin, doxorubicin	1	—	1	6

years and that, of the patients with recurrence, it developed more than 13 years after initial treatment in 23%. Since that report, evaluation of the group has shown more patients with recurrent disease at 8, 8, 12, 13, 17, and 22 years. To date, 3 of these 6 patients have died of their disease, and 3 have been treated with cyclophosphamide and doxorubicin; cyclophosphamide, doxorubicin, and cisplatin; and cyclophosphamide and cisplatin with responses of 2, 4, and 6 years. The patients with 4- and 6-year responses have had multiple recurrences, including intrahepatic lesions. After 1 year of chemotherapy, a remaining solitary intrahepatic lesion was resected from each patient, and they were alive 3 and 5 years later, apparently free of disease. Margolin et al. (31) emphasized the development of intrahepatic recurrence and evaluated the hemorrhagic problems associated with these recurrences. We found intrahepatic recurrences but no hemorrhagic problems.

As follow-up data accumulate, the need for breast examination has been documented by the presence of breast carcinoma in 5.5% (6), 6.4% (7), 20% (32), and 3.7% (33) of patients. Of a particularly ominous nature is the report by Lack et al. (32), in which 2 of 10 premenarchal patients with granulosa cell tumors subsequently developed breast cancer. The three other series involved adult granulosa cell tumors. Accordingly, our follow-up examinations include periodic abdominal–pelvic computed tomography and mammography in addition to a complete physical evaluation.

Juvenile Type

This type of granulosa cell tumor was first delineated by Scully (5), and subsequent data have warranted its separation both pathologically and clinically. It accounts for 85% of the granulosa cell tumors that occur before puberty, and 82% of these are associated with the rapid development of isosexual pseudoprecocity (1). Young and Scully (1) detailed the difference in this type of precocity as being due to estrogen excess as opposed to the more common constitutional central precocity caused by early activation of the hypothalamus or anterior pituitary gland. In a series of 125 cases, Young et al. (34) reported that 3% of the tumors were bilateral at initial operation and 2% became bilateral within 1 year postoperatively. This observation seems to suggest that the latter tumors had been present at the initial operation.

According to the reported experiences with these tumors (Table 4), 33% to 82% are associated with precocity; 44% to 80% occur during the first decade of life, and, at most, 22% occur beyond age 20 years; and 73.6% to 100% are Stage I at diagnosis. Only one series (34) reported a 5-year survival rate of less than 100%, that being 94.4%. To date, no series has reported late recurrences, unlike the adult type of tumor. Lack et al. (32) reported that 2 of 10 patients with juvenile granulosa cell tumor had breast cancer at 33 and 39 years of follow-up, one of whom died of metastatic breast cancer. These breast lesions occurred in relatively young women (one in her 30s and the other in her early 40s), a point worth noting as patients are followed up.

Histologically, these tumors are distinct from their adult counterparts in that they show immature follicles rather than mature ones, the follicles contain much mucin as opposed to little or none, the number of Call–Exner bodies is minimal, and the cell nuclei are dark and rarely grooved whereas grooved and pale nuclei are common in adult granulosa cell tumors. This immature histologic appearance does not correlate with the clinical behaviour of the tumor. Young et al. (34) reported a 5-year survival of 99% for patients with Stage IAi tumors. However, in patients with tumors that were Stage IAii or higher, the mortality rate was 26% (6 of 23 patients). The deaths occurred 7 to 36 months after the initial operation and despite radiation therapy and chemotherapy. The drug combinations used were bleomycin, vinblastine, and cisplatin in two patients; cyclophosphamide, hexamethylmelamine, doxorubicin, and cisplatin in one patient; actinomycin, fluorouracil, and cyclo-

TABLE 4 STUDIES OF JUVENILE GRANULOSA CELL TUMOR

Reference, year	No. of patients	No. of patients with precocity	Decade of life (% of patients)				Stage I disease (%)	5-yr survival (%)	Late recurrence (%)
			1st	2nd	3rd	>3rd			
Young et al., 1984 (34)	125	82	44	34	19	3	73.6	94.4	0
Roth et al., 1979 (35)	3	33	66	33	—	—	100	100	0
Zaloudek and Norris, 1982 (36)	26	75	62.5	37.5	—	—	100	—	0
Lack et al., 1981 (32)	10	70	80	20	—	—	100	100	0

phosphamide in two patients; fluorouracil, cyclophosphamide, mitomycin, and chromomycin in one patient; and vincristine, actinomycin, and cyclophosphamide in two patients. Bleomycin and cisplatin were used alone in one patient each. Some patients received more than one drug combination during the course of therapy.

Young and Scully (1) reported that 2 of 125 cases were associated with enchondromatosis (Ollier's disease). Tamimi and Bolen (37) reported a third case of enchondromatosis associated with juvenile granulosa cell tumor and stated that two cases in the literature were associated with Maffucci's syndrome. A search of Mayo Clinic records for cases of enchondromatosis or enchondromatosis associated with subcutaneous hemangiomatosis revealed no cases of associated ovarian lesions over a 10-year period. Roth et al. (35) reported a bilateral lesion in an infant with Potter's syndrome.

To date, no cases of associated endometrial carcinoma have been reported.

Treatment for Stage IAi disease is unilateral oophorectomy or unilateral salpingo-oophorectomy. However, from cases reported in the literature, total abdominal hysterectomy and bilateral salpingo-oophorectomy is appropriate for any higher stage of disease. Experience with radiation therapy immediately postoperatively to appropriate fields is scarce. If it is to be of use, it should be administered at this point and not after recurrence, as should multiple-agent chemotherapy.

THECOMAS

Thecomas are defined as containing mainly theca cells with a small fibroblastic component. At what point the fibroblastic component makes the lesions 'fibrothecomas' and, still further, fibromas is arbitrary.

In a Mayo Clinic review of 24 patients with thecomas treated from 1976 to 1984, the average age was 57 years (range, 16 to 83 years). Of these 24 patients, 5 were premenopausal or perimenopausal, and the rest were postmenopausal. The average parity was 2.8, and 9% of the patients were nulliparous. Presenting symptoms were abnormal bleeding in 23%, a pelvic mass in 36%, and an incidental finding at operation for other reasons in 27%. At operation, the lesion was Stage IAi in 83% and IAii in the remainder. The lesions were more than 10 cm in diameter in 25%, 6 to 10 cm in 33%, and less than 6 cm in the rest. Associated uterine lesions were adenomatous endometrial hyperplasia in 4 patients, endometrial carcinoma in 3, endometrial carcinoma associated with mixed mesodermal tumor in one, and atrophic endometrium in 6. Two patients died: one of endometrial carcinoma at 9 months postoperatively (which was Stage III at the original operation) and one of pancreatic carcinoma 11 months postoperatively (the thecoma was an incidental ovarian finding).

Gusberg and Kardon (26) noted endometrial carcinoma in 19%, adenomatous hyperplasia in 34.7%, and cystic hyperplasia in 20%

of 46 patients with thecomas. The malignant lesions all occurred in postmenopausal patients, but 25% of the cases of adenomatous hyperplasia were in premenopausal patients. Because the cells of thecomas have been considered a neoplastic variant, Fienberg (38) studied the ovaries of 11 patients with endometrial carcinoma and found that 10 had stromal theca cells. Other than the presence of these cells, he drew no particular conclusions.

The operations in our series ranged from resection of the tumor with conservation of the ovary in the 2 teenage patients to total abdominal hysterectomy and bilateral salpingo-oophorectomy in the postmenopausal patients.

The recent series reported in the literature (Table 5) indicate that these tumors are few in number, are associated with a 5-year survival rate of 100%, are almost entirely unilateral, and are associated with endometrial hypertrophy in 13% to 66% of cases and with endometrial carcinoma in 4% to 34% of cases. The percentage of associated endometrial carcinoma emphasizes the need for dilatation and curettage in any patient who has treatment that is less extensive than a total abdominal hysterectomy and bilateral salpingo-oophorectomy.

Gee and Russell (20) noted that an associated finding in the contralateral ovary was stromal hyperplasia in 16% of cases. Evans et al. (6) described 2 patients with theca cell tumors who had associated ovarian malignancies: one malignant teratoma and one epithelial serous cystadenocarcinoma. They also reported two deaths from associated endometrial carcinoma in their series of 82 theca cell tumors.

Thecomas have been associated with pregnancy (1, 39, 40), and they are highly luteinized in such cases. Gillibrand (40) summarized the 27 pregnancy-related granulosa–theca cell cases in the literature and noted that, among the 14 patients in the third trimester, 3 died because of rupture, 1 had rupture, 6 had premature labor, 3 had cesarean sections because of obstructed labor, and 1 had no problems. Two of three hormonally active tumors were masculinizing in character.

Gaffney et al. (41) studied three ovarian thecomas by ultrastructural and immunohistochemical techniques and found that a few cells stained for estradiol. They hypothesized that the small number of cells that showed localization of estrogen suggested that they were capable of steroid synthesis.

Yaghoobian and Pinck (42) and Diakoumakis et al. (43) reported what they considered sonographic findings diagnostic of an ovarian thecoma, specifically, 'very poor penetration of the mass with acoustic shadowing corresponding to most of the tumor' in combination with a noncalcified ovarian mass. Woo and Ghosh (44) reported that ultrasonic evaluation of a thecoma showed primarily cystic characteristics. With due respect to these reports, ultrasonic findings for either solid or cystic ovarian masses remain nonspecific and nondiagnostic for the histologic type of tumor.

By virtue of their behaviour, treatment of ovarian thecomas is dilatation and curettage and, in young patients, resection of the lesion if

TABLE 5 STUDIES OF THECOMA

Reference, year	No. of patients	5-yr survival (%)	Unilateral lesions (%)	Associated endometrial lesions	
				Malignant (%)	Hyperplastic (%)
Anikwue et al., 1978 (9)	39	100	92	4	38
Björkholm and Pettersson, 1980 (33)	35	100	100	34	13
Antolič et al., 1980 (25)	46	100	100	15	16
Gee and Russell, 1981 (20)	12	100	100	8	66
Evans et al., 1980 (6)	81	100	100	26.8	36.6

the ovary can be preserved or resection of the involved ovary if the lesion has destroyed it. Total abdominal hysterectomy and bilateral salpingo-oophorectomy is reserved for patients with associated endometrial carcinoma or other associated ovarian lesions or for post-menopausal patients. There is no need for adjuvant radiation or chemotherapy for ovarian thecomas.

SEX CORD TUMORS WITH ANNULAR TUBULES

At one time, approximately 10% of sex cord stromal tumors were unclassified. The sex cord tumors with annular tubules have been separated from the unclassified group; three were first described by Scully in 1970 (45), and a body of literature has slowly developed. He thought the tumor arose from granulosa cells and then proceeded to grow in a pattern more closely observed in Sertoli cells. Norris and Chorlton (46), in fact, regarded these tumors as a variant of the Sertoli cell tumors. Should this be the case, one might expect to find a virilizing variant of sex cord tumors with annular tubules in the female population with Peutz–Jeghers syndrome. Hertel and Kempson (47) evaluated the ultrastructure of two sex cord tumors with annular tubules and concluded that 'the striking similarity between the predominant cell type and granulosa cells, as well as the presence of fibrillary material of the type seen in Call–Exner bodies, suggests a granulosa cell origin for these neoplasms.' Hart et al. (48) stated more strongly than others their belief that the lesion is a variant of granulosa cell tumor and should in fact be listed as such and not as a separate entity. Their first three cases were reported to occur in association with Peutz–Jeghers syndrome, an autosomal dominant disorder characterized by multiple gastrointestinal polyps and mucocutaneous pigmentation.

As more cases have been reported, it has been evident that not all such tumors are associated with Peutz–Jeghers syndrome; at present, about 30% to 35% are associated and the rest are not. Scully (45) reported that sex cord tumors with annular tubules are the most frequent ovarian tumor in women with Peutz–Jeghers syndrome. Christian (49) pointed out that 1 in 10 women with this syndrome has ovarian tumors and that patients with the syndrome have a risk 20.4 times that of the general female population. In a review of women with Peutz–Jeghers syndrome who had gynecologic tumors (50), 16 of 28 had sex cord tumors with annular tubules, which were bilateral in 10 of 13 cases in which both ovaries were examined.

According to the recent literature (Table 6), although some of the cases may represent dual reporting, (1) 32.6% of cases are associated with Peutz–Jeghers syndrome, and if only Young's series is evaluated, 36%; (2) the bilateral lesions are associated with Peutz–Jeghers syndrome; (3) 47% of cases associated with Peutz–Jeghers syndrome are bilateral; (4) in young patients the lesions may be associated with sexual precocity; (5) the lesion causes menstrual disturbances during the reproductive years; (6) the lesion can cause bleeding in postmenopausal patients; and (7) the lesion has been shown to have malignant potential in only 3 patients, 2 of whom had recurrences 7.5 and 10.5 years after the initial treatment—a behavior similar to that of granulosa cell tumors.

The diagnosis of sex cord tumor with annular tubules in women with Peutz–Jeghers syndrome should be considered when problems such as irregular uterine bleeding, hyperplasia on dilatation and curettage, or postmenopausal bleeding are present. It should be included in the differential diagnosis of girls with precocious puberty. The lesions tend to be small and, therefore, palpation, ultrasound testing, or computed tomography cannot necessarily rule them out. Although the symptoms and physical findings suggest estrogen production, few cases are documented as having increased serum estrogen levels such that they could be used as a diagnostic instrument.

Although Young and Scully (1) stated that sex cord tumors with annular tubules not

TABLE 6 STUDIES OF SEX CORD TUMORS WITH ANNULAR TUBULES

Reference, year	No. of patients	PJS[a] present (no. of patients)	Ovarian involvement (no. of patients)		Hormonal activity (no. of patients)				
			Unilateral	Bilateral	Endometrial hyperplasia	Menstrual irregularity	Amenorrhea	Precocious puberty	Malignant activity
Mayo, 1986	1	Yes 1	—	LSO[b] 1973 RO[b] 1985	—	—	—	—	0
Rodu and Martinez, 1984 (51)	1	Yes 1	1	—	—	—	—	—	1 (died of tumor)
Young et al., 1983 (52)	2	Yes 2	2	—	—	—	—	2	0
Young et al., 1982 (53)	74	Yes 27	—	13	7	12	—	2	0
		No 47	47	—	—	22	4	5	—
Anderson et al., 1980 (54)	5	Yes 0	—	—	—	—	—	—	—
		No 5	5	—	—	2	1	2	—
Hart et al., 1980 (48)	6	Yes 0	—	—	—	—	—	—	—
		No 6	6	—	—	5	1	—	2 (7.5 and 10.5 yr later)
Purohit and Alam, 1980 (55)	2	Yes 1	1	1	1	1	—	—	0
		No 1	—	—	—	—	—	—	—
Hertel and Kempson, 1977 (47)	2	Yes 0	—	—	1	—	—	1	—
		No 2	2	—	—	—	—	—	—
Scully, 1970 (45)	10	Yes 3	1	2	2	—	—	—	0
		No 7	6 (1 unknown)	—	2	—	1	—	0

[a] PJS, Peutz–Jeghers syndrome.
[b] LSO, left salpingo-oophorectomy; RO, right oophorectomy.

associated with Peutz–Jeghers syndrome are clinically malignant in at least 20% of cases, the cases reported in the literature do not bear out this figure. In fact, the literature suggests malignant behaviour in about 2% of such cases.

Treatment of Stage IAi lesions in patients who do not have Peutz–Jeghers syndrome could safely be unilateral oophorectomy associated with appropriate peritoneal washings and biopsies. However, if such an operation is considered in patients with Peutz–Jeghers syndrome, careful evaluation of the contralateral ovary is necessary. The one Mayo Clinic patient had two operations 12 years apart for identical lesions in each ovary. Should the stage of the lesion be higher than IAi, then total abdominal hysterectomy and bilateral salpingo–oopherectomy with omentectomy, peritoneal cytology, and peritoneal biopsy are in order. Radiation has not been shown to be efficacious: the one patient described by Rodu and Martinez (51) failed to respond, and one described by Hart et al. (48) did respond. The significant difference in these cases was the point in the course of the disease at which the radiation was used—Rodu and Martinez administered it at diagnosis and Hart et al., 10.5 years after initial treatment. In the only report of chemotherapy (51), actinomycin, vincristine, and cyclophosphamide were without effect.

REFERENCES

1 Young RH, Scully RE. Ovarian sex cord-stromal tumours: recent advances and current status. Clin Obstet Gynecol 1984; 11: 93.
2 Fox H. Sex cord-stromal tumours of the ovary. J Pathol 1985; 145: 127.
3 Malkasian GD Jr, Hawks BL. Granulosa-cell tumor of the ovary: report of a case. Obstet Gynecol 1964; 23: 122.
4 Malkasian GD Jr, Dockerty MB, Wilson RB, Faber JE. Functioning tumors of the ovary in women under 40. Obstet Gynecol 1965; 26: 669.
5 Scully RE. Sex Cord-Stromal Tumors. In: Blaustein A ed Pathology of the Female Genital Tract. New York: Springer-Verlag, 1977: 505.
6 Evans AT III, Gaffey TA, Malkasian GD Jr,
Annegers JF. Clinicopathologic review of 118 granulosa and 82 theca cell tumors. Obstet Gynecol 1980; 55: 231.
7 Ohel G, Kaneti H, Schenker JG. Granulosa cell tumors in Israel: a study of 172 cases. Gynecol Oncol 1983; 15: 278.
8 Young RH, Dudley AG, Scully RE. Granulosa cell, Sertoli–Leydig cell, and unclassified sex cord-stromal tumors associated with pregnancy: a clinicopathological analysis of thirty-six cases. Gynecol Oncol 1984; 18: 181.
9 Anikwue C, Dawood MY, Kramer E. Granulosa and theca cell tumors. Obstet Gynecol 1978; 51: 214.
10 Nakashima N, Young RH, Scully RE. Androgenic granulosa cell tumors of the ovary: a clinicopathologic analysis of 17 cases and review of the literature. Arch Pathol Lab Med 1984; 108: 786.
11 Demopoulos RI, Bell DA. The fine structure of a virilizing human granulosa–theca cell tumor: observations on the nature of the hormone producing cell. Cancer 1983; 51: 1858.
12 Young PCM, Grosfeld JL, Ehrlich CE, Roth LM. Progestin- and androgen-binding components in a human granulosa–theca cell tumor. Gynecol Oncol 1982; 13: 309.
13 Meyer JS, Rao BR, Valdes R Jr, Burstein R, Wasserman HC. Progesterone receptor in granulosa cell tumor. Gynecol Oncol 1982; 13: 252.
14 Bergqvist A, Kullander S, Thorell J. A study of estrogen and progesterone cytosol receptor concentration in benign and malignant ovarian tumors and a review of malignant ovarian tumors treated with medroxyprogesterone acetate. Acta Obstet Gynecol Scand (Suppl) 1981; 101: 75.
15 Schwartz PE, MacLusky N, Sakamoto H, Eisenfeld A. Steroid-receptor proteins in nonepithelial malignancies of the ovary. Gynecol Oncol 1983; 15: 305.
16 Hamilton TC, Davies P, Griffiths K. Androgen and oestrogen binding in cytosols of human ovarian tumours. J Endocrinol 1981; 90: 421.
17 Holt JA, Lyttle CR, Lorincz MA, Stern SD, Press MF, Herbst AL. Estrogen receptor and peroxidase activity in epithelial ovarian carcinomas. J Natl Cancer Inst 1981; 67: 307.
18 Schwartz PE, Smith JP. Treatment of ovarian stromal tumors. Am J Obstet Gynecol 1976; 125: 402.
19 Björkholm E, Silfverswärd C. Prognostic factors in granulosa-cell tumors. Gynecol Oncol 1981; 11: 261.
20 Gee DC, Russell P. The pathological assessment of ovarian neoplasms. IV: The sex cord-stromal tumours. Pathology 1981; 13: 235.

21 Björkholm E. Granulosa cell tumors: a comparison of survival in patients and matched controls. Am J Obstet Gynecol 1980; 138: 329.

22 Teyssier J-R, Adnet J-J, Pigeon F, Bajolle F. Chromosomal changes in an ovarian granulosa cell tumor: similarity with carcinoma. Cancer Genet Cytogenet 1985; 14: 147.

23 Fox H, Agrawal K, Langley FA. A clinicopathologic study of 92 cases of granulosa cell tumor of the ovary with special reference to the factors influencing prognosis. Cancer 1975; 35: 231.

24 Slayton RE. Management of germ cell and stromal tumors of the ovary. Semin Oncol 1984; 11: 299.

25 Antolič ZN, Kovačič J, Rainer S. Theca and granulosa cell tumors and endometrial adenocarcinoma. Gynecol Oncol 1980; 10: 273.

26 Gusberg SB, Kardon P. Proliferative endometrial response to theca–granulosa cell tumors. Trans Am Gynecol Soc 1971; 94: 184.

27 Jacobs AJ, Deppe G, Cohen CJ. Combination chemotherapy of ovarian granulosa cell tumor with cis-platinum and doxorubicin. Gynecol Oncol 1982; 14: 294.

28 Malkasian GD Jr, Webb MJ, Jorgensen EO. Observations on chemotherapy of granulosa cell carcinomas and malignant ovarian teratomas. Obstet Gynecol 1974; 44: 885.

29 Neville AJ, Gilchrist KW, Davis TE. The chemotherapy of granulosa cell tumors of the ovary: experience of the Wisconsin Clinical Cancer Center. Med Pediatr Oncol 1984; 12: 397.

30 Camlibel FT, Caputo TA. Chemotherapy of granulosa cell tumors. Am J Obstet Gynecol 1983; 145: 763.

31 Margolin KA, Pak HY, Esensten ML, Doroshow JH. Hepatic metastasis in granulosa cell tumor of the ovary. Cancer 1985; 56: 691.

32 Lack EE, Perez-Atayde AR, Murthy ASK, Goldstein DP, Crigler JF Jr, Vawter GF. Granulosa theca cell tumors in premenarchal girls: a clinical and pathologic study of ten cases. Cancer 1981; 48: 1846.

33 Björkholm E, Pettersson F. Granulosa-cell and theca-cell tumors: the clinical picture and long-term outcome for the Radiumhemmet series. Acta Obstet Gynecol Scand 1980; 59: 361.

34 Young RH, Dickersin GR, Scully RE. Juvenile granulosa cell tumor of the ovary: a clinicopathological analysis of 125 cases. Am J Surg Pathol 1984; 8: 575.

35 Roth LM, Nicholas TR, Ehrlich CE. Juvenile granulosa cell tumor: a clinicopathologic study of three cases with ultrastructural observations. Cancer 1979; 44: 2194.

36 Zaloudek C, Norris HJ. Granulosa tumors of the ovary in children: a clinical and pathologic study of 32 cases. Am J Surg Pathol 1982; 6: 503.

37 Tamimi HK, Bolen JW. Enchondromatosis (Ollier's disease) and ovarian juvenile granulosa cell tumor: a case report and review of the literature. Cancer 1984; 53: 1605.

38 Fienberg R. The stromal theca cell and postmenopausal endometrial adenocarcinoma. Cancer 1969; 24: 32.

39 Gough HM, Walther GL. Thecoma in pregnancy. Can Med Assoc J 1973; 108: 595.

40 Gillibrand PN. Granulosa-theca cell tumors of the ovary associated with pregnancy: case report and review of the literature. Am J Obstet Gynecol 1966; 94: 1108.

41 Gaffney EF, Majmudar B, Hewan-Lowe K. Ultrastructure and immunohistochemical localization of estradiol in three thecomas. Hum Pathol 1984; 15: 153.

42 Yaghoobian J, Pinck RL. Ultrasound findings in thecoma of the ovary. J Clin Ultrasound 1983; 11: 91.

43 Diakoumakis E, Vieux U, Seife B. Sonographic demonstration of thecoma: report of two cases. Am J Obstet Gynecol 1984; 150: 787.

44 Woo JSK, Ghosh A. Sonographic appearance of the ovarian thecoma (letter to the editor). Am J Obstet Gynecol 1985; 152: 361.

45 Scully RE. Sex cord tumor with annular tubules: a distinctive ovarian tumor of the Peutz–Jeghers syndrome. Cancer 1970; 25: 1107.

46 Norris HJ, Chorlton I. Functioning tumors of the ovary. Clin Obstet Gynecol 1974; 17: 189.

47 Hertel BF, Kempson RL. Ovarian sex cord tumors with annular tubules: an ultrastructural study. Am J Surg Pathol 1977; 1: 145.

48 Hart WR, Kumar N, Crissman JD. Ovarian neoplasms resembling sex cord tumors with annular tubules. Cancer 1980; 45: 2352.

49 Christian CD. Ovarian tumors: an extension of the Peutz–Jeghers syndrome. Am J Obstet Gynecol 1971; 111: 529.

50 Young RH, Welch WR, Scully RE, Dickersin GR. The distinctive gynecologic neoplasms of the Peutz–Jeghers syndrome (abstract). Lab Invest 1980; 42: 162.

51 Rodu B, Martinez MG Jr. Peutz–Jeghers syndrome and cancer. Oral Surg Oral Med Oral Pathol 1984; 58: 584.

52 Young RH, Dickersin GR, Scully RE. A distinctive ovarian sex cord-stromal tumor causing sexual precocity in the Peutz–Jeghers syndrome. Am J Surg Pathol 1983; 7: 233.

53 Young RH, Welch WR, Dickersin GR, Scully RE. Ovarian sex cord tumor with annular tubules: review of 74 cases including 27 with

Peutz–Jeghers syndrome and four with adenoma malignum of the cervix. Cancer 1982; 50:
1384.

54 Anderson MC, Govan ADT, Langley FA,
Woodcock AS, Tyagi SP. Ovarian sex cord

tumours with annular tubules. Histopathology
1980; 4: 137.

55 Purohit RC, Alam SZ. Sex cord tumour of the
ovary with annular tubules (SCTAT). Histopathology 1980; 4: 147.

Chapter **2**

Sertoli–Leydig Cell Tumor, Gynandroblastoma, and Lipid Cell Tumors of the Ovary

F.J. Montz and C.P. Morrow

Division of Gynecologic Oncology, Women's Hospital, Los Angeles, California, USA

INTRODUCTION

Gonadal stromal tumors in women are classified according to their differentiation towards ovarian follicles, testicular tubules, Leydig cells or adrenal cortical cells. The majority are tumors of 'female directed' cells classified as granulosa–theca tumors. A smaller percentage of gonadal stromal tumors are 'male directed', belonging in the Sertoli–Leydig category. The gynandroblastoma contains elements of both female and male directed cells. Lipid cell tumors encompass a group of neoplasms consisting primarily of Leydig (hilus) like cells, adrenal cortical like lipoid cells or both. Not infrequently gonadal stromal tumors are not sufficiently well differentiated to allow exact classification.

SERTOLI–LEYDIG CELL TUMORS

History

The Sertoli–Leydig cell tumors are unusual ovarian neoplasms initially described by Pick and labelled 'testicular adenomas' (1). Much of the early work on differentiating the histologic types of these stromal tumors was completed by Meyer (2–5). He utilized the trivial term 'arrhenoblastoma' (from Greek: *arrhenos*,

male). The World Health Organization has stated that the term 'Sertoli–Leydig cell tumor' (SLCT) is a more appropriate title (6). Reasons cited include: (1) 'Arrhenoblastoma' and 'androblastoma' connote masculinization whereas many of these tumors are hormonally inert or occasionally estrogenic, (2) multiple other types of ovarian neoplasms may be androgenic; (3) the morphologic designation 'Sertoli–Leydig cell' is parallel to that used for sex-stromal tumors that exhibit an ovarian direction of differentiation, the granulosa–theca cell tumors.

Epidemiology and Etiology

SLCT comprise approximately 1% of all ovarian tumors (7). A specific etiology of these neoplasms has not been discerned. The fact that the average age at diagnosis of the SLCT is significantly less than that of all ovarian neoplasms (25 years versus 57 years) is probably related to the cell line of origin of the SLCT and reflects a lack of a specific carcinogen.

The occurrence of these tumors is higher than the population average in three groups of individuals:

1. Patients with thyroid nodules (8–13).

2. Familial occurrence (9, 10, 14–17).
3. Patients with sarcoma botyroides (13).

Biology and Pathology

Biology

The existence of these neoplasms testifies to the sexual bipotentiality of the embryonic gonad. The parenchyma of the ovary and testicle are derived from the same primitive gonadal stroma, with granulosa and Sertoli cells as well as theca and Leydig cells being homologous (18). Adrenal and gonadal anlagen develop in adjacent areas of the embryo. Together these areas have been titled the 'steroid ridge'. The proximity of these embryologic precursors may account for certain ovarian stromal tumors resembling adrenal neoplasm (19).

Pathology

Gross. SLCTs lack a significant gross finding that would easily differentiate them from other solid ovarian neoplasms (20). Their size ranges from microscopic (21) to greater than 25 cm (20), with the average of the major series being approximately 10 cm. The well differentiated tumors as a whole are the smallest (average 5 to 6 cm), the poorest differentiated the largest (average 16 to 17 cm) and those of intermediate differentiation being between the two extremes (average 12 to 13 cm) (13, 20, 21).

These tumors are predominantly mixed solid and cystic (55–60%) with pure cystic tumors being uncommon (4–5%). On cross section the solid components are usually yellow-orange, reflecting a high lipid content. These masses are often lobulated (Figure 1).

Microscopic. Histologically, Sertoli–Leydig cell tumors are classified in four categories (6):

i) *Well differentiated*—tumors containing more than a small component of Leydig cells as well as Sertoli cells arranged in tubular patterns (Figures 2 and 3).

ii) *Intermediately differentiated*—tumors in

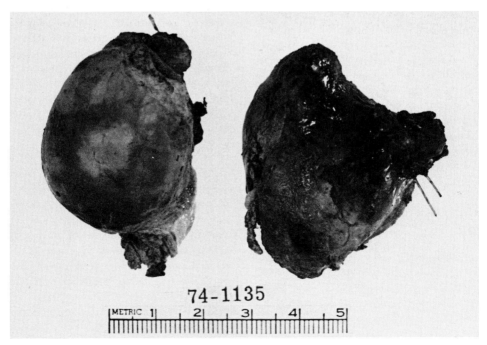

Figure 1 Sertoli–Leydig cell tumor of the ovary.

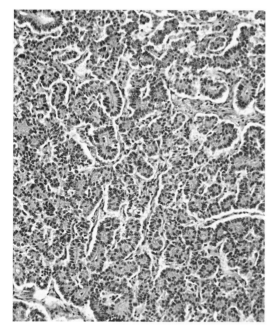

Figure 2 Sertoli–Leydig tumor, well differentiated. Leydig cells scanty.

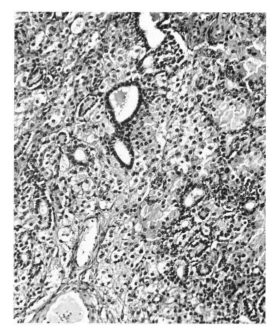

Figure 4 Sertoli–Leydig cell tumor intermediate differentiation (Leydig cells conspicuous).

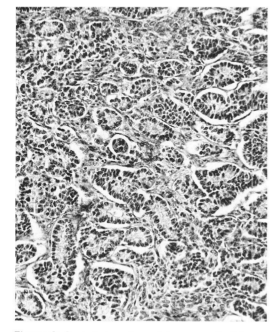

Figure 3 Sertoli–Leydig cell tumor well to intermediately differentiated.

which immature Sertoli cells are typically arranged diffusely, in islands, or in cords resembling embryonic testicular sex cords. Well defined tubules may be present and mature Leydig cells are usually identifiable (Figures 4 and 5).

iii) *Poorly differentiated*—tumors composed of tissue resembling that of the undifferentiated gonad. These tumors may resemble sarcomas (Figures 6 and 7).

iv) *Heterologous tumours*—tumors of intermediate or poor differentiation that contain, in addition, cell types foreign to the developing gonad. These include tubules and cysts lined by mucus filled epithelial cells and argentaffin cells, cartilage and skeletal muscle (Figure 8).

Young and Scully's review of 207 patients with SLCT, the largest to date, consisted of 11% well differentiated, 54% intermediately differentiated, 13% poorly differentiated and 22% of tumors demonstrating heterologous elements (13). This statistical separation is

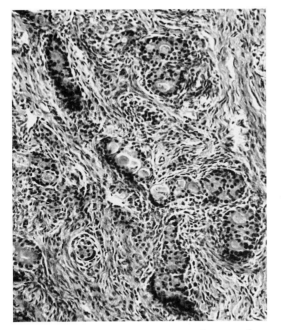

Figure 5 Sertoli–Leydig cell tumor. Intermediate differentiation. (original magnification: ×200)

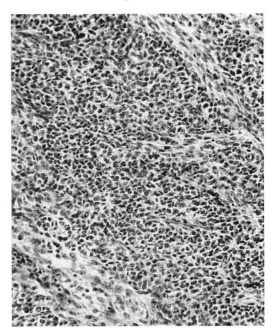

Figure 7 Poorly differentiated Sertoli–Leydig tumor (sarcomatoid pattern). (original magnification: ×200)

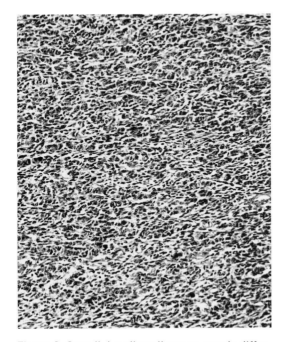

Figure 6 Sertoli–Leydig cell tumor, poorly differentiated.

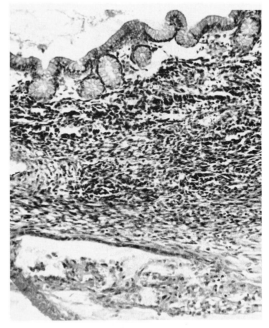

Figure 8 Sertoli–Leydig tumor with heterologous component (mucus epithelium and glands). (original magnification ×200)

2 Sertoli–Leydig cell tumor, gynandroblastoma, and lipid cell tumors

consistent with that reported by other compilations (12, 20, 21).

Pure Sertoli cell tumors are also a recognized entity (6) comprising approximately 5% of SLCT (22). Histologically pure Sertoli cell tumors are composed exclusively of Sertoli cells or contain only a minor component of steroid hormone-secreting elements consistent with Leydig cells (6) (Figure 9). The Sertoli cell tubules may be predominantly hollow or chiefly solid, the variants occurring with equal frequency (22, 23). Cell differentiation encompasses the gamut from poor to well with the latter appearing in the majority of cases (22–25).

Young and Scully assert that the microscopic differential diagnosis of SLCT varies with the degree of differentiation, as well as the presence of heterologous or retiform components (13). The differential diagnosis for the well differentiated tumors and those intermediate tumors that are better differentiated includes well differentiated endometrioid car-

cinomas (26, 27) tubular Krukenberg tumors (28), and carcinoid tumors of the insular type (29) (Figure 10).

The explanation given by Young and Scully as to why these neoplasms may be confused is that the glands and solid epithelial formations may mimic the hollow and solid tubules of SLCT (13). They state that SLCT may also be lined by hobnail cells that could suggest the diagnosis of a clear cell carcinoma.

Separating SLCT of intermediate and poor differentiation from the granulosa cell tumors (GCT) may be a histopathologic challenge. Young and Scully claim that the appearance of heterologous elements is specific for a SLCT. The same is true for a retiform pattern, while the majority of the other features which are typical for SLCT may occasionally be evident in GCT.

Those tumors interpreted as containing both SLCT and GCT components have been termed as 'gynandroblastomas' (30–32). The World Health Organization recommends that

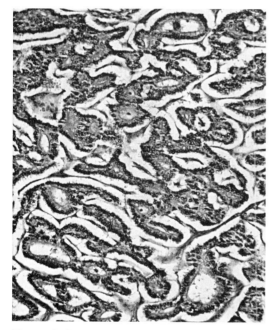

Figure 9 Sertoli cell tumor (Pick's adenoma). (original magnification: ×200)

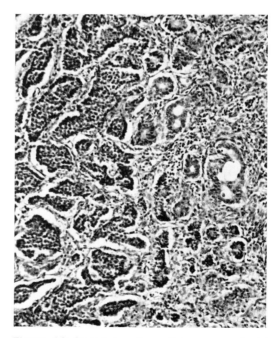

Figure 10 Sertoli–Leydig cell tumor carcinoid variant. (original magnification: ×200)

the diagnosis of gynandroblastoma be reserved for those neoplasms with substantial amounts of easily recognizable ovarian and testicular elements, as extensive sampling of a GCT or SLCT frequently demonstrates small foci of cells that are more characteristic of the opposing cell type (6).

Intermediate forms of SLCT have a differential diagnosis including, granulosa cell tumors (13), carcinoid tumor of the trabecular type (33), and endometrioid stromal sarcomas of ovary (34).

The heterologous SLCT (containing gastrointestinal epithelium (35) skeletal muscle or cartilage (36), and the poorly differentiated SLCT contain in their differential diagnosis, mixed mesodermal sarcoma of ovary (13), ovarian teratomas (37, 38), and pure mucinous cystic tumors (13).

Young and Scully state that the retiform variant of SLCT causes specific problems in differential diagnosis. These tumors are most often confused with an *endodermal sinus tumor*. However, by appreciating a variety of clinical and pathologic differences, the correct diagnosis can be ascertained (13).

The differential diagnosis for the pure Sertoli cell tumors encompass lipid cell tumors (22), well differentiated endometrioid tumors (28), metastatic tubular Krukenberg tumors (28), carcinoid tumors (39), and ovarian tumors of probable Wolffian origin (40).

Meticulous histopathologic technique interfaced with information on clinical presentation allows discernment of the appropriate diagnosis (22).

In those cases where the differentiation of SLCT from other histologic types of ovarian neoplasm is difficult, Young and Scully propose that electron microscopic and immunocytochemical examination should be implemented. These modalities may yield the essential findings to confirm a provisional diagnosis. Electron microscopy may reveal the Charcot–Bottcher crystals of Sertoli cells or the crystalloids of Reinke associated with Leydig cells. Similarly, the typical cytologic features of steroid hormone secreting cells or the charac-

teristic findings of other cell lines may be identified (41–43). The present experience employing immunocytochemistry is limited but this modality appears to be a valuable tool (44).

Clinical Features

The specific features of a given patient with a SLCT will vary with the degree of histologic differentiation. The mean age of all subjects is approximately 25 years (12, 13, 21, 22). Well differentiated tumors appear on the whole in the older patient (Roth et al.: 41 years (21), Zaloudek and Norris: 40 years (12), while Young and Scully showed a mean of 35 years (13). Tumors with a prominent retiform pattern or low grade of differentiation occur in significantly younger patients (13, 21). This is also the case in patients with pure Sertoli tumors (22, 23). Most lesions are palpable on bimanual examination, having an average diameter of 10 cm, and appreciated prior to celiotomy.

The paramount and prototypical clinical features of SLCT are defeminization and virilization. During the reproductive years, defeminization usually precedes virilization, but these two features may occur in a disorderly fashion. The former process includes oligo-amenorrhea with atrophy of the breast and genital tissues. More reliable indications of excessive androgen production are the signs of virilization. These include clitorimegaly, hirsutism, acne, changes in voice characteristics, and increased libido. Less often the body muscle mass increases and temporal balding occurs. These changes often develop over a period of several years before diagnosis, although a rapid onset of virilization is more specific for a neoplastic origin. The changes of androgen excess are usually less obtrusive in the postmenopausal female, but, even in young women these signs and symptoms may be insidious. Instances of heterosexual precocity due to SLCT have rarely been reported (45–47). In the series by Roth et al., 39% of patients with SLCT were virilized and 11% were hirsute (21). Similarly, Zaloudek and Norris noted virilization in 38% of patients with SLCT (12) while Young and Scully reported similar findings in 34% of their patients (13). Roth et al. (21), as well as O'Hearn and Neubecker (20) demonstrated an increased incidence of virilization in patients with histologically less well differentiated neoplasms. Neither the Zaloudek and Norris (12) series nor the Young and Scully (13) series concurred. The latter authors did show that patients with a prominent retiform component had a lower incidence of these side effects (13).

The classic aberration in the hormonal milieu of patients with SLCT and virilization is an elevation of plasma testosterone (48–56). Elevated levels of plasma androstenedione (13), 17-ketosteroids (12), and corticosteroids (57) have also been reported. It has been repeatedly emphasized that patients with SLCT traditionally have higher levels of testosterone than those with non-neoplastic causes of androgen excess (i.e. stromal hyperthecosis, polycystic ovary syndrome, and testosterone secreting adrenal adenoma) (58–62). The clinician should recall that SLCTs are not the sole ovarian neoplasm which may be androgenic GCTs have been documented as being androgenic (63–66), and, as will be discussed later in this chapter, both gynandroblastomas and the lipid cell tumors may be androgenic. Reported cases of Krukenberg tumors have been demonstrated to be responsible for virilization (67–70) particularly in relationship to pregnancy.

Sixty-five per cent of patients with pure Sertoli cell tumors manifest symptoms of hyperestrogenism (22). SLCTs have also been associated with estrogenic effects (12, 13, 20–21, 71, 72). The presence of androgen excess is evidence against the diagnosis of a pure Sertoli cell tumor since androgen production is the province of Leydig cells (22). Symptoms of estrogen excess include isosexual precocious puberty, menstrual irregularities and post-menopausal bleeding. Histologic diagnosis at time of evaluation of endometrial specimens has shown all stages of hyperplasia including well differentiated adenocarcinoma (12, 13).

A paraneoplastic syndrome of resistant hypertension has been demonstrated in patients with pure Sertoli cell tumors. Etiology of this hypertension is reportedly due to aldosteronism (25) or excessive non-renal renin production (73). Unfortunately, when Ehrlich et al. reported their case in 1962, renin assays were unavailable. In reviewing the case history it is probable that the patient's hypertension was related to excessive non-renal renin production.

SLCT may be associated with elevated alpha-fetoprotein (APF) levels (11, 74, 75). AFP is an oncofetal antigen normally produced in early fetal development by cells of the yolk sac, liver and upper gastrointestinal tract, and is useful as a tumor marker while following patients with endodermal sinus (yolk sac) tumor (EST), embryonal carcinoma or a mixed germ cell neoplasm of the ovary containing one of these elements. It is purported that in the process of tumorogenesis derepression of genes coding for AFP production occurs and this may account for AFP production by these non-germ cell tumors (74). The value of routine AFP screening has not been documented in patients with SLCT. If an elevated AFP is demonstrated it should motivate the pathologist to re-evaluate the surgical specimen to guarantee that a component of EST has not been overlooked.

Investigation

SLCT should be the primary diagnostic consideration in the patient who presents with symptoms of androgen excess and a unilateral adnexal mass (76, 77). In contradistinction, the preoperative diagnosis of SLCT is impossible in those patients lacking physical or laboratory findings consistent with androgen excess. When evaluating the patient with androgen excess the clinician must remember that very small SLCTs which could not be appreciated on physical examinations have been responsible for androgen excess (21, 78).

In the patient lacking the above mentioned 'classic' clinical presentation, the differential diagnosis will vary depending upon the presence or absence of signs of androgen excess. If these signs are present the differential diagnosis should include:

1. Anovulation.
2. Polycystic ovary disease.
3. Stromal thecosis.
4. Cushing's syndrome.
5. Acromegaly.
6. Pregnancy (with possible associated luteoma).
7. Exogenous source of androgens:
   a. Methyltestosterone.
   b. Anabolic agents.
   c. Dilantin (phenytoin).
   d. Danazol.
   e. Oral contraceptive (17-nor ketosteroids).
8. Congenital adrenal hyperplasia.
9. Genetic abnormalities:
   a. Y-containing mosaic.
   b. Incomplete testicular feminization.

Should signs of androgen excess be lacking, the differential diagnosis is that of any other solid or solid–cystic adnexal mass with a primary ovarian neoplastic process being foremost.

Characterizing the etiology of androgen excess appears initially to be a complex, time consuming procedure. However, following the orderly sequence described by Speroff et al. (79) it can be completed without undue stress (Table 1, Figures 11 and 12, used with permission).

Recent reports have highlighted the value of selected ovarian and adrenal vein steroid sampling in evaluating the patient with androgen excess (80, 81). Realizing that catherization is an invasive procedure which is not without risk, we would recommend its implementation only in the patient where a diagnosis has been unobtainable using tools short of surgical exploration (82–85).

SLCT in Pregnancy

SLCT, being found predominantly in the reproductive age female, may occur in association with pregnancy (17, 86–91). Many of these patients will present with the classic symptoms of virilization (17) which may progress during the gestation (87, 73). This scenario can occur in patients who are routinely judged to be anovulatory. It has been well documented that ovulation and subsequent conception may occur despite an abnormally high serum testosterone of long standing (90). If the fetus is a female infant, the infant is at risk of virilization (88).

Management mimics that of the non-pregnant female and will be described later in this chapter. Five-year survival rates are comparable stage for stage with the non-pregnant patient (17).

Staging

The staging of ovarian cancer most widely used is that adopted by the General Assembly of the International Federation of Gynaecology and Obstetrics (FIGO) in New York City, April 12, 1970 (modified September 1985). Significant to note is that ovarian malignancy, in contradistinction to the other gynecologic malignancies, is staged at time of surgical exploration. The final cytology and

TABLE 1 PROCEDURE FOR CHARACTERIZING THE ETIOLOGY OF ANDROGEN EXCESS

1 History and physical examination
2 Radioimmunoassay (RIA) for serum levels of:
   A Testosterone (Figure 12)
   B DHEAS (Figure 11)
   C Prolactin
   D Thyroid function tests
3 Screen for Cushing's syndrome/disease if suspicion is high:
   A 24 hours free cortisol excretion
   B Late evening plasma cortisol level
   C Single dose overnight dexamethasone suppression test
   D If C abnormal: low dose dexamethasone suppression test

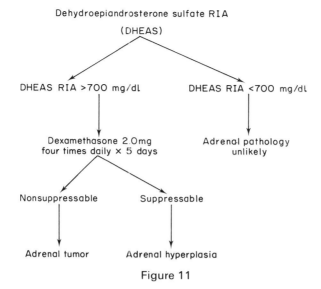

Figure 11

histology is to be considered in the staging (Table 2).

The majority of reported cases demonstrate SLCT confined to the ovary (97–100%) (12, 13, 20, 21). Bilaterality occurs rarely. Neither Roth et al. (21) nor Zaloudek and Norris (12) reported this occurrence. Young and Scully (13) noted bilaterality in 1.5% of SLCT. Bilaterality has also been reported by Okun (92). Young and Scully state that several of the purported examples of bilateral SLCT in the literature are tumors of other cell types (13) such as Krukenberg tumors (38, 45–48, 93–94), luteinized thecomas (86) or a testicular tumor in a patient with androgen insensitivity (95). Those neoplasms that have spread to other pelvic structures or beyond (FIGO Stage II and III) are usually of poor differentiation or contain heterologous elements (12, 13).

Management and Prognosis

Surgery

The great majority of these lesions are unilateral, solid and limited to the ovary (FIGO Stage IA). Therefore surgical management is the mainstay of therapy. In the young repro-

ductive age patient, the preferred operation is a unilateral adnexectomy. Women beyond childbearing are best treated with a bilateral salpingo-oophorectomy and total abdominal hysterectomy. This recommendation is given independent of cell type or malignant potential. A fractional dilatation and curettage is indicated prior to laparotomy in the patient with abnormal uterine bleeding. Information as to the presence of premalignant or malignant endometrial neoplasia is essential before performing a conservative operation.

The SLCT, as has been discussed earlier, is frequently difficult to identify histologically. Frozen section may be helpful in certain instances. Should the tumor be predominantly solid and not deeply pigmented, dysgerminoma, mixed germ cell tumor or metastatic tumor to the ovary must be ruled out. Intraoperative identification is helpful since lymph node involvement and occult bilaterality are common in dysgerminoma, for example. Similarly, a search for a primary malignancy must be performed if the lesion is felt to be a metastasis. In all cases peritoneal washings for cytology (pelvis and abdomen) are to be obtained. A careful exploration of the abdomen and pelvis for evidence of intra- and

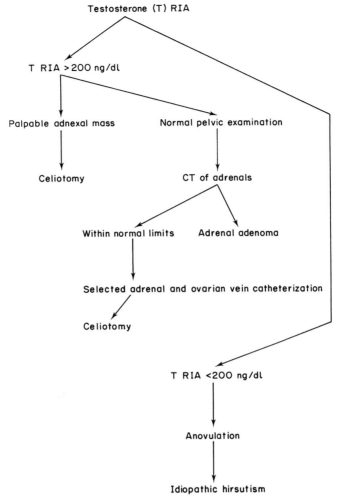

Figure 12

retroperitoneal metastasis is performed. Target peritoneal biopsies, omental biopsy (dependent, adherent or clinically suspicious portion) and biopsy of any suspect areas of the opposite ovary should be carried out.

Prognosis for long term survival is intimately related to degree of differentiation and stage at time of diagnosis (13, 77). In the major studies none of the well differentiated tumors, all of which were Stage IAi, behaved in a malignant fashion (12, 13, 20–23). Only 20% of Stage I tumors are clinically malignant whereas the reported cases of Stage III tumors have been universally fatal (13, 21). Those tumors that have ruptured are more likely to be malignant and of poorly differentiated cell types (12, 13). The mitotic rate of tumors is also predictive of prognosis. Scully and Young (13) use the finding of 15 mitotic figures per 10 high power fields (HPFs), while Zaloudek and Norris found that the mitotic rate had prognostic significance when it was over 10 mitotic figures per 10 HPFs (12). Tumors with high mitotic rates are generally of the poorly differentiated type. However, intermediate cell types have been identified with similar high mitotic

TABLE 2 STAGING OF OVARY CARCINOMA (Based on findings at clinical examination and surgical exploration. The final histology (and cytology when required) *after surgery* is to be considered in the staging.)

Stage I	Growth limited to the ovaries.
Stage IA	Growth limited to one ovary; no ascites. No tumor on the external surface: capsule intact.
Stage IB	Growth limited to both ovaries; no ascites. No tumor on the external surfaces; capsules intact.
Stage IC[a]	Tumor either Stage IA or IB but with tumor on surface of one or both ovaries; or with capsule ruptured; or with ascites present containing malignant cells or with positive peritoneal washings.
Stage II	Growth involving one or both ovaries with pelvic extension.
Stage IIA	Extension and/or metastases to the uterus and/or tubes.
Stage IIB	Extension to other pelvic tissues.
Stage IIC[a]	Tumor either Stage IIA or IIB, but with tumor on surface of one or both ovaries; or with capsule(s) ruptured; or with ascites present containing malignant cells or with positive peritoneal washings.
Stage III	Tumor involving one or both ovaries with peritoneal implants outside the pelvis and/or positive retroperitoneal or inguinal nodes. Superficial liver metastasis equals Stage III.
Stage IIIA	Tumor grossly limited to the true pelvis with negative nodes but with histologically confirmed microscopic seeding of abdominal peritoneal surfaces.
Stage IIIB	Tumor of one or both ovaries with histologically confirmed implants of abdominal peritoneal surfaces none exceeding 2 cm in diameter. Nodes are negative.
Stage IIIC	Abdominal implants greater than 2 cm in diameter and/or positive retroperitoneal or inguinal nodes.
Stage IV	Growth involving one or both ovaries with distant metastases. If pleural effusion is present, there must be positive cytology to allot a case to Stage IV. Parenchymal liver metastasis equals Stage IV.

[a] To evaluate the impact on prognosis of the different criteria for allotting cases to Stage IC or IIC, it would be a value to know: (1) if rupture of the capsule was (a) spontaneous or (b) caused by the surgeon or (2) if the source of malignant cells detected was (a) peritoneal washings or (b) ascites.

counts (12, 13). In Young and Scully's series, the size of the tumor also correlated with prognosis when the Stage IAi tumors of intermediate differentiation were evaluated. Only one of 50 tumors under 15 cm in diameter was malignant compared to four of 16 larger tumors (13).

Recurrence of the SLCT classically occurs early (66–70% in 1 year) and locally (12, 13). However, distant metastases including the lung, scalp, and supraclavicular lymph node have been reported. Recurrence of SLCT has been accompanied with recurrence of signs and symptoms of androgen excess (21, 96, 97). The value of serial postoperative androgen/testosterone serum levels has not, however, been confirmed.

Adjunctive Therapy

Postoperative adjunctive therapy is indicated for those patients who have SLCT with greater than 15 mitoses/10 HPFs of heterologous elements: gastrointestinal mucosa, skeletal muscle or cartilage. Similarly any patient whose SLCT is more advanced than Stage IAi should receive adjunctive therapy. The decision in these cases, therefore, is not whether adjunctive therapy is indicated, but in what form it should be implemented. Due to the rarity of these neoplasms and the fact that the majority are of early stage and low or intermediate grade, there is no adequate series to date for determining the best modality. At present a combination of multiagent chemotherapy or radiation is the most frequently implemented adjunct.

In 1976 Schwartz and Smith (98) recommended radiation therapy alone if the residual tumor after surgical debulking consisted of nodules smaller than 2 cm. Patients with larger residual implants were treated with a combination of vincristine, actinomycin D, and cyclophosphamide (VAC). Of 3 patients treated with VAC, 2 had an objective response and were alive at 20 months and 3 years. The latter patient had also received pelvic radiation therapy.

Cisplatin, bleomycin and etoposide (VP-16) (11) or triosulfan (21) have been employed by other authors with only short term responses. Pride et al (89) reported a patient with Stage III SLCT who was treated by extensive cytoreductive surgery followed by 11 courses of bleomycin, vincristine, cyclophosphamide, doxorubicin and cisplatin chemotherapy. Clinically the patient was free of disease after two courses of chemotherapy, and after eight courses, underwent a negative second look celiotomy (see Table 3). Three further courses of chemotherapy were given and the patient was clinically free of disease 22 months after the initial therapy. Zaloudek and Norris presented a patient with Stage III disease who was treated with a bilateral salpingo-oophorectomy, omentectomy, 5000 cGy whole pelvis radiation and VAC chemotherapy. The patient underwent second look celiotomy 2 years later and was found to be free of disease. She was clinically free of tumor when last evaluated by the authors 3 years after instituting therapy.

In the largest collection to date (Young and Scully (13)), 13 of 22 patients with clinically malignant SLCT of intermediate or poor differentiation received chemotherapy, 8 received radiation therapy and chemotherapy, and 2 had radiation therapy alone. The authors claim benefit in 5 of the treated patients (38%). However, follow-up was short, and 2 of the 5 patients died from complications of the therapy. One, a 16 year old with a poorly differentiated, ruptured tumor (Stage IAii), received doxorubicin and chlorambucil postoperatively. Six months later a recurrent pelvic mass was resected and radiation and chemotherapy were administered. Doxorubicin was given again, followed by cyclophosphamide, actinomycin D, cisplatin, vinblastine, and bleomycin. She died 28 months postoperatively of *Pneumocystis carinii* pneumonia. An autopsy was not performed, but the patient was clinically free of tumor at the time of her death. The second case was a 19 year old with a

TABLE 3 RESTAGING CELIOTOMY

Indications	(1) To assess completeness of response (2) To reduce resectable tumor volume
Timing	After completion of six cycles of VAC chemotherapy, patients exhibiting a complete response or a partial response with respectable disease will undergo a restaging laparotomy.
Incision	Midline vertical
Ascites	If present, must be examined cytologically
Washings	If no ascites, washings must be obtained immediately upon opening the peritoneal cavity from: (a) pelvis (b) right and left paracolic gutters (c) subdiaphragmatic space The separate specimens should be examined cytologically
Exploration	All peritoneal surfaces must be visually examined including direct inspection of the diaphragm. The location and exact size of tumor node must be described. Biopsy proof of residual disease is necessary. If no visual tumor is seen, routine biopsies must be obtained from: (a) pelvic peritoneum (b) cul-de-sac peritoneum (c) right and left abdominal gutter peritoneum (2 biopsies) (d) undersurface of the right diaphragm (e) remaining omentum (f) adhesive bands, abnormally scarred areas (g) retroperitoneum—the spaces on both sides of the pelvis should be opened and selected lymph nodes from the pelvic and para-aortic chains removed.
Laparoscopy	Laparoscopic evaluation of the peritoneal cavity is acceptable as a second-look procedure if disease can be seen and biopsied through the laparoscope. If no disease is seen, then exploratory operation is mandatory.

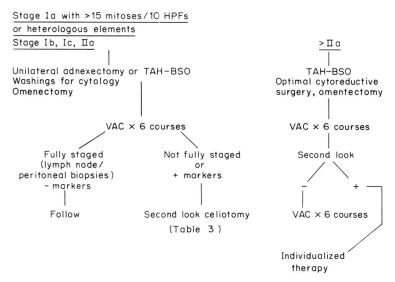

Figure 13 Adjunctive therapy of SLCT.

poorly differentiated Stage IA(i) tumor which was recurrent in the pelvis and omentum 8 months postoperatively. The tumor was excised and VAC chemotherapy followed by bleomycin was administered postoperatively. The patient was well for the next year but then developed progressive respiratory failure and died clinically free of disease 2 years after her initial diagnosis.

Our recommendation is that candidates for adjunctive therapy be managed as illustrated in Figure 13.

GYNANDROBLASTOMA

History

Meyer first described the gynandroblastoma in 1930 (99). Since that time there have been sporadic reports of these rare neoplasms. Furthermore, extensive discussions as to whether they truly are a separate entity and what pathologic criteria allow a stromal neoplasm to qualify as such have been held.

Epidemiology and Etiology

These tumors are excessively rare, comprising less than 1% of all ovarian stromal tumors (100, 101). Etiology, as in the case of the other gonadal stromal tumors, is unknown.

Biology and Pathology

The origin of gynandroblastoma is still debated. At present the most popular theory is that these tumors are derived from undifferentiated gonadal mesenchyme which has a bisexual potential (102). The neoplastic insult occurs and the common precursor cell differentiates into both 'female directed' and 'male directed' cell lines.

Gross

These lesions are ordinarily 7 and 10 cm in size, solid yellow-white with cystic areas commonly being present. Size may vary greatly, however, with a remarkable case of a 37 lb tumor reported (103).

Microscopic

Histopathologically, this neoplasm manifests a 'paradoxical combination of elements' (104) of

both male and female directed cells. To fulfill
the World Health Organization requirements
for classification as a gynandroblastoma rigid
pathologic, not clinical, criteria must be fulfilled (105–107) Identification of unequivocal
granulosa–theca cell elements and Sertoli–
Leydig cell elements is essential. The tumor
must be fairly well differentiated (101) so that
these are readily distinguished (Figure 14). In

addition, all the constituent cell types must be
intimately mixed (6) as separate SLCT and
GCT have been found in the same ovary (100).
Fulfillment of these criteria is imperative, as
production of both estrogen and androgen by
an ovarian tumor is not diagnostic, despite the
fact that early authors have claimed such
(108). Testicular elements may be feminizing
and ovarian elements masculinizing (109).

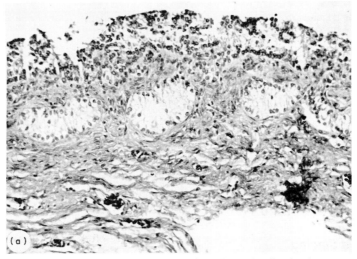

Figure 14a Gynandroblastoma. Surfacing Call–Exner bodies in close apposition
to tubules composed of Sertoli cells. (original magnification: ×200)

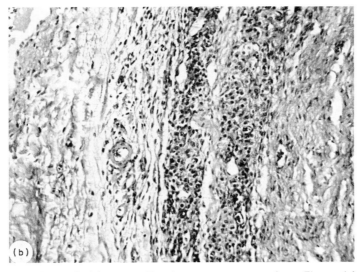

Figure 14b Gynandroblastoma. Ovarian stroma remote from Figure 14a exhibiting clusters of interstitial cells. (original magnification: ×200)

Clinical Features

Gynandroblastomas were first described as presenting with signs and symptoms of both estrogen and androgen over production (99), and may be expected to behave according to the nature of their constituent elements.

Review of reported cases shows that the majority of these tumors occur in patients in their third, fourth or fifth decade (30, 31, 99, 104, 107, 110). Sixty percent of patients have symptoms of androgen excess as described for SLCT. It has been reported that where male and female cellular elements coexist, the androgenic stimulus overrides the estrogenic effects as far as the general body pattern is concerned, so that virilization is the presenting picture. Yet the estrogenic influence predominates at its specific end organ site so that endometrial hyperplasia is commonly noted in those patients whose endometrium is sampled (110). Due to the large average size of these lesions, the majority are palpable preoperatively.

Investigation and Staging

As was highlighted under the discussion of SLCT, patients with symptoms of androgen excess and a unilateral adnexal mass have a diagnosis of an androgen producing ovarian neoplasm until proven otherwise. Gynandroblastomas due to their excessively rare occurrence, are uncommonly the primary preoperative diagnosis.

Hormonal analysis preoperatively in those patients who have histopathologically confirmed gynandroblastoma conventionally demonstrates elevated circulating testosterone (102, 101, 110) or urinary 17-ketosteroids (31). Lesser elevations of androstenedione, dehydroepiandrosterone and dihydrotestosterone have also been noted (112, 111) with or without associated elevation of serum testosterone or urinary 17-ketosteroids. Elevated serum estradiols have also been confirmed (113). Hormonal evaluation was not completed in all reported cases (31, 32) and in a very unusual case of an 18 year old mentally retarded patient with marked virilization and a 37 lb gynandroblastoma the testosterone and androsteredione levels were normal preoperatively (103). After oophorectomy the testosterone and androstenedione levels fell dramatically.

For the patient presenting with symptoms of androgen excess but lacking significant physical findings on pelvic/abdominal examination, the workup is as described under the SLCT.

Management and Prognosis

The principles of management of gynandroblastoma follow those set forth for SLCT. Surgery is the mainstay, with the emphasis on unilateral adnexectomy in the young reproductive age female with early (FIGO IA) disease. More extensive and radical surgery is indicated in the postreproductive patient and those with more advanced disease. Adequate surgical staging is essential. Those unusual gynandroblastomas that have ruptured, spread beyond the ovary or are associated with ascites are often fatal (32) and require aggressive management. Intraperitoneal ^{32}P has been implemented as adjunctive therapy, but reported cases are few and indications limited (103). Our recommendation is vincristine, actinomycin D and cyclophosphamide chemotherapy as with the other specialized gonadal stromal tumors. In the patient with elevated serum estrogen or androgen levels we would serially measure these as they may be useful tumor markers.

LIPID CELL TUMORS

History

These heterogeneous stromal tumors were first grouped by Barzilai (114) in 1943 and first labelled as a generic class by Scully in 1963 (115) who included all tumors composed of large, rounded polyhedral cells that resemble Leydig, lutein and adrenal cortical cells.

Synonymous titles used for these tumors include:

hilar cell tumor (116–118),
Leydig cell tumor (119, 120),
stromal luteoma (121, 122),
adrenal rest tumor (123),
adrenal like tumor (124),

as well as others (125).

Epidemiology and Etiology

Lipid cell tumors comprise less than 0.1% of ovarian neoplasms, being one of the least common tumors arising from the female gonad (127, 126). The etiology of these, as with the other ovarian stromal tumours, is unknown.

Biology and Pathology

Hughesdon has proposed that fibromas, fibrothecomas, thecomas, lipid cell thecomas and lipid cell tumors form a series of related 'stromatogenous tumors' (129, 128). Previously, certain authors preferred to distinguish hilar cell tumors from lipid cell tumors classifying those with demonstrable Reinke's crystalloids into the former category (127). In 1973, the World Health Organization committee on histologic classification of tumors elected to include the hilar cell tumor with lipid cell tumors (6). Scully has subdivided lipid cell tumors into two categories: the hilus cell type with Reinke's crystalloids and the stromal type lacking these (100). We will follow Scully's lead and subsequently discuss these two groups separately.

The cell of origin of these tumors is still in question. Kempson suggested that the lipid cell tumor was derived from ovarian stromal cells (130). Taylor and Norris (127) as well as Hiura et al. (131) agree. Koss et al. concluded that the lipid cell tumor they studied was related to the adrenal cortex and may have arisen from an adrenal rest in the ovary (132). Hughesdon (128) and Sobrinko and Kase (123) were of a similar opinion. Origin from hilar cells (Leydig cells) also has been proposed (133, 134). These

hypotheses of origin reflect different primary cell lines of the tumors evaluated rather than different levels of histopathologic diagnostic competency.

Hilus Cell Type with Reinke's Crystalloids (Leydig Cell)

These tumors are predominantly unilateral, solid yellow-orange in color with the majority being less than 6 cm in diameter. Leydig cell tumors are composed entirely of Leydig cells. The designation 'hilus cell tumor' is usually reserved for those tumors located in the ovarian hilus and composed entirely of Leydig cells. The pure Leydig cell tumor differs from the SLCT in that it lacks a sex cord (Sertoli cell) component and differs from the stromal-Leydig cell tumor in that it lacks the thecoma like stromal component (126).

These tumors are distinguished from the lipoid cell tumors primarily by the presence of Reinke's crystalloids the pathognomonic microscopic feature of Leydig cells (121, 135).

Lipoid Cell Tumors (Hilus Stromal Type without Reinke Crystalloids)

Grossly, these lesions are small (50% < 5 cm (124), solid unilateral and yellow-orange in color. The lipoid cell tumors are characterized by large, rounded or polyhedral cells resembling Leydig cells, luteinized ovarian stromal cells and adenocortical cells (128). Crystalloids of Reinke must be absent for inclusion in this subcategory.

Clinical Features

The published literature demonstrates that Leydig cell tumors occur predominantly in the postmenopausal female while lipoid cell tumors occur most frequently during the reproductive years. Presentation in postmenopausal females and children, however, has been confirmed in the lipoid tumors (136).

Characteristically, this group of tumors is virilizing, with only 10% having normal androgen profiles and lacking signs of excess androgen production (124). The Leydig cell tumors classically produce testosterone (83, 117, 133, 137). They have been reported to produce high levels of estrogen with patients developing subsequent endometrial hyperplasia and adenocarcinoma (138–141). The lipoid tumors which produce androgens are, unlike the Leydig cell tumor and SLCT, often associated with a substantial increase in serum androstenedione (142). This is reflected in elevated urinary 17-ketosteroids. However, the steroid pattern of these tumors has a wide interpatient variance (143–147).

Paraneoplastic syndromes have been associated with the lipid cell tumors. Cushingoid features have been demonstrated (57, 127) and recently a well documented case of an ovarian lipid cell tumor causing Cushing's syndrome with elevated serum cortisol was reported (148). Paraneoplastic erythrocytosis associated with production of erythopoietin and testosterone by a malignant lipid cell tumor has also been reported (125).

The lipid cell tumors are frequently not appreciated preoperatively due to their small average size (149). Should a lesion be clinically androgenic, the differential diagnosis is as that outlined for the SLCT. If the tumor is hormonally inert, a preoperative clinical diagnosis more specific than ovarian neoplasia is impossible.

Investigation and Staging

The investigation and staging of the lipid cell tumors are the same as that of SLCT. Recently a NP59 ([6-^{131}I]iodomethyl nor-cholesterol) scan was instrumental in diagnosing a lipid cell tumor in a 36 year old patient with a 30 year history of virilization of unknown etiology (135).

Management and Prognosis

Leydig cell tumors are almost invariably benign while perhaps 20% of lipoid cell tumors are malignant (127, 136, 143, 144). Those tumors with pleomorphism, increased mitoses and a maximal diameter greater than 8 cm should be considered malignant. Early stage tumors (FIGO IAi) in the reproductive age patient may be managed by unilateral adnexectomy. Patients not desirous of future fertility and those with more advanced stage disease are best treated by total abdominal hysterectomy, bilateral salpingo-oophorectomy with extensive tumor reductive surgery when indicated.

Lipid cell tumors which are metastatic have been treated in a variety of fashions (125, 136, 143, 144) and due to the lack of a large series in the literature, anecdotal information is pervasive. Echt and Hadd treated a metastatic hilus cell tumor (probable FIGO III) with surgery and radiation (136). Not all the tumor was primarily removed and progression of disease was noted early in the postoperative course. The tumor was refractory to aggressive radiation therapy and continued to grow while the patient was treated with chlormadinone acetate and high dose Premarin. The patient died from her disease 3 years after diagnosis.

Lipsett et al. reported a virilizing lipoid cell tumor which recurred 14 years after unilateral adnexectomy (143). The lesion was not surgically debulked and was treated as an adrenal cortical cell tumor with hCG (human chorionic gonadotropin) and op′-DDD (2,2-bis-[p-chlorophenyl]-1,1-dichloroethane). 17-Ketosteroid excretion, plasma testosterone and androstenedione levels dropped remarkably, but after 21 days of treatment therapy was stopped because of clinical progression of disease. The patient died 14 days later.

A case of probable Stage III lipoid cell tumor in a XXX female was reported by Khoo and Buntine (144). The patient was treated by surgical resection with no gross residual tumor remaining. Postoperatively she was treated with melphalan and was disease free when last seen 9 months after surgery.

Montag, Murphy and Belinson treated a Stage IV lipoid cell tumor with suboptimal surgical debulking followed by Cytoxan, Adriamycin and cis-platinum chemotherapy, with the patient failing after three courses (125). Attempts at rescue with hexamethylmelamine, 5-FU, methotrexate as well as vinblastine and actinomycin D were unsuccessful and the patient succumbed to her disease.

Our present recommendation is that every attempt at aggressive cytoreductive surgery be made. The patient should then be treated with triple chemotherapeutic agents, our preference being vincristine, actinomycin D and Cytoxan. If the patient has elevated serum androgens we recommend that these be followed monthly until normal for 3 months and then re-determined every 3 months. Chemotherapy should be continued for a minimum of eight courses. In the patient who did not have optimal tumor reduction at initial surgery, responders should be re-explored to resect any residual disease at the completion of six to eight courses.

REFERENCES

1 Pick L. Uber Adenoma der mannlicken und weiblichen Keimdrüse. Berl Klin Wehn 1905; 42: 502.
2 Meyer R. Uber Adenoma malignum ovarii. Z Geburtsch Gynak 1915; 76: 616.
3 Meyer R. Tubulare (testikulare) und solide Formen des Andreiblastoma ovarii und ihre Beziehung zur Vermannlichung. Beitr Path Anat 1930; 84: 485.
4 Meyer R. Zur Pathologie der zur Vermannlichung fuhrenden Tumoren der Ovarien (Arrhenoblastoma ovarii). Verhandl Deutsch Path Gesellsch 1930; 25: 328.
5 Meyer R. Pathology of some special ovarian tumors and their relation to sex characteristics. Am J Obstet Gynecol 1931; 22: 657.
6 Serov SF, Scully RE, Soblin LH. International histological classification of tumors No. 9. Histological typing of ovarian tumors. Geneva: World Health Organization, 1973.
7 Hughesdon PE. Raver non-germinal ovarian malignancies. In: Hudson CN. ed, Ovarian Cancer. Oxford: Oxford Medical Publications, 1985: 119.
8 Javert CT, Finn WF. Arrhenoblastoma. The incidence of malignancy and the relationship to pregnancy, sterility and treatment. Cancer 1951; 4: 60.
9 Jensen RD, Norris HJ, Fraumen JF. Familial arrhenoblastoma and thyroid adenoma. Cancer 1974; 33: 218.
10 O'Brien PK, Wilansky DL. Familial thyroid nodulation and arrhenoblastoma. Am J Clin Pathol 1981; 75: 578.
11 Benfield GEA, Taper-Jones L, Stout GV. Androblastoma and raised serum-fetoprotein with familial multinodular goitre. Case report. Br J Obstet Gynecol 1982; 89: 323.
12 Zaloudek C, Norris HJ. Sertoli–Leydig tumors of the ovary. A clinicopathologic study of 64 intermediate and poorly differentiated neoplasms. Am J Surg Pathol 1984; 8: 405.
13 Young RH, Scully RE. Ovarian Sertoli–Leydig cell tumors: A clinicopathological analysis of 207 cases. Cancer (in press).
14 Henderson DN. The malignancy of special ovarian tumors. Am J Obstet Gynecol 1957; 62: 816.
15 Goldstein DD, Lamb EJ. Arrhenoblastoma in first cousins. Report of 2 cases. Obstet Gynecol 1970; 35: 444.
16 Murad J, Mancini R, Georg J. Ultrastructure of a virilizing ovarian Sertoli–Leydig cell tumor with familial incidence. Cancer 1973; 31: 1440.
17 Kristenen GB, Baunsgaard P, Hesseldahl H. Androblastoma associated with pregnancy in two sisters: Case report. Br J Obstet Gynecol 1984; 91: 592.
18 Teilum G. Special Tumors of Ovary and Testis and Related Extragonadal Lesions: Comparative Pathology and Histological Identification, 2nd edition. Philadelphia: JB Lippincott, 1977.
19 Pinkerton JHM, McKay DG, Adams EC, Hertig AT. Development of the human ovary, a study using histochemical technics. Obstet Gynecol 1961; 18: 152.
20 O'Hearn TM, Neubecker RD. Arrhenoblastoma. Obstet Gynecol 1962; 19: 758.
21 Roth LM, Anderson MC, Guvano ADT, Langley FA, Gowing NFC, Woodcock AS. Sertoli–Leydig cell tumors: A clinicopathologic study of 34 cases. Cancer 1981; 48: 187.
22 Young RH, Scully RE. Ovarian Sertoli cell tumors: A report of 10 cases. Int J Gynecol Pathol 1984; 2: 349.
23 Tavassoli FA, Norris HJ. Sertoli tumors of the ovary. A clinicopathologic study of 28 cases with ultrastructural observations. Cancer 1980; 46: 2281.
24 Solh HM, Azoury RS, Najjar SS. Peutz–Jeghers Syndrome associated with precocious puberty. J Pediatr 1983; 103: 593.
25 Ehrlich RN, Doninquez OV, Samuels LT, Lynch D, Oberhelman H, Warner NE. Aldosteronism and precocious puberty due to an ovarian androblastoma (Sertoli cell tumor). J Clin Endocrinol Metab 1963; 23: 358.

26 Roth LM, Liban E, Czernobilsky B. Ovarian endometrioid tumors mimicking Sertoli and Sertoli–Leydig cell tumors. Sertoliform variant of endometrioid carcinoma. Cancer 1982; 50: 1322.

27 Young RH, Prat J, Scull RE. Ovarian endometrioid carcinomas resembling sex cord-stromal tumors. A clinicopathologic analysis of 13 cases. Am J Surg Pathol 1982; 6: 513.

28 Bullon A, Arseneau T, Prat J, Young RH, Scully RE. Tubular Krukenberg tumor. A problem in histopathologic diagnosis. Am J Surg Pathol 1981; 5: 225.

29 Robboy SJ, Norris HJ, Scully RE. Insular carcinoid primary in the ovary: A clinicopathologic analysis of 48 cases. Cancer 1975; 36: 404.

30 Emig OR, Hertig AT, Rowe FJ. Gynadroblastoma of the ovary. Review and report of a case. Obstet Gynecol 1959; 13: 135.

31 Neubecker RO, Breen JL. Gynadroblastoma: A report of five cases with discussion of the histogenesis and classification of ovarian tumors. Am J Clin Pathol 1962; 38: 60.

32 Novak ER. Gynadroblastoma of the ovary. Review of 8 cases from the ovarian tumor registry. Obstet Gynecol 1967; 30: 709.

33 Robboy SJ, Scully RE, Norris HJ. Primary trabecular carcinoid of the ovary. Obstet Gynecol 1977; 49: 202.

34 Young RH, Prat J, Scully RE. Endometrioid stromal sarcomas of the ovary: A clinicopathologic analysis of 23 cases. Cancer 1984; 1143.

35 Young RH, Prat J, Scully RE. Ovarian Sertoli–Leydig cell tumor with heterologous elements: (1) gastrointestinal epithelium. Cancer 1982; 50: 2448.

36 Prat J, Young RH, Scully RE. Ovarian Sertoli–Leydig cell tumors with heterologous elements (II) cartilage and skeletal muscle. Cancer 1982; 50: 2465.

37 Fox H, Langley FA. Tumors of the Ovary. Chicago: Year Book Medical Publisher, 1976: 156–157.

38 Reddick RL, Walton LA. Sertoli–Leydig cell tumor of the ovary with teratomatous differentiation. Cancer 1982; 50: 1171.

39 Young RH, Scully RE. Ovarian sex cord-stromal tumors: Recent progress. Int J Gynecol Pathol 1982; 1: 101.

40 Young RH, Scully RE. Ovarian tumors of probably wolffian origin. A report of eleven cases. Am J Surg Pathol 1983; 7: 125.

41 Astengo-Asuno C. Ovarian sex cord tumor with anular tubules. Case report with ultrastructural findings. Cancer 1984; 54: 1070.

42 Salazar H, Gonzalez-Angulo A. Ultrastructural diagnosis in gynecological pathology. Clin Obstet Gynecol 1984; 11: 25.

43 Tavassoi FA, Norris HJ. Sertoli tumors of the ovary. A clinicopathologic study of 28 cases with ultrastructural observation. Cancer 1980; 46: 2281.

44 Kurman RJ, Andrade D, Goebelsmann U, Taylor CR. An immunohistological study of steroid localization in Sertoli–Leydig tumors of the ovary and testis. Cancer 1978; 42: 1772.

45 Moore JC, Schifrin BS, Erez S. Ovarian tumors in infancy, childhood and adolescence. Am J Obstet Gynecol 1967; 99: 913.

46 Novak ER, Long JH. Arrhenoblastoma of the ovary: A review of the ovarian tumor registry. Am J Obstet Gynecol 1965; 92: 1082.

47 Serment H, Laffargue P, Piana L, Blanc B. Ovarian hormone tumors of female children. Int J Gynecol Obstet 1970; 8: 409.

48 Sato T, Shinada T, Matsumoto S. A clinical and metabolic study of masculinizing arrhenoblastoma. Am J Obstet Gynecol 1969; 104: 1124.

49 Mahesh VB, McDonough PG, Deleo CA. Endocrine studies in the arrhenoblastoma. Am J Obstet Gynecol 1970; 107: 183.

50 Radman HM, Bhagavan BS, Strummer D. Arrhenoblastoma of the ovary—presentation of a case and a discussion of the differential diagnosis. Am J Obstet Gynecol 1970; 106: 1187.

51 Latikainen T, Pelkonen R, Vihko R. Plasma steroids in 2 subjects with ovarian androgen producing tumors, arrhenoblastoma and gynadoblastoma. J Clin Endocrinol Metab 1972; 34: 580.

52 Tucci RJ, Zah W, Kaloeron AE. Endocrine studies in an arrhenoblastoma responsive to dexamethason, ACTH and human chorionic gonadotropin. Am J Med 1973; 55: 687.

53 Maidman JE, Chatterton RT, Arrata WSM, Schifano J, Lueck JA. Steroid metabolism in arrhenoblastoma. Obstet Gynecol 1974; 44: 333.

54 Samaan A, Gates RB, Hickey RC, Rutledge FH. Endocrine studies during stimulation—suppression in hirsutism. Obstet Gynecol 1975; 46: 104.

55 Soules MR, Abraham GE, Bossen EH. The steroid profile of a virilizing ovarian tumor. Obstet Gynecol 1978; 52: 73.

56 Munemur M, Nakamura T, Matsuura K, Maeyama M, Iwamasa T. Endocrine profile of an ovarian androblastoma. Obstet Gynecol 1982; 59: 1005.

57 Baylin SB, Mendelsohn G. Ectopin (inappropriate) hormone production by tumors:

Mechanisms involved and the biological and clinical implications. Endocrine Rev 1980; 1: 45.

58 Easterling WE Jr, Talbert LM, Potter HD. Serum testosterone levels in polycystic ovary syndrome. Am J Obstet Gynecol 1974; 120: 385.

59 Meldrum DR, Abraham GE. Peripheral and ovarian venous concentrations of various steroid hormones in virilizing ovarian tumors. Obstet Gynecol 1979; 53: 36.

60 Gabrilove JL, Seman AT, Sabet R, Mitty HA, Nicolis GL. Virilizing adrenal adenoma with studies on the steroid content of the adrenal venous effluent and a review of the literature. Endrocrine Rev 1981; 2: 462.

61 Wiebe RH, Morris CV. Testosterone/androstenedione ratio in evaluation of women with ovarian androgen excess. Obstet Gynecol 1983; 61: 279.

62 Friedman CI, Schmidt GE, Kim MN, Powell J. Serum testosterone concentration in the evaluation of androgen producing tumors. Am J Obstet Gynecol 1985; 153: 44.

63 Norris HJ, Taylor HB. Virilization associated with cystic granulosa cell tumor. Obstet Gynecol 1969; 34: 629.

64 Hatjis CG, Polin JI, Wheele JE et al. Amenorrhea–galactorrhea associated with testosterone producing solid granulosa cell tumor. Am J Obstet Gynecol 1978; 131: 226.

65 Demoponlos RI, Bell DA. The structure of a virilizing human granulosa–theca cell tumor: Observation on the nature of the hormone producing cell. Cancer 1983; 51: 1858.

66 Nakashima N, Young RH, Scully RE. Androgenic granulosa cell tumors of the ovary. Arch Pathol Lab Med 1984; 108: 786.

67 Fox LP, Stamm WJ. Krukenberg tumor complicating pregnancy: Report of a case with androgenic activity. Am J Obstet Gynecol 1965; 92: 702.

68 Ances IG, Ganis FM. Metabolism of testosterone by virilizing Krukenberg tumor of the ovary. Am J Obstet Gynecol 1968; 100: 1062.

69 Connor TB, Ganis FM, Levin HS, Migeon CJ, Marton LG. Gonadotropin-dependent Krukenberg tumor causing virilization during pregnancy. J Clin Endocrinol Metab 1968: 28: 198.

70 Forest MG, Orgiazz J, Tranchant D, Mornex R, Bertrano J. Approach to the mechanism of androgen over production in a case of Krukenberg tumor responsible for virilization during pregnancy. J Clin Endocrinol Metab 1978; 47: 428.

71 de Torres EF. Feminization in tumors of Sertoli–Leydig cells. Acta Cytol 1974; 18: 187.

72 Genton CY, Schmid J. Ovarian Sertoli–Leydig cell tumor with hyperoestrinism. Virchows Path (Pathol Anat) 1981; 390: 243.

73 Korzets A, Nouriel H, Steiner Z, Griffel B, Kraus L, Freund U, Klajman A. Resistant hypertension associated with renin producing ovarian Sertoli Cell Tumor. Am J Clin Pathol 1986; 85: 242.

74 Chumas JC, Rosenwaks Z, Mann WJ, Finkel G, Pastore J. Sertoli Leydig Cell Tumor of the ovary producing alpha fetoprotein. Int J Gynecol Pathol 1984; 3: 213.

75 Mann WJ, Chumas JC, Rosenwaks Z, Merrill JA, Davenport D. Elevated serum alpha fetoprotein associated with Sertoli–Leydig cell tumors of the ovary. Obstet Gynecol 1986; 67: 141.

76 Young RH, Scully RE. Ovarian sex cord stromal tumors. Recent advance and current status. Clin Obstet Gynecol 1984; 11: 93.

77 Young RH, Scully RE. Well differentiated ovarian Sertoli–Leydig cell tumors: A clinicopathological analysis of 23 cases. Int J Gynecol Pathol 1984; 7: 277.

78 Jones GS, Goldberg B, Woodruff DJ. Enzyme histology of a masculinizing arrhenoblastoma. Obstet Gynecol 1967; 29: 328.

79 Speroff L, Glass RH, Kase NG. Hirsutism. In: Clinical Gynecologic Endocrinology and Infertility, 3rd edition. Baltimore/London: Williams and Wilkins, 1983: 201–224.

80 Moltz L, Schwartz U, Sorensen R, Pickartz H. Hammerstein J. Ovarian and adrenal vein steroids in patients with non neoplastic hyperandrogenism: Selective catheterization findings. Fertil Steril 1984; 42: 69.

81 Moltz L, Pickartz H, Sorensen R, Schwartz U, Hammerstein J. Ovarian and adrenal vein steroids in patients with androgen secreting ovarian neoplasms: Selected catheterization findings. Fertil Steril 1984; 42: 585.

82 Casthely S, Diamandis HP, Piere-Louis R. Hilar cell tumor of the ovary: Diagnostic value of plasma testosterone by selected ovarian vein catheterization. Am J Obstet Gynecol 1977; 129: 108.

83 Weiland AJ, Bookstein JJ, Cleary RE, Judd HL. Preoperative localization of virilizing tumors by selected venous sampling. Am J Obstet Gynecol 1978; 131: 797.

84 Aleem FA, Spenillo AR, Oberlander S, Surks MI. Hilar cell tumor of the ovary preoperative localization by selective retrograde venous sampling. Obstet Gynecol 1980; 56: 99.

85 Judd HL, Spore WW, Talner LB, Rigg LA, Yen SSC, Benirschke K. Preoperative localization of a testosterone secreting ovarian tumor

by retrograde venous catheterization and selective sampling. Am J Obstet Gynecol 1974; 120: 91.

86 Brenthal CP. A care of arrhenoblastoma complicated pregnancy. J Obstet Gynaecol Br Common 1945; 52: 235.

87 Young WR. Association of masculinizing tumor of the ovary and pregnancy. Illinois Med J 1951; 100: 263.

88 Galle PC, McColl JA, Elsner CW. Arrhenoblastoma during pregnancy. Obstet Gynecol 1978; 51: 359.

89 Pride GL, Pollock WJ, Norgard MJ. Metastatic Sertoli–Leydig cell tumor of the ovary during pregnancy treated by BV-CAP chemotherapy. Am J Obstet Gynecol 1982; 143: 231.

90 Barkan A, Cassorla F, Loriauk DL, Marshall JC. Pregnancy in a patient with virilizing arrhenoblastoma. Am J Obstet Gynecol 1984; 149: 909.

91 Young RH, Dudley AG, Scully RE. Granulosa cell, Sertoli–Leydig cell, and unclassified sex cord-stromal tumors associated with pregnancy: A clinicopathological analysis of thirty-six cases. Gynecol Oncol 1984; 18: 181.

92 Okun LE. Bilateral arrhenoblastoma of the ovary. Obstet Gynecol 1965; 25: 448.

93 Curtis AH. Another case of arrhenoblastoma. Am J Obstet Gynecol 1946; 52: 128.

94 Kreines KL, Garancis JC, Esselborn VM. Arrhenoblastoma of the ovary. Surg Gynecol Obstet 1963; 116: 328.

95 Langley FA. "Steroli" and "Leydig" cells in relation to ovarian tumors. J Clin Pathol 1954; 7: 10.

96 Krock F, Wolferman SJ. Arrhenoblastoma of the ovary. Ann Surg 1941; 114: 78.

97 Widholm O, Ikonen M. A case of malignant arrhenoblastoma. Ann Chir Gyn Fenn 1975; 64: 55.

98 Schwartz PE, Smith JP. Treatment of ovarian stromal tumors. Am J Obstet Gynecol 1976; 125: 402.

99 Meyer R. Tubulare (testikulare) und solide Formen des Andreioblastoma ovarii und ihre Beziehungen zur Vermannlichung. Beitr Path Anat 1930; 84: 485.

100 Dougherty GM, Thompson WB, McCall ML. Obstet Gynecol 1958; 76: 653.

101 Anderson MC, Rees DA. Gynandroblastoma of the ovary. Br J Obstet Gynecol 1975; 82: 68.

102 Chalvardjian A, Derzko C. Gynandroblastoma: Its ultrastructure. Cancer 1982; 50: 710.

103 Cantor B, Pierson KK, Kalra PS. Hormone studies in a gynandroblastoma. Fertil Steril 1978; 29: 681.

104 Neubecker RD, Breen JL. Gynandroblastoma. Am J Clin Pathol 1962; 38: 60.

105 Hughesdon PE and Fraser IT. Arrhenoblastoma of the ovary: case report and histological review. Acta Obstet Gynecol Scand 1953; 32 Suppl 4: 1.

106 Scully RE. An unusual ovarian tumor containing Leydig cells but associated with endometrial hyperplasia in a postmenopausal women. J Clin Endocrinol 1953; 13: 1254.

107 Emig OR, Hertis AT, Rowe FJ. Gynandroblastoma of the ovary. Obstet Gynecol 1959; 13: 135.

108 Mechler EA, Black WC. Gynandroblastoma of the ovary. Am J Pathol 1943; 19: 633.

109 Govan ADT. In: Fox H, Langley FA eds Postgraduate Obstetrical and Gynecological Pathology. Oxford: Pergamon Press 1973: 245.

110 Novak ER. Gynandroblastoma of the ovary: Review of 8 cases from the Ovarian Tumor Registry. Obstet Gynecol 1967; 30: 709.

111 Soules MR, Abraham GE, Bossen EH. The steroid profiles of a virilizing ovarian tumor. Obstet Gynecol 1978; 52: 73.

112 Laatikainen T, Pelkonen R, Vihko R. Plasma steroids in two subjects with ovarian androgen producing tumors, arrhenoblastoma, gynandroblastoma. J Clin Endocrinol Metab 1972; 34: 580.

113 Luca V, Halalau F, Obresui I, Palos N, Florea O. Gynandroblastoma of the ovary. Morph Embryol 1983; 29: 117.

114 Barzilai G. Atlas of Ovarian Tumors. New York: Grune and Stratton, 1943.

115 Scully RE. Androgenic lesions of the ovary. In: Grady HE, Smithy DE eds The Ovary. International Academy of Pathology Monograph. Baltimore: Williams and Wilkins, 1963: 143–174.

116 Green JA, Maqueo M. Histopathology and ultrastructure of an ovarian hilar cell tumor. Am J Obstet Gynecol 1966; 96: 478.

117 Echt CR, Hadd HE. Androgen excretion pattern in a patient with metastatic hilus cell tumor of the ovary. Am J Obstet Gynecol 1968; 100: 1055.

118 Huang TY, Holiday WJ. An ovarian hilus cell tumor associated with endometrial carcinoma: report of a case. Am J Clin Pathol 1970; 54: 147.

119 Sternberg WH, Roth LM. Ovarian stromal tumors containing Leydig cells I. Stromal Leydig cell tumors and non-neoplastic transformation of ovarian stroma to Leydig cells. Cancer 1973; 32: 940.

120 Sternberg WH, Roth LM. Ovarian stromal tumors containing Leydig cells II. Pure Leydig cell tumor, non hilar type. Cancer 1973; 32: 952.

121 Scully RE. Stromal luteoma of the ovary: A

distinctive type of lipoid-cell tumor. Cancer 1964; 17: 763.

122 Sandberg AA, Slaunwhite WR, Jackson JE et al. Androgen biosynthesis by ovarian lipoid cell tumor. J Clin Endrocrinol 196 ; 22: 929.

123 Sobrinko LG, Kase NC. Adrenal rest cell tumor of the ovary: Report of a case. Obstet Gynecol 1970; 36: 895.

124 Pepowitz P, Pomeranes W. Adrenal like tumors of the ovary: Review of the literature and report of two new cases. Obstet Gynecol 1962; 19: 183.

125 Montag TW, Murphy RE, Belinson JL. Virilizing malignant lipid cell tumor producing erythropoietin. Gynecol Oncol 1984; 19: 98.

126 Young RH, Perez-Atayde AR, Scully RE. Ovarian Sertoli–Leydig cell tumor with retiform and heterologous components. Am J Surg Pathol 1984; 8: 709.

127 Taylor HB, Norris HJ. Lipid cell tumor of the ovary. Cancer 1967; 20: 1953.

128 Hughesdon PS. Ovarian lipoid and theca cell tumors: Their origin and interrelations. Obstet Gynecol Surv 1966; 21: 245.

129 Hughesdon PE. Lipid cell thecomas of the ovary. Histopathology 1983; 7: 681.

130 Kempson RL. Ultrastructure of ovarian stromal cell tumors Sertoli–Leydig cell tumor and lipid cell tumor. Arch Pathol 1968; 86: 492.

131 Hiura M, Muta M, Noguna T, Nagai N, Katoh K, Fujiwara A. Histogenesis, cytodifferentiation and its subcellular steroidogenic sites in the virilizing ovarian Leydig cell tumor. Gynecol Oncol 1984; 17: 175.

132 Koss LG, Rothchild EO, Fleisher M, Francis JE. Masculinizing tumor of the ovary apparently with adreno-cortical activity. Cancer 1965; 23: 1245.

133 Boivin Y, Richart RM. Hilus cell tumors of the ovary. Cancer 1965; 18: 231.

134 Corral-Gallardo J, Aceuado HA, Perez de Salazar J et al. A hilus cell tumor of the ovary associated with polycystic ovarian disease: In vivo and in vitro studies. Acta Endocrinol (Kbh) 1966; 52: 425.

135 Ishida T, Okagaki T, Tagatz GE et al. Lipid cell tumor of the ovary: An ultrastructural study. Cancer 1977; 40: 234.

136 Echt GR, Hadd HE. Androgen excretion patterns in a patient with a metastatic holus

tumor of the ovary. Am J Obstet Gynecol 1968; 100: 1055.

137 Anderson MC. Hilar cell tumor of the ovary. J Clin Pathol 1965; 25: 106.

138 Scully RE. An unusual ovarian tumor containing Leydig cells but associated with endometrial hyperplasia in a post-menopausal woman. J Clin Endocrinol 1953; 13: 1254.

139 Huang T-Y, Holaday WJ. An ovarian hilus cell tumor associated with endometrial carcinoma: Report of a case. Am J Clin Pathol 1970; 54: 147.

140 Salm R. Ovarian hilus cell tumors: Their varying presentation. J Pathol 1974; 113: 117.

141 Mohamed NC, Cardenas A, Villasanta U et al. Hilus cell tumor of the ovary and endometrial carcinoma. Obstet Gynecol 1977; 52: 486.

142 Nagamani M, Gonzalez-Vitale JC. Steroid secretion pattern of a hilus cell tumor of the ovary. Obstet Gynecol 1981; 58: 521.

143 Lipsett MD, Kirschner MA, Wilson H et al. Malignant lipid cell tumors of the ovary: Clinical, biochemical, etiologic consideration. J Clin Endocrinol 1970; 30: 336.

144 Khoo SK, Buntine D. Malignant stromal tumor of the ovary with vivilizing effects in a XXX female with streak ovaries. Aust NZ J Obstet Gynecol 1980; 20: 123.

145 Imperato-McGinley J, Peterson RE, Dawood MY et al. Steroid hormone secretion from a virilizing lipoid cell tumor of the ovary. Obstet Gynecol 1981; 57: 535.

146 Davidson BJ, Waisman J, Judd HL. Long standing virilism in a woman with hyperplasia and neoplasia of ovarian lipidic cells. Obstet Gynecol 1981; 58: 753.

147 Barkan AL, Cassarla F, Loriaux DL et al. Steroid and gonadotropin secretion in a patients with a 30 year history of virilization due to lipoid cell ovarian tumor. Obstet Gynecol 1984; 64: 287.

148 Marieb NJ, Spangler S, Kashgarian M et al. Cushing's syndrome secondary to ectopic cortisol production by an ovarian carcinoma. J Clin Endocrinol Metab 1983; 57: 737.

149 Bryson MJ, Dominquez OV, Kaiser IH et al. Enzymic steroid conversion in a masculinovoblastoma. J Clin Endocrinol Metab 1962; 22: 773.

Textbook of Uncommon Cancer
Edited by C.J. Williams, J.G. Krikorian, M.R. Green and D. Ragharan
© 1988 John Wiley & Sons Ltd

Chapter **3**

Management of Ovarian Germ Cell Tumours

E.S. Newlands,
P.J. Southall,
F.J. Paradinas and
L. Holden
Charing Cross Hospital, London, UK

INTRODUCTION

Malignant germ cell tumours (GCT) of the ovary are rare and account for approximately 1% of all ovarian tumours. Their incidence is approximately one-tenth of the incidence of malignant GCT of the testis and therefore information on their management has been correspondingly less. In common with testicular GCTs, the incidence of malignant GCT of the ovary may be rising (1). The average age at presentation is less than 20 years. However, with improvements in management and the development of modern chemotherapy, it should be rare for these patients to succumb from their disease and in most cases it should be possible to preserve fertility.

In contrast to malignant ovarian GCTs benign ovarian teratomas are much more common, constituting approximately 25% of all ovarian tumours (2). Benign ovarian teratomas reach a peak incidence in the fourth and fifth decades of life and usually present with a pelvic mass and without abdominal pain. It should be noted that patients presenting at an older age with apparently benign ovarian teratomas have a higher incidence of malignancy developing within their tumour (3).

Overall, the incidence of malignancy in a large series of benign cystic ovarian teratomas is low (0.46%) (3). The management of benign ovarian teratomas is by surgical resection.

PATHOLOGY

Classification

Based on the World Health Organization histological typing of ovarian tumours (4) (Table 1), the GCTs are divided into different categories, including neoplasms containing both germ cells and sex cord stroma derivatives.

Histogenesis

In the embryo, germ cells first appear in the wall of the yolk sac, then migrate to the genital ridge and become incorporated into the developing gonad. As with testicular GCTs, ovarian GCTs are derived from differentiation of these totipotential germ cells towards (a) somatic tissues (teratoma), (b) germinal epithelium (dysgerminoma), (c) extra-embryonic

37

TABLE 1 CLASSIFICATION OF OVARIAN GERM
           CELL TUMOURS

Tumours of one single type
Dysgerminoma
Endodermal sinus tumour (yolk sac tumour)
Embryonal carcinoma
Polyembryoma
Choriocarcinoma
Teratoma:
   mature
   cystic (dermoid cyst)
   solid
   immature
   with malignant transformation

Mixed forms

Monodermal
Struma ovarii
Carcinoid
Struma ovarii and carcinoid
Others

Tumours of germ and sex cord stromal cells
Gonadoblastoma
Gonadoblastoma with dysgerminoma or other GCT
Others

TABLE 2 INCIDENCE OF OVARIAN TUMOURS

Type	% Incidence (approx.)
Epithelial tumours (benign and malignant)	50–70
Germ cell tumours	20–30
Benign cystic teratomas	25
Solid teratomas	2
Anaplastic and mixed germ cell tumours	1
Dysgerminomas	1
Monodermal teratomas	1
Sex cord stromal tumours	2
Mixed germ cell–stromal tumours	1
Lipid cell tumours	0.1

of blocks. With GCTs, combinations of histologically different tumour types may occur (Figure 1). Identification of these various components is of importance since they may influence subsequent treatment.

Dysgerminoma

This is the ovarian counterpart of the testicular seminoma. Although usually unilateral, there is in 10–17% of cases, involvement of both ovaries (6). They are often solid masses which, if not confined to the ovary, may be adherent to surrounding structures including uterine ligaments, fallopian tubes and the retroperitoneum. Dissemination to retroperitoneal, mediastinal and supraclavicular lymph nodes and haematogenous spread to liver, lungs and bones may occur.

Histologically, the appearances are often identical with the classic seminoma of the testis (Figure 2). Variants homologous to spermatocytic seminoma have not been described. Typically, the parenchymal cells are large, uniform, round or polygonal and resemble germ cells. The nuclei are round and vesicular, containing one or more nucleoli. Abundant glycogen dispersed in a clear cytoplasm is commonly present and there may also be some lipid. Mitoses are invariable and a lymphocytic infiltrate is characteristic. Variable quantities of connective tissue septa surround the tumour cells. Granulomas are frequently noted and

trophoblast (choriocarcinoma) and (d) yolk sac (yolk sac tumour) (Figure 1) (5).

Incidence

With the exception of 'dermoid cysts', all other GCTs comprise less than 5% of ovarian tumours (Table 2). Certainly, in comparison with ovarian epithelial neoplasms, malignant GCTs are rare.

Thorough examination of the gross specimen combined with extensive sampling is important with these tumours. Some of them may be enormous when excised and there is potential sampling error. This can be reduced to some extent by taking an adequate number

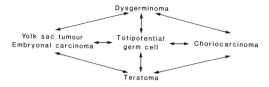

Figure 1 Presumed derivation of ovarian germ cell tumours. Mixed forms, common in the testis, are uncommon in the ovary.

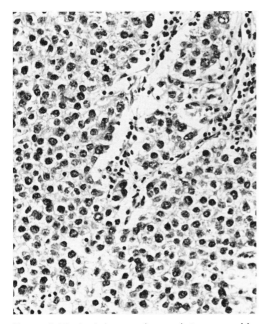

Figure 2 Typical dysgerminoma interspersed by thin connective tissue septa and a mild lymphocytic infiltrate (haematoxylin and eosin, original magnification: ×300).

usually contain foreign-body and Langhans' type giant cells. Other giant cells resembling syncytiotrophoblast and associated with human chronic gonadotrophin (hCG) production are found in a few cases (7). Other germ cell elements may be an uncommon accompaniment with dysgerminoma (8). These include teratoma, yolk sac tumour, embryonal carcinoma and choriocarcinoma (2). The presence of large, round, calcified bodies in a dysgerminoma should initiate a search for foci of gonadoblastoma (9). The association of dysgerminoma with gonadoblastoma will be discussed later.

Yolk Sac Tumour and Embryonal Carcinoma

In the ovary these are rare, highly malignant tumours, mainly occurring in children and adolescents. The majority are yolk sac tumours. A review of 42 tumours identified 38 as yolk sac and 4 as embryonal carcinoma (10). In up to 60% of cases, they exist as pure

tumours but can also occur in association with teratoma and dysgerminoma.

Macroscopically, these are large tumours and the grey cut surface may display extensive haemorrhagic necrosis. Cysts containing gelatinous material may also be present. Local involvement of the pelvic peritoneum and spread to the other ovary is frequently noted at initial presentation.

Embryonal carcinoma is recognized histologically as consisting of large, primitive and pleomorphic epithelial-like cells that are arranged as sheets, cords, tubules or papillae. hCG-secreting giant cells, some resembling synctiotrophoblast, may be present and alpha-fetoprotein (AFP) expression has also been observed (10).

Morphologically, yolk sac tumours manifest differentiaton towards structures similar to those normally identified in the developing ovum, especially extra-embryonic endoderm normally found in the yolk sac.

The patterns of yolk sac tumour that have been described include reticular, pseudopillary (containing numerous Duval–Schiller bodies), polyvesicular vitelline, glandular and solid patterns (Figure 3) (10). Varying amounts of globular, hyaline basement-membrane-like material may be associated with any of these patterns (11).

AFP can almost always be demonstrated by immunohistochemistry within yolk sac tumours and in embryonal carcinoma containing recognizable yolk sac structures (10).

Choriocarcinoma

As different therapeutic strategies may be utilized, it is important to differentiate choriocarcinoma of gestational origin from that of non-gestational, germ cell derivation. It may be particularly difficult to exclude gestational choriocarcinoma when pure choriocarcinoma is found in patients of child-bearing age. An admixture of cytotrophoblast and syncytiotrophoblast with other germ cell tumour structures is indicative of a non-gestational origin. Where only choriocarcinoma is identified,

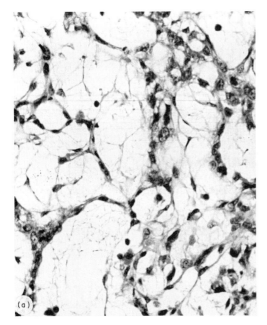

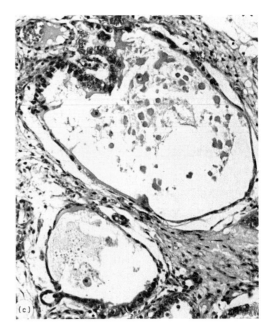

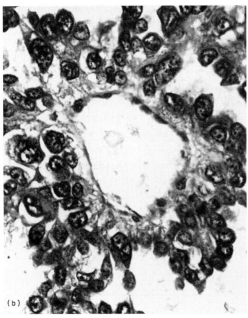

Figure 3 Examples of structures found in yolk sac tumours: (a) reticular pattern (haematoxylin and eosin, original magnification: ×350), (b) Duval–Schiller body (haematoxylin and eosin, original magnification: ×500), (c) polyvesicular–vitelline pattern (haematoxylin and eosin, original magnification: ×200).

Necrosis and haemorrhage are usual features. One or both ovaries may contain multiple lutein cysts.

The diagnosis of choriocarcinoma can be made when both cytotrophoblast and syncytiotrophoblast are present. The appearances often recapitulate that of villous trophoblast.

Teratomas

Cystic teratomas ('dermoid cysts') account for up to 25% of all ovarian neoplasms. They are benign and consist of mature tissues, which may be derived from all three germ cell layers. Malignant transformation in some of the mature tissues occurs in between 1 and 2%. Although younger women may be affected, this sinister development is more usual in postmenopausal women (3, 12).

The most frequent malignant neoplasm is squamous cell carcinoma and over three-

chromosomal analysis of fresh unfixed tumour may help if this is available, since paternal HLA antigens have been identified in gestational choriocarcinoma.

Germ cell choriocarcinomas tend to be large, having a predilection for the right ovary.

quarters of the malignancies are of this type. Less common forms of malignant change described are adenocarcinoma including thyroid carcinoma, carcinoids, melanoma and a variety of sarcomas (2). The malignant change may only be represented by a focal area of thickening and it is imperative to sample any localized thickening in the wall of a benign cystic teratoma. Local infiltration into pelvic structures may occur and lymph node involvement may occasionally be observed. Haematogenous dissemination is uncommon.

Solid teratomas are rare and may be composed of mature or a mixture of mature and immature tissues. They are usually unilateral and large, and penetration of the capsule by tumour may be apparent. Although mainly solid, the cut surface may show cystic spaces, of which the largest are the result of haemorrhage and necrosis (Figure 4).

Neoplasms composed entirely of fully differentiated mature elements such as bone, tooth buds, cartilage, adipose tissue, squamous epithelium, skin appendages and neuroglia are uncommon. Such tumours can be expected to show no malignant potential (13), provided sampling has been meticulous. It is more usual for tissues to be less well differentiated and it is often primitive neuroectodermal tissue that is susceptible to malignant change. For example, neuroblastoma, medulloblastoma, ependyoma or astrocytoma may be recognized. It should be remembered, however, that the implants in patients with peritoneal gliomatosis comprise mature neuroglia and that the prognosis is excellent if the ovarian tumour is excised. Opinions vary as to how these nodules develop (14, 15).

Of course, apart from neuroectoderm, other elements derived from the three germ layers may be present and in various stages of maturity. The range of tissues is extensive and some may be seen more frequently than others. A rare feature of teratomas, benign or malignant, is hepatoid differentiation. We have recently seen in a solid ovarian teratoma

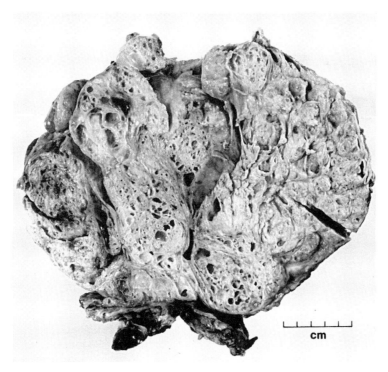

Figure 4 Solid ovarian teratoma.

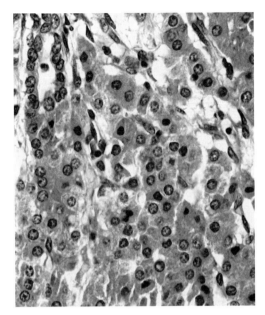

Figure 5 Hepatoid differentiation in a solid ovarian teratoma. Cells resembling hepatocytes
appear to line sinusoids and a bile duct like
structure is seen in the lower left corner of the
picture (haematoxylin and eosin, original magnification: ×500).

arising in a 20 year old woman structures
resembling liver tissue including hepatocytes
producing bile and portal tracts containing
bile ducts (Figure 5).

Embryoid bodies may be present and if
numerous such tumours have been called
polyembryos. However, such a classification is
probably unnecessary (2, 16).

The prognosis is influenced by the nature
and quantity of the embryonal (immature)
component (17) and is improved when the
latter is predominantly neural. The size and
stage of the tumours are related to survival but
it is the histological grading of the primary
tumour that correlates best with extra-ovarian
dissemination (18). Likewise, the grade of the
metastases correlates best with the subsequent
course. The grading system recommended by
Norris and Adams (19) is a modification of that
originally proposed by Thurlbeck and Scully
(20):

Grade 0:
   Wholly mature teratoma.

Grade I:
   Abundance of mature tissues, intermixed
   with loose mesenchymal tissue with occasional mitoses; immature cartilage; tooth buds.
Grade II:
   Fewer mature tissues: rare foci of neuropith-
   elium with common mitoses, not exceeding
   three low-magnification (× 40) fields in any
   one slide.
Grade III:
   Few or no mature tissues; numerous neuro-
   pithelial elements, margins with a cellular
   stroma occupying four or more low-magnification fields.

Teratomas associated with anaplastic extra-
embryonic germ cell tumours such as yolk sac
tumours, choriocarcinoma or embryonal carcinoma must be clearly separated from this
group of somatic malignancies since in patients
with extra-embryonic germ cell elements the
prognosis previously has been markedly worse
(13).

Monodermal or Monophyletic Teratomas

These are tumours that consist predominantly
of one type of tissue and are regarded as
teratomatous since they are often associated
with a tissue of different type. Thus, a germ cell
origin is tenable. However, in the absence of
other tissue, the histogenesis of these tumours is
contentious.

Struma ovarii are tumours composed of
thyroid tissue that usually appears mature.
Under half the cases consist purely of thyroid
tissue. The others are combined with benign
cystic teratoma, mucinous cystadenomas or
carcinoids (strumal carcinoid). Unusual features are the development of hyperthyroidism
and malignancy. Unequivocal evidence of the
latter are metastases which may not become
manifest until several years following the excision of the primary tumour.

Carcinoid tumours may be associated with
the typical carcinoid syndrome. Microscopically, the appearance is similar to carcinoid

tumours elsewhere, where solid nests of small round regular cells alternate with ribbon and acinar patterns. They may resemble carcinoid tumours of midgut derivation (insular) or those of foregut or hindgut origin (travecular). The argentaffin reaction is usually positive.

Other monodermal teratomas include mucinous cysts with argentaffin cells (2), epidermoid cysts (21) and malignant neuroectodermal tumours (22).

Gonadoblastomas

These tumours contain a combination of germ cells and derivatives of the gonadal stroma that resemble either immature granulosa or Sertoli cells. In the majority of cases, these cells are arranged as solid nests surrounding spaces containing basement-membrane-like material, reminiscent of Call–Exner bodies. In a few gonadoblastomas, clusters of germ cells are surrounded by stromal cells. Frequently, Ley-

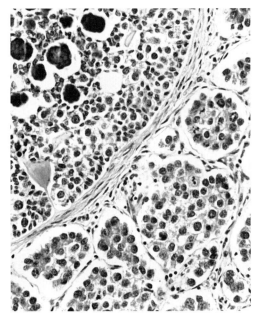

Figure 6 Dysgerminoma arising in a gonadoblastoma. Calcified material surrounded by small stromal and germ cells in the upper part of the picture separated by a band of connective tissue from the larger cells of dysgerminoma in the lower half (haematoxylin and eosin, original magnification: ×300).

dig cells and luteinized stromal cells are present. Calcification is common, the calcospherites being located within the tubules. Almost all the patients have gonadal dysgenesis and most of the tumours arise in phenotypic females. The prognosis for pure gonadoblastoma is excellent. Dysgerminoma, resulting from overgrowth of the germ cells, is common (23) (Figure 6) and other germ cell tumour elements may also occur.

Differential Diagnosis of Ovarian Germ Cell Tumours

Paradinas (5) has given a recent account of the problems faced by the pathologist in this regard. They may be enumerated as follows:

1. Differentiation of choriocarcinoma from that of gestational origin (clinical history, identification of other germ cell components and chromosomal studies).
2. Differentiation of ovarian adenocarcinoma, especially mesonephroid type, from embryonal carcinoma and yolk sac tumour (the former is not associated with APP production).
3. Differentiating malignant teratomas from mixed mesodermal (mullerian) tumours. The latter occurs most frequently in postmenopausal women and structures derived from the three germ layers are absent. Neuroectodermal tissues are not seen and although there may be squamous metaplasia and a variety of mesodermal tissues, the cartilage component is often poorly differentiated, resembling chondrosarcoma.
4. Differentiating dysgerminomas from ovarian lymphomas. Glycogen is more common within the dysgerminoma cells. Monoclonal antibodies reactive with the leucocyte common antigen should also help in diagnosis.
5. Primary carcinoid tumours in the ovary must be distinguished from metastatic carcinoid. The latter are usually bilateral and often associated with metastases elsewhere.

6. The diagnosis of gonadoblastoma may be overlooked if the stromal cells are abundant with only a minimal germ cell contribution. The existence of a 'burnt out' gonadoblastoma in a mainly dysgerminomatous tumour is suggested by the presence of calcification (9).

DIAGNOSIS AND STAGING

Despite their rarity, it should be borne in mind that the age of a patient presenting with a pelvic mass is important. In women less than 20 years, ovarian GCTs comprise 58% of all tumours and 65% of these are malignant (24). The incidence of malignancy in GCTs increases the younger the patient and is 81% in girls less than 10 years old (24).

The clinical presentation depends on the rate of tumour growth. In more slowly growing tumours such as pure dysgerminomas, abdominal symptoms may be non-specific with the patient noting abdominal enlargement and a varying degree of pain. Menstrual irregularities may occur, particularly in those tumours producing placental hormones such as hCG. In rapidly growing malignant germ cell tumours the clinical history is frequently short with the patient presenting with lower abdominal pain which may be acute if haemorrhage has occurred and a lower abdominal or pelvic mass. This presentation frequently results in an early laparotomy without extensive preoperative staging. It should now be recognized at laparotomy on a young patient presenting with an ovarian tumour which may be of germ cell origin that the preservation of fertility is an important consideration. Particularly in patients less than 20 years of age, where the chance of the tumour being of germ cell origin is more common, the surgery should be limited to removal of the primary tumour with preservation of the contralateral ovary and uterus if possible. In addition to removal of the primary tumour, it is important to stage the patient for intra-abdominal spread. These patients are usually classified using the FIGO staging for the more common adenocarcinomas of the ovary.

Once the diagnosis of malignant ovarian germ cell tumour has been made, additional staging procedures are necessary. The radiological investigations that are essential include a chest x-ray and, if this is normal, a thoracic computed tomography (CT) scan. In the abdomen, a CT scan is also important to detect disease in the liver and para-aortic region. Ultrasound is now the most sensitive means of detecting hepatic metastases and in these thin young patients can be more sensitive in detecting para-aortic nodes than CT scanning. Obviously, if a pelvic mass remains postoperatively, ultrasound is also useful in monitoring this. Given the quality of CT scanning and ultrasound, we have now stopped doing lymphography in these patients.

It is now well recognized that malignant germ cell tumours produce a range of tumour markers, the most important of which are hCG, AFP, placental alkaline phosphatase (PLAP) and lactate dehydrogenase (LDH). Dysgerminomas commonly produce both PLAP and LDH and these can be used for monitoring this tumour. Some patients with histologically pure dysgerminoma have a raised hCG in the serum. Significantly raised hCG probably indicates that the tumour in fact is a mixed germ cell tumour containing trophoblast and therefore should not be managed as a pure dysgerminoma. The majority of patients with the other histological variants of malignant germ cell tumour have raised serum levels of both hCG and/or AFP (25). In these cases initial PLAP and LDH estimations should be made and if these are raised they can also be used for monitoring the disease In those patients with raised tumour markers, they provide one of the most sensitive methods of detecting residual tumour after surgical resection. Serial estimations need to be made to determine whether the tumour has been completely excised or not. More recently, new applications of these tumour markers have been made. These markers can be detected by immunohistochemistry on the pathological specimen and it is also possible to localize the residual tumour using the technique of anti-body localization. This entails injecting ^{131}I-labelled antibody to the tumour marker which localizes on the tumour cell surface and sub-tracting the blood background using techne-tium-labelled albumin. Although this tech-nique is not simple and there are problems from artefact, it is possible to localize tumour masses down to approximately 2 cm in size by this technique. In certain cases it can detect tumour which is not seen on CT scanning or ultrasound. The specificity of this technique can be improved using a numerical analysis comparing the area under suspicion with a control area (26).

The pattern of spread of malignant ovarian GCTs includes local pelvic infiltration, intra-peritoneal spread, para-aortic nodal spread, pulmonary metastases and hepatic metastases. Although pulmonary metastases are less com-mon in patients with malignant ovarian germ cell tumours than they are in those with malignant testicular germ cell tumours, it is important to consider the possibility of central nervous system spread in those patients with pulmonary metastases and/or trophoblastic tumours. Patients should have a lumbar punc-ture performed to estimate the concentrations of hCG and AFP in the cerebrospinal fluid (CSF). When the blood/brain barrier is intact, the serum:CSF hCG ratio should be greater than 60:1 (27). In those patients at risk of developing central nervous system (CNS) metastases (those with pulmonary metastases and/or a serum hCG of greater than 1000 IU/litre) we have given CNS prophylaxis with intrathecal methotrexate since the penetration of many cytotoxic drugs into the CNS is poor. Details of the management of patients with brain metastases is discussed in more detail elsewhere (28, 29).

MANAGEMENT OF DYSGERMINOMAS

Initial treatment here is a laparotomy and oophorectomy with biopsy of the contralateral ovary since bilateral involvement is not uncommon. In the series of Asadourian and Taylor (30), the risk of recurrence after unila-teral oophorectomy was about 20%. In our view the advances in chemotherapy are such that those patients who relapse can be salvaged with further treatment. The earlier approach by Brody (31) of following a unilateral oophor-ectomy with local radiation to the site of the tumour in an attempt to preserve fertility does involve considerable scatter of radiation to the uterus and contralateral ovary.

There is no doubt that pure dysgerminomas are highly radiosensitive and even quite wide-spread disease can be controlled using this approach (32, 33). In our view, dysgermino-mas are so chemosensitive that virtually all patients can be salvaged with chemotherapy if this is necessary. For patients who are Stage I and where all tumour has been removed, we have followed these carefully without further treatment (see below). So far none of these patients has relapsed and required additional treatment. Given these points, the role of radiotherapy in dysgerminomas should be carefully questioned and should be restricted to selected cases such as patients where the preservation of fertility is not important or there is some contraindication to giving modern chemotherapy.

MANAGEMENT OF TERATOMA (IMMATURE, SOLID)

These tumours are derived from any of the three germ layers and do not contain either yolk sac or trophoblast. In those presenting with low grade malignancy (grade 0 or 1) the prognosis is good with surgical resection alone (19). As the grade of malignancy increases, there is an increase in the incidence of progres-sive and/or recurrent disease. We have staged these patients carefully and if there is no evidence of metastatic disease they have been followed closely (see below). The results with current chemotherapy in patients with metas-tatic disease are such that adjuvant chemo-therapy is not indicated. However, it is important when reading articles about malignant ovarian germ cell tumours, to identify those papers which include prophylactic chemotherapy since this will artificially improve the figures in those series.

MANAGEMENT OF ANAPLASTIC GERM CELL TUMOUR (AGCT)

The usual management of these patients is by laparotomy and removal of the primary tumour if possible or removal of as much bulk of tumour as is compatible with preservation of the uterus and contralateral ovary. Clearly the laparotomy should include staging the patient for any sites of metastatic disease and biopsy of secondary deposits if these are present. Given the explosive growth of some of the AGCTs, it may only be possible to biopsy the tumour at initial surgery. For these patients, a better course of action is to treat the patient with effective chemotherapy and to plan for second-look surgery at the end of treatment. AGCTs are not very sensitive to radiotherapy and results before the introduction of effective chemotherapy were poor (34, 35).

It has been recognized for several decades that malignant ovarian germ cell tumours can respond dramatically to cytotoxic chemotherapy. However, prior to the introduction of cis-platinum and etoposide the chance of developing drug resistance was high and the majority of patients with metastases succumbed from their disease. Various drug combinations were used including methotrexate, actinomycin D, cyclophosphamide, vinblastine, bleomycin and mithramycin. Using various combinations of these drugs, we have 3 long-term survivors at 11 +, 15 + and 17 + years out of 12 patients treated.

During the 1970s the most widely used combination of cytotoxic drugs was vincristine, actinomycin D and cyclophosphamide (VAC). Representative of the results that were obtained using this combination were those of Slayton et al. (35) where in 39 patients the survival fell from 16 out of 23 patients with Stage I and IIA disease to 8 out of 16 in

patients with Stages IIB to IV. Cangir et al. (36) also confirmed that the survival declined progressively with advancing stage of disease and time of starting treatment. Gershenson (37) analysed 41 patients with yolk sac tumours of the ovary treated with VAC chemotherapy. Again the survival dropped from 12 out of 13 patients with Stage I disease to 2 out of 5 with Stage III disease. More recently Slayton et al. (38) have analysed 76 patients treated with VAC chemotherapy. Of these 54 were treated after removal of all gross disease and, despite this, 15 (28%) developed progressive disease. Where residual tumour was left after surgery, the results were unsatisfactory in that 15 (68%) of 22 patients developed progressive disease. Gershenson et al. (39) analysed 80 patients who were treated with VAC chemotherapy. Again the survival was directly related to stage in that 32 (86%) of 37 patients with Stage I disease remain in remission but this fell to 4 (57%) of 7 patients with Stage II disease and 10 (50%) out of 20 patients with Stage III disease and 0 to 2 patients with Stage IV disease. There is now a consensus among those with adequate experience of treating malignant ovarian germ cell tumours that VAC chemotherapy is inadequate for two reasons: (1) it cannot deal with major metastatic disease and many of the long term survivors may not have required treatment at all (Stage I patients); and (2) many groups have continued chemotherapy for up to 2 years and alkylating agent therapy of this duration increases the risk of second malignancies (40).

During the 1970s two new highly active cytotoxic drugs, cis-platinum and etoposide (VP 16-213), were introduced in the management of malignant germ cell tumours. A number of centres have used the combination of cis-platinum, vinblastine, bleomycin (PVB) Williams et al. (41) reported a series of 30 patients and at the time of this report 54% were in complete remission. Carlson et al. (42) also used this combination and had 9/9 survivors but it should be noted that the majority of their patients had Stage I disease. Wiltshire et al. (43) obtained 7/8 complete remissions using PVB. Slayton (44) reported (1/16 patients with yolk sac tumours were free of disease following PVB therapy. However, in those patients with immature teratomas only 4/11 achieved complete remission. Gershenson et al. (39) have recently reported a group of 15 patients treated with PVB and obtained 6/7 remissions in patients where this was the primary treatment. However, in the patients where this was used as salvage chemotherapy only 3/8 had a complete response to this therapy alone. A recurring point that applies not only to this last series but to many others is that malignant germ cell tumours from any site while initially chemosensitive to modern chemotherapy can develop drug resistance if the tumour is not eliminated rapidly as part of the primary treatment. As with all cancer therapy the time to achieve the maximum survival is to use the optimum treatment as first line and not to rely on salvage therapy at a later stage.

At the Charing Cross Hospital we have developed an alternative approach to VAC and PVB therapy. In 1977 we had identified the activity of etoposide (VP 16–213) against malignant germ cell tumours (45) and we have integrated this into an alternating chemotherapy schedule which includes cis-platinum (POMB/ACE) (Table 3). Between 1977 and 1986 we have treated over 200 male patients with this drug combination and the results have been previously published (28, 46). Detailed analysis of these patients has identified patients with a poor prognosis. These were patients with an initial serum tumour marker concentration of hCG > 50000 IU/l and/or AFP > 500 KU/l and patients who had received prior radiotherapy (28, 46, 47). Using POMB/ACE chemotherapy, the stage of disease at the time of starting treatment, the volume of metastatic disease and the presence of liver and brain metastases were not major adverse prognostic factors in this large group of male patients.

We have also treated patients with metastatic malignant GCTs of the ovary with POMB/

TABLE 3 POMB/ACE CHEMOTHERAPY

POMB
Day 1   vincristine 1 mg/m^2 intravenously; methotrexate 300 mg/m^2 as a 12-h infusion.
Day 2   bleomycin 15 mg as a 24-h infusion; folinic acid rescue started at 24 h after the start of methotrexate in a dose of 15 mg 12-hourly for four doses.
Day 3   bleomycin infusion 15 mg by 24-h infusion.
Day 4   cisplatin 120 mg/m^2 as a 12-h infusion, given together with hydration and 3 g magnesium sulphate supplementation.

ACE
Etoposide (VP 16-213) 100 mg/m^2 days 1 to 5; actinomycin D 0.5 mg intravenously days 3, 4 and 5; cyclophosphamide 500 mg/m^2 intravenously day 5.

OMB
Day 1   vincristine 1 mg/m^2 intravenously; methotrexate 300 mg/m^2 as a 12-h infusion.
Day 2   bleomycin 15 mg by 24-h infusion; folinic acid rescue started at 24 h (after the start of methotrexate) in a dose of 15 mg 12-hourly for four doses.
Day 3   bleomycin 15 mg by 24-h infusion.

The chemotherapy schedules have been reported previously (25, 28, 46).

ACE chemotherapy. Early analyses of this series have been previously presented (25, 48). We have analysed the 43 patients (5 dysgerminomas and 38 anaplastic and combined GCTs who have completed treatment to 1.3.86. In most cases the primary tumour had been removed but in all cases metastatic disease was identified at the time of starting chemotherapy. A small number of the patients had received prior radiotherapy and a limited amount of chemotherapy. The sequence of POMB/ACE chemotherapy is shown in Figure 7. Two courses of POMB are followed by ACE and then POMB is alternated with ACE until the patients are in biochemical remission as determined by serial estimations of hCG, AFP, PLAP and LDH. We have previously shown that in order to obtain stable remissions in patients with advanced metastatic disease it was necessary to have a minimum of three courses of POMB (28). After biochemical remission has been obtained patients alternate

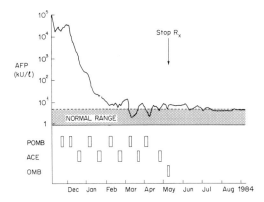

Figure 7 Patient (aged 21 years) with a presacral yolk sac tumour presenting with a high AFP (>500 kU/l). Due to loss of high frequency hearing after two courses of POMB the dose of cisplatin was dropped to 60 mg/m² per course and so she received the equivalent of four courses of POMB in full dose. With this adjustment, no further hearing loss recurred.

OMB with ACE until biochemical, clinical and radiological remission has been maintained for 12 weeks. At this point patients are restaged with CT scanning and ultrasound and if there is a major mass lesion still present at the end of chemotherapy it is our policy to excise this. It is now well recognized that certain elements within a malignant GCT can change on effective cytotoxic chemotherapy into cystic differentiated teratoma. Although this tissue can remain biologically inert for long periods there is the risk of local pressure from the cystic mass and the possibility of dedifferentiation into malignant tissue again. It is therefore our policy to remove this tissue whenever possible.

POMB/ACE chemotherapy differs in several respects from other schedules that have been used in this disease. First, it introduces seven drugs in the initial management of the tumour which is intended to minimize the chances of developing drug resistance (this is particularly relevant in patients with massive metastatic disease). Second, the POMB schedule is only moderately myelosuppressive and so the intervals between each course of chemotherapy can be kept to a maximum of 14 days

(usually 9–14 days) which minimizes the time for tumour recovery between each course. Third, while the alternating schedule is primarily designed to minimize the development of drug resistance having courses of ACE between those containing cis-platinum makes the chemotherapy psychologically easier to tolerate. Fourth, when bleomycin is given by infusion over 48 hours this reduces the pulmonary toxicity and no case of clinically significant bleomycin toxicity has been seen in 250 patients treated with this schedule.

We have performed multi-variate analyses of these patients and the overall survival of 43 patients treated since 1977 is 81% (Figure 8). However, two sub-groups within the 43 patients have a poor prognosis. The first is those patients who had received prior radiotherapy, where the survival was only 40% in 5 patients (Figure 9). If these patients are omitted from the group the survival of patients who have not received prior therapy apart from surgery rises to 86%, which is close to the survival in the male patients, which is currently 92%. In figure 10 patients are analysed by age. In those patients presenting at > 30 years the survival is poor which may be related to other cell elements (squamous cell carcinoma, adenocarcinoma and sarcoma) occurring within their tumour.

In the larger series of male patients we have been able to compensate for the patients presenting with high initial serum tumour markers (an hCG concentration > 50000 IU/l and/or AFP > 500 kU/l) by increasing the number of courses of POMB to a minimum of three. In the male patients there is now no difference in survival in 82 sequential patients presenting with low serum tumour markers who have a survival of 92% and those presenting with markers of a higher concentration where the survival is 91% in 38 patients. However, in the female patients (Figure 11) there is still a trend to a poorer prognosis in those presenting with high tumour markers. However, this difference is not at present significant and the numbers in this group are quite small. In most series using cytotoxic

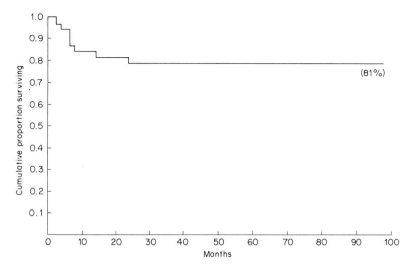

Figure 8 Overall survival of 43 female patients with ovarian (plus one presacral) germ cell tumours treated with POMB/ACE chemotherapy 1977–1986.

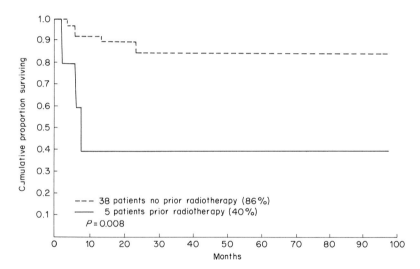

Figure 9 Survival of patients with ovarian germ cell tumours by whether or not they had received prior radiotherapy (1977–1986).

chemotherapy to treat metastatic malignant germ cell tumours both in the male and female, the presence of hepatic metastases has carried a bad prognosis. Using POMB/ACE chemotherapy in the male patients the survival in patients with large liver metastases is 82% and in patients with CNS metastases is 80%. In Figure 12 the survival in the 8 female patients

with hepatic metastases is very close to the survival of the whole group.

These results indicate that metastatic malignant germ cell tumours of the ovary behave in a very similar biological manner to those arising in the testicles. With appropriate chemotherapy it should be rare for any of these patients to succumb from their disease. How-

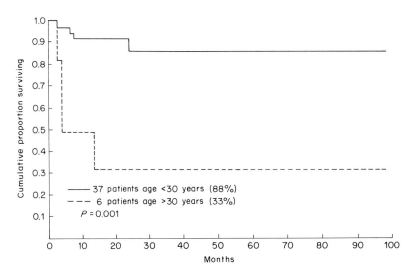

Figure 10 Analysis of survival of patients with ovarian germ cell tumours by age > or <30 years (1977–1986).

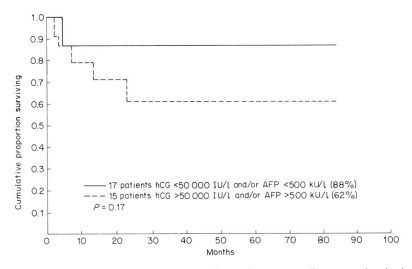

Figure 11 Analysis of survival of patients with ovarian germ cell tumours by the initial serum concentration of human chorionic gonadotrophin (hCG) and alpha-fetoprotein (AFP) (1979–1986).

ever, it needs emphasizing again that prior therapy with either chemotherapy and/or radiotherapy will compromise the chances of obtaining a complete remission since these tumours develop drug resistance if they are not rapidly eliminated.

So far with a maximum of a 9 year follow-up

no long term side effects have been identified in patients treated with POMB/ACE chemotherapy. The children treated are developing normally and going through puberty without any evidence of endocrine dysfunction. Menstruation is normal in patients who have not received radical surgery and several have

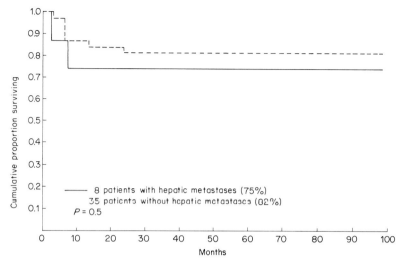

Figure 12 Analysis of survival of patients with ovarian germ cell tumours by whether or not they had hepatic metastases at the time of starting treatment (1977–1986).

completed normal pregnancies. Cytotoxic chemotherapy given intermittently over a limited period does not usually have a major effect on ovarian function. In a parallel series of patients treated for gestational choriocarcinoma (with different chemotherapeutic regimens) analysis of 445 patients showed that 86% of those who wanted to become pregnant were successful (49).

STAGE I PATIENTS AND FOLLOW-UP

Patients who have had a primary malignant GCT resected require careful staging (see above). If serial estimations of tumour markers, CT scanning of thorax and abdomen, ultrasound of liver and para-aortic region and pelvis are all normal, confirming that the patient has Stage I disease, we have not treated them with adjuvant chemotherapy. So far we have followed 11 patients with Stage I ovarian GCT and to date none have relapsed. However, if this surveillance policy is going to be used then patients do need to be followed very carefully. Patients should be seen for a clinical check-up at monthly intervals during the first year together with a chest x-ray. CT scanning

and ultrasound should be repeated as indicated. The follow-up sequence for both male and female patients with GCTs is shown in Table 4. In addition to the 11 female patients, we have a larger experience in male patients with Stage I disease following testicular GCT. Although the relapse rate in these patients is approximately 25% all of these patients have been salvaged with POMB/ACE chemotherapy. These results confirm that it is not

TABLE 4 FOLLOW-UP OF PATIENTS WITH GERM CELL TUMOURS OF THE OVARY AND TESTIS AT CHARING CROSS HOSPITAL

From completion of treatment—Stage I from normalization of markers.

Serum tumour markers (beta hCG and AFP):

Year 1	weekly × 10
	2-weekly × 21
Year 2	monthly
Year 3	2-monthly
Years 4 and 5	3-monthly
Subsequent years	6-monthly

Clinical examination with chest x-ray (unless CT scan is available):

Year 1	monthly
Year 2	2-monthly
Years 3 and 4	3-monthly
Subsequent years	6-monthly

necessary to subject these patients to chemotherapy unless metastatic disease has been
clearly identified.

The rarity of ovarian GCTs and the complexity of their management, together with the
experience that is needed to get the optimum
results from cytotoxic chemotherapy make it
imperative that these patients are referred to
centres with special experience in managing
this group of diseases.

ACKNOWLEDGEMENTS

We would like to thank Professor K.D. Bagshawe, Dr R.H.J. Begent and Dr G.J.S. Rustin
who have been closely involved in the development of the management of germ cell tumours
at Charing Cross Hospital and to the gynaecologists, surgeons and physicians who have
referred patients. This work has been supported in part by the Cancer Research Campaign and Medical Research Council.

REFERENCES

1 Walker AH, Ross RK, Pike MC, Henderson BE.
   A possible rising incidence of malignant germ
   cell tumours in young women. Br J Cancer 1984;
   49: 669–72.
2 Fox H, Langley FA. In: Tumours of the Ovary.
   London: William Heinemann Medical Books,
   1976: 173–261.
3 Stamp GHW, McConnell EM. Malignancy
   arising in cystic ovarian teratomas. A report of
   24 cases. Br J Obstet Gynaecol 1983; 90: 671–5.
4 Serov SF, Scully RE, Sobin LH. Histological
   typing of ovarian tumours. International Histological Classification of Tumours. Geneva:
   WHO, 1973: 46–50.
5 Paradinas FJ. Pathology. Clin Oncol 1983; 2:
   17–50.
6 Mueller CW, Topkins P, Lapp WA. Dysgerminoma of the ovary. An analysis of 427 cases. Am
   J Obstet Gynecol 1950; 60: 153–9.
7 Castleman B, Scully RE, McNeely BU. Case
   records of the Massachusetts General Hospital.
   N Engl J Med 1972; 286: 594–600.
8 Abell MR, Johnson VJ, Holtz F. Ovarian
   neoplasms in childhood and adolescence, I.
   Tumours of germ cell origin. Am J. Obstet
   Gynecol 1965; 92: 1059–81.
9 Scully R.E. Gonadoblastoma. A review of 74
   cases. Cancer 1970; 25: 1340–56.
10 Langley FA, Govan ADT, Anderson MC, Gowing NFC, Woodstock AS, Hanilal KR. Yolk sac
   and allied tumours of the ovary. Histopathology
   1981; 5: 389–401.
11 Nogales FF, Silverberg SG, Bloustein PA, Mar-
   tinez-Hernandez A, Pierce B. Yolk sac carcinoma (endodermal sinus tumour). Ultrastructure and histogenesis of gonadal and
   extragonadol tumours in comparison with normal human yolk sac. Cancer 1977; 39: 1462–74.
12 Peterson WF. Malignant degeneration of
   benign cystic teratomas of the ovary: a collective
   review of the literature. Obstet Gynecol Surv
   1957; 12: 793–830.
13 Beilby JOW, Parkinson C. Features of prognostic significance in solid ovarian teratoma.
   Cancer 1975; 36: 2147–59.
14 Fortt RW, Mathie IK. Gliomatosis peritonei
   caused by ovarian teratoma. J Clin Pathol 1969;
   22: 348–53.
15 Robboy SJ, Scully RE. Ovarian teratoma with
   glial implants on the peritoneum. An analysis of
   12 cases Hum Pathol 1970; 1: 643–53.
16 Beck JS, Fulmer HF, Lee ST. Solid malignant
   ovarian teratoma with "embryoid bodies" and
   trophoblastic differentiation. J Pathol 1969; 99:
   67–73.
17 Nogales FF, Favara BE, Major FJ, Silverberg
   SG. Immature teratoma of the ovary with a
   neural component ("solid" teratoma). Hum
   Pathol 1976; 7: 625–42.
18 Norris HJ, Zirkin HJ, Benson WL. Immature
   (malignant) teratoma of the ovary. A clinical
   and pathologic study of 58 cases. Cancer 1976;
   37: 2359–72.
19 Norris HJ, Adams AE. Malignant germ cell
   tumours of the ovary. In: Coppleson M ed
   Gynecological Oncology, Ch. 51. Edinburgh:
   Churchill Livingstone, 1981: 680–96.
20 Thurlbeck WM, Scully RE. Solid teratoma of
   the ovary: a clinicopathological analysis of nine
   cases. Cancer 1960; 13: 804–11.
21 Young RM, Prat J, Scully RE. Epidermoid cyst
   of the ovary. A report of three cases with
   comments on histogenesis. Am J Clin Pathol
   1980, 73: 272–6.
22 Aguirre P, Scully RE. Malignant neuroectodermal tumour of the ovary, a distinctive form of
   monodermal teratoma: report of five cases. Am J
   Surg Pathol 1982; 6: 283–92.
23 Hart WR, Burkons DM. Germ cell neoplasms
   arising in gonadoblastomas. Cancer 1979; 43:
   669–78.
24 Norris HJ, Jensen RD. Relative frequency of
   ovarian neoplasms in childhood and adolescence. Cancer 1979; 30: 713–19.
25 Newlands ES, Begent RHJ, Rustin GJS, Bagshawe KD Potential for cure in metastatic

ovarian teratomas and dysgerminomas. Br J Obstet Gynaecol 1982, 89: 555–60.

26 Green AJ, Begent RHJ, Keep PA, Bagshawe KD. Analysis of radioimmunodetection of tumours by substraction technique. J Nucl Med 1986; 25: 96–100.

27 Bagshawe KD, Harland S. Detection of intra-cranial tumours with special reference to immu-nodiagnosis. Proc Soc Med 1976; 69: 51–3.

28 Newlands ES, Begent RHJ, Rustin GJS, Parker D, Bagshawe KD. Further advances in the management of malignant teratomas of the testis and other sites. Lancet 1983; i: 948–51.

29 Rustin GJS, Bagshawe KD, Newlands ES, Begent RHJ, Crawford SM. Successful manage-ment of metastatic and primary germ cell tumours in the brain. Cancer 1986; 57: 2108–13.

30 Asadourian LA, Taylor HB. Dysgerminoma, an analysis of 105 cases. Obstet Gynecol 1969; 33: 370–5.

31 Brody S. Clinical aspects of dysgerminoma of the ovary. Acta Radiol 1961; 56: 209–30.

32 Krepart G, Smith JP, Rutledge F, Delclos L. The treatment for dysgerminoma of the ovary, Cancer 1978; 41: 986–90.

33 Lucraft HL. A review of 33 cases of ovarian dysgerminoma emphasising the role of radio-therapy. Clin Radiol 1979; 30: 385–9.

34 Thurlbeck WM, Scully RE. Teratoma of the ovary. Cancer 1960; 13: 804–8.

35 Slayton RE, Hreshcyhshyn MM, Silverberg SG. et al. Treatment of malignant ovarian germ cell tumours. Response to vincristine, dactinomycin and cyclophosphamide. Cancer 1978; 42: 390–8.

36 Cangir A, Smith J, Van Eys J. Improved prognosis in children with ovarian cancers fol-lowing modified VAC (vincristine sulfate, dacti-nomycin and cyclophosphamide) chemo-therapy. Cancer 1978; 42: 1234–8.

37 Gershenson DM, Del Junco G, Herson J, Rut-ledge FN. Endodermal sinus tumour of the ovary: The M.D. Anderson experience. Obstet Gynecol 1983; 61: 194–202.

38 Slayton RE, Park RC, Silverberg SG, Shingle-ton H, Creasman WT, Blessing JA. Vincristine, dactinomycin and cyclophosphamide in the treatment of malignant germ cell tumors of the ovary. A gynecologic oncology group study (A final report). Cancer 1985; 56: 243–8.

39 Gershenson DM, Copeland LJ, Kavanagh JJ, Cangir A, del Junco G, Saul PB, Stringer A, Freedman RS, Edwards CL, Taylor Wharton J. Treatment of malignant nondysgerminomatous germ cell tumors of the ovary with vincristine, dactinomycin and cyclophosphamide. Cancer 1985; 56: 2756–61.

40 Greene MH, Boice JP, Greer BE, Blessing JA, Demoo A. Acute non-lymphoblastic leukaemia after therapy with alkylating agents for ovarian cancer. N Engl J Med 1982; 307: 1416–21.

41 Williams S, Blessing J, Adcock C, Homesberg H. Treatment of ovarian germ cell tumours with cisplatin, vinblastine and bleomycin (PVB). Proc Am Soc Clin Oncol 1984; 3: 175.

42 Carlson RW, Sikic BI, Turbow MM, Ballon SC. Combination cis-platin, vinblastine and bleo-mycin chemotherapy (PVB) for malignant germ cell tumours of the ovary. Clin Oncol 1983; 1: 645–51.

43 Wiltshaw E, Stuart-Harris R, Barker GH, Gow-ing NFC, Raju S. Chemotherapy of endodermal sinus tumour yolk sac tumour) of the ovary: Preliminary communication. J R Soc Med 1982; 75: 888–92.

44 Slayton RE. Management of germ cell and stromal tumours of the ovary. Sem Oncol 1984; 11: 299–313.

45 Newlands ES, Bagshawe KD. Epipopophyllin derivative (VP 16–213) in malignant teratomas and choriocarcinomas. Lancet 1977; ii: 87.

46 Newlands ES, Bagshawe KD, Begent RHJ, Rustin GJS, Crawford SM, Holden L. Current optimum management of anaplastic germ cell tumours of the testis and other sites Br J Urol 1986; 58: 307–14.

47 Germa-Lluch JR, Regent RHJ, Bagshawe KD Tumour marker levels and prognosis in malig-nant teratomas of the testis. Br J Cancer 1980; 42: 850–5.

48 Bagshawe KD, Begent RHJ, Glaser M, House M, Newlands ES. The ovary. In: Bagshawe KD, Begent RHJ, Newlands ES. eds Germ Cell Tumours. London: WB Saunders, 1983; 215–32.

49 Rustin GJS, Booth M, Dent J, Salt S, Rustin F, Bagshawe KD. Pregnancy after cytotoxic chemotherapy for gestational trophoblastic tumours. Br Med J 1984; 288: 103–6.

Textbook of Uncommon Cancer
Edited by C.J. Williams, J.G. Krikorian, M.R. Green and D. Raghavan
© 1988 John Wiley & Sons Ltd

Chapter 4

Mixed Mullerian Tumours of the Corpus Uteri

Ian Vellacott* and
Robert W. Shaw†
*Lecturer and †Professor, Academic Department of Obstetrics and Gynaecology, Royal Free Hospital, London, UK

HISTORY

Wagner in 1854 first described a tumour that contained both epithelial and stromal elements. The first case arising in endometrium was subsequently described by Virchow (1) in 1864, and in 1870 a case was reported which involved the corpus uteri. Two years later the first well documented case of a carcinosarcoma was reported.

Over the subsequent decades a confusing variety of terminology has been applied to these tumours depending on their site of origin, naked eye appearance and histological structure, including mixed mesodermal tumours (or mesodermal mixed tumours), carcinosarcoma, sarcoma botryoides, carcinosarcomatoides, mesenchymal sarcoma, etc. In an extensive review of the literature McFarland (2) found 119 names to describe these tumours.

The term mesodermal mixed tumour was first suggested in 1906 to describe those tumours in which heterologous elements such as muscle and cartilage can be found, and this terminology has been widely accepted since that time. The term carcinosarcoma has been reserved for a homologous mixture of carcinomatous and sarcomatous elements, all of which

are derived from elements normally developing in the mullerian system. The overall term 'mullerian mixed tumour' has been recommended by the World Health Organization (3), subdivided into these two groups. The term sarcoma botryoides, often used for the polypoidal form of this tumour, is best confined to the more truly grape-like tumours of younger patients, usually embryonal rhabdomyosarcomas.

A number of series of cases have been reported over the years, and early references to this tumour have been reviewed. (4, 5).

EPIDEMIOLOGY AND AETIOLOGY

The incidence of mixed mullerian tumours varies in different series. In 1905 it was stated that the ratio of this tumour to other malignancies of the corpus uteri was 1:7500. Many other studies (6–8) quote an incidence of between 2 and 5%. A further study (9) reported that 0.8% of 26114 gynaecological admissions present with a mixed mullerian tumour. However, as many patients were referred to that institute with a suspicion of malignancy, the high incidence noted is perhaps not representative of the population as a whole.

An incidence of 0.99 per 100000 females over the age of 20 has been reported (10) and another study (11) found one mullerian mixed tumour for every eight with adenocarcinoma of the corpus uteri and concluded they are not as rare as was previously thought, particularly when endometrial malignancies are extensively pathologically reviewed.

Attempts have been made to try to bring the total number of cases up to date but this has, and has continued to be, a very difficult task as the classification of these tumours has been so variable. Many authors do not specify the exact histological findings or the criteria under which they accept or exclude cases under the heading of mixed mullerian tumour.

The majority of mixed mullerian tumours occur between the ages of 50 and 70, nearly all being postmenopausal, but examples in much younger and much older women have been recorded (12). The mean age at diagnosis varies between 61.3 and 67.3 years (5, 8, 13–15).

The mean age of the menopause does not seem to show a difference from that expected in the normal population (11), and the median interval from menopause to presentation appears to be between 15 and 17 years (10, 13, 15).

Constitutional risk factors associated with endometrial carcinoma (diabetes mellitus, hypertension and nulliparity) appear to be present in comparable proportions with mixed mullerian tumours (13, 16). One study (17) reported that 50% of their cases were nulliparous and another 40% (13). However, other studies have shown significantly lower numbers of nulliparous patients, reporting only 11% (9) and 12% (13).

Some authors have reported a higher incidence of mixed mullerian tumours in black women. In one series of 21 cases (14), there were 17 black patients against a background population ratio of 2:1 black to white. In a further later study of the same population, a ratio of 3:1 was noted (18). Other studies, however, suggest the opposite. Only 1 black patient was seen in a series of 49 cases (2%) (5), although his unit admitted 4% black patients.

In another series (13) the ratio of black to white was 2.5:1, in contrast to adenocarcinoma of the uterus where the ratio was 0.8:1. These authors also made several suggestive associations. White women had significantly more homologous tumours than black women and were significantly older at diagnosis, although black women tended to have more advanced disease. This may suggest a different biological origin in the two races.

The question as to whether prior exposure of the uterine cavity to radiation predisposes to the development of mixed mullerian tumours is still a controversial topic. It has been suggested (19) that irradiation to the endometrium predisposed to the development of malignant disease. An incidence of previous irradiation in 11 of 29 cases of uterine carcinosarcoma has been quoted (20). Another study on the other hand (14) had no patients with previous irradiation in a series of 21 cases, and in a further report only 2 in a series of 51 (18). In one report 17% of the cases with mullerian mixed tumour had received radiotherapy but all for other gynaecological malignancies (9). Another study had 5 patients in their series (17.8%) who had received intracavity radium for benign conditions to induce a radium menopause (11). In addition 6 patients had received surgical treatment for dysfunctional bleeding during the perimenopausal period and they postulated that it may not be the radium per se which resulted in the tumour process but the underlying cause for the dysfunctional haemorrhage (11).

A recent study compared 9 cases of mixed mullerian tumour associated with prior pelvic irradiation with 8 non-irradiation associated (21). Their conclusions were that patients with post-irradiation tumours presented at a younger age and with symptoms of much more extensive disease. Two-thirds were heterologous whereas the same proportion in the non-irradiation group were homologous. Prognosis, however, did not significantly differ, and was very poor, in both groups.

In view of the recent interest in the role of unopposed oestrogens in endometrial malignancies, this has been examined in two recent series. In one, only 3 (10.7%) had received hormone replacement therapy at any time (11), whilst in the other series of 61 patients only one had oestrogen therapy in the past (16). These data do not support the theory for a role of exogenous oestrogens in induction of the tumour.

PATHOLOGY

The mullerian ducts fuse across the midline to form the uterus, and thus the cavity will be lined from fundus to cervix with endometrium that is derived from mullerian mesoderm from which arises both the stroma and epithelium of the formed endometrium.

The term mesenchymal sarcoma of the uterus has been used (22) to include tumours featuring malignant mesenchymal tissue (leiomyosarcomas excluded). Mesenchymal tumours can be subdivided into pure (one cell type only) or mixed (more than one cell type), and to whether they are homologous—containing elements indigenous to the uterus, or heterologous—containing elements foreign to the uterus, e.g. striated muscle or cartilage.

The distinction was made by Symmonds and Dockerty (23) between the homologous carcinosarcoma which consisted of intermingled carcinomatous and sarcomatous elements and the heterologous mixed mesodermal tumours which may contain such tissues as cartilage, striated muscle or bone. Norris and Taylor (15) also advocated the separation of the mixed mullerian tumours into these two groups and in their study suggested that carcinosarcoma had a better prognosis. Many other workers (9, 16) did not demonstrate any difference in terms of prognosis between the two groups and since the distinction is based only on the presence or absence of heterologous elements, the recognition of which depends on many variable factors, the subclassification seems unhelpful.

The gross appearance of the tumour is not that dissimilar to that of other malignant neoplasms of the uterus. The size of the uterus may range from small and atrophic to enlarged and fused to all the other pelvic organs as a large mass. In some cases the pelvic organs are not identifiable and are replaced by a large friable mass (17).

In one series the uterine weight ranged between 85 and 4050 g with a mean of 1157 g and a median of 500 g (13). The length of the uterus ranged from 9 to 30 cm. The mean diameter was 8.5 cm, ranging from 3 to 20 cm, compared to another series (15) where it was 5.6 cm but with a similar range.

Typically, the tumour is polypoid and located at the fundus of the uterus, most commonly on the posterior wall but also on the anterior wall. It may be attached at multiple sites to the endometrium.

Norris and Taylor (15) found that the tumour was polypoid or pedunculated in 81% and soft in 76%, with areas of necrosis (48%) haemorrhage (36%) and cystic change (23%) being present. They also noted that the colour and consistency was variable in view of the various areas of necrosis and haemorrhage (Figures 1 and 2).

As the tumour grows, it fills the uterus and distends the cavity, and it may dilate the cervix to allow the growth to project into the vagina (Figure 3). The intact tumour may be mistaken for a fibroid polyp. When the tumour is cut, the surface is less firm than a fibroid, the cut surface lacks the whorling appearance and there are often areas of haemorrhage. The tumour can occasionally be shelled out of its bed. The endometrium adjacent tends to be thinned and atrophic but sometimes is the site of an endometrial carcinoma.

Histological assessment of these tumours is less straightforward than that of pure adenocarcinoma, the presence of multiple tissues making it hard to find reproducible criteria, for example the degree of differentiation.

Microscopically there is a bewildering variety of tissue patterns. Lebowich and Ehrlich (24) proposed that the presence of embryonal

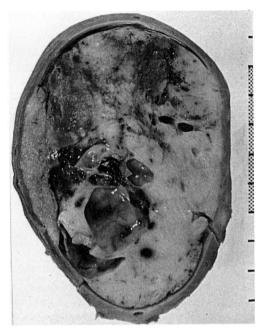

Figure 1 The cavity of the uterus is filled with partly necrotic and haemorrhagic tumour which arises from a limited area of endometrium (1 and 5 cm markers). (*Reproduced by permission of the British Journal of Obstetrics and Gynaecology.*)

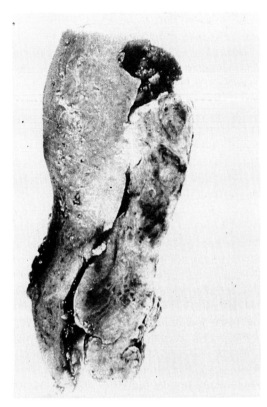

Figure 3 Necrotic tumour filling the uterine cavity and extruding from the cervical os.

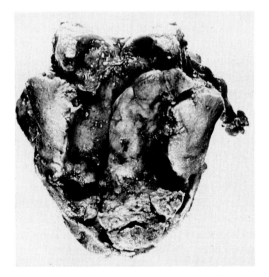

Figure 2 Localized tumour mass distorting but not filling the uterine cavity.

myoblasts was mandatory for the diagnosis of mesodermal mixed tumours, presenting typically longitudinal and transverse striations (24). In addition smooth muscle, mature or immature hyaline cartilage, bone, osteoid, myxomatous tissue and adipose tissue may be present. Other observers feel that the presence of two or more heterotopic elements where the appearance and clinical characteristics are typical should be sufficient for diagnosis.

The carcinosarcoma is a diffuse admixture of the two neoplastic elements; one being epithelial elements ranging from well differentiated to undifferentiated elements and the other malignant mesenchymal elements of homologous sarcoma. These may be independent or resemble a collision tumour, or features of sarcomatous growth may invade the pervading adenocarcinoma.

In the 28 patients in the series of Shaw et al. (11), cells accepted as myoblasts were found in 22 and cartilage in 4, but in 4 patients neither were detected.

Two other fine structures are worthy of closer investigation, the degree of differentiation as shown by mitotic activity, and the reaction between the epithelial and mesodermal components, particularly where there is a local predominance of one.

Mitotic activity varies greatly within the tumours; in most cases the stroma and epithelium can be assessed separately but more attention has been given to the former for it is this that distinguishes the mixed tumour from endometrial adenocarcinoma. In the series of Shaw et al. (11) material mitoses were counted per 20 oil immersion fields, an area of approximately 0.25 mm^2, and counts ranged between 1 and 44 with no correlation to clinical outcome.

Pure mixed sarcoma is rare but when it occurs its open pattern may raise problems of differentiation from stromal sarcoma, the recognition of heterotopic structures becoming of particular importance. However, all the tumour examined contained epithelial elements. While the relation between the two varies there are four basic patterns. The first suggests an 'organoid' relation between sarcoma and carcinoma possibly implying better differentiation; there are patterns often papillary in which masses of sarcomatous tissue are covered by epithelium (Figure 4), and those in which gland-like structures within the tumour are mantled by stroma in a concentric arrangement (Figure 5). In the third (Figure 6), presumably less well differentiated, the two types are more intimately mixed with increasingly irregular epithelial masses forming cell groups that can be recognized with certainty only where the reticulum pattern of the surrounding sarcoma has been preserved. Finally, (Figure 7) there are those in which pure carcinoma exists alongside typical mixed mullerian tumour. In the series of Shaw et al. (11) areas of pure adenocarcinoma were seen in 14 of the 24 hysterectomy specimens, two indeed

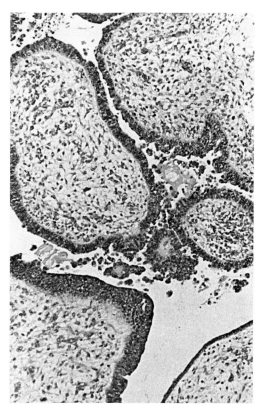

Figure 4 A mixed tumour of papillary structure in which the epithelial element covers sarcomatous tissue (haematoxylin and eosin, original magnification: ×160). (*Reproduced by permission of the British Journal of Obstetrics and Gynaecology.*)

were predominantly carcinoma with the localized foci only of typical mixed mullerian tumour. The latter is more likely to occur in the polypoidal part of the tumour, and several had what appeared to be pure carcinoma at their bases, at the point of contact with normal tissue. Differentiation was usually glandular but the squamous foci were not uncommon and several showed massive squamous differentiation.

The structure of the endometrium of the body varies. In Shaw's series (11), of the 16 specimens with endometrium available or unaltered by radium, 12 were atrophic, with active proliferation in one, cystic proliferation in another and atypicalities in the adjacent endometrium in two of those with atrophy.

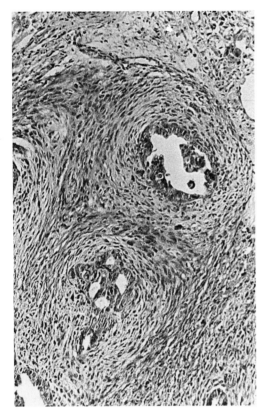

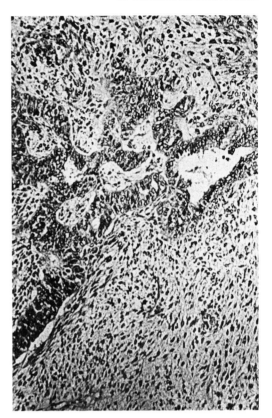

Figure 5 Malignant glands are surrounded by sarcoma by varying texture in places forming concentric layers (haematoxylin and eosin, original magnification: ×160). (*Reproduced by permission of the British Journal of Obstetrics and Gynaecology.*)

Figure 6 An apparently random mixture of epithelial and mesenchymal elements (haematoxylin and eosin, original magnification: ×160).

It has been stated that extension of the tumour is mostly local and that distant metastases rarely occur (25) but most reports do suggest that distant metastases are the rule rather than the exception. In one series, only 2 patients of the 51 died without some evidence of metastatic disease (18).

Early metastatic spread occurs by direct extension to the cervix and to the vagina. In some cases the bladder and rectum may be involved. Extension to the abdomen is frequent. Distant lymphatic spread may occur to all the pelvic nodes, pre-aortic nodes, and occasionally medistinal nodes.

Generalized dissemination of growth is noted at most post-mortem examinations (26). Metastases to the lung, brain, chest wall, lumbar muscles and even the eye-lid have been reported. Extension to the parotid has been demonstrated in one case (12), and in another to the tenth dorsal vertebra. Other studies have also reported metastases to the spine (8, 14).

The histology of the secondary deposits is often unpredictable. They may be the same as the primary, or may consist entirely of carcinoma or sarcoma, or a mixture with or without heterotopic elements.

CLINICAL FEATURES

In all recorded series of mixed müllerian tumours by far the most common presenting symptom is abnormal vaginal bleeding. In one

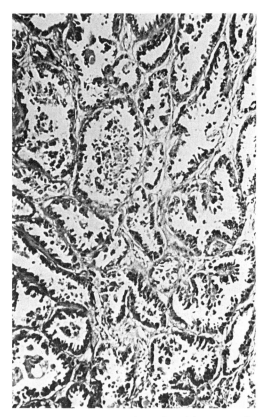

Figure 7 At the base of a polypoid tumour the epithelial elements predominates to give the pattern of a carcinoma (haematoxylin and eosin, original magnification: ×160).

series 93.7% but in nearly all series at least 80% present in this way.

Abnormal bleeding can present as a bloody discharge, intermenstrual bleeding, post-coital bleeding, menorrhagia or most commonly postmenopausal bleeding. In the series of Shaw et al. 25 of 28 patients presented with postmenopausal bleeding, the duration being 1 to 6 months (11). Other authors found a mean duration of bleeding before treatment was sought of 2 months (8), and 2.8 months (15). Macasaet et al. (13) noted a duration of between 8 and 19 months in their series.

Vaginal discharge and lower abdominal pain are the next most frequently found symptoms. In one series 27.5% of the patients complained of a vaginal discharge, two-thirds

of these being purulent, and the rest watery in nature, and an equal number with abdominal pain were also noted. In another series, this was as high as 41.3% (17).

Other symptoms include weight loss, urinary and intestinal symptoms, anorexia, weakness or the presence of an abdominal mass.

In many cases bimanual examination reveals an enlarged uterus. One series noted that finding in 64% of their cases (11), and other series show similar figures. Extrusion of the tumour is frequently seen through the cervical os. Shaw et al. (11) noted this in 4 of their 28 cases. Other series have shown this more commonly, indeed one series reported this sign in 40% of their cases (15).

INVESTIGATION AND STAGING

Definitive diagnosis of mixed mullerian tumour in the series of Shaw et al. (11) was made from uterine curettings in 20 to 28 cases, plus cervical biopsy—2, vault biopsy—2, peritoneal biopsy—1, and hysterextomy specimen—1. In the remaining 3 patients the curettings were reported as adenocarcinoma in the first instance, the true diagnosis being made on section of the uterus. In another series, of the 38 cases in which dilatation and curettage were performed, the initial diagnosis was correct in 29 (75%) and inacurrate in 9 instances; 3 being endometrial sarcoma, 5 adenocarcinoma of the endometrium and 1 atypical glandular hyperplasia.

Other series, however, have found curettings or punch biopsy less accurate. Masterson and Kremper (8) found that punch biopsy only diagnosed 4 out of 9 cases, and curettage 8 out of 16. Bartisch et al. (17) found that diagnostic curettage and biopsies were only effective in establishing diagnosis in 31.3% of cases.

Recent studies have investigated the use of cytology as an aid to diagnosis. Shaw et al. (11) performed cervical and/or vault cytology in 21 out of 28 patients. The smears were reported as follows: positive with malignant cells of endometrial origin—9, atypical or suspicious glandular cells—6, atypical squamous cells—1 and negative (grade I or II)—5. Even on careful retrospective review of the slides no specific cytological abnormalities to differentiate these cases from endometrial carcinomas were apparent.

Macasaet et al. (13) had cervical cytology available in 27 of their 35 patients; 30% had negative smears, while 15% had atypical smears and 55% positive. They also noted that amongst the patients presenting with an endo-cervical mass, only 40% showed abnormal cervical cytology, although biopsies of all masses were positive.

There is no staging peculiar to mixed mul-lerian tumours of the corpus uteri. Most recent studies have used the International Federation of Gynaecology and Obstetrics staging for adenocarcinoma of the uterus.

Macasaet et al. (13) used three different staging systems in an attempt to determine the most discriminating in determining outcome. The first was the clinical staging used by FIGO for endometrial carcinoma. The second they called the 'pathologic staging': using FIGO pathological criteria but applying them to the extent of the disease as determined by the surgical and pathological findings. The third system proposed upstaging subjects with lymph vascular invasion by one stage. They looked at 2-year and mean survival rates and concluded that the clinical staging was a relatively poor determinator of outcome. There was a statistically significant difference between Stages I–II and Stages III–IV but the numbers were too small to determine whether the proposed staging was more discriminating than the FIGO pathological staging.

MANAGEMENT AND PROGNOSIS

Surgery

No one form of treatment has proven to be definitive in the treatment of mixed mullerian tumours. There are no recorded cases of 5-year survival with radiotherapy or chemotherapy alone and the mainstay therefore is surgery. The extent of the surgery, or whether it is

combined with radiotherapy, depends in many series on the individual choice of the surgeon involved.

In the series of Ober and Tovill (22), total abdominal hysterectomy and bilateral salp-ingo-oophorectomy was considered to be the primary method of treatment. They also sug-gested that the removal of necrotic tissue from the cervical canal by preoperative curettage would facilitate definitive surgery. Krupp et al. (18) recommended that the minimal surgical procedure should be a Wertheim's hysterec-tomy and pelvic gland dissection with or without vaginectomy, and in many cases recommended complete exenteration because of invasion into the bladder or rectum.

Ober and Tovill (22) recommended that in younger women in whom the growth is con-fined to the uterus it may not be necessary to perform a bilateral salpingo-oophorectomy as metastases to these structures had not been reported and there is no evidence that ovarian secretion has a growth-promoting effect on the neoplasm. Other series since, however, have reported metastases to the fallopian tubes and ovaries (11), and this conservative approach has not found favour.

Radiotherapy and Chemotherapy

Henderson (27) recommended total abdomi-nal hysterectomy followed by pelvic irradia-tion and has shown a long term survival in 5 cases despite incomplete surgical removal of the tumour. Others (23) have also emphasized the value of irradiation. One author, however, commented that performing preliminary irra-diation would delay the performance of sur-gery and could therefore worsen the prognosis (9).

In the literature no 5-year survival has been reported with radiotherapy alone although one series (28) reported an irradiation cure of a patient with primary mixed mesodermal tumour who died from pulmonary metastases 32 months later. There was no sign at post-mortem of tumour in the pelvis.

One recent series compared the survival of

25 patients with disease confined to the uterus and followed up for 2 years or more and found no significant difference in survival whether radiotherapy was used or not. Similarly in 16 patients with disease outside the uterus and followed up for a similar period, no therapeutic differences could be seen (16).

Other workers (29, 30) feel that a combined approach of surgery and radiotherapy may provide some improvement in survival rates and better local control. This may be especially so when the metastases are predominantly adenocarcinomatous. Although chemotherapeutic agents have been tried in a number of series, no therapeutic benefit has been proven. In the series of Shaw et al. both radiotherapy and chemotherapeutic agents were used only in patients with advanced disease at the time of surgery or when recurrences occurred (11).

Prognosis

Mixed mullerian tumours are one of the most malignant in the entire field of encology. One author (18) reported no 5-year survivors in his series of 51 patients. The average survival was 8.5 months.

Other reports, however, are somewhat more favourable; one reported 42.2% 5-year survival and another 41.1%. Of Lotocki's series of 61, in the 28 who had tumour confined to the uterus there was a 76% 2-year survival whereas of the 33 with extrauterine involvement there was only a 16.5% 2-year survival (16). Other studies concur that the survival is much improved if the disease has not spread beyond the uterus.

In the series of Shaw et al. (11), 7 of their 28 patients (25%) were alive and tumour free at follow-up after 5 years. Fifteen of the 21 who died did so within the first year, another 3 within 2 years and the remainder within 3 years. In one-half of their patients the tumour had spread beyond the uterus at diagnosis and only one of these was alive and well after 5 years.

Although one author suggested an improved prognosis with carcinosarcoma compared to mixed mesodermal tumour (15); other studies do not agree (5, 12).

In the series of Chuang et al. (5) there was a 30% 5-year survival with Stage I. In their 24 patients treated by surgery alone 5 (21%) survived 5 years, in their 8 with radiotherapy only 1 survived. They also noted that the number of mitoses per high power field did not correlate to survival rate. Macasaet et al. (13) had 7 survivors in 35 (20%) after 2 years, the cause of death in all but 4 due to tumour spread.

CURRENT SITUATION

Unfortunately, there are no specific markers at present to aid in the diagnosis of mixed mullerian tumours. Cytology has proven to be of only very limited use, even dilatation and curettage is misleading, and the diagnosis is very often only made at direct sectioning of the uterus. If a marker could be found, then this would undoubtedly help to improve the prognosis as all studies suggest that the earlier the diagnosis the better the long term survival. Surgical removal before there is evidence of extrauterine spread is the treatment of choice, the tumour being relatively radioinsensitive and chemotherapy being of no use. If the patient is disease free after 2 years there appears to be a favourable prognosis.

This tumour continues to present a challenge regarding diagnosis, classification and effective treatment. It is perhaps not as uncommon as was once thought, and failure of diagnosis amongst endometrial carcinoma patients may account for the poor results achieved in some of these cases. Careful vigilance by the pathologist is thus called for.

ACKNOWLEDGEMENTS

Our thanks to Dr Tom Wade-Evans, Department of Pathology, Birmingham and Midland Hospital for Women, who took the original pathology photographs.

REFERENCES

1 Virchow R. Die Krankhaften Geschwulste, Vol. 2. Berlin: August Hirschwald, 1864; 182.

2 McFarland J. Dysontogenetic and mixed tumours of the urogenital region. Surg Gynecol Obstet 1935; 63: 42.

3 Poulsen HE, Taylor CW. International Histological Classification of Tumours No. 15: Histological typing of the female genital tract tumours. Vol. 69. Geneva: WHO.

4 Taylor CW. Mesodermal mixed tumours of the female genital tract. J Obstet Gynaecol Br Emp 1958; 65: 177.

5 Chuang JT, Van Velden DJJ, Graham JB. Carcinosarcoma and mixed mesodermal tumour of the uterine corpus. Obstet Gynecol 1970; 35: 769.

6 Falkinburg LW, Hoey WO, Savran J, Stuart JR. Mesodermal mixed tumour of the corpus uteri. Am J Obstet Gynecol 1964; 90: 450.

7 Edwards DL, Sterling LN, Keller RH, Nolan JF. Mixed heterologous mesenchymal sarcomas (mixed mesodermal sarcomas) of the uterus. Am J Obstet Gynecol 1963; 85: 1002.

8 Masterson JG, Kremper J. Mixed mesodermal tumours. Am J Obstet Gynecol 1969; 104: 693.

9 Sternberg WH, Clark WH. Malignant mixed mullerian tumour (mixed mesodermal tumour of the uterus). Cancer 1954; 7: 704.

10 Williamson EO, Christopherson WM. Malignant mixed mullerian tumours of the uterus. Cancer 1972; 29: 585.

11 Shaw RW, Lynch PF, Wade-Evans T. Mullerian mixed tumour of the uterine corpus: a clinical histopathological review of 28 patients. Br J Obstet Gynaecol 1983; 90: 562.

12 Taylor CW. Mullerian mixed tumours. Acta Pathol Microbiol Scand (A) 1972; 233: 48.

13 Macasaet MA, Waxman M, Fruchter RG, Boyce J, Hong P, Nicastri AD, Remy JC. Prognostic factors in malignant mesodermal (mullerian) mixed tumours of the uterus. Gynecol Oncol 1985; 20: 32.

14 Hayes D. Mixed mullerian tumour of the corpus uteri. J Obstet Gynaecol Br Emp 1974; 81: 160.

15 Norris HJ, Taylor HB. Mesenchymal tumours of the uterus III. A clinical and pathological study of 31 carcinosarcomas. Cancer 1966; 19: 1459.

16 Lotocki R, Rosenshein NB, Grumbine F, Dillon M, Parmley T, Woodfuff JD. Mixed mullerian tumours of the uterus: clinical and pathological correlations. Int J Gynecol Obstet 1982; 20: 237.

17 Bartisch EG, O'Leary JA, Moore JG. Carcinosarcoma of the uterus. Obstet Gynecol 1967; 30: 518.

18 Krupp PJ, Sternberg WH, Clark WH, St Romain MJ, Smith RC. Malignant mixed mullerian neoplasms (mixed mesodermal tumours). Am J Obstet Gynecol 1961; 81: 959.

19 Speert H, Peightal TC. Malignant tumours of the uterus fundus subsequent to irradiation for benign pelvic conditions. Am J Obstet Gynecol 1949; 57: 261.

20 Klein J. Carcinosarcoma of the endometrium. Am J Obstet Gynecol 1953; 65: 1212.

21 Varela-Duran J, Nochomovitz LE, Prem KA, Dehner LP. Postirradiation mixed mullerian tumours of the uterus. Cancer 1980; 45: 1625.

22 Ober WB, Tovill HMM. Mesenchymal sarcomas of the uterus. Am J Obstet Gynecol 1959; 77: 246.

23 Symmonds RE, Dockerty MB. Sarcoma and sarcoma-like proliferations of the endometrial stroma 1. Clinicopathologic study of 19 mesodermal mixed tumours. Surg Gynecol Obstet 1955; 100: 232.

24 Lebowich RJ, Ehrlich HE. Mesodermal mixed tumours of the corpus uteri. Surgery 1941; 10: 411.

25 Amolsch AL. Mixed mesodermal tumours of the uterus and vagina with a report of six cases. Am J Cancer 1939; 37: 435.

26 Alznauer RL. Mixed mesodermal sarcoma of the corpus uteri. Arch Pathol 1955; 60: 329.

27 Henderson DN. Endolymphatic stromal meiosis. Am J Obstet Gynecol 1946; 52: 1000.

28 Heinrichs WL, Climie ARW, Cook JC. Cure of mesodermal mixed tumours by radiotherapy. Obstet Gynecol 1962; 19: 537.

29 Badib AO, Vontgama V, Kurohara SS, Webster JH. Radiotherapy in the treatment of sarcomas of the corpus uteri. Cancer 1969; 24: 724.

30 Belgrad R, Elbadawi N, Rubin P. Uterine sarcoma. Radiology 1975; 114: 181.

Textbook of Uncommon Cancer
Edited by C.J. Williams, J.G. Krikorian, M.R. Green and D. Raghavan
© 1988 John Wiley & Sons Ltd

Chapter **5**

Mixed Mullerian Tumours of the Gynaecological System other than Endometrial Tumours

Robert J. Marshall

Department of Histopathology, Royal Cornwall Hospital (Treliske), Truro, Cornwall, UK

INTRODUCTION

Mixed mullerian tumours (MMT) occur in the body of the uterus, the ovary, fallopian tube and cervix. There are also reports of mullerian sarcomas and one MMT outside the female genital tract. They are composed of an epithelial and a stromal component, both of which are malignant. Because tumours occur in which both components are benign—adenofibromas—and in order to avoid any possible misunderstanding, 'malignant' should be prefixed to the title. Adenosarcomas are tumours with a benign epithelial component in a sarcomatous stroma. Histogenetically, they are related to MMTs, but are not embraced by that title and are not considered further here.

The sarcomatous component of the tumours may show differentiation towards cell types found normally in the tissue of origin, or towards components such as bone or cartilage. The former is called homologous, the latter heterologous differentiation.

Any examination of MMTs is bedevilled by the variety of names under which these tumours masquerade. The commonest alternative is carcinosarcoma, which is generally used to refer to the homologous type of MMT.

A name so different misleadingly suggests a far greater division between the two tumours than is warranted. Either mixed mullerian tumour or carcinosarcoma is an acceptable name, but not both.

The literature is replete with statements that MMTs outside the body of the uterus are commonest in the cervix or vagina (1–6). This is because early reports include pure sarcomas, including embryonal rhabdomyosarcoma (sarcoma botryoides), among the MMTs (7, 8). In fact, the commonest extra-uterine site is the ovary, followed by the fallopian tube and then the cervix. MMTs have not been reported in the vulva or vagina.

They are rare tumours in the uterus, and exceedingly rare outside it. Approximately 200 cases have been reported in the ovary, 27 in the fallopian tube and 12 in the cervix. Even of these few, some must be rejected as unsuitable. MMTs account for 1% of ovarian malignancy (9, 10). Any primary malignancy in the fallopian tube is a rare event and it is possible that MMTs form a higher percentage of these. In the cervix, criteria for establishing such a tumour as primary were given by Abell and Ramirez (11). For all these extra-uterine sites, the uterus should be available for pathological examination to exclude a uterine primary. A uterus of normal size, from which normal curettings are obtained, can also reasonably be assumed not to harbour tumour, though normal curettings can be obtained from a uterus containing MMT.

These aggressive tumours often obliterate the organ in which they arise. This may have led to an underestimate of Stage III and IV tumours and falsely increased survival statistics in what are already tumours of very poor prognosis.

The following account describes the features of ovarian MMT before those of the tube and cervix and then deals with theories of histogenesis.

OVARY

Epidemiology and Aetiology

The great majority of ovarian MMTs occur in postmenopausal women. About 65% occur in the sixth and seventh and 85% after the age of 50. There are two reports of MMT in young women (12, 13). One, in a woman aged 18, is described as predominantly a mucinous cystadenocarcinoma with a focal sarcomatous component (12). However, there is no reason to doubt either diagnosis.

About 35% of women with ovarian MMT are nulliparous. A similar association has been found with uterine MMT. There is no evidence of a racial predisposition (2, 14).

A significant number of patients with uterine MMT have received prior pelvic irradiation. The proportion varies between different series, but is about 20% (15–17). The association is more remote in patients with ovarian tumours, only two of whom are reported to have received previous irradiation (10, 18).

Pathology

Grossly, the tumours vary greatly in size, from 5 cm to as great as 30 cm diameter (1, 2, 13, 19). Weights over 2.5 kg are exceptional, though tumours of 8 and 9.5 kg are recorded (12, 20).

MMTs are often found to have spread widely at the time of laparotomy. There is frequently involvement of both ovaries and omentum, with seedlings over the peritoneal surface (14, 21). Adhesions are often present between tumour and omentum, loops of bowel or bladder (12, 14, 22, 23).

Nearly all tumours are composed of multilocular cysts (1, 2, 10, 12, 13, 19, 21, 24), and contain areas of haemorrhage and necrosis (1, 2, 13, 22). Solid areas may have a mucoid appearance or show papillary projects into the cysts (23). Torsion of the tumour is a rare event (25). There is one report of a right pleural effusion which cleared after operative removal of a left ovarian tumour (25).

Microscopically, these tumours may have a very varied appearance. The essential criterion for diagnosis is the presence of both a carcinomatous and sarcomatous component. The proportion of each varies greatly between tumours and between different areas of the same tumour. Both components may be so undifferentiated as to blend almost imperceptibly with one another, causing diagnostic difficulty (10). Usually, however, there are at least some areas of evident glandular differentiation, and often a papillary growth pattern (1, 2, 19), sometimes with psammoma bodies (1). Areas of carcinoma commonly show endometrioid or serous differentiation (1, 9, 13). Clear cell or mucinous differentiation is often present (1, 9, 10). Squamous differentiation occurs, often with keratinization, but is more often described as metaplastic within glandular elements (9, 13), than arising de novo within surrounding sarcoma (12).

The sarcomatous component may be homologous or heterologous. the majority of tumours, about 60% to 70%, show heterologous differentiation, though there is considerable variation between larger series, from about 50% (9, 13) to 80% (12). Homologous elements may be composed of small, round or spindle-shaped cells with hyperchromatic nuclei and little cytoplasm, resembling the stroma of proliferative endometrium. Myxoid areas are a common component (3, 12, 19), and there is frequently very marked pleomorphism within the stromal element. Smooth muscle differentiation, probably rarely sought, is rarely reported; there seems no justification for saying that it is heterologous to the ovary (10).

True heterologous elements consist of cartilage, bone, striated muscle and fat. The last may also often be ignored and is certainly very rarely reported (1, 12). Care should be taken to identify genuine lipoblasts in such areas, and not be misled by vacuolated cells which can be present in myxoid areas. Cartilage is the commonest component, reported in about 60% heterologous tumours, while osteoid has been found in about 20%. Though both these components usually show differentiation towards the adult tissue, they also have clearly malignant features. The reported proportion of heterologous tumours showing striated muscle differentiation varies from 10% to 50%. The considerable difference between those finding frequent striated muscle differentiation (12, 13), and those finding it rarely (10), is probably due to different criteria used for identifying striated muscle. Dictor, for example, found one case among 17 heterologous tumours having cells with cross-striations, the strictest definition; two further cases showed cells with abundant eosinophilic cytoplasm (1). It has been objected that the latter definition is too loose, since similar cells may be found in carcinomas, leiomyosarcomas, and even leiomyomas (16).

Cytoplasmic myoglobin can now be detected immunohistochemically. One study has examined 25 cases of MMT and reclassified three cases as heterologous because immunochemical staining for myoglobin was present (26). The technique was particularly useful in the ovarian cases examined. Electron microscopy may also reveal striated muscle differentiation not evident on light microscopy. This distinction is of more than academic interest, since the presence of heterologous components may have prognostic significance (13). The criteria used in striated muscle differentiation should be stated and should include cross-striations visible on light microscopy, the presence of myoglobin detected immunohistochemically or myofilaments seen by electron microscopy.

Apart from the detection of myoglobin, immunohistochemistry has little to offer diagnostically, but much of interest. Dictor pointed out the presence of hyaline droplets in most ovarian MMTs, which stained immunohistochemically for alpha$_1$ antitrypsin (27). These droplets probably represent aggregates of alpha$_1$ antitrypsin which can be detected in most MMTs of the uterine corpus and of the ovary (28). Epithelial antigens are detected in the carcinomatous component of these tumours, as expected. They can also be detected in some cells of the sarcomatous components, however (29). This has important implications for tumour histogenesis and also, in a negative sense, diagnostically, for such markers do not therefore give a definitive answer in the differential diagnosis of mixed mullerian tumours from those carcinomas in which the glandular areas merge with undifferentiated carcinoma. Vimentin, the intermediate filament found predominantly in mesenchymal cells, is unhelpful for similar reasons; it is found in both components of MMT, as it is in the epithelial and stromal component of normal endometrium (personal observation).

Post mortem studies have been performed in a number of cases (12, 13, 19, 23), and illustrate the pattern of metastasis. Transcoelomic spread predominates, though lymphatic and haematogenous metastases occur. Widespread involvement of the peritoneal cavity is a universal finding with ascites and involvement of small and large bowel mesentery and omentum. The para-aortic nodes are often involved (12, 23). Liver involvement is common and the spleen may be involved (13). Some descriptions suggest that involvement of these visceral organs is rather an extension of the generalized peritoneal spread than haematogenous metastasis. Although the lung is often mentioned as a possible metastatic site, specific instances are not common (13, 19). The histology of the metastases may show pure adenocarcinoma

(19), or sarcoma (23), but usually both, with the sarcoma predominating (12, 13).

There are several cases in which the contralateral ovary contained carcinoma (1, 2, 23, 30), and some of these, at least, may reflect the capacity of MMT to metastasize as a single component. However, Dehner et al. (13), reported benign tumours in the contralateral ovary in 3 of their 27 cases, and there may be an increased risk of ovarian neoplasia in these patients.

Endometriosis is reported in some cases (1, 10, 30, 31), either closely associated with the tumour or elsewhere in the genital tract. This finding is considered further with the histogenesis of MMT.

MMT, though very diverse histologically, nevertheless has a characteristic appearance. The main differential diagnosis is with malignant teratoma. This tumour occurs in young women, a quite different age group from MMT. Neural tissue, such as neuroglia, ependyma and choroid plexus, is often present in teratomas, but is not found in MMT. The epithelial and mesenchymal components that may be shared by the two tumours characteristically show more differentiation to normal fetal or adult tissue in the teratoma, whereas in MMT they are frankly malignant.

Carcinomas with a reactive, sarcomatoid stroma must also be differentiated from MMT. It is rare that such a reactive stroma forms a major component of the tumour. Mitoses can be numerous, but are rarely atypical. Paradoxically, diversity of the cell types in a reactive stroma is a clue to its benign nature; a more monomorphic stroma should be regarded with suspicion. Usually, the pleomorphism of sarcomatous elements prevents any problem, but the diagnosis can be very difficult (13).

Clinical Features

There is nothing in the mode of presentation of patients with MMT that distinguishes this tumour from other forms of ovarian carcinoma. The commonest presenting syptoms are increased abdominal girth, abdominal pain,

loss of weight, and anorexia (10–14, 19–21, 23). Gastrointestinal symptoms, such as nausea, vomiting and dyspepsia are also common (12, 19, 21), as are urinary symptoms (2, 4, 19, 22). There may be a vaginal discharge (10, 19), but several reports comment on the absence or rarity of vaginal bleeding (12, 13, 18). The duration of symptoms is variable from one week to one year and is said to be shorter for heterologous than homologous tumours (13).

Examination is equally non-specific. An abdominal mass is usually palpable and can be distinguished from the uterus on examination per vaginam. Nodules of metastatic tumour may be palpated in the pouch of Douglas (21). Ascites, though said to be uncommon (13, 21), is not infrequently reported (10, 14, 19, 21, 23, 25) and may obscure the tumour mass (1). The patient may be anaemic (2, 4, 13).

Investigation and Staging

The diagnosis of a pelvic mass, probably of ovarian origin, can usually be made on physical examination and further investigations may delay surgery. Intravenous pyelography and barium enema have revealed displacement of normal structures (3), or other pathology not likely to affect management (23, 32). Ultrasonography and CT scan now offer non-invasive techniques to visualize tumours but virtually no experience in their use for MMT is reported, and again they may only be postponing an inevitable laparotomy.

Clinically, the only diagnostic problem arises in the new premenopausal women, in whom an ectopic pregnancy may be suspected (24).

The cytology of ascitic fluid is not likely to provide a definitive diagnosis. Malignant cells may be observed (21), but the observation of malignant epithelial cells with a separate spindle cell component only seems to have led to a diagnosis already made histologically (32).

The staging of MMT follows the same criteria as defined for ovarian carcinoma by the International Federation of Gynaecology and Obstetrics (FIGO) (33). Few reports state tumour stage and allocating a stage from their descriptions is not always possible. Of approximately 110 tumours whose stage is given, or can be calculated, 15% were Stage I, 22% Stage II, and 63% Stage III or IV, (1, 2, 9, 10, 12, 14, 21, 23, 25, 30, 34, 35). These figures agree closely with Hanjani et al. (2), and emphasize the advanced nature of the disease at presentation. It has been suggested that heterologous tumours are more advanced at presentation than homologous (1). This is supported by the findings of Dehner et al. that 7 of 13 patients with homologous tumours had no evidence of extension of disease or metastases at surgery, compared with only 4 of 14 patients with heterologous tumours (13).

Management and Prognosis

Surgery offers the best hope of cure. Its extent is determined by the stage of the tumour. Bilateral salphingo-oophorectomy and hysterectomy are the ideal, but only less extensive surgery may be possible for advanced tumours, when pelvic clearance may be impossible and only de-bulking can be attempted (1, 2, 12). Omentectomy is often performed (2, 14).

Radiotherapy has been given in most cases, though these tumours are said to be resistant (4, 21). Doses of 3000 to 5000 rad have been administered, often divided between the whole abdomen and the pelvis. Radiotherapy is often combined with chemotherapy. Vincristine, actinomycin D, and cyclophosphamide are the combination used most frequently (2, 18), with other drugs, such as Adriamycin and cisplatin, used for recurrent tumour.

It is virtually impossible to assess the efficacy of these treatments, since numbers are inevitably small, the tumour stage is often not given and there is no control group with which to compare results. Carlson et al. reported 12 patients treated postoperatively with radiotherapy and vincristine, actinomycin D and cyclophosphamide (18). Four of these patients showed a complete response, 1 being well at 5 years, 1 dying at 55 months and the other 2

during therapy at 8 and 12 months, all of unrelated causes. No tumour was found at post mortem in any of the 3 patients who died. Tumour stage was not given, but presumably was III in at least 3 patients whose tumours were incompletely resected. Carlson and Day later reported a further patient whose recurrent tumour in the pelvis was resected and treated as above with continuing remission at 5 years (35). This at least gives grounds for hoping that aggressive therapy can produce a significant response. Adriamycin alone was evaluated in 31 patients, most Stage III or IV (36). Only 1 of 10 with measurable disease showed a partial response, 8 others dying between 2 and 10 months. Few of the other 21 patients without measurable disease showed a positive response to treatment, and the authors concluded that Adriamycin alone was not a useful agent.

Lele et al. carried out a retrospective assessment of 35 cases of ovarian MMT treated with different regimens (37). Only patients with residual disease were considered evaluable. No patient responded to single agent chemotherapy. There was only a 12% response to first line chemotherapy and a 7% response to second line agents; no particular combination was more successful than the others.

There are isolated case reports in which chemotherapy was of benefit (10). Though these give little reason for therapeutic optimism, it is no longer true to say that further therapy following surgery fails to alter prognosis (23). However, it is a recurrent theme that the side effects of such aggressive therapy lead to cessation of treatment and not infrequently to the death of the patient (2, 14, 18, 36). Carlson et al. recommend possible treatment modifications to reduce toxicity (18).

While there may be disagreement as to the best form of therapy, there is none that these are tumours with a dismal prognosis. Tumour stage is the best single prognostic indicator, but a significant number with Stage I tumours are dead within 6 months. Overall, though, Stage I tumours are the only ones offering any chance of reasonable survival (Table 1). About

TABLE 1 OVARIAN MIXED MULLERIAN
TUMOURS: SURVIVAL
RELATED TO STAGE

| Stage | Survival (months) | |
	Mean	Range
I	28.5	(4–168)
II	7	($\frac{1}{2}$–24)
III	6.5	(1–19)
IV	5	($\frac{1}{2}$–18)

50% of patients are dead within 6 months, and 65% within a year (1, 2, 9, 14). These tumours occur in elderly women, some of whom die of unrelated causes but these deaths do not significantly alter survival figures. Survival for more than 2 years is nearly always associated with Stage I tumours (2, 9, 12), though long survival is possible with Stage III tumours (9, 18). Survival is therefore worse than for ovarian carcinoma (38), and for MMT in the uterine corpus (16, 17).

It has been argued that heterologous tumours in the uterus have a worse prognosis than homologous (17). Data on tumour stage and type are not available in sufficient numbers of ovarian tumours to allow meaningful comparison. The claim that such a difference does exist for ovarian tumours rests largely on the results of Dehner's series, which compared 13 homologous with 14 heterologous tumours (13). The median survival in the first group was 12 months, in the second 6. A greater proportion of heterologous tumours presented at a more advanced stage, but there was also a marked difference in survival when women with metastatic tumours only were compared. Nevertheless, numbers in this series were small and the difference in survival between the two types is denied by some authors, though sometimes on even scantier evidence (2, 9, 13).

FALLOPIAN TUBE

MMTs of the fallopian tube are very rare. An intraluminal growth pattern reasonably establishes a tubal neoplasm as primary, but more extensive tumours involving tube and other structures, such as the tubo-ovarian mass described in Case 3 of Acosta et al. (50) are more dubious. An early case report by Motta (39) of a tumour in a 14 year old girl was rejected by Manes and Taylor because there was extensive pelvic disease and the primary site could not be determined (40). Two of their own cases were questioned by Hanjani et al. because possible primary uterine tumours were not excluded (41).

About 25 reported cases remain. Tubal MMTs occur between 35 and 76 years of age (40, 42), having a very similar age distribution to ovarian MMT. About 35% of patients are nulliparous. Previous irradiation is not reported. Two patients had previously received anti-syphilitic therapy (42, 43).

Grossly there is usually hydrosalpinx or haematosalpinx (40, 44), which is occasionally bilateral (42, 43, 45). Any part of the tube may be involved. Sections across the involved area show a pale, fleshy tumour, often with areas of haemorrhage or necrosis, projecting as a polypoid mass into the tubal lumen (44–46), or filling and distending the tube (6, 40, 43). Invasion into the wall can be so extensive as to cause rupture (47). Tumours up to 15 cm maximum dimension and 500 g are recorded (47).

Heterologous tumours are twice as common as homologous, with cartilage being by far the commonest component of the heterologous types (5, 6, 43, 47–49). Striated muscle is the only other component recorded, being present in 2 cases (46, 47). the microscopic pattern is similar to ovarian tumours, though a papillary pattern is often prominent (6, 40, 44), suggesting that the epithelial component is 'homologous to the oviduct epithelium' (6). Tumour giant cells are often a prominent feature (5, 43, 46).

Metastatic spread is to other pelvic organs, to the peritoneum and omentum (5, 6, 41). The contralateral tube and both ovaries are frequently involved (47, 49). Metastases to lymph node (41, 49, 50), lung and liver (42) are described. They may be composed of either or both components (42, 49).

The mode of presentation is variable and non-specific. Vaginal bleeding and abdominal pain are common (6, 40, 43, 44, 48–50); nausea, vomiting and fever also occur (5, 50). Tumours may be found incidentally in patients undergoing hysterectomy for prolapse, though there is usually also a history of previous bleeding (48). A further patient presented with an inguinal mass, which proved to be a lymph node containing adenocarcinoma on biopsy (41).

On examination there is often ascites (5, 49, 50) and an adnexal mass palpable per vaginam which may extend to be palpable in the abdomen. Cytological examination may reveal adenocarcinoma (48, 49) but is more often negative (6, 46).

Nearly all patients have been treated with hysterectomy and bilateral salpingo-oophorectomy with pelvic or mesenteric lymphadenoctomy in 2 cases (41, 49) and omentectomy in another, when there was obvious omental involvement (6). Most patients were given postoperative radiotherapy. Three patients received chemotherapy (6, 41, 43).

About half of these tumours were confined to the tube at operation. It has been suggested that fimbrial fusion prevents spread of tumour into the peritoneal cavity (43). Five such patients were alive and well at intervals of 1 to 5 years (40, 43, 46, 48); 1 was alive with disease at $4\frac{1}{2}$ years (40) and 3 had died at 6, 7 and 8 months (40, 49, 50). Three patients with extension into the pelvis died, 2 at 6 months (45, 47), the third postoperatively (50). Of 4 patients with abdominal disease, 1 was alive and well at 15 months (6), 1 died in the postoperative period (5) and the other 2 at 26 and 29 months (41, 50). There is no evidence that radiotherapy improves the prognosis of these tumours, though most case reports date from an era when radiotherapy lacked many of its modern refinements. Two of the patients receiving chemotherapy had Stage III tumours; one was treated with Adriamycin, actinomycin D and cyclophosphamide and

was alive without evidence of disease at 15 months (6); the other was treated with vincristine, actinomycin D and cyclophosphamide and showed marked tumour regression before dying at 26 months (41). The third, with Stage I tumour, received similar therapy and was alive without evidence of disease at 5 years (43). No conclusions can be drawn from so few cases, but these reports do at least argue for an aggressive chemotherapeutic approach following surgery.

CERVIX

MMTs of the cervix are exceedingly rare. The requirement that tumours extending to the body of the uterus be assumed to have arisen in it is correct, but must have led to an underestimate of cervical MMT. Rotmensch et al. (51) reported 9 cases of cervical MMT but 4 of these at least are dubious: Bashour et al. (52) reported a case occurring in a 16 year old following cyclophosphamide therapy for nephrotic syndrome. However, the tumour involved the vagina, was described as soft and gelatinous and no pathological description beyond 'mixed mullerian tumour' was given. Other cases were pure sarcomas (53) or extended to the body of the uterus (8) or were simply inadequately described (54, 55).

About 9 genuine cases remain (56–58), the longest series being the 6 cases reported by Abell and Ramirez (11). The age distribution is similar to ovarian tumours, though 3 patients were only in their fifth decade. Parity is rarely mentioned. One patient developed MMT in a cervical stump, having undergone a supracervical hysterectomy for benign leiomyomas 37 years previously (57). Another had been irradiated 12 years previously for an invasive cervical carcinoma (11). It is impossible to know the significance of one such instance among so few tumours. It is, though, interesting that this patient was the youngest, at 44, to develop MMT.

Grossly, these tumours are usually polypoid masses (11, 51, 56–58) but may present as irregular, corrugated lesions on the cervix (11, 51). Microscopically, four were homologous tumours and five heterologous. Striated muscle differentiation was detected in all the latter tumours and cartilage in three. Other types of differentiation were not reported. Though the microscopic appearance was generally very similar to MMT elsewhere, the carcinomatous component was of endocervical type in one case (58) and at least partially squamous in most of the cases of Abell and Ramirez (11). This suggests that not only is differentiation of the epithelial component limited to the potential of the mullerian tract, but has a specific preference towards the epithelium from which it arises.

Electron microscopy has been used in one case to demonstrate the endocervical nature of the glandular cells and also to show convincing evidence of smooth muscle differentiation in some cells of the sarcomatous component of a homologous tumour (58).

The mode of spread is not well recorded, but local extension to the pelvis is common and metastases to the lung occur (11). The sarcomatous component again usually predominates in these metastases (11).

Most patients present with vaginal bleeding (11, 56–58) or discharge (11). One patient passed tumour tissue per vaginam, from which the diagnosis was made (11). Physical examination is more likely to mislead than help. The erosive, necrotic and obviously malignant tumours are the minority; the polypoid tumours are frequently mistaken for endocervical polyps or polypoid leiomyomas.

Most patients are treated with hysterectomy and bilateral salpingo-oophorectomy. Pelvic lymphadenectomy and aortic node sampling were carried out in one case (56). Most tumours were irradiated and one patient was treated with vincristine, Adriamycin and cyclophosphamide (57).

It might be hoped that a polypoid lesion on the cervix would present at an early stage and have a reasonable prognosis. Unfortunately, cervical MMTs are as lethal as elsewhere. Abell and Ramirez donot give the stages of

their 6 cases, but all died between 10 and 15 months after presentation (11). One patient with a Stage I tumour was alive and well at 30 months (56) and another with a Stage III tumour was alive and well at 9 months (57). Though the latter is not a long survival, it may be significant that this was the only patient given chemotherapy.

TUMOURS OUTSIDE THE GENITAL TRACT

Two cases of so-called carcinosarcoma were reported by Ober and Black, which had arisen in pelvic tissues outside the uterus, tubes and ovaries (59). It is clear from their description, however, that these were sarcomas with no malignant epithelial component. They belonged to a similar category as the sarcoma arising in an omental endometrial cyst reported by Ginzler and Herrera (60) and the so-called endometriotic sarcoma reported by Ferraro et al. in a woman with long standing pelvic endometriosis (61). Though these tumours are outside the scope of this chapter, their association with endometriosis is relevant to a discussion of the histogenesis of MMT.

One convincing case of MMT remains (62). This was a pericaecal mass in a 77 year old woman who presented with rectal bleeding and died shortly after operation. The tumour was a heterologous MMT. The uterus and ovaries were normal and no endometriosis was found. The authors argued that in areas the mesothelium over the surface of the tumour-dipped into clefts and there became multilayered and malignant, but their illustration suggests only reactive hyperplasia.

HISTOGENESIS

Theories concerning the histogenesis of these tumours have been a matter of art rather than science, as one attractive, unprovable hypothesis has replaced another.

The earliest theory that MMTs were derived from 'cell rests' displaced from elsewhere

(55) has long been discredited. It is still argued that some cases are 'collision tumours'—separate primaries arising and intermingling in the same site. This is argued as a possibility by Abell and Ramirez for one of their cervical tumours, whose epithelial component was composed only of squamous carcinoma (11). Given the extreme rarity of sarcomas of the female genital tract, the chances of such a collision are remote.

It has also been argued that carcinomas can induce malignant transformation in their supporting stroma. Though this has been suggested as the possible histogenesis of some tumours (12), more evidence is required than the form and composition of the tumour.

For uterine tumours, probably the most popular hypothesis is that MMTs derive from a primitive stromal cell that retains the capacity for divergent differentiation towards epithelial and mesenchymal derivatives (16, 17). It is but a step from this hypothesis, given the concept of the unity of tumours of the mullerian system, to argue the same histogenesis outside the body of the uterus. This is certainly defensible for fallopian tube and cervix, but ignores the fact that the ovary is not derived from the mullerian duct. Proponents of the theory bypass this difficulty by arguing that mesothelium coating the ovary is ultimately derived from the coelomic epithelium, from which the mullerian duct is also ultimately formed, and that MMTs are derived from these multipotential cells and their subcapsular connective tissue (13). However, this is invoking two potential cells of origin for the one tumour. There is no evidence to suggest that ovarian stroma has such a potential. The surface mesothelium may have, but the steps it must take in carcinogenesis would be much more complex than those of its postulated equivalent in the endometrium.

It has often been suggested that these tumours arise in foci of endometriosis. The origin of sarcomas from such foci outside the genital tract has been mentioned (60, 61) and would be the only sensible theory even without the evidence of adjacent endometriosis.

Several true MMTs have also been shown to arise in endometriosis (1, 4, 23, 30, 31, 34) as have various carcinomas (63). Opponents of this theory argue that in most tumours no evidence of endometriosis exists and that the tumours arise at an age when endometriosis is inactive (2, 10, 12, 13). Neither argument holds water. Firstly, one would expect a malignant tumour to overgrow and destroy the tissue in which it arose. This fact should long ago have called into question Sampson's strict criteria for postulating the origin of a tumour in endometriosis, namely that there should be continuity between tumour and endometriosis (64). Secondly, if MMT of the uterine body arises at an age when the endometrium is inactive, it would be strange if tumours arising in endometriosis failed to do likewise.

Science has not resolved this issue. Tissue culture studies have shown two morphologically distinct lines with no intermediate forms, suggesting that these are not carcinomas with areas of dedifferentiation (65, 66). Two different hyperdiploid cell populations have also been demonstrated on flow cytometry, and presumed to represent the two different components (66).

Epithelial antigens in the stromal cells of these tumours have been shown in the uterus (29) and confirmed in ovarian tumours (personal observation). Invasion of stroma by single epithelial cells is certainly partly responsible but in virtually all cases, typical spindle-shaped stromal cells can also be shown to express epithelial antigens. These findings support the theory that MMTs originate from a primitive precursor cell with the capacity for differentiation to epithelium and mesenchyme.

In summary, there are three feasible, histogenetic theories. The notion of a multipotential precursor cell in the endometrium, tube and cervix is acceptable, bearing in mind the unity of the epithelium and adjacent stroma in these three areas. This does not exclude the possibility of some cases in tube and cervix originating in endometriosis. An origin in endometriosis certainly offers a simple histogenetic theory for ovarian MMT but an origin from ovarian surface mesothelium is also possible.

REFERENCES

1 Dictor M. Malignant mixed mesodermal tumor of the ovary. Obstet Gynecol 1985; 65: 720–4

2 Hanjani P, Petersen RO, Lipton SE, Nolte SA. Malignant mixed mesodermal tumors and carcinosarcoma of the ovary: Report of eight cases and review of literature. Obstet Gynecol Surv 1983; 38: 537–45.

3 Elbers JRJ, Wagenaar SS. Malignant mixed mesodermal tumor of the ovary. Europ J Obstet Gynec Reprod Biol 1980; 10: 47–53.

4 Cooper P. Mixed mesodermal tumor and clear cell carcinoma arising in ovarian endometriosis. Cancer 1978; 42: 2827–31.

5 O'Toole RV, Tuttle SE, Shah NT. Heterologous carcinosarcoma of the fallopian tube: A case report. J Reprod Med 1982; 27: 749–52.

6 Holst N, Erichsen A. Mixed mesodermal tumour of the fallopian tube: A case report. Ann Chir Gynaecol 1981; 70: 207–9.

7 Taylor CW. Mesodermal mixed tumors of the female genital tract. J Obstet Gynaecol Br Comm 1958; 65: 177–88.

8 Marcella LC, Cromer JK. Mixed mesodermal tumors: A report of 11 cases. Am J Obstet Gynecol 1959; 77: 275–85.

9 Morrow CP, d'Ablaing G, Brady LW, Blessing JA, Hreshchyshyn MM. A clinical and pathologic study of 30 cases of malignant mixed Mullerian epithelial and mesenchymal ovarian tumors: A gynecologic oncology group study. Gynecol Oncol 1984; 18: 278–92.

10 Barwick KW, Livolsi VA. Malignant mixed mesodermal tumors of the ovary: A clinicopathologic assessment of 12 cases. Am J Surg Pathol 1980; 4: 37–42.

11 Abell MR, Ramirez JA. Sarcomas and carcinosarcomas of the uterine cervix. Cancer 1973; 31: 1176–92.

12 Fenn ME, Abell MR. Carcinosarcoma of the ovary. Am J Obstet Gynecol 1971; 110: 1066–1074.

13 Dehner LP, Norris HJ, Taylor HB. Carcinosarcomas and mixed mesodermal tumors of the ovary. Cancer 1971; 27: 207–16.

14 Hernandez W, Disaia PJ, Morrow CP, Townsend DE. Mixed mesodermal sarcoma of the ovary. Obstet Gynecol 1977; 49: 59–63.

15 Norris HJ, Taylor HB. Postirradiation sarcomas of the uterus. Obstet Gynecol 1965; 26: 689–94.

16 Norris HJ, Roth E, Taylor HB. Mesenchymal tumors of the uterus: II A clinical and pathologic study of 31 mixed mesodermal tumors. Obstet Gynecol 1966; 28: 57–63.

17 Norris HJ, Taylor HB. Mesenchymal tumors of the uterus III: A clinical and pathologic study of 31 carcinosarcomas. Cancer 1966; 19: 1459–1465.

18 Carlson JA, Edwards C, Wharton JT, Gallager HS, Delclos L, Rutledge F. Mixed mesodermal sarcoma of the ovary. Cancer 1983; 52: 1473–77.

19 Anderson C, Cameron HM, Neville AM, Simpson HW. Mixed mesodermal tumours of the ovary. J Path Bact 1967; 93: 301–7.

20 Decker JP, Hirsch NB, Garnet JD. Mixed mesodermal (Mullerian) tumor of the ovary: Report of two cases. Cancer 1968; 21: 926–32.

21 Grover V, Dhall K, Grover RK, Choudhry T. Malignant mixed mesodermal tumor of ovary. Europ J Obstet Gynec Reprod Biol 1985; 20: 241–46.

22 Orchard NP. Mixed mesodermal tumours of the ovary. Med J Aust 1972; 2: 151–5.

23 Czernobilsky B, LaBarre GC. Carcinosarcoma and mixed mesodermal tumor of the ovary: A clinicopathologic analysis of 9 cases. Obstet Gynecol 1968; 31: 21–32.

24 Edghill AR, Gardiner J, Hayes JA. Mixed mesodermal tumor of the ovary. Am J Obstet Gynecol 1967; 97: 578–9.

25 Fathalla MF. Primary mesodermal mixed tumours in the ovary: A report of two cases. J Obstet Gynaecol Brit Comm 1967; 74: 605–7.

26 Mukai K, Varela-Duran J, Nochomovitz LE. The rhabdomyoblast in mixed Mullerian tumors of the uterus and ovary. Am J Clin Pathol 1980; 74: 101–4.

27 Dictor M. Ovarian malignant mixed mesodermal tumor: The occurrence of hyaline droplets containing A-l-antitrypsin. Hum Pathol 1982; 13: 930–3.

28 Marshall RJ, Braye SG. A-l-antitrypsin, A-l-antichymotrypsin, actin and myosin in uterine sarcomas. Int J Gynecol Pathol 1985; 4: 346–54.

29 Ramadan M, Goudie RB. Epithelial antigens in malignant mixed Mullerian tumors of endometrium. J Pathol 1986; 148: 13–18.

30 Marchevsky AM, Kaneko M. Bilateral ovarian endometriosis associated with carcinosarcoma of the right ovary and endometrioid carcinoma of the left ovary. Am J Clin Pathol 1978; 70: 709–12.

31 Macfarlane KT, Pritchard JE. Two cases of Mullerian carcinosarcoma. Am J Obstet Gynecol 1954; 68: 652–8.

32 Silverman JF, Gardner J, Larkin EW, Finley JL, Norris HT. Ascitic fluid cytology in a case of metastatic malignant mixed mesodermal tumor of the ovary. Acta Cytol 1986; 30: 173–6.

33 International Federation of Gynaecology and Obstetrics. Classification and staging of malignant neoplasms of the female pelvis. J Int Gynec Obstet 1965; 3: 204.

34 Saunders P, Price AB. Mixed mesodermal tumor of the ovary arising in pelvic endometriosis. Proc R Soc Med 1970; 63: 44–5.

35 Carlson JA, Day TG. Five-year survival following combination radiotherapy and chemotherapy for recurrent mixed mesodermal sarcoma of the ovary. Gynecol Oncol 1985; 22: 129–2.

36 Morrow CP, Bundy BN, Hoffman J, Sutton G, Homesley H. Adriamycin chemotherapy for malignant mixed mesodermal tumor of the ovary. Am J Clin Oncol 1986; 9: 24–26.

37 Lele SB, Piver MS, Barlow JJ. Chemotherapy in management of mixed mesodermal tumors of the ovary. Gynecol Oncol 1980; 10: 298–302.

38 Fox H, Langley FA. Tumours of the Ovary. London: William Heinemann, 1976: 61–9.

39 Motta G. Contributto alla conoscenza dei tumori misti rari dell'apparato genitale feminile (carcinosarcoma della salpinge). Ann Obstet Ginecol 1926; 48: 611–33.

40 Manes JL, Taylor HB. Carcinosarcoma and-mixed Mullerian tumors of the fallopian tube: Report of four cases. Cancer 1976; 38: 1687–93.

41 Hanjani P, Petersen RO, Bonnell SA. Malignant mixed Mullerian tumor of the fallopian tube: Report of a case and review of literature. Gynecol Oncol 1980; 9: 381–93.

42 Williams TJ, Woodruff JD. Malignant mixed mesenchymal tumor of the uterine tube. Obstet Gynecol 1963; 21: 618–21.

43 Kahanpaa KV, Laine R, Saksela E. Malignant mixed Mullerian tumor of the fallopian tube: Report of a case with 5-year survival. Gynecol Oncol 1983; 16: 144–9.

44 Jain U. Mixed mesodermal tumor of the fallopian tube: Report of a case and review of literature. Md State Med J 1977; 43–46.

45 Malnasy J, Gaal M. Primary carcinosarcoma of the fallopian tube. Gynaecologia 1963; 154: 203–8.

46 Viniker DA, Mantell BS, Greenstein RJ. Carcinosarcoma of the fallopian tube: a case report and review of the literature. Br J Obstet Gynaecol 1980; 87: 530–4.

47 McQueeney AJ, Carswell BL, Sheehan WJ. Malignant mixed Mullerian tumor primary in uterine tube. Obstet Gynecol 1964; 23: 338–42.

48 Wu JP, Tanner WS, Fardal PM. Malignant mixed Mullerian tumor of the uterine tube. Obstet Gynecol 1973; 41: 707–12.

49 De Queiroz AC, Roth LM. Malignant mixed Mullerian tumor of the fallopian tube. Obstet Gynecol 1970; 36: 554–7.

50 Acosta AA, Kaplan AL, Kaufman RH. Mixed Mullerian tumors of the oviduct. Obstet Gynecol 1974; 44: 84–90.

51 Rotmensch J, Rosenshein NB, Woodruff JD. Cervical sarcoma: A review. Obstet Gynecol Surv 1983; 38: 456–60.

52 Bashour BN, Mancer K, Rance CP. Malignant mixed Mullerian tumor of the cervix following cyclophosphamide therapy for nephrotic syndrome. J Pediatr 1973; 82: 292–3.

53 Ferreira HP. A case of mixed mesodermal tumour of the uterine cervix. J Obstet Gynaecol Br Emp 1951; 58: 446–8.

54 Vellios F, Stander RW, Huber CP. Carcinosarcoma (malignant mixed mesodermal tumor) of the uterus. Am J Clin Pathol 1963; 39: 496–505.

55 Sternberg WH, Clark WH, Smith RC. Malignant mixed Mullerian tumour (mixed mesodermal tumour of the uterus). Cancer 1954; 7: 704–24.

56 Miyazawa K, Hernandez E. Cervical carcinosarcoma: a case report. Gynecol Oncol 1986; 23: 376–80.

57 Waxman M, Waxman JS, Alinovi V. Heterologous malignant mixed Mullerian tumor of the cervical stump. Gynecol Oncol 1983; 16: 422–8.

58 Hall-Craggs M, Toker C, Nedwich A. Carcinosarcoma of the uterine cervix: a light and electron microscopic study. Cancer 1981; 48: 161–9.

59 Ober WB, Black MB. Neoplasms of the subcoclomic mesenchyme. Arch Pathol 1955; 59: 698–705.

60 Ginzler AM, Herrera NE. Sarcoma arising in omental endometrial cyst. J Mount Sinai Hosp NY 1957; 24: 869–74.

61 Ferraro LR, Hetz H, Carter H. Malignant endometriosis. Pelvic endometriosis complicated by polypoid endometrioma of the colon and endometriotic sarcoma; report of a case and review of the literature. Obstet Gynecol 1956; 7: 32–9.

62 Weisz-Carrington P, Bigelow B, Schinella RA. Extragenital mixed hererologous tumor of Mullerian type arising in the cecal peritoneum: report of a case. Dis Colon Rectum 1977; 20: 329–33.

63 Scully RE, Richardson GS, Barlow JF. The development of malignancy in endometriosis. Clin Obstet Gynecol 1966; 9: 384–411.

64 Sampson JA. Endometrial carcinoma of the ovary arising in endometrial tissues in that organ. Arch Surg 1925; 10: 1–72.

65 Rubin A. The histogenesis of carcinosarcoma (mixed mesodermal tumor) of the uterus as revealed by tissue culture studies. Am J Obstet Gynecol 1959; 77: 269–74.

66 Centola GM. Long-term in vitro growth of a heterologous mixed Mullerian tumor of the ovary. Invasion Metastasis 1986; 6: 123–32.

Textbook of Uncommon Cancer
Edited by C.J. Williams, J.G. Krikorian, M.R. Green and D. Raghavan
© 1988 John Wiley & Sons Ltd

Chapter **6**

Fallopian Tube Cancer

Mahmood Yoonessi

Associate Professor of Gynecology-Obstetrics, State University of New York at Buffalo School of Medicine, Buffalo, New York, USA

INTRODUCTION

The fallopian tube, though frequently involved in non-neoplastic pathology, is an uncommon site for malignancy. Most often, fallopian tube cancers are secondary to uterine and/or ovarian neoplasias. Primary tubal cancers, predominantly adenocarcinomas, are rarely seen. Isolated cases of malignant mixed mullerian tumors, other sarcomas, choricarcinomas and teratomas have been reported, however.

FALLOPIAN TUBE ADENOCARCINOMA

Historical Notes

Primary carcinoma of the fallopian tube is one of the rarest female genital cancers. It was first described by Renaud at a meeting of the Manchester, Pathological Society in 1847 and later by Rokitansky in 1861 (1). In spite of these earlier descriptions, the first genuine case report of primary fallopian tube carcinoma has been attributed to Orthmann (2), who described the disease in 1888. In 1950, Hu et al., reviewed 466 reported cases and added 12 of their own (3). By 1981, approximately 1100 cases had been collected from the literature (4) and at least 250 cases have subsequently been reported.

Incidence

The relative incidence of fallopian tube cancer among gynecologic malignancies has varied from a low of 0.16% to a high of 1.61% with a mean of 0.60% (5). Among all clinically treated gynecologic patients, an estimated 0.006% to 0.14% with a mean of 0.04% have had tubal carcinomas (5). Multifocal primary genital tract malignancies involving the uterus, ovaries and fallopian tubes are not included in these statistics and are often reported as ovarian and/or uterine carcinomas with tubal metastasis.

Epidemiology

Few communications have dealt with the epidemiology of fallopian tube cancer and thus far no significant world-wide variation in the incidence rate of fallopian tube carcinoma has been observed or reported. Kruijff (5) noted variations in the incidence rate of fallopian tube cancer in different parts of Netherlands. However, from correlation calculations, these variations appeared to relate to regional differences in aging of the female population and density of reporting gynecologists. He reaffirmed the reportedly higher incidence of fallopian tube carcinoma in patients with a history of infertility problems. Furthermore, he noted that the incidence rate of fallopian tube cancer in Netherlands remained constant during the postwar era at a time of the declining hospital morbidity of genital tuberculosis and a rising incidence of non-tuberculous adnexitis.

Risk Factors

There are no demographic or personal characteristics that clearly identify the individuals at a higher risk for developing fallopian tube carcinoma. The following frequently made observations are worthy of consideration, however.

1 Age. Although isolated cases of fallopian tube carcinoma have been encountered in patients as young as 17 years (6), the vast majority have occurred in the fourth and fifth decade of life. This must be, therefore, considered a disease of post- and perimenopausal years. In our own series, the average age of patients was 52.7 years an age similar to that reported by Sedlis (7, 8) and others. Ninety-eight percent of patients in our series were over 35 years old.

2 Race. Unavailability of information regarding race in many reported series makes a comparative analysis or meaningful conclusion regarding racial predictions very difficult. However, the majority of our patients (90%) were Caucasian and of 34 reported cases in the literature where the race was known, only 5 (15%) were black.

3 Parity and menstrual history. Infertility and sterility have commonly occurred in women who later develop this malignancy. The incidence of the former conditions has varied between a low of 21% and a high of 74% (9). This is higher than the rate expected in the North American and European population. Hanton had observed more survivors of fallopian tube carcinoma among nulliparous than among those with multiple pregnancies (10).

Sixty-four percent of our patients and approximately 50% of those in other reported series have been postmenopausal.

4 Coexistent pathologic conditions. The common occurrence of chronic nonspecific salpingitis and occasional cases of coexistent tuberculous salpingitis in patients with fallopian tube carcinoma has led some to believe that these infectious processes may be casually related to the development of neoplasia. Sedlis noted, however, that the incidence rate of the pelvic tuberculosis in these patients is not higher than that in the general population and the association of fallopian tube carcinoma with chronic tubal infection appears to represent the coexistence of an infrequent malignancy with a common pelvic pathology. Four of our 47 and 3 of Engstrom's (11) 39 patients with fallopian tube carcinoma had coexistent pelvic endometriosis. Engstrom furthermore, had observed histological support of malignancy originating from endometriosis.

Although cases of fallopian tube carcinoma have been observed in patients with prior history of breast carcinoma and the two conditions at times have coexisted, there is no indication that individuals with breast carcinoma are more prone to develop fallopian tube malignancies.

Early Diagnosis

The diagnosis of fallopian tube carcinoma is seldom made early or preoperatively. Dammreuter is said to have been the first to make a correct diagnosis prior to the surgery. McGoldrick (12) in reviewing 376 cases, found one correctly diagnosed preoperatively, that of Martzloff (13). Israel et al. (14) in 1954 estimated that less than half of the 499 cases reported up to that time had symptoms that in retrospect could have led to a correct preoperative diagnosis and that no more than 5% were so recognized. Boutselis and Thompson (15) noted that most, if not all, of their 14 patients had features suggestive of the disease, but only one had been diagnosed. Chalmers and Marshall's observation (16) of no correct preoperative diagnosis in their series reported in 1976, attests to the fact that this malignancy, unfortunately, was not suspected more often in the 1970s than in the first half of the century.

The most important reason for a failure to diagnose tubal carcinoma preoperatively appears to be the lack of a high index of suspicion. It is generally agreed that despite the lack of specificity of the symptoms and signs, this malignancy in most instances does not remain as silent as ovarian carcinoma. The triad of (1) pain, (2) sero-sanguineous discharge, and (3) pelvic mass is considered characteristic of this disease and was encountered in 11% of the cases in the series of Hanton et al. (10). Similar findings were noted in 17% of our patients with earlier stages, and 13% of those with a Stage III disease (overall 15%).

Abnormal uterine bleeding (pre- or postmenopausal with or without associated findings), pain (with or without other symptoms or signs), vaginal discharge (alone or otherwise) are other common presenting features. Only 2 of our 47 patients were asymptomatic. Pain and pressure symptoms had been reported by more than 26% of 423 reported cases reviewed by Sedlis. These symptoms are considered to be the result of distention of the tumor-containing tube.

Intermittent vaginal discharge with a diminishing adnexal mass on bimanual examination, the so called 'hydrops tubae profluens' has been considered to be pathognomenic of tubal cancer. However, as noted by Besserer (17), this syndrome neither appears early nor is common. Furthermore, it can be seen in conjunction with other tubal pathologies. The frequent association of the tubal carcinoma with some of the most common pelvic pathologies (uterine leiomyoma, chronic salpingitis, endometriosis) and the well known fact that the gross appearance of the diseased tube might be misleading must be remembered. If and when in doubt, the tubes should be visualized and/or removed for proper histologic diagnosis.

Abnormal cervical cytology appears to be an inadequate diagnostic aid for early diagno-

sis of fallopian tube carcinoma, although isolated cases of primary carcinoma of the fallopian tube along with suspicious or positive Pap smears in patients with fallopian tube carcinoma was reported by Sedlis. This rate appears to be higher than that observed by other investigators and is certainly higher than that found in our own series. A 0–20% accuracy rate is considered to be a more realistic figure. Some investigators have unsuccessfully tried to define cytologic clues characteristic of fallopian tube carcinoma. Special collection techniques, i.e. the use of a cervical cap, have been recommended to improve the yield of abnormal cytology. Hysterosalpingography has been recommended as a diagnostic aid. Others have expressed concern over the risk of spreading cancer with this procedure. Lack of specific diagnostic criteria to differentiate chronic infectious tubal pathology from neoplastic lesions further points to the inadequacy of this technique.

Cul de sac aspiration and culdoscopy have been used and recommended but have never gained widespread acceptance and/or popularity. Chalmers and Ingram, among others, have recommended the use of laparoscopy. The available information indicates that at least in the following circumstances, the disease should be suspected and patients must be subjected to appropriate diagnostic evaluation.

a. In the presence of previously mentioned diagnostic triad.

b. Persistence of unexplained abnormal uterine bleeding in spite of negative cytology and dilatation and curettage, particularly in patients 35 years of age or older.

c. Persistence of an abnormal and otherwise unexplainable vaginal discharge. If the discharge is bloody, and/or patient is 35 years of age or older, this, suspicion should be heightened.

d. Persistence of an otherwise unexplainable pelvic, lower abdominal and/or low back pain.

e. An abnormal, otherwise unexplainable,

cervical cytology, particularly if it is suggestive of an adenocarcinoma.

f. Presence of an adnexal mass in the peri- and postmenopausal woman.

Additional diagnostic work-up should preferably include laparoscopy with or without hysteroscopy. A histologic diagnosis must be established if the tubes are grossly abnormal.

Immunobiology

Little is known about the immunobiology of this malignancy. England and Davidson demonstrated that the isoantigens A, B and H which are normally present in the fallopian tube mucosa are lost in the process of malignant transformation (18). It is suggested that these subtle immunological changes of transformation may precede histological dedifferentiation. Whether or not the presence of this cancer is associated with the assayable antigens (specific or otherwise) or if any tumor marker (immunologic or otherwise) can be identified and used for early detection of this malignancy remains to be seen. We have, however, observed elevated levels of CA-125 in a patient with fallopian tube carcinoma.

Histopathology

Proliferative abnormalities have been observed and reported by Moore and Enterline (19) and their significance remains undetermined. Preinvasive (in situ) carcinomas of the fallopian tube have been described by Greene and Scully (20), Hayden and Potter (21), Ryan (22), Woodruff and Pauerstein (23) and other investigators. Invasive lesions are often secondary to the more common ovarian and/or uterine adenocarcinomas.

Fallopian tube adenocarcinoma can present grossly in misleading forms such as hematosalpinx or hydrosalpinx or as an exophytic lesion protuding through the ostium. Bilateral involvement of the fallopian tubes has been observed in up to 31.1% (Wechsler, 1926) (24) of the cases, with a mean of 16.8%. The

following criteria are established for the diagnosis of primary fallopian tube adenocarcinoma:

1. The main tumor is in the tube and arises from the endosalpingeal.
2. Histologically the pattern reproduces the epithelium of the mucosa and often shows a papillary pattern.
3. If the wall is involved, the transition between benign and malignant tubal epithelium should be demonstrable.
4. Extension or metastasis from a primary ovarian or endometrial adenocarcinoma must be excluded.

Various grading systems have been proposed and the following, which was originally adopted by Hu et al. (3) is popular; Grade 1 papillary, Grade 2 papillary alveolar, Grade 3 alveolar medullary.

Classification and Staging

The approach to the staging of this disease has not been uniform. Several classifications have been proposed, but none have been endorsed by the International Federation of Gynaecologists and Obstetricians (FIGO). It has been demonstrated that this malignancy may spread by contiguous invasion, transluminal migration, transcelomic, hematogenous and lymphatic dissemination.

Similarity of pathways followed in the spread of this disease with those observed in ovarian carcinoma encourages speculation that lessons learned regarding adequacy and standardization of surgical staging procedures in ovarian cancer are applicable to this malignancy.

Therefore, after an approach through an adequate incision, cytologic specimens of the peritoneal fluid, should be obtained and careful inspection and palpation of all intra-abdominal structures, peritoneal surfaces and lymph node bearing areas carried out. Some investigators have recommended the use of a classification and staging system similar to the one accepted by the FIGO for ovarian neoplasms. Others have stressed the similarity of the fallopian tube and gastrointestinal tract and prognostic significance of serosal extension.

Although in our review of this malignancy, we used a classification and staging system that had been used by Sedlis and originally proposed by Erez, we now use a modification of the FIGO staging system for ovarian carcinoma similar to that proposed by Kruijff. This classification and staging system is as follows:

Stage 0	Carcinoma in situ
Stage I	Carcinoma confined to the tubes whether in the mucosa, submucosa or invading the muscularis
Stage IA	Growth limited to one tube
Stage IB	Growth limited to both tubes
Stege IC	Tumor, either Stage IA or IB with ascites and/or positive peritoneal washings
Stage II	Tumor growth involving one or both tubes with pelvic extension
Stage IIA	Tumor has extended through the serosa (IIA1) or has invaded the ovary and/or uterus (IIA2)
Stage IIB	Extension and/or metastases to other pelvic tissues
Stage IIC	Tumor, either Stage IIA or IIB, with ascites and/or positive peritoneal washings
Stage III	Tumor involving one or both tubes with intraperitoneal and/or retroperitoneal nodal metastasis
Stage IV	Tumor growth with metastatic disease outside of the abdomen (parenchymal liver metastasis included)
Special category	Multi-focal primary tumors involving the fallopian tube, uterus and ovaries

Treatment

The optimal method of treatment has not been established particularly with regard to the extent of surgery, the role of adjuvant radio-therapy, chemotherapy and/or hormonal therapy.

The incidence of bilaterality in our series was 13%, a rate higher than the 5% reported by Frick (25) and one in agreement with that reported by Hanton and others (14.8%). Sedlis noted a high incidence of bilaterality (26% in 176 cases).

The high frequency of bilateral involvement of the tubes with potential for early dissemination to the uterus and ovaries provides justification for the removal of both tubes, ovaries and uterus even in early cases. This has been the surgical treatment of choice for many authors. In a series of 38 patients reported by Engstrom in 1957, the uterus had been retained in 24 cases (11). These patients received postoperative radiotherapy including intrauterine radium sources. The authors observed that the survival in this group did not differ from those who had a hysterectomy. Their approach, which preserves the uterus for use as a reservoir for radium sources, never gained popularity.

The value of routine omentectomy in early stages has not been clearly established, although omental biopsies provide for a more factual staging. Removal of regional lymph nodes has been recommended by some authors. The true incidence of pelvic and peri-aortic nodal metastases in various stages of this disease and the value of pelvic and peri-aortic lymphadenectomy remain undetermined. Some autopsy series, including our own, have demonstrated the appreciable frequency of lymphatic disemination but others have not yielded similar data.

Sedlis's review of 56 patients in whom lymphadenectomy was performed yielded a low incidence (5.4%) of nodal metastases (8). Resection of suspicious and/or grossly positive nodes as well as sampling of high peri-aortic and pelvic nodes would appear to be justifiable. This would allow for more accurate staging and prognosis and may aid the clinician in the proper design of adjuvant therapy.

More extensive surgery (with removal of the involved segments of the bowel and a portion of the abdominal wall) has produced gratifying results and is recommended for selective locally advanced and technically resectable cases. Clark and Brunschwig (26) reported a $6\frac{1}{2}$-year survival after pelvic exenteration for extensive but localized recurrent fallopian tube carcinoma (26). The accumulated experience in patients with ovarian cancer seems to indicate that adequate cytoreductive tumor surgery may increase the chances of response to other modalities of therapy, and therefore improve the outcome. The same may be true in patients with tubal carcinoma.

Radiotherapy

Postoperative radiotherapy has been recommended by some investigators, whereas others have questioned the value of routine postoperative radiation. The combination of external radiotherapy and vaginal radium was recommended by Hobbs (27), Hu et al. (3), Hartvigsen and Blom (28) and Engstrom (11). Benedet et al. (29, 30), among others, used intraperitoneal radioactive substances (gold-198 and phosphorus-32) with or without external radiation and/or radium. Engstrom believed that the expected 5-year survival in non-irridiated groups is 5% and he attributed an achievement of 36% 5-year survival rate to postoperative radiation. Sedlis's initial review revealed 20.3% 5-year survivals among 128 irradiated and 14.8% in the non-irradiated group (61 cases). However, in his subsequent analysis he concluded that there was no evidence to indicate that postoperative radiotherapy improved survival.

Clearly, no conclusion can be drawn from the available data regarding the value of postoperative adjuvant radiotherapy. Variations in surgical staging procedures, sources of radiation, field sizes, fractionations, and total tumor dose, makes meaningful comparison difficult if not impossible. The accumulated experience with radiotherapy of ovarian cancer and fallopian tube malignancy allows one to postulate that postoperative intraperitoneal chromium phosphate (^{32}P) instillation may have a place in the treatment of patients with minimal residual intraperitoneal disease. Selected patients with small residual disease in the pelvis may benefit from postoperative pelvic radiotherapy.

Chemotherapy and Hormonal Therapy

Limited information is available regarding chemotherapy and/or hormonal therapy in fallopian tube carcinoma.

1 Single agent therapy. Various alkylating agents (chlorambucil, thiotepa, melphalan, nitrogen mustard, cyclophosphamide) were used in our series—(Table 1). or have been used by other investigators (Table 2). Partial responses have been observed to treatment with chlorambucil and thiotepa. In 1973, Boronow (31) reviewed the available literature of the previous decade and reported a case of objective complete response to melphalan for 13 months. Smith (32) reported 1 of 3 patients treated with thiotepa with a complete response lasting 15 months, and 2 of 11 patients treated with melphalan with partial responses.

Other investigators have observed objective and subjective responses in patients treated with intermittent high doses of cyclophosphamide. Occasional short term responses have been observed with 5-FU (Table 2). We have observed good partial responses to doxorubicin, and others have reported transient partial responses to iphosphamide. Transient complete responses have been reported to platinum analogs (33) (CHIP = *cis*-dihydro, *trans*-dihydroxy, bis-isopropylamine platinum) (Table 3). Morphological changes of the tubal epithelium during the menstrual cycle or under the influence of exogenous hormones (34–36) tend to indicate that the endosalpingeal mucosa is hormone responsive. We have observed estrogen receptors in some cases of fallopian tube adenocarcinoma. Nevertheless, the question of presence or absence of steroid receptors in fallopian tube cancer and the value of hormonal therapy remains unresolved. Progestatio-

TABLE 1 SINGLE AGENT CHEMOTHERAPY IN PATIENTS WITH FALLOPIAN TUBE
CARCINOMA RECURRENT AND/OR KNOWN RESIDUAL DISEASE

Drugs	No. of patients	Prior RT Yes	No	No. of courses 2	>2	Response CR	PR	NC	Prog.	Original 1 yr	>1 yr
Alkylating agents											
Chlorambucil	6	1	5	6	0	0	1	1	4	3	3
Melphalan	2	2	0	2	0	0	0	0	2	1	1
Thiotepa	1	0	1	1	0	0	0	0	1	1	1
Thiotepa–CMB	2	1	1	2	0	0	1	0	1	0	2
Thiotepa, intraperitoneal	2	2	0	0	2	0	0	0	2	2	0
HN^2 intraperitoneal	1	1	0	0	1	0	0	0	1	1	0
Hexamethylmelamine	1	1	0	1	0	0	0	0	1	0	1
Antibiotics											
Adriamycin	3	3	0	3	0	0	1	0	2	1	2
Antimetabolites											
Methotrexate, high dose with LCV	1	1	0	0	1	0	0	0	1	0	1
Hormones											
Megace	1	1	0	1	0	0	0	0	1	0	1
Oreton	1	1	0	1	0	0	0	0	1	0	1
Dapsone	2	1	1	2	0	0	0	0	2	0	2

RT   = radiotherapy.
CR   = complete response: disappearance of all measurable disease lasting at least 2 months.
PR   = greater than 50% reduction in size of measurable disease.
NC   = No change: static disease.
PR   = partial response.
Prog.= progression.
CMB= chlorambucil.
LCV = leucovorin.

nal agents have been empirically added to some therapeutic regimens.

2 Combination therapy. We have previously reported partial responses to combination chemotherapy using 5-FU with an alkylating agent or nitrosourea (CCNU) (Table 4). Other drug combinations have been tried and some impressive responses have been observed (Table 5).

Platinum containing combinations have yielded gratifying results. In our own institution, the best results were obtained with a combination chemotherapy using cisplatin, leucovorin–5-FU, doxorubicin, high dose methotrexate/leucovorin rescue, Cytoxan and Provera.

Interpretation of the data regarding combinations of radiotherapy and chemotherapy is even more difficult, if not impossible. Griffiths (37) treated 2 patients with pelvic spread and inguinal nodal metastases with postoperative pelvic radiotherapy and chlorambucil (for 12 months) and they both reportedly were alive and well at 6 and 9 years. Combination of melphalan and a synthetic progestin used by Smith in 8 cases resulted in 2 complete responses for 9 and 19 months and a partial response lasting for 5 months (Table 5). Although no firm conclusion can be drawn, it can be stated that in patients with recurrent fallopian tube carcinoma and those with large residual disease after surgery, trials of combination drug therapy are justifiable.

Prognosis and Survival

The prognostic value of histological characteristics of adenocarcinoma has been debated. Hu et al (3) found consistent correlations of grading with survival.

In the series of Momtazee and Kempson

TABLE 2 SINGLE ALKYLATING AGENT CHEMOTHERAPY IN PATIENTS WITH FALLOPIAN TUBE CARCINOMA

Drugs	Author and year	No. of patients	Results CR	PR	NB	No follow-up or not evaluable	Comments
Unspecified	Greene and Scully 1962 (20)	1			1		
Intra-arterial HN²	Hurlbutt and Nelson 1963 (38)	1				1	
HN²	Hanton et al., 1966 (10)	2			2		
	Houghton 1970 (39)	1			1		
	Jahshan et al., 1973 (40)	1			1		
Thiotepa	Hanton et al., 1966 (10)	2			2		
	Erez et al., 1967 (41)	2			2		
	Cohn et al., 1969 (42)	1			1		
	Smith, 1975 (32)	3	1		2		CR for 15 mos.
Chlorambucil	Steele, 1967 (43)	1				1	Patient alive, no evidence
	Blaikley, 1973 (44)	1	1				of disease
	Jahshan et al., 1973 (40)	1				1	after 5 yrs
Cytoxan high dose	Pigatto, 1967 (45)	1		1			Response lasting 6 mos.
	Tukianen, 1968 (46)	Un-specified		Un-specified			Some response reported
Cytoxan	Weber et al., 1970 (47)	1ª			1		
	Farber, 1973 (48)	1				1	Drug given intraperitoneally and intravenously at surgery; well at 8 mos.
Total		20	2	1	14	3	

ª Patient had leukemia and keratoacanthoma.
CR = clinical response; PR = partial response; NB = no benefit.

(64), Grade 3 lesions had the worst outcome (16.7% 3-year cure rate) but little difference was shown between histological Grade 1 and Grade 2. The relationship between histological grading and survival has been inconsistent. Furthermore, observations made by Hayden and Potter (21) and Hanton et al. (10) have clearly shown that admixtures of patterns can be seen in the same lesion and this casts further doubt on the prognostic significance of the histological grading. Better survivals have been reported in patients with tubal ostial closure often due to coexistent infectious process. This presumably interferes with translu-minal migration, thereby preventing dissemi-nation of the disease. Most authors have noted that the extent of the disease at the time of discovery is the most important prognostic factor. The overall 5-year survival of patients in Sedlis's review (7, 8) 38.1%. This figure has varied in different reported series, i.e. 5% (19), 21.6% (15), 40% (3) and 44% (10). Eight of 9 patients with Stages I and II in the series of Phelps and Chapman (59) survived but 6 patients with Stage III disease died.

In our own previously reported series, all 5-year survivors had Stage I and II disease. A short period of follow-up does not allow us to draw conclusions regarding the eventual effect of our newer combination chemotherapeutic regimen on the survival of patients with Stage III and IV disease. It has been noted that half

TABLE 3 SINGLE AGENT DRUG TRIALS IN PATIENTS WITH FALLOPIAN TUBE CARCINOMA

		No. of patients	CR	PR	NB	No follow-up or not evaluable	Comments
Cytoxan	Chalmers and Marshall 1976 (16)	2			2		1 patient died 2 wks post CT
	Benedet et al., 1977 (29)	2			2		
Alkeran	Boronow, 1973 (31)	1	1				Response lasted 13 mos.
	Smith, 1975 (32)	11		2	9		
Subtotal		16	1	2	13		
5 FU	Hanton et al., 1966 (10)	2			?		
	Erez et al., 1967 (41)	1		1			Response lasted 2 mos.
	Kinzel, 1976 (49)	1			1		
Subtotal		4	0	1	3		
Delalutin	Hreshchyshyn and Graham, 1969 (50)	1			1		
Progesterone	Chalmers and Marshall 1976 (16)	1				1	
Colprone	Kinzel, 1976 (49)	1				1	
Subtotal		3			1	2	
Vinglycinate (VGL)	Armstrong et al., 1967 (51)	2			2		
Isophosphamide	Cohen et al., 1975 (52)	1		1			Transient response
CHIP	Wong et al., 1985 (33)	2	1	1			
Total		18	2	5	19	2	

TABLE 4 COMBINATION CHEMOTHERAPY IN PATIENTS WITH FALLOPIAN TUBE CARCINOMA (RECURRENT AND/OR KNOWN RESIDUAL DISEASE)

Combination chemotherapy	No. of patients	Prior RT Yes	Prior RT No	No. of courses 2	No. of courses >2	Response Good	Response Partial	Response Prog.	Survival (yrs) 1	Survival (yrs) >1
1. CCNU+chlorambucil			x			x				
2. Azauridine+5-FU					x		x			x
3. 6-Azauridine+5-FU+Hydrea Ara C+6-thioguanine	1		x	x			x			
4. Iphosphamide					x		x			
Dactinomycin+5-FU+Cytoxan	1		x				x		x	
Chlorambucil+5-FU	2	2		2			2			2
5-FU+vincristine	1	x		x			x	x		
Depo-Provera+chlorambucil	2	1	1	2			2	2		
Thiotepa, RT, 5-FU, Chlorambucil	1		x				x			x

RT=Radiotherapy.

TABLE 5 OTHER DRUG THERAPEUTIC REGIMENS IN PATIENTS WITH FALLOPIAN TUBE CARCINOMA

Author	Treatment regimen	No. of patients	Results	Comments
Hanton et al., 1966 (10)	Cytoxan and HN^2	1	No significant regression	
Dodson et al., 1970 (53)	L-Sarcolysin+5-FU or progesterone	3	1 patient survived 4–5 yrs; 2 patients. died within 2 yrs	Patient had surgery+ RT+CT or RT
Merkov, 1970 (54)	Cytoxan RT+	1	Patient well 5 mos. after treatment	
Trelford, 1970 (56)	Unspecified	4	No benefit	Review of some published studies
Boutselis and Thompson, 1971 (15)	5-FU, methotrexate, L-Sarcolysin perfusion	1	No response	
Meng and Yu, 1972 (57)	Endoxan, 5-FU, Mitomycin-C Toyomycin, vit B6	1	Adjunctive therapy. No evidence of disease after 2 mos	
Griffiths, 1973 (37)	Chlorambucil+RT following surgery	2	Both patients well after 6 and 9 yrs	
Jashan et al., 1973 (40)	HN^2–Alkeran–Endoxan Intraperitoneal TEM+Endoxan	1	Progressive disease	
Karag'Ozova, 1973 (55)	Endoxan+RT Intraperitoneal TEM+Endoxan	1	Progressive disease	
Phelps and Chapman, 1974 (59)	Chlorambucil	1	3 patients with Stage III disease survived 2 yrs	
	Alkeran post RT	1		
	Chlorambucil+5-FU	1		
	Hydrea+CCNU used after previous therapy failed			
Susann and Franklin, 1974 (60)	(HN^2–Alkeran–chlorambucil) Surgery+CT	3	Mean survival 26.7 mos.	
	Surgery+RT+CT	8	Mean survival 35.9 mos.	
Smith, 1975 (32)	Alkeran+synthetic progestin	8	2 complete responders 9 and 19 mos. 1 partial response 5 progressions	
Chalmers and Marshall, 1976 (16)	Intraperitoneal thiotepa followed by Cytoxan+ progesterone	1	Patient well at 12 mos. Partial responders	
Kinzel, 1976 (49)	Chlorambucil+RT	2	1 Patient well at 8 yrs 1 patient no evaluable	(DOD) Original Stage I disease
	Cytoxan+RT	1	Survived 4 yrs, 5 mos.	(DOD) Both original Stage I disease
	Cytoxan +^{32} P. instillation	1	Survived 4 yrs 2 mos.	Original Stage III disease
	5-FU, vincristine, ext. RT+ ^{32}P	1	No follow-up. DOD	
Benedet et al., 1977 (29)	Cytoxan+RT	3	2 DOD in 7 and 21 mos. 3rd no evidence of disease at 5 mos.	Original Stages IIB and III Original Stage IV disease
	Alkeran+RT	1	DOD in 14 mos.	Original Stage IIB disease
	Alkeran and Cytoxan+RT	1	DOD in 7 mos.	Original Stage IV disease
Deppe et al., 1980 (61)	Cis-platinum, Adriamycin– progesterone	1	Complete response	Surgically proven complete response
	Cis-platinum, Adriamycin– progesterone+CT	1	Complete response	
Raju et al., 1981(62)	Cis-platinum+CMB HMM, Depo-Provera	1	NB	
	Cis-platinum+CMB Depo-Provera	1	NB	
Guthrie and Cohen, 1981 (63)	Adriamycin, CT CT=gestronal	1	Complete response	

CR=complete response; CT=chemotherapy; DOD=died of disease, NB=no benefit; RT=radiotherapy. HMM=hexamethylmela-mine. CMB=chlorambucil.

or more of patients dying of this disease will do so within the first 2 years. The overall survival figures in Stages I, II and III have been reported as 60%, 40% and 10% respectively.

FALLOPIAN TUBE SARCOMAS

Sarcomas of the female genital tract are rare and the fallopian tube appears to be the least common primary site.

The modification of the original Ober and Tovell's classification of mesenchymal tumors of the uterus has commendably been applied to fallopian tube lesions. Mesenchymal tumors could be pure, mixed, homologous and/or heterologous. Malignant mixed mullerian tumors and carcinosarcomas are the most commonly reported (1–6). Deppe et al. (7) estimated that by 1984, 26 patients with primary mixed mesodermal tumors of the fallopian tube had been reported in the world's literature. The primary site of tumor in some of these cases has been disputed.

The mean age of patients with malignant mixed mullerian tumors at the time of diagnosis has been 55. Most patients have had a low fertility index, presented late in the course of their disease and have had negative cervical cytology.

Gross appearance of the tubes in mixed mesodermal sarcomas is similar to that in cases of fallopian tube adenocarcinoma. The histological appearance of these lesions is identical with that of their counterparts in the uterus and ovaries (Chapter 5).

The diagnostic criteria set by Finn and Javert (8) might be helpful in determining the primary tubal or ovarian origin. The routes of metastatic spread are similar to fallopian tube adenocarcinoma. Surgery (removal of the uterus, tubes and ovaries and all grossly visible and resectable tumor, omental and nodal biopsies) remains the backbone of the treatment of patients with this malignancy. The value of adjuvant radiotherapy remains undetermined. Deppe was able to identify three reported cases in which the patients had responded to combination chemotherapy using vincristine–dactinomycin–cyclophosphamide doxorubicin and DTIC, or cyclophosphamide and 5-FU. He additionally reported a case of complete remission using cyclophosphamide and cisplatin chemotherapy. Other combination chemotherapies (i.e. CYVADIC regimen using Cytoxan, vincristine, doxorubicin and DTIC) used in ovarian mixed mesodermal tumors may prove useful in fallopian tube lesions.

OTHER FALLOPIAN TUBE MALIGNANCIES

Malignant teratomas and choriocarcinomas of the fallopian tube have been observed and reported (1–5). One can only speculate that these lesions are biologically similar to those encountered in the ovary or uterus and may respond to currently available effective chemotherapeutic regimens (i.e. vinblastine, etoposide, bleomycin, cisplatin for teratomas and methotrexate, dactinomycin with or without alkylating agent or Bagshawe regimen for choriocarcinomas).

REFERENCES

1 Yoonessi M. Carcinoma of the fallopian tube. Obstet and Gynecol Surv 1979; 34: 257–70.
2 Orthmann EG. Ueber Carcinoma tubae. Geburtsh Gynakol 1888; 15: 212 14.
3 Hu CY, Taymor ML, Hertig AT. Primary carcinoma of the uterine tube. Obstet Gynecol 1950; 21: 730–6.
4 Hershey DW, Fennell RH, Major FJ. Primary carcinoma of the Fallopian tube. Obstet Gynecol 1981; 57: 367–70.
5 Kruijff H. Primary carcinoma of the Fallopian Tube. Drukkering De Kempenoer Oegstgeest. 1983.
6 Blaustein A. Tubal adenocarcinoma coexistent with other genital neoplasms. Obstet Gynecol 1963; 21: 61–6.
7 Sedlis A. Primary carcinoma of the Fallopian tube. Obstet Gynecol Surv 1961; 16: 209–26.
8 Sedlis A. Carcinoma of the fallopian tube. Surg Clin North America 1978; 58: 121–9.
9 Engeler V, Reinisch E, Schreiner WE. Das primare Tubenkarzinom—Eine klinische Studie an 37 Patientinne. Geburtsh Frauenheilk 1981; 41: 325–9.

10 Hanton EM, Malkasian Jr, GD, Dahlin DC, Pratt JH. Primary carcinoma of the fallopian tube. Am J Obstet Gynecol 1966; 94: 832–9.

11 Engstrom L. Primary carcinoma of the Fallopian tube. Acta Obstet Gynecol Scand 1957; 36: 289–305.

12 McGoldrick JL, Strauss H, Rao J. Primary carcinoma of the fallopian tube. Am J Surg 1943; 59: 555–62.

13 Martzloff KH. Primary carcinoma of the Fallopian tube. A consideration of its incidence, clinical diagnosis, and treatment, with the report of a case diagnosed before operation. Am J Obstet Gynecol 1940; 40: 804–21.

14 Israel SL, Crisp WE, Adrian DC. Preoperative diagnosis of primary carcinoma of the Fallopian tube. Am J Obstet Gynecol 1954; 68: 1589–93.

15 Boutselis JG, Thompson JN. Clinical aspects of primary carcinoma of the Fallopian tube. A clinical study of 14 cases. Am J Obstet Gynecol 1971; 111: 98–101.

16 Chalmers JA, Marshall AT. Carcinoma of the fallopian tube. Br J Obstet Gynaecol 1976; 83: 580–3.

17 Besserer G. Was leistet zytodiagnostik bei der Erkennung des primaren Tubenkarzinomas? Geburtsh Frauenheil 1953; 13: k660–3.

18 England D, Davidson I. Isoantigens A, B, and H in carcinoma of the fallopian tube. Arch Pathol 1973; 96: 350–4.

19 Moore SW, Enterline HT. Significance of proliferative epithelial lesions of the uterine tube. Obster Gynecol 1975; 45: 385–90.

20 Greene TH Jr, Scully RE. Tumors of the Fallopian tube. Clin Obstet Gynecol 1962; 886–906.

21 Hayden GE, Potter EL. Primary carcinoma of the Fallopian tube. With report of 12 new cases. Am J Obstet Gynecol 1960; 79: 24–31.

22 Ryan GM. Carcinoma in situ of the Fallopian tube. Am J Obstet Gynecol 1962; 84: 198.

23 Woodruff JD, Pauerstein CJ. The Fallopian Tube. Structure, Function, Pathology, and Management. Baltimore: Williams & Wilkins 1969: 1–37, 266–306.

24 Wechsler HF. Primary carcinoma of the Fallopian tubes. Arch Pathol Lab Med 1926; 2: 161–205.

25 Frick II, HC. Cancer of the fallopian tube. In: Gusberg SB, Frick II HC eds Corscaden's Gynecologic Cancer, Baltimore: Williams & Wilkins, 1978: 368–74.

26 Clark DGC, Brunschwig A. Total pelvic exenteration for recurrent carcinoma of the uterine tube. Obst Gynecol 1964; 24: 569–71.

27 Hobbs JE. Primary carcinoma of the fallopian tube. South Med J 1942; 35: 733.

28 Hartvigsen FR, Blomm, Primary carcinoma of the Fallopian tube. Nord Med 1950; 43: 708–10.

29 Benedet JL, White GW, Fairey RN, Boyes DA. Adenocarcinoma of the fallopian tube. Experience with 41 patients. Obstet Gynecol 1977; 50: 654–7.

30 Benedet JL, White GW. Malignant tumors of fallopian tube. In: Coppleson M ed Gynecologic Oncology, Edinburgh: Churchill Livingstone, 1981: 621–629.

31 Boronow RC. Chemotherapy for disseminated tubal cancer. Obstet Gynecol 1973; 42: 62–6.

32 Smith JP. Chemotherapy in gynecologic cancer. Clin Obstet Gynecol 1975; 4: 109–24.

33 Wong WS, Tindall VR, Wagstaff J, Bramwell V, Crowther D. Primary carcinoma of the fallopian tube: Favourable response to new chemotherapeutic agent. CHIP. J R Soc Med 1985; 78 (3): 203–6.

34 Pauerstein CJ, Woodruff JD. Cellular patterns in proliferative and anaplastic disease of the fallopian tube. Am J Obstet Gynecol 1966; 96: 486–92.

35 Pauerstein CJ. The Fallopian Tube, A Reappraisal. Philadelphia: Lea and Febiger, 1974: 1–158.

36 Pauerstein CJ, Eddy CA. Morphology of the fallopian tube. In: Beller FK, Schumacher GFB eds The Biology of the Fluids of Female Genital Tract. New York: Elsevier North Holland, 1979: 299–317.

37 Griffiths CT. Ovary and Fallopian tube. In: Holland JF, Frei III E eds Cancer Medicine. Philadelphia: Lea & Febiger, 1973: 1710–20.

38 Hurlbutt FR, Nelson HB. Primary carcinoma of the uterine tube. Am J Obstet Gynecol 1963; 59: 58–67.

39 Houghton RC. Bilateral adenocarcinoma of the fallopian tube: Report of a case. N Carolina Med J 1970; 31: 347.

40 Jahshan EA, Nahhas AW, Azoury SR. Primary papillary carcinoma of the fallopian tubes: a clinical study of 7 patients. J Med Lib 1973; 26: 315–22.

41 Erez S, Kaplan AL, Wall JA. Clinical staging of carcinoma of the uterine tube. Obstet Gynecol 1967; 30: 547–50.

42 Cohn S, Rossano RW, Fenton AN. Primary carcinoma of the fallopian tube. New York State J Med 1969; 10: 1321–8.

43 Steele SJ. Carcinoma of the Fallopian tubes. Proc R Soc Med 1967, 60 (9): 884.

44 Blaikley JB. Advanced adenocarcinoma of the fallopian tube. J Obstet Gynaecol Brit Commonw 1973; 80 (8): 757–8.

45 Pigatto JC. Chemotherapy of malignant tumors with high intermittent doses of Endoxan.

Munch Med Wochenschr 1967; 109 (40); 2082–2084.

46 Tukianen P. High doses of cyclophosphamide in the treatment of female genital tumors. Duodecim 1968; 84 (10): 763–77.

47 Weber G, Stetter H, Pliess G, Stickl H. Simultaneous occurrence of eruptive kerato-acanthomas, carcinoma of the Fallopian tube and paramyeloblastic leukemia. Arch Klin Exp Dermatol 1970; 238 (2): 107–19.

48 Farber SA. Carcinoma of the Fallopian tube. S Afr Med J 1973; 47 (29): 1321–4.

49 Kinzel GE. Primary carcinoma of the Fallopian tube. Am J Obstet Gynecol 1976; 125 (6): 816–20.

50 Hreshchyshyn MM, Graham RM. 17 Alpha-Hydroxyprogesterone caproate treatment of gynecologic cancer. Am J Obstet Gynecol 1969; 104 (6): 916–18.

51 Armstrong JG, Dyke RW, Fouts PJ, Hawthorne JJ, Jansen CJ, Peabody AM. Initial clinical experience with new derivative of the *Vinca rosea* alkaloids. Cancer Res 1967; 27 (Pt 2) 221–7.

52 Cohen MH, Creaven PJ, Tejada F, Hansen HH, Muggia F, Mittelman A, Selawry OS. Phase I clinical trial of isophosphamide (NSC-109724). Cancer Chemotherapy Rep 1975; 59 (4): 751–5.

53 Dodson MG, Ford JH, Averette HE. Clinical aspects of fallopian tube carcinoma. Obstet Gynecol 1970; 36: 935–9.

54 Merkov L. Report of two cases of primary carcinoma of the fallopian tubes. Akush Ginekol (Sofiia) 1970; 9 (6): 506–8.

55 Karag'Ozova. Case study of primary carcinoma of the fallopian tube. Akush Ginekol (Sofiia) 1973; 12 (2): 166–8.

56 Trelford JD. A Discussion of the Results of Chemotherapy on Gynecological Cancer and the Host's Immune Response. Sixth National Cancer Conference Proceedings. Philadelphia: JB Lippincott, 1970.

57 Meng, HC, Yu MP. Primary carcinoma of the Fallopian tube with report of a case. Chin Med J 1972; 18 (3): 162–5.

58 Karag'Ozova. Case study of primary carcinoma of the Fallopian tube. Akush Ginekol (Sofiia) 1973; 12 (2): 166–8.

59 Phelps MH, Chapman EK. Role of radiotherapy in treatment of primary carcinoma of the uterine tube. Obstet Gynecol 1974; 43 (5): 669–73.

60 Susann PW, Franklin EW. Adenocarcinoma of the fallopian tube. Abdom Surg 1974; 16 (8): 223–30.

61 Deppe G, Bruckner HW, Cohen CJ. Combination chemotherapy for advanced carcinoma of the fallopian tube. Obstet Gynecol 1980; 56 (4): 530–2.

62 Raju KS, Barker GH, Wiltshaw E. Primary carcinoma of the fallopian tube. Report of 22 cases. Br J Obstet Gynaecol 1981; 88 (11): 1124–9.

63 Guthrie D, Cohen S. Carcinoma of the fallopian tube treated with a combination of surgery and cytotoxic chemotherapy. Case report. Br J Obstet Gynaecol 1981; 88 (10): 1051–3.

64 Momtazee S, Kempson RL. Primary adenocarcinoma of the fallopian tube. Obstet Gynecol 1968; 32: 649–56.

Selected Papers: Mixed Mullerian Tumor

1 Hanjani P, Petersen RO, Bonnell SA. Malignant mixed mullerian tumor of the fallopian tube. Report of a case and review of the literature. Gynecol Oncol 1980; 9 (3): 381–93.

2 Jain U. Mixed mesodermal tumor of the fallopian tube: report of a case and review of literature. Md State Med J 1977; 26 (11): 432–6.

3 Manes JL, Taylor HB. Carcinosarcoma and mixed mullerian tumors of the fallopian tube: Report of four cases. Cancer 1976; 38 (4): 1687–93.

4 Pickel H, Thalhammer M. Chondrosarcoma of the fallopian tube. Geburtsh Frauenheilkd 1971; 31 (12): 1243–8.

5 Ullman AS, Kallet MB. Primary mixed myosarcoma of the uterine tube: A case report and review of the literature. Can Med Assoc J 1968; 98 (5): 258–61.

6 Viniker DA, Mantell BS, Greenstein RJ. Carcinosarcoma of the fallopian tube: A case report and review of the literature. Br J Obstet Gynaecol 1980; 87 (6): 530–4.

7 Deppe G, Zbella E, Friberg J, Thomas W. Combination chemotherapy for mixed mullerian tumor of the fallopian tube. Cancer 1984; 54 (8) 1517–20.

8 Finn WJ, Javert C. Primary and metastatic cancer of the fallopian tube. Cancer 1949; 2: 803–14.

Selected Papers: Choriocarcinoma and Teratoma

1 Chapero L, Martinez V. Pregnancy choriocarcinoma of the fallopian tube. Rev Child Obstet Ginecol 1974; 39 (6): 279–87.

2 Davidenko AA, Ilina IG. Chorioepithelioma of the fallopian tubes. Vopr Onkol 1972; 18 (2): 89–91.

3 Mazzarella P, Okagaki T, Richart RM. Tera-

toma of the uterine tube. A case report and
review of the literature. Obstet Gynecol 1972; 39
(3): 381–8.

4 Ober WB, Maier RC. Gestational choriocarcinoma of the fallopian tube. Diagn Gynecol
Obstet 1981; 3 (3): 213–31.

5 Soulier A, Chasseray JE, Riquet M, Bellamy J,
Aurosseau R. Tubal choriocarcinoma. A case
report (author's transl). J Chir (Paris) 1982; 119
(4): 267–70.

SUPPLEMENTARY REFERENCES

dAloya P, Segala V, Agnello G, Rainaldi V.
Adenocarcinoma of the Fallopian tube. Reexa-
mination of 5 cases observed during the period
of 1961–1980 in the Department of Obstetrics
and Gynecology, University of Ferrara. Eur J
Gynaecol Oncol 1982; 3 (1): 42–5.

Alessandrini G. Le cancer de la trompe. Rev Méd
Suisse 1969; 89: 589–98.

Amendola BE, LaRouere J, Amendola MA,
McClatchey KD, Han IH, Morley GW. Adenocarcinoma of the fallopian tube. Surg Gynecol Obstet 1983; 157 (3): 223–7.

Anbrokh YM. Macroscopic characteristics of
cancer of the fallopian tube. Neoplasma
(USSR) 1970; 17: 557–64.

Anderson HE, Bantin CF, Giffen HK, Olson LJ,
Schack CB. Primary carcinoma of the fallopian
tube. Obstet Gynecol 1954; 3: 89–92.

Antonowitsch, E. Die Diagnose des primaren
Tubenkarzinomas in Rontgenbild (mit 35%
igem Perabrodil). Fortschritte auf dem Gebiete
der Rontgenstrahlen und der Nuclearmedizin
1950; 73: 189–94.

Atlas of Cancer Mortality in the Netherlands 1969–
1978. Netherlands Central Bureau of Statistics.
The Hague: Staatsuitgeverij, 1980.

Ayre JE, Bauld WAG, Kearns PJ. Primary carcinoma of the Fallopian tube. Am J Obstet
Gynecol 1945; 50: 196–202.

Baak JPA, Kurver PHJ, Snoo-Niewlaat AJE,
DeGraef S, De Makkink B, Boon ME. Prognostic indications in breast cancer—morpho-
metric methods. Histopathology 1982; 6: 327–
39.

Baak JPA, Oort J. Applications of morphometry in
tumour pathology. In: Baak and JP, Oort J eds
A Manual of Morphometry in Diagnostic
Pathology. Heidelberg: Springer Verlag, 1983:
48–203.

Barnert G. Zur Klinik und Pathologie primar
maligner Tubengeshwulste unter besonderer
Auswertung des gleichzeitig doppelseitigen
Befalls. Zentralb Gynäkol 20: 1977; 1243–8.

Bartl W, Feichtinger, W, Breitenecker G. Clinical
and pathological aspects of primary carcinoma
of the fallopian tube (author's transl). Wien
Klin Wochenschr 1980; 92 (10): 360–4.

Benson PA. Cytologic diagnosis in primary carcinoma of fallopian tube. Case report and
review. Acta Cytol (Baltimore) 1974; 18 (5):
429–34. (Review).

Benson PA. Psammoma bodies found in cervico-
vaginal smears. Acta Cytol (Baltimore) 1973;
17: 64–6.

Boschann HW. Zur Klinik und Pathologie des
primaren Tubenkarzinomas. Geburtshilfe
Gynäkol 1952; 136: 58–83.

Brewer JI, Guderian AM. Diagnosis of uterine-tube
carcinoma by vaginal cytology. Obstet Gynecol 1956; 8: 664–72.

Broeders GHB. Moeilijkheden big de diagnostiek
van het primaire tubacarcinoom. Ned Tijdschr
Verlosk Gynaecol 1965; 65: 347–357.

Brown MD, Kohorn EI, Kapp DS, Schwartz PE,
Merino M. Fallopian tube carcinoma. Int J
Radiat Oncol Biol Phys 1985; 11 (3): 583–90.

Brux J De, Hafez ESE. Histophysiologie de la
Trompe. In: Brosens J, Cognet M, Constantin
A, Thibler M eds Oviducte et Fertilité. Paris:
Masson, 1979: 29–49.

Burgdorf F. Ein Beitrag zur Diagnostic des primaren Tubenkarzinomas. Zentralb Gynäkol
1949; 12: 1182–5.

Chen W, Calame R, Tricomi V. Primary adenocarcinoma of oviduct with hydrothorax. New
York State J Med 1971; 1765–7.

Cole P. Epidemiology. In: Gusberg SB, Frick II HC
eds Corscaden's Gynecologic Cancer. Baltimore: Williams & Wilkins, 1978: 466–82.

Compendium Health Statistics of the Netherlands.
Netherlands Central Bureau of Statistics;
Ministry of Public Health and Environmental
Hygiene (2980). The Hague: Staatsuitgeverij,
1979: 196.

Cruttenden LA, Taylor CW. Primary carcinoma of
Fallopian tube. Report of a case superimposed
on tuberculous salpingitis. J Obstet Gynaecol
Br Com 1950; 57: 937–40.

Csomor S, Toth F, Szeker J. Clinical problems of
primary tubal carcinoma. Strahlentherapie
1970; 139 (4): 404–9.

Diamond SB, Rudolph SH, Lubicz SS, Deppe G,
Cohen CJ. Cerebral blindness in association
with cis-platinum chemotherapy for advanced
carcinoma of the fallopian tube. Obstet Gynecol 1982; 59 (6, Suppl): 84S–86S.

Dietrich AH. Die Neubildungen der Eileiter. In:
Halban J, Seitz L, eds Biologie und Pathologie
des Weibes. Ein Handbuch der Frauenheil-
kunde und Geburtshilfe, Band 5, Teil 1. Berlin,

Vienna: Urban & Schwarzenberg, 1926, 13–25.

Dodson MG, Ford JH. Jr, Averette HE. Clinical aspects of fallopian tube carcinoma. Obstet Gynecol 1970; 36 (6): 935–9.

Doran A. An unreported case of primary cancer of the Fallopian tubes in 1847, with notes on primary tubal cancer. Transactions of the Obstetrical Society, London, 1896; 38: 322–6.

Doran A. Carcinoma of the fallopian tube: 100 cases. J Obstet Gynaecol Br Empire 1910; 17: 1.

Dougherty CM, Cotten NM. Proliferative epithelial lesions of the uterine tube. I. Adenomatous hyperplasia. Obstet Glynecol 1964; 24: 849–54.

Dougherty CM, Cotten NM, Braby HH. Proliferative epithelial lesions of the uterine tube. II. Adenocarcinoma. Obstet Gynecol 1965; 25: 37–42.

Dukes CE. The classification of cancer of the rectum. J Pathol Bacteriol 1932; 35: 323–32.

Eddy GL, Copeland LJ, Gershenson DM. Second look laparotomy in Fallopian tube carcinoma. Gynecol Oncol 1984; 19 (2): 182–6.

Eddy GL, Copeland LJ, Gershenson DM, Atkinson EN, Wharton JT, Rutledge FN. Fallopian tube carcinoma. Obstet Gynecol 1984; 64 (4): 546–52.

Emge LA. Six cases of primary carcinoma of the fallopian tube. Western J Surg 1948 56: 344–5.

Engeler V, Reinisch E, Schreiner WE. Primary carcinoma of the fallopian tube. A clinical study of 37 cases. 1981.

Ennker J. Zur praoperativen Diagnose des Tubenkarzinoms. Geburtshilfe Frauenheil 1951; 15: 898–907.

Fathalla MF. Factors in the causation and incidence of ovarian cancer. Obstet Gynecol Surv 1972; 27: 751–68.

Ferko S. Cytostatic attack therapy for incurable carcinoma of the cervix and for carcinoma of the uterine tube (author's transl). Strahlentherapie 1980; 156 (4): 234–9.

Finn WF, Javert CT. Primary and metastatic cancer of the fallopian tube. Cancer 1949; 2: 803–14.

Fogh I. Primary carcinoma of the fallopian tube. Cancer 1969; 23 (6): 1332–5.

Fogh I. Primary carcinoma of the fallopian tube. In: Ariel IM ed Progress in Clinical Cancer. New York: Grune & Stratton, 1973: 263–6.

Fox H, Langley FA. Tumours of the Ovary. London: William Heinemann Medical Books, 1976; 19–28.

Franek K, Zielonka I, Kwasniewska-Rokicinska C. Primary carcinoma of the fallopian tubes in the records of the Institute of Oncology in Gliwice. Nowotwory 1976; 26 (2): 141–4.

Frank R. Gynecological and Obstetrical Pathology. New York: Appleton, 1922: 353.

Frankel AN. Primary carcinoma of the fallopian tube. Am J Obstet Gynecol 1956; 131–42.

Franque O Von. Ueber das gleichzeitige Vorkommen von Karzinom und Tuberkulose an den weiblichen Genitalien, insbesondere Tube und Uterus. Geburtshulfe Gynäkol 1911; 69: 409–452.

Freese U. Ein Beitrag zur Zytologie des Tubenkarzinoms. Geburtshilfe Frauenheilk 1957; 17: 173–80.

Garret R. Extrauterine tumor cells in vaginal and cervical smears. Obstet Gynecol 1959; 14: 21–7.

Goldman JA, Gans B, Eckerling B. Hydrops tubae profluens—A symptom in tubal carcinoma. Obstet Gynecol 1961; 18: 631–4.

Golubev LN. Primary cancer of the fallopian tubes. Feldsher Akush 1984; 49 (8): 28–30.

Greene RR, Gardner GH. A preinvasive carcinoma of the uterine tube. Obstet Gynecol Surv 1950; 5: 734–44.

Guttner V, Dvorak O. Primary oviductal cancer at the 1st Department of Gynaecology, Prague, in 1953–1973 (author's transl). Cesk Gynekol 1978; 43 (10): 749–51.

Helo A. Carcinoma of the fallopian tube with special reference to the yellow discharge which appears with it. Acta Obstet Gynecol Scand 1960; 39: 259–66.

Henderson SR, Harper RC, Salazar OM, Rudolph JH. Primary carcinoma of the fallopian tube: Difficulties of diagnosis and treatment. Gynecol Oncol 1977; 5 (2): 168–79.

Hershey DW, Fennell RH, Major FJ. Primary carcinoma of the Fallopian tube. Obstet Gynecol 1981; 57 (3): 367–70.

Hertig AT, Gore H. Tumors of the Female Sex Organs. Part III. Tumors of the Ovary and Fallopian Tube. (Atlas of Tumor Pathology, Section IX—Fascicle 33) Washington DC.: Armed Forces Institute of Pathology, 1961; 166–76.

Hilfrich HJ, Tagisade M. Report of cases of primary tubal carcinoma. Zentralbl Gynäkol 91 (52): 1689–94.

Holland WW. Primary carcinoma of the fallopian tubes. Surg Gynecol Obstet 1930; 51: 683–91.

Hop WCJ, Hermans J. Statistische analyse van koverlevingsduren. Tijdschr Soc Geneeskd 59: 279–88.

Hoynck Van Papendrecht HPCM, Os WAAA Van. Primair tubacarcinoom gecombineerd met salpingitis tuberculosa. Ned Tijdschr Verlosk Gynaecol 1962; 62: 133–42.

Jamaludin A. Het primaire carcinoom van de tuba Fallopii. Thesis, Rotterdam, 1971.

Johnston GA Jr. Primary malignancy of the fallopian tube. A clinical review of 13 cases. J Surg Oncol 1983; 24 (4): 304–9.

Jones OV. Primary carcinoma of the uterine tube. Obstet Gynecol 1965; 26: 122–9.

Jowett M. The phosphatide and cholesterol contents of normal and malignant human tissues. Biochemical J 1931; 25: 1991–8.

Kadziora MB, Srinivasan R. Primary carcinoma of the fallopian tube. Can J Surg 1981; 24 (4): 425–6.

Kanbour AI, Stock RJ. Squamous cell carcinoma in situ of the endometrium and fallopian tube as superficial extension of invasive cervical carcinoma. Cancer 1978; 42 (2): 570–80.

Kaplan EL, Meier P. Nonparametric estimation from incomplete observations. J Am Statistical Assoc 1958; 53: 457–81.

Kapp D, Schwartz PE. Gynecologic oncology: Cancer update (second of two parts). Conn Med 1980; 44 (9): 557–63.

Kneale BL, Attwood HD. Primary carcinoma of the fallopian tube. Report of 13 cases. Am J Obstet Gynecol 1966; 94 (6): 840–8.

Kokhanovska KI, Sakhenko ML. Fallopian tube cancer according to data from the Chernovtsy Province Oncological Dispensary over 15 years (1961–1975). Pediatr Akush Ginekol 1979; 5: 50–1.

Kruijff H. Het primaire carcinoom van de tuba Fallopii. Ned Tijdschr Geneesk 1980; 124: 1825–7.

Kubista E, Kupka S. Clinical problems, therapy and prophylaxis of primary carcinoma of the fallopian tube (author's transl). Geburtshilfe Frauenheilkd 1937; 37 (12): 1044–9.

Latzko, W. Linkseitiges Tubenkarzinom, rechseitige karzinomatose Tubo-ovarialcyste. Zentralb Gynäkol 1916; 30: 599–600.

Lippes J. Analysis of human oviductal fluid for low molecular weight compounds. In: Beller FK, Schumacher GFB eds The Biology of the Fluids of the Female Genital Tract. Amsterdam: Elsevier North Holland Inc, 1979, 373–87.

Lofgren KA, Dockerty MB. Primary carcinoma of the fallopian tubes. Surg Gynecol Obstet 1946; 82: 199–206.

Maclean KS. Tubal malignancy—A method for collecting specimens for cytologic study. Science 1951; 114: 181.

Madsen V. Hysterosalpingograms in genital tuberculosis in women. Acta Radiolog 1947; 28: 812–23.

Malinconico LL. Primary carcinoma of the fallopian tube. Cytologic diagnosis. Connecticut State Medical J 1956; 20: 521–3.

Malkasian GD Jr, Decker DG, Mussey E, Johnson CE. Observations of gynecologic malignancy treated with 5-fluorouracil. Am J Obstet Gynecol 1968; 100 (7): 1012–17.

Malkov IM, Kulinich SI. Assessment of modern methods of diagnosing and treating Fallopian tube cancer. Akush Ginekol (Mosk) 1980; 1: 52–4.

Momtazee S, Kempson RL. Primary adenocarcinoma of the Fallopian tube. Obstet Gynecol 1968; 32 (5): 649–56.

Morrison J, Yon JL. Acute leukemia following chlorambucil therapy of advanced ovarian and fallopian tube carcinoma. Gynecol Oncol 1978; 6 (1): 115–20.

Moutquin JM, Dery JP, Boivin Y. Néoplasies primitives de la trompe de Fallope. L'Union Médicale du Canada 1973; 102: 1664–9.

Mukhina EP, Zeldovich DR. Cancer of the oviducts. Vopr Onkol 1970; 16 (12): 61–3.

Novak ER, Woodruff JD. Gynecologic and Obstetric Pathology, 7th edition. Philadelphia: WB Saunders, 1974; 313–27.

Olesen H, Albeck V. Primary tubal carcinoma with metastasis to the endometrium and the mesovarium. Acta Obstet Gynecolog Scand 1949; 29: 245–54.

Ooms ECM, Essed E, Veldhuizen RW, Alons CL, Kurver PHJ, Boon ME. The prognostic significance of morphometry in T 1 bladder tumours. Histopathology 1980; 5: 311–18.

Orthmann EG. Zur Kenntnis der malignen Tubenneubildungen. Z Geburtshulfe Gynäkol 1906; 58: 376–424.

Page EW. Human Reproduction. Philadelphia: WB Saunders 1972; 28–34.

Papanicolaou GN. Diagnostic value of exfoliated cells from cancerous tissues. JAMA 1946; 131: 372–8.

Park RC, Parmley TH. Fallopian tube cancer. In: McGowan Led Gynecologic Oncology. New York: Appleton-Century-Crofts, 1978; 274–80.

Parsons L, Sommers SC. Gynecology, 2nd edition. Philadelphia: WB Saunders, 1978; 1571–81.

Pascu F, Muller P, Kracht J. Fruherkennung eines Tubenkarzinoms durch Exfoliativ-Zytologie. Dtsche Med Wochenschr 1975; 100: 1476–7.

Passchier J, Walta HF. Gynaecologen in ziekenhuispraktijken. Publication no. 80.190, National Ziekenhuisinstituut, Utrecht, 1981.

Persaud V, Burkett G. A case of primary carcinoma of the Fallopian tube with a review of the literature. West Indian Med J 1971; 20 (1): 46–50.

Picha E, Weghaupt K. Report on 20 primary tubal carcinomas from the years 1950–1963. Zentralbl Gynäkol 1973; 92 (19): 596–600.

Plentle A, Friedman EH. Lymphatic System of the

Female Genitalia. Philadelphia: WB Saunders, 1971: 153–67.

Puflett D. Tuberculous salpingitis resembling adenocarcinoma. Med J Aust 1972; 2: 149–51.

Reiffenstuhl G. Das Lymphystem des Weiblichen Genitale. Berlin, Vienna: Urban & Schwarzenberg, 1957; 9, 30–1, 108–9, 149–57.

Richtlijnen ex artikel 3 van de Wet Ziekenhuisvoorzieningen voor het ontwerpen van plannen; tevens becordelingskader bij de toepassing van artikel 29, errste lid, van de Wet Ziekenhuisvoorzieningen. Ministry of Public Health and Environmental Hygiene. The Hague: Staatsuitgeverij, 1981.

Roberts JA. Management of gynecologic tumors during pregnancy. Clin Perinatol 1983; 10 (2): 369–82 (Review).

Robey M Goiran JP, Robey F, Salleron A. Fallopian tube adenocarcinoma. J Gynecol Obstet Biol Reprod (Paris) 1972; 1 (6): 581–90.

Ross WM. Primary tumours of the fallopian tube: A report of eight cases of adenocarcinoma and one case of unusual carcinoma. Can Med Assoc J 1967; 96 (6): 328–31.

Sampson JA. The lymphatics of the mucosa of the fimbriae of the fallopian tube. Am J Obstet Gynecol 1937; 33: 911–30.

Sanger M, Barth J. Die Neubildungen der Eileiter. In: Martin AE ed Krankeiten der Eileiter. Leipzig: Eduard Besold, 1895: 240–94.

Santamaria-Urrego A. Primary carcinoma of the fallopian tubes. Review of national occurrence. Rev Colomb Obstet Ginecol 1968; 19 (4): 247–57.

Schiller HM, Silverberg SG. Staging and prognosis in primary carcinoma of the fallopian tube. Cancer 1971; 28 (2): 389–95.

Schulz BO, Hof K, Friedrich HJ, Weppelmann B, Krebs D. Platin-containing cytostatic combinations in the therapy of advanced gynecologic carcinomas. Geburtshilfe Fraunheilkd 1984; 44 (1): 34–8.

Senapad S. Primary carcinoma of the fallopian tube. J Med Assoc Thai 1973; 56 (9): 552–7.

Skinha AC. Hydrops tubae profluens as a presenting symptom in primary carcinoma of the fallopian tube. Report of two cases and review of literature. Br Med J 1959; ii: 996–1001.

Smith JP. Chemotherapy in gynecologic cancer. Clin Obstet Gynecol 1975; 18 (4): 109–24.

Song YS. The significance of positive vaginal smears in extrauterine carcinomas. Am J Gynecol 1957; 73: 341–8.

Sontag S. Illness as Metaphor. New York: Vintage Books, 1979.

Stern BD, Hanley BJ. Primary carcinoma of the Fallopian tube. Am J Obstet Gynecol 1949; 58: 517–23.

Sturmans F. Epidemiologie en ziekte-oorzaken. Van monocausaal naar multicausaal. Medisch Contact 1977; 32: 343–9.

Tamimi HK, Figge DC. Adenocarcinoma of the uterine tube: Potential for lymph node metastases. Am J Obstet Gynecol 1981; 141 (2): 132–7.

Vermeulen ACM. Besmetting en herbesmetting bij Tuberculose. Thesis, Leiden, 1961.

Vinall PS, Buxton N, Cowen PN. Primary carcinoma of the Fallopian tube associated with tuberculous salpingitis. A case report. Br J Obstet Gynaecol 1979; 86: 984–9.

Wachtel E. The cytology of tumors of the ovary and fallopian tubes. Clin Obstet Gynecol 1961; 4: 1159–71.

Way S. Malignant Disease of the Female Genital Tract. London: J & A Churchill, 1951: 218–22.

Weekes LR, Anz UE, Whiting EB. Primary carcinoma of the fallopian tube. J Obstet Gynecol 1952; 64: 62–71.

Wharton LR, Krock FH. Primary carcinoma of the fallopian tube. Arch Surg 1929; 19: 848–70.

Wolf A, Vahrson H. Die Radiogoldtherapie des primaren Tubenkarzinoms. Geburtshilfe Frauenheilk 1976; 36: 178–83.

Wu AR. Management of primary carcinoma of the fallopian tube. Chung Hua Chung Liu Tsa Chih 1982; 4 (3): 197–9.

Wynder EL, MacCornack FA, Stellman SD. The epidemiology of breast cancer in 785 United States caucasian women. Cancer 1978; 41: 2341–54.

Yeung HH, Bannatyne P, Russell P. Adenocarcinoma of the fallopian tubes: A clinicopathological study of eight cases. Pathology 1983; 15 (3): 279–86.

Young JA, Kossman CR, Green MR. Adenocarcinoma of the Fallopian tube: Report of a case with an unusual pattern of metastasis and response to combination chemotherapy. Gynecol Oncol 1984; 17 (2): 238–40.

Zielinski J, Sablinska B. Primary cancer of the oviduct. Ginekol Pol 1971; 42 (8): 1031–5.

Chapter **7**

Unusual Tumours of the Uterine Corpus

John H. Malfetano* and
Rudolfo Florentin†

*Associate Professor of Obstetrics and Gynecology, Albany Medical College, Albany, New York, USA and
†Professor, Department of Pathology, Albany Medical Center Hospital, Albany, New York, USA

INTRODUCTION

Primary cancers of the uterine corpus are the most common gynecologic malignancies with an estimated 36 000 new cases to be reported in the United States in 1986 (1). These lesions can arise from either the endometrium or the myometrium. Primary neoplasms arising from the cervix will not be included since treatment and routes of metastases differ from endometrial lesions.

Generally, primary endometrial cancers occur in the postmenopausal female and will present with uterine bleeding, pain or an abdominal/pelvic mass. The diagnosis is readily made by an endometrial biopsy, aspirate or formal dilatation and curettage.

Endometrial cancers are staged according to the International Federation of Gynaecology and Obstetrics (FIGO) classifications reported in 1974 (2). The staging process and clinical assessment depends on the history and physical examination, chest and x-ray roentgenograms. The mainstay of treatment for uterine cancers remains surgery with removal of the uterus, tubes and ovaries, surgical staging and

attempts at reduction of extrauterine metastases. Staging should include peritoneal cytology and sampling of the retroperitoneal pelvic and para-aortic nodes. Further therapy will include radiation therapy, chemotherapy or both depending on the histopathologic review of the surgical specimens. This approach to the patient with cancers of the uterus will allow individualization of therapy when unusual tumors are encountered either preoperatively or intraoperatively. For the majority of the unusual corpus cancers there is no uniformly accepted therapy since the number of reported cases are small with no randomized clinical studies. Only with adequate surgical and pathologic information can gynecologist, radiotherapist and chemotherapist formulate treatment plans.

Ninety percent of endometrial cancers are carcinomas arising from the endometrial epithelium with adenocarcinoma being the most common histologic form (3). The yearly incidence to annual mortality ratio approximates 13 to 1 and is now responsible for the sixth most common cancer death in females in the United States. The low mortality from

TABLE 1   CARCINOMA OF THE CORPUS UTERI

Stage 0	Carcinoma in situ. Histologic findings are suspicious of malignancy; cases of Stage 0 should not be included in any therapeutic statistics
Stage I	The carcinoma is confined to the corpus
Stage IA	The length of the uterine cavity is 8 cm or less
Stage IB	The length of the uterine cavity is more than 8 cm

It is desirable that the Stage I cases be subgrouped with regard to the histologic type of the adenocarcinoma as follows:

G1	Highly differentiated adenomatous carcinoma
G2	Differentiated adenomatous carcinoma with partly solid areas
G3	Predominantly solid or entirely undifferentiated carcinoma
Stage II	The carcinoma has involved the corpus and the cervix but has not extended outside the uterus
Stage III	The carcinoma has extended outside the uterus but not outside the true pelvis
Stage IV	The carcinoma has extended outside the true pelvis or has obviously involved the mucosa of the bladder or rectum. A bullous edema as such does not permit a case to be allotted to Stage IV
Stage IVA	Spread of the growth to adjacent organs
Stage IVB	Spread to distant organs

corpus cancer is related to the fact that 75–80% are confined to the uterus at initial diagnosis (FIGO Stage I) (Table 1) (2).

Risk factors, natural history, diagnosis and management of endometrial adenocarcinoma are well published and beyond the scope of this chapter (4–12). A brief review of the embryologic development of the uterus is important to understand how unusual variants of cancer can present with the uterus being the primary site.

EMBRYOLOGY

The paramesonephric (mullerian) ducts fuse in the mid-line to form the genital duct. The cranial and intermediate portions give rise to the fallopian tubes. The caudal portion becomes the uterus. The epithelial cell types seen in these organs having arisen from the mullerian duct maintain a metaplastic potential throughout life. The cuboidal cell lining of the genital duct gives rise to the epithelial lining of the uterus. The musculature of the genital tract is derived from the mesenchyme surrounding the paramesonephric ducts. According to some investigators, the upper part of the vagina is derived from the fused paramesonephric ducts and the lower part from the sinovaginal bulbs (13). Abnormalities in the fusion of the caudal portion of the paramesonephric ducts result in various malformations of the uterus and vagina. The close relationship in the development in the mesonephric (wolffian) and paramesonephric (mullerian) ducts can explain the anomalies in which the mesonephric derivatives open into the uterus or vagina.. Thus, the uterus is composed of an epithelial lining and a stroma derived from mesenchyme. This will help explain how the uterus is vulnerable to the development of some unusual cancers.

ADENOCARCINOMA (TYPICAL)

The most common form of invasive endometrial cancer is adenocarcinoma of primary origin constituting about 95% of all endometrial neoplasms (5, 6). Endometrial adenocarcinoma may be localized or diffuse. The localized form is polypoid and friable often superficially ulcerative. In the diffuse form the endometrium is thickened and indurated. Microscopically, there is excessive proliferation and crowding of glands with only a few strands or no stromal cells between the glands. The gland sizes are varied and lined by stratified epithelium. The epithelial cells show nuclear atypia with prominent nucleoli, chromatin clumping and mitoses. The stroma is generally vascular and contains leukocytic infiltrates. The well differentiated adenocarcinoma can be difficult to distinguish from atypical endometrial hyperplasia. Unlike atypical hyperplasia, adenocarcinoma shows intra-glandular epithelial bridging; stromal fibrous reaction and stromal foamy cells may be prominent (14).

The current grading is according to the system developed by FIGO (15). These tumors are graded 1–3 on the basis of their proportions of glandular and solid growth. In general, the degree of nuclear atypia and mitotic activity increases correspondingly to the degree of undifferentiation in the carcinoma. Well differentiated adenocarcinomas have only glandular, intra-glandular epithelial cribriform bridging and papillary patterns. Moderately differentiated adenocarcinomas are dominantly glandular but contain a lesser amount of solid cell nests. Poorly differentiated adenocarcinoma is composed dominantly of solid masses of cells and gland formation is less evident or barely seen. At times the carcinoma will show wide variation in differentiation. The tumor is then graded according to the most poorly differentiated pattern to reflect its most malignant potential.

Treatment remains exploratory laparotomy, total abdominal hysterectomy, bilateral salpingo-oophorectomy, cytologic washings from the peritoneal cavity and para-aortic and pelvic lymph node sampling. Adjuvant therapy is tailored to the histologic findings. The tumor grade, depth of invasion into the myometrium, cytology and status of the retroperitoneal nodes will dictate further therapy (4, 7). Generally, pelvic radiotherapy is indicated in Stage I patients with deeply invasive lesions, cervical involvement or Grade 3 lesions. The addition of para-aortic nodal radiation therapy may improve survival in patients with metastasis to those nodes (16). The treatment for advanced endometrial cancer (Stages III/IV) will include multiple modalities with combinations of surgery, radiation and chemotherapy.

Adenocarcinoma within Adenomyosis

Depth of tumor penetration into the myometrium is a known prognostic factor for endometrial adenocarcinoma. The unusual occurrence of adenocarcinoma within a foci of adenomyosis must be distinguished from myometrial invasion. Adenomyosis is frequently an incidental finding within a hysterectomy specimen regardless of the indication with an incidence varying from 30 to 50% (17, 18). A distinction between tumor invasion into the myometrium and involving adenomyosis is often difficult but must be ascertained for the prognostic significance is vastly different.

At least 19 cases of adenocarcinoma in adenomyosis have been reported with adequate follow-up 1970 (19, 20). In the 11 patients reported by Hernandez and Woodruff, all tumors were Grade 1 (20). There is no mention of tumor grade in the series by Hall et al (19). However, in both series, there have been no recurrences and all 19 patients were alive without evidence of disease at 5 years. These two entities, tumor invasion into the myometrium and adenocarcinoma involving foci of adenomyosis must be differentiated from one another since the latter has an excellent prognosis.

ATYPICAL ENDOMETRIAL ADENOCARCINOMAS

Less than 10% of adenocarcinomas of the endometrium have atypical patterns. Clear cell carcinomas of the endometrium account for 3–5.5% of endometrial adenocarcinomas (21–23). Only isolated reports of endometrial clear cell carcinoma appeared in the literature until 1973. After came two series of 12 and 21 patients (21, 22). They are composed of numerous cells with clear cytoplasm frequently alternating with 'hobnail' cells and arranged in papillary, tubular, cystic and/or solid patterns. The clear cytoplasm contains glycogen which stains positive with periodic acid–Schiff (PAS) and is diastase sensitive. The nuclei of the hobnail cells protrude into the gland lumina where the cytoplasm is attenuated (Figure 1). Intracytoplasmic and intraluminal eosinophilic bodies that are PAS positive and

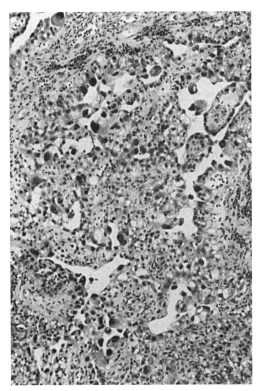

Figure 1 Clear cell carcinoma: clear cells containing glycogen and hobnail cells that project into lumina, papillary pattern.

diastase resistant are seen in the majority of cases previously regarded as of mesonephric origin. Because of its histologic similarity to renal cell carcinoma, it is currently considered of mullerian derivation as evidenced by its occurrence as a primary tumor of the endometrium and its counterpart in the ovary, vagina and cervix. This tumor has been previously designated mesonephroma, mesonephric carcinoma and mesonephroid carcinoma (21–23). Histologically the clear cell adenocarcinoma of the endometrium has many of the features of the more common clear cell adenocarcinoma of the ovary (21). Histologic grading of clear cell carcinoma is very difficult due to the frequent combinations of the various histologic patterns of this tumor and, therefore the surgical staging and depth of myometrial invasion are most important for prognostic considerations (21–31). From the largest series

of clear cell carcinoma in the literature, it appears that these endometrial cancers occur in a slightly older postmenopausal woman than the usual adenocarcinomas. These lesions are generally poorly differentiated and highly aggressive with poor survival rates of 20–55% (21–33). The use of adjuvant pelvic radiation appears indicated.

Secretory carcinoma of the endometrium has been included in reports of clear cell endometrial cancers (21, 32). The reason for discussing this subtype atypical adenocarcinoma of the endometrium is to describe its unique histologic appearance and to differentiate it from secretory hyperplasia. Its incidence is not known. It is composed of well differentiated glands lined by infrequently stratified columnar cells with cytoplasmic vacuoles resembling the early secretory phase of the menstrual cycle. Unlike normal secretory endometrium, the glands are crowded and back to back with very little or no stroma between glands. These tumors generally present at an earlier age than the usual adenocarcinomas and are generally well differentiated lesions. The prognosis from this atypical adenocarcinoma is generally favorable, with only 2 deaths out of 15 patients at 5 years in the series of Christopherson et al. (23). Although the number of cases is small, 2 additional patients died from recurrent disease after 5 years suggesting longer follow-up is necessary with these lesions (23, 32).

Mucinous adenocarcinoma of the endometrium is very rare and is histologically similar to those occurring in the endocervix, ovary and gastrointestinal tract. They secrete large amounts of mucin and are PAS positive after diastase digestion. This tumor is seen more often as a component of typical adenocarcinoma. If the rare, dominant or pure mucinous adenocarcinoma is seen on uterine curettings, primary endocervical and metastatic ovarian or gastrointestinal carcinoma should be excluded (33). This lesion should be regarded as a morphologic variant of the typical adenocarcinomas of the endometrium and treated accordingly (33–37).

Small cell carcinoma, argyrophil cell carcinoma or adenocarcinoma with neuroendocrine differentiation is an unusual primary tumor of the endometrium. It is presumed that these neoplasms arise from argyrophilic cells and are part of the family of neoplasms that arise from the diffuse epithelial endocrine system originally described by Feyreter in 1938 (38). These cells have been referred to as being part of the APUD cell system (cells capable of amine precursor uptake and decarboxylation since they can synthesize and secrete amines of polypeptide hormones). This tumor is characterized by the presence of neuroendocrine granules by the NES (neuron specific enolase PAP) or Gremiluis stains or dense core neurosecretory granules, similar to those of pulmoary oat cell carcinoma by electron microscopy (Figures 2 and 3). These granules have been demonstrated in typical adenocarcinomas, adenosquamous carcinomas and in undifferentiated carcinomas of the endometrium. In the edenosquamous carcinoma the neuroendocrine granules were localized in the glandular and squamous compartments. The histogenesis is unclear since neurosecretory granules have not been demonstrated in normal endometrium. The behavior of argyrophil cell carcinoma is unknown because of the limited

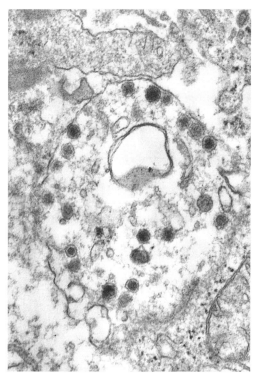

Figure 2 Electron micrograph showing intracytoplasmic neurosecretory granules from small cells in left of Figure 3.

number of cases (39–43). Only three pure small cell carcinomas of the endometrium have

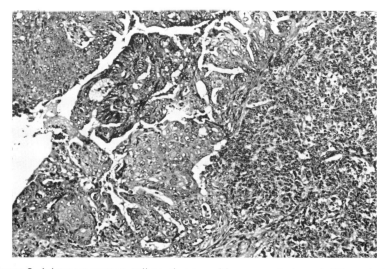

Figure 3 Adenosquamous cell carcinoma with neuroectodermal differentiation.

been reported with inadequate follow-up (39, 41, 43). It appears that these lesions are highly aggressive and have a poor prognosis because of hematogenous spread to bone, liver and brain. Aggressive therapy for these lesions should include not only surgery but radiation and probably chemotherapy. Active antineoplastic agents include the combination of vincristine, Adriamycin and Cytoxan as well as CisDDP and VP-16 (44–47).

ADENOACANTHOMA AND ADENOSQUAMOUS (MIXED CARCINOMAS)

Adenocarcinomas with squamous metaplasia (adenoacanthoma) and mixed tumors or adenosquamous carcinoma are adenocarcinomas with squamous differentiation. These tumors have been separated into separate clinicopathologic entities based on the histologic appearance of the squamous elements (48). Prior to 1950, adenoacanthoma was a rare entity with a frequency of between 2.3 and 3.3% of all adenocarcinomas (49). As squamous elements were found to be more common in endometrial adenocarcinomas, the diagnosis of adenocanthoma increased in the 1960s to a frequency of 15.7–43.7% (50–53).

Ng in 1968 reported on a series of 368 adenocarcinomas and suggested for the first time that these cases of adenocarcinoma with a squamous component be divided into two categories: (48). Those with histologically benign squamous foci—adenoacanthomas; and those with malignant appearing squamous elements—adenosquamous or mixed carcinomas. In the adenoacanthoma the histologic appearance of the squamous elements is benign and intercellular bridges and keratin can be seen (Figure 4). In the mixed tumors, the squamous elements appear malignant and resemble either keratinizing or large cell nonkeratinizing squamous cell carcinoma of the cervix, and frequently invade the stroma (Figure 5). The relative frequencies of these two carcinomas in Ng's series was 24.2% and 6.9% respectively. In a later series by Ng of 542

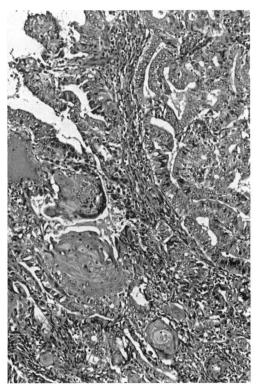

Figure 4 Adenoacanthoma (adenocarcinoma with squamous metaplasia): malignant glands and benign squamous epithelium.

cases, the poor prognosis with mixed tumors was realized (54). The 5-year survival for mixed carcinomas was 19.2% versus 79% for adenocarcinoma and 71.1% for adenoacanthomas. The aggressiveness of the adenosquamous carcinomas was related to the fact that most tumors had Grade 3 (poorly differentiated) glandular elements and frequent vascular space involvement in 50% of the specimens. These poorly differentiated areas of a high grade pure adenocarcinoma may be difficult to distinguish from the poorly differentiated squamous component of a mixed adenosquamous carcinoma. Also, the squamous component may have spindle shaped squamous cells and be misinterpreted as sarcoma. Therefore, adequate tissue sampling and at times ultrastructural studies may be necessary for diagnosis. In contrast, the adenocanthomas have a glandular epithelium which is usually well

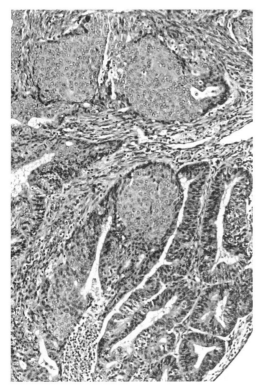

Figure 5 Adenosquamous cell carcinoma: malignant glands and malignant squamous component.

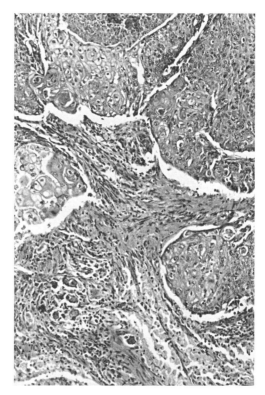

Figure 6 Squamous cell carcinoma invading myometrium.

differentiated (Grade 1) and therefore the prognosis is as favorable as similar pure adeno-carcinomas of the endometrium (55–58). The prognosis is significantly worse for patients with mixed carcinomas largely because of the poorly differentiated glandular epithelium (49, 54, 59). However, when mixed carcino-mas are compared to poorly differentiated adenocarcinomas, their survivals are similar suggesting that it is the glandular and not the squamous elements which portend the poor prognosis.

Treatment modalities for adenoacanthoma should be as those of pure adenocarcinomas of the endometrium. However, the treatment of adenosquamous carcinoma is somewhat more difficult. Since frequently these tumors are outside of the uterus at diagnosis and because of the poor survival rates, aggressive adjuvant therapy should be considered (60–62).

Patients with disease apparently confined to the uterus should be treated with adjuvant postoperative pelvic radiotherapy and those with disease outside of the uterus, with whole abdominal radiation or pelvic radiation and chemotherapy.

SQUAMOUS CELL CARCINOMA

Primary pure squamous cell carcinoma of the endometrium is extremely rare with 29 cases reported in the literature (63–77). It is thought to originate from squamous metaplasia of the reserve cell between the glandular columnar cells and basement membrane (Figure 6). The following diagnostic criteria established by Fluhamann in 1956 have to be satisfied to prove that the squamous cell carcinoma is of endometrial origin: (1) absence of adenocarci-noma in the endometrium (this requires examination of multiple sections); (2) no evidence of a primary cervical squamous cell carcinoma with spread to the corpus; (3) the endometrial squamous cell carcinoma does not have any connection with the cervical squamous mucosa (72). With such few cases in the world's literature, the prognosis is not known but presumably corresponds to the grade and depth of myometrial invasion of the tumor.

The presenting symptoms are very similar to adenocarcinoma, uterine bleeding. The occurrence of a pyometria has been noted in 8 out of 29 cases but in only 2 out of 16 since 1967 and therefore its significance is suspect (66, 73). This rare tumor appears to present at a more advanced stage and with myometrial invasion. After appropriate surgery and staging, implementation of pelvic radiotherapy, chemotherapy or both should be considered since this tumor may spread via lymphatics and hematogenously

One case of verrucous carcinoma of the endometrium has been reported in the world's literature (74). This is a variant of squamous cell carcinoma and is identical to the more commonly found lesions in the larynx, esophagus, skin and anogenital regions of males and females (74, 75). The one reported case was treated with TAH/BSO and has been a long term survivor of greater than 5 years without subsequent adjuvant therapy (74).

GLASSY CELL CARCINOMA

Endometrial glassy cell carcinoma is histologically similar to the more common glassy cell carcinoma of the cervix (76–78). It is considered a variant of adenosquamous carcinoma occurring as nests of large cells, finely granular to homogeneous (ground glass) cytoplasm with pleomorphic nuclei containing prominent nucleoli. A few reported cases behaved more aggressively than the usual endometrial adenosquamous carcinoma. Glassy cell carcinomas of the cervix are also known to have a much worse prognosis than the usual cervical adenosquamous carcinomas (76).

UTERINE PAPILLARY SEROUS CARCINOMA

This relatively new morphologic variant of adenocarcinoma of the endometrium is extremely aggressive since it invades the myometrium frequently and metastasizes very early. This adenocarcinoma very closely resembles ovarian papillary serous carcinoma. These lesions typically feature a high degree of cytologic anaplasia as well as papillary growth and psammoma bodies (79). The papillary architecture is complex with broad and sometimes hyalinized papillae with vascular cores (Figure 7). The lining epithelium is frequently tufted and composed of pleomorphic and hyperchromatic cells with macronucleoli, and abnormal mitoses are often seen. Tumor necrosis is also often present. The differential diagnosis includes papillary foci in typical

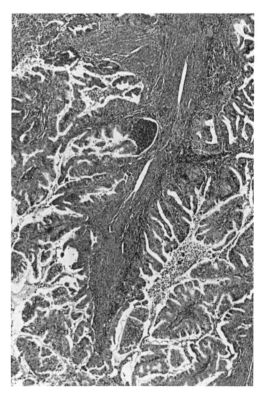

Figure 7 Uterine papillary serous carcinoma: broad papillae with fibrovascular core and secondary papillae.

endometrial carcinomas and papillary meta-plasia without fibrovascular cores usually found at or near the endometrial surface. Distinct epithelial stratification and marked nuclear anaplasia and foci of necrosis are not seen in papillary areas of well differentiated typical adenocarcinomas.

The first 2 cases of this variant of endome-trial carcinoma were reported in 1963 (80) and again in 1972 (81). The unusual feature of both of these lesions was the large number of psammoma bodies found in the uterine speci-men. It really was not until 1982 that the terms uterine papillary serous carcinoma were estab-lished in a series of 26 cases that were reported (82).

The initial symptoms of patients with uter-ine papillary serous carcinoma are very similar to those of any uterine cancer, uterine bleed-ing. Nearly 50% of these patients at the time of surgery will have extrauterine disease. The spread patterns are very typical of those of serous carcinoma of the ovary, namely miliary disease on all peritoneal surfaces, including the omentum and retroperitoneal nodes. These tumors frequently have deep myometrial inva-sion in nearly 40% of presumed Stage I cases. Invasion of lymphatic and capillary like spaces is another frequent finding and may help explain why nearly 50% of these patients with Stage I disease will develop recurrence (82–85).

Since this lesion has a tendency for early recurrence and upper abdominal spread, treatment must consist of TAH/BSO and surgical staging as in ovarian carcinoma. Con-sideration should then be given for adjuvant therapy consisting of either whole abdominal radiation or chemotherapy as for ovarian carcinoma. The most active agents appear to be the combination of platinum, cyclophos-phamide and Adriamycin.

UTERINE SARCOMAS
(Chapter 10)

Homologous

Uterine sarcomas account for 2–6% of all uterine tumors (86–87). These mesenchymal tumors can arise from the endometrial glands and stroma, the uterine muscle (myometrium) and in supporting structures of the uterus such as blood vessels, nerves and fibroadipose tis-sues. The capacity of corporal neoplasms to form heterologous elements may be explained by the potentiality of the uterine primordium to form heterologous mesodermal tissues since the analage of the mullerian duct and its surroundings mesenchyme is coelomic and therefore of mesodermal origin (88). These tumors are classified on the basis of their cell type and site of origin. These include smooth muscle cell tumors, endometrial stromal tumors and mixed mesodermal tumors. Pure sarcomas are composed of one cell type while mixed sarcomas are made up of more than one cell type. Tumors that contain tissue elements from the uterus are called homologous tumors and those with tissue elements not normally found in the uterus such as bone, cartilage and striated muscle are heterologous tumors. There is much confusion in the literature on the criteria for the diagnosis of sarcomas. Macro-scopic appearance, degree of cellular differen-tiation and mitotic rate are important con-siderations in diagnosis.

The most important prognostic and diag-nostic criterion for sarcomas appears to be the mitotic rate, cellular atypia, pleomorphism and the extent of disease at initial presentation. Those lesions with less than five mitotic figures per ten high power fields appear to behave in a benign fashion, while those with greater than ten mitotic figures per ten high power fields are highly malignant. The lesions with five to ten mitotic figures per ten high power fields and moderate to severe cellular atypia may recur late and therefore must be considered low grade or borderline sarcomas (86, 89, 90).

Leiomyosarcoma is the most common uter-ine sarcoma accounting for 45% of all sarco-mas. This is followed by mixed mesodermal tumors (35%), endometrial stromal sarcomas (15%) and all others accounting for approxi-mately 5% (86, 91–100). The role of previous pelvic or intracavitary radiation therapy for benign menstrual disorders and subsequent uterine sarcoma has been a subject of debate. Aaro et al. in 1966 noted that 6.5% of patients with previous radiation therapy developed leiomyosarcoma while 26% developed an endometrial stromal sarcoma (92). However, Fehr and Prem in their series of 2294 patients treated with radiation therapy for carcinoma of the cervix noted only 5 patients developing uterine sarcomas in the follow-up period (101). Boyce et al in their reports of 15 cancer registries in eight countries in whom women were treated for carcinoma of the cervix found only 162 (5%) of 3324 second cancers that could be attributed to radiation therapy. This series encompassed 182040 patients (102). Therefore, although there appears to be a relationship with prior radiation therapy for benign gynecologic disease and uterine sarcomas, this relationship does not hold true for patients being treated for cervical cancer or among atomic bomb survivors.

Leiomyosarcoma generally occurs in women in the fifth and sixth decades of life. This appears to occur at an earlier age than the other endometrial sarcomas. Generally, the diagnosis is made on the histologic examination of the uterus operated upon for suspected uterine fibroids. The incidence of sarcomatous degeneration in leiomyomas is between 0.13 and 0.81% (87, 103–105). Presenting symptoms include abdominal pain, an enlarging uterus, uterine hemorrhage and a myomatous uterus (105–109). The diagnostic confusion occurs in differentiating leiomyosarcoma from cellular leiomyoma and bizarre leiomyomas. The two lesions are distinguished from leiomyosarcoma on the basis of the mitotic count and generally have less than five mitotic figures per ten high power fields but may have cellular atypia. The prognosis with surgery alone is usually excellent in these two variants of leiomyosarcoma. The exception may be with the bizarre leiomyomas also called leiomyoblastoma, epithelioid muscle tumors, clear cell leiomyomas and plexiform tumorlets, where 6 out of 32 tumors have recurred or metastasized (110–113). These lesions, therefore, should be

considered as low grade malignancies and therapy should include TAH/BSO and surgical staging. The follow-up period is extremely important since recurrences may occur late. There is no apparent indication for adjuvant therapy.

Nearly 33–50% of all patients with leiomyosarcoma have extrauterine disease at the time of diagnosis (86, 90, 109, 114). This tumor spreads through the myometrium via lymphatics and blood vessels as well as to contiguous pelvic structures. The most frequent sites of metastases include the lung and pleura in 80%, kidneys in 33%, liver 20% and regional lymph nodes in 47%. The survival ranges from 20 to 63% with a mean of 47% at 5 years (90, 116). The survival appears to be related to the number of mitoses with lesions having greater than ten mitotic figures per ten high power fields having a worse survival (86, 90, 100, 106, 109, 114–119). Adjuvant therapy, either pelvic radiotherapy, whole abdominal radiotherapy or systemic chemotherapy has not prevented the occurrence of metastatic lesions (120). Further trials are ongoing to establish the benefit of one of the treatment modalities as an adjuvant modality in Stage I/II lesions.

Three other rare clinical pathologic variants of leiomyosarcoma must be considered. Intravenous leiomyomatosis is a histologically benign appearing lesion in which the uterine and iliac veins as well as the broad ligament are frequently visibly filled with benign leiomyomatous tissue (121–123). Microscopic vascular invasion within a leiomyoma and no extension outside the tumor is not clinically important and should not be classified as intravenous leiomyomatosis. Frequently, this tissue extends all the way to the pelvic sidewalls. The treatment should consist of TAH/BSO and attempts at tumor reductive surgery; however, frequently tumor is left behind within the pelvic vessels. The prognosis, however, remains excellent. Both local and late recurrences can occur with extension to the vena cava or metastasis to the heart. Recent data suggest that estrogen may stimulate the proliferation of these lesions and, therefore, bila-

teral salpingo-oophorectomy may be beneficial (124). These lesions must be considered as
a low grade leiomyosarcoma and follow-up for
long periods of time is necessary. the role of
adjuvant therapy has not been established and
therefore not indicated.

The second variant of leiomyosarcoma is
metastasizing leiomyoma (see Chapter 20).
These lesions also should be classified as low
grade malignant potential with occurrences 5
years or more after TAH/BSO for uterine
fibroids. These recurrences are generally single
or multiple within the lung or retroperitoneal
nodes. These nodules histologically contain
benign smooth muscle similar to the uterine
leiomyomas (125–130). Treatment should
consist of further tumor reductive surgery if
pelvic disease occurs or possibly segmental
resection of pulmonary lung nodules (131–
136).

The final varaint of leiomyosarcoma is leiomyomatosis peritonealis disseminata (see
Chapter 9). This condition is characterized by
sub-peritoneal nodules of benign smooth
muscle, decidua and fibroblasts within the
peritoneal cavity associated with uterine or
ovarian leiomyomas (137). This entity is frequently associated with pregnancy and generally in non-white females suggesting an estrogen dependency for this disorder (138–142).
The explanation for these benign metastases is
metaplasia of the peritoneal mesenchymal cells
rather than metastasis from leiomyomas (143).
The literature suggests appropriate therapy to
be TAH/BSO and attempts at tumor reductive
surgery of these implants. The prognosis for
these lesions appears excellent with and without complete resection (144, 145).

ENDOMETRIAL STROMAL SARCOMA

Stromal sarcomas are polypoid endometrial
tumors or nodular intramural tumors that
resemble leiomyomas. They nearly always
present with abnormal vaginal bleeding and
pelvic pain. Benign stromal nodules are well
circumscribed tumors confined to the endome-

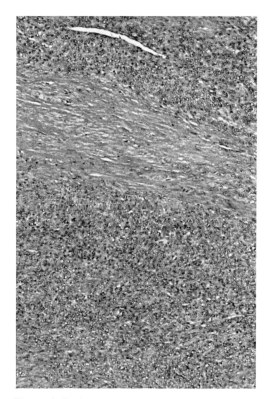

Figure 8 Endometrial stromal sarcoma invading myometrium.

trium; stromal sarcomas invade the endometrium and angioinvasion is a frequent finding
(Figure 8). Most of the tumor is extra-vascular
in contrast to endolymphatic stromal myosis.
All endometrial stromal tumors histologically
resemble the normal proliferative endometrial
stroma but are less differentiated. High grade
stromal sarcomas histologically are more atypical and pleomorphic and frequently show
foci of hemorrhage and necrosis compared to
the low grade stromal sarcomas. Low grade
stromal sarcomas show mild to moderate cellular atypia and less than ten mitotic figures per
ten high power fields in the most active areas
(86, 89).

At least 37 cases of pure endometrial stromal
sarcoma have been reported. This is a rapidly
lethal sarcoma with a 27% 5-year survival rate

(86, 89, 146). Treatment must consist of total abdominal hysterectomy, bilateral salpingo-oophorectomy and sampling of regional and para-aortic nodes. Further consideration should be given for the use of adjuvant radiotherapy and/or chemotherapy. As with most uterine sarcomas even when the disease is localized recurrences occur in over half the cases and 50% of these recurrences are outside of the pelvis. The most common distant failures are in the upper abdomen and the lungs (115–146).

Mixed Mesodermal (Mullerian) Tumors (see Chapter 4)

These tumors are composed of admixtures of epithelial and mesenchymal neoplastic tissues. These highly malignant neoplasms exhibit histologically malignant epithelial and mesenchymal components. The homologous mixed mesodermal tumors are those with mesenchymal components homologous (contains only tissue normally found in the uterus) to the uterus and are also identified as carcinosarcomas (Figure 9) (147). The heterologous mixed mesodermal tumors are those with mesenchymal components heterologous (contains tissues foreign to the uterus such as striated muscle, cartilage, bone or fat) to the uterus (Figure 10). These sarcomas are nearly always found in postmenopausal women averaging between 60 and 70 years of age. The most common presenting symptoms are postmenopausal bleeding and lower abdominal pain. The uterus is often enlarged and felt to be irregular in contour. The tumor is frequently bulky, polypoid and may protrude through the endocervical canal. In a high proportion of patients the tumor rapidly invades adjacent tissues and organs and may be palpated within the adnexal areas.

These are pleomorphic tumors. The epithelial component is commonly adenocarcinoma in 95% and occasionally squamous cell carcinoma. The mesenchymal component is dominantly endometrial stromal sarcoma and rarely leiomyosarcoma. The constituents of the

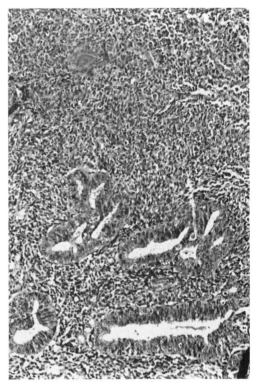

Figure 9 Carcinosarcoma (homologous malignant mixed mesodermal tumor): malignant glands and malignant homologous stroma.

heterologous component in order of frequency are rhabdomyoblasts, chondroblasts, osteoblasts, and lipoblasts.

The prognosis for carcinosarcoma and mixed mesodermal tumors is universally poor (147, 148). The treatment as with other sarcomas is total abdominal hysterectomy, bilateral salpingo-oophorectomy, surgical staging if the disease is confined to the uterus or attempts at debulking all extrauterine disease. Consideration has to be given for adjuvant chemotherapy or whole abdominal radiation therapy for these lesions.

Adenosarcoma (see Chapter 4)

In 1974 Clement and Scully reported on 10 cases of an unusual type of mullerian mixed tumor of the uterus, they designated as mullerian adenosarcoma (149). This polypoid and

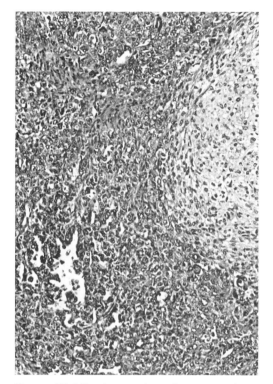

Figure 10 Mixed mesodermal tumor: adeno-carcinoma and heterologous sarcoma (stromal sarcoma with chondrosarcoma).

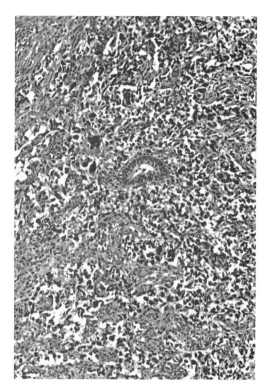

Figure 11 High grade adenosarcoma, heter-ologous: benign glandular component and malignant mesenchymal component with giant rhabdomyoblastic element.

papillary biphasic tumor is characterized by a malignant endometrial stroma resembling homologous or heterologous stromal sarcoma and a benign appearing epithelial component (Figure 11). The epithelium is proliferative and sometimes hyperplastic but not carcino-matous. Originally, these tumors were differ-entiated from the aggressive mixed mesoder-mal sarcomas by being considered to have low malignant potential, with occurrences gener-ally being local. These lesions must also be differentiated from the benign uterine adenofi-bromas which have histologically benign stro-mal and epithelial components (150–153).

The most common presenting symptom is postmenopausal bleeding. These tumors often fill the endometrial cavity and are bulky and polypoid appearing growths. Treatment should be TAH/BSO and surgical staging of the neoplasm. Optimal adjuvant therapy has not been substantiated to date. However, these

tumors are more aggressive than originally described with not only local (vaginal) occur-rence being more common in 30% but with a mortality rate of 24%. The median interval between diagnosis and recurrence approaches 5 years suggesting long periods of observation are needed to produce cures (154, 159). Over 90 cases of adenosarcoma have now been reported including extra-endometrial tumors in the cervix, ovary, round and broad liga-ments (160–166). The use of a postoperative vaginal cylinder to treat the apex of the vagina has reduced local recurrence rates. The role of adjuvant pelvic radiotherapy or systemic chemotherapy still awaits further trials.

Endolymphatic Stromal Myosis (ESM)

Endolymphatic stromal myosis is a low grade

uterine sarcoma which has perplexed gynecologists and oncologists for years due to confusing terminology and to a benign histologic
appearance coupled to a malignant clinical
behaviour. Duran and Lockyer described the
first case of endolymphatic stromal myosis in
the English literature and called it uterine
stromatosis (167). In 1946 Henderson suggested the name endolymphatic stromal myosis for this entity based on the pathologic
feature of growth within dilated venous and
lymphatic channels (168). TeLind on a review
of Henderson's paper felt a more appropriate
term would be stromatosis (169). Since these
early descriptions came a miriad of terms
including proliferative stromatosis, stromal
adenomyosis, malignant stromatosis, endometriosis interstitial, stromatoid mural sarcoma,
endometrial stromatosis, and finally low grade
endometrial stromal sarcoma. Low grade
endometrial stromal sarcoma appears to be the
most appropriate term because of the lesion's
benign appearance. There is little or no cellular atypia and a low mitotic rate (170). The
uterus is moderately enlarged and on sectioning shows yellowish tan worm-like tissue projecting into vessels, the myometrium and
broad ligament. This lesion generally shows
irregular nests and sheets of spindle stromal
cells with ovoid vesicular nuclei and little
cytoplasm invading the full length of the
myometrium and protruding into vascular
and lymphatic spaces within the uterus and
often in extrauterine sites (Figure 12).

The diagnosis of ESM is rarely made preoperatively. The patient generally presents
with abnormal uterine bleeding or a myomatous uterus and only at surgery and on histologic review is the diagnosis confirmed. Seventy
to eighty per cent of patients with this lesion are
initially felt to have Stage I disease although
extension beyond the uterus and to contiguous
structures is found in about 30–40% of patients
(170–172). Recurrent disease both locally and
distant occurs in nearly 50% of patients.
Recurrences beyond 5 years after initial surgery are common with recurrences as late as 25
years having been reported (173, 174).

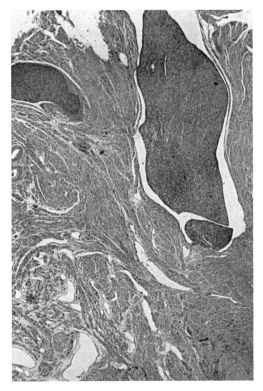

Figure 12 Endolymphatic stromal myosis: neoplastic endometrial stromal tissue within vessels
of myometrium.

Optimal therapy for this lesion consists of
laparotomy, TAH/BSO and surgical staging.
Adjuvant therapy should consist of pelvic
radiation to prevent the local recurrences and
consideration should be given to progesterone
therapy since there is evidence that this lesion is
hormonally dependent. Complete responses to
progesterone therapy have been reported (173,
174).

Mesenchymal Tumors—Heterologous Sarcomas

This group of sarcomas is extraordinarily rare.
It has been suggested that these lesions arise
from the endometrial stromal cells which are
felt to be multi-potential and by a process of
metaplasia produce these heterologous elements. The most frequent albeit rare heterolo-

gous sarcoma is the rhabdomyosarcoma with some 50 reported (175–178), followed by chrondrosarcomas with 13 being (179–181) reported, and 8 cases of uterine osteosarcoma (182–186).

Generally, these lesions present with uterine bleeding or an abdominal–pelvic mass in the postmenopausal patient. They form large polypoid masses which fill the endometrial cavity often invading the myometrium and frequently prolapsing through the cervix. Histologically all of these sarcomas look identical to those occurring in the more common sites of origin. With few such cases being reported but with the extremely aggressive behavior, treatment must consist of TAH/BSO and attempts at cytoreduction of tumor beyond the uterus. Consideration must be given for whole abdominal radiation and adjuvant chemotherapy.

Angiosarcoma

Uterine hemangiosarcomas are extremely unusual with only 9 cases in the current literature (187, 188). Benign vascular tumors, hemangiomas, have been frequently reported.

These patients as with other sarcomas present with vaginal bleeding and have a high recurrence rate despite surgery and radiation therapy since they metastasize mainly through the blood stream. Future treatment of these tumors should continue to be surgical staging and extirpation of the pelvic organs with consideration of chemotherapy and/or a combination of radiation therapy and chemotherapy (189).

Fibrosarcomas

Three cases of fibrosarcoma have been reported in the literature with no survivor whether treatment consisted of surgery or surgery and irradiation therapy. Consideration must be given towards systemic chemotherapy with or without radiation therapy in these patients (190).

Uterine Tumors Resembling Ovarian Sex Cord Tumors

These uterine tumors closely resemble histologically the ovarian sex cord tumors and are frequently interpreted as granulosa cell tumors although some have been reported as of the Sertoli cell type. Generally these patients present with an enlarged uterus or abnormal bleeding. The majority of these tumors appear benign; however, a few cases have been reported with metastasis (191). Origin of these lesions is unknown, though it has been suggested that they arise from displaced ovarian tissue. Clement and Scully reported uterine tumors histologically resembling gonadal stromal tumors with prominent tubular, trabecular and plexiform patterns. They decided that these lesions were of endometrial stromal origin (191). Foci suggestive of epithelial differentiation are frequently seen in stromal sarcomas and should not be confused with poorly differentiated endometrial adenocarcinoma. There is only a small number of cases being reported to date. Larger series are necessary to establish the potential malignancy of these lesions. It does appear that the small well differentiated and circumscribed lesions are benign. However, these patients should be followed at regular intervals until more data are available. Optimal therapy depends on the age of the patient. Generally, total abdominal hysterectomy, bilateral salpingo-oophorectomy for localized disease (Stage I and II) and consideration of radiotherapy with chemotherapy for the more advanced lesions is appropriate therapy.

Treatment of Uterine Sarcomas

Treatment of uterine sarcomas remains very difficult since these lesions spread not only to contiguous pelvic structures but via lymphatics and hematogenously. Even when the disease appears localized to the uterus (Stage I and II) nearly 50% will recur and of those 50% will recur outside of the pelvis with the lung being the primary site. The initial step should be exploratory laparotomy with TAH/BSO and sampling of regional and para-aortic nodes. Attempts at tumor reduction should be made if the disease is extrauterine at surgery. Adjuvant therapy or additional therapy consisting of irradiation and/or chemotherapy can only be rationally planned after a review of the surgical and histological findings (192–209). The role of pelvic radiotherapy alone remains controversial in that some of the uterine sarcomas are radio resistant (120, 192, 193, 196). It would appear that surgery and pelvic radiotherapy for mixed mesodermal tumors and endometrial stromal tumors (Stage I and II) probably increases the disease free progression interval and increases pelvic control of recurrence; however, it may not improve survival. Therefore, it is necessary to consider chemotherapy for metastatic lesions and for localized Stage I and II sarcomas. Several agents including cyclophosphamide, vincristine, Adriamycin, and DTIC appear to be active as single agents and perhaps in combination against sarcomas (194, 195, 197, 199, 210–209). Recent interests in etoposide, ifosfamide and cis-platinum (207, 208) have provided three more agents for use against uterine sarcomas. Future trials must consider these agents for use both in metastatic lesions and in an adjuvant fashion for localized disease in order to improve upon the dismal survival for these extremely aggressive and lethal endometrial lesions.

LYMPHOMAS

Secondary genital tract involvement by lymphoma occurs in nearly 40% of patients and in almost 41% of patients with leukemia. However, primary malignant lymphoma of the uterus is extremely rare with only some 28 cases reported (210–220). Criteria for primary lymphoma were specified by Fox and Moore and consist of localization of the disease to the uterus at initial diagnosis, the absence of the leukemic blood picture and survival for at least several months without appearance of lymphoma at other sites (220). 'Histiocytic lymphoma' or 'reticulum cell sarcoma' appears to

be the most common histologic diagnosis accounting for 68% followed by lymphocytic lymphoma in 18% and Hodgkin's disease in 14% (212). In the majority of these recorded cases the cervix is the most common site of involvement although the endometrium or uterus is involved in nearly 11%.

The majority of patients present with abnormal uterine or vaginal bleeding and diagnosis is made on cervical and endometrial biopsies. This is in distinct contrast to those patients that are found to have disseminated lymphoma involving the genital tract in which case they are usually asymptomatic. With such a small number of cases and no universal therapy, treatment must be individualized. Exact extent of disease must be defined prior to any form of therapy which will usually include radiation and chemotherapy.

PLACENTAL SITE TROPHOBLASTIC TUMOR

This lesion deserves some attention as being an unusual tumor of the endometrium with only about 42 cases reported to date (221). Originally the term trophoblastic pseudotumor was proposed by Kurman et al. in 1976 (222) because of the allegedly benign behavior of this tumor. The prognosis in those 12 reported cases was excellent. It was not until further reports were available in which deaths occurred, some with metastases, that Scully and Young proposed the name of placental site trophoblastic tumor for these lesions since they are clinically malignant (223).

These unusual lesions may occur or follow normal pregnancy, abortion or hydatidiform mole. Histologically these tumors appear as polypoid firm masses projecting into the endometrial cavity almost appearing like a placental polyp. Other lesions may occupy the myometrium appearing like adenomyosis. Extension and infiltration of tumor into the parametrium and to the broad ligament resembling uterine sarcomas is not uncommon. This lesion is generally cellular with mononuclear and multinuclear cells infiltrating the uterus and blood vessels. Unlike the bimorphic cell components (syncytiotrophoblasts and cytotrophoblasts) of choriocarcinoma, placental site trophoblastic tumor is composed of only one cell type with deciduoid cytology and strains positive for human placental lactogen by the immunoperoxidabe method favoring its trophoblastic nature. Chorionic villi are not found. Hypercellularity, foci of necrosis, clear or slightly granular cytoplasm and eight to twelve mitoses per ten high power fields are the histologic features (223). Frequently these lesions spontaneously regress or if bleeding persists can be cured with curettage or hysterectomy. A more malignant form of this lesion occurs with extension into contiguous structures, distant metastasis or uterine perforation.

These lesions must be considered as potentially malignant and therefore follow-up as with gestational trophoblastic disease is mandatory (223–229). This relatively new lesion must be considered in the differential diagnosis of persistent uterine bleeding after an antecedent pregnancy event and HCG titers must be appropriately followed.

METASTATIC LESIONS TO THE UTERINE CORPUS

The uterus as harboring metastasis from extragenital tumors is very unusual. The most common extrapelvic tumors metastasizing to the uterus are from the breast, followed by the stomach or colon, pancreas, gall bladder, lung, melanoma, kidney or bladder and the thyroid (230). These lesions generally effect the myometrium rather than the endometrium. In only about 25% cases does the uterus harbor the first signs and symptoms of the malignancy (231). Usually the uterus is involved only at the time of widespread dissemination of the extragenital lesion. These metastatic lesions spread to the uterus via lymphatic or hematogenous pathways (232–236). Carcinomas of the cervix, rectosignoid colon, urinary bladder and ovary invade the uterus directly or by lymphatic channels. Treatment for these lesions obviously must be individualized and

control of the primary tumor is most important.

SIMULTANEOUS OVARIAN AND UTERINE MALIGNANCY

Synchronous primary neoplasms of the endometrium and ovary are uncommon but well recognized. Difficulty frequently arises in whether to classify these lesions as Stage III adenocarcinoma of the endometrium or FIGO Stage II ovarian carcinoma. FIGO has ruled that cancers involving both organs should be staged according to the organ where the original symptoms developed (237). It appears that endometrioid carcinomas of the ovary and a simultaneous adenocarcinoma of the endometrium is the most common occurrence in about 15% of patients (237). These lesions appear to have a better prognosis than the non-endometrioid ovarian lesions with simultaneous occurrence of adenocarcinoma of the endometrium (238, 239).

Appropriate therapy includes TAH/BSO and surgical staging. Pelvic radiotherapy should be considered if the ovarian lesion is confined to the pelvis, if extrapelvic disease is found consideration should be given to systemic chemotherapy or a combination of radiation and systemic chemotherapy.

ENDOMETRIAL MALACOPLAKIA

At least 3 cases of endometrial malacoplakia have been described. The first was in 1969 followed by a second report in 1978 and most recently in 1983 (240–242). These patients have all presented with uterine bleeding and curettage produces yellowish nodular material with fragments of necrotic material. The importance of this lesion is to differentiate it from an endometrial carcinoma for which it is frequently clinically mistaken. This is probably a lesion caused from bacilliform microorganisms (243). Histologically it is a xanthogranulomatous inflammatory lesion with large numbers of histiocytes, lymphocytes and other leukocytes; intracellular and extracellular

Michaelis–Gutmann bodies (bacterial parts by electron microscopy) are present. Generally, these lesions can be treated with antibiotics after appropriate cultures and no further therapy is indicated.

REFERENCES

1 Cancer Statistics. American Cancer Society Publication. 1986; 36: 9–41.
2 Classification and staging of malignant tumors in the female pelvis. ACOG Tech Bull 47: June 1977.
3 Scully RE. Cancer of uterine corpus—pathologic types. radiat Oncol Biol Phys 1980; 6: 361–3.
4 Boronow RC, Morrow CP, Creasman WT, et al. Surgical staging in endometrial cancer: clinical–pathologic findings of a prospective study. Obstet Gynecol 1984; 63: 825–32.
5 Piver MS, Malfetano JH. Natural history, investigation, and staging of carcinoma of the endometrium. In Williams CJ, Whitehouse JMA, eds Cancer of the Female Reproductive System, Vol 3. Chichester: John Wiley & Sons, 1985; 207–16.
6 Piver MS, Malfetano JH. Management of carcinoma of the endometrium. In: Williams CJ, Whitehouse JMA eds Cancer of the Female Reproductive System, Vol 3. Chichester: John Wiley & Sons, 1985; 217–37.
7 Piver MS, Lele S, Barlow JJ, Blumenson LE. Paraaortic lymph node evaluation in Stage I endometrial carcinoma. Obstet Gynecol 1982; 59: 97–100.
8 Creasman WT, Boronow RC, Morrow CP et al. Adenocarcinoma of the endometrium: its metastatic lymph node potential. Gynecol Oncol 1976; 4: 239–43.
9 Lewis BV, Stallworthy JA, Cowdell R. Adenocarcinoma of the body of the uterus. J Obstet Gynaecol Br Commonw 1970; 77: 343–8.
10 Onsrud M, Kolstad P, Mormann T. Postoperative external pelvic irradiation in carcinoma of the corpus Stage I: a controlled unilateral trial. Gynecol Oncol 1976; 4: 222–31.
11 Ng APB, Regan JW. Incidence and prognosis of endometrial carcinoma by histologic grade and extent. Obstet Gynecol 1970; 35: 437–43.
12 Jones HW. Treatment of adenocarcinoma of the endometrium. Obstet Gynecol Surv 1975; 30: 147–69.
13 McKelvey JL, Baxter JS. Abnormal development of the vagina and genitourinary tract. Am J Obstet Gynecol 1935; 29: 267–71.
14 Danagne MP, Silverberg SG. Foam cells in endometrial carcinoma: a clinico-pathologic study. Gynecol Oncol 1982; 13: 67–75.
15 Beahs OH. Manual for Staging of Cancer, 2nd edition. American Joint Committee on Cancer. Philadelphia: JB Lippincott, 1983.
16 Potish RA, Twiggs LB, Adcock LL et al. Paraaortic lymph node radiotherapy in cancer of the uterine corpus. Obstet Gynecol 1985; 65: 251–6.
17 Benson RC, Sneedon VD. Adenomyosis: A reappraisal of symptomatology. Am. J. Obstet Gynecol 1958; 76: 1044–61.
18 Bird CC, McElin TW, Manalo-Estrella P. The elusive adenomyosis of the uterus-revisited. Am. J. Obstet. Gynecol 1972; 112: 583–93.
19 Hall JB, Young RH, Nelson JH. The prognostic significance of adenomyosis in endometrial carcinoma. Gynecol Oncol 1984; 17: 32–40.
20 Hernandez ZE, Woodruff JD. Endometrial adenocarcinoma arising in adenomyosis. Am J Obstet Gynecol 1980; 138: 827–32.
21 Kurman RJ, Scully RE. Clear cell carcinoma of the endometrium. An analysis of 21 cases. Cancer 1976; 37: 872–82.
22 Silverberg SG, DeGiorgi LS. Clear cell carcinoma of the endometrium, clinical, pathological and ultrastructional findings. Cancer 1973; 31: 1127–40.
23 Christopherson WM, Alberhasky RC, Connelly, PJ. Carcinoma of the endometrium I—A clinicopathologic study of clear cell carcinoma and secretory carcinoma. Cancer 1982; 49: 1511–22.
24 Eastwood J. Mesonephroid (clear cell) carcinoma of ovary and endometrium. A comparative prospective clinicopathological study and review of literature. Cancer 1978; 41: 1911–28.
25 Brufman G, Biran S, Milwidsky A, Behar AJ. Solitary lung involvement from clear cell carcinoma of the endometrium. Int Surg 1978; 63: 86–8.
26 Carinelli SG, Senzani F. Clear cell carcinoma of endometrium. Tumor 1979; 65: 201–5.
27 Fechner RE. Endometrium with pattern of mesonephroma. Report of a case. Obstet Gynecol 1968; 31: 485–90.
28 Kay S. Clear cell carcinoma of the endometrium. Cancer 1957; 10: 124–30.
29 Photopulos GJ, Carney CN, Edelman DA et al. Clear cell carcinoma of the endometrium. Cancer 1979; 43: 1448–56.
30 Rovat E, Ferenczy A, Richart RM. The ultrastructure of clear cell adenocarcinoma of endometrium. Cancer 1974; 33: 880–7.
31 Rutledge F, Kotz HL, Chang SC. Mesonephric adenocarcinoma of the endometrium. Obstet Gynecol 1965; 25: 362–70.

32 Elton NW. Morphologic variations in adeno-carcinoma on the fundus of the uterus with reference to secretory activity and clinical interpretations. Am J Clin Pathol 1942; 12: 32–47.

33 Tiltman AJ. Mucinous carcinoma of the endometrium. Obstet Gynecol 1980; 55: 244–7.

34 Solomon C, Polishuk W. Myxometra resulting from mucous metaplasia of the endometrium. Am J Obstet Gynecol 1954; 68: 1600–3.

35 Salm R. Mucin production of normal and abnormal endometrium. Arch Pathol 1962; 73: 30–9.

36 Moore RB, Reagan JW, Schoenberg MD. The mucins of the normal and cancerous uterine mucosa. Cancer 1959; 12: 215–21.

37 Liu CT. A study of endometrial adenocarci-noma with emphasis on morphologically variant types. Am J Clin Pathol 1972; 57: 562–73.

38 Feyreter F. Uber Diffuse Endokrinen Epithaliale Organe. Leipzig: Johann Amlorosius Barth, 1938.

39 Albones-Saayedra J, Rodriquez-Martinez HA, Hernandez D. Carcinoid tumors of the cervix. Pathol Annu 1979; 14: 273–91.

40 Ueda G, Sato Y, Yamasaki M, et al. Argyro-phil cell adenocarcinoma of the endometrium. Gynecol Oncol 1978; 6: 467–73.

41 Olson N, Twiggs L, Sibley R. Small cell carcinoma of the endometrium: light micro-scopic and ultrastructural study of a case. Cancer 1982; 50: 760–5.

42 Prade M, Gadenne C. Duvillard P et al. Endometrial carcinoma with argyrophil cells. Hum Pathol 1982; 13: 870–1.

43 Kumar NB. Small cell carcinoma of the endometrium in a 23 year-old woman: light micro-scopic and ultrastructural study. Am J Clin Pathol 1984; 81: 98–101.

44 Weiss RB. Small cell carcinoma of the lung: Therapeutic management. Ann Intern Med 1979; 88: 522–31.

45 Greco FA, Oldham RK. Current concepts in cancer: small cell lung cancer. New Engl. J. Med. 1979; 301: 355–8.

46 Oldham RK, Greco FA. Small cell lung cancer, a curable disease. Cancer Chemo-therapy Pharm 1980; 4: 173–7.

47 Livingston RB, Moore TN, Heilburn L et al. Small cell carcinoma of the lung: combined chemotherapy and radiation. Ann Intern Med 1978; 88: 194–9.

48 Ng AB. Mixed carcinoma of the endometrium. Am J Obstet Gynecol 1968; 102: 506–15.

49 Sliverberg SG. Significance of squamous ele-ments in carcinoma of the endometrium: a review. Prog Surg Pathol 1982; 4: 115–36.

50 Chanen W. A clinical and pathological study of adenoacanthoma of the uterine body. J Obstet Gynaecol 1960; 67: 287–93.

51 Charles D. Endometrial adenoacanthoma. A clinicopathologic study of 55 cases. Cancer 1967; 18: 737–50.

52 Liggins GC, Way S. Comparison of the prog-nosis of adenoacanthoma and adenocarcinoma of the corpus uteri. J Obstet Gynaecol 1960; 67: 294–96.

53 Novak ER, Nalley WB. Uterine adenoacan-thoma. Obstet Gynecol 1957; 9: 396–402.

54 Ng AB, Reagan JW, Storaasli JP, Wentz WB. Mixed adeno squamous carcinoma of the endo-metrium. Am J Clin Pathol 1973; 59: 765–81.

55 Marcus SL. Adenoacanthoma of the endome-trium: a report of 24 cases and a review of squamous metaplasia. Am J Obstet Gynecol 1961; 81: 259–67.

56 Morrison DL. Adenocanthoma of the uterine body. J Obstet Gynaecol Br Commonw 1966; 72: 605–10.

57 Ayne JE. Adenoacanthoma of the uterus. Am J Obstet Gynecol 1945; 49: 261–4.

58 Pojoly TA. A comparison of the clinical be-havior of uterine adenocarcinomas and ade-noacanthomas. Am J Obstet Gynecol 1970; 108: 1080–4.

59 Salazar OM, Deppapp EW, Bonfiglio TA, Feldstein ML, Rubin P, Rudolph JH. Adeno squamous carcinoma of the endometrium. An entity with an inherent poor prognosis? Cancer 1977; 40: 119–30.

60 Haqqani MT, Fox H. Adenosquamous carci-noma of the endometrium. J Clin Pathol 1976; 29: 959–66.

61 Julian CG, Daikoku NH, Gillespie A. Adeno epidermoid and adenosquamous carcinoma of the uterus. A clinicopathologic study of 118 cases. Am J Obstet Gynecol 1977; 128: 106–16.

62 Silverberg SG, Bolin MG, DeGiorgi LS. Adenoacanthoma and mixed adenosquamous carcinoma of the endometrium. A clinicopath-ologic study. Cancer 1972; 30: 1307–14.

63 Lifshitz S, Schuberger CW, Platz CA, Robert VA. Primary squamous cell carcinoma of the endometrium. J Reprod Med 1981; 26: 25–7.

64 Datta CK, Gordon PE. Primary squamous cell carcinoma of the endometrium: A case report. W Va Med J 1980; 76: 109–10.

65 Vyas MCR, Joshi KR, Mathur DR, Sharma MM, Mathur A. Primary squamous cell carci-noma of the endometrium: Report of a case and review of literature. Indian J Pathol Microbiol 1980; 23: 289–92.

66 Yamashina M, Robara T. Primary squamous cell carcinoma with its spindle cell variant in

the endometrium: A case report and review of literature. Cancer 1986; 57: 340–5.

67 Bibro C, Kapp D, Livolsi V, Schwartz P. Squamous carcinoma of the endometrium with ultrastructural observations and review of the literature. Gynecol Oncol 1980; 10: 217–23.

68 White AJ, Buchsbaum HJ, Macasaet MA. Primary squamous cell carcinoma of the endometrium. Obstet Gynecol 1973; 41: 912–19.

69 Kay S. Squamous-cell carcinoma of the endometrium. Am J Clin Pathol 1974; 61: 264–9.

70 Melin JR, Wanner L, Schutz DM, Cassel EE. Primary squamous cell carcinoma of the endometrium. Obstet Gynecol 1979; 53: 115–19.

71 Baggish MS, Woodruff JD. The occurrence of squamous epithelium in the endometrium. Obstet Gynecol Surg 1967; 22: 69–115.

72 Fluhmann CF. Squamous epithelium in the endometrium in benign and malignant conditions. Surg Gynecol Obstet 1928; 46: 309–16.

73 Levine S, Scirsci EF. Squamous cell carcinoma of the uterine corpus and its relation to pyometra. Cancer 1966; 19: 485–8.

74 Ryder DE. Verrucous carcinoma of the endometrium—A unique neoplasm with long survival. Obstet Gynecol 1982; 59: 785–805.

75 Karus FT, Perez-Mesa C. Verrucous carcinoma: clinical and pathologic study of 105 cases involving oral cavity, larynx and genitalia. Cancer 1966; 19: 26–38.

76 Littman P, Clement PB, Hendrickson B. Glassy cell carcinoma of the cervix. Cancer 1976; 37: 22–38.

77 Swan DS, Roddick JW. A clinical–pathological correlation of cell type classification for cervical cancer. Am J Obstet Gynecol 1973; 116: 666–70.

78 Christopherson WM, Alberhasky RC, Connelly PJ. Glassy cell carcinoma of the endometrium. Hum Pathol 1982; 13: 418–21.

79 Factor SM. Papillary adenocarcinoma of the endometrium with psammoma bodies. Arch Pathol 1974; 98: 201–5.

80 Karpas CM, Bridge MF. Endometrial adenocarcinoma with psammomatous bodies. Am J Obstet Gynecol 1963; 87: 935–41.

81 Hameed K, Morgan DA. Papillary adenocarcinoma of the endometrium with psammoma bodies: histology and fine structure. Cancer 1972; 29: 1326–35.

82 Hendrickson M, Ross J, Eifel P et al. Uterine papillary serous carcinoma. A highly malignant form of endometrial adenocarcinoma. Am J Surg Pathol 1982; 6: 93–108.

83 Lauchlan SC. Tubel (serous) carcinoma of the endometrium. Arch Pathol 1981; 105: 615–18.

84 Walker AN, Mills SE. Serous papillary carci-

noma of the endometrium: a clinicopathologic study of 11 cases. Diagn Gynecol Obstet 1982; 4: 261.

85 LiVolsi VA. Adenocarcinoma of the endometrium with psammoma bodies. Obstet Gynecol 1977; 50: 725–8.

86 Kempson RL, Bari W. Uterine sarcomas: classification, diagnosis and prognosis. Hum Pathol 1970; 1: 331–50.

87 Montague ACW, Swartz DP, Woodruff JD. Sarcoma arising in a leiomyoma of the uterus. Am J Obstet Gynecol 1965; 92: 421–7.

88 Gruenwald P. Developmental basis of regenerative and pathological growth in the uterus. Arch Pathol 35: 53–65, 1943.

89 Norris HJ, Taylor HB. Mesenchymal tumors of the uterus I. A clinical and pathologic study of 53 endometrial stromal tumors. Cancer 1966; 19: 755–66.

90 Taylor HB, Norris HJ. Mesenchymal tumors of the uterus IV. Diagnosis and prognosis of leiomyosarcomas. Arch Pathol 1966; 82: 40–4.

91 Gudgeon DH. Leiomyosarcoma of the uterus. Obstet Gynecol 1968; 32: 96–100.

92 Aaro LA, Symmonds RE. Dockerty MD. Sarcoma of the uterus: a clinical and pathological study of 177 cases. Am J Obstet Gynecol 1966; 94: 101–9.

93 Badib AO, Vongtama V, Kurohara SS, Webster JH. Radiotherapy in the treatment of sarcomas of the corpus uteri. Cancer 1969; 24: 724–9.

94 Bartsich EG, O'Leary JA, Moore JG. Carcinosarcoma of the uterus: a 50-year review of 32 cases (1917–1966). Obstet Gynecol 1967; 30: 518–23.

95 Chuang JT, Van Velden JJ, Graham JR. Carcinosarcoma and mixed mesodermal tumor of the uterine corpus: review of 49 cases. Obstet Gynecol 1970; 35: 769–80.

96 Giarratano RC, Slate TA. Sarcomas of the uterus. Obstet Gynecol 1971; 38: 472–7.

97 Nieminen U, Soderlin E. Sarcoma of the corpus uteri: Results of the treatment of 117 cases. Strahlentherapie 1974; 148: 57–61.

98 Norris HJ, Taylor HB. Postirradiation sarcomas of the uterus. Obstet Gynecol 1965; 26: 689–94.

99 Salazar, OM, Bonfiglio TA, Patten SE, Keller BE, Feldstein ML, Dunne ME, Rudolf JH. Uterine sarcomas: Natural history, treatment and prognosis. Cancer 1978; 42: 1152–60.

100 Saksela E, Lampinen V, Procope BJ. Malignant mesenchymal tumors of the uterine corpus. Am J Obstet Gynecol 1974; 120: 452–60.

101 Fehr PE, Prem KA. Malignancy of the uterine corpus following irradiation therapy for squa-

mous cell carcinoma of the cervix. Am J Obstet Gynecol 1974; 119: 685–92.

102 Boyce JD, Day NE, Anderson A et al. Second cancers following radiation treatment for cervical cancer. An international collaboration among cancer registries. JNCI 1985; 74: 955–75.

103 MacFarlane KT. Sarcoma of the uterus: an analysis of 42 cases. Am J Obstet Gynecol 1950; 59: 1304–20.

104 Persaud V, Arjoon PD. Uterine leiomyoma: Incidence of degenerative change and a correlation of associated symptoms. Obstet Gynecol 1970; 35: 432–6.

105 Persaud V, Knight LP. Malignant mesenchymal tumors of the corpus uteri. W Indian Med J 1968; 17: 96.

106 Christopherson WM, Williamson EO, Gray LA. Leiomyosarcoma of the uterus. Cancer 1972; 29: 1512–17.

107 Bartsich EG, Bowe ET, Moore JG. Leiomyosarcoma of the uterus: a 50-year review of 42 cases. Obstet Gynecol 1968; 32: 101–6.

108 Bazzocchi F, Brandi G, Pileri S et al. Clinical and pathologic prognostic features of Leiomyosarcoma of the uterus. Tumor 1983; 69: 75–7.

109 Barter JF, Smith EB, et al. Leiomyosarcoma of the uterus: clinicopathologic study of 21 cases. Gynecol Oncol 1985; 21: 220–7.

110 Lavin P, Hajdu SI, Foote FW. Gastric and extragastric leiomyoblastomas. Clinicopathologic study of 44 cases. Cancer 1972; 29: 305–11.

111 Kurman RJ, Norris HJ. Mesenchymal tumors of the uterus. VI. Epithelial smooth muscle tumors including leiomyoblastoma and clear-cell leiomyoma. A clinical and pathologic analysis of 26 cases. Cancer 1976; 37: 1853–6.

112 Chang V, Aikawa M, Druet R. Uterine leiomyoblastoma. Ultrastructural and cytological studies. Cancer 1977; 39: 1563–9.

113 Rywlin AM, Recher L, Benson J. Clear cell leiomyoma of the uterus. Report of 2 cases of a previously undescribed entity. Cancer 1964; 17: 100–4.

114 Hendrickson MR, Kempson RL. Smooth muscle neoplasms. In: Surgical Pathology of the Uterine Corpus. Philadelphia: WB Saunders, 1980: 468–529.

115 Hart WR, Billman JK. A reassessment of uterine neoplasms originally diagnosed as leiomyosarcomas. Cancer 1978; 41: 1902–10.

116 Fleming WP, Peters WA et al. Autopsy findings in patients with uterine sarcoma. Gynecol Oncol 1972; 19: 168–72.

117 Silverberg SG. Leiomyosarcoma of the uterus. A clinicopathologic study. Obstet Gynecol 1971; 38: 613–28.

118 Dinh TV, Woodruff JD. Leiomyosarcoma of the uterus. Am J Obstet Gynecol 1982; 144: 817–23.

119 Peters WA, Kvmar NB, Fleming WP, Morley GW. Prognostic feature of sarcomas and mixed tumors of the endometrium. Obstet Gynecol 1984; 63: 550–6.

120 Vongtama V, Karlan J, Piver S et al. Treatment, results and prognostic factors in Stage I and II sarcomas of the corpus uteri. Am J Roent Rad Ther Med 1976; 126: 139–47.

121 Norris HJ, Parmley T. Mesenchymal tumors of the uterus, V. Intravenous leiomyomatosis. A clinical and pathological study of 14 cases. Cancer 1975; 36: 2164–78.

122 Scharfenberg JC, Geary WL. Intravenous leiomyomatosis. Obstet Gynecol 1974; 43: 909–14.

123 Thompson JW, Symmonds RE, Dockerty MB. Benign uterine leiomyoma with vascular involvement. Report of 3 cases. Am J Obstet Gynecol 1962; 84: 182–6.

124 Miller JN. Pregnancy complicated by intravenous leiomyomatosis. Am J Obstet Gynecol 1975; 122: 485–9.

125 Bachman D, Wolff M. Pulmonary metastases from benign-appearing smooth muscle tumors of the uterus. Am J Roentgenol 1976; 127: 441–6.

126 Barnes HM, Richardson PJ. Benign metastasizing fibroleiomyoma. Br J Obstet Gynaecol 1973; 80: 569–73.

127 Boyce CR, Buddhdev HN. Pregnancy complicated by metastasizing leiomyoma of uterus. Obstet Gynecol 1973; 42: 52–8.

128 Clark DH, Weed JC. Metastasizing leiomyoma: a case report. Am J Obstet Gynecol. 1977; 127: 672–3.

129 Horstmann JP, Pietra GG, Harman JA, Cole NG, Grinspan S. Spontaneous regression of pulmonary leiomyomas during pregnancy. Cancer 1977; 39: 314–21.

130 Idelson MG, Davids AM. Metastases of uterine fibroleiomyomata. Obstet Gynecol 1963; 21: 78–85.

131 Kaplan C, Katoh A, Shamoto M, Rogow E, Scott JH, Cushing W, Cooper J. Multiple leiomyomas of the lung: benign or malignant. Am Rev Respir Dis 1973; 108: 656–9.

132 Konis EE, Belsky RD. Metastasizing leiomyoma of the uterus. Report of a case. Obstet Gynecol 1966; 27: 442–6.

133 Pocock E, Craig JR, Bullock WK. Metastatic uterine leiomyomata. A case report. Cancer 1976; 38: 2096–100.

134 Spiro RH, McPeak CJ. On the so-called metastasizing leiomyoma. Cancer 1966; 19: 544–8.

135 Tench WD, Dail D, Gmelich JT. Benign

metastasizing leiomyomas: a review of 21 cases (abstract). Lab Med 1978; 38: 37.

136 Abell MR, Littler ER. Benign metastasizing uterine leiomyoma: multiple lymph node metastases. Cancer 1975; 36: 2206–13.

137 Goldberg MF, Hurt WG, Frable WJ. Leiomyomatosis peritonealis disseminata. Report of a case and review of the literature. Obstet Gynecol. 1977; 49: 465–525.

138 Aterman K, Fraser GM, Lea RH. Disseminated peritoneal leiomyomatosis. Virchows Arch (A Pathol Anat Histol) 1977; 374: 13–26.

139 Crosland DB. Leiomyomatosis peritonealis disseminata: A case report. Am J Obstet Gynecol. 1973; 117: 179–81.

140 Nogales FF, Matilla A, Carrascal E. Leiomyomatosis peritonealis disseminata. An ultrastructural study. Am J Clin Pathol 1978; 69: 452–7.

141 Parmley TH, Woodruff JD, Winn K, Johnson JWC, Douglas PH. Histogenesis of leiomyomatosis peritonealis disseminata (disseminated fibrosing deciduosis). Obstet Gynecol 1975; 46: 511–16.

142 Taubert H, Wissner SE, Haskins AL. Leiomyomatosis peritonealis disseminata. An unusual complication of genital leiomyomata. Obstet Gynecol 1965; 25: 561–74.

143 Winn KJ, Woodruff JD, Parmley TH. Electronmicroscopic studies of leiomyomatosis peritonealis disseminata. Obstet Gynecol 1976; 48: 225–7.

144 Edwards DL, Peacock JF. Intravenous leiomyomatosis of the uterus. Report of 2 cases. Obstet Gynecol 1966; 27: 176–181.

145 Harper RS, Scully RE. Intravenous leiomyomatosis of the uterus. A report of 4 cases. Obstet Gynecol 1961; 18: 519–29.

146 Yoonessi M, Hart WR. Endometrial stromal sarcomas. Cancer 1977; 40: 898–906.

147 Doss LL, Clovens AS, Henriquez EM: Carcinosarcoma of the uterus: a 40 year experience from the state of Missouri. Gynecol Oncol 1984; 18: 43–53.

148 Kahadpaa KV, Wahlstrom T, Grohn P, et al. Sarcomas of the uterus: a clinicopathologic study of 119 patients. Obstet Gynecol 1986; 67: 417–24.

149 Clement PB, Scully RE. Mullerian adenosarcoma of the uterus. A clinicopathologic analysis of 10 cases of a distinctive type of mullerian mixed tumor. Cancer 1974; 34: 1138–49.

150 Zalouder CJ, Norms HJ. Adenofibroma and adenosarcoma of the uterus: a clinicopathologic study of 35 cases. Cancer 1981; 48: 354–66.

151 Abell MR. Papillary adenofibroma of the uterine cervix. Am J Obstet Gynecol 1971; 110: 990–3.

152 Grimalt M, Arguelles M, Ferenczy A. Papillary cystadenofibroma of endometrium: a histochemical and ultrastructural study. Cancer 1975; 36: 137–144.

153 Vellios F, Ng ABP, Reagan JW. Papillary adenofibroma of the uterus: a benign mesodermal mixed tumor of mullerian origin. Am J Clin Pathol 1973; 60: 543–51.

154 Clement PB, Scully RE. Extrauterine mesodermal (mullerian) adenosarcoma. A clinicopathologic analysis of five cases. Am J Clin Pathol 1978; 9: 276–83.

155 Katzenstein ALA, Askin FB, Feldman PS. Mullerian adenosarcoma of the uterus. An ultrastructural study of four cases. Cancer 1977; 40: 2233–42.

156 Bibro MC, LiVolsi VA, Schwartz PE. Adenosarcoma of the uterus. Ultrastructural observations. Am J Clin Pathol 1978; 71: 112–17.

157 Borello DJ, Wood WG, Newman RL. Mullerian adenosarcoma: Two additional cases with ultrastructural observations. Am J Diag Gynecol Obstet 1979; 1: 275–82.

158 Gloor E. Mullerian adenosarcoma of the uterus. Clinicopathologic report of five cases. Am J Surg Pathol 1979; 3: 203–9.

159 Fox H, Havilal KR, Youell A. Mullerian adenosarcoma of the uterine body: a report of nine cases. Histopathology 1979; 3: 167–80.

160 Fayem AO, Ali M, Braun EV. Mullerian adenosarcoma of the uterine cervix. Am J Obstet Gynecol 1978; 130: 734–5.

161 Roth LM, Pride GL, Sharma HM. Mullerian adenosarcoma of the uterine cervix with heterologous elements. A light and electron microscopic study. Cancer 1976; 37: 1725–36.

162 Valdex VA, Planas AT, Lopez VF et al. Adenosarcoma of uterus and ovary. A clinicopathologic study of two cases. Cancer 1979; 43: 1439–47.

163 Bard ES, Bard DS, Vargas-Cortez F. Extrauterine mullerian adenosarcoma; a clinicopathologic report of a case with distant metastases and review of the literature. Gynecol Oncol 1978; 6: 261–74.

164 Kao GF, Norris HJ. Benign and low grade variants of mixed mesodermal tumor (adenosarcoma) of the ovary and adnexal region. Cancer 1978; 42: 1314–24.

165 Czernogilsky B, Gillespie JJ, Roth L. Adenosarcoma of the ovary. A light and electron-microscopic study with review of the literature. Diag Gynecol Obstet 1982; 4: 25–36.

166 Czernobilsky B, Hohlneg-Majert P, Dallenbach-Hellneg G. Uterine adenosarcoma: a clinicopathologic study of 11 cases with a reevaluation of histologic criteria. Arch Gynecol 1983; 233: 281–94.

167 Doran AHG, Lockyer C. Two cases of uterine
    fibroids showing peritheliomatous changes;
    long immunity from recurrence after oper-
    ation. Proc R Soc Med 1908; 2: 25–39.
168 Henderson DN. Endolymphatic stromal myo-
    sis. Am J Obstet Gynecol 1946; 52: 1000–2.
169 TeLind RW. Discussion of Henderson: endo-
    lymphatic stromal myosis. Am J Obstet Gyne-
    col 1946; 52: 1000–12.
170 Kreiger PD, Gusberg SB. Endolymphatic stro-
    mal myosis—A Grade I endometrial sarcoma.
    Gynecol Oncol 1973; 1: 299–313.
171 Hart WR, Yoonessi M. Endometrial stromato-
    sis of the uterus. Obstet Gynecol 1977; 49: 393–
    403.
172 Piver MS, Rutledge RN, Copeland L, Webster
    K, Blumenson L, Suh O. Uterine endolym-
    phatic stromal myosis: a collaborative study.
    Obstet Gynecol 1984; 64: 173–8.
173 Pellillo D. Proliferative stromatosis of the uter-
    us with pulmonary metastases. Remission fol-
    lowing treatment with a longacting synthetic
    progestin: a case report. Obstet Gynecol 1968;
    31: 33–9.
174 Gloor E, Schnyder P, Cikes M et al. Endolym-
    phatic stromal myosis: surgical and hormonal
    treatment of extensive abdominal recurrence
    20 years after hysterectomy. Cancer 1982; 50:
    1888–93.
175 Donkers B, Kazzaz BA, Meijering JH. Rhab-
    domyosarcoma of the corpus uteri. Am J
    Obstet Gynecol 1972; 114: 1025–30.
176 Hart WR, Craig JR. Rhabdomyosarcoma of
    the uterus. Am J Clin Pathol 1978; 70: 271–3.
177 Gliazali S. Embryonic rhabdomyosarcomas of
    the urogenital tract. Br J Surg 1973; 60: 120–8.
178 Middlebrook LF, Tennant R. Rhabdomyosar-
    coma of the uterine corpus. Obstet Gynecol
    1968; 32: 537–41.
179 Clement PB. Chondrosarcoma of the uterus:
    report of a case and review of the literature.
    Hum Pathol 1978; 9: 726–32.
180 Hartfall SJ. Chondro-sarcoma of the uterus. J
    Obstet Gynecol Brit Emp 1931; 38: 593–600.
181 Pena EF. Primary chondrosarcoma of the
    uterus. Am J Obstet Gynecol 1951; 61: 461–4.
182 Amromin GD, Gildenhorn HL. Review of
    pathogenesis of primary osteogenic sarcoma of
    the uterus and adnexa. Report of 2 cases. Am J
    Obstet Gynecol 1962; 83: 1574–8.
183 Carleton CC, Williamson JW. Osteogenic sar-
    coma of the uterus. Arch Pathol Lab Med
    1961; 72: 121–5.
184 Karpas CM, Menendino JJ. Uterine osteoge-
    nic sarcoma: histochemical studies and report
    of a case. Obstet Gynecol 1964; 24: 629–33.
185 Scheffey LC, Levinson J, Herbert PA, et al.

Osteosarcoma of the uterus. Report of a case.
    Obstet Gynecol 1956; 8: 444–50.
186 Crum LP, Rogers BH, Andersen W. Osteosar-
    coma of the uterus: case report and review of
    the literature. Gynecol Oncol 1980; 9: 256–68.
187 Ongkasuwan C, Raylor JE, Tang CK, Prem-
    pree T. Angiosarcomas of the uterus and ovary:
    clinicopathologic report. Cancer 1982; 49:
    1469–75.
188 Ehrmann RL, Griffiths CT. Malignant
    hemangioendothelioma of the uterus. Gynecol
    Oncol 1979; 8: 376–83.
189 Gerbie AB. Hirsch MR, Greene RR. Vascular
    tumors of the female genital tract. Obstet
    Gynecol 1955; 6: 499–507.
190 Mantravadi RVP, Bardawil WA, Lochman
    OT et al. Uterine sarcomas: an analysis of 69
    patients. Int J Rad Oncol Biol Phys 1981; 7:
    917–22.
191 Clement PB, Scully RE. Uterine tumors resem-
    bling ovarian sex cord tumors. A clinicopatho-
    logic analysis of fourteen cases. Am J Clin
    Pathol 1976; 66: 512–25.
192 Salazar OM, Bonfiglio TA, Patten SE, et al.
    Uterine sarcomas. Analysis of failures with
    special emphasis on the use of adjuvant radia-
    tion therapy. Cancer 1978; 42: 1161–70.
193 Salazar OM, Dunne ME. The role of radiation
    therapy in the management of uterine sarco-
    mas. Int J Rad Oncol Biol Phy 1980; 6: 899–
    902.
194 Azizi F, Bitran J, Javehari G, Herbst AL.
    Remission of uterine leiomyosarcomas treated
    with vincristine, Adriamycin and dimethyl-
    triazeno-imidazole carboxamide. Am J Obstet
    Gynecol 1979; 133: 379–81.
195 Barlow JJ, Piver MS, Chnang JR et al. Adria
    mycin and bleomycin, alone and in combina-
    tion in gynecologic cancers. Cancer 1973; 32:
    735–43.
196 Perez CA, Askin F, Baglan RJ et al. Effects of
    irradiation on mixed mullerian tumors of the
    uterus. Cancer 1979; 43: 1274–84.
197 Thigpen JT, Shingleton H, Homesley H. A
    phase II trial of cisdiamminedichloroplatinum
    (CDDP) in treatment of advanced or recurrent
    mixed mesodermal sarcoma of the uterus. Proc
    ASCO 1982; 1: 110, (Abstract).
198 DiSaia PJ, Morrow CP, Boronow R et al.
    Endometrial sarcoma: lymphatic spread pat-
    tern. Am J Obstet Gynecol 1978; 130: 104–5.
199 Piver MS, DeEulis TG, Lele SB et al. Cyclo-
    phosphamide, vincristine, adriamycin and
    dimethyltriazen imidazole carboxamide
    (CYVADIC) for sarcomas of the female genital
    tract. Gynecol Oncol 1982; 14: 319–23.
200 Edwards CL. Undifferentiated tumors in

Cancer of the Uterus and Ovary: A Collection of Papers Presented at the 11th Annual Clinical Conference on Cancer at the MD Anderson Hospital and Tumor Institute, Chicago. Year Book Medical Publishers, 1969; 89.

201 Omura GA, Major FJ, Blessing JA, et al. A randomized study of Adriamycin with and without Dimethyltriazenoimidazole carboxamide in advanced uterine sarcomas. Cancer 1983; 52: 626–32.

202 Blum RH, Carter SK. Adriamycin: a new anticancer drug with significant clinical activity. Ann Intern Med 1974; 80: 249–59.

203 Jacobs EM. Combination chemotherapy of metastatic testicular germ cell tumors and soft part sarcomas. Cancer 1970; 25: 324–32.

204 Hannigan EV, Freedman RS, Elder FW et al. Treatment of advanced uterine sarcoma with vincristine, actinomycin-D and cyclophosphamide. Gynecol Oncol 1983; 15: 224–9.

205 Smith JP, Rutledge F, Delclos L, Suton W. Combined irradiation and chemotherapy for sarcomas of the pelvis in females. Am J. Roentgenol. 1976; 123: 571–6.

206 Yazigi R, Piver MS, Barlow JJ. Stage III uterine sarcoma: case report and literature review. Gynecol. Oncol. 1979; 8: 92–6.

207 Thigpen JT, Blessing JA, Orr JW, DiSaia, PJ. Phase II trial of cisplatin in the treatment of patients with advanced or recurrent mixed mesodermal sarcomas of the uterus: a gynecologic oncology group study. Cancer Treat Rep 1986; 70: 271–4.

208 Piver MS, Lele SB, Patsner B. Cis-diamminedichloroplatinum plus dimethyl-triazenoimidazole carboxamide as second and third line chemotherapy for sarcomas of the female pelvis. Gynecol Oncol 1986; 23: 371–5.

209 Gottlieb JA, Benjamin RS, Barus LH, et al. Role of (NSC-45388) in the chemotherapy of sarcoma. Cancer Treat Rep 1976; 60: 199–203.

210 Gall JA, Sartiano G, Deutsch M. Primary reticulum cell sarcoma of the uterus. Oncology 1975; 31: 157–63.

211 Johnson CE, Soule EH. Malignant lymphoma as a gynecologic problem. Obstet Gynecol 1957; 9: 149–57.

212 Lathrop JC. Malignant pelvic lymphomas. Obstet Gynecol 1967; 30: 137–45.

213 Kapadia SB, Krause JR, Kanbour AI, Hartsock RJ. Granulocytic sarcoma of the uterus. Cancer 1978; 41: 687–91.

214 Cihak RW, Hamada J. Primary reticulum cell sarcoma of the uterus. A case report and review of the literature. Cancer 1974; 33: 1039–44.

215 Anderson GG. Hodgkin's disease of the uterine cervix. Obstet Gynecol 1967; 29: 170–2.

216 Welch JW, Helwig CA. Reticulum cell sarcoma of the uterine cervix. Obstet Gynecol 1963; 22: 293–4.

217 Chorlton I, Karnei RF, King FM, Norris HJ. Primary malignant reticuloendothelial disease involving the vagina, cervix and corpus uteri. Obstet Gynecol 1974; 44: 735–48.

218 Hahn GA. Gynecologic consideration in malignant lymphomas. Am J Obstet Gynecol 1958; 75: 673–83.

219 Wright WE. Solitary malignant lymphoma of the uterus. Am J Obstet Gynecol 1973; 117: 114–20.

220 Fox H, Moore JRS. Primary malignant lymphoma of the uterus. J Clin Path 1965; 18: 723–8.

221 Young RH, Scully RE, McCluskey RT. A distinctive glomerular lesion complicating placental site trophoblastic tumor: report of two cases. Hum Pathol 1985; 16: 35–42.

222 Kurman RJ, Scully RE, Norris HJ. Trophoblastic pseudotumor of the uterus: an exaggerated form of "syncytial endometritis" simulating a malignant tumor. Cancer 1976; 38: 1214–26.

223 Scully RE, Young RH. Trophoblastic pseudotumor: a reappraisal. Am J Surg Pathol 1981; 5: 75–6.

224 Driscoll SG. Placental-site chorioma. The neoplasm of the implantation site trophoblast. J Reprod Med 1984; 29: 821–5.

225 Blackwell JB, Papadimitrion JM. Trophoblastic pseudotumor of the uterus. Cancer 1979; 43: 1734–41.

226 Eckstein RP, Paradinas FJ, Bagshore KD. Placental site trophoblastic tumour (trophoblastic pseudotumor): a study of four cases requiring hysterectomy including one fatal case. Histopathology 1982; 6: 211–26.

227 Gloor E, Hurlimann J. Trophoblastic pseudotumor of the uterus: clinicopathologic report with immunohistochemical and ultrastructural studies. Am J Surg Pathol 1981; 5: 5–13.

228 Rossenshein NB, Wijhen H, Woodruff JD. Clinical importance of the diagnosis of trophoblastic pseudotumors. Am J Obstet Gynecol 1980; 136: 635–8.

229 Twiggs LB, Okagaki T, Phillips GL et al. Trophoblastic pseudotumor: evidence of malignant disease potential. Gynecol Oncol 1981; 12: 238–48.

230 Kumar NB, Hart WR. Metastases to the uterine corpus from extragenital cancers. A clinicopathologic study of 63 cases. Cancer 1982; 50: 2163–9.

231 Mazur MT, Hsueh S, Gersell DJ. Metastases to

the female genital tract. Analysis of 325 cases. Cancer 1984; 53: 1978–84.

232 Charache H. Metastatic carcinoma in the uterus. Am J Surg 1941; 53: 152–7.

233 Stemmerman GN. Extrapelvic carcinoma metastatic to the uterus. Am J Obstet Gynecol 1961; 82: 1261–6.

234 Weingold AB, Boltuch SM. Extragenital metastases to the uterus. Am J Obstet Gynecol 1961; 82: 1267–72.

235 Goldstein J, Mazor M, Leiberman JR. Primary carcinoma of the cecum with uterine metastases. Hum Pathol 1981; 12: 1139–40.

236 Aleghat E, Taluman A. Adenocarcinoma of the veriform appendix presenting as a uterine tumor. Gynecol Oncol 1982; 13: 265–8.

237 Czernobilsky B, Silverman BB, Mikutan JJ. Endometrioid carcinoma of the ovary. A clinicopathologic study of 75 cases. Cancer 1970; 26: 1141–52.

238 Eifel P, Hendrickson M, Ross J et al. Simulta-neous presentation of carcinomas involving the ovary and the uterine corpus. Cancer 1982; 50: 163–70.

239 Ulbright TM, Roth LM. Metastatic and independent cancers of the endometrium and ovary: a clinicopathologic study of 34 cases. Hum Pathol 1985; 16: 28–34.

240 Rao NR. Malacoplakia of Broad Ligament, Inguinal Region and Endometrium. Arch Pathol 1969; 88: 85–8.

241 Thomas W, Sadeghieh B, Fresco R, et al. Malacoplakia of endometrium: a probable cause of post menopausal bleeding. Am J Clin Pathol 1978; 69: 637–41.

242 Molnar JJ, Poliak A. Recurrent endometrial malakoplakia. Am J Clin Pathol 1983; 80: 762–4.

243 Lewin KJ, Fair WR, Steigbigel RT et al. Clinical and laboratory studies in the pathogenesis of malacoplakia. J Clin Pathol 1976; 29: 354–63.

Textbook of Uncommon Cancer
Edited by C.J. Williams, J.G. Krikorian, M.R. Green and D. Raghavan
© 1988 John Wiley & Sons Ltd

Chapter **8**

Uncommon Vaginal Cancers

J.M. Monaghan
Queen Elizabeth Hospital, Gateshead, Tyne and Wear,
UK

INTRODUCTION

Most cancers in the vagina are secondary tumours arising from the cervix and corpus uteri, the vulva, ovary, bladder, rectum, sigmoid colon and kidney.

Primary carcinoma of the vagina is rare and represents only 1–2% of all genital malignancies. It is consequently difficult for individual practitioners to build up a large series; hence most reports are the accumulated experience of large institutions over a long period of time (1–6). Most primary cancers are of squamous origin and will not be dealt with in detail. However, there are some rare squamous cancers which will be discussed.

Aetiology

No single aetiological agent has been incriminated in the development of vaginal carcinoma. In previous series veneral disease, chronic infection and the chronic irritation associated with procidentia and prolapse and the wearing of vaginal pessaries were commonly impugned. There is no doubt that carcinoma of the vagina does occur in these circumstances, but the author (7) has shown the rarity of these factors. In more recent times greater significance has been placed on the role of previous radiotherapy (6, 8), although this aetiological factor has been discounted by

Perez and Camel (9). Wharton et al. (2) in their series noted that 48% of patients had had a preceding total abdominal hysterectomy for unrelated disease; 16.7% had had previous cervical intraepithelial neoplasia (CIN) or clinical carcinoma of the cervix. Peters et al. (6) noted that in 35 of their reported series of 68 patients there had been 37 previous malignancies, 32 of which had been invasive or preinvasive carcinomas of the cervix. Other authorities have noted a similar association with previous cervical disease (4). The possibility of a multicentric origin for vaginal carcinoma has been discussed, but is not as clear as the relationship between vulval neoplasia (both intraepithelial and invasive) and carcinoma of the cervix (10). Recent interest in viral aetiological factors for genital cancers has focused attention on the herpes simplex type II and the papova virus family, particularly types 16 and 18. These may be involved in the development of multifocal neoplasia of the genital tract (11).

RARE SQUAMOUS CANCERS

Verrucous Carcinoma

History

This extremely rare variation of carcinoma of the vagina has been reported less than 20 times (12). It was said to have been first described by Martens and Tilesius in 1804, (13).

Epidemiology and Aetiology

There does not appear to be a clear aetiological agent although the tumour probably develops due to stimulation by the papovavirus and may be similar to the large condyloma acuminatum found in the male, the giant condyloma of Buschke–Löwenstein. Verruccous carcinoma of the mouth is related to tobacco usage and of the penis to poor hygiene.

Pathology and Biology

The disease is characterized by a relatively benign pattern of growth virtually never metastasizing and involving other organs in the pelvis only very late in its growth. The gross appearance is of a fungating, verrucous, brown, trabeculated tissue. Microscopically the tumour is markedly acanthotic with prominent rounded rete ridges, pushing into surrounding tissues but rarely showing clear invasive appearances. The cellular pattern is characterized by abundant oesinophilic cytoplasm. The nuclei are generally round with prominent nucleoli. Mitotic figures are few. There is often a marked tissue reaction to be found along the margins of the tumour, including giant cells exhibiting a foreign body response to the keratotic material in the carcinoma.

Clinical Features (Including Special Features Differentiating from Common Tumours of the Same Organ)

Bleeding does not commonly occur as a primary symptom the tumour being most frequently diagnosed following routine examination when a massive fungating mass in the vagina is noted. Procidentia and a mass appearing at the vulva is a frequent presentation.

Investigation and Staging

The most important and valuable investigation is to perform an adequate biopsy. This should be carried out as a formal procedure under anaesthetic when a large piece of tissue to include the growing edge of the tumour should be taken.

Management and Prognosis

Surgery. The optimal management appears to be to perform a wide local excision. Unfortunately because of the large size of these tumours the margin is frequently found to be inadequate and recurrence occurs. In the author's experience the patient may have had a large series of small procedures before presenting to an oncologist. Extensive surgery may then be necessary to effect a cure. It seems that lymphadenectomy is a debatable part of the primary management, (14).

Radiotherapy. This is not advised as there is a poor cure rate (15) and a significant risk of malignant transformation of the tumour into an anaplastic carcinoma (16).

Chemotherapy. There is currently no effective chemotherapeutic agent available. It is often found that the tumour has been treated ineffectually in the past with podophyllin.

Major Differences from Common Tumours of that Organ

The most important feature of this tumour is its relatively benign course in spite of enormous growth potential. However, the tumour is frequently undertreated and has a great tendency to recur.

Current Biological Research Likely to Affect Future Management

Considerable interest has been shown in identifying papovavirus capsids in the cancer. They are not a constant feature and a direct relationship has not been firmly established.

Basal Cell Carcinoma

History

This tumour is extraordinarily rare in the vagina; Blaustein records only one case of 'basal cell-like carcinoma', reported by Naves et al. (17).

Epidemiology and Aetiology

Naves et al. discussed the possibility that the tumour which they had described may have arisen from a group of cell rests and may have had features of the 'cylindromas or basal adenoid carcinomas' of the cervix reviewed by Rosen and Dolan (18).

Management and Prognosis

Surgery. Wide local excision is all that is required to cure the cancer. Widespread metastases do not occur.

Radiotherapy. This modality is of value when the vagina has to be preserved.

Squamous Cell Carcinoma with Sarcoma-like Stroma

This extremely rare cancer is also known as pseudosarcoma, carcinosarcoma and spindle cell carcinoma. This unusual variant is well described by Steeper et al. (19), two out of their four cases arising in the vagina.

Carcinoma Arising in a Neovagina

This extremely rare event has been reported on a number of occasions, the first squamous carcinoma occurring in a grafted vaginal epithelium in 1959 (20). Over the years a number of other reports have been made; recently even a verrucous carcinoma has been reported to arise in a split thickness skin grafted vagina (21).

ADENOCARCINOMA OF THE VAGINA

History

Primary adenocarcinoma of the vagina is rare and represents only 4–5% of cases of vaginal carcinoma. In recent years considerable interest has been shown in clear cell adenocarcinomas of the genital tract, including those of the vagina, occurring in young women with a history of maternal ingestion of diethyl stilboestrol during pregnancy. However, there does appear to have been an overall increase in prevalence of clear cell adenocarcinomas, both related and unrelated to stilboestrol ingestion. This increase has been observed in patients of all age groups (2).

Even rarer adenocarcinomas do also occur including mixed intestinal adenocarcinoma–argentaffin carcinoma, which appears to arise from aberrant intestinal cells present in the vagina (22).

Epidemiology and Aetiology

Although clear cell carcinoma of the vagina occurs rarely, in 1970 Herbst and Scully (23) reported an unusually high frequency in a short space of time in Boston, United States. They reported 7 young women who had developed the tumour, and in 6 they were able to show that their mothers had taken diethyl stilboestrol (DES) during the course of their pregnancies (24). Many more reports followed from the United States where DES had been used extensively to maintain high risk pregnancies, especially those with a past history of abortion, diabetes and twin pregnancies.

It was not until 1977 that the first case was seen in Britain (25), and since that time 4 more cases have been reported (26, 27). Herbst and Scully (28) have maintained a registry of cases; to date more than 500 cases of clear cell carcinoma of the vagina and cervix have been recorded.

In very rare circumstances adenocarcinoma of the vagina and cervix has been noted in association with congenital anomalies, including double uterus and vagina and unilateral agenesis (29, 30). Thus it appears that the carcinoma may develop de novo, from adenosis and from endometriosis (31, 32).

Pathology and Biology

The tumour has a very characteristic appearance with sheets of cells, tubules and cysts (Figure 1). The most common cell types are 'clear cells' with vacuolated or clear areas in the cells and 'hob nail' nuclei. Occasionally the 'clear' cells may be absent and the tumour appears poorly differentiated. Interestingly it is this poorly differentiated group of adenocarcinomas which have been reported by Ireland and Monaghan (33) to occur on the cervix and carry a very poor prognosis.

Stilboestrol is known to be a teratogenic, the characteristic stigmata in the female being vaginal and cervical adenosis, coxcombing and hooding of the cervix and the development of a transverse ridge in the vagina. This teratogenic effect will only occur if the stilboestrol is given prior to 18 weeks gestation (34). There is no solid evidence that the drug is carcinogenic, but the tumour probably develops because the ectopic columnar epithelium in the vagina is of an endocervical type and is susceptible to carcinogens present within the vaginal environment. Prins et al. in 1976 (35) suggested that initiation of the cancer may be by endoge-

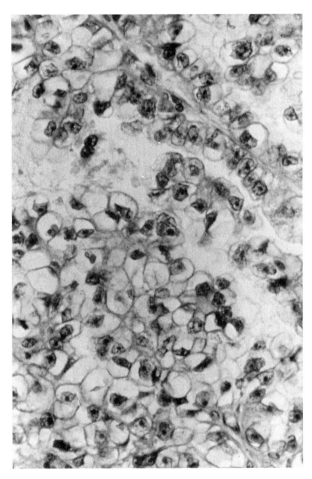

Figure 1 High power (original magnification: ×40) photomicrograph of clear cell carcinoma of the vagina.

nous oestrogens. The cancer risk to those females with the stigmata appears to be very low, of the order of 1:1000–1400 (28).

Clinical Features (Including Special Features Differentiating from Common Tumours of the Same Organ)

The carcinoma presents in a similar manner to other malignancies of the lower genital tract with abnormal bleeding and discharge. Often an abnormal cervical smear may institute referral, dysplastic cells having been picked up from a high vaginal lesion. Unlike squamous carcinomas it occurs predominantly in young women in their teens and twenties, although the age range spreads widely.

Investigation and Staging

As with all carcinomas of the vagina it is very easy to miss the lesion in the vagina as it is often covered by the speculum. It is worthwhile reiterating the caveat to always examine the whole vagina in patients who have abnormal smears particularly when no obvious lesion can be identified on the cervix.

Management and Prognosis

Surgery. Many different modalities of treatment have been used but it appears that local excision is inferior to more radical methods. Lymph node metastases are of the same order Stage for Stage as carcinoma of the cervix, 18% for Stage I and 30% for Stage II. Five-year actuarial survivals of 90% Stage I, 80% Stage II and 37% Stage III have been reported (28). Recurrences occur more commonly after local treatments and are best treated by surgery or radiotherapy. Unfortumately if surgical management is radical, loss of much or all of the vagina is inevitable. A neovagina should be planned for patients wishing to be sexually active. This problem is of great relevance as most of the patients with adenocarcinoma of the vagina are young.

If a vaginectomy is performed it is feasible to perform a McIndoe procedure, replacing affected vaginal epithelium with a graft. If a larger procedure such as an exenteration is performed then a neovagina formed from bilateral gracilis myocutaneous grafts will not only produce a new functioning vagina but will also bring a new blood supply to the pelvis. This neovascularization is of great importance where the patient has previously been treated with radiotherapy.

Radiotherapy. Radiotherapy is a satisfactory option for primary treatment although the consequent vaginal morbidity can produce serious long term problems. For Stage III and IV disease radiotherapy is the best treatment although there are a small percentage of patients with localized Stage IV disease where an exenterative procedure will give the best prospect of survival (1).

Chemotherapy. To date no effective chemotherapeutic agent has been reported.

Major Differences from Common Tumours of that Organ

The most striking characteristic of adenocarcinomas of the vagina when compared with squamous carcinoma has been the remarkable increase in prevalence since 1970 and the possibility of other sequelae of the use of exogenous hormonal agents.

Current Biological Research Likely to Affect Future Management

For a number of years there has been confusion and disagreement over the risk of cervical and vaginal dysplasia developing in DES exposed young women. Matingly and Stafl in 1974 (36) predicted that exposed women would be at increased risk of the development of dysplasia. Since that time a variety of comments have been made. Robboy et al. in 1984 (37), reviewing the experience of the National Collaborative DES Project, stated that the incidence of dysplasia and carcinoma in situ was significantly higher in the exposed group than in a matched cohort. These higher rates only occurred if the squamous metaplasia extended to the outer half of the cervix or onto the vagina. The possibility of a precancerous atypical vaginal adenosis has been mooted by Davis et al. (27) and more recently by Robboy et al. (38). This appears to be characterized by tuboendometrial glandular epithelium consisting of mucin free from ciliated cells. Documentation is sketchy and unclear.

SARCOMA OF THE VAGINA
(Chapter 10)

Sarcomas of the vagina may occur in both young and old patients. Leiomyosarcomas, spindle cell sarcomas, alveolar soft part sarcomas, angiosarcomas, fibrosarcomas, neurofibrosarcomas and mixed mesodermal tumours of the vagina occur predominantly in older patients but are extremely rare (2% of all malignant vaginal tumours).

Embryonal rhabdomyosarcomas (sarcoma botryoides), develop in young girls between 6 months and 16 years of age.

Sarcomas of the Elderly

History

Leiomyosarcomas are the most common of the adult sarcomas. They often grow slowly and the tumour may occasionally be responsive to wide local excision.

Epidemiology and Aetiology

There are no clear aetiological agents but Peters et al. (39) report that one-third of 17 patients had previous pelvic irradiation for carcinoma of the cervix.

Pathology and Biology
Clinical Features (Including Special Features Differentiating from Common Tumours of the Same Organ)

The tumour generally develops alongside the vaginal epithelium presenting as a lump which may cause problems with micturition, defecation or intercourse. Because they are subdermal, bleeding and discharge are late features.

Investigation and Staging

As with many cancers the biopsy is extremely important and must include the growing edge of the cancer if possible. It is important not to underestimate the subdermal extent of the cancer.

Management and Prognosis

Surgery. Extremely wide local excision is essential. The tumour mass often has a false compression capsule consisting of cancer tissue. This 'capsule' must be widely excised with a good margin of normal tissue. As the vagina is so close to other vital organs this wide excision will often dictate that an exenterative procedure is performed. In the series of Peters et al. (39), this form of treatment produced the only long term survivals.

Radiotherapy. This has only rarely been used mainly by Rutledge (40) from the M.D. Anderson Hospital with mixed results.

Chemotherapy. Unfortunately treatment of adult sarcomas with chemotherapy does not produce the excellent results found in paediatric sarcomas. Chemotherapy may possibly be useful as a tumour reductive agent prior to extensive surgery.

Sarcomas of the Young

History

These rare tumours develop in young infants with a mean age of 2 years (41). They present with bleeding or bloody discharge and a rapidly growing mass presenting at the introitus.

Epidemiology and Aetiology

There are no clear features which have been consistently established.

Pathology and Biology

The prospect of cure is closely related to the size of the tumour stage of the disease and the degree of differentiation. The histology may appear deceptively benign. There is a loose myxomatous stroma below and intact epithelium. Two characteristic features are the presence of rhabdomyoblasts and striated muscle fibres.

Clinical Features (Including Special Features Differentiating from Common Tumours of the Same Organ)

Delay in seeking advice is a common feature.

The sarcoma botryoides is characteristically described as a mass of grape like structures. The clinician should be very suspicious of any polypoid growth in the vagina as simple polyps are extraordinarily rare (42). Unlike other sarcomas these vaginal lesions tend to spread locally initially and then later by lymphatic rather than haematogenous routes, the patient reaching a late stage in the disease before distant metastases occur.

Investigation and Staging

As with all cancers an adequate biopsy is essential. This should be performed under the same anaesthetic as the staging. For all young patients examination without anaesthetic is distressing so it is vital that a planned approach is made and all necessary examinations and biopsies are carried out under one anaesthetic. Access to the vagina may be limited and it is recommended that in these circumstances vaginoscopy using a cystoscope is of value. The bladder and rectum must be examined to determine whether spread has occurred to either of these organs.

Management and Prognosis

Surgery. The treatment of sarcoma botryoides has traditionally been by radical surgery including exenteration, but survival figures are poor. Huffman (43) found only 12 out of 150 cases survived 5 years.

Radiotherapy. There appears to be no advantage in using radiotherapy. In exceptional circumstances where there is persistent disease in the lower vagina radiotherapy may be indicated. However, the most important problem is the damage which radiotherapy does to the epiphyses of the pelvic bones in the small child.

Chemotherapy. In recent years aggressive chemotherapy has revolutionized the management of this disease, resulting not only in long term survival but preservation of the pelvic organs. The use of VAC (vincristine, actinomycin D and cyclophosphamide) has revolutionized the management of this disease (44, 45).

Often the disease will completely regress during the prolonged chemotherapy. If regression is not complete surgery is usually used as an adjunct. Rarely will this be an exenteration, the most frequent procedure being a Wertheim hysterectomy with vaginectomy.

Angiosarcoma of the Vagina

The first case to be claimed was reported in 1983 by Prempree et al. (46). They advocated treating the cancer with a combination of external and intracavitary radiation, their decision being based on experience of the treatment of cervical angiosarcomas. Most of the angiosarcoma had been removed at surgical biopsy.

RETICULOENDOTHELIAL CANCERS

This group of very rare tumours will include the reticulum cell sarcomas which are now considered lymphomas.

History

The genital tract including the vagina may not infrequently be involved in metastatic lymphomas. However, it is rare for the vagina to be the primary site.

Epidemiology and Aetilogy

Little is known about aetiological factors.

Pathology and Biology

The pathological features are the same as lymphomas of other sites in the body.

Clinical Features (Including Special Features Differentiating from Common Tumours of the Same Organ)

The tumours can occur in both pre- and postmenopausal patients. Bleeding is the most frequent presenting symptom, with pain (dyspareunia) also occurring. Masses may be noted at routine pelvic examination.

Investigation and staging

Lymphomas are staged using both the International Federation of Gynaecology and Obstetrics (FIGO) and the Ann Arbor methods.

Management and Prognosis

Surgery. This is almost entirely reserved for the performance of biopsies, except where the tumour is very small and localized.

Radiotherapy. This modality is frequently used to treat both the primary site and the routes of metastases to the pelvic side wall. It has been combined with chemotherapy with some early success.

Chemotherapy. A variety of chemotherapeutic combinations have been used including CVP (cyclophosphamide, vincristine and prednisone) and CHOP (cyclophosphamide,

Adriamycin, vincristine and prednisone). Both partial and complete regressions have been reported (47).

ENDODERMAL SINUS TUMOURS

History

This rare cancer of the vagina affects infants of 2 years or younger (48).

Epidemiology and Aetiology

The controversy as to whether this is an extragonadal germ cell tumour or a tumour of mesonephric remnants is unsolved.

Pathology and Biology

The histological pattern of the tumour shows glomeruloid formations, hobnail patterns and the presence of PAS positive hyaline globules allowing a clear distinction to be made between it and clear cell adenocarcinoma. Alpha-fetoprotein levels in the blood are also elevated.

Clinical features (Including Special Features Differentiating from Common Tumours of the Same Organ)

Delay in seeking advice is a common feature. The endodermal sinus tumour is characteristically a polypoid lesions and consequently is often mistaken for a sarcoma botryoides.

Investigation and Staging

The use of PAS staining and immunohistochemistry allows the diagnosis to be made and differentiates the tumour from sarcoma botryoides.

Management and Prognosis

Surgery. Endodermal sinus tumours have been treated by surgery, the longest reported survival following this form of treatment being 7 years (49).

Radiotherapy. This modality may have a place in combination with chemotherapy. Unfortunately the damage to the infantile bony pelvis may produce major problems in the surviving child.

Chemotherapy. More recently it has been shown that chemotherapy is of great value (45). Ortega (50) showed that preliminary or complete treatment with chemotherapy was at least equal to radical surgical treatment without the very significant morbidity and mutilation. His group used VAC vincristine, actinomycin D and cyclophosphamide) initially, later adding Adriamycin to the regimen.

   Chemotherapeutic agents are now showing clear benefits and greater hope for long term cures. Patients are monitored using the serum alpha-fetoprotein tumour markers; the chemotherapy is given first, followed by local excision of the lesion and then a further series of chemotherapeutic courses. This combination has been shown to preserve fertility in selected cases (51).

MELANOMAS

History

Malignant melanomas of the vagina are extraordinarily rare representing less than 1% of all melanomas affecting the female. In 1975 Pomante (52) had collected 39 cases and in 1980 the author added 2 more (53): Lee et al. (54), in a major review, have updated the world's collected series to 106.

Epidemiology and Aetiology

The disease follows the age distribution of the other carcinomas of the vagina with a wide age distribution from the third to the ninth decade with a mean age in the sixth decade of life. There is no known aetiological agent and

obviously because of its position there is no relationship to exposure to ultraviolet light.

Pathology and Biology

The tumour is said to arise from vaginal melanocytes which are thought to be present in 3% of normal females (55).

Clinical Features (Including Special Features Differentiating from Common Tumours of the Same Organ)

Vaginal bleeding and discharge are the commonest presenting symptoms. It is important to make an adequate biopsy of the lesion as occasionally the abnormality may still be confined to the epithelium (melanomatous intraepithelial neoplasia), and an excision biopsy is all that is required.

   The tumour is usually black or blue-black, affecting the lower third of the vagina, particularly the anterior wall.

Management and Prognosis

Surgery. Unfortunately when the lesion is invasive the prospects for cure are very poor; both radical surgery and radiotherapy have been used and with little success. If the lesion is of the lower one-third of the vagina radical excision combined with radical vulvectomy is the treatment of choice (53).

Radiotherapy. This modality has a significant place in the treatment of melanomas in sites which mitigate against wide surgical excision. Recurrences are controlled by the use of implantation techniques.

Chemotherapy. Recent evidence suggests that it is important to consider the disease as a systemic problem; therefore adjuvant therapy should be used (54). Chemotherapy has been used but with relatively little success; of the drugs used dacarbazine (DTIC) and hydroxyurea probably are the most effective. Immunotherapy may improve the effectiveness of drug treatments.

Miscellaneous

The propensity for melanomas to metastasize widely by both the lymphatic and haematological routes makes them a lethal and unpredictable cancer. They also appear to have a capacity to lie dormant for a number of years and then to reappear after minor stress especially surgical procedures.

HAEMANGIOPERICYTOMA

History

This extraordinarily rare tumour of the genital tract appears to have been reported to occur in the vagina on only one occasion by Buscema et al. 1985 (56).

Epidemiology and Aetiology

There is no current information available.

Pathology and Biology

The tumour is characterized by proliferation of capillaries surrounded by a cell population derived from the 'myoepithelial' pericyte. It can be mistakenly be diagnosed as a leiomyosarcoma.

Clinical Features (Including Special Features Differentiating from Common Tumours of the Same Organ)

The cancer develops as an ulcerating mass of the vaginal epithelium with bleeding occurring both spontaneously and after trauma.

Investigation and Staging

A biopsy and careful pathological assessment is essential including the use of electron microscopy.

Management and Prognosis

Surgery. Exenterative surgery is probably the best option though the extent of surgery required will ultimately depend on the site and size of the tumour.

Radiotherapy. This modality does not appear to have a place in treatment.

Chemotherapy. No chemotherapeutic agent or combination has been shown to be effective.

Major Differences from Common Tumours of that Organ

The equivalent cancer in other sites of the body is extremely aggressive. However, this has not been the general experience when the cancer occurs in the genital tract.

REFERENCES

1 Al-Kurdi M, Monaghan JM. Thirty-two years experience in management of primary tumours of the vagina. Br J Obstet Gynaecol 1981; 88: 1145–50.
2 Wharton JT, Fletcher GH, Delclos L. Invasive tumors of vagina: clinical features and management. Gynecol Oncol 1981; 27: 345–9.
3 Ball HG, Berman ML. Management of primary vaginal carcinoma. Gynecol Oncol 1982; 14: 154–63.
4 Benedet JL, Murphy KJ, Fairey RN, Boyes DA. Primary invasive carcinoma of the vagina. Obstet Gynecol 1983; 62: 715–9.
5 Kucera H, Langer M, Smekal G, Weghaupt K. Radiotherapy of primary carcinoma of the vagina: management and results of different therapy schemes. Gynecol Oncol 1985; 21: 87–91.
6 Peters WA, Kumar NB, Morley GW. Carcinoma of the vagina. Factors influencing treatment outcome. Cancer 1985; 55: 892–7.
7 Monaghan JM. The management of carcinoma of the vagina. In: Shepherd JS, Monaghan JM eds Clinical Gynaecological Oncology. Oxford: Blackwell 1985; 155.
8 Pride GL, Schultz AE, Chuprevich TW, Buchler DA. Primary invasive squamous carcinoma of the vagina. Obstet Gynecol 1979; 53: 2, 218–25.
9 Perez CA, Camel HM. Long term follow-up in

radiation therapy of carcinoma of the vagina. Cancer 1982 49: 1308–15.

10 Hammond IG, Monaghan JM. Multicentric carcinoma of the female lower genital tract. Br J Obstet Gynaecol 1983; 90: 557–61.

11 Weed JC, Lozier C, Daniel SJ. Human papilloma virus in multifocal, invasive female genital tract malignancy. Obstet Gynecol 1983; 62: 83s–87s.

12 Jones MJ, Levin HS, Ballard LA. Verrucous squamous cell carcinoma of the vagina. Case report. Cleve Clin Q 1981; 48: 305–13.

13 Ramzy I, Smout MS, Collins JA. Verrucous carcinoma of the vagina. Am J Clin Pathol 1976; 65: 644–53.

14 Powell JL, Franklin EW, Nickerson IF, Burrell MO. Verrucous carcinoma of the female genital tract. Gynecol Oncol 1978; 6: 565–73.

15 Goethals PL, Harrison EG Jr, Devine KD. Verrucous squamous carcinoma of the oral cavity. Am J Surg 1963; 106: 845–51.

16 Kraus FT, Perez-Mesa C. Verrucous carcinoma; Clinical and pathological study of 105 cases involving oral cavity, larynx and genitalia. Cancer 1966; 19: 26–38.

17 Naves AE, Monti JA, Chichoni E. Basal cell-like carcinoma in the upper third of the vagina. Am J Obstet Gynecol 1980; 137: 136.

18 Rosen Y, Dolan TE. Carcinoma of the cervix with cylindromatous features believed to arise in mesonephric duct. Cancer 1975; 36: 1739.

19 Steeper TA, Piscioli F, Rosai J. Squamous cell carcinoma with sarcoma like stroma of the female genital tract. Cancer 1983; 52: 890–8.

20 Jackson GW. Primary carcinoma of an artificial vagina. Obstet Gynecol 1959; 14: 534.

21 Abrenio JK, Chung HI, Pomante R. Verrucous carcinoma arising from an artificial vagina. Obstet Gynecol 1977; 50: 18s–21s.

22 Fukushima M, Twiggs LB, Okagaki T. Mixed intestinal adenocarcinoma-argentaffin carcinoma of the vagina. Gynecol Oncol 1986; 23: 387–94.

23 Herbst AL, Scully RE. Adenocarcinoma of the vagina in adolescence; a report of seven cases including six clear cell carcinomas (so called mesonephromas). Cancer (Philad) 1970; 25: 745–7.

24 Herbst AL, Ulfelder H, Poskanzer DC. Adenocarcinoma of the vagina: association of maternal stilboestrol therapy with tumour appearance in young women. N Engl J Med 1971; 284: 878.

25 Monaghan JM, Sirisena LAW. Stilboestrol and vaginal clear cell adenocarcinoma syndrome. Br Med J 1978; i: 1588–90.

26 Dewhurst Sir J, Ferreira HP, Dalley VM, Staffurth JF. Stilboestrol associated vaginal carcinoma treated by radiotherapy. J Obstet Gynaecol 1980; 1: 63–4.

27 Davis JA, Wadehra V, McIntosh AS, Monaghan JM. A case of clear cell adenocarcinoma of the vagina in pregnancy. Br J Obstet Gynecol 1981; 88: 322–7.

28 Herbst AL, Scully RE. (1983) Newsletter—Registry for Research on Hormonal Transplacental Carcinogenesis.

29 Nordquist SRB, Fidler WJ, Woodruff JM, Lewis JL. Clear cell adenocarcinoma of the cervix and vagina. Cancer 1976; 37: 858–71.

30 Hall SW, Monaghan JM. Clear cell carcinoma of the cervix in a woman with subseptate vagina, double cervix and uterus. J Obstet Gynaecol 1983; 1: 62–3.

31 Kapp DS, Merino M, Livolsi V. Adenocarcinoma of the vagina arising in endometriosis: long-term survival following radiation therapy. Gynecol Oncol 1982; 14: 271–8.

32 Granai CO, Walters MD, Safaii H, Jelen I, Madoc-Jones H, Moukhtar M. Malignant transformation of vaginal endometriosis. Obstet Gynecol. 1984; 64: 592–5.

33 Ireland D, Monaghan JM. Mucin production in cervical intraepithelial neoplasia and in Stage Ib carcinoma of cervix with pelvic lymph node metastases. Br J Obstet Gynaecol (in press).

34 Ulfelder H. The stilboestrol–adenosis–carcinoma syndrome. Cancer 1976; 38: 426–31.

35 Prins RP, Morrow CP, Townsend DE, Disaia PJ. Vaginal embryogenesis estrogens and adenosis. Obstet Gynecol 1976; 48: 246–50.

36 Mattingly R, Stafl A. Cancer risk in diethylstilbestrol-exposed-offspring. Am J Obstet Gynecol 1976; 126: 543–8.

37 Robboy SJ, Noller KL, O'Brien P, Kaufman RH, Townsend DE, Barnes AB, Gundersen J, Lawrence WD, Bergstrahl E, McGorray S, Tilley BC, Anton J, Chazan G. Increased incidence of cervical and vaginal dysplasia in 3980 diethylstilbestrol-exposed young women. JAMA 1984; 252: 2979–83.

38 Robboy SJ, Young RH, Welch WR, Truslow GY, Prat J, Herbst AL, Scully RE. Atypical vaginal adenosis and cervical ectropion. Cancer 1983; 54: 869–75.

39 Peters WA, Kumar NB, Anderson WA, Morley GW. Primary sarcoma of the adult vagina: A clinicopathological study. Obstet Gynecol 1985; 65: 699–704.

40 Rutledge F. Cancer of the vagina. Am J Obstet Gynecol 1967; 97: 635.

41 Hilgers RD. Prenatal oncogenesis and the development of malignant tumours in the infant and adolescent vagina—a review and hypothesis. Gynecol Oncol 1977; 5: 262–72.

42 Dewhurst Sir J. Malignant diseases of the genital organs in childhood. In: Shepherd JS, Monaghan JM eds Clinical Gynaecological Oncology. Oxford: Blackwell, 1985; 270.

43 Huffman JW. The Gynecology of Childhood and Adolescent. Philadelphia: WB Saunders, 1968.

44 Hilgers RD, Malkasian GD, Soule EH. Embryonal rhabdomyosarcoma (botryoid type) of the vagina. Am J Obstet Gynecol 1970; 107: 484–502.

45 Hilgers RD, Ghavimi F, D'Angio GJ et al. Memorial Hospital experience with pelvic exenteration and embryonal rhabdomyosarcoma of the vagina. Gynecol Oncol 1973; 1: 262–70.

46 Prempree T, Tang C, Hatef A, Forster S. Angiosarcoma of the vagina: A clinicopathological report. Cancer 1983 51: 618–22.

47 Harris NL, Scully RE. Malignant lymphoma and granulocytic sarcoma of the uterus and vagina. Cancer 1984; 53: 2530–45.

48 Allyn DL, Silverberg SG, Salzberg AM. Endodermal sinus tumour of the vagina. Report of a case with 7 year survival and literature review of so-called 'mesonephromas'. Cancer 1971; 27: 1231–8.

49 Dewhurst Sir J, Ferreira HP. An endodermal sinus tumour of the vagina in an infant with seven year survival. Br J Obstet Gynaecol 1981; 88: 859–62.

50 Ortega JA. A therapeutic approach to childhood pelvic rhabdomyosarcoma without pelvic exenteration. J Pediat 1979; 94: 205–9.

51 Copeland LJ, Sneige N, Ordonez NG, Hancock KC, Gershenson DH, Saul PB, Kavanagh JJ. Endodermal sinus tumour of the vagina and cervix. Cancer 1985; 55: 2558–65.

52 Pomante RG. Malignant melanoma—primary in the vagina. Gynecol Oncol 1975; 3: 15–20.

53 Edington PT, Monaghan JM. Malignant melanoma of the vulva and vagina. Br J Obstet Gynaecol 1980; 87: 422–4.

54 Lee RB, Buttoni L, Dhru R, Tamini H. Malignant melanoma of the vagina: a case report of progression from preexisting melanosis. Gynecol Oncol 1984; 19: 238–45.

55 Nigogosyan G. De La Pava S, Picken JW. Melanoblasts in vaginal mucosa: origin for primary malignant melanoma. Cancer 1964; 17: 912–13.

56 Buscema J, Rosenhein NB, Taqi F, Woodruff JD. Vaginal hemangiopericytoma: A histopathologic and ultrastructural evaluation. Obstet Gynecol 1985; 66: 82s–85s.

Textbook of Uncommon Cancer
Edited by C.J. Williams, J.G. Krikorian, M.R. Green and D. Raghavan
© 1988 John Wiley & Sons Ltd

Chapter **9**

Leiomyomatosis Peritonealis Disseminata

Shingo Fujii

*Department of Gynecology and Obstetrics, Faculty of
Medicine, Kyoto University, Sakyo-ku, Kyoto, Japan*

HISTORY

Leiomyomatosis peritonealis disseminata (LPD) is an unusual entity that occurs in women and is characterized by multiple nodules of varying size scattered throughout the abdominal cavity. The nodules are microscopic in size to 10.0 cm in diameter. They occur on the surfaces of abdominal and pelvic organs, in the omentum, the mesenteries, and the parietal peritoneum. The discovery of this multiplicity of nodules during laparotomy or laparoscopy often gives rise to a false impression of carcinomatosis, but the nodules are composed of either benign smooth muscle cells or an admixture of smooth muscle cells, fibroblasts, myofibroblasts, and decidual cells.

LPD was first clearly described and named by Taubert et al. (1) in 1965. However, the first case of LPD associated with a granulosa cell tumor of the ovary was reported by Wilson and Peale (2) in 1952. In the view of Taubert et al. (1), 3 women with multiple benign intraperitoneal leiomyomas were initially mistaken for disseminated lesions of low grade leiomyosarcoma. Nevertheless, a laparotomy performed on a woman at 14 weeks of gestation to evaluate a pelvic mass revealed the lesion and resection of several seedlings resulted in the disappearance of the residual nodules documented at a subsequent postpartum exploratory laparotomy. Although the majority of the lesions were left behind, all 3 women showed no evidence of further growth of the remaining nodules after oophorectomy. As 2 of the patients were pregnant and possessed an unusual degree of peritoneal decidualization, they concluded that the lesion was a clinically and histologically benign condition, presumably the result of an abnormal endocrine status or an enhanced tissue sensitivity and reactivity to circulating placental hormones (1).

Until 1980, 22 cases of LPD (1–18) were reported, predominantly in black women. They were found incidentally at the time of cesarean section or during oral contraceptive use. Although the histogenesis of LPD has been a matter of controversy, these reports confirmed the clinical observations and assumptions of Taubert et al. (1) and concluded that LPD was a clinically benign condition characterized by a subperitoneal mesenchymal proliferation under the stimulation of reproductive steroids.

Although thought to be quite rare, LPD has been reported with increasing frequency in recent years. An additional 39 cases (19–35) were reported after 1980, and resulted in a shift of the clinicopathological spectrum of LPD. Now, there is no evidence of a racial predilection observed in earlier series. The majority of the recent reports are not directly related to pregnancy or to oral contraceptive steroids. Such cases now comprise 36% of the total. A few cases (22, 32, 43) have been reported in women without any evidence of elevated reproductive steroids. An unusual predisposition or selective sensitivity of subperitoneal mesenchymal cells to normal levels of reproductive steroids has been suggested to explain these cases (12, 13, 25, 30, 32).

In many cases, an apparent relationship exists between the presence of the disease and the elapsed time since the pregnancy or ingestion of oral contraceptive steroids. After the withdrawal of such hormonal stimuli, regression of the lesions is observed (1, 7, 13, 16, 25, 29). Therefore, when LPD is observed without apparent hormonal stimulation, it may represent persistent disease that developed at some prior time.

LPD is usually found incidentally, and has not often produced symptoms. However, a patient reported by Brumback et al. (33), at the age of 55 with very low levels of sex hormones manifested symptoms of blood loss caused by mucosal ulceration of the bowel wall adjacent to an LPD nodule. The nodules measured 10 cm in diameter without degenerative features. Their relationship to neighboring organs seemed to suggest growth and not regression even in the face of postmenopausal hormonal status. This case suggests that LPD or an entity histologically similar to it, may rarely acquire the capacity to grow autonomously. This is an exception to the earlier description suggesting that LPD will regress after the menopause and will not affect neighbouring organs.

Etiology

Of 61 reported cases of LPD, 49% were white, 42% were black, and 9% were oriental.

Although a few women are postmenopausal, LPD remains primarily a condition of the reproductive years (average age, 35 years) and 79% of the women are younger than 40 years

of age. The youngest was 22. Three women aged 50, 54, and 55 had the disease and an example of LPD was found incidentally at autopsy in a 69 year old woman.

Twenty-four women (39%) were diagnosed during or soon after the termination of a pregnancy, and 14 women (23%) were on oral contraceptive steroids at the time of diagnosis. The average age of the former group was 31, and of the latter 35. One woman had a granulosa cell tumor of the ovary (2). The remaining 22 women (36%) were not recently pregnant or taking oral contraceptive steroids. The average age of this group was 41 years and the majority (50% were older than 40 years of age. This is older than the group of women pregnant or on oral contraceptives. This implies that the lesion may have been present for some time in these patients.

Three had a history of oral contraceptive use (12, 33, 34). Only 3 (2, 26, 34) were nulliparous, one of whom (2) had a granulosa cell tumor of the ovary, while another (34) had had two pregnancies that terminated early. Only one case reported by Borel et al. (26) had no history of either pregnancy or oral contraceptives.

In 1941, animal experiments performed by Lipschutz and Vargas (36, 37) in an attempt to understand the histogenesis of uterine leiomyomas, resulted in the production of multiple nodules located under the peritoneal mesothelium. Large doses of estrogen produced this result in guinea pigs. The nodules regressed when the steroids were withdrawn. The nodules were composed of fibroblasts. LPD nodules are mainly composed of smooth muscle cells, but they are located under the peritoneal mesothelium. LPD nodules, associated with pregnancy or oral contraceptive steroids, regress postpartum (1, 7, 16, 25, 30), after withdrawl of oral contraceptive steroids (13), and after surgical castration (25). The clinical entity therefore shows features with the model.

LPD nodules are characteristically covered by the mesothelium and are in various stages of development suggesting multifocal origin of the lesion. The mesothelium and the associated mesenchyme of the fetal intraembryonic coelom, both elements of mesodermal origin, develop into the adult peritoneum and its subjacent stroma. Invagination of this intraembryonic coelom gives rise to the paramesonephric (mullerian) ducts which are represented in the adult by the uterine tube, the fundus of the uterus, the cervix, and a portion of the vagina (4, 38). The embryonic kinship between the mullerian duct and the peritoneum is reflected in the similarity of the responses of the peritoneum and its underlying stroma to the response of the endometrium when both are stimulated by estrogen and progesterone (4, 38). Clinically, the sensitivity of subcoelomic mesenchyme to hormones is manifested in an ectopic decidual reaction in the ovaries, the peritoneum including the omentum and even in pelvic lymph nodes (38). Decidual nodules can be detected microscopically in almost 100% of ovaries at term (39, 40). Also exogenous hormones can cause changes in tissues outside the endometrium. The use of norethindrone has been associated not only with the rapid atypical proliferation of a uterine leiomyoma, but also with the formation of decidual nodules on the uterine serosa, and on the surfaces of the ovary and appendix (41). Therefore, in general, the subcoelomic mesenchyme responds to appropriate reproductive steroids with the formation of decidual nodules.

LPD nodules are reportedly composed of either smooth muscle cells, or an admixture of smooth muscle cells, fibroblasts, myofibroblasts, and decidual cells (25). The frequency of blood vessels in LPD nodules has suggested that the smooth muscle cells arise from small blood vessels (6). However, an intimate relationship between the smooth muscle cells of the nodules and those of the blood vessels has not been demonstrated (7, 25).

The subcoelomic mesenchyme, as discussed by Ober (38) may give rise to endometrial stromal type cells, decidual cells, and smooth muscle cells via a metaplastic process (42). As the mesothelium is capable of undergoing

metaplasia to endometrial, endosalpingeal, or rarely endocervical epithelia, the subcoelomic mesenchyme can achieve mullerian stromal differentiation (12, 42–46). Accordingly, the cells constituting LPD nodules probably arise from the subcoelomic mesenchyme via metaplasia. How this occurs has been controversial.

Some investigators have thought that the cells of LPD are smooth muscle and are derived from a primitive mesenchymal stem cell via direct metaplasia (12). Others have postulated that LPD develops from stem cells that differentiate predominantly into myofibroblasts (11). A slightly different view is the thesis of Parmley et al. (4), and Winn et al. (47). On the basis of ultrastructural observations of nodules removed from pregnant women, they described the initial step in the development of LPD as the transformation of cells in the subcoelomic mesenchyme into decidual cells. The decidual cells are then either replaced by fibroblasts or myofibroblasts, which then become smooth muscle (4, 47). Most other observers (9, 12, 16, 17, 21, 25, 27, 29, 35), however, have demonstrated primarily ultrastructural evidence of smooth muscle differentiation in the nodules in women who are pregnant and in women who are not pregnant. Nevertheless, whether or not a primary step is the development of decidua, is undecided.

The use of oral contraceptive drugs, often prolonged use, in women who are not pregnant, may produce 'pseudodecidual' changes in the subcoelomic mesenchyme. There are 4 cases of LPD nodules intermingled with the glands and stroma of endometriosis (12, 14, 25, 31). This suggests that pre-existing multifocal nests of peritoneal endometriosis, particularly the endometrial stromal cells, might be a precursor of LPD nodules. After the phase of decidual transformation, the cells may further transform into myofibroblasts and/or smooth muscle cells. Tavassoi and Norris (25) reported that decidual cells and smooth muscle cells have some ultrastructural features in common, and they suggested the possibility that a range of transformation forms occur between the two. The relative frequency of endometriosis and the rarity of LPD suggests that the conversion of metaplasia of a differentiated cell type like a smooth muscle cell or a myofibroblast (25, 40) from an endometrial stromal cell is not common. At the endomyometrial junction, metaplasia of endometrial stroma has been felt to contribute to the increased mass that occurs in hyper-estrogenic states and pregnancy (47). However, it is not clear whether an endometrial stromal cell per se or a primitive mesenchymal stem cell is the precursor of smooth muscle cells.

Tavassoli and Norris (25) studying LPD nodules by transmission electron microscopy confirmed an intimate relationship between fibroblasts, myofibroblasts, and smooth muscle cells. They proposed that the origin of all these cell types was from a multi-potential primitive mesenchymal stem cell. Since decidual cells were not found during the first trimester either in their cases or in the literature (3), they suggested that decidual cells in the LPD nodules were most probably coincidental and resulted from the elevated serum progesterone levels in pregnancy. As smooth muscle cells show decidual changes during pregnancy, LPD cells with variable degrees of smooth muscle differentiation may also show decidual changes during pregnancy. This may constitute the range of transformation forms between decidual cells and smooth muscle cells reported by Tavassoli and Norris (25). Such a concept is supported by the recent experimental work of Fujii's group (49) who reproduced the animal model of Lipschutz and Vargas (36) and induced peritoneal nodules in guinea pigs with high levels of estrogen. Peritoneal nodules resembling LPD were produced when estrogen was given alone. Ultrastructurally they were fibroblasts. The addition of low doses of progesterone induced both smooth muscle cells and decidual cells. These results imply that the initial step in nodule formation is the proliferation of the subcoelomic mesenchymal cells which respond to estrogen. Decidual cell differentiation is most likely the result of the synergistic action of estrogen and progesterone on these cells. Therefore, an estrogenic stimulus to

the cells of the subcoelomic mesenchyme, probably to a multi-potential primitive mesenchymal stem cell, is a likely initial step in the development of LPD. The synergistic action of estrogen and progesterone then produces differentiation into decidual cells, myofibroblasts, and smooth muscle cells (48, 49).

Hormonal stimulation is apparent in patients who are pregnant or taking oral contraceptive steroids, and is the likely initiator or promoter of LPD. LPD may occur in asymptomatic form more frequently than is realized. However, considering the number of women who are pregnant or taking contraceptive steroids, the rarity of LPD is striking. In the tissues of LPD, receptors for estrogen and progesterone have been detected (13, 34). Sutherland et al. (13) reported increased levels of estrogen and progesterone receptors in the smooth muscle of LPD compared to those of normal myometrium, and a decrease in progesterone receptors after castration. Accordingly, an unusual predisposition, or selective sensitivity of the subperitoneal mesenchymal cells to reproductive steroids, may be the explanation for its development (2, 13, 25, 30, 32).

The development of LPD in normal women who are neither pregnant nor taking oral contraceptive steroids has also been explained in this way (25). In such instances, except for the case of Wilson and Peale (2) which was associated with a granulosa cell tumor of the ovary, the ovaries are unlikely sources of excess hormone production. The ovaries are histologically normal in appearance and the patients usually have normal menstrual cycles (25). The levels of circulating ovarian steroids are either normal (22, 34) or low (33). Therefore, an unusual predisposition, or selective sensitivity of the subperitoneal mesenchymal cells to even normal levels of ovarian steroids, is a plausible cause of LPD in these cases. This type of lesion is discovered predominantly after 40 years of age and the size of the nodules is usually larger than that of those associated with pregnancy or oral contraceptives. The difference is assumed to be due to long latency between the time of onset of the disease and its discovery. In cases of repeated cesarean section, LPD has been observed to possibly recur or progress with subsequent pregnancy (15, 25). This raises the possibility that a lesion produced in a prior pregnancy or by prior oral contraceptive use might have persisted until discovery. Except for the case of Borel et al. (26), all reported cases have had a history of pregnancy or oral contraceptive use. The cases of Kuo et al. (12) and Brumback et al. (33) are assumed to be triggered by previous oral contraceptive use.

After the menopause, LPD appears to regress completely or to persist as atrophic remnants (32). However, the recent case of Brumback et al. (33), aged 55 with very low levels of circulating sex steroids, seems inconsistent with the view. In this case, LPD was assumed to have been initiated by the use of oral contraceptive steroids for 2 years at age 48. However, nodules large enough to cause intestinal ulceration without atrophic features seem to have grown autonomously even in a postmenopausal hormonal milieu. This implies that some LPD may acquire the potential to grow autonomously even in a low sex steroid milieu or some other factor may control the growth of nodules. Beta-adrenergic mimetic drugs have been reported to produce mesovarial leiomyomas in experimental animals (52, 53). Among LPD patients, some cases (3, 28) including the case of Brumback et al. (33), are complicated by hypertensive disease (3, 28, 33). Therefore, in the future, the effect of adrenergic stimuli should be considered in the pathogenesis of LPD.

In general then, due to an unusual predisposition, or selective sensitivty of subperitoneal mesenchymal cells to reproductive steroids, LPD is produced multifocally in subperitoneal locations via a metaplastic process. However, most of the time, the sensitivity of the subperitoneal mesenchymal cells to reproductive steroids is variable but too low to result in the disease. LPD occurring in the excessive hormonal environment of pregnancy or oral contraceptive use shows regression soon after the withdrawal of these environments. This implies that the cells require higher hormone levels than those of normal ovarian cycles in order to respond. In contrast, LPD discovered in a woman experiencing normal ovarian cycles regresses with castration. In these cases, the subperitoneal mesenchymal cells are sensitive enough to respond to cyclic hormone levels. In patients of this type, nodules may grow continuously like uterine leiomyomas under the prolonged stimulation of ovarian steroids. Consequently, they may affect neighbouring organs like the case of Brumback et al. (33) and rarely they may acquire the capacity to grow autonomously.

In order to define the full spectrum of LPD, it is necessary to get more information about any unusual predisposition, or selective sensitivity of subperitoneal mesenchymal cells to reproductive steroids. It is also necessary to keep in mind that other factors may control the growth of LPD. In order to choose appropriate therapy it is also important to know whether or not LPD will change into a genuine neoplasm.

PATHOLOGY AND BIOLOGY

Gross Appearance

Numerous firm gray-white nodules are scattered all over the peritoneal cavity. The nodules vary from being microscopic in size to 10.0 cm in diameter, and are usually discrete, solid and round. The nodules are sessile, or pedunculated with short stalks, and occasionally show prominent vascularity on their surface or around them (Figures and 1 and 2). They occur predominantly in the omentum (Figure 1), which often forms a matted nodularity or an ill-defined thickening. They are studded diffusely over the pelvic peritoneum (Figure 2), on the uterine serosa, the surface of the ovary, the serosa of the large and small intestine, the mesentery (Figure 2), the peritoneal surface of the fallopian tube, the cul-de-sac, and even the subdiaphragmatic surfaces. The liver is sometimes involved on its surface, and involvement of retroperitoneal (19) and

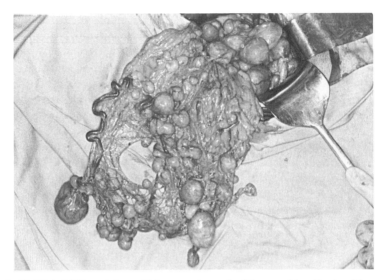

Figure 1 Multiple LPD nodules within omentum of a 37 year old patient neither recently pregnant nor taking oral contraceptive steroids. (*Reproduced by permission of Drs T. Isono and Y. Takeda*).

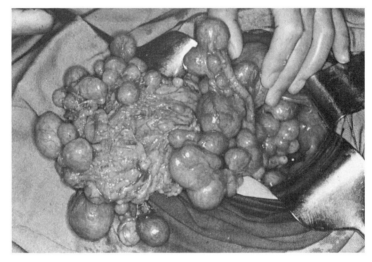

Figure 2 Multiple LPD nodules within omentum and pelvic cavity. Note nodules along appendix vermiformis and prominent vascularity on their surface. (*Reproduced by permission of Drs T. Isono T. and Y. Takeda*).

omental (16) lymph nodes are also reported. The cut surface of the nodules usually shows a whorled appearance. It sometimes is accompanied by a central hemorrhagic area.

LPD is rarely accompanied by ascites (12).

One case developed signs of an acute abdomen 6 days postpartum due to intraperitoneal hemorrhage from multiple areas of endometriosis (25). Leiomyomas are reported in the uterus in the majority of cases.

Light Microscopic Findings

The majority of nodules are well circumscribed and covered by the mesothelium (Figures 3 and 4). Spindle cells with elongated nuclei often containing small distinct nucleoli characteristic of smooth muscle are arranged in whorls (Figures 4 and 5). The cells have abundant eosinophilic cytoplasm, in which parallel longitudinal fibrils are stained with PTAH or Gomori's trichrome. Pleomorphism or atypia is usually not found, and mitotic figures are rare. In the most active areas of nodules, mitotic figures do not exceed more

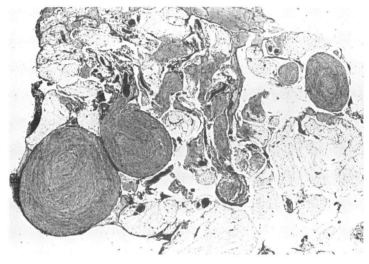

Figure 3 Light microscopic section of LPD nodules within omentum incidentally found during pregnancy. Note several nodules containing smooth muscle cells arranged in whorls. (Gomori's trichrome stain, original magnification: ×10)

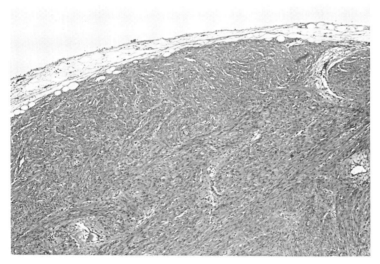

Figure 4 Light microscopic section of LPD nodules which is not directly related to pregnancy or to oral contraceptive steroids. Note spindle cells' proliferation arranged in whorls under the peritoneum. (Hematoxylin and eosin, original magnification: ×40)

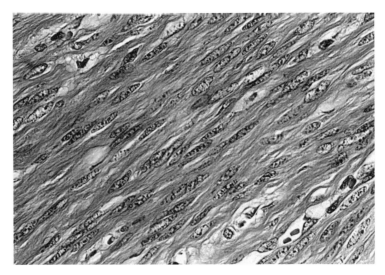

Figure 5 High power view of Figure 4. Note spindle cells with abundant eosinophilic cytoplasm and elongated nuclei often containing small distinct nucleoli characteristic of smooth muscle. (Hematoxylin and eosin, original magnification: ×400)

than three in ten high power fields. Some nodules show focal areas of fibrosis or hyalinization.

Although the majority of the nodules are composed of smooth muscle cells, the cellular composition of nodules varies particularly in pregnant cases. Collagen, fibroblastic cells, and decidual cells are mixed with smooth muscle. During pregnancy, a miniature nodule shows an accumulation of irregular, large, decidualized cells (Figure 6) under the mesothelium. These cells possess a low nuclear–cytoplasmic ratio and granular eosinophilic, and often vacuolated, cytoplasm. They blend

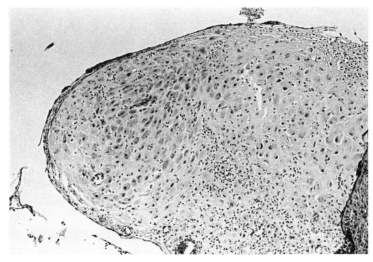

Figure 6 Light microscopic section of a miniature nodule found in LPD patient during pregnancy. Note an accumulation of irregular, large, decidualized cells under the mesothelium. (Gomori's trichrome stain, original magnification: ×100)

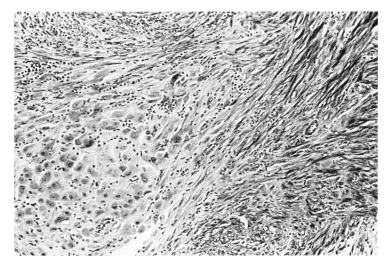

Figure 7 Light microscopic section of a miniature LPD nodule found during pregnancy. Note decidualized cells blend gradually with the adjacent fibroblastic, and smooth muscle proliferation. (Gomori's trichrome stain, original magnification: ×100)

gradually with the adjacent fibroblastic and smooth muscle proliferation (Figure 7). A relatively large nodule is mainly composed of smooth muscle and fibroblastic cells (Figure 8). Edema and lymphatic infiltrates are often present, but necrosis is rare.

LPD nodules often show prominent vascularity, but there is no consistent relationship between the smooth muscle of nodules and that of vessel walls.

Glandular structures of various sizes resembling endometrial glands are reported in some peritoneal nodules (12, 14, 25, 31). They are lined by low columnar cells and some are ciliated. Some of the glands contain cellular debris and are hemorrhagic; hemosiderin pig-

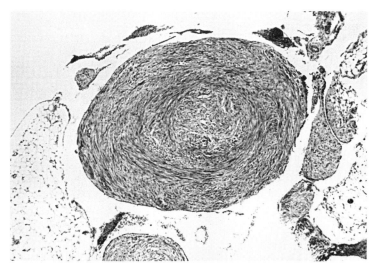

Figure 8 Light microscopic section of a relative large nodule found during pregnancy. Nodule is mainly composed of smooth muscle cells and fibroblastic cells arranged in whorls. (Gomori's trichrome stain, original magnification: ×40)

ments are found in adjacent tissues. Peritoneal endometriosis is usually co-existent in such instances.

Ultrastructural Findings

The spindle cells show features typical of smooth muscle cells (Figure 9). They are surrounded by a thin basal lamina, and are separated from each other by a narrow band of collagen fibrils. The cell membrane shows numerous pinocytotic vesicles scattered along the cytoplasmic border. The cytoplasm is filled with abundant longitudinally oriented myofilaments with dense bodies. A thin rim of rough endoplasmic reticulum (rER), Golgi complexes, occasional mitochondria, and lysosomal granules are present in perinuclear areas. Nuclei are irregularly shaped with deep and shallow indentations, and contain a prominent nucleolus. Some typical smooth muscle cells are closely apposed to each other forming junctions characterized by an electron dense submembranous material, at the interfaces between adjacent cells.

Instead of these typical smooth muscle cells, some nodules are composed of cells interpreted as modified smooth muscle cells or myofibroblasts. These spindle shaped cells contain smaller amounts of intracytoplasmic filaments, more prominent rER, and less distinct pinocytotic vesicles compared with typical smooth muscle cells. Intermingled with these myogenic cells, cells resembling fibroblasts also exist. All three cell types are reported to show a close association with collagen fibers and seem capable of producing collagen.

During pregnancy, typical decidual cells with abundant cytoplasm and shallow convoluted margins with numerous cytoplasmic protrusions and microvillous processes are present. A round-to-oval centrally located nucleus contains one or two nucleoli. The cytoplasmic matrix is pale or electron dense. Rough endoplasmic reticulum, small inconspicuous tubular mitochondria, and fine microfilaments are

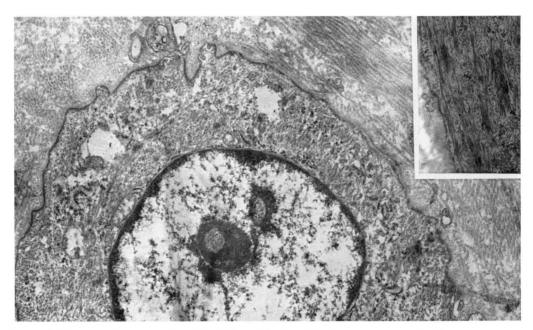

Figure 9 Electron micrograph of cell in LPD nodule found during pregnancy. A cell cut transversely shows features of smooth muscle cells surrounded by a thin basal lamina. The cytoplasm is filled with abundant longitudinally oriented myofilaments with dense bodies (inset shows longitudinal section). (original magnifications: ×15000, inset×9000)

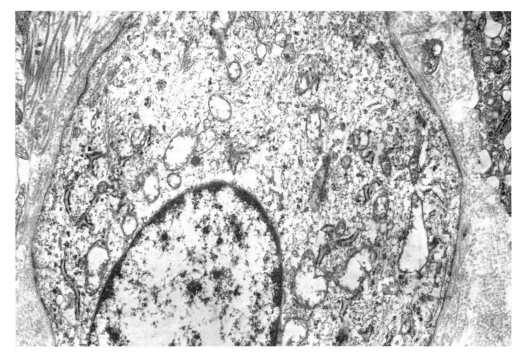

Figure 10 Electron micrograph of a decidual cell with abundant cytoplasm and fine microfilaments diffusely distributed throughout the cytoplasm (original magnification: ×15000).

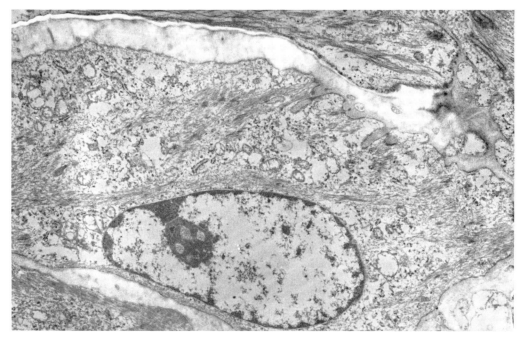

Figure 11 Electron micrograph of cells intermediate between smooth muscle cells and decidual cells. Note a cell with the configuration of decidual cells and an increased density of cytoplasmic filaments with some dense body formation. (original magnification: ×15000)

diffusely distributed throughout the cytoplasm (Figure 10). In addition to typical decidual cells, cells intermediate between smooth muscle cells and decidual cells are noted (Figure 11). These cells have the configuration of decidual cells, but exhibit an increased density of cytoplasmic filaments with some dense body formation at the periphery of the cytoplasm. Pincytotic vesicles are prominent, and the cells are invested by a patchy, fine basal lamina.

Regressive Features of Nodules

Aterman et al. (7) observed at a second-look operation a reduction in the size of nodules after the hormonal stimulus of pregnancy had ceased. Histologically, the cytoplasm was reduced to barely visible rims, so that the nodules seemed to consist almost of naked, uniform nuclei distinctly reduced in size. No decidual cells were seen.

Williams and Pavlock (17), who also did a second-look operation, reported that after surgical castration the cells of the nodules showed the features of atrophic smooth muscle. Ultrastructurally, the cells had only a few cytoplasmic organelles and myofilaments that were focally condensed into numerous dense bodies.

Endocrinological Aspects

Although abnormal endocrine status has been suggested in LPD patients, hormonal studies are rare among published cases.

Serum Estrogen and Progesterone Levels

There are five reports in which the levels of serum reproductive steroids are reported. During pregnancy, Fujii et al. (16) found normal estrogen but low progesterone levels in their patient, and they suggested that a hormonal imbalance precipitated the development of the LPD nodules.

In the patient taking oral contraceptive steroids, Kuo et al. (12) reported normal estradiol levels before surgery, and low levels after oophorectomy.

Of the 3 patients neither pregnant nor taking oral contraceptive steroids, Isono et al. (34) reported normal estrogen and progesterone levels both in the folicular and luteal phases in a 37 year old; in the 50 year old patient Pearse (22) reported normal estrogen levels before surgery and Brumback et al. (33) found very low levels of sex hormones and little estrogenic effect on the uterine cervix in the 55 year old.

Therefore, there is no convincing evidence that abnormal levels of circulating reproductive steroids are associated with LPD.

Estrogen and Progesterone Receptors

In a patient taking oral contraceptive steroids, Sutherland et al. (13) found that the concentration of estrogen and progesterone receptor proteins in tissues obtained at the time of hysterectomy was 120 and 434 fmol/mg cytosol protein, respectively. This represents a ninefold increase in the concentration of estrogen receptors and a twofold increase in the concentration of progesterone receptors when compared to normal myometrium from the same patient (13 and 215 fmol/mg protein, respectively). Progesterone receptors were not detectable in the leiomyomatous tissues obtained at the time of laparoscopy 6 months following surgical castration.

In contrast, Walley (31) reported that estrogen receptors were 17, 41, and 9 fmol/mg and progesterone receptors were 252, 518, and 11 fmol/mg in normal myometrium, mural leiomyoma, and peritoneal nodules, respectively, in a 49 year old patient neither recently pregnant nor taking oral contraceptive steroids.

In a 37 year old patient, Isono et al. (34) found that estrogen receptors were 41.2 fmol/mg protein and progesterone receptors were 208.7 fmol/mg protein in the peritoneal nodule.

These receptor studies are few, but compared to the levels of estrogen receptors, the levels of progesterone receptors are relatively lower in LPD nodules..

CLINICAL FEATURES

LPD as an incidental finding has been reported in 60 women. None of these had signs or symptoms referable to it. One 55 year old woman (33) had a 2-week history of dizziness, anorexia, nausea, and marked weakness. Suspected gastrointestinal bleeding was evaluated radiologically and a highly vascular abdominal and/or pelvic tumor discovered.

Of the 61 women, 24 were discovered during pregnancy or immediately postpartum; 12 of these at the time of cesarean section, 4 at the time of laparoscopic tubal ligation, 1 at laparotomy to exclude broad ligament hematoma. Two were found at myomectomy during pregnancy, and 4 at laparotomy for evaluation of a pelvic mass detected during early pregnancy. One developed signs of an acute abdomen 6 days postpartum and laparotomy disclosed hemorrhage from multiple areas of endometriosis.

The 37 women who were not pregnant had complaints of pelvic discomfort or pain. Hypermenorrhea, dysmenorrhea, and menometrorrhagia were noted. Of the 37 women, 33 had co-existing uterine leiomyomas. Therefore, the symptoms may be due to uterine leiomyomas rather than to LPD.

One case was found incidentally at autopsy in a 69 year old woman.

INVESTIGATION

On physical examination, the masses of LPD were usually difficult to identify abdominally. Pelvic examination may reveal multiple nodules in the cul-de-sac, similar to endometriosis or peritoneal carcinomatosis. Therefore, preoperatively, the diagnosis of the very rare LPD is not suggested.

However, in the case of Brumback et al. (33) with suspected gastrointestinal bleeding, a radiologic study was helpful in locating the lesion. A radionuclide angiography, per-

formed in order to localize a possible bleeding site, demonstrated LPD to be hypervascular. Because of the highly vascular nature of the LPD nodules, it was suggested that a radionuclide angiogram or an intravenous digital subtraction angiogram might be valuable as a diagnostic method. Since complete resection of nodules may not be possible, these studies may also be valuable in the follow-up of patients. In addition, computerized tomography might be considered. However, as one-third of LPD patients are pregnant or immediately postpartum, there is limitation on the usefulness of radiologic studies.

For final diagnosis, laparoscopy with biopsy is necessary. Frozen section is also important and omission of this procedure can be hazardous. Clearly, the frozen section may help avoid unnecessary surgery.

MANAGEMENT AND PROGNOSIS

Since LPD is a widely disseminated condition, complete resection of the nodules may not be possible. None of the patients reported had complete excision. In the earlier series, more extensive surgery including total hysterectomy with bilateral salpingo-oophorectomy and partial omentectomy was performed. However, LPD is a benign condition which does not affect the neighbouring organs and characteristically regresses after hormone withdrawal. It does not require extensive surgery, nor does it compromise future childbearing. More recently only biopsies have been performed. There are no reports of a fatal outcome due to LPD. As patients have variable pathogenetic hormonal backgrounds, however, management is potentially different.

Patients who have a background of excess hormonal stimulation can be expected to demonstrate regression when hormones are withdrawn. They do not require extensive surgery. Biopsy of the nodules is required for diagnosis and it has been recommended that levels of both estrogen and progesterone receptors should be measured. After the withdrawal of a pathogenetic stimulation, clinical assessment of whether the nodules regress or not is the most important point of management. Usually, the nodules will regress soon after the withdrawal of the stimulation. Although there are no reports of further growth after that, there is a report that the nodules persisted 1.2 years later at repeated laparotomy (25). In such instance, the nodules might have a sensitivity to grow under the normal ovarian cycles and may require more treatment to further regress nodules either by surgery or drug therapy. Castration may be indicated, but if the nodules have some levels of estrogen receptors and progesterone receptors, treatment with either anti-estrogenic agents or progesterone, or combination of both, will be a choice.

In patients with hormone producing ovarian tumors, the removal of the ovarian tumors and biopsy of the nodules are recommended. However, the age of such patients is usually high. Therefore, total hysterectomy with bilateral salpingo-oophorectomy will be a usual procedure.

In the patients of reproductive age having ambiguous pathogenetic hormonal stimulation it can be considered that the nodules of LPD are under the control of normal ovarian cycles. In such cases, LPD is predominantly accompanied by uterine leiomyomas with symptoms of dysmenorrhea, hypermenorrhea, or menometrorrhagia. Therefore, in patients who have no desire for further childbearing total abdominal hysterectomy with bilateral salpingo-oophorectomy can be recommended. However, treatment using anti-estrogenic agents or progesterone, or combination of both, is also a choice if the nodules may have measurable levels of estrogen and/or progesterone receptors.

In patients discovered after menopause, the lesion itself may be regressing or a remnant, but as in the case of Brumback et al. (33), some lesions may affect the neighbouring organs. Histological assessment of degenerative features will be helpful to avoid extensive surgery. However, if the nodules do not show degenerative features and are affecting neighbouring organs, resection of nodules which affect the neighbouring organs may be necessary. Since these patients are supposed to have low levels of reproductive steroids, castration or anti-estrogenic agents would not seem likely to cause regression of nodules. However, castration would at least detect any ovarian factors.

Prognosis

All reported women with follow-up were alive from 3 months to 10 years after the diagnosis. Despite a variable treatment, there are no reports of a fatal outcome referable to LPD.

DIFFERENTIAL DIAGNOSIS

Leiomyomatosis of the Colon

Freni and Keeman (54) described what they termed leiomyomatosis of the colon in a 30 year old woman who 1 week after delivery of her child was found to have multiple benign leiomyomas both intramurally and on the serosal surface of the right colon without nodules on the other serosal surfaces including the uterus and adnexae. Although the surgical resection incompletely removed the tumor nodules from the colon, a second-look operation 4 months later revealed no further evidence of the leiomyomas. This case is assumed to be a variant example of LPD in which there was predominantly bowel involvement (33).

Primary Leiomyosarcoma of the Gastrointestinal Tract and Peritoneum (25, 55)

This usually presents as a solitary mass at least 5 cm in diameter (mostly more than 10 cm) and it may have accompanying satellite nodules. The low mitotic activity (rarely exceeding two mitotic figures per ten high power fields) and lack of atypia help distinguish LPD from leiomyosarcoma, which usually has prominent mitotic activity. Some leiomyosarcomas show a paucity of mitoses; however, they have prominent tumor cell necrosis which LPD lacks. The large numbers and the small size of LPD nodules are unlike the findings in leiomyosarcoma. The nodules of leiomyosarcoma are progressive.

Benign Metastasizing Leiomyoma (25, 56)

Microscopically, the distinction of LPD from benign metastasizing leiomyoma may be very difficult. The distinction is mainly based on the distribution and the composition of the lesions. Benign metastasizing leiomyoma generally presents as one or more pulmonary nodules, but when it occurs in the pelvis, there are only a few nodules, the nodules are usually larger than those of LPD, and they tend to be positioned in the region of the round ligament or near the iliac veins. The nodules of benign metastasizing leiomyomas persist without diminution in size.

Intravenous Leiomyomatosis (56, 57)

Microscopically, LPD nodules are not associated with blood vessels although they may be in some foci. Unlike LPD, intravenous leiomyomatosis generally involves large pelvic veins.

CURRENT BIOLOGICAL AND CLINICAL RESEARCH

With regard to LPD, information about current biological or clinical research is few. However, as described in the etiology, in order to define the full spectrum of LPD, it is necessary to get more information about any unusual predisposition, or selective sensitivity of subperitoneal mesenchymal cells to reproductive steroids. At least, more data are needed on the levels of estrogen and progesterone receptors in the nodules. Biochemical research work which has been done on uterine leiomyoma, such as the measurement of the activity of 17-β-hydroxysteroid dehydrogenase

(58, 59) or cytochrome P-450 (60) may also be necessary. In addition, the studies of growth potential under hormonal supplementation as performed in uterine leiomyoma (51, 61), shall provide some information about the sensitivity of LPD nodules to reproductive steroids.

ACKNOWLEDGEMENT

I wish to express thanks to Dr Tim H. Parmley for editing the chapter.

REFERENCES

1 Taubert HD, Wissner SE, Haskins AL. Leiomyomatosis peritonealis disseminata. An unusual complication of genital leiomyoma. Obstet Gynecol 1965; 25: 561.

2 Wilson JR, Peale AR. Multiple peritoneal leiomyomas associated with a granulosa cell tumor of the ovary. Am J Obstet Gynecol 1952; 48: 225.

3 Crosland DB. Leiomyomatosis peritonealis disseminata. A case report. Am J Obstet Gynecol 1973; 117: 179.

4 Parmley TH, Woodruff JD, Winn K, Johnson JWC, Douglas PH. Histogenesis of leiomyomatosis peritonealis disseminata (disseminating fibrosing deciduosis). Obstet Gynecol 1975; 46: 511.

5 Bettendorf U, Stelter U. Leiomyomatosis peritonealis disseminata. Arch Gynecol 1975; 220: 179.

6 Goldberg MF, Hurt WG, Frable WJ. Leiomyomatosis peritonealis disseminata. Report of a case and review of the literature. Obstet Gynecol 1977; 49: 46s.

7 Aterman K, Fraser GM, Lea RH. Disseminated peritoneal leiomyomatosis. Virchows Arch Pathol Anat 1977; 374: 13.

8 Altinger HP, Atkins BJ. Leiomyomatosis peritonealis disseminata in a non-pregnant female: A case report. Med J St Joseph Hospital (Houston) 1977; 12: 179.

9 Nogales Jr FF, Matilla A, Carrascal E. Leiomyomatosis peritonealis disseminata: An ultrastructural study. Am J Clin Pathol 1978; 69: 452.

10 O'Sullivan BT. Leiomyomatosis peritonealis disseminata. Aust NZ J Obstet Gynecol 1978; 18: 94.

11 Piesler PC, Orenstein JM, Hogan DL, Breslow A. Ultrastructure of myofibroblasts and decidualized cells in leiomyomatosis peritonealis disseminata. Am J Clin Pathol 1979; 72: 875.

12 Kuo T, London SN, Dinh TV. Endometriosis

occurring in leiomyomatosis peritonealis disseminata: ultrastructural study and histogenetic consideration. Am J Surg Pathol 1980; 4: 197.

13 Sutherland JA, Wilson EA, Edger DE, Powell D. Ultrastructure and steroid binding studies in leiomyomatosis peritonealis disseminata. Am J Obstet Gynecol 1980; 136: 992.

14 Kaplan D, Bernischke K, Johnson KC. Leiomyomatosis peritonealis disseminata with endometrium. Obstet Gynecol 1980; 55: 119.

15 Lim OW, Segal A, Ziel HK. Leiomyomatosis peritonealis disseminata associated with pregnancy. Obstet Gynecol 1980; 55: 122.

16 Fujii S, Okamura H, Nakashima N, Ban C, Aso T, Nishimura T. Leiomyomatosis peritonealis disseminata. Obstet Gynecol 1980; 55: 79s.

17 Williams LJ, Pavlick FJ. Leiomyomatosis peritonealis disseminata: Two case reports and a review of the medical literature. Cancer 1980; 45: 1726.

18 DelCastillo H, Rubio PA, Farrel EM. Leiomyomatosis peritonealis disseminata in a non-pregnant female: A case report. Int J Gynecol Obstet 1980; 17: 428.

19 Hsu YK, Rosenshein NB, Parmley TH, Woodruff JD, Elberfeld H: Leiomyomatosis in pelvic lymph nodes. Obstet Gynecol 1981; 57: 91s.

20 Strom H, Jacobson L, Hedberg K. Leiomyomatosis peritonealis disseminata. Acta Obstet Gynecol Scand 1981; 60: 421.

21 Cecacci L, Jacobs J, Powell A. Leiomyomatosis peritonealis disseminata: Report of a case in a non-pregnant woman. Am J Obstet Gynecol 1982; 144: 105.

22 Pearce PH: Leiomyomatosis peritonealis disseminata. Am J Obstet Gynecol 1982; 144: 133.

23 Donovan DC, Morani JG, Boria MC. Leiomyomatosis peritonealis disseminata following hysterotomy. Md State Med J 1982; 31: 48.

24 Chen KTK, Hendriks EJ, Freeburg B. Benign glandular inclusion of the peritoneum associated with leiomyomatosis peritonealis disseminata. Diagn Gynecol Obstet 1982; 4: 41.

25 Tavassolu FA, Norris HJ. Peritoneal leiomyomatosis (leiomyomatosis peritonealis disseminata): A clinico pathologic study of 20 cases with ultrastructural observations. Int J Gynecol Pathol 1982; 1: 59.

26 Borel B, Herlicoviez M, Raffy P, Rousselot P. Leiomyomatose péritonealie disséminée: à propos d'une observation. Ann Pathol 1982; 2: 60.

27 Cremer H, Totovic V, Citoler P. Die Leiomyomatosis peritonealis disseminata. Eine lichtund elektronen mikroskopische Studie. Geburtsh Frauenheilkd 1982; 42: 616.

28 Erbstoesser E, Lessel W. Leiomyomatosis peritonealis disseminata. Zentralbl Chir 1982; 107: 223.

29 Frappart L, Berger G, Vernevaut, Y, Mallet-Guy Y, Palayer C, Spay G, Feroldi J. La leiomyomatose péritoneale disséminée: Etude anatomoclinique et ultrastructurale d'un cas associé à un hemangiome caverneux du fioe. Arch Anat Cytol Pathol 1982; 30: 117.

30 Hoynck Van Papendrecht HPCM, Gratama S. Leiomyomatosis peritonealis disseminata. Eur J Obstet Gynecol Reprod Biol 1983; 14: 251.

31 Walley VM. Letter to the editor. Int J Gynecol Pathol 1983; 2: 222.

32 Valente PT. Leiomyomatosis peritonealis disseminata: A report of two cases and review of the literature. Arch Pathol Lab Med 1984; 108: 669.

33 Brumback RA, Brown BS, Sobie P, Shapiro MJ, Wallinga HA. Leiomyomatosis peritonealis disseminata. Surgery 1985; 97: 707.

34 Isono T, Yokoo I, Adachi T, Kasai H, Wada Y, Iguchi T, Yoshida S, Takeda Y. A case report of leiomyomatosis peritonealis disseminata. Nippon San Fujinka Gakkai Kanto Rengo 1985; 41: 1.

35 Dreyer L, Simson IW, Sevenster CBVO, Dittrich DC. Leiomyomatosis peritonealis disseminata. A report of two cases and review of the literature. Br J Obstet Gynecol 1985; 92: 856.

36 Lipschutz A, Vargas L. Structure and origin of uterine and extragenital fibroids induced experimentally in the guinea pig by prolonged administration of estrogens. Cancer Res 1941; 1: 236.

37 Lipschutz A. Experimental fibroids and the antifibromatogenic action of steroid hormones. JAMA 1942; 120: 171.

38 Ober WB, Black MD. Neoplasms of the subcoelomic mesenchyme. Arch Pathol Lab Med 1955; 59: 695.

39 Herr JC, Heidger PM, Scott JR, Anderson JW, Curet LB, Mossman HW. Decidual cells in the human ovary at term. 1. Incidence, gross anatomy and ultrastructural features of merocrine secretion. Am J Anat 1978; 152: 7.

40 Herr JC, Platz CE, Heidger PM, Curet LB. Smooth muscle within ovarian decidual nodules: A link to leiomyomatosis peritonealis disseminata? Obstet Gynecol 1979; 53: 451.

41 Parakash S, Scully RE. Sarcoma-like pseudopregnancy changes in uterine leiomyomas. Obstet Gynecol 1964; 24: 106.

42 Scully RE. Smooth muscle differentiation in genital tract disorders. Arch Pathol Lab Med 1981; 105: 505.

43 Lauchlan SC. The secondary müllerian system. Obstet Gynecol Surv 1972; 27: 133.

44 Fujii S, Konishi I, Ban C, Okamura H. Adenomatoid tumor-like structures in the subperitoneal nodules produced by sex steroids. Am J Obstet Gynecol 1983; 145: 850.

45 Rohlfing MB, Kao KJ, Woodard BH. Endo-

myometriosis: possible association with leiomyomatosis disseminata and endometriosis. Arch Pathol Lab Med 1981; 105: 556.

46 Cozzutto C. Uterus-like mass replacing ovary. Arch Pathol Lab Med 1981; 105: 508.

47 Winn KJ, Woodruff JD, Parmley TH. Electronmicroscopic studies of leiomyomatosis peritonealis disseminata. Obstet Gynecol 1976; 48: 225.

48 Bird CC, Williams RA. The production of smooth muscle by the endometrial stroma of the adult human uterus. J Pathol Bacteriol 1965; 90: 75.

49 Konishi I, Fujii S, Okamura H, Mori T. Development of smooth muscle in the human fetal uterus: An ultrastructural study. J Anat 1984; 139: 239.

50 Fujii S, Nakashima N, Okamura H, Takenaka A, Kanzaki H, Okuda Y, Morimoto K, Nishimura T. Progesterone-induced smooth muscle-like cells in the subperitoneal nodules produced by estrogen. Experimental approach to leiomyomatosis peritonealis disseminata. Am J Obstet Gynecol 1981; 139: 164.

51 Kawaguchi K, Fujii S, Konishi I, Okamura H, Mori T. Ultrastructural study of cultured smooth muscle cells from uterine leiomyoma and myometrium under the influence of sex steroids. Gynecol Oncol 1985; 21: 32.

52 Nelson LW, Kelly WA. Mesovarial leiomyomas in rats in a chronic toxicity study of soterenol hydrochloride. Vet Path 1971; 8: 452.

53 Jack D, Poynter D, Spurling NW. Beta-adrenocepter stimulants and mesoovarian leiomyomas in the rat. Toxicology 1983; 23: 315.

54 Freni SC, Keeman JN. Leiomyomatosis of the colon. Cancer 1977; 39: 263.

55 Ranchod M, Kempson RL. Smooth muscle tumors of the gastrointestinal tract and retroperitoneum. Cancer 1977; 39: 255.

56 Norris HJ, Zaloudek CJ. Mesenchymal tumors of the uterus. In: Blaustein A ed Pathology of the Female Genital Tract. New York: Springer-Verlag, 1982: 352.

57 Norris HJ, Parmley T. Mesenchymal tumors of the uterus. V. Intravenous leiomyomatosis. Cancer 1975; 36: 2164.

58 Pollow K, Sinnerker G, Boquol E, Pollow B. In vitro conversion of estradiol-17β into estrone in normal human myometrium and leiomyoma. J Clin Chem Clin Biochem 1978; 16: 493.

59 Newton CJ, James VHT. 17β-hydroxysteroid dehydrogenase activity in leiomyoma and myometrium and its relationship to concentrations of estrone, estradiol and progesterone throughout the menstrual cycle. J Steroid Biochem 1985; 22: 487.

60 Senler TI, Hofmann GE, Sanfilippo JS, Barrows GH, Dean WL, Wittliff JL. Cytochrome p-450 activity in human leiomyoma and normal myometrium. Am J Obstet Gynecol 1985; 153: 551.

61 Cramer SF, Robertson AL, Ziats NP, Pearson OH. Growth potential of human uterine leiomyomas: some in vitro observations and their implications. Obstet Gynecol 1985; 66: 36.

Textbook of Uncommon Cancer
Edited by C.J. Williams, J.G. Krikorian, M.R. Green and D. Raghavan
© 1988 John Wiley & Sons Ltd

Chapter **10**

Management of Gynecologic Sarcomas

David L. Marchetti* and
M. Steven Piver†

Clinician II, Department of Gynecologic Oncology, Roswell Park Memorial Institute, Buffalo, New York, Assistant Professor, State University of New York at Buffalo, Buffalo, New York, USA and † Chief, Department of Gynecologic Oncology, Roswell Park Memorial Institute, Buffalo, New York, Clinical Professor, State University of New York at Buffalo, Buffalo, New York, USA

INTRODUCTION

Of 70 000 new cases per year of carcinoma of the uterus, cervix and ovary, approximately 1% of malignant neoplasms of the female genital tract will involve sarcomatous change. Consequently, in view of the uncommon occurrence of these tumors, optimal management is often difficult to determine. In many situations, clearer treatment protocols can be defined; in others, too few cases have been compiled to delineate clear treatment recommendations. This chapter will review gynecologic sarcomas, excluding mixed mesodermal tumors and adenosarcomas, which are discussed elsewhere (Chapters 4 and 5).

UTERINE SARCOMA
(Chapter 7)

This discussion follows the classification of uterine sarcoma outlined by Kempson and Bari (1) (Table 1), which represents modification of the earlier Ober classification (2). Patients are staged according to the International Federation of Gynaecology and Obstetrics (FIGO) classification for adenocarcinomas of the uterus (Table 2).

Leiomyosarcoma

Any description of leiomyosarcoma reflects histologic criteria utilized in determining histopathologic diagnosis. This feature was well recognized by Taylor and Norris (3). A discrepancy in 5-year survival of 8% to 68% reflected the difficulty in the diagnosis of leiomyosarcoma of the uterus (4–11). Their study concluded that lesions with fewer than ten mitoses per ten high power fields were benign regardless of cytologic atypia, whereas tumors of ten or more mitotic figures per ten high power fields were very likely to recur. Subsequent studies did not find any formal agreement, as indicated by the report of Kempson and Bari (1), who concluded tumors with less than five mitoses per ten high power fields should be interpreted as benign. Silverbag (12) was the strongest opponent of the utilization of mitotic count as the sole criteria for histologic diagnosis. He proposed a grading system which included such features as atypical mitoses, nuclear inclusions, hyperchromatic nuclei, the presence or absence of multinucleated giant cells and dense cellularity. More recently, Van Dinh and Woodruff (13) made an effort to combine both diagnostic

TABLE 1 CLASSIFICATION OF UTERINE SARCOMAS

I Pure sarcomas
  A Pure homologous
    1 Leiomyosarcoma
    2 Stromal sarcoma
    3 Endolymphatic stromal myosis
    4 Angiosarcoma
    5 Fibrosarcoma
  B Pure heterologous
    1 Rhabdomyosarcoma (including sarcoma botryoides)
    2 Chondrosarcoma
    3 Osteosarcoma
    4 Liposarcoma
II Mixed sarcomas
  A Mixed homologous
  B Mixed heterologous
    Mixed heterologous sarcomas with or without homologous elements
III Malignant mixed müllerian tumors (mixed mesodermal tumors)
  A Malignant mixed müllerian tumor, homologous type
    Carcinoma plus leiomyosarcoma, stromal sarcoma, or fibrosarcoma, or mixtures of these sarcomas
  B Malignant mixed müllerian tumor, heterologous type
    Carcinoma plus heterologous sarcoma with or without homologous sarcoma
IV Sarcoma, unclassified
V Malignant lymphoma

From Kempson and Bari (1).
(Reprinted with permission from W.B. Saunders Co.)

TABLE 2 CLINICAL STAGING OF UTERINE SARCOMAS

Stage I: The sarcoma is confined to the corpus uteri.
    Stage 1A: The length of the uterine cavity is 8 cm or less.
    Stage 1B: The length of the uterine cavity is more than 8 cm.
Stage II: The sarcoma has involved the corpus and the cervix.
Stage III: The sarcoma has extended outside the uterus but not outside the true pelvis.
Stage IV: The sarcoma has extended outside the true pelvis or has invaded the mucosa of the bladder or rectum. Bullous edema alone does not establish Stage IV disease.

approaches, and in addition, proposed the use of a single high power field as a third type of methodology.

Taylor and Norris (3) reviewed 63 highly cellular uterine tumors with 31 recurrences in

TABLE 3 COMPARISON OF TUMOR GRADE AND SURVIVAL

Grade	Mitotic count/10 HPEs[a]		Outcome	
	Mean	Range	Alive	Dead
I	5.2	1–13	4	0
II	9.8	3–28	7	2
III	6.6	0–23	6	4
IV	23.3	[b]	1	6

[a]HPF=High power fields.
[b]=2 patients with 3+7 mitoses/10 HPs.

the 36 patients interpreted to have leiomyosarcoma. Kempson and Bari (1) reviewed 29 cases which were previously diagnosed as cellular atypical leiomyoma and leiomyosarcoma. Twelve patients were found to have more than ten mitoses per ten high power fields, with 7 patients dying from recurrence and 2 living with metastasis. Seven patients comprised a group of five to nine mitoses per ten high power fields, with 5 patients dead secondary to recurrence. There were 10 patients with less than five mitoses per ten high power fields, with one recurrence 7 years following initial surgery with a similar tumor removed from the fifth lumbar vertebra. Following this, she remained without evidence of further metastasis. The remaining patients are all alive without evidence of disease. It was concluded that presence or absence of giant cells did not correlate with survival, and atypical stromal cells were not a reliable sign of malignancy. Silverberg (12) evaluated mitotic count and grade. Table 3 compares tumor grade, mean mitotic count and outcome. When mitotic count alone was compared to survival, there was one recurrence among 10 patients with nought to four mitoses per ten high power fields. There were 11 deaths and one recurrence among 20 patients with five or more mitotic figures. It was Silverberg's conclusion that histologic grading was equal to mitotic count as an indicator of prognosis (1, 3, 12, 13).

Survival

Five-year survivals range from 0 to 73% (1, 3,

13–17). Of reports that differentiate Stage I from more advanced stage patients, Salazar (18) reported 5-year survival of 58% for Stage I uterine leiomyosarcoma treated by surgery alone. This probably represents the most reliable figure.

Prior Pelvic Radiotherapy

In Taylor and Norris's series (3) none of the 39 patients with leiomyosarcoma had prior pelvic radiotherapy; while the study of Aaaro et al. (17) revealed a history of prior radiotherapy in 7 of 105 patients. From those and several other series (3, 12–15, 17), only 8 of 270 patients were treated with prior pelvic radiotherapy. Data accumulated from the more recent studies suggest radiotherapy does not play a significant role in the etiology of this malignancy.

Sarcomatous Degeneration of Benign Leiomyoma

In Silverberg's review (12), he described 8 cases in which the focus of sarcoma was clearly within the boundaries of a leiomyoma. In 3 other patients, it was felt that the focus of origin occurred in a leiomyoma, but the malignant growth had extended beyond the myomatous boundary. In nine patients with follow-up data, 6 were free of recurrence. Taylor and Norris (3) reported that none of the tumors in their report had originated in a benign leiomyoma. In Hart and Billman's review (15) of leiomyosarcoma, origin from pre-existing leiomyoma was apparent in only one patient. This was a large solitary tumor that extended into the adnexa. This patient died with widespread metastatic leiomyosarcoma within one year following her initial surgery. In Van Dinh and Woodruff's series (13), 9 patients were discovered to have leiomyosarcoma after myomectomy. Three of these patients underwent subsequent hysterectomy, while there was no further surgical treatment in the remaining patients. Eight of 9 patients remained free of disease from 1 to 13 years following the initial treatment. Three of the 6 patients treated by

myomectomy only, for infertility, achieved pregnancy and remained free of disease 3–13 years after their initial surgical management.

From the available data, the prognosis appears to be somewhat improved for those leiomyosarcomas which are confined within a myoma.

Ideally, when myomectomy is performed as the initial operation, subsequent management should include total abdominal hysterectomy and bilateral salpingo-oophorectomy. If for reasons of fertility, the patient desires no further surgical intervention, the risks, although less, still remain significant.

As to the question and incidence of sarcomatous degeneration of benign smooth muscle tumors of the uterus, there was no formal agreement in the above notated studies.

Menopausal Status

In Silverberg's series (12), there were 21 premenopausal and 13 postmenopausal patients. Of 18 premenopausal patients with follow-up, 3 developed recurrent disease. In 12 postmenopausal patients, 10 died of recurrent disease. In Hart's collection of 15 patients (15), all died of tumor within $7\frac{1}{2}$ years. No correlation is seen between increased length of survival and premenopausal status. Vardi and Tovell (16) reported 5-year survival in 63 patients as 3% and 5.5% in pre- and postmenopausal patients respectively. In the study of Bazzocchi et al. (19), 8 of the 10 surviving patients were premenopausal. It is noteworthy that 6 of these 8 patients had fewer than ten mitoses per ten high power fields. In Van Dinh and Woodruff's study (13), 15 of 17 patients were free of disease with 5-year follow-up as compared to 7 of 14 postmenopausal patients.

Van Dinh and Woodruff's data (13) are probably the most substantial available to suggest that preservation of ovaries does not affect subsequent outcome in patients with sarcoma confined within leiomyoma. However, as the ovaries can represent occult site of metastasis, the ideal recommendation for minimal surgical treatment would include total abdominal hysterectomy and bilateral salpingo-oophorectomy.

Endometrial Stromal Sarcoma

Norris and Taylor (20) analyzed 53 patients with endometrial stromal tumors. Pathologic features evaluated included cellular atypia, pushing or infiltrating borders and mitotic count. This evaluation of endometrial stromal tumor resulted in the following pathologic designations; endometrial stromal nodules, endometrial stromal myosis and endometrial stromal sarcoma. Endometrial stromal nodules were characterized by lack of recurrence, pushing margins, singularity, with cells similar to those found in the normal endometrial stroma. There was no vascular invasion and mitotic activity was reported as a median of two per ten high power fields. Infiltrating tumors were divided into two groups on the basis of mitotic activity: tumors containing fewer than ten mitoses per ten high power fields were designated as endolymphatic stromal myosis; and those containing ten or more mitotic figures were designated as endometrial stromal sarcoma.

Ten-year actuarial survival for endometrial stromal myosis was 100%. However, follow-up beyond 10 years revealed that 53% of patients were alive without evidence of disease, 11% had died of other causes, 31% were living with tumor, and 5% had died secondary to tumor. In 15 patients with endometrial stromal sarcoma, 5-year actuarial survival was 55%, although only 4 patients (26%) were without evidence of disease.

Cellular features such as atypia were marked in endometrial stromal nodules, and tended to be more severe with endometrial stromal sarcoma; however, there was considerable overlap and no correlation could be found between the degree of cellular atypia and recurrence.

Salazar's review of the literature, based on more than 900 cases including 73 from his own series, reported only 65 patients with endometrial stromal sarcoma (21). Five-year survival for 23 patients with Stage I disease was 55%,

and was similar to that of leiomyosarcoma and mixed mesodermal tumors. Patients with Stage II to IV disease revealed a 5-year survival of 12%.

Kempson and Bari (1) evaluated 17 patients with infiltrating stromal lesions. Two groups were identified. In the first group, 10 tumors were identified containing more than 20 mitoses per ten high power fields; with 9 of the 10 having either died or suffered recurrences. The second group consisted of 7 patients with five or fewer mitoses per ten high power fields, all of whom were alive 3 to 15 years following their initial treatment without evidence of recurrence. No tumors were identified with mitotic counts between six and 20 mitoses per ten high power fields.

Radiation Therapy

Radiation therapy as the sole treatment for uterine sarcoma has clearly been shown to be inferior to the surgical approach. Although reports (18, 22) have suggested the addition of radiation therapy to surgery, no improvement in survival has been demonstrated. The most thorough review of the role of radiation therapy in the treatment of uterine sarcoma was reported by Salazar (21). This included retrospective analysis of 73 cases from his own files, in addition to thorough review of the literature of over 900 cases. The series included 49 Stage I leiomyosarcoma patients treated with surgery alone, with a demonstrated 5-year survival of 49%; compared to 13 patients treated with surgery plus pelvic radiotherapy, with a demonstrated 5-year survival of 77% (p > 0.05). Fifteen patients with stage I endometrial sarcoma revealed a 5-year survival of 47% with surgery alone as compared to 88% for 7 patients treated with surgery and radiation (p > 0.05). These data illustrate the difficulty of any comment concerning the effectiveness of adjuvant radiation therapy in the treatment of uterine sarcoma. Even in this tremendous review of over 900 cases, there were only a small number of evaluable patients treated with combined modalities of surgery and radiation. When these patients were analyzed, there were no isolated pelvic failures (23). Thirty-five per cent of these patients presented with both pelvic and distant recurrence, and 65% with distant recurrence alone. In those patients treated with surgery alone, there was an 11% incidence of pelvic failure, 33% pelvic distant, and 37% distant. Most reports concerning the utilization of adjuvant radiotherapy in the treatment of uterine sarcoma have been retrospective and lack any clear cut criteria for the addition of this treatment modality. The role of radiation therapy needs to be more clearly defined in future prospective studies (see chemotherapy).

Chemotherapy

As already discussed, most patients who die from uterine sarcoma will succumb to distant or distant and local metastases. To evaluate the role of adjuvant chemotherapy in Stage I and II uterine sarcoma, the United States Gynecologic Oncology Group (24) performed a prospective randomized study in which patients were treated with 60 mg/M^2 of Adriamycin (doxorubicin) every 3 weeks for eight doses as adjuvant treatment. The recurrence rate in the Adriamycin arm was 41%, compared to 53% in the observation arm, which was not statistically significant. The addition of optional pelvic radiotherapy added a bias to the study. In another randomized study of the Gynecologic Oncology Group (25), Adriamycin was compared with Adriamycin and dacarbazine in patients with Stages III and IV or recurrent sarcoma of the uterus. The response rate for Adriamycin alone was 16.3%; for Adriamycin plus dacarbazine 24.2%, which was not clinically significant. There was a suggestion that better responses were seen in patients with leiomyosarcoma. There are data (26) to suggest, however, that such doses of Adriamycin may need to approach 70–90 mg/M^2 if this agent is to be used alone. Treatment of other soft tissue sarcomas (27) suggest regimens consisting of cyclophosphamide, vincristine, Adriamycin and dacarba-

zine (CYVADIC) offer an improved response rate of 47–56%. Piver et al. (28) had a 23% response rate when using CYVADIC for sarcomas of the female genital tract. This was achieved in patients who had extensive prior treatment with other chemotherapeutic regimens and/or radiation therapy, suggesting that treatment with CYVADIC may achieve greater success when utilized as first-line chemotherapy.

Hannigan et al. (29) reported the use of adjuvant chemotherapy in early uterine sarcoma in 34 patients treated with vincristine, actinomycin D and cyclophosphamide (VAC) or Adriamycin alone or in combination with vincristine and cyclophosphamide. It was their conclusion that the drug regimens utilized were not effective as adjuvant treatment. Hannigan et al. (30) also evaluated the effectiveness of VAC in 74 patients with metastatic or advanced sarcoma of uterine origin. The response rate was 28.9% overall, with a 15.6% partial response. Mean duration of complete response was 15 months; that of partial response was 5.5 months. The most dramatic report to date comes from the Norwegian Radium Hospital, in which Kolstad (31) revealed in preliminary data on 18-month survival of 85% for those patients treated with surgery plus Adriamycin (50 mg/M^2), as compared to 55% in those patients treated with surgery, actinomycin D and radiation.

In conclusion, active regimens in the treatment of uterine sarcoma have been identified. Reported response rates have been low. As yet, no improvement has been demonstrated with the use of adjuvant chemotherapy for early uterine sarcoma. However, to date, no study has reported the use of CYVADIC as adjuvant treatment in early stage uterine sarcoma. Currently, an ongoing prospective study at Roswell Park Memorial Institute (United States) utilizes this regimen in all patients with Stage I uterine sarcoma. Hopefully, this regimen, which has been shown to be effective in the treatment of soft tissue sarcomas, will result in improved survival for those patients with Stage I uterine sarcoma. The ideal study would compare patients with Stage I uterine sarcoma treated with surgery alone to patients treated with surgery plus adjuvant chemotherapy and surgery plus pelvic radiotherapy plus adjuvant chemotherapy utilizing CYVADIC.

Endolymphatic Stromal Myosis

Endolymphatic stromal myosis differs histologically from endometrial stromal sarcoma primarily in the number of mitotic figures per high power field. In the former there are less than ten mitoses per ten high power fields, and frequently even fewer than five. In 20 patients evaluated by Norris and Taylor (20) actuarial survival of 10 years was reported as 100%; however, 7 patients developed recurrent disease with one death at 12 years following initial therapy. Six patients were living with tumors 3.5 to 19 years following treatment. Reported recurrences were both local and distant. Hart and Yoonessi (32) reported 9 patients, 3 of whom died with recurrent tumor 5.8 to 9.0 years following initial surgery. In Baggish and Woodruff's (3) report of 12 patients, 2 were treated with surgery and pelvic radiotherapy, with one patient dying 20 years later with recurrent disease, the second having died 2 years after initial treatment with recurrent hepatic and pulmonary metastases. One patient with pulmonary recurrences was treated with progesterone with complete response. This study was characterized by locally invasive disease, late and distant recurrences, and tumor sensitivity to hormonal treatment.

Thatcher and Woodruff (34) reviewed an additional 33 cases and observed that lack of differentiation and depth of myometrial invasion were the most significant criteria for diagnosis of this malignancy. Of 24 patients treated with surgery alone, two died of recurrence and two were living with disease. Nine patients were treated with surgery and progestins, 5 having extension of disease beyond the uterus and all were living without evidence of disease.

Piver et al. (35), in the largest single series with 52 patients, demonstrated a significant level of recurrence of 50% for Stage I disease, characterizing again the long 5- and 10-year survivals which were reported for 88% of surgical Stage I patients. Median survival was 178 months. Of the 56% surgical Stage I patients who developed recurrent disease, 37% were alive without evidence of tumor following treatment. Twenty-one percent were alive with cancer, and 42% had died of disease. Data also indicated that there was some benefit in preventing pelvic recurrence with adjuvant pelvic radiotherapy, although these patients were still at risk for distant recurrence. Hormonal sensitivity and the curative effects of hormonal therapy were also demonstrated. Lack of responsiveness to systemic chemotherapy was highly suggested. Given the high recurrence rate of this disease, it would appear that initial therapy should be total abdominal hysterectomy, bilateral salpingo-oophorectomy and indefinite hormonal therapy with progesterone. The exact role of postoperative pelvic radiation remains unclear. Certainly, these tumors have been shown to be radiosensitive and in specific clinical situations residual disease following surgery would suggest the need for the addition of this modality.

CERVIX
(Chapter 11)

Cervical sarcoma is rarely seen (36). Abell and Ramirez (37) report 26 primary cervical sarcomas. Six patients presented with carcinosarcoma, with all succumbing to their disease. Twelve patients had endocervical stromal sarcoma with 4 survivors 2 to 18 years after initial therapy. Eight patients were treated for leiomyosarcoma of the cervix; 6 with surgery and 2 with radiation, with only 2 patients in the surgery group alive 5 years following treatment.

Jawalekar et al. (38) reviewed the literature and compiled a total of 13 cases of leiomyosarcoma of the cervix. Based on this review, it was their conclusion that initial therapy should include surgery, accompanied by adjuvant radiation therapy and chemotherapy. This conclusion was based on the fact that treatment failure occurred at the primary site, as well as at sites of distant metastasis.

Ortner et al. (39) described a case of embryonal rhabdomyosarcoma of the cervix treated with hysterectomy and left salpingo-oophorectomy. Surgical margins were negative, radiation therapy was omitted and treatment with vincristine, actinomycin D and cyclophosphamide was continued over a 2-year period. At the time of this report, the patient was free of disease 13 months following completion of her initial therapy. Botryoid sarcoma originating in the cervix is rare with its true incidence difficult to estimate, as the primary site of origin is not always exactly stated in the literature.

Other reports (40–42) of embryonal rhabdomyosarcoma have demonstrated improved survival utilizing a combination of surgery, radiation therapy and chemotherapy, as opposed to earlier treatment with ultraradical surgery.

LYMPHOMA

In contrast to ovarian lymphoma, reported survivals for lymphoma of the uterine cervix are significantly better. Charlton et al. (43) reviewed the United States Armed Forces Institute of Pathology files. The incidence of malignant lymphoma arising from the female genital tract was one in 730. Komaki et al. (44) reviewed the literature and reported 25 cases of malignant lymphoma originating from the uterine cervix. Abnormal vaginal bleeding was seen in 70% of patients, pelvic discomfort in 40% and vaginal discharge in 20%. Malignant lymphoma presented as an expansile lesion with a smooth enlargement of the cervix, endocervix and uterine body. Pap smears were positive in 4 of 10 reported cases. In 4 patients with Stage IB disease treated with surgery alone, the average survival was 70 months, with one patient dead of disease. The average survival of 12 patients treated by irradiation was 47 months, despite more advanced stage. Patients treated with extended field irradiation did better than those treated by pelvic irradia-

tion alone. Average survival of 5 patients treated by surgery and radiation was 29 months, with one death due to disease. Twelve of 51 known patients treated with radiation therapy were without evidence of disease. It was their conclusion that lymphoma of the cervix is a highly radio-curable disease, even with advanced stages, that can be effectively treated with a moderate amount of radiation (4000 to 5000 rad). It was also observed that the regression rate can be slow, sometimes taking several months to see a complete regression. In the presence of recurrence chemotherapy was advocated.

Delgado et al. (45) reported 4 patients with reticulum cell sarcoma of the cervix with radiation therapy as primary treatment in 3 of the patients, and radical hysterectomy in the fourth. The latter patient was the only patient to have disease confined to the cervix. Of the patients treated with radiation therapy, one was treated with pelvic radiotherapy alone, while the other 2 received pelvic radiotherapy and radium. The patient treated with surgery died of metastatic disease shortly after initial therapy, at which time pelvic lymph nodes were noted to contain metastasis. Of the 3 patients treated with radiation therapy, surgical evaluation in 2 of the patients revealed no metastatic disease, and both patients were alive without disease at 3 and 10 years following initial treatment. A third patient treated by radiation therapy alone without surgical evaluation died 2 years following initial treatment without evidence of disease. This study emphasized the importance of complete staging and the advantage of radiation therapy in the treatment of this disease entity.

From the limited data available, it appears that the best initial treatment is radiation therapy for localized disease, as determined by preoperative diagnostic evaluation and staging lymphadenectomy. The data also suggest that the presence of positive pelvic nodes is associated with a poor prognosis, even with the addition of postoperative radiation therapy. In the presence of this finding, chemotherapy should entail part of the initial treatment.

VAGINAL SARCOMA
(Chapter 8)

Hilgers et al. (46) reviewed the United States Mayo Clinic experience of 10 cases of sarcoma botryoides of the vagina, and compared these histopathologically with 17 botryoid sarcomas of extravaginal origin. Seventy-one cases of sarcoma botryoides of the vagina were reviewed from the literature as well. Histologically, each tumor exhibited embryonal rhabdomyoblasts, an intact overlying epithelium, undifferentiated round and spindle cells, and myxoid stroma. Bone, cartilage, fat and malignant epithelial features associated with mixed mesodermal tumors were not observed. Presenting symptoms of vaginal sarcoma were vaginal mass or vaginal bleeding or both. Delay in the diagnosis was the rule rather than the exception with physician delay accounting for 12 months, as compared to patient delay of 2 months. Initially, the tumor arose in subepithelial fashion, and was either unicentric or multicentric. Its growth pattern caused the vaginal epithelium to bulge, with initial growth being expansile and later growth infiltrative. The most common site was the anterior vaginal wall, with the posterior vaginal wall being the second most common site.

Fifteen cases in the literature review had autopsy performed, with confinement to the pelvis in 50% of these patients. Fifteen percent of the 49 patients treated survived; none of those not treated were long-term survivors. Nine of the 10 Mayo Clinic patients with vaginal embryonal rhabdomyosarcoma died of their disease. Of 14 patients treated with primary hysterectomy and vaginectomy 5 were 10-year survivors, while there were 3 10-year survivors among the 6 patients treated with exenteration. Of patients treated with local excision and radiation, there were no 10-year survivors. Recurrences after pelvic exenteration were both local and distant. It was the conclusion of this study that minimal treatment should include exenteration and pelvic lymphadenoectomy. Since this study, the concepts of therapeutic management have changed. Kumar et al. (41) reported 3 children with rhabdomyosarcoma of the vagina managed by modified resection and treated with chemotherapy and radiation. These patients were free of tumor at 32, 44 and 54 months following their initial treatment. The feeling of this group was that hysterectomy and vaginectomy, coordinated with chemotherapy and radiation, was an acceptable alternative to the exenterative procedure.

The Intergroup Rhabdomyosarcoma Study was established in 1972 to evaluate the use of radiation therapy in patients with completely resected disease, who were also treated with adjuvant chemotherapy (40). In addition, the evaluation of different chemotherapy regimens was also performed. Fifty-eight children with genitourinary sarcomas were evaluated with 22 tumors of the bladder, 14 of the prostate, 6 of the vagina and uterus, and 16 of paratesticular tissues. When radiation therapy was utilized, 5000 to 6000 rad were delivered in children older than 5, while the dose did not exceed 4000 rad in younger children, due to believed increased sensitivity of growing tissues.

Radiation therapy was utilized in patients with positive nodes (Table 4), and all patients received systemic chemotherapy. Fifteen patients had positive nodes, of which 11 were treated with radiation, with 9 of these 11 remaining disease free. Two of 4 patients with positive nodes not treated with radiation also remained disease free. Of 23 patients with negative nodes, 15 of 17 patients not treated

TABLE 4 INTERGROUP RHABDOMYOSARCOMA
STUDY (40): NODES SAMPLED

	Radiation therapy	Disease free	No radiation therapy	Disease free
Patients with positive nodes (15)	11	9	4	2
Patients with negative nodes (23)	6	4	17	15

TABLE 5 INTERGROUP RHABDOMYOSARCOMA STUDY (40): NODES NOT SAMPLED

Number of patients	Radiation therapy	Disease free	No radiation therapy	Disease free
20	10	9	10	7

with radiation were disease free. Of 6 who received radiation therapy, 4 were disease free. There was another group of 20 patients (Table 5) who did not have node sampling, with 16 of these patients disease free. Nine of the 10 treated with radiation therapy are free of disease, while 7 of 10 not treated with radiation therapy are free of disease.

It was the conclusion of this study to utilize radiation therapy when nodes were involved. However, if nodes were negative, radiation was withheld. It was felt that if subsequent disease did exist in unsampled tissue, systemic chemotherapy was sufficient treatment. Extrapolating from data (40–42, 46–53) concerning treatment of all embryonal rhabdomyosarcomas in children, radiation and chemotherapy in combination with surgery provided effective treatment for this virulent tumor. In an attempt to avoid exenteration, surgery should entail tumor resection with evaluation of regional nodes. If the nodes are positive or if there is residual disease following surgery, radiotherapy should be added, in conjunction with chemotherapy. Reports suggest that VAC (vincristine, actinomycin-D, cyclophosphamide) is effective. If the surgical margins are negative and the nodes are not involved, effective treatment is surgery plus chemotherapy. Data suggest that radiation therapy in the range of 3000 to 4000 rad is sufficient to control microscopic disease, while doses of 4000 to 5000 rad are effective for the control of larger amounts of residual disease.

SMOOTH MUSCLE TUMORS OF THE VAGINA

Tavassoli and Norris (54) provide an extensive review of 60 smooth muscle tumors of the vagina. Clinically, the median age was 40 years, with only 10 patients greater than 50 years of age. Recent enlargement of tumor was seen in 7 patients, while 6 complained of pain, and 2 complained of vaginal bleeding. Three patients had the tumor detected during pregnancy. The size of the lesion varied from 0.5 to 15 cm, with a median of 3 cm. Only 6 neoplasms were greater than 5 cm. Fourteen neoplasms were reported to demonstrate cellular atypia. There was no recognizable mitotic activity in 35 neoplasms, while in the remaining 25, mitotic activity varied, with only 7 neoplasms demonstrating five or more mitotic figures per ten high power fields. Tumor margin was circumscribed in all but one patient.

Five patients demonstrated tumor recurrence, and mitotic count in all 5 neoplasms was equal to or greater than five mitotic figures per ten high power fields. Four had moderate or marked atypia. All were greater than 3 cm in size. Only one patient developed distant recurrence and died, and this was the only neoplasm characterized by an infiltrating margin. Mitotic count in this neoplasm was 15 mitotic figures per ten high power fields. The remaining 4 patients who developed recurrence were alive from 4 to 7.5 years after initial diagnosis. Mitotic activity was the most reliable indicator of recurrence, with 5 of 7 neoplasms with five or more mitotic figures per ten high power fields developing recurrence. Four of these also had moderate or marked atypia. Neoplasms with five or more mitotic figures per ten high power fields and marked atypia were designated as leiomyosarcomas. Tavassoli and Norris recommended that treatment by local excision with re-excision of recurrence was adequate treatment for these low grade leiomyosarcomas. Individualized therapeutic approach was recommended for the highly malignant infiltrating type lesion.

Sarcomas of the adult vagina represent a rare form of adult gynecologic malignancy and have generally been associated with poor clinical outcome. Recently Peters et al. (55) reported 17 cases of primary sarcoma of the adult vagina and compiled an additonal 68 cases from the literature. This study utilized the same histologic criteria advocated by Tavassoli and Norris (54). Leiomyosarcoma was the histologic type in 68% of reported cases. In their own 17 cases, exenteration was their most effective modality. Review of cases compiled from the literature suggested that therapeutic success could be achieved with less radical surgery; however, the histologic criteria for diagnosis of this entity has not been uniform, and interpretation of these results is difficult. Numerous studies (53–60) utilizing variable treatment methods have provided variable results. Initial treatment should include surgical resection. Exenterative surgery is indicated in specific clinical settings. Radiation therapy appears to be of limited value.

VULVA
(Chapter 13)

Tavassoli and Norris (61) reviewed a series of 32 smooth muscle tumors of the vulva. The median age in the study was 35 years. In 14 patients, the area of involvement was the labia majora. Eleven were adjacent to the Bartholin gland. Seven patients were pregnant. Microscopic evaluation revealed some degree of cellular atypia in 14 neoplasms, with bizarre tumor giant cells in 5. Mitotic figures ranged from nought to two per ten high power fields in 25 of the patients, with only 6 patients demonstrating five or more mitotic figures per ten high power fields. Enucleation was the initial therapy in 28 of the patients. Four of the 32 patients developed recurrence and all 4 were without evidence of disease 6 years following treatment for recurrence. It was concluded that neoplasms greater than 5 cm with infiltrating margins and five or more mitotic figures per ten high power fields were most likely to recur, and were therefore designated as leiomyosarcomas. Of 3 patients with infiltrating margins, 2 recurred. Only one of 6 patients with five or more mitotic figures recurred. One of their 4 recurrences was

characterized by an expansile lesion with one or two mitotic figures 1 + atypia and a lesion size of 1.5 cm. The study also indicates that cellular atypia did not correlate with mitotic activity or with recurrence. The study was not able to demonstrate microscopic feature of features as definite criteria for the diagnosis of leiomyosarcoma. This study provided guidelines for the diagnosis of sarcomatous change in smooth muscle tumors of the vulva.

Davos and Abell (62) reported 15 cases of vulvar sarcoma, comprising 5 cases of leiomyosarcoma, 2 malignant fibrous histiocytomas, and a variety of other sarcomas, ranging from dermatofibrosarcoma to embryonal stromal sarcoma. Specifically, the leiomyosarcomas ranged from 4 to 10 cm in diameter. Mitotic counts were evaluated, and were noted to be well above the level of ten per ten high power fields. Three of the leiomyosarcomas were treated with local excision, with all 3 requiring treatment for recurrent tumors with one patient dying 9 years later with distant metastasis. Of the 2 patients treated with wide local excision, one developed disseminated metastasis 6 months after initial treatment, while the other was without evidence of disease 28 months after her initial treatment. All the other lesions were treated with local excision or wide local excision with recurrence characterizing their future course. One patient with dermatofibrosarcoma was without evidence of disease 20 years later. Another patient with malignant mesothelioma was without evidence of disease 5 years later. It was Davos and Abell's impression that the majority of these tumors were relatively slow growing, insidiously infiltrative with a tendency to recur and metastasize by hematogenous spread. Results of treatment were generally more favorable when extensive or radical surgical procedures were employed soon after diagnosis.

DiSaia et al. (63) reported the M.D. Anderson Tumor Institute (United States) experience with 12 cases of vulvar sarcoma, of which leiomyosarcoma was the most prevalent lesion (5), with 3 cases of rhabdomyosarcoma and neurofibrosarcoma, and one patient with fibrosarcoma. There were 5 patients surviving without evidence of disease. Initial treatment involved radical vulvectomy, although all patients did not undergo inguinal lymphadenectomy.

Epithelioid sarcomas of the vulva (64, 65) have rarely been reported, Piver et al. (66) provided the first description with sarcomatous growth of the spindle cells and polygonal cells which bear a resemblance to squamous cells. Most previously reported cases occurred on the extremities or the scalp, with tendency to invade along dense fibrous structures, such as tendons, fascia, or periosteum. These tumors were characterized by 85% recurrence rate, which was attributed to under-treatment (67). The tumor from this report was treated with wide local excision of a 10 cm area, and had not recurred following 15-year follow-up. Treatment was limited in this situation to wide excision, rather than radical vulvectomy, based on the parallel data from other epithelioid sarcomas.

Vulvar sarcomas are characterized by regional and late recurrences and disseminated metastasis after recurrence. Once the diagnosis is established, radical vulvectomy and inguinal lymphadenectomy would be the treatment of choice in most clinical situations.

OVARY

Ovarian sarcomas constitute less than 1% of all ovarian malignancies. Of the 2400 cases of ovarian malignancy in the Emil Novak Ovarian Tumor Registry (Johns Hopkins University, United States), only 43 were primary ovarian sarcomas (68). They occurred primarily in postmenopausal women with low parity and were characterized by rapid growth. The majority of patients presented with an abdominal mass on initial examination. These neoplasms were classified as teratoid, stromal or mesenchymal sarcomas, and müllerian sarcomas (mixed mesodermal tumors, carcinosarcoma).

Teratoid sarcomas are represented by two categories: (a) undifferentiated embryonic sarcomatoid lesions, or (b) neoplasms arising secondarily from an initially benign adult teratoma. Ten were diagnosed as sarcomas arising in ovarian teratomas. Patients ranged in age from 7 to 56; however, the latter was the only patient over the age of 25. Sarcomas varied from rhabdomyosarcoma to leiomyosarcoma, chondrosarcoma and undifferentiated sarcomas. All patients died within 6 months. None received adjuvant chemotherapy.

Fourteen patients were diagnosed to have primary mesenchymal sarcomas. Mesenchyme was defined to include both connective tissue or supporting matrix of the undifferentiated theca-like stroma. Seven sarcomas were designated as stromal cell tumors, and 5 of these designated as low grade sarcomas, with all patients living without evidence of disease 6 to 14 years following initial surgery. The 2 patients designated to have stromal cell sarcoma both died within 2 years following their initial surgery. There were 7 patients designated as fibroleiomyosarcoma, ranging in age from 35 to 67 years. All patients died from 1 months to $2\frac{1}{2}$ years following initial treatment, except for one patient with low grade fibrosarcoma who died 8 years later with metastasis.

The third category of müllerian sarcomas included 23 patients from the Registry. These patients ranged in age from 39 to 85 years, with 7 of the 23 patients greater than 70 years of age. Only 4 patients survived more than 1 year.

Pratt and Scully reviewed 17 cases (69) of atypical fibromatous tumors, to establish criteria for histologic diagnosis and prognosis. These atypical fibromatous tumors were subdivided as fibrous (one to three mitotic figures per ten high power fields) which were usually benign; and fibrosarcomas, which were characterized by higher mitotic counts and were always malignant. Of those patients with cellular fibromas, the average age was 49 years (14–82). Seven of the patients were postmenopausal. There was no clinical evidence of estrogen overproduction by the tumor in any of the patients. In 3 cases where the tumor has ruptured, there was associated hemorrhagic ascites. Nine of the 11 patients were without evidence of disease from 3 to 13 years following their initial surgery. Two patients recurred 3 to 7 years after the initial surgery, although the former case actually represented progression of disease following incomplete resection of the tumor. Of the 6 patients with fibrosarcoma, the average age at diagnosis was 58 years. Tumors ranged from 9 to 35 cm in diameter and were associated with a unilocular cystadenoma. Cellular pleomorphism was moderate in 2 and marked in 4. The number of mitotic figures ranged from four to 25 per ten high power fields. All 6 patients recurred 1–44 months after the initial surgery. Four of these recurrences were within 6 months. Tumors designated as cellular fibromas were characterized by one to three mitotic figures per ten high power fields, and Grade 1 to 2 nuclear pleomorphism, while fibrosarcomas revealed four or more mitotic figures per ten high power fields and Grade 2 to 3 nuclear pleomorphism. This classification would allow for conservative surgery in the younger patient.

Carcinosarcoma (Chapter 5)

Ober (70) reviewed 77 cases of carcinosarcoma of the ovary with mean age of 60 years at diagnosis (20% less than age 50). Patients were frequently nulliparous with clinical presentation of abdominal pain and swelling, associated with lower abdominal mass. Five-year survival was 4%. Histogenesis suggested the epithelial component arises from the surface mesothelium, and stromal components arise from the subcoelomic mesenchyme. Fenn and Abell (71) reported 23 cases of carcinosarcoma of the ovary with 22 of the 23 patients dead of disease at the time of the report. Only one patient survived longer than 2 years.

Prat and Scully (72) reviewed 2 cases of sarcoma arising as distinct solitary nodules in the walls of ovarian mucinous cystic tumors. In one patient the tumor was a fibrosarcoma associated with the mucinous cystadenoma. The other was undifferentiated sarcoma asso-

ciated with a mucinous cystadenocarcinoma. Both patients died within $1\frac{1}{2}$ years of surgery. Seven cases (73) of mucinous ovarian tumors with sarcoma-like nodules in the wall of the cyst were reported. Each of the patients at exploration had Stage IA cystic ovarian tumor. All of the specimens contained one or more distinct nodules in their walls, most of which were dark brown in color and hemorrhagic in nature. Microscopically, four of the tumors had a borderline malignant epithelial component and three had a well differentiated epithelial component. Six of the patients are alive without evidence of disease, with one patient dead secondary to coronary thrombosis 10 years after initial surgery with no evidence of recurrence. Tumors ranged in size from 12 to 40 cm with all specimens containing one or more mural nodules, 0.6 to 5 cm in diameter. Nodules protruded into the lumina of the locules. These nodules were solitary in 3 patients, and multiple in 4. Nodules were characterized by pleomorphism and the presence of histiocytic type giant cells. Mononucleated cells were markedly pleomorphic, with hyperchromatic nuclei, abnormal chromatin patterns and atypical mitoses ranging from four to ten per ten high power fields. It was their conclusion that the nodules reflected a reactive response, the nature of which was not clarified. In an effort to detect early stages of these nodules, slides were reviewed of 40 other mucinous tumors. Three showed foci of histiocytic reaction, occasionally with the formation of multinucleated giant cells. It was concluded that these sarcoma-like mural nodules did not alter the prognosis as determined by microscopic evaluation of the epithelial components.

Treatment

As the above suggest, sarcomas are highly malignant tumors, associated with an extremely poor prognosis. Smith and Rutledge (74) reported 38 patients with advanced recurrent or metastatic sarcomas of the pelvis treated with irradiation and chemotherapy. Fourteen of the 38 patients were without evidence of disease from 10 to 65 months following initial therapy. Leiomyosarcomas were the most successfully treated with 7 of 8 patients without evidence of disease. The majority of patients were treated with vincristine, actinomycin D and cyclophosphamide.

Because of the highly lethal nature of these tumors, all patients should be treated with systemic chemotherapy. The most effective chemotherapy for soft tissue sarcomas has been cyclophosphamide, vincristine, Adriamycin and imidazole carboxamide (CYVADIC). Gottlieb et al. (27) reported a 55% response rate in 136 women with soft tissue and bone sarcomas, suggesting that this is the most effective chemotherapy for sarcomas in general. At Roswell Park Memorial Institute (United States) (75), of 1275 cases of ovarian cancer, 35 (2.6%) were found to be primary ovarian sarcomas. This report included treatment with multiple regimens, with 5 of 42 patients demonstrating a response. Two of 9 patients responded to VAC chemotherapy (vincristine, actinomycin D, cyclophosphamide) with 3 other patients responding to varied regimens, which included methotrexate, cis-platinum, dacarbazine, cyclophosphamide and 5-fluorouracil.

From 1977 to 1981, 26 patients were treated with CYVADIC chemotherapy for sarcomas of the female genital tract (28). An overall response rate of 23% was achieved in patients who had extensive prior treatment with chemotherapy and/or radiation therapy. A combination of decarbazine and cis-platinum has also been shown to be effective as second-line chemotherapy. Current prospective studies at Roswell Park Memorial Institute (United States) have combined these two agents with Adriamycin as a potentially effective regiment for the treatment of pelvic sarcomas.

Ovarian Lymphoma

Woodruff et al. (76) reported 35 cases of ovarian lymphomas from the Ovarian Tumor Registry (Johns Hopkins University, United States). Eighteen of the 35 patients were between 21 and 45 years of age. Pain and abdominal swelling were the most common symptoms. Only 4 patients in this study had previously known sites of lymphoma. Treatment usually consisted of hysterectomy and bilateral or unilateral adenexectomy. Seven patients received radiation therapy in addition to surgery. At the time of this report, only 3 patients were alive from 1 to 16 years after the initial treatment.

In regard to the origin of the lymphoma, the authors noted that lymphoid tissue was not found in the ovary, but may be present in the hilus or medulla.

Chorlton et al. (77) reported 19 cases of ovarian lymphoma in the files of the Armed Forces Institute of Pathology. Ten patients presented with disease limited to the ovary. Only one patient was alive without evidence of disease at 17 years. Of the remaining patients with disease present outside the ovary, all were dead of tumor. The poor survival contrasts sharply with other reports of early stage I lymphoma arising from extranodal sites where survivals of 45% to 68% have been reported (78). Poor survival may be explained by a more aggressive disease process, or may present inaccurate staging. In Fox's review of the literature (79), it is his recommendation that radical surgery and external radiation offer the greatest hope for successful treatment. His conclusions were based, in part, on the work of Lathrop (80) and Hahn (81), where this treatment has been effective in other extranodal sites of lymphoma.

Crisp reported 6 cases of pelvic lymphoma (82), in which patients were characterized as presenting with a rapidly enlarging asymptomatic pelvic mass, chylous ascites, or a pelvic mass and a Pap smear read as chronic inflammation with many lymphocytes. He pointed out that surgical therapy in gynecologic extranodal disease is not considered curative and that there was no indication for radical surgery in extranodal pelvic lymphoma. Radiation therapy was felt to be potentially curative in localized disease. However, it was his feeling that the localized findings were uncommon. Chemotherapy could be used for patients with more extensive disease.

In conclusion, surgery plays a limited role in the treatment of ovarian lymphoma, as poor survivals for even so-called Stage I ovarian lymphomas would dictate against a radical surgical approach. Radiation therapy and/or chemotherapy represent the most reasonable treatment modalities.

REFERENCES

1 Kempson RL, Bari W. Uterine sarcomas: classification, diagnosis and Prognosis. Hum Pathol 1970; 1: 331–49.
2 Ober WB. Uterine sarcomas: histogenesis and taxonomy. Ann NY Acad Sci 1959; 75: 568.
3 Taylor HB, Norris HJ. Mesenchymal tumors of the uterus. IV. Diagnosis and prognosis of leiomyosarcomas. Arch Pathol 1966; 82: 40–4.
4 Kneale B, Barter R. Leiomyosarcoma of the uterus. Aust NZ J Obstet Gynaec 1961; 12: 17–23.
5 Leberge J. Prognosis of uterine leiomyosarcomas based of histopathological criteria. Am J Obstet Gynec 1962; 84: 1833–7.
6 Evans N. Malignant myomata and related tumors of the uterus. Surg Gynecol Obstet 1920; 30: 225–39.
7 Kimbrough RA. Sarcoma of the uterus. Am J Obstet Gynec 1934; 28: 723–30.
8 Aaro LA, Dockerty MB. Leiomyosarcoma of the uterus. Am J Obstet Gynec 1959; 77: 1187–98.
9 Spiro RH, Koss LG. Myosarcoma of the uterus. Cancer 1965; 18: 571–88.
10 Bosse MD, Stanton JN. Sarcoma of the uterus. Am J Obstet Gynec 1943; 45: 262–8.
11 Novak E, Anderson DF. Sarcoma of the uterus. Am J Obstet Gynec 1937; 34: 740–61.
12 Silverberg SG. Leiomyosarcoma of the uterus: A clinicopathologic study. Obstet Gynecol 1971; 38: 613–28.
13 Van Dinh T, Woodruff JD. Leiomyosarcoma of the uterus. Am J Obstet Gynecol 1982; 144: 817–3.
14 Barter JF, Smith EB, Szpak CA, Hinshaw W, Clarke-Pearson DL, Creasman WT. Leiomyosarcoma of the uterus: Clinicopathologic study of 21 cases. Gynecol Oncol 1985; 21: 220–7.
15 Hart WJ, Billman JK. A reassessment of uterine neoplasms originally diagnosed as leiomyosarcomas. Cancer 1978; 41: 1902–10.
16 Vardi JR, Tovell HM. Leiomyosarcoma of the uterus: Clinicopathologic study. Obstet Gynecol 1980; 56: 428–34.
17 Aaro LA, Symmonds RE, Dockerty MB. Sarcoma of the uterus: A clinical and pathologic study of 177 cases. Am J Obstet Gynecol 1966; 94: 101–9.
18 Salazar OM, Bonfiglio TA, Patten SF, Keller BE, Feldstein M, Dunne ME, Rudolph J. Uterine sarcomas: Natural history, treatment and prognosis. Cancer 1978; 42: 1152–60.
19 Bazzochi F, Brandi G, Pileri S, Mancuso A, Massaro A, Martinelli G. Clinical and pathologic prognostic features of leiomyosarcoma of the uterus. Tumori 1983; 69: 75–7.
20 Norris HJ, Taylor HB. Mesenchymal tumors of the uterus. I. A clinical and pathological study of 53 endometrial stromal tumors. Cancer 1966; 19: 755–66.
21 Salazar OM, Dunne ME. The role of radiation therapy in the management of uterine sarcomas. Int J Radiat Oncol Biol Phys 1980; 6: 899–902.
22 Vongtama V, Karlen JR, Piver MS, Tsukada Y, Moore RH. Treatment, results and prognostic factors in stage I and II sarcomas of the corpus uteri. Am J Roent Rad Ther Nuclear Med 1976; 126: 139–47.
23 Salazar OM, Bonfiglio TA, Patten SF, Keller BE, Feldstein M, Dunne ME, Rudolph JH. Uterine sarcomas: Analysis of failures with special emphasis on the use of adjuvant radiation therapy. Cancer 1978; 42: 1161–70.
24 Omura GA, Blessing JA, Major F, Lifshitz S, Ehrlich CE, Mangan C, Beecham J, Park R, Silverberg S. A randomized clinical trial of adjuvant adriamycin in uterine sarcomas: A gynecologic oncology group study. J Clin Oncol 1985; 3: 1240–45.
25 Omura GA, Major FJ, Blessing JA, Sedlacek TV, Thigpen JT, Creasman WT, Zaino RJ. A randomized study of adriamycin with and without dimethyl triazenoimidazole carboxamide in advanced uterine sarcomas. Cancer 1983; 52: 626–32.
26 Rosenbaum C, Schoenfeld D. Treatment of advanced soft tissue sarcomas. Proc AACR/ASCO 1977; 18: 287.
27 Gottlieb JA, Baker LH, O'Bryan RM, Sinkovics JG, Hoogstraten B, et al. Adriamycin (NSC-123127) used alone and in combination for soft tissue and bony sarcomas. Cancer 1975; 6: 271–82.
28 Piver MS, DeEulis TG, Lele SB, Barlow JJ. Cyclophosphamide, vincristine, adriamycin, and dimethyl-triazeno imidazole carboxamide (CYVADIC) for sarcomas of the female genital tract. Gynecol Oncol 1982; 14: 319–23.
29 Hannigan EV, Freedman RS, Rutledge FN. Adjuvant chemotherapy in early uterine sarcoma. Gynecol Oncol 1983; 15: 56–64.

30 Hannigan EV, Freedman RS, Elder KW, Rutledge FN. Treatment of advanced uterine sarcoma with vincristine, actinomycin D and cyclophosphamide. Gynecol Oncol 1983; 15: 224–9.

31 Kolstad P. Adjuvant chemotherapy in sarcoma of the uterus: A preliminary report. In: Morrow CP ed Recent Clinical Developments in Gynecologic Oncology. New York: Raven Press, 1983: 123–9.

32 Hart WR, Yoonessi M. Endometrial stromatosis of the uterus. Obstet Gynecol 1977; 49: 393–403.

33 Baggish MS, Woodruff JD. Uterine stromatosis. Clinicopathologic features and hormone dependency. Obstet Gynecol 1972; 40: 487–98.

34 Thatcher SS, Woodruff JD. Uterine stromatosis. A report of 33 cases. Obstet Gynecol 1982; 59: 428–34.

35 Piver MS, Rutledge FN, Copeland L, Webster K, Blumenson L, Suh O. Uterine endolymphatic stromal myosis: A collaborative study. Obstet Gynecol 1984; 64: 173–8.

36 Rotmensch J, Rosenshein NB, Woodruff JD. Cervical sarcoma: A review: Obstet Gynecol Surv 1983; 38: 456–60.

37 Abell MR, Ramirez JA. Sarcomas and carcinosarcoma of the uterine cervix. Cancer 1973; 31: 1176–92.

38 Jawalekar KS, Zacharopoulou M, McCaffrey RM. Leiomyosarcoma of the cervix uteri. Southern Med J 1981; 74: 510–11.

39 Ortner A, Weiser G, Haas H, Resch R, Dapunt O. Embryonal rhabdomyosarcoma (botryoid type) of the cervix: A case report and review. Gynecol Oncol 1982; 13: 115–19.

40 Tefft M, Hays D, Raney RB, Lawrence W, Soule E, Donaldson MH, Sutow WW, Gehan E. Radiation to regional nodes for rhabdomyosarcoma of the genitourinary tract in children: Is it necessary? Cancer 1980; 45: 3065–8.

41 Kumar APM, Wrenn EL, Fleming ID, Hustu HO, Pratt CB. Combined therapy to prevent complete pelvic exenteration for rhabdomyosarcoma of the vagina or uterus. Cancer 1976; 37: 118–22.

42 Weichselbaum RR, Cassady JR, Jaffe N, Filler R. The evolution of combination therapy of genitourinary rhabdomyosarcoma in children: A preliminary report. Int J Radiat Oncol Biol Phys 1977; 2: 267–72.

43 Charlton I, Karnei RF, King FM, Norris HJ. Primary malignant reticuloendothelial disease involving the vagina, cervix, and corpus uteri. Obstet Gynecol 1974; 44: 735–48.

44 Komaki R, Cox JD, Hansen RM, Gunn WG, Greenberg M. Malignant lymphoma of the uterine cervix. Cancer 1984; 54: 1699–1704.

45 Delgado G, Smith JP, Luis D, Gallagher S.

46 Hilgers RD, Malkasian GD, Soule EH. Embryonal rhabdomyosarcoma (botryoid type) of the vagina. Am J Obstet Gynecol 1970; 107: 484–02.

Reticulum-cell sarcoma of the cervix. Am J Obstet Gynecol 1976; 125: 691–4.

47 Hays DM. Pelvic rhabdomyosarcomas in childhood: Diagnosis and concepts of management reviewed. Cancer 1980; 45: 1810–14.

48 Jereb B, Ghavimi F, Exelby P., Zang E. Local control of embryonal rhabdomyosarcoma in children by radiation therapy when combined with chemotherapy. Int J Radiat Oncol Biol Phys 1980; 6: 827–33.

49 Exelby PR, Ghavimi F, Jereb B. Genitourinary rhabdomyosarcoma in children. J Pediat Surg 1978; 13: 746–52.

50 LaVecchia C, Draper GJ, Franceschi S. Childhood nonovarian female genital tract cancers in Britain, 1962–1978. Cancer 1984; 45: 188–92.

51 Weichert KA, Bove KC, Aron BS, Lampkin B. Rhabdomyosarcoma in children: A clinicopathologic study of 35 patients. Am J Clin Pathol 1976; 66: 692–701.

52 Crosfeld JL, Smith JP, Clatworthy HW. Pelvic rhabdomyosarcoma in infants and children. J Urol 1972; 107: 673–5.

53 Piver MS, Barlow JJ, Wang JJ, Shah NK. Combined radical surgery, radiation therapy and chemotherapy in infants with vulvovaginal embryonal rhabdomyosarcoma. Obstet Gynecol 1973; 42: 522–6.

54 Tavassoli FA, Norris HJ. Smooth muscle tumors of the vagina. Obstet Gynecol 1979; 53: 689–93.

55 Peters WA, Kumar NB, Andersen WA, Morley GW. Primary sarcoma of the adult vagina: A clinicopatholigic study. Obstet Gynecol 1985; 65: 699–704.

56 Davos I, Abell MR. Sarcomas of the vagina. Obstet Gynecol 1976; 47: 342–50.

57 Malkasian GD, Welch JS, Soule EH. Primary leiomyosarcoma of the vagina: Report of 8 cases. Am J Obstet Gynecol 1963; 86: 730–6.

58 Rastogi BL, Bergman B, Angervall L. Primary leiomyosarcoma of the vagina: A study of five cases. Gynecol Oncol 1984; 18: 77–86.

59 Diehl WK, Haught JS. Sarcoma of the vagina. Am J Obstet Gynecol 1946; 52: 302.

60 Palmer JP, Biback SM. Primary cancer of the vagina. Am J Obstet Gynecol 1954; 67: 377.

61 Tavassoli FA, Norris HJ. Smooth muscle tumors of the vulva. Obstet Gynecol 1979; 53: 213–17.

62 Davos I, Abell MR. Soft tissue sarcomas of the vulva. Gynecol Oncol 1976; 4: 70.

63 DiSaia PJ, Rutledge F, Smith JP. Sarcoma of the vulva: Report of 12 patients. Obstet Gynecol 1971; 38: 180–4.

64 Gallup DG, Abell MR, Morley GW. Epithelioid sarcoma of the vulva. Obstet Gynecol 1976; 48: 14S–17S.

65 Hall DJ, Grimes MM, Goplerud DR. Epithelioid sarcoma of the vulva. Gynecol Oncol 1980; 9: 237–46.

66 Piver MS, Tsukada Y, Barlow JJ. Epithelioid sarcoma of the vulva. Obstet Gynecol 1976; 40: 839–42.

67 Enzinger FM. Epithelioid sarcoma. Cancer 1970; 26: 229–36.

68 Azoury RS, Woodruff JD. Primary ovarian sarcomas. Obstet Gynecol 1971; 37: 920–41.

69 Prat J, Scully RE. Cellular fibromas and fibrosarcomas of the ovary: A comparative clinicopathologic analysis of seventeen cases. Cancer 1981; 47: 2663–70.

70 Ober WB. Carcinosarcoma of the ovary. Am J Diagnostic Gynecol Obstet 1979; 1: 73–81.

71 Fenn ME, Abell MR. Carcinosarcoma of the ovary. Am J Obstet Gynecol 1971; 110: 1066–4.

72 Prat J, Scully RE. Sarcomas in ovarian mucinous tumors: A report of two cases. Cancer 1979; 44: 1327–1.

73 Prat J, Scully RE. Ovarian mucinous tumors with sarcoma-like mural nodules: A report of seven cases. Cancer 1979; 44: 1332–4.

74 Smith JP, Rutledge F. Advances in chemotherapy for gynecologic cancer. Cancer 1975; 36: 669–74.

75 Lele SB, Piver MS, Barlow JJ. Chemotherapy in management of mixed mesodermal tumors of the ovary. Gynecol Oncol 1980; 10: 298–302.

76 Woodruff JD, Noli Castillo RD, Novak ER. Lymphoma of the ovary. Am J Obstet Gynecol 1963; 85: 912–18.

77 Chorlton I, Norris HJ, King FM. Malignant reticuloendothelial disease involving the ovary as a primary manifestation. Cancer 1974; 34: 397–407.

78 Freeman C, Berg JW, Cutter SJ. Occurrence and prognosis of extranodal lymphomas. Cancer 1972; 29: 252–60.

79 Fox HD, Cartnick EN, Shohov P, Zaino E. Lymphoma of the ovary: A case report and a review of the literature: Gynecol Oncol 1975; 3: 347–53.

80 Lathrop JC. Malignant pelvic lymphoma. Obstet Gynecol 1967; 30: 137–45.

81 Hahn GA. Gynecologic considerations in malignant lymphomas. Am J Obstet Gynecol 1958; 75: 673–83.

82 Crisp WE, Surwit EA, Grogan TM, Freedman MF. Malignant pelvic lymphoma. Am J Obstet Gynecol 1982; 143: 69–74.

Textbook of Uncommon Cancer
Edited by C.J. Williams, J.G. Krikorian, M.R. Green and D. Raghavan
© 1988 John Wiley & Sons Ltd

Chapter **11**

Rare Tumours of the Cervix

David Lowe* and C. N. Hudson†

*Senior Lecturer/Honorary Consultant in Histopathology,
St Bartholomew's Hospital Medical College, London,
UK., and †Consultant Gynaecologist, St Bartholomew's
and Homerton Hospitals, London, UK

INTRODUCTION

Cancer of the cervix is a condition relatively commonly encountered by gynaecologists, for which there is usually a well defined management policy on diagnosis, staging and therapy. The occurrence of rare tumours or tumour-like conditions of the cervix may therefore easily be overlooked. As the biological behaviour of such conditions can be very different from that of typical cervical squamous cell carcinoma, it is very important that their existence is appreciated. The need for a tissue diagnosis before embarking upon therapy is paramount.

AETIOLOGY AND EPIDEMIOLOGY

The aetiology of the various tumours in this group is largely a matter of speculation. By extrapolation of data from uterine or other commoner primary tumours, a few tentative associations can be drawn. In young women whose mothers were treated with diethylstilboestrol (DES) during pregnancy, clear cell adenocarcinoma of the lower genital tract can arise. Gestational choriocarcinoma of the cervix is rare, but is more likely to be seen in those geographic areas where gestational choriocarcinoma of the uterine corpus is common.

The role of infection in the aetiology of cervical neoplasia now excites very consider-able interest, and this may extend to rare mesenchymal tumours of the cervix when associated with chronic immunosuppression, such as may be seen in transplant recipients or patients who have been treated for reticuloendothelial neoplasms like Hodgkin's disease with chemotherapy (Figure 1).

DIFFERENTIAL DIAGNOSIS OF CERVICAL CANCER
(Table 1)

Developmental Abnormalities

The anatomy of the cervix can be distorted by developmental abnormalities, especially those arising in the stroma of the ectocervix. Congenital malformations include 'cock's comb' cervix, a growth disturbance induced by maternal DES ingestion (1, 2). Other variants of congenital abnormality can occasionally be confusing; for example if there is hypoplasia of one side of the müllerian system which results in a rudimentary horn of the corpus, the abnormal mass can be mistaken for a neoplasm.

Cysts of the cervix arising from mesonephric and paramesonephric ducts can occasionally be mistaken for metastatic adenocarcinoma. The presence of a collection of glandular remnants of the mesonephric (wolffian) duct

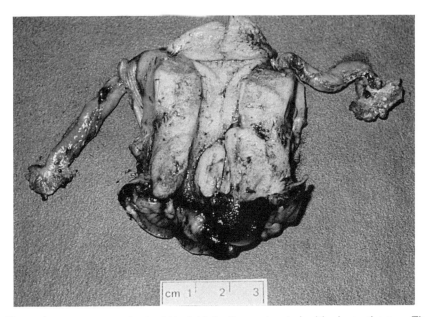

Figure 1 Uterus from a woman who had Hodgkin's disease treated with chemotherapy. There was a leiomyoasarcoma of the cervix, cervical intraepithelial neoplasia Grade 3 and early invasive adenocarcinoma of the cervix.

can be mistaken by the unwary for neoplasia (Figure 2). Mesonephric duct remnants are lined by cuboidal, faintly eosinophilic cells with regular nuclei (3); they were found in about 8% of cervices which were specifically examined for these structures (4) but are rarely encountered in routine histopathological practice. Distinguishing features are that mitoses are usually absent, and the cysts or small glandular structures usually contain dense inspissated colloidal secretion; there is little cellular pleomorphism and no stromal destruction. Congenital cysts are often difficult to classify, and a purely descriptive diagnosis such as 'a developmental cyst of the anterior cervix lined by tubal epithelium' is probably best (5). True mesonephric carcinoma is discussed below.

Endocervical Polyps

Any structure protruding through the cervix can be mistaken for a malignant neoplasm, and certainly hyperplastic endocervical polyps,

adenomyomatous polyps, decidual cervical polyps and submucosal leiomyoma can all mimic malignancy.

Hyperplastic endocervical polyps, especially those which are large and extend through the external cervical os, can have very disturbing clinical appearances. They are composed of hyperplastic but not atypical endocervical glands and stroma, and there is often a dense infiltrate of lymphocytes and plasma cells. The much rarer decidual or pseudodecidual polyp can have similar gross features. Both of these reactive conditions can be mistaken clinically for epithelial neoplasms such as squamous papilloma and adenocarcinoma, for connective tissue neoplasms like leiomyoma and sarcoma, and for mixed tumours composed of both glandular and connective tissue elements such as adenomyoma and adenofibroma. The distinction is usually readily apparent on histological examination.

Carcinoma arising in a hyperplastic endocervical polyp is rare, and has a prevalence of only 0.2–0.4% (6). Non-neoplastic polypoid

TABLE 1 FLOW DIAGRAM OF RARE TUMOURS OF THE CERVIX, CLASSIFIED BY HISTOLOGICAL FEATURES

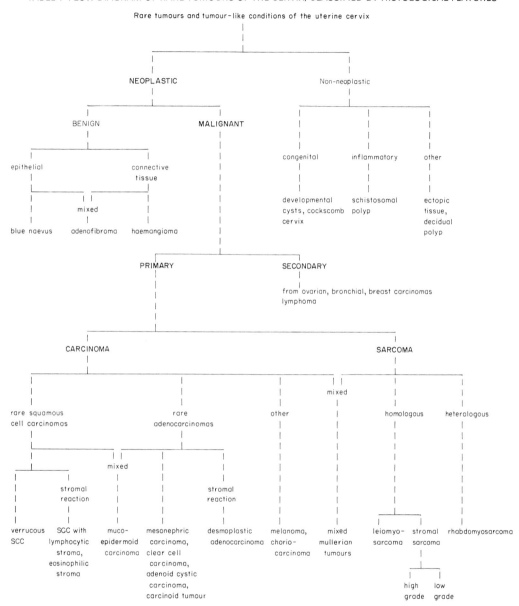

surface epithelium can be involved by direct extension of endocervical carcinoma arising in the adjacent, non-polypoid cervix; the diagnosis of malignant change in a previously benign polyp can therefore be made only when the base or stalk of the polyp is involved by tumour.

Hyperplastic Endometrial Polyp and Adenomyomatous Polyp

The soft glossy appearance of a hyperplastic endometrial polyp presenting at the external cervical os is usually characteristic. When a hyperplastic polyp has smooth muscle in its

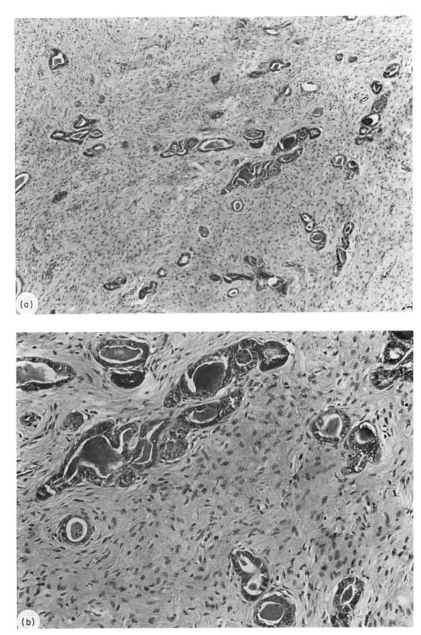

Figure 2 Wolffian duct remnants. In the deep endocervical stroma there are collections of irregular ducts and glands lined by cuboidal and flattened cells and containing dense, inspissated secretion. The cytology of the lining cells is bland and no mitoses are present. (Haematoxylin and eosin, original magnifications: ×100 (a) and ×250 (b))

stroma (adenomyomatous polyp) it has a much firmer consistency. The clinical differential diagnosis of these polyps is seldom from cervical carcinoma but from sarcoma. Histolo-

gical confirmation is essential, especially in young women, and any cervical polyp in a child should be regarded with the greatest suspicion.

Submucosal Leiomyoma (Submucosal Fibroid)

The serosanguineous discharge and iron deficiency anaemia associated with this condition can be clinically suggestive of malignancy and, especially if the tumour is ulcerated, the appearance can be equally disturbing. The texture of the lesion on palpation will often help, the tough resilience being a useful diagnostic feature.

Decidua and Products of Conception

Polypoid masses presenting at the external cervical os may consist of decidua (decidual or pseudodecidual polyp), trophoblast (placental polyp) (7) or rarely fetal tissues implanted at parturition or termination of pregnancy (e.g. glial polyp) (8, 9). In addition, a very low uterine pregnancy or the much rarer true cervical ectopic pregnancy can bleed profusely on digital examination and be mistaken clinically for malignancy.

Endocervical crypts can develop an Arias-Stella pattern (10, 11) which can be misdiagnosed histologically and cytologically as adenocarcinoma. Similarly, the epithelial abnormalities induced in cervical mucosa by folate and vitamin B12 deficiencies can lead to a cytological misdiagnosis of malignancy (12, 13).

Other Lesions

Solitary cervical condyloma acuminatum to the naked eye can mimic an exophytic neoplasm. Characteristically, a condyloma is softer and does not have the friability of carcinoma. Psammoma bodies (calcospherites) in cervical smears and biopsies may be associated with malignancy, especially adenocarcinoma of the endometrium or fallopian tubes (14), but can also be found in patients with intrauterine contraceptive devices and are therefore not pathognomonic of malignancy (15, 16).

Chronic inflammatory conditions of the ectocervix such as granulomatous inflammation can mimic the clinical appearance of invasive carcinoma and cause considerable diagnostic difficulty. The two most common conditions, tuberculosis and schistosomiasis, are largely confined to the tropics (17). Schistosomal infection of the cervix (18) can result in profound reactive hyperplasia ('pseudoepitheliomatous' hyperplasia) of the ectocervical epithelium, which can cause diagnostic difficulties because of its resemblance to well differentiated carcinoma. Histologically, ova in various stages of degeneration are numerous and occasionally the adult cestodes can be found. Infection is usually by *Schistosoma haematobium*.

Rarely, a syphilitic chancre can be confused with carcinoma macroscopically (19); in tertiary syphilis gumma of the cervix can ulcerate and form fungating mass which can be mistaken clinically for carcinoma (20) but this is now extremely rare in Western countries.

Secondary Malignancy in the Cervix

Involvement of the cervix by a primary tumour arising elsewhere is rare but the possibility should not be overlooked. Direct extension to the cervix may occur from endometrial carcinoma or from carcinoma involving the pouch of Douglas, such as from a primary tumour in the ovary or sigmoid colon. In fact, any intra-abdominal malignancy can produce transcoelomic spread to the pouch of Douglas (Blumer's prerectal shelf) and therefore by extension present in the cervix via the posterior cervical stroma or the posterior vaginal fornix. The cervix may rarely be involved by blood-borne metastases (21), a situation which can give rise to considerable diagnostic confusion.

RARE PRIMARY MALIGNANT TUMOURS

Rare Squamous Cell Tumours of the Cervix

Verrucous Carcinoma

The term verrucous carcinoma was coined by

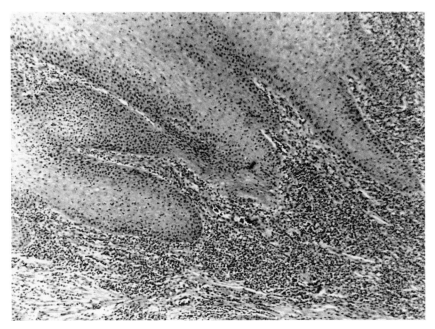

Figure 3 Verrucous carcinoma of the cervix. The deep border of the tumour is composed of very well differentiated squamous cells which invade the stroma in a 'pushing' fashion. The islands of tumour are for the most part devoid of fibrovascular cores. (Haematoxylin and eosin, original magnification: ×150)

Ackerman in 1948 (22) to describe well differentiated, warty, indolent but locally aggressive squamous cell carcinoma of the oral cavity. Similar tumours have been reported on the penis (23), bladder, nasal spaces and larynx, rectum and scrotum (24). The entity is almost certainly the same as giant condyloma of Buschke and Löwenstein (23) and carcinoma cuniculatum, both similar indolent well differentiated squamous cell tumours; the latter tends to occur in heavily keratinized epithelium such as on the foot (25). The first cervical verrucous carcinoma was described by Jennings and co-workers in 1972 (26), and other cases have since been reported (24, 27–30) (Figure 3).

Verrucous carcinoma of the cervix appears macroscopically as a pale pink or white mass which grows superficially over the mucosa and also has a deep growth component. Histologically, there is proliferation of very well differentiated squamous epithelium without formation of central fibrovascular cores, as are usually seen in condylomata acuminata (31). Surface keratinization is variable but in some cases is dense. The endophytic growth pattern also helps to distinguish the condition from a viral wart. Verrucous carcinoma invades the stroma in a 'pushing' fashion by blunt, rounded projections, and irregular, infiltrative islands of tumour cells are absent (32).

Unusual Stromal Reactions to Squamous Cell Carcinoma of the Cervix

Most cases of cervical carcinoma have a mixed inflammatory cell infiltrate of lymphocytes, plasma cells, occasional histiocytes, and eosinophils but sometimes there is a dense infiltrate in which one inflammatory cell type predominates. A heavy lymphocyte infiltrate around invasive cervical carcinoma has been found to have a good prognosis (33, 34) and a dense plasma cell infiltrate has similarly been found to be beneficial (33, 35). However, in a review of reports of lymphoreticular infiltration in

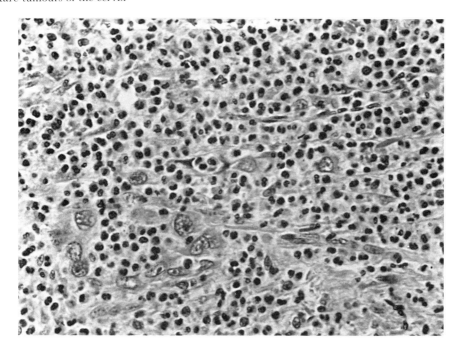

Figure 4   Carcinoma of the cervix with massive eosinophilia. The tumour cells are widely separated by a very dense infiltrate of eosinophils, which can lead to diagnostic difficulties on small biopsies of these tumours. (Haematoxylin and eosin, original magnification: ×450).

tumours, no distinct prognostic advantage was apparent (36).

About 2% of cases of cervical carcinoma (which are almost always large cell non-keratinizing tumours) have a massive stromal and intramural infiltrate of eosinophils (Figure 4) (37). The length of history before presentation is similar in these cases to that of non-eosinophilic cervical carcinoma, but patients with tumours with eosinophilia have a mean age approximately ten years lower than those with non-eosinophilic tumours, and have a better prognosis (38). A further histological feature of importance is that occasionally the eosinophil infiltrate can be so intense that the presence of tumour cells is obscured; when a massive eosinophil infiltrate in the cervix is found, therefore, a search must be made to exclude carcinoma before a diagnosis of eosinophilic cervicitis is accepted.

In the absence of circulating eosinophilia, tissue eosinophilia around the tumour is a good prognostic sign (37, 39, 40); patients with this

rare inflammatory reaction have a significantly better 5-year survival than those with the more usual mild and non-specific inflammatory response. Circulating eosinophilia, on the other hand, is associated with metastatic tumour spread and a poor prognosis (37, 41).

Rare Varieties of Adenocarcinoma of the Cervix

Cervical adenocarcinoma composed of tall, clear, mucus-secreting endocervical cells is the most common type of cervical adenocarcinoma (42). The rarer varieties of adenocarcinoma arising from endocervical columnar cells include clear cell adenocarcinoma, papillary serous adenocarcinoma, endometrioid adenocarcinoma and the intestinal type of mucus-secreting cervical adenocarcinoma. The histological features of these tumours are the same in the cervix as in endometrial primary tumours.

Diagnosis of one of these rare tumours as a

primary adenocarcinoma of the endocervix is contingent upon there being no tumour in the endometrium. When there is, because of the much greater likelihood of origin in the uteriner body, the cervix is deemed to be involved by downward spread from a primary tumour in the endometrium.

Clear Cell Carcinoma of the Cervix

The obsolescent term for this tumour, mesonephroid carcinoma, has been abandoned, partly because it is now considered to be derived from paramesonephric (müllerian) structures (43) and partly to avoid confusion with the much rarer mesonephric carcinoma (see below).

Clear cell carcinoma of the cervix accounted for about 40% of the cases reviewed by the Registry of Clear Cell Adenocarcinoma of the Genital Tract (44) and occurs principally in children and young women, with a mean age of 17 years. Half of the cases in the Registry collection occurred in the children of women treated with DES during pregnancy.

Macroscopically, clear cell carcinoma is similar to typical endocervical adenocarci-

noma. the tumours may be polypoid and friable, and invade the stroma of the endocervix and later ectocervix to a variable depth. Histologically the tumours are composed of clear cuboidal cells and flattened cells which form sheets, papillae and tubules; the latter two structures may also be formed from cells which have their nuclei positioned well away from the basement membrane and which appear to have a waisted or 'hobnail' appearance (Figure 5) (45, 46). Other neoplastic cell types, such as typical endocervical adenocarcinoma or endometrioid carcinoma, are often present in some areas of the tumour. Clear cell carcinoma of the endocervix has a better prognosis than typical endocervical adenocarcinoma (47, 48).

Mesonephric Tumours of the Cervix

Benign and malignant tumours can arise from the mesonephric (Wolffian) duct as it passes through the lateral cervical wall. Papillary adenoma probably of mesonephric origin has been described (49) but is very rare. Adenocarcinoma is commoner, though still very rare (50). It is important to establish that the

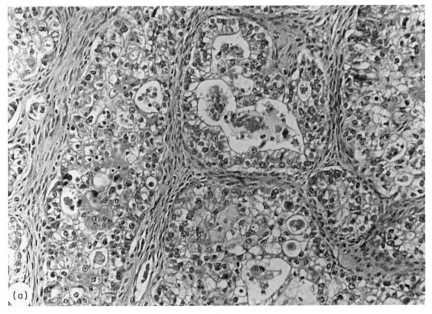

Figure 5a (see legend on facing page).

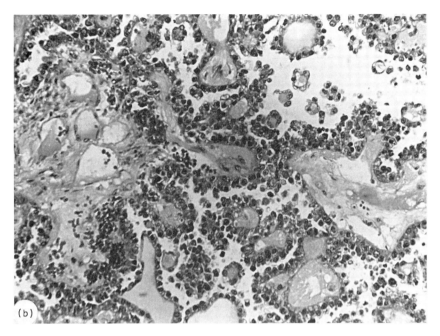

Figure 5 Clear cell ('mesonephroid') carcinoma of the cervix. The tumour has areas of clear polyhedral cells arranged in islands and irregular cords (a) and papillary areas in which the tumour cells are more eosinophilic and have their nuclei high in the apical poles of the cells ('hobnail cells') (b). (Haematoxylin and eosin, original magnification: ×250)

carcinoma is confined to the lateral cervical stroma (51); it is otherwise not possible to be certain that the tumour is not in fact a clear cell carcinoma arising from paramesonephrically derived surface epithelium.

Adenoid Cystic Carcinoma of Cervix

Adenoid cystic carcinoma of the cervix occurs predominantly in postmenopausal women and is rare; elderly multiparous black women appear to be particularly affected (52). The tumour is usually an exophytic, firm nodule which may be friable and ulcerated on the surface.

Histologically, adenoid cystic carcinoma of the cervix (53–61) closely resembles adenoid cystic carcinoma of salivary gland, breast, and lung (57, 62). In some cases the tumours are associated with cervical intraepithelial neoplasia or invasive carcinoma of the adjacent mucosa (55). As at other sites, perineural

invasion is a quite frequent finding (56) and metastases to regional and distant lymph nodes, adjacent pelvic structures, bones and viscera occur rarely (54).

Carcinoid Tumours of the Cervix

These rare tumours (63, 64) are thought to arise from the argyrophil cells of the normal endocervix (65). The histological appearance of these tumours varies from a typical well differentiated, easily recognizable tumour similar to carcinoid of the small bowel to poorly differentiated carcinoma resembling oat cell carcinoma of the bronchus (65, 66). Silver stains for argyrophilia and electron microscopical examination for neurosecretory granules are usually positive (67) and cervical carcinoid has been reported as a cause of the carcinoid syndrome (68). The prognosis of these tumours is very poor (69).

Some classifications of cervical carcinoma

include a category of undifferentiated small cell carcinoma thought to arise from subcolumnar reserve cells (70). Some of these tumours have been found to have argyrophilic cytoplasmic granules and to secrete adrenocorticotrophic hormone (71) and insulin (72), and the points of distinction between these tumours and poorly differentiated carcinoids are therefore unclear. It would seem best to reserve the term undifferentiated small cell carcinoma of reserve cell type for those tumours which do not have neurosecretory granules.

Carcinoma of Cervix of Mixed Patterns

Glassy Cell Carcinoma of the Cervix

These tumours form large, exophytic and fungating masses on the cervix which usually grow rapidly and cause extensive destruction. They are composed of diffuse sheets and strands of large, polyhedral, finely granular cells with large open nuclei and prominent nucleoli (73–75). Differentiation towards squamous elements is usually sparse; intercellular bridges are not seen and there is usually little keratinization. Only occasional glandular structures are present, and mucin production is not a feature, though small amounts of glycogen may be demonstrable (76). Glassy cell carcinoma is therefore classified as a poorly differentiated mixed adenoaquamous carcinoma (77). The prognosis is very poor (78).

Mucoepidermoid Carcinoma

Mucoepidermoid carcinoma of the cervix closely resembles the counterpart arising in salivary glands (79, 80). These tumours are composed of islands of malignant squamous cells of variable differentiation in which are scattered goblet or signet-ring cells containing mucin. Gland formation is rarely seen, a feature which helps to distinguish mucoepidermoid carcinoma from the much commoner adenosquamous carcinoma. This distinction is important as mucoepidermoid carcinoma has a very poor prognosis (70).

Other Rare Types of Carcinoma of the Cervix

Gestational choriocarcinoma involving the cervix alone, with no disease of the endometrium or ovaries, is extremely rare.

Malignant melanoma of the cervix is also extremely rare (81, 82). The tumour is identical to malignant melanoma elsewhere in the body, and diagnosis of a cervical primary requires both the exclusion of any possible origin in the skin or other organs and also evidence of melanocytic atypia at the junction of the involved cervical epithelium and stroma. The pathogenesis of malignant melanoma of the cervix is presumably the same as that of the relatively more common vaginal melanoma.

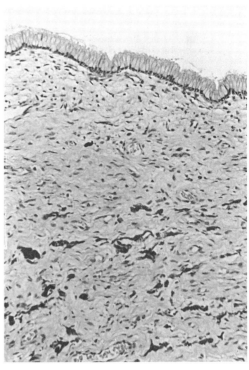

Figure 6 Cervical melanosis. Dendritic melanocytes containing large amounts of melanin are present in the superficial stroma of the endocervix. (Haematoxylin and eosin, original magnification: ×200).

Origin from cervical melanosis ('blue naevus of the cervix' (Figure 6) (83–85) has also been suggested.

Sarcoma of the Cervix (see Chapter 10 for a fuller description)

Primary cervical sarcoma can arise as malignant change in a benign neoplasm or de novo. Diagnosis of a primary cervical neoplasm, as with rare adenocarcinoma, depends on there being no malignancy in the uterine corpus.

Except for embryonal rhabdomyosarcoma, cervical sarcoma usually occurs after the age of 50 years (86, 87). Most form fungating polypoid masses which bleed easily, and it is seldom possible to identify the tumour cell type confidently from the macroscopical features alone. Histologically, cervical leiomyosarcoma, stromal sarcoma, and mixed mesodermal tumours all have the same morphology as similar tumours of the body of the uterus (88, 89).

Embryonal rhabdomyosarcoma is a rare tumour of the cervix arising in children and adolescents. The terms botryoid rhabdomyosarcoma and sarcoma botryoides are often used as synonyms for embryonal rhabdomyosarcoma, but should strictly be reserved for such of these tumours as are polypoid and translucent, and resemble a bunch of grapes (Figure 7). Botryoid rhabdomyosarcoma is composed of sparse, stellate or polygonal tumour cells widely separated from each other by myxoid stroma. Rhabdomyoblasts are difficult to find and intracytoplasmic cross-striations are rarely apparent.

Non-botryoid embryonal rhabdomyosarcoma has a range of histological appearances, varying from well differentiated tumours resembling fetal muscle to very poorly differentiated spindle cell neoplasms which might be impossible to diagnose with certainty without electron microscopic or immunocytological techniques (90) to demonstrate myoglobin (91, 92) or myosin (93). Most cases are comprised of areas of parvicellular, oedema-

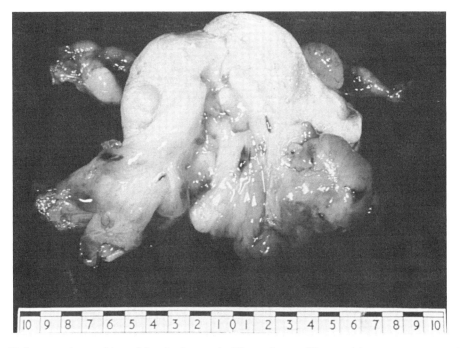

Figure 7   Sarcoma botryoides arising in the cervix. The patient, a 23 year old woman, presented with vaginal discharge.

tous or myxoid tissue and collections of hyperchromatic cells with eosinophilic cytoplasm, some of which may be characteristic of rhabdomyoblasts. Cross-striations may be found in the tumour cell cytoplasm in well differentiated tumours but are not essential for the diagnosis to be made. Intracellular glycogen is usually present.

Malignant lymphoma arising in the cervix is less common than involvement of the cervix by systemic lymphoma (94). Primary cervical lymphomas include both Hodgkin's and non-Hodgkin's lymphomas (95–99). Lymphoma tends to replace the stroma of the cervix without obliterating the epithelial structures, unlike carcinomas and other sarcomas.

Other very rare sarcomas of the cervix, which have been recorded as case reports only, include alveolar soft part sarcoma (100), Wilms' tumour (101) and yolk sac tumour (102).

CLINICAL FEATURES AND INVESTIGATIONS

Many of the clinical features of rare cervical tumours will inevitably be those of the more common malignant tumours of the cervix. Some rare neoplasms will arise within the stroma of the cervix and have intact ectocervical and vaginal epithelium, and in these cases extensive tissue sampling for histological diagnosis is essential.

The group of patients in whom the symptoms are often the mot bizarre and misleading is that of young women, adolescent girls and children. Prepubertal vaginal bleeding must always be investigated fully and will often require examination under anaesthesia. An adapted endoscope, the simplest being an adult nasal speculum, can be used to display the infant vagina. Benign adenomatous polyps are virtually unknown in prepubertal girls, and cervical polyps should be considered to be malignant until proved otherwise.

Exfoliative cytology is particularly difficult in children and adolescents, and may be misleadingly normal when the mucosa over a malignant stromal lesion is uninvolved. Nevertheless cytology should be performed regularly in girls exposed in utero to materanl diethylstilboestrol.

Colposcopic examination, in essence, provides information on the microvascular architecture of the lesion. Superficial extension of a tumour over the endocervical or ectocervical epithelium will obliterate the normal pattern of capillary loops and stimulate the formation of telangiectatic and bizarre vessels in the underlying stroma. The appearances may therefore easily be mistaken for cervical intraepithelial neoplasia or invasive squamous cell carcinoma. When feasible, colposcopy should be part of the surveillance of young women at risk from DES-induced malignancy.

Biochemical alteration in serum constituents is only likely to be found in cases of obstructive urinary tract disease. Serum examination for β-hCG should be performed if cervical pregnancy or choriocarcinoma are suspected. Both β-hCG and alpha-fetoprotein levels should be measured when a teratoma or a yolk sac tumour is suspected; the latter in infancy usually arises in the vagina, and may be confused with the DES-related clear cell tumour. Carcinoembryonic antigen may be elevated in many cases of genital malignancy and is not specific: very high levels should arouse the suspicion of secondary involvement by tumour from the gastrointestinal tract.

STAGING OF CERVICAL NEOPLASMS

The principles of staging of rare cervical malignancy are the same as those applied to common tumours. The heterogeneity of rare tumours makes it unlikely that visualization by monoclonal antibody techniques would be useful.

Examination under anaesthesia is very important in staging the disease, especially in the very young. Careful examination is essential to determine whether a malignant tumour is arising in or merely involving the cervix. Endoscopical examination of the bladder and large bowel may also be necessary and can be carried out at the same time.

Chest radiographs and intravenous urography are traditionally used in the investigation of cervical tumours but have largely been superseded by computed tomography (CT) scanning. CT is the most widely available technique for the visualization of lesions spreading to or involving the retroperitoneal tissues, although for intraperitoneal disease it is no more efficient than ultrasound examination; both of these techniques lack sufficient resolution to demonstrate small tumour deposits. Magnetic resonance imaging is a new technique which may prove effective at this stage, but there are only anecdotal data at present. Lymphography is of limited value but should be performed in conjunction with CT when a germ cell tumour or a lymphoma is suspected. Fine needle aspiration of a tumour deposit, possibly directed by CT, will provide material for cytological examination.

TREATMENT

The primary objective in the treatment of all pelvic cancer is the achievement of local disease control. Cure is a secondary though laudable objective. The local symptoms of uncontrolled pelvic malignancy, however, are so unpleasant that their prevention or relief must in some cases be of paramount importance. A further major therapeutic consideration is the effect of treatment on reproductive and sexual functions, and on the adjacent urinary and alimentary systems.

Both surgery and radiotherapy effectively eliminate most of the possibilities for future reproduction. With advances in techniques for assisted reproduction, however, preservation of ovarian function may be important even if the uterus is removed. The patient's oocytes could then be used in an artificial reproductive situation.

Chemotherapy, even in combination, is capable of allowing preservation of reproductive function in younger women. The regimen used for choriocarcinoma has often been followed

by successful pregnancy. The same has been achieved in germ cell tumours of the ovary, even when metastatic. There are no reports that chemotherapy is effective in rare tumours of the cervix.

Major extirpative surgery may have a role in the management of cervical sarcoma provided that the disease is localized. A careful search for metastatic disease is therefore important. In the treatment of genital malignancy of childhood, a combination of chemotherapy and radiotherapy has greatly reduced the need for exenterative surgery (102). In practice, effective use of combination chemotherapy (usually a vinca alkaloid, actinomycin D and an alkylating agent) can obviate the need for radiotherapy. For sarcoma in older women there is no specific, obviously effective therapy. There is thus no drug regimen which could justifiably be used as adjuvant therapy after major extirpation, and radiotherapy and chemotherapy should be reserved for cases with recurrent or metastatic disease.

SUMMARY

The firm diagnosis of a cervical origin for most of the rare tumours of the cervix depends on the exclusion of a primary site elsewhere. Most of the rare cervical tumours have the same pathological features as, and behave in a similar manner to, their more common counterparts in the uterine corpus, and their management follows the same principles.

REFERENCES

1 Robboy SJ, Kaufman RH, Prat R et al. Pathological findings in young women enrolled in the National Cooperative Diethylstilbestrol Adenosis (DESAD) project. Obstet Gynecol 1979; 53: 309–17.
2 Sandberg EC. Benign cervical and vaginal changes associated with exposure to stilbestrol in utero. Am J Obstet Gynecol 1976; 125: 777–89.
3 Buerger PT, Petzing HE. Congenital cysts of the corpus uteri. Am J Obstet Gynecol 1954; 67: 143–51.
4 Sneeden VD. Mesonephric lesions of the cer-

vix: a practical means of demonstration and a suggestion of incidence. Cancer 1958; 11: 334–6.

5 Sherrick JC, Vega JG. Congenital intramural cysts of the uterus. Obstet Gynecol 1962; 19: 486–93.

6 Aaro LA, Jacobson LJ, Soule EH. endocervical polyps. Obstet Gynecol 1963; 21: 659–65.

7 Rosen Y, Giannattasio CR, Boyce JG. Implantation of placental tissue in the cervix: complication of simultaneous cone biopsy and abortion. JAMA 1977; 237: 767.

8 Niven PA, Stansfeld AG. 'Glioma' of the uterus: a fetal homograft. Am J Obstet Gynecol 1973; 115: 534–8.

9 Roca AN, Guajardo M, Estrada WJ. Glial polyp of the cervix and endometrium. Report of a case and review of the literature. Am J Clin Pathol 1980; 73: 718–20.

10 Cove H. The Arias-Stella reaction occurring in the endocervix in pregnancy. Am J Suirg Pathol 1979; 3567–8.

11 Schneider V. Arias-Stella reaction in the endocervix: frequency and location. Acta Cytol 1981; 25: 224–8.

12 Van Nierkerk WA. Cervical cytological abnormalities caused by folic acid deficiency. Acta Cytol 1966; 10: 67–73.

13 Whitehead N, Reyner F, Lindenbaum J. Megaloblastic changes in the cervical epithelium. JAMA 1973; 226: 1421–2.

14 Beyer Boon ME. Psammoma bodies in cervical vaginal smears: an indicator of the presence of ovarian carcinoma. Acta Cytol 1974; 78: 41–4.

15 Highman WJ. Calcified bodies and the intrauterine device. Acta Cytol 1971; 15: 473–5.

16 Qizilbach AH. Psammoma bodies in cercicovaginal smears. Acta Cytol 1974; 18: 355.

17 Nogales-Ortiz F, Taracon I, Nogales PF. The pathology of female genital tract tuberculosis. Obstet Gynecol 1979; 53: 422–8.

18 Lucas SB. Bladder tumours in Malawi. Br J Urol 1982; 54: 275–9.

19 Tchertkoff V, Ober WB. Primary cancer of cervix uteri. NYJ Med 1966; 66: 1921–4.

20 Crossen R. A case of gumma of the testis. Am J Obstet Gynecol 1920; 19: 708.

21 Lemoine NR, Hall PA. Epithelial tumour metastatic to the uterine cervix. A study of 33 cases and review of the literature. Cancer 1986; 57: 2002–5.

22 Ackerman LV. Verrucous carcinoma of the oral cavity. Surgery 1948; 23: 670–8.

23 Lowe D, McKee PH. Verrucous carcinoma of the penis (Buschke–Löwenstein tumour): a clinicopathological study. Br J Urol 1983; 55: 427–9.

24 Degefu S, O'Quinn AG, Lacey CG, Merkel M, Barnard DE. Verrucous carcinoma of the cervix: a report of two cases and literature review. Gynecol Oncol 1986; 25: 37–47.

25 Aird I, Johnson D, Lennox B, Stansfeld AG. Epithelioma cuniculatum: variety of squamous carcinoma peculiar to the foot. Br J Surg 1954; 42: 245–50.

26 Jennings RH, Barclay DL. Verrucous carcinoma of the cervix. Cancer 1972; 30: 430–4.

27 Lucas WE, Benirschke K, Lebherz TB. Verrucous carcinoma of the female genital tract. Am J Obstet Gynecol 1974; 119: 435–440.

28 Spratt DW, Lee SC. Verrucous carcinoma of the cervix. Am J Obstet Gynecol 1977; 126: 699–700.

29 Raheja A, Katz DA, Dermer MS. Verrucous carcinoma of the endocervix. Obstet Gynecol 1983; 62: 535–8.

30 Maeyama M, Fukuma K, Tanaka N, Inoue S, Tohya T. A case of verrucous carcinoma of the uterine cervix: clinical, light and electron microscopic, and immunohistological observations. Gynecol Oncol 1985; 22: 244–9.

31 Kraus FT, Perez-Mesa C. Verrucous carcinoma—clinical and pathological study of 105 cases involving oral cavity, larynx and genitalia. Cancer 1966; 19: 26–38.

32 Crowther M, Lowe DG, Shepherd JH. Verrucous carcinoma of the female genital tract. Obstet Gynecol Surv (in press).

33 Bailar JC, Thomas LB, Thomson AD, Eisenberg H, Vick RM. Morphology and survival rates of cervical cancer in Connecticut and Southwest England. Natl Cancer Inst monogr 1966; 19: 385–400.

34 Sidhu GS, Koss LG, Barber HRK. Relation of histologic factors to the response of stage I epidermoid carcinomas of the cervix to surgical treatment: analysis of 115 patients. Obstet Gynecol 1970; 35: 329–38.

35 Lauder I, Aherne W, Stewart J, Sainsbury R. Macrophages infiltration of breast tumours: a prospective study. J Clin Pathol 1977; 30: 563–8.

36 Underwood JCE. Lymphoreticular infiltration of human tumours: prognostic and biological implications: a review. Br J Cancer. 1974; 30: 538–48.

37 Lowe D, Jorizzo J, Hutt MSR. Tumour-associated eosinophilia: a review. J Clin Pathol 1981; 34: 1343–8.

38 Lowe D. Tumour eosinophilia in cervical carcinoma: clinical aspects and prognostic implications. Br J Obstet Gynaecol, 1987 (in press).

39 Pastrnák A, Jansa P. Local eosinophilia in

stroma of tumors related to prognosis. Neoplasma 1984; 31: 323–6.

40 Kapp DS, LiVolsi VA. Intense eosinophilic stromal infiltration in carcinoma of the uterine cervix: a clinicopathological study of 14 cases. Gynecol Oncol 1983; 16: 19–30.

41 Isaacson NH, Rapoport P. Eosinophilia in malignant tumours: its significance. Ann Intern Med. 1946; 25: 893–902.

42 Anderson MC, Fraser AC. Adenocarcinoma of the uterine cervix: a clinical and pathological appraisal. Br J Obstet Gynecol 1976; 83: 320–5.

43 Roth LM, Hornback NB. Clear-cell adenocarcinoma of the cervix in young women. Cancer 1074; 34: 1761–8.

44 Herbst AL, Robboy SL, Scully RE, Poskanzer DC. Clear cell adenocarcinoma of the vagina and cervix in girls: analysis of 170 registry cases. Am J Obstet Gynecol 1974; 119: 713–24.

45 Inoue S, Matsuo I, Shemokawa K, Tohya T, Maeyama M. A case of clear cell adenocarcinoma of the cervix uteri in pregnancy. Gynecol Oncol 1986; 24: 120–5.

46 Senekjian EK, Hubby M, Bell DA, Anderson D, Herbst AL. Clear cell adenocarcinoma (CCA) of the vagina and cervix in association with pregnancy. Gynecol Oncol 1986; 24: 207–19.

47 Fawcett KJ, Dockerty MB, Hunt AB. Mesonephric carcinoma of the cervix uteri: a clinical and pathological study, Am J Obstet Gynecol 1966; 95: 1068–79.

48 Hameed K. Clear cell carcinoma of the uterine cervix. Am J Obstet Gynecol 1968; 101: 954–8.

49 Mackles A, Wolfe SA, Neigus I. Benign and malignant mesonephric lesions of the cervix. Cancer 1958; 11: 292–305.

50 McGee CT, Cromer DW, Green RR. Mesonephric carcinoma of the cervix: differentiation from endocervical adenocarcinoma. Am J Obstet Gynecol 1962; 84: 358–66.

51 Rosen Y, Dolan TE. Carcinoma of the cervix with cylindromatous features believed to arise in mesonephric duct. Cancer 1975; 36: 1739–47.

52 Gallagher HS, Simpson CB, Ayala AG. Adenoid cystic carcinoma of the uterine cervix: report of four cases. Cancer 1971; 27: 1398–1402.

53 Miles PA, Norris HJ. Adenoid cystic carcinoma of the cervix. An analysis of 12 cases. Obstet Gynecol 1971; 38: 103–10.

54 Ramzy I, Yuzpe AA, Hendleman J. Adenoid cystic carcinoma of uterine cervix. Obstet Gynecol 1975; 45: 679–83.

55 Shingleton HM, Lawrence WD, Gore H. Cervical carcinoma with adenoid cystic pattern: a light and electron microscopic study. Cancer 1977; 40: 1112–21.

56 Hoskins WJ, Averette HE, Ng ABP, Yon JL. Adenoid cystic carcinoma of the cervix uteri: report of six cases and review of the literature. Gynecol Oncol 1979; 7: 371–84.

57 Lawrènce JB, Mazur MT. Adenoid cystic carcinoma: a comparative pathologic study of tumors in salivary gland, breast, lung, and cervix. Hum Pathol 1982; 13: 916–24.

58 Gonzales S. Adenoid cystic pattern in uterine cervical carcinoma: report of three cases. J Miss State Med Assoc 1984; 25: 207–9.

59 Berchuck A, Mullin TJ. Cervical adenoid cystic carcinoma associated with ascites. Gynecol Oncol 1985; 22: 201–11.

60 Musa AG, Hughes RR, Coleman SA. Adenoid cystic carcinoma of the cervix: a report of 17 cases. Gynecol Oncol 1985; 22: 167–73.

61 van Dinh T, Woodruff JD. Adenoid cystic and adenoid basal carcinomas of the cervix. Obstet Gynecol 1985; 65: 705–9.

62 Koss LG, Brannan CD, Ashikari R. Histologic and ultrastructural features of adenoid cystic carcinoma of the breast. Cancer 1970; 26: 1271–9.

63 Alborez-Saavedra J, Larraza O, Poucell S, Rodriguez-Martinez HD. Carcinoid of the uterine cervix: additional observations on a new tumor entity. Cancer 1976; 38: 2328–42.

64 Habib A, Kaneko M, Cohen CJ, Walker G. Carcinoid of the uterine cervix: a case report with light and electron microscopic studies. Cancer 1979; 43: 535–8.

65 Tateishi R, Wada A, Hayakawa K, Hongo J, Ishii J, Terakaira N. Argyrophil cell carcinomas (apudomas) of the uterine cervix: light and electron microscope observations of 5 cases. Virchow Arch Path Anat 1975; 366: 257–74.

66 Yamasaki M, Tateishi R, Hongo J, Ozaki Y, Inoue M, Ueda G. Argyrophil small cell carcinomas of the uterine cervix. Int J Gynecol Pathol 1984; 3: 146–52.

67 Turner WA, Gallup DG, Talledo OE, Otken LB, Guthrie TH. Neuroendocrine carcinoma of the uterine cervix complicated by pregnancy: case report and review of the literature. Obstet Gynecol 1986; 67: 80S–83S.

68 Stockdale AD, Leader M, Phillips RH, Henry K. The carcinoid syndrome and multiple hormone secretion associated with a carcinoid tumour of the uterine cervix. Br J Obstet Gynaecol 1986; 93: 397–401.

69 Silva EG, Kott MM, Ordonez NG. Endocrine carcinoma intermediate cell type of the uterine cervix. Cancer 1984; 54: 1705–13.

70 Ferenczy A. In: Blaustein A (ed) Pathology of

the Female Genital Tract, 2nd edition. New York: Springer Verlag, 1982: 210.

71 Jones HW, Plymate S, Gluck FB, Miles FA, Green JF. Small cell non-keratinizing carcinoma of the cervix associated with ACTH production. Cancer 1976; 38: 1629–35.

72 Kiang DT, Bauer GE, Kennedy BT. Immunoassayable insulin in carcinoma of the cervix associated with hypoglycaemia. Cancer 1973; 31: 801–5.

73 Littman P, Clement PB, Henriksen B, Wang CC, Robboy SJ, Taft PD, Ulfelder H, Scully RE. Glassy cell carcinoma of the cervix. Cancer 1976; 37: 2238–46.

74 Seltzer V, Sall S, Castadot MJ, Muradian-Davidian M, Sedlis A. Glassy cell cervical carcinoma. Gynecol Oncol 1979; 8: 141–51.

75 Nuñez C, Abdul-Karim FW, Somrak TM. Glassy cell carcinoma of the uterine cervix. Cytopathologic and histopathologic study of five cases. Acta Cytol (Baltimore) 1985; 29: 303–9.

76 Maier RC, Norris HJ. Glassy cell carcinoma of the cervix. Obstet Gynecol 1982; 60: 219–24.

77 Ulbright TM, Gersell DJ. Glassy cell carcinoma of the uterine cervix. A light and electron microscopic study of five cases. Cancer 1983; 51: 2255–63.

78 Pak HY, Yokota SB, Paladugu RR, Agliozzo CM. Glassy cell carcinoma of the cervix. Cytologic and clinicopathologic analysis. Cancer 1983; 52: 307–12.

79 Papadia S. Mucinous patterns in epidermoid carcinomas of the uterine cervix. Gynecologia 1962; 153: 337–48.

80 Dougherty CM, Cotten N. Mixed squamous cell and adenocarcinoma of the cervix. Combined, adenosquamous and mucoepidermoid types. Cancer 1964; 17: 1132–43.

81 Jones HW, Droegmueller W, Makowski EL. A primary melanocarcinoma of the cervix. Am J Obstet Gynecol 1971; 111: 959–63.

82 Krishnamoorthy A, Desai A, Simanowitz M. Primary malignant melanoma of the cervix. Br J Obstet Gynaecol 1986; 93: 84–6.

83 Majundar B, Ross RJ, Gorelkin L. Benign blue nevus of the uterine cervix. Am J Obstet Gynecol 1979; 134: 600–1.

84 Walter A. Blue nevus of the endocervix. Br J Obstet Gynaecol 1982; 89: 1059–61.

85 Patel DS, Bhagavan BS. Blue nevus of the uterine cervix. Hum Pathol 1985; 16: 79–86.

86 Abell MR, Ramirez JA. Sarcomas and carcinosarcomas of the uterine cervix. Cancer 1973; 31: 1176–92.

87 Rotmensch J, Rosenstein NB, Woodruff JD. Cervical sarcoma: a review. Obstet Gynecol Surv 1983; 38: 456–60.

88 Jaffe R, Altaras M, Bernheim J, Ben Aderet N. Endocervical stromal sarcoma—a case report. Gynecol Oncol 1985; 22: 105–8.

89 Miyazawa K, Hernandex E. Cervical carcinosarcoma: a case report. Gynecol Oncol 1986; 23: 376–80.

90 Sarnat HB, de Mello DE, Siddiqui SY. Diagnostic value of histochemistry in embryonal rhabdomyosarcoma. Am J Surg Pathol 1979; 3: 177–83.

91 Mukai K, Rosai J, Hallaway BE. Localization of myoglobin in normal and neoplastic human skeletal muscle cells using an immunoperoxidase method. Am J Surg Pathol 1979; 3: 373–6.

92 Corson JM, Pincus GS. Intracellular myoglobin—a specific marker for skeletal muscle differentiation in soft tissue sarcomas. An immunoperoxidase study. Am J Pathol 1981; 103: 384–9.

93 Koh EJ, Johnson WW. Antimyosin and antirhabdomyoblastic sera: their use for the diagnosis of childhood rhabdomyosarcoma. Arch Pathol Lab Med 1980; 104: 118–22.

94 Lathrop JC. Malignant pelvic lymphomas. Obstet Gynecol 1967; 30: 137–45.

95 Chorlton I, Karnei RF, King FM, Norris HJ, Primary malignant reticuloendothelial disease involving the vagina, cervix and corpus uteri. Obstet Gynecol 1974; 44: 735–48.

96 Castaldo TW, Ballon SC, Lagasse LD, Petrilli ES. Reticuloendothelial neoplasia of the female genital tract. Obstet Gynecol 1979; 54: 167–70.

97 Komaki R, Cox JD, Hansen RM, Gunn WG, Greenberg M. Malignant lymphoma of the uterine cervix. Cancer 1984; 54: 1699–1704.

98 Taki I, Aozasa K, Kurokawa K. Malignant lymphoma of the uterine cervix. Cytological diagnosis of a case with immunocytochemical corroboration. Acta Cytol (Baltimore) 1985; 29: 607–11.

99 Bowen DC, Grant MC. Primary lymphoma of the cervix. S Afr Med J 1985; 68: 889–90.

100 Flint A, Gikas PW, Roberts JA. Alveolar soft part sarcoma of the uterine cervix. Gynecol Oncol 1985; 22: 263–7.

101 Bell DA, Shimm DS, Gang DL. Wilms' tumor of the endocervix. Arch Pathol Lab Med 1985; 14: 543–4.

102 Copeland LJ, Sneige N, Ordonez NG, Hancock KC, Gershenson DM, Saul PB, Kavanagh JJ. Endodermal sinus tumor of the vagina and cervix. Cancer 1985; 55: 2558–65.

103 Malpas JS. Paediatric malignancy. In: Medicine Illustrated, 1987: 1660–3.

Textbook of Uncommon Cancer
Edited by C.J. Williams, J.G. Krikorian, M.R. Green and D. Raghavan
© 1988 John Wiley & Sons Ltd

Chapter **12**

Aggressive Cervical Carcinoma in Young Women

Mary E. Crowther* and
John H. Shepherd†
*Gynaecological Oncology Fellows, St Bartholomew's
Hospital, London, UK, and †Consultant Gynaecological
Surgeon, St Bartholomew's Hospital, London, UK

INTRODUCTION

It is rare to find cervical carcinoma in women under 20; the youngest case reported in the world literature was a 15 year old virgin with a squamous cell carcinoma (1). Tumours in younger children are rare and tend to be adenocarcinoma (2).

In recent years the biological behaviour of cervical carcinoma seems to have changed in that:

1. the incidence and mortality is increasing in women less than 35 years of age;
2. these women are said to have more 'bad-prognosis' factors than older women;
3. the proportion of adenocarcinoma, traditionally 5–10%, is increasing in younger women;
4. a significant proportion of women have negative cytology in the 3 years prior to diagnosis, suggesting a greater number of more rapidly progressive cases;
5. the incidence of precursor lesions (cervical intraepithelial neoplasia—CIN) has increased dramatically in all age groups, but particularly in teenage and younger women.

This review aims to discuss the evidence for each of these points in turn and suggests ways in which diagnosis and treatment may be improved.

EPIDEMIOLOGY—INCIDENCE AND MORTALITY

Epidemiological studies and their interpretation are plagued by the small size of populations on which data are often based. Mortality rates are more reliable to review than incidence rates as the latter are influenced by incomplete registration, cytological screening, hysterectomies and removal from the population of women with precursor lesions treated before they become malignant (3).

It is assumed that pre-malignant disease of the cervix (dysplasia or CIN) progresses slowly over 15–20 years to invasive cancer. It is not known what proportion of CIN becomes invasive or indeed whether all cases of invasive disease have a precursor phase. It is assumed that many of the minor lesions regress spontaneously (4), although most subsequently recur (5); and that most CIN 3 lesions become invasive over 5–10 years (6). The only factor which might indicate which lesions are likely to progress is the presence of certain types of human papillomavirus (see below). Currently, there is confusion about the appropriate management of CIN.

Most studies suggest that cervical screening campaigns have had a beneficial impact on both the mortality and incidence of invasive disease, although Green (7) disagrees. Data from British Columbia (8), Scotland (9), the Nordic countries (10) and the United States (11, 12) all provide evidence that comprehensive screening of the female population has a dramatic effect on the disease incidence.

An increase in mortality in the United Kingdom was first reported in 1978. Yule (13) showed that the overall mortality had decreased in England and Wales by 11.8%, but in women aged less than 35 (from whom 70% of all smears came) mortality had doubled in 6 years. Macgregor and Teper (9) confirmed these figures for Scotland, England and Wales and noted a doubling of the mortality rate in women under 35 from 11/million to 17.7/

million. In real terms the increase in mortality was from about 37 women per year in 1968 to 67 per year in 1976. That has now increased to just over 100 per year (Table 1).

Similar data have been reported from other countries (Table 2). In Alberta the incidence of carcinoma of the cervix trebled over 20 years from 12/100000 to 40/100000 in women aged 20–34 while the incidence had been falling in older women. This was in association with a massive increase in CIN 3 (8). Mortality rates in New Zealand doubled in women aged 20–34 (7) and in Australia, mortality which had been steadily falling since 1908 showed a levelling off in women aged 20–39 between 1970 and 1978, followed by an increase (14–16). In America, similar pictures are emerging (11, 17).

More detailed analysis of the United Kingdom mortality rates shows that the increase which began in the mid-60s for women aged 25–29, was followed by a similar rise about 5 years later for women aged 30–34, a pattern then repeated about 5 years later for

TABLE 1 MORTALITY DATA FOR CANCER OF THE CERVIX IN ENGLAND AND WALES (OFFICE OF POPULATION CENSUSES AND SURVEYS): TOTAL NUMBER OF DEATHS SINCE 1964

Year	15–24	25–34	35–44	45–54	55–64	>65	Total
1964	3	32	337	627	561	1017	2577
1965	3	33	330	596	604	887	2453
1966	0	27	280	555	599	1021	2472
1967	1	32	241	628	574	971	2449
1968	3	32	226	630	618	925	2434
1969	5	32	205	564	607	1003	2417
1970	5	34	170	566	625	943	2343
1971	2	41	184	580	594	924	2315
1972	4	46	164	510	604	890	2218
1973	7	39	137	542	605	919	2249
1974	5	50	122	443	524	924	2068
1975	9	68	136	412	597	921	2143
1976	7	60	128	455	669	915	2206
1977	2	71	166	396	570	940	2145
1978	1	93	163	358	572	966	2153
1979	6	83	168	317	585	948	2107
1980	10	104	161	309	548	956	2088
1981	7	111	198	275	510	933	2034
1982	8	103	202	259	468	907	1947
1983	3	121	196	282	449	908	1932
1984	4	107	214	241	493	840	1899

TABLE 2 STUDIES ON THE INCREASED INCIDENCE* AND MORTALITY OF
YOUNG WOMEN WITH CERVICAL CARCINOMA

Reference	Years of study	Age group	Findings
Cramer (11)	1947–70	20–29	89 to 138 per million (*)
Green (7)	1959–76	<35	Doubling in incidence and mortality
Macgregor and Teper (4)	1968–76	15–34	110 to 177 per million
Yule (13)	1970–76	<35	Doubling in mortality
Anello and Lao (17)	1970–76	<25	0.39 to 0.54 per million
Armstrong and Holman (14)	1972–76	20–39	107 to 146 per million (*) Increased mortality
Walton (8)	1956–76	20–34	120 to 400 per million (*)
Fay et al. (114)	1965–79	20–34	27.2 to 73.1 per million
Cook and Draper (18)	1963–80	15–24	3 to 12 per million (*)
		25–34	53 to 135 per million (*)
	1950–82	15–24	0.6 to 2.2 per million
		25–34	18 to 30 per million
Bourne and Grove (16)	1974–80	20–44	Increased incidence Mortality stable
Carmichael et al. (81)	1971–80	>35	30.3 to 89.4 per million (*)

women aged 35–39 and so on (18) (Figure 1). This birth-cohort effect, first described by Hill and Adelstein (19), is seen in both mortality and incidence rates (3). In other words rates vary according to the year of birth of the women concerned. Women born around 1921 have high mortality rates, those born between 1926 and 1931 low rates, and women born since 1935 have shown steady increases. In fact women born around 1951 have death rates double those of women born 10 years earlier. This cohort effect has also been observed in the Nordic countries (10) and Australia (14) where the increasing mortality involves women born after 1935 and is only for cervical carcinoma and not other cancers of the uterus.

Incidence rates for invasive cancer are more difficult to interpret for the reasons mentioned above. Nevertheless, there has been a marked increase in registration of the disease for women under 35 with a four-fold increase in women aged 15–24 (Table 3). Although this does not reflect the true incidence rates, it can not all be explained by earlier diagnosis through screening. The cohort effect is also apparent here with a marked increase for women born in the years around 1931, 1941 and 1951. Parkin et al. (3) have shown an

interesting change in the incidence curve in the past 15 years. In 1963 the curve was unimodal with the peak incidence years 45–49. Since this time there has been a progressive flattening of the curve for the age range 35–39 until by 1978 the curve is bimodal with peaks at 35–39 and 55–59 (Figure 2). The decrease in the 40–49 age range is nearly 50%. Other authors noticing this bimodal pattern, have suggested that carcinoma of the cervix has two forms, one which affects young women and one older women (20), but Parkin et al. (3) attribute this pattern to the removal of precursor lesions (CIN 3) in women aged 25–44 since the mid-1960s. Incidence curves for Denmark and Sweden show the same effect, and this bimodal pattern has also been observed on a local scale in a Yorkshire population (21).

It has become popular in Britain to criticize the efficacy of exfoliative cervical cytology, which has never been the subject of a nationally organized programme, let alone one with 'public-health' in mind (22, 23). Indeed in 1969 Lees (24) published cohort mortality rates for England and Wales showing that the death rate had been falling for all ages until 1945–50, i.e. before the introduction of cytology. Nevertheless, both Draper and Cook (25)

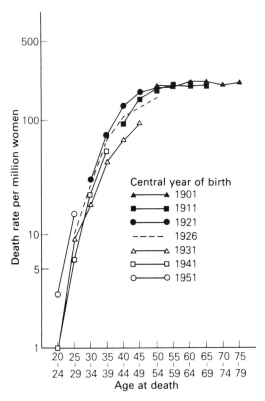

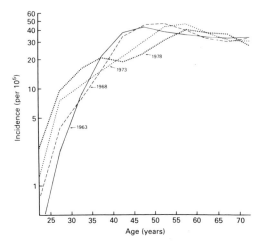

Figure 2 Observed incidence of clinical cervical cancer in 1963, 1968, 1973 and 1978. (*From Parkin et al. (3), reprinted by kind permission of Blackwell Scientific Publications.*)

Figure 1 Cohort mortality rates for carcinoma of the cervix in England and Wales 1951–1980. Rates are plotted for women dying at specified ages and born in years centred on 1 January 1901, 1911, etc. Each point is based on mortality date for 5 years. (*From Cook and Draper (18), reprinted by kind permission of Macmillan Press.*)

and Parkin et al. (3) have suggested that screening has prevented up to 50% of the potential cases in young women in the past 15 years, and therefore hidden the huge rise in incidence in this group.

AETIOLOGY

The traditional epidemiological factors which are correlated with the development of this disease such as high parity and low socio-

TABLE 3 INCIDENCE DATA FOR CANCER OF THE CERVIX IN ENGLAND AND WALES (OFFICE OF POPULATION CENSUSES AND SURVEYS): TOTAL REGISTRATIONS SINCE 1971

Year	15–24	25–34	35–44	45–54	55–64	>65	Total
1971	34	258	557	1219	960	1062	4090
1972	34	240	472	1081	1050	1066	3943
1973	24	298	489	1052	1081	1121	4065
1974	30	323	438	1008	1065	1178	4042
1975	26	318	480	942	1071	1194	4031
1976	30	361	456	875	1092	1150	3964
1977	47	414	472	806	1077	1200	4016
1978	46	445	514	691	1003	1173	3872
1979	35	469	553	646	982	1193	3879
1980	44	492	609	609	1005	1203	3962
1981	43	568	636	622	926	1229	4024
1982	42	504	672	580	920	1193	3911

economic class may be less important than age of first coital activity, poor genital hygiene, multiple sexual partners, genital tract infection, smoking and the sexual behaviour of the woman's consort (26, 27). It is postulated that viruses (herpes simplex II and human papillomavirus) act in conjunction with protein from the sperm head to initiate carcinogenic change in the cells of the transformation zone. This is a particularly dynamic area in the adolescent and post-partum woman, where encroaching columnar epithelium undergoes squamous metaplasia and it is here that squamous cell carcinoma and its precursor CIN lesions develop.

Whilst much attention has been paid to the sexual behaviour of women who get this disease, it is also clear that the sexual behaviour of men is important (27) and Singer et al. (28) suggest that there is a 'high-risk' male.

Certainly, there has been a massive increase in the number of abnormal smears, and the incidence of CIN 3 in all age groups but particularly in young women. Lappaluoto (29) reported an 800% increase in the number of suspicious smears from young women since 1970, and two factors were present in most of the patients—promiscuity and the oral contraceptive pill. Throughout the 70s this has been the trend in Canada (30), Italy (31) and the United Kingdom (13, 32–35). Andrews et al. (33) noted with some concern that in 10 years the mean age of women presenting with invasive cancer had fallen from 50 to 35. Wolfendale et al. (35) reported an increased rate of abnormal smears in women who were already in screening programmes and who were from non-manual, middle class and professional backgrounds. Even Jewish women, traditionally protected from this disease, are displaying a significant number of abnormal smears (36).

Incidence rates for CIN 3 are highly unreliable, since many cases may not be registered, and rates reflect to a large extent the number of smears taken. Nevertheless, between 1973 and 1979, the number of smears notified to the DHSS increased by about 19% and two-thirds were re-screens for women already screened. One would therefore expect with this level of re-screening that the detection of precursor lesions would have removed them from the study population. Yet registrations for CIN 3 have steadily increased and in women aged 25–34 by 131% (25).

Changes in Sexual Behaviour

It is difficult to escape the conclusion that changes in sexual behaviour are one aspect of the increase in cervical carcinoma. Teenagers now are more sexually active than pre-war teenagers (37), and there has been a disturbing increase in the number of abnormal smears in this group (38, 39). Delke et al. (38) reported that 13.7% of teenagers referred to his Dysplasia Unit had CIN 3. Analysis of all smears taken in the United States during 1981 (39) showed prevalence rates for CIN of 18.8/1000 for teenagers and 28.8/1000 for women aged 20–24. The majority of the 3651 teenagers with dysplasia gave a history of sexual intercourse before 15, and more than half had had more than one partner.

Sexually Transmitted Organisms

Beral (40) showed that the increased mortality in certain cohorts of women in the United Kingdom paralleled the cohort-specific increases in rates of gonorrhoea at the age of 20. There has been a doubling of attendances to Special Clinics in the past 10 years with over 590 000 new cases of sexually transmitted diseases in 1983, nearly 10% of which were genital warts (41). In 1981, one-third of all recorded cases of gonorrhoea in women in Britain occurred in teenagers. It is of some concern that these diseases may be asymptomatic in women for some time. Saltz et al. (42) studied 100 sexually active middle-class teenagers attending an Adolescent Health Clinic; *Chlamydia trachomatis* was cultured in 22% and gonorrhoea in 3%. Of these girls, whose mean age was 17 years, 30% had had six or more sexual partners.

Herpes Simplex Virus II (HSV-2)

Antibodies to HSV-2 (43) and virus specific antigen (44) have been found in up to 90% of patients and their cervical biopsies. Zur Hausen (45) has postulated that the virus acts as a cofactor with human papillomavirus (HPV), initiating the transformation process in the cell towards malignancy but not replicating further.

Human Papillomavirus (HPV)

Koilocytic atypia in cells and flat non-condylomatous lesions on the cervix are pathognomonic of infection (46), and about one-third of the routine smears from women between 21 and 25 may have evidence of HPV infection. About 60% of the lesions resolve spontaneously or with treatment and 5% progress to dysplasia over 21–60 months.

HPV can be detected in cervical lesions, with decreasing frequency as the dysplasia becomes more severe (47), Zur Hausen (48) has shown that the majority of cases of cervical and vulval carcinoma contain HPV 16 and 18 integrated into the host cell DNA, whereas HPV 6, 10 and 11 are not integrated. He has suggested that the former carry a high risk for the development of cancer in the female genital tract.

Epidemiological studies on HPV infection in teenagers (49) demonstrate the increased incidence of dyskariotic smears, and progression to CIN 3. The consorts of men with penile warts are also at high risk of contracting warts and developing dyskariotic smears (50). There are well known associations between vulvo-vaginal warts (51), penile cancer (52) and cervical cancer.

Other Organisms

Cytomegalovirus (53), *Chlamydia trachomatis* (54) and *Irichomonas vaginalis* (55) have all been implicated in the aetiology of dysplasia and cervical cancer, on the basis of serological tests in affected women (53) or the high incidence of dysplastic smears in association with these infections.

The assumption that there is a causal link between cervical cancer, dysplasia and these venereally transmitted diseases is not necessarily incorrect simply because infective agents are not found in all cases. One only has to recall the pathology of leprosy to realize that signs of contagion may be minimal.

There are two other social changes which have occurred to women born after 1935 and which may have some bearing on the observed cohort effect. These are smoking and steroid contraception.

Smoking

Case-control studies have shown that women who smoke are 13 times more likely to get cervical cancer than non-smokers (27, 56), even when sexual characteristics between the two groups have been standardized. The risk appears to be dose-related and is increased in 'passive' smokers. Nicotine and tar products have been found concentrated in cervical epithelium (Singer, personal communication), where they may lead to an immune disturbance of Langerhans' cells, and so increase the risk of HPV super-infection.

Contraception and Diethylstilboestrol

Barrier methods of contraception would appear to offer some protection to women from the development of cervical dysplasia and malignancy (56, 57), although a more recent study on the factors which may cause lesions to progress did not confirm this (58).

In 1977 Stern et al. (59) noted that dysplasia progressed more rapidly to CIN 3 in women taking the oral contraceptive pill (OCP), although Bamford's study again has not confirmed this (58). Many studies, some of them prospective and based on large numbers of participants, have suggested that duration of use is important (56, 60, 61).

Vessey's prospective study (61) on the

women entered into the Oxford Family Planning Association Contraceptive study, noted
that 13 women using the OCP developed an
invasive squamous cell cervical carcinoma,
compared with none of the users of an intrauterine contraceptive device (IUCD). Their
risk of dysplasia and invasive disease doubled
after 8 years of oral contraceptive use to 2.2 per
1000-woman years. Seven of the cancers were
'occult' and only 2 advanced and aggressive.

This risk has not been confirmed by others
(62, 63) but follow-up less than 6 years may be
insufficient (61). Criticism of the Vessey study
emphasizes the confounding effects of smoking
and sexual behaviour on any results which
may be obtained, even though he tried to
document similar sexual histories from both
groups of women. To try and avoid this the
WHO Collaborative Study of Neoplasia and
Steroid Contraceptives (64) limited its report
to women from developing countries only and
attempted to screen for 23 variables of sexual
behaviour, including age of first coitus,
number of sexual relationships (of wife only)
and parity. They found a relative risk of 1.19 in
women who had taken the OCP, increasing to
1.53 after 5 years' usage. The study did not
take into account smoking habits, or the sexual
behaviour of the male consorts.

If steroid usage does have an influence on
this disease, it may be by its propensity to cause
cervical ectopy, with subsequent squamous
metaplasia (29). Cellular atypia and intense
mitotic activity sufficient to simulate the
appearances of adenocarcinoma has been
reported to resolve when contraceptive usage
stops (65). There are anecdotal reports of
women on the OCP developing cervical adenocarcinoma (66–68), the incidence of which
appears to be increasing (see below) and
Dallenbach-Hellweg (67) has postulated a
connection between this cancer and progesto-
gen usage. The epidemiology is different from
that of squamous cell carcinoma in that women
tend to be nulliparous (69).

There is certainly a well established association between clear cell adenocarcinoma of the
vagina and cervix in teenage girls whose

mothers ingested diethylstilboestrol (DES)
during pregnancy. Herbst (70), who first
brought the world's attention to this in 1971,
has calculated the risk to be 0.14–1.4/1000
exposed girls up to the age of 24. In America up
to two million females were exposed to the
drug, in the United Kingdom 7000–8000. To
date 429 of these tumours have been registered
in the United States (150 of which involve the
cervix) and 4 in the United Kingdom (71).

It is unclear whether these girls have an
increased risk of developing squamous cell
carcinoma of the cervix in the future. Orr et al.
(72) noted that 4.7% of 300 DES-exposed
females had CIN 3. If the model of a long
transformation period from dysplasia to cancer
is correct, it is still too early to say whether
there will be an increased risk. Their small
numbers have had no influence on the current
increase in incidence in young women.

PATHOLOGY

It is controversial whether the pathology of this
disease is different in younger women, and
reports of aggressive behaviour by tumours are
usually based on individual case reports or
small numbers of patients.

Clinical Features

Most women with cervical carcinoma present
with abnormal vaginal discharge or inappropriate vaginal bleeding (e.g. intermenstrual
loss, menorrhagia and post-coital bleeding),
but early stages of the disease are generally
symptomless (73).

The cervix may look normal (occult carcinoma), or the lesion be mistaken for benign
cervical ectopy. This leads to delay in diagnosis
and inappropriate treatment such as dia-
thermy to supposed benign lesions. An endocervical lesion may cause no other abnormality
than an enlarged 'barrel-shaped' cervix.

Disease which has spread causes pain from
perineural or periosteal involvement, or leg
oedema from lymphatic obstruction. Enlarged
para-aortic nodes may cause hypogastric pain.

Haematuria or rectal bleeding and malignant fistulae to the vagina signify involvement of the bladder and rectum, and uraemia may occur from bilateral ureteric obstruction. Metastatic involvement of the lungs may give rise to chronic cough, chest pain and haemoptysis; deposits in the liver, brain, skin and bone lead to jaundice, cerebral symptoms and pain. The supraclavicular (scalene) nodes maybe enlarged.

Diagnostic Cytology

Cervical smears have an inherent false nega- tive rate of about 20–60% depending on quality control in individual laboratories (74). The problem is equally divided between labor- atory error, faulty technique in taking the smear and variations in the rate at which malignant cells exfoliate when covered with necrotic slough. Taking smears in pairs reduces the false-negative rate by nearly 20% (74).

Rylander (75) and Berkeley et al. (76) have suggested that CIN becomes invasive more quickly in young women, resulting in a high incidence of 'negative' smears (Table 4). There is a tendency to undercall abnormal smears in young women (8, 81), but false reading of smears is also disturbingly high (21, 75, 76).

Paterson et al. (21) reported that over 50% of 'negative' smears in younger women were in fact abnormal and a further 20% were unsatis- factory. Berkeley et al. (76) reported that of 10 women with advanced and aggressive disease within 10 months of a negative smear, 5 had slides showing frankly malignant or dysplastic cells. The problem of negative smears is not, however, confined to younger women and up to 60% of smears in older women may be negative within 3 years of invasive disease (81). It is not clear that the biological behaviour of this tumour is different in young women; it may simply be that the intense screening in young women and poor uptake in older women distorts the figures.

Adenocarcinoma is more likely to be missed on cytological screening than squamous cell carcinoma (30, 82). In a study (80) of women who had been screened within 3 years of diagnosis, 28% of women with negative smears had an adenocarcinoma and 20% an adenos- quamous carcinoma.

A further problem, highlighted by the recent publicity of a woman who died from cervical carcinoma in Oxford, is human error and failure to respond adequately to a positive cytology report. Elwood et al. (83) noted that only 59% of over 1000 women with abnormal

TABLE 4 INCIDENCE OF FALSE NEGATIVE SMEARS IN WOMEN WITH CERVICAL CARCINOMA

Reference	Percentage negative smears	Percentage false[a] negative smears	Years before diagnosis	Age group mainly affected
Rylander (75)	36	62.5	5	<40 yrs
Berkeley et al. (76)	10 cases	50	10 mos.	20–39
Dunn and Schweitzer (12)	29	18.5	5	—
Morrell et al. (77)	20	28	3	—
Bain and Crocker (78)	28	—	3	30–35
Bamford et al. (79)	27	—	2	Young[b]
Benoit et al. (80)	31	—	1	—
Paterson et al. (21)	26	73.7	5	<45
Carmichael et al. (81)	71.4	—	3	<35

[a]On review of all 'negative' smears, the proportion with cytological abnormality, i.e. malignant or dysplastic cells.
[b]Women in a Family Planning Clinic.

cytology had received appropriate follow-up and treatment, and this could rarely be attributed to the patient.

Histological Diagnosis

Any woman with an abnormal smear or a suspicious lesion of the cervix should be advised colposcopic examination regardless of cytology (84). This is highly accurate, particularly with occult lesions. Early invasive disease can only be diagnosed from a formal cone biopsy. A wedge biopsy from a clinically invasive lesion assesses the depth of stromal invasion. Adenocarcinoma is diagnosed from a fractional curettage. Tru-Cut biopsies can be taken of other masses and needle aspiration of supraclavicular or other accessible nodes is very accurate (85, p. 56).

Histology (Chapter 11)

Approximately 90% of cervical tumours are squamous cell carcinoma and 10% are adenocarcinoma which show the full range of müllerian differentiation. Other types of neoplasia are rare. Three groups of squamous cell carcinoma are recognized: large cell non-keratinizing (50–60%), large cell keratinizing (35–45%), which are thought to be less differentiated, and small cell tumours (10–15%), which contain abundant mitotic figures.

The proportion of patients with adenocarcinoma is increasing (Tables 5 and 6), particularly in younger women (68, 88, 89, 91, 93). It seems that this may be a genuine increase in the incidence (88) rather than a reflection of the decrease in the proportion of squamous cell carcinoma. Adenocarcinoma in situ of the cervix is described, often in association with CIN (69, 95) but many authorities feel that this is a difficult diagnosis as criteria of invasion are subjective.

There are a variety of different histological appearances. The commonest pattern is malignant endocervical glands, but two others may be important in young women: the 'glassy cell' carcinoma, said to be highly malignant particularly in pregnancy (96, 97), and the clear cell carcinoma (mesonephroid) found in adolescent girls and young women (see above). These tumours occur half as often in the cervix as in the vagina. Shingleton et al. (90), however, have found no evidence for the 'glassy cell' tumour nor an association with pregnancy (69, 90).

TABLE 5 INCIDENCE DATA FOR ENDOCERVICAL CARCINOMA IN ENGLAND AND WALES (OFFICE OF POPULATION CENSUSES AND SURVEYS): TOTAL REGISTRATIONS SINCE 1971

Year	15–24	25–34	35–44	45–54	55–64	>65	Total
1971	1	—	9	32	29	31	102
1972	2	3	14	35	37	41	132
1973	—	6	19	45	41	52	163
1974	—	5	16	45	36	31	133
1975	—	6	16	34	49	48	143
1976	—	11	17	29	45	42	144
1977	—	9	9	25	45	34	122
1978	—	9	15	31	42	58	155
1979	1	21	33	58	57	70	240
1980	4	29	33	54	76	71	267
1981	1	27	41	47	68	80	264
1982	2	30	43	33	71	75	254

TABLE 6 STUDIES ON THE INCREASE IN INCIDENCE OF CERVICAL
ADENOCARCINOMA

Reference	Years of study	Percentage of adenocarcinoma	Effect of age
Tasker and Collins (86)	1953–72	6.9	—
Davis and Moon (87)	28 months	34[a]	—
Gallup and Abell (88)	1965–70	9.6	33% <40 yrs; 5 patients <32 on OCP
Hurt et al. (82)	1954–71	3	—
Berkowitz et al. (89)		13.6	26% <35 yrs
Shingleton et al. (90)	1969–80	8.2 to 18.6	
Tamimi and Figge (91)	1963–79	7.7 to 15.5	48% <40 yrs
Milsom and Friberg (92)	1965–74	6.2	—
Benoit et al. (80)	1976–81	14.9	—
Carmichael et al. (30)	1973–82	11.4	—
Gallup et al. (93)	1974–82	15.7	50% <40 yrs
Ireland et al. (94)	1969–83	4.1 to 12.5	—
Peters et al. (68)	1972–82	8.8 to 13.9	Increase in women <35 at rate of 8.2% per year

[a] Only 14/41 patients.

CLINICAL STAGING (FIGO CLASSIFICATION)

Cervical carcinoma spreads locally onto the vaginal fornices and into the cardinal ligaments towards the pelvic side walls. Eventually it involves the ureters, bladder, rectum and nerves of the lumbo-sacral plexus. It disseminates via the pelvic lymphatics to the pelvic, lumbar, para-aortic nodes and supraclavicular (scalene) nodes, and metastasizes to liver, skin, bone, the lungs and brain.

The FIGO classification (Table 7) for staging the disease is clinical and not surgical, and does not take into account lymph node involvement, tumour size, or depth of invasion, all of which affect survival. Compared with surgical staging it has been shown to be incorrect in up to 40% of cases (98).

There is some confusion about very early invasive disease, so-called Stage IA. In 1974 the Society of Gynecologic Oncologists suggested a definition of invasion less than 3 mm depth into the stroma with no evidence of lymph-vascular space invasion. In 1981, the Royal College of Obstetricians and Gynae-

cologists Study Group on Preclinical Carcinoma of the Cervix (99) revised this definition to include two groups:

1. Early stromal invasion—invasive buds are present either in continuity with a CIN 3 lesion or as apparently separated cells not more than 1 mm from the nearest surface basement membrane or crypt.

2. Micro-invasion—a measurable lesion in two dimensions, no more than 5 mm from the epithelial base, and with its largest surface dimension no greater than 10 mm. The confluent nature of the lesion and any invasion into capillary or lymphatic spaces should be noted.

The diagnosis of micro-invasive disease can only be accurately made on a full cone sample and not colposcopic biopsies.

'Occult' invasive carcinoma may be colposcopically overt but is diagnosed on cone biopsy. Regrettably, as with micro-invasive disease, many are only diagnosed retrospectively after cone biopsy or simple hysterectomy for benign pathology. Occult tumours are grouped with Stage IB lesions.

TABLE 7 INTERNATIONAL FEDERATION OF GYNAECOLOGY AND OBSTETRICS STAGING SYSTEM FOR INVASIVE CERVICAL CANCER

STAGE I	Carcinoma strictly confined to the cervix (extension to the corpus should be disregarded).
Stage IA	Micro-invasive carcinoma.
Stage IB	All other cases of Stage I. Occult cancer should be marked 'occ'.
STAGE II	The carcinoma extends beyond the cervix, but has not extended on to the pelvic wall. The carcinoma involves the vagina but not the lower third.
Stage IIA	No obvious parametrial involvement.
Stage IIB	Obvious parametrial involvement.
STAGE III	The carcinoma has extended on to the pelvic wall and on rectal examination there is no cancer-free space between the tumour and the pelvic wall. The tumour involves the lower third of the vagina. All cases with a hydronephrosis or non-functioning kidney should be included, unless they are known to be due to another cause.
Stage IIIA	No extension on to the pelvic wall.
Stage IIIB	Extension on to the pelvic wall and/or hydronephrosis or non-functioning kidney.
STAGE IV	The carcinoma has extended beyond the true pelvis or has clinically involved the mucosa of the bladder or rectum. A bullous oedema as such does not permit a case to be allotted to Stage IV.
Stage IVA	Spread of the growth to adjacent organs.
Stage IVB	Spread to distant organs.

Clinical staging is performed under anaesthetic with cystoscopy to exclude malignant involvement of the bladder, although this is rare in early disease. Nodularity and tethering from pelvic sepsis or endometriosis may well lead to misdiagnosis of ligament involvement. Ureteric obstruction on intravenous urography (IVU) assigns a case to Stage IIIB.

PRE-TREATMENT INVESTIGATIONS

A full blood count, urea and electrolytes and liver function tests will detect anaemia, renal compromise, liver involvement, malignant hypercalcaemia and poor nutritional and protein status. Pelvic recurrence is commoner in women with an initial haemoglobin less than 10 g per cent (100).

Radiological tests include a chest x-ray and IVU to detect ureteric obstruction and other renal disease which may influence treatment, e.g. congenital abnormalities. Forty per cent of women with Stage III disease have abnormal IVUs (85, p. 57). A computed tomography (CT) scan may demonstrate liver metastases and hydronephrosis (101). Para-aortic nodes larger than 1 cm are clearly shown but pelvic nodes are more difficult to define because of the pelvic vessels. Lymphangiography is only indicated if a CT scan is negative and is associated with a high incidence of both false negative and false positive results (98).

In the absence of a CT scan, an ultrasound scan may show enlarged lymph nodes, liver metastases and hydronephrosis. Neither test is accurate in assessing parametrial involvement (101). A bone scan may be required to aid in the diagnosis of bony lesions.

PROGNOSTIC FEATURES

Squamous Cell Carcinoma

Tumours greater than 2–3 cm in size or those which extend into the endometrium or more than two-thirds of the way through the cervix are associated with a higher risk of lymph node metastases (102), lymph-vascular space invasion (103), worse response to radiotherapy (102) and recurrence (104). It is controversial whether cell type influences prognosis, although Van Nagell et al. (105) noted that a third of their patients with small cell tumours developed recurrence within 6 months, and others have noted the association between poorly differentiated tumours and a worse survival (106, 107).

Lymph-vascular space invasion (108) and lymph node involvement (109) decreases survival significantly and varies from 15% in Stage IB disease to nearly 50% in Stage III disease (85, p. 68). Para-aortic node involvement is associated with very poor survival, and ranges from 6% in IB to 40% in advanced disease. Bilateral node involvement or positive common iliac nodes are ominous (85, p. 93, 110).

Attempts to assess nodal disease by a retroperitoneal surgical approach to the para-aortic nodes (98) is associated with significant complications if radiotherapy is given afterwards. There is no evidence that this procedure ultimately alters the prognosis (111) and it does not allow for adequate exploration of the pelvic nodes.

It is unclear whether young age is associated with poor prognostic features and worse survival (Table 8). Yule (reported in 'GP' 21.9.84) has stated that cells in abnormal smears look far less differentiated than they were 10 years ago. Prempree et al. (107) noted that women aged 23–29 years with Stage I disease had a 5-year survival of 43% compared with 75% for women aged 30–39, and 87% for all the other women. These young women had a 30% incidence of poorly differentiated and anaplastic tumours compared with 14% of older women, a finding confirmed by others (112–114). Forty per cent had local or distant recurrence compared with 13% of older patients. Furthermore only 35% presented with Stage I disease compared with 54% of older women. Stanhope et al. (113) noted the worse survival, stage for stage, in young women. Most failures occurred in Stage IIB disease where metastases were distant in 80%

TABLE 8 EFFECT OF AGE ON THE SURVIVAL OF WOMEN WITH CERVICAL CARCINOMA

Reference	Proportion of women <35 years	5-year survival	Comments on prognosis
Truelsen (116)	2.8%	59.1%[a]	No diff.
Lindell (117)	4%	54.3%[a]	Slightly worse
Decker et al. (118)	11.6%	85.7%[a]	No diff.
Randall et al. (119)	19.4%[b]	38.1	Worse (54.9% for older women)
Dodds and Latour (120)	3%	62.2%[a]	No diff.
Diddle and Watts (121)	6%	—	Mis Diagnosis commoner in younger women
Blomfield et al. (122)	10.9%[b]	—	No diff.
Sidhu et al. (123)	53%[c]	82%	Worse; more positive nodes
Kyriakos et al. (124)	—	82.4%[a]	No diff.
Futoran and Nolan (125)	—[b]	—	No diff.
Kjorstad (126)	6.9%	83%[a]	No diff.
Cullhed (127)	—[c]	83.5%[a]	Better survival
Berkowitz et al. (89)	24.5%	—	Earlier stage disease
Stanhope et al. (113)	12.3%	85.7%[a]	Worse
Hankey and Steinhorn (128)	16.5%	—	No diff. Less regional disease
Bouma and Crane-Elders (129)	10.1%	78%	Better survival
Hall and Monaghan (112)	11.4%	—	Poor; more positive nodes Tumours anaplastic
Prempree et al. (107)	16.7%	43–75%	Poor; more advanced tumours; poorly differentiated
Gauthier et al. (103)	—	—	No diff.
Carmichael et al. (81)	—	—	Better survival; more early stage disease

[a]=Stage IB disease.   [b]=<40 years.   [c]=<45 years.

of cases, in spite of central control. Other studies have suggested that young women treated with radiotherapy alone respond less favourably than older women (115, 117, 119).

In the United Kingdom, Hall and Monaghan (112) noted the increasing proportion of young women over a period of 7 years. Survival was less than 50% and one-third had pelvic node metastases. Forty per cent of the women had had a negative smear within 6 years of diagnosis. Only 6% had well differentiated tumours, compared with 25% of the women over 40 years, and most of the women who died had anaplastic or poorly differentiated tumours.

In sharp contrast, Bouma and Crane-Elders (129) found no evidence that their young patients did worse than their older patients. In fact two-thirds of their young patients had Stage IB disease compared with only 42% of their older patients. The most definitive paper to date comes from Carmichael et al. (81) who reviewed the cytological and clinical histories of 121 women less than 35 years. The proportion of young women presenting to their hospital with clinical disease has increased from 6.8% in 1975 to 13.6% by 1983. Seventy-one per cent of the young women had had a negative smear within 3 years of diagnosis compared with 61.1% of the older women. However, they presented with less advanced disease (64.5% with Stage IB compared with only 43% of older women; 14.9% with Stage III or IV compared with 26% older women) and had better overall survival rates because they presented earlier, but stage for stage the survival rates were the same.

On a larger scale, Hankey and Steinhorn (128) have used four cancer registers in the United States from 1950 to 1973 to calculate survival rates of women with cervical cancer. Women under 35 years with Stage I disease were not more likely to die than older women (489/2965 patients) and they had a lower incidence of regional disease (8.5%) compared with 42.4% of women aged 35–49, and 49.1% of women aged 50–65.

Stage of disease is still the single most important prognostic factor which dictates survival. Although clinical staging may be inaccurate, there is no evidence that surgical staging to improve the detection of postive nodes actually improves survival (111). In all age groups the proportion of women diagnosed with early disease has increased substantially since cytological screening, and this is especially so for young women.

In micro-invasive (IA) disease depth of stromal invasion is the most important prognostic factor. When this is less than 3 mm from the basement membrane, with no large confluent tongues of tumour, or lymph-vascular invasion, there are rarely lymph node metastases (130). A third of patients with capillary space involvement or invasion greater than 5 mm may have lymph node metastases (131), and in occult carcinoma a fifth of all patients may have lymph node involvement (130).

Adenocarcinoma

It is taught that this tumour is radioresistant, metastasizes quickly to lymph nodes and carries a worse prognosis than squamous cell carcinoma although not all agree (119). Shingleton et al. (90) found that 77% of the patients in their study presented with Stage I disease. Lesions less than 2 cm in size were associated with a 5-year survival of 85% compared with 40% when lesions were over 3 cm. The lesion may be difficult to diagnose colposcopically and smears may be negative (see above). Adenosquamous carcinoma carries a poor prognosis (93).

Clear Cell Carcinoma

Herbst et al (132) noted that girls under 15 years had more aggressive tumours and a higher proportion of papillary or solid tumours than girls over 19 years, who had a better survival and a higher proportion of tubulocystic tumours. The overall 5-year survival is 78% (133).

TREATMENT

The aims of therapy are to treat the tumour and its regional lymph nodes. Women with cervical carcinoma have traditionally received radiotherapy but there is increasing awareness of the benefits of radical surgery, especially in the young.

Micro-invasive Disease—Stage IA

These patients can be treated with a simple hysterectomy and selective node biopsy, or large cone biopsy if fertility is required, as the incidence of node involvement is very low (134). Incomplete excision or doubtful margins on a cone or hysterectomy specimen are associated with a significant risk of recurrence (73), because additional micro-invasive or even frankly invasive lesions may have been left behind.

Radical treatment is not necessary when the extent of invasion is less than 3 mm (131) and excision complete. On the other hand, patients with invasion greater than 5 mm, lymphatic space involvement (135), or incomplete excision should be treated as having Stage IB disease. When the diagnosis is made after hysterectomy for benign pathology, re-operation and selective lymphadenectomy, or radiotherapy should be given.

Early Advanced Disease—Stage IB and Early IIA

Radiotherapy

Almost identical 5-year survival rates of 70–90% have been achieved using either radiotherapy or primary radical surgery (136–138), and for many years radiotherapy has been the treatment of choice. Small tumours less than 2 cm can be treated with intracavitary caesium-137 but larger lesions and positive nodes are irradiated from external sources. Irradiation of involved para-aortic nodes has not been shown to significantly prolong survival (139). Complete regression of the tumour by the end of treatment is associated with a good prognosis

(140). Joslin (141) has reported an improved 5-year disease-free interval when a combination of intracavitary and external beam radiotherapy is used.

Significant complications (Table 9) occur in

TABLE 9 ADVANTAGES, DISADVANTAGES AND COMPLICATIONS OF THERAPY

Advantages

Radiotherapy
  can be given to all patients
  can be given as out-patient treatment
  survival rates equal to surgery

Surgery
  psychological effect
  spares ovaries
  infected adnexae can be removed
  surgical staging accurate
  vagina shortened, but more pliable

Disadvantages

Radiotherapy:
  vaginal stenosis, dryness and rigidity, loss of sensation
  urinary tract complications;
    acute haemorrhagic cystitis
    low capacity bladder, frequency
    chronic haematuria
    ureteric stricture
    fistula (ureteric; vesico-vaginal)
  bowel complications:
    chronic diarrhoea
    flatulence, proctitis
    strictures and obstruction
    malabsorption from terminal ileum
    fistula (small bowel; recto-vaginal)
  avascular necrosis to femoral head
  pyometra from cervical stenosis
  destruction of ovaries
  secondary malignancy, e.g. oesteogenic sarcoma

Surgery:
  complications from prolonged operating time;
    anaesthesia
    haemorrhage
  infection in chest, wound, urinary tract, pelvic sepsis and abscess
  urological complications;
    atonic bladder
    frequency, low capacity bladder
    fistula (ureteric; vesico-vaginal)
  lymphocyst formation, lymphoedema
  obturator nerve damage during lymphadenectomy
  paralytic ileus
  thrombo-embolism
  sexual dysfunction from shortened vagina
  may still require postoperative radiotherapy

about 6% of women (142) and in about 22% of those under 35 years (143). Surgical management of fistula formation or strictures is then difficult as the tissues are poor and urinary diversion or colostomy may be required. Complications are increased in small women, those who have previously had pelvic sepsis or abdominal surgery, and those who are malnourished (105). The pathological changes on mucous membranes in particular may continue for some years after treatment and sexual dysfunction almost always occurs in young women (144, 145).

Surgery

A radical hysterectomy and pelvic lymphadenectomy (after Wertheim and Meig) offers the psychological advantage of tumour removal, and adequate surgical staging. Diseased organs from pelvic sepsis or endometriosis can be removed and ovarian function preserved, as carcinoma of the cervix rarely metastasizes to the ovaries (146). The incidence of immediate operative complications is low (147, 148) and mortality less than 1% (106, 147, 149).

Combined Therapy

It is controversial whether combined therapy results in a better survival than either modality alone (85, p. 146, 136). However, when the tumour is greater than 5 cm preoperative radiotherapy has been shown to lower the recurrence rate (105). Other retrospective studies have generally shown no advantage to radiotherapy postoperatively because it does not prevent distant metastases in women with surgically proven positive nodes (110, 150, 151). Morbidity can be high (150) as the anatomy of the pelvis is altered by surgery.

Locally Advanced Disease—Stages IIB to IVA

Patients with Stages IIB (unless very early), III and IVA (bladder or rectal involvement) are normally treated with radiotherapy. We do not recommend exenteration as a primary procedure in women with Stage IVA disease as 30% of patients survive when given radiotherapy alone (152), and the incidence of fistula formation is very low.

Metastatic Disease

Chemotherapy offers the only hope of remission of symptoms and prolongation of life to these unfortunate women (see below).

Adenocarcinoma

Adenocarcinoma is treated in the same way as squamous cell carcinoma. The primary therapy of bulky endocervical lesions more than 3 cm in diameter should be radiotherapy (153, 154), as surgery is associated with a higher incidence of recurrence (90). It may be that bulky barrel-shaped lesions should be classified as IIB rather than IB.

Clear Cell Adenocarcinoma of the Cervix and Vagina

Local excision has been attempted in these young women and teenagers, but has not been successful and Herbst now recommends a radical hysterectomy and lymphadenectomy with vaginectomy (133). At times a total pelvic exenteration may be necessary, with vaginal reconstruction subsequently; the functional results are good (155). Such an approach allows conservation of ovarian function and avoids the complications of radiotherapy, although this may be necessary preoperatively for extensive disease or as palliation if there is recurrence. Chemotherapy has not been shown to be helpful.

In conclusion, we offer radical surgery as the treatment of choice to women with Stage IB and IIA disease if they are fit for anaesthetic, and use radiotherapy in the following situations:

1. Patients in whom surgery is not appropriate, or where the woman refuses surgery.

2. Intracavitary caesium when micro-invasive disease or occult invasive disease is found unexpectedly in a cervix after a hysterectomy; with external beam therapy added if the surgical margins are not clear or the lesion is greater than 1 cm given the poorer prognosis (156, 157).
3. Preoperative intracavitary and/or external beam radiotherapy in Stage IB disease where the lesion is greater than 5 cm in size or there is a bulky endocervical lesion.
4. Stages IIA to IVA.
5. Postoperative external beam radiotherapy in patients with multiple lymph node metastases found at surgery, in those where the disease is found to be too extensive at operation, and where there is proximity of tumour to the resection line.
6. Patients with pelvic recurrence following surgery who may well have a 25% survival (158)—see below.

SURVIVAL

Shingleton and Orr (85, p. 117) have extensively reviewed the survival figures. Tumour size and stage are the single most decisive factors; hence the need for rigorous preoperative selection of patients. Large tumours are associated with a higher incidence of node metastases and when surgical excision margins are within 1 cm of the tumour, recurrence is high (159). Local failure from radiotherapy is also highest in those with the largest tumours (160).

Survival rates in the United States are 87–92% in Stage I, 66–77% in Stage II, and 28–60% in Stage III disease (143). Survival in Stage IA disease is 99% (135), and in Stage IV disease 1–30% (152). These results are much the same in Europe.

It is not clear that young women survive less than older women given the same prognostic factors, and results of large studies on survival are conflicting. The most recent figures from the Office of Population Censuses and Surveys show no evidence for a worse survival (Table 10), and if anything a better overall survival.

TABLE 10 CANCER SURVIVAL REGISTRATIONS 1971–79 (OFFICE OF POPULATION CENSUSES AND SURVEYS): 5-YEAR RELATIVE SURVIVAL RATES (AGE-ADJUSTED)

Year	15–24	25–34	35–44	45–54	55–64	65–74
1971	—	74.2	65.9	52.7	51.7	42.0
1972	—	77.5	71.3	53.8	48.7	40.4
1973	—	77.7	66.8	52.9	52.5	40.8
1974	—	73.2	64.5	52.5	52.4	40.3
1975	—	75.3	67.6	53.5	50.0	36.8
1976	—	77.0	62.3	55.4	46.6	41.7
1977	89.2	74.4	61.6	53.3	51.8	42.2
1978	79.3	77.6	68.0	53.7	51.9	40.9
1979	68.7	73.3	72.3	56.0	54.3	45.9

This may well be because the disease is diagnosed at an earlier stage than in older women.

It is also not clear that women with adenocarcinoma survive less than women with squamous cell carcinoma although Korhonen (153) found lower survivals for each stage than one would expect for patients with squamous cell carcinoma.

CERVICAL CARCINOMA IN PREGNANCY

The true incidence of this sad occurrence is difficult to ascertain but is about 1:1000–5000 pregnant women (161). The incidence may be increasing, in line with the genuine increase in CIN 3 in younger women (162, 163) and the greater use of cytological screening in antenatal clinics. The average age of affected women is 33 years (163).

Diagnosis

This is made in the same way as in the non-pregnant women, but 20% are asymptomatic and mis-diagnosis is frequent (163). Vaginal examination should be a routine part of antenatal care, and should be performed on any woman with bleeding during pregnancy which is not due to placenta praevia. Colposcopic directed biopsies of suspicious lesions are of minimal risk to the woman; vaginal bleeding is not excessive and the risk of abortion is not increased (164). If an invasive lesion is suspected, a wedge or formal cone biopsy must be done. This carries a morbidity of 50% (165), particularly in the first trimester, and includes fetal loss, pre-term delivery, haemorrhage, and cervical laceration at delivery.

Investigations can not include a CT scan or lymphangiogram, but a single-shot IVU exposes the fetus to a very small dose of radiation.

Prognostic Features

It is controversial whether there is a higher incidence of anaplastic tumours in pregnancy, including the 'glassy-cell' type (90, 96, 114, 166). A higher proportion of pregnant women are diagnosed with early disease than non-pregnant women (96, 166) although Sablinska et al. (162), found that young women did not come for antenatal care as often as older women, and were more likely to have advanced disease at presentation, often because of mis-diagnosis. Patients diagnosed and treated post-partum may have a worse prognosis (114, 162, 163).

Treatment

This depends very much on the stage of the disease, the gestational age of the fetus and the parents' wishes. Great care and sensitivity is needed in counselling a couple once the diagnosis has been made. As in the non-pregnant patient, either surgery or radiotherapy may be appropriate.

Stage IA Disease

A cone biopsy may be sufficient but a caesarean hysterectomy is preferred. Delays of up to 28 weeks before treatment have not been shown to be harmful (167).

Surgical Management—Stage IB and Early IIA Disease

This is the same as in the non-pregnant woman although after 26–28 weeks a classical caesarean section is performed prior to the radical hysterectomy with a short delay if the fetus is nearing viability (24 weeks). Vaginal delivery, whilst not jeopardizing survival (166), is associated with haemorrhage, sepsis, and cervical laceration. Surgery is not technically difficult (168, 169).

Advanced Lesions and Situations where Surgery Is Not Appropriate

Radiotherapy leads to abortion within 3–6 weeks of 3000 rads, and is associated with a high incidence of sepsis and gastrointestinal and urinary fistulae (167). A hysterotomy may be necessary after 20 weeks as abortion of a potentially viable fetus is variable and may damage the cervix. A normal fetus can be born after intracavitary radiation (170) but fetal abnormality is always a risk (171).

Survival

It is not clear that pregnant women have an overall worse survival than non-pregnant women (163, 166), although some individual reports suggest that they have more bad prognostic features and post-partum cases are more advanced than intra-partum cases when diagnosed (114, 162). In early disease it appears that pregnant women have survival rates similar (163) or better (162) than non-pregnant women. On the other hand, in advanced disease their survival is worse because of treatment difficulties (163). Radiotherapy is more difficult to administer as sepsis leads to interruptions, and the altered anatomical configurations make dosimetry calculations unreliable.

CHEMOTHERAPY

Chemotherapy has not been extensively evaluated in cervical carcinoma because in early disease other treatment modalities are successful, and in recurrent disease few studies have shown lasting or significant benefit. Its use is limited by poor renal function, poor bone marrow reserve following radiotherapy and poor pelvic vascular perfusion. Response in the pelvis is difficult to assess when woody fibrosis has resulted from irradiation.

There are four areas in which chemotherapy may be useful:

1. In women who present with Stage IVB disease (Figure 3).
2. In women with recurrence following previous radiotherapy, sometimes given before exenterative procedures.
3. In women with early disease who have additional risk factors such as lymphatic involvement, extensive infiltration through the cervix and uterine cavity, and poor tumour differentiation.
4. As a radiosensitizer to enhance the effect of radiotherapy.

Various single agents have been used in recurrent and disseminated disease, including cyclophosphamide, 5-fluorouracil, methotrexate, doxorubicin, bleomycin and cis-platinum. The response rates vary between 10 and 90% but remissions tend to be short-lived with a median survival of 6–9 months (172). Although progestogens and bromocriptine have been used, there is no evidence that cervical carcinoma is hormone-dependent.

Combinations of drugs have not improved the response rates although Friedlander et al. (173) used a combination of cis-platinum, bleomycin and vinblastine to achieve remission rates of 67%; in those with a complete response the median survival was 40 weeks, compared with 12 weeks in those with no response. More recently iphosphamide has been shown to achieve remissions in 25% of patients, but haematological and central nervous system toxicity is great (190, 191).

Chemotherapy in the primary treatment of women with locally advanced disease is gaining interest (174, 175) but in the primary management of women with poor prognostic factors in early disease is still experimental.

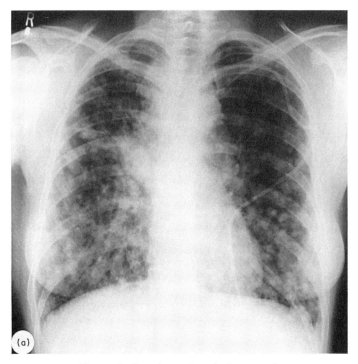

Figure 3a (see legend on facing page).

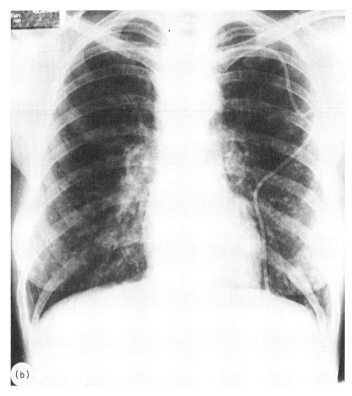

Figure 3 (a and b) Effect of chemotherapy on pulmonary metastases in a 33 year old woman who presented with Stage IVB disease. A smear and curettings for post-coital bleeding were negative 3 months prior to diagnosis.

Only one trial so far has compared surgery with surgery and chemotherapy. Patients with involved nodes and more than half the cervix replaced by tumour showed a survival advantage (104).

The value of radiopotentiating agents, such as hydroxyurea is unproven (176, 177). Overall, chemotherapy for metastatic and recurrent disease has proved disappointing and has little potential for cure.

RECURRENT DISEASE

Following treatment about one-third of patients have residual or recurrent disease, and this increases to about two-thirds when nodes are involved (178). Sixty per cent of patients who develop recurrence do so in the first year, and a further 25% in the second year (105,

158). This risk is influenced by the poor prognostic features mentioned before. About equal numbers of patients have central disease, disease with spread to the pelvic side walls and distant metastases (158), although it has been suggested (179) that young women are more likely to develop distant metastases. The faster the recurrence the worse the prognosis and 80% of patients die within 2 years (158). Central recurrence has a better survival because it is surgically treatable.

Diagnosis

Diagnosis may be difficult in patients who have previously had radiotherapy. Suspicion should be aroused by vaginal bleeding or discharge, rectal pain, tenesmus, bony or nerve pain in the legs and pelvis, lymphoedema and venous obstruction in the legs. Disease beyond the pelvis gives rise to bony pain, skin nodules, cough, jaundice and cerebral symptoms. Weight loss is difficult to assess as it may occur with radiation damage to the bowel. Examination may reveal obvious lesions in the pelvis or fibrosis and nodularity which is difficult to assess after radiotherapy.

The slightest suspicion of recurrence should be investigated with a CT scan, IVU, lymphangiography, barium enema, bone scan, ultrasound scan of the liver and other x-rays as required. Lesions are biopsied under anaesthetic, at which time a cystoscopy and sigmoidoscopy can be performed. Bullous oedema and nodularity of the bladder base are diagnostic of bladder involvement with disease and are quite different from radiation changes.

Biopsies may sometimes be negative since:

1. there is no recurrent disease but other pathology such as progressive radiation damage or pelvic sepsis;
2. small rests of malignant cells are scattered through areas of radiation-induced fibrosis.

In this situation the only way of making an adequate diagnosis may be by laparotomy.

Treatment

Radiotherapy is futile if the patient has previously received a full course of radiotherapy (180). It may have a small curative role in the woman who has previously been surgically treated and presents with pelvic side wall disease not suitable for surgical resection (105). It can also be used for the palliation of pain from bony metastases or symptoms from cerebral involvement. Chemotherapy is only palliative (see above).

Exenterative surgery in certain situations offers the chance of cure with a 5-year survival of 20–60% (181, 182). Only a small proportion of women referred for this are suitable (105) and its only indication is that macroscopic disease, whether persistent or recurrent can be completely excised. On occasion persistent disease after radiotherapy can be managed

with a radical hysterectomy alone (102), illustrating the difficulty in differentiating between radiation-induced fibrosis and extensive recurrence.

Details of this procedure and its absolute contraindications are given elsewhere (179, 181). Full discussion is essential between the doctor, the patient and her husband about the alteration in body image, the change in sexual relations and the realities of one if not two stomas. Women should also be prepared for the fact that the final diagnosis may only be made at operation, and that they may be found to have inoperable disease.

We give all patients two courses of chemotherapy preoperatively and create a neovagina from amnion (183) some days after exenteration if coital function is required. The complication rate, which is about 60%, is mugh higher when disease is not eradicated, and rapidly leads to the patient's demise.

SOCIAL ASPECTS OF CERVICAL CANCER

The diagnosis of cervical cancer in young women is particularly distressing. For the woman without children, treatment will of necessity destroy any hope she may have of bearing children in the future. In most women treatment is followed by some degree of reactive depression which is aggravated if there are physical sequelae to treatment such as bladder dysfunction, dyspareunia, lymphoedema or unpleasant symptoms from oophorectomy. Women treated with radiotherapy almost always have significant sexual dysfunction (144, 145) which is difficult to rectify. Vaginoplasty is often not successful as healing is poor in the irradiated area, and the Williams 'copulation pouch' (184) may not be found satisfactory by the male partner.

An additional factor with a profound and sometimes devastating effect is the sense of guilt engendered in women by sensational and misleading comments on the 'sexual transmission' of this disease. The idea that female genital cancer is evidence for past sexual 'misconduct' by either partner is counter-productive and we are increasingly aware of couples who question each other's fidelity and past sexual lives in the light of this. A further misconception is that the disease can be 'caught' by intercourse and that further coitus is harmful or wrong. Sexual difficulties are also likely to arise if vaginal discharge or bleeding are activated or worsened by intercourse; or if women who have had exenterative surgery are embarrassed by their stomas. Ideally, these conflicts should be discussed and resolved as part of preoperative counselling.

Many young women already have families when the diagnosis is made, and their treatment may cause disruption of the family, particularly if they require extensive hospitalization for exenterative surgery, chemotherapy or terminal care. In this regard, considerable symptomatic relief must be given for pain, depression, anorexia, and fistula formation. A palliative colostomy should be performed to allow a women comfort from the misery of a recto-vaginal fistula; and urinary diversion via percutaneous mephrostomy stents should be performed when there is a vesico-vaginal fistula. Whether a woman chooses to die at home, in a hospice or in the hospital, her family should be encouraged and permitted to be with her, and her end as peaceful as possible.

CONCLUSIONS AND RESOLUTIONS

The incidence and mortality from cervical cancer is increasing in young women under the age of 35 years, although it seems as if this trend may also appear in cohorts of older women in the future. One of the aetiological factors may be the increasing incidence of sexually transmitted diseases, particularly human papillomavirus, which in conjunction with other variables such as nicotine or herpes simplex virus, may generate the malignant transformation of cells.

It is not clear that the prognosis in young women is significantly worse than in older women and the Office of Population Censuses and Surveys figures suggest, if anything, a better overall survival (Table 10). The pathology is the same, although there may be an increase in the incidence of adenocarcinoma and the oral contraceptive pill has been implicated in this (68).

A number of resolutions may help to limit this increase, and improve treatment:

1. All women should have regular smears after the onset of sexual activity. Although it has been suggested that smears should be done annually (8), there is little difference in the protection afforded by screening every year compared with every 3 years (185) and the age of women does not affect the sensitivity of the test. Women who are not sexually active should have regular smears after the age of 25 for detection of adenocarcinoma.

2. Approximate action when a smear is reported as abnormal must be undertaken; computerized recall-systems may alleviate the burden of follow-up, but responsibility should be delegated to either the clinician or cytologist to notify patients of abnormal findings (83).

3. The clinician should have a high index of suspicion when faced with a young woman with suspicious symptoms or an abnormal looking cervix, regardless of the smear results. Colposcopy and biopsy are required (84), even in pregnancy (164).

4. An emphasis on barrier methods of contraception may be appropriate in the future, if the association between the OCP and carcinoma becomes more obvious (59, 61, 66, 68).

5. More education on the relative risks of smoking would be advisable.

6. Adequate surgical staging and determination of bad prognostic features in the tumour are important in the management of the woman. Step-sectioning of lymph nodes rather than random sectioning leads to greater histological accuracy in the diagnosis of micro-metastases (104).

7. More appropriate selection of patients for

radiotherapy should mean that most women are treated with radical surgery with a subsequent decrease in significant complications, particularly sexual dysfunction.

8. Consideration should be given to the use of chemotherapy as part of primary treatment when women do have bad prognostic features.

9. A greater awareness of exenterative surgery as a treatment option with central recurrent disease is needed.

10. Research into vaccination against herpes virus and papillomavirus in the future is required. Screening of genital warts to detect HPV types associated with a high risk of malignant change may facilitate more aggressive treatment of precursor CIN lesions likely to become malignant (45, 48).

In our own practice the proportion of young women presenting with this disease has increased dramatically in the past few years, but most of these women are referred from outside the area. The majority have Stage IA or IB disease,and they do not appear to have a worse survival than older women presenting for the first time. We also see a significant number of young women who have been treated with radiotherapy for early disease and present with recurrence soon after. Often they are treated with caesium only, to avoid the problems of external beam radiotherapy, and this suggests that their initial treatment may be sub-optimal. The wider use of radical surgery should obviate this in the future.

Aggressive cervical cancer in young women is not a new problem. Henrietta Lacks, who immortalized the world's first continuous human cell line of tumour cells, was 31 years old when she presented to her gynaecologist with intermenstrual bleeding. That was in 1951, and she died from disseminated disease 8 months later. A national multi-centre study of the clinical and pathological features of young women with this disease, perhaps organized by the Royal College of Obstetricians and Gynae-

cologists in the UK, would do much to verify or refute the commonly held view that this disease is becoming more aggressive.

ACKNOWLEDGEMENTS

With grateful acknowledgement to Mr Christopher Hudson for helpful discussion.

REFERENCES

1 Dekel A, Van Iddekinge B, Leiman G. Invasive squamous carcinoma of the cervix in a 15 year old girl. S Afr Med J 1982; 61: 628–9.

2 Dalley VM, Dewhurst CJ, Flood CM. Carcinoma of the cervix in childhood. J Obstet Gynaecol Br Comm 1971; 78: 1133–6.

3 Parkin DM, Nguyen-Dinh X, Day NE. The impact of screening on the incidence of cervical cancer in England and Wales. Br J Obstet Gynaecol 1985; 92: 150–7.

4 Macgregor JE, Teper S. Uterine cervical cytology and young women. Lancet 1978; i: 1029–31.

5 Stern E. Epidemiology of dysplasia. Obstet Gynecol Surv 1969; 24: 711–23.

6 Boyes DA, Morrison B, Knox EG, Draper GJ, Miller AB. A cohort study of cervical cancer screening in British Columbia. Clin Invest Med 1982; 5: 1–29.

7 Green GH. Cervical cancer and cytology screening in New Zealand. Br J Obstet Gynaecol 1978; 85: 881–6.

8 Walton RJ (Chairman). Cervical cancer screening programs: summary of the 1982 Canadian Task Force Report. Can Med Assoc J 1982; 581–9.

9 Macgregor JE, Teper S. Mortality from carcinoma of cervix uteri in Britain, Lancet 1978; ii: 774–6.

10 Hakama M, Trends in the incidence of cervical cancer in the Nordic countries. In: Magnus K ed. Trends in Cancer Incidence, Causes and Practical Implications. Washington: Hemisphere Publishing, 1982: 279–92.

11 Cramer DW. The role of cervical cytology in the declining morbidity and mortality of cervical cancer. Cancer 1974; 34: 2018–27.

12 Dunn JE, Schweitzer V. The relationship of cervical cytology to the incidence of invasive cervical cancer and mortality in Alameda County, California, 1960–1974. Am J Obstet Gynecol 1981; 139: 868–76.

13 Yule R. Mortality from carcinoma of the cervix. Lancet 1978; i: 1031–2.

14 Armstrong B, Holman D. Increasing mortality from cancer of the cervix in young Australian women. Med J Aust 1981; May 2: 460–2.

15 Armstrong BK. The falling, rising incidence of invasive cancer of the cervix. Med J Aust 1983; Feb 19: 147–8.

16 Bourne RG & Grove WD. Invasive carcinoma of the cervix in Queensland. Change in incidence and mortality, 1959–1980. Med J Aust 1983; Feb 19, 156–8.

17 Anello C, Lao C. US Trends in mortality from carcinoma of the cervix. Lancet 1979; i: 1038 (letter).

18 Cook GA, Draper GJ. Trends in cervical cancer and carcinoma in situ in Great Britain. Br J Cancer 1984; 50: 367–75.

19 Hill GB, Adelstein AM. Cohort mortality from carcinoma of the cervix. Lancet 1967; ii: 605–6.

20 Hakama M, Penttinen J. Epidemiological evidence for two components of cervical cancer. Br J Obstet Gynaecol 1981; 88: 209–14.

21 Paterson MEL, Peel KR, Joslin CAF. Cervical smear histories of 500 women with invasive cervical cancer in Yorkshire. Br Med J 1984; 289: 896–8.

22 Chamberlain J. Failure of the cervical cytology screening programme. Br Med J 1984; 289: 853–4.

23 Editorial. Cancer of the cervix: death by incompetence. Lancet 1985; ii: 363–4.

24 Lees TW. Failure of cervical cytology? Lancet 1969; i: 1020 (letter).

25 Draper GJ, Cook GA. Changing patterns of cervical cancer rates. Br Med J 1983; 287: 510–12.

26 Rotkin ID. A comparison review of key epidemiological studies in cervical cancer related to current searches for transmissible agents. Cancer Res 1973; 33: 1353–67.

27 Buckley JD, Harris RWC, Doll R, Vessey MP, Williams PT. Case control study of the husbands of women with dysplasia or carcinoma of the cervix uteri. Lancet 1981; ii: 1010–14.

28 Singer A, Reid BL, Coppleson M. A hypothesis: The role of a high-risk male in the etiology of cervical carcinoma. Am J Obstet Gynecol 1976; 126: 110–15.

29 Lappaluoto P. Promiscuity and Pill: etiologic agents in the genesis of cervical malignancy? Acta Cytol 1977; 21: 182 (letter).

30 Carmichael JA, Jeffrey JF, Steele HD, Ohlke ID. The cytologic history of 245 patients developing invasive cervical carcinoma. Am J Obstet Gynecol 1984; 148: 685–90.

31 Cecchini S. Cervical intraepithelial neoplasia in younger women. Lancet 1982; ii: 926–7 (letter).

32 Davies SW, Kelly RM. Intraepithelial carcinoma of the cervix uteri in women aged under 35 years. Br Med J 1971; iv: 525–6.

33 Andrews FJ, Linehan JJ, Melcher DH. Cervical cancer in younger women. Lancet 1978; ii: 776–8.

34 Bamford PN, Barber M, Beilby JOW. Changing pattern of cervical intraepithelial neoplasia seen in a Family Planning Clinic. Lancet 1982; i: 747 (letter).

35 Wolfendale MR, King S, Usherwood MM. Abnormal cervical smears: are we in for an epidemic? Br Med J 1983; 287: 526–8.

36 Baram A, Schachter A. Cervical carcinoma: disease of the future for Jewish women. Lancet 1982; i: 747–8 (letter).

37 Schofield M. Sexual Behaviour of Young People. Harmondsworth: Penguin, 1965.

38 Delke IM, Veridiano NP, Russell S, Tancer ML. Abnormal cervical cytology in adolescents. J Ped 1981; 98: 985–7.

39 Sadeghi SB, Hsieh EW, Gunn SW. Prevalence of cervical intraepithelial neoplasia in sexually active teenagers and young adults. Am J Obstet Gynecol 1984; 148: 726–9.

40 Beral V. Cancer of the cervix: a sexually transmitted infection? Lancet 1974; i: 1037–40.

41 Chief Medical Officer, DHSS. Sexually transmitted diseases; extract from annual report for 1982. Br J Vener Dis 1984; 60: 199–203.

42 Saltz GR, Linnemann CC, Brookman RR, Rauh JH. Chlamydia trachomatis cervical infections in female adolescents. J Ped 1981; 98: 981–5.

43 Vass-Sorensen M, Abeler V, Berle E, Pedersen B, Davy M, Thorsby E, Norrild B. Prevalence of antibodies to herpes simplex virus and frequency of HLA antigens in patients with preinvasive and invasive cervical cancer. Gynecol Oncol 1984; 18: 349–58.

44 Eglin RP, Sharp F, Maclean AB, Macnab JC, Clements JB, Wilkie NM. Detection of RNA complementary to herpes simplex virus DNA in human cervical squamous cell neoplasms. Cancer Res 1981; 41: 3597–603.

45 Zur Hausen H. Human genital cancer: synergism between two virus infections or synergism between a virus infection and initiating events? Lancet 1982; ii: 1370–72.

46 Meisels A, Morin C, Casas-Cordero M. Human papillomavirus infection of the uterine cervix. Int J Gynecol Pathol 1982; 1: 75–94.

47 Reid R, Crum CP, Herschman BR, Fu YS, Braun L, Shah KV, Agronow SJ, Stanhope CR. Genital warts and cervical cancer. III Subclinical papillomaviral infection and cervical neoplasia are linked by a spectrum of

continuous morphologic and histologic change. Cancer 1984; 53: 943–53.

48 Zur Hausen H. Exploring the link between condyloma virus and cervical cancer. Diagnostic Medicine, September 1984: 31–35.

49 Franceschi S, Doll R, Gallwey J, La Vecchia C, Peto R, Spriggs AI. Genital warts and cervical neoplasia: an epidemiological study. Br J Cancer 1983; 48: 621–8.

50 Campion MJ, Singer A, Clarkson PK, McCance DJ. Increased risk of cervical neoplasia in consorts of men with penile condylomata acuminata.

51 Schmauz R, Claussen CP, Cordes B, Owor R. Condylomata acuminata and their possible relation to cancer of the uterine cervix. Case report and geographic observations. Acta Cytol 1983; 27: 533–9.

52 Martinez I. Relationship of squamous cell carcinoma of the cervix uteri to squamous cell carcinoma of the penis among Puerto Rican women married to men with penile carcinoma. Cancer 1969; 24: 777–80.

53 Melnick JL, Lewis R, Wimberly I, Kauffman RH, Adam E. Association of cytomegalovirus (CMV) infection with cervical cancer: isolation of CMV from cell cultures derived from cervical biopsy. Intervirology 1978; 10: 115–9.

54 Paavonen J, Vesterinen E, Meyer B, Saikku P, Suni J, Purola E, Saksela E. Genital chlamydia trachomatis infections in patients with cervical atypia. Obstet Gynecol 1979; 54: 289–91.

55 Meisels A. Microbiology of the female reproductive tract as determined in the cytologic specimen. III In the presence of cellular atypias. Acta Cytol 1969; 13: 64–71.

56 Harris RWC, Brinton LA, Cowdell RH, Skegg DCG, Smith PG, Vessey MP, Doll R. Characteristics of women with dysplasia or carcinoma in situ of the cervix uteri. Br J Cancer 1980; 42: 359–69.

57 Wright NH, Vessey MP, Kenward B, McPherson K, Doll R. Neoplasia and dysplasia of the cervix uteri and contraception: a possible protective effect of the diaphragm. Br J Cancer 1978; 38: 273–9.

58 Bamford PN, Forbes-Smith PA, Rose GL, Beilby JOW, Inskip H, Guillebaud J. An analysis of factors responsible for progression or regression of mild and moderate cervical dyskariosis. Br J Fam Plann 1985; 11: 5–8.

59 Stern E, Forsythe AB, Youkeles L. Steroid contraceptive use and cervical dysplasia: increased risk of progression. Science 1977; 196: 1460–2.

60 Ory HW, Conger SB, Naib Z, Taylor CW, Hatcher RA. Preliminary analysis of oral contraceptive use and risk of developing premalig-

nant lesions of the uterine cervix. In: Garattini S, Berendes HW eds Pharmacology of Steroid Contraceptive Drugs. New York: Dover Press, 1977: 211–8.

61 Vessey MP, Lawless M, McPherson K, Yeates D. Neoplasia of the cervix uteri and contraception: a possible adverse effect of the pill. Lancet 1983; ii: 930–4.

62 Worth AJ, Boyes DA. A case control study into the possible effects of birth control pills on preclinical carcinoma of the cervix. L Obstet Gynaecol Br Comm 1972; 79: 673–9.

63 Boyce JG, Lu T, Nelson JH, Fruchter RG. Oral contraceptives and cervical carcinoma. Am J Obstet Gynecol 1977; 128: 761–6.

64 WHO collaborative study of neoplasia and steroid contraceptives. Invasive cervical cancer and combined oral contraceptives. Br Med J 1985; 290: 961–5.

65 Filotico M, Grasso S. Atypical reserve cell hyperplasia of cervical glands, simulating adenocarcinoma. An undescribed reversible lesion in a woman taking oral contraceptives. Tumori 1981; 67: 491–6.

66 Czernobilsky B, Kessler I, Lancet M. Cervical adenocarcinoma in a woman on long-term contraceptives Obstet Gynecol 1974; 43: 517 21.

67 Dallenbach-Hellweg G. On the origin and histological structure of adenocarcinoma of the endocervix in women under 50 years of age. Path Res Pract 1984; 179: 38–50.

68 Peters RK, Chao A, Mack TM, Thomas D, Bernstein L, Henderson BE. Increased frequency of adenocarcinoma of the uterine cervix in young women in Los Angeles County. J Nat Cancer Inst 1986; 76: 423–8.

69 Korhonen MO. Epidemiological differences between adenocarcinoma and squamous cell carcinoma of the uterine cervix. Gynecol Oncol 1980; 10: 312–7.

70 Herbst AL, Cole P, Colton T, Robboy SJ, Scully RE. Age-incidence and risk of diethylstilbestrol-related clear cell adenocarcinoma of the vagina and cervix. Am J Obstet Gynecol 1977; 128: 43–50.

71 Emens M. Vaginal adenosis and diethylstilboestrol. Br J Hosp Med 1984; 31: 42–8.

72 Orr JW, Shingleton HM, Gore H, Austin JM, Hatch KD, Soong S. Cervical intraepithelial neoplasia associated with exposure to diethylstilbestrol in utero: a clinical and pathologic study. Obstet Gynecol 1981; 58: 75–82.

73 Larsson G, Alm P, Gullberg B, Grundsell H. Prognostic factors in early invasive carcinoma of the uterine cervix. Am J Obstet Gynecol 1983; 146: 145–53.

74 Beilby JOW, Bourne R, Guillebaud J, Steele

SJ. Paired cervical smears: a method of reducing the false-negative rate in population screening. Obstet Gynecol 1982; 60: 46–8.

75 Rylander E. Negative smears in women developing invasive cervical cancer. Acta Obstet Gynecol Scand 1977; 56: 115–8.

76 Berkeley AS, Livolsi VA, Schwartz PE. Advanced squamous cell carcinoma of the cervix with recent normal Papanicolaou tests. Lancet 1980; ii: 375–6 (letter).

77 Morell ND, Taylor JR, Snyder RN, Ziel HK, Saltz A, Willie S. False-negative cytology rates in patients in whom invasive cervical cancer subsequently developed. Obstet Gynecol 1982; 60: 41–5.

78 Bain RW, Crocker DW. Rapid onset of cervical cancer in an upper socioeconomic group. Am J Obstet Gynecol 1983; 146: 366–71.

79 Bamford PN, Beilby JOW, Steele SJ, Vlies R. The natural history of cervical intraepithelial neoplasia as determined by cytology and colposcopic biopsy. Acta Cytol 1983; 27: 482–4.

80 Benoit AG, Krepart GV, Lotocki RJ. Results of prior cytologic screening in patients with a diagnosis of Stage I carcinoma of the cervix Am J Obstet Gynecol 1984; 148: 690–4.

81 Carmichael JA, Clarke DH, Moher D, Ohlke ID, Karchmar EJ. Cervical carcinoma in women aged 34 and younger. Am J Obstet Gynecol 1986; 154: 264–9.

82 Hurt FG, Silverberg SG, Frable WJ, Belgrad R, Crooks LD. Adenocarcinoma of the cervix: histopathologic and clinical features. Am J Obstet Gynecol 1977; 129: 304–15.

83 Elwood JM, Cotton RE, Johnson J, Jones GM, Curnow J, Beaver MW. Are patients with abnormal cervical smears adequately managed? Br. Med. J. 1984; 289: 891–4.

84 Dolan TE, Boyce J, Rosen Y, Lu T. Cytology, colposcopy and directed biopsy: what are the limitations? Gynecol Oncol 1975; 3: 314–24.

85 Shingleton HM, Orr JW. Cancer of the Cervix. Diagnosis and Treatment. Edinburgh: Churchill Livingstone, 1983.

86 Tasker JT, Collins JA. Adenocarcinoma of the uterine cervix. Am J Obstet Gynecol 1974; 118: 344–8.

87 Davis JR, Moon LB. Increased incidence of adenocarcinoma of uterine cervix. Obstet Gynecol 1975; 45: 79–83.

88 Gallup DG, Abell MR. Invasive adenocarcinoma of the uterine cervix. Obstet Gynecol 1977; 49: 596–603.

89 Berkowitz RS, Ehrmann RL, Lavizzo-Mourey R, Knapp RC. Invasive cervical carcinoma in young women. Gynecol Oncol 1979; 8: 311–6.

90 Shingleton HM, Gore H, Bradley DH, Soong

SJ. Adenocarcinoma of the cervix. I Clinical evaluation and pathological features. Am J Obstet Gynecol 1981; 139: 799–814.

91 Tamimi HK, Figge DC. Adenocarcinoma of the uterine cervix. Gynecol Oncol 1982; 13: 335–44.

92 Milsom I, Friberg LG. Primary adenocarcinoma of the uterine cervix. A clinical study. Cancer 1983; 52: 942–7.

93 Gallup DG, Harper RH, Stock RJ. Poor prognosis in patients with adenosquamous cell carcinoma of the cervix. Obstet Gynecol 1985; 65: 416–422.

94 Ireland D, Hardiman P, Monaghan JM. Adenocarcinoma of the uterine cervix: a study of 73 cases. Obstet Gynecol 1985; 65: 82–5.

95 Teshima S, Shimosato Y, Kishi K, Kasamatsu T, Ohmi K, Uei Y. Early stage adenocarcinoma of the uterine cervix. Histopathologic analysis with consideration of histogenesis. Cancer 1985; 56: 167–72.

96 Cherry CP, Glucksmann A. Histology of carcinoma of the uterine cervix and survival rates in pregnant and non-pregnant patients. Surg Gynecol Obstet 1961; 113: 763–76.

97 Littman P, Clement PB, Henriksen B, Wang CC, Robboy SJ, Taft PD, Ulfelder H, Scully RE. Glassy cell carcinoma of the cervix. Cancer 1976; 37: 2238–46.

98 Lagasse LD, Ballon SC, Berman ML, Watring WG. Pretreatment lymphangiography and operative evaluation in carcinoma of the cervix. Am J Obstet Gynecol 1979; 134: 219–24.

99 Jordan JA, Sharp F, Singer A (eds). Preclinical Neoplasia of the Cervix. London: Royal College of Obstetricians & Gynaecologists, 1982, 240.

100 Vigario G, Kurohara SS, George FW. Association of haemoglobin levels before and during radiotherapy with prognosis in uterine cervix cancer. Radiology 1973; 106: 649–52.

101 Brenner de, Whiteley NO, Prempree T, Villasanta U. An evaluation of the computed tomographic scanner for the staging of carcinoma of the cervix. Cancer 1982; 50: 2323–8.

102 Piver MS, Chung WS. Prognostic significance of cervical lesion size and pelvic node metastases in cervical carcinoma. Obstet Gynecol 1975; 46: 507–10.

103 Gauthier P, Gore I, Shingleton HM, Soong SJ, Orr JW, Hatch KD. Identification of histopathologic risk groups in Stage IB squamous cell carcinoma of the cervix. Obstet Gynecol 1985; 66: 569–74.

104 Ward BG, Shepherd JH, Monoghan JM. Occult advanced cervical cancer. Br Med J 1985; 290: 1301–2.

105 Van Nagell JR, Rayburn W, Donaldson ES, Hanson M, Gay EC, Yoneda J, Marayuma Y, Powell DF. Therapeutic implications of patterns of recurrence in cancer of the uterine cervix. Cancer 1979; 44: 2354–2361.

106 Underwood PB, Wilson WC, Kreutner A, Miller MC. Radical hysterectomy: a critical review of twenty-two years' experience. Am J Obstet Gynecol 1979; 134: 889–98.

107 Prempree T, Patanaphan V, Sewchand W, Scott RM. The influence of patients' age and tumor grade on the prognosis of carcinoma of the cervix. Cancer 1983; 51: 1764–71.

108 Barber HRK, Sommers SC, Rotterdam H, Kwon T. Vascular invasion as a prognostic factor in Stage IB cancer of the cervix. Obstet Gynecol 1978; 52: 343–8.

109 Lagasse LD, Smith ML, Moore JG, Morton DG, Jacobs M, Johnson GH, Watring WG. The effect of radiation therapy on pelvic lymph node involvement in Stage I carcinoma of the cervix. Am J Obstet Gynecol 1974; 119: 328–34.

110 Martimbeau PW, Kjorstad KE, Iversen T. Stage IB carcinoma of the cervix, the Norwegian Radium Hospital. II Results when pelvic nodes are involved. Obstet Gynecol 1982; 60: 215–8.

111 Kademian MT, Bosch A. Is staging laparotomy in cervical cancer justifiable? Int. J Radiol Oncol Biol Phys 1977; 2: 1235–8 (letter).

112 Hall SW, Monaghan JM. Invasive carcinoma of the cervix in younger women. Lancet 1983; ii: 731 (letter).

113 Stanhope CR, Smith JP, Wharton JT, Rutledge FN, Fletcher GH, Gallager HS. Carcinoma of the cervix: the effect of age on survival. Gynecol Oncol 1980; 10: 188–93.

114 Fay RA, Crandon AJ, Hudson CN, Langlands AO, Tiver KW. Cervical carcinoma associated with pregnancy. Lancet 1982; ii: 1213 (letter).

115 Glucksmann A. Can radiosensitivity and histopathology of cervical cancer be correlated? JAMA 1965; 193: 823–7.

116 Truelsen F. Cancer of the Uterine Cervix. Copenhagen: Rosenkilde & Bagger, 1949.

117 Lindell A. Carcinoma of the uterine cervix; incidence and influence of age; statistical study. Acta Radiol 1952; Suppl 92: 1–101.

118 Decker DG, Fricke RE, Pratt JH. Invasive carcinoma of the cervix in young women. JAMA 1955; 158: 1417–20.

119 Randall JH, Elkins HB, Goddard WB. Carcinoma of the cervix. Treated during the years 1942 to 1951 at the State university of Iowa Hospitals. Radiology 1958; 70: 713–9.

120 Dodds JR, Latour JPA. Relationship of age to survival rate in carcinoma of the cervix. Am J Obstet Gynecol 1961; 82: 33–6.

121 Diddle AW, Watts J. Cervical carcinoma in women under 30 years of age. Delay in diagnosis. Am J Obstet Gynecol 1962; 84: 745–8.

122 Blomfield GW, Cherry CP, Glucksmann A. Biological factors influencing the radiotherapeutic results in carcinoma of the cervix. Br J Radiol 1965; 38: 241–54.

123 Sidhu HS, Koss LG, Barber KRK. Relation of histologic factors to the response of Stage I epidermoid carcinoma of the cervix to surgical treatment. Analysis of 115 patients. Obstet Gynecol 1970; 35: 329–38.

124 Kyriakos M, Kempson RL, Perez CA. Carcinoma of the cervix in young women. Obstet Gynecol 1971; 38: 930–44.

125 Futoran RJ, Nolan JF. Stage I carcinoma of the uterine cervix in patients under 40 years of age. Am J Obstet Gynecol 1976; 125: 790–7.

126 Kjorstad K. Carcinoma of the cervix in the young patient. Obstet Gynecol 1977; 50: 28–30.

127 Cullhed S. Carcinoma cervicis uteri. Stage I and IIA. Acta Obstet Gynecol Scand 1978; Suppl. 75: 1–149.

128 Hankey B, Steinhorn SC. Long-term patient survival for some of the more frequently occurring cancers. Cancer 1982; 50: 1904–12.

129 Bouma J, Crane-Elders ABF. Cervical carcinoma in younger patients. Lancet 1983; i: 248 (letter).

130 Boronow RC. Stage I cervix cancer and pelvic node metastasis. Special reference to the implications of the new and the recently replaced FIGO classifications on Stage IA. Am J Obstet Gynecol 1977; 127: 135–7.

131 Creasman WT, Fetter BF, Clarke-Pearson DL, Kaufmann L, Parker RT. Management of Stage IA carcinoma of the cervix. Am J Obstet Gynecol 1985; 153: 164–72.

132 Herbst AL, Cole P, Norusis MJ, Welch WR, Scully RE. Epidemiological aspects and factors related to survival in 384 Registry cases of clear cell adenocarcinoma of the vagina and cervix. Am J Obstet Gynecol 1979; 135: 876–86.

133 Herbst AL, Norusis MJ, Rosenow PJ, Welch WR, Scully RE. An analysis of 346 cases of clear cell adenocarcinoma of the vagina and cervix with emphasis on recurrence and survival. Gynecol. Oncol. 1979; 7: 111–122.

134 Morgan LS, Nelson JH. Surgical treatment of early cervical cancer. Semin Oncol 1982; 9: 312–30.

135 Yajima A, Noda K. The results of treatment of microinvasive carcinoma (Stage IA) of the

uterine cervix by means of simple and extended hysterectomy. Am J Obstet Gynecol 1979; 135: 685–8.

136 Perez CA, Camel HM, Kao MS, Askin F. Randomized study of preoperative radiation and surgery or irradiation alone in the treatment of Stage IB and IIA carcinoma of the uterine cervix: preliminary analysis of failures and complications. Cancer 1980; 45: 2759–68.

137 Roddick JW, Greenelaw RH. Treatment of cervical cancer. A randomized study of operation and radiation. Am J Obstet Gynecol 1971; 109: 754–64.

138 Newton M. Radical hysterectomy or radiotherapy for Stage I cervical cancer. A prospective comparison with 5 and 10 year follow-up. Am J Obstet Gynecol 1975; 123: 535–42.

139 Piver MS, Barlow JJ, Krishnamsetty R. Five-year survival (with no evidence of disease) in patients with biopsy-confirmed aortic node metastases from cervical carcinoma. Am J Obstet Gynecol 1981; 139: 575–8.

140 Marcial VA, Bosch A. Radiation-induced tumor regression in carcinoma of the uterine cervix: prognostic significance. Am J Roentgenol 1970; 108: 113–23.

141 Joslin CAF. Radiotherapy of the cervix, uterine corpus and ovary. In: Shepherd JH, Monaghan JM eds. Clinical Gynaecological Oncology. Oxford: Blackwell, 1985, 303–15.

142 Strickland P. Complications of radiotherapy. Br J Hosp Med 1980; 23: 552–61.

143 Hanks GE, Herring DF, Kramer S. Patterns of care outcome studies. Cancer 1983; 51: 959–67.

144 Abitbol MM, Davenport JH. Sexual dysfunction after therapy for cervical carcinoma. Am J Obstet Gynecol 1974; 119: 181–9.

145 Seibel M, Freeman MG, Graves WL. Sexual function after surgical and radiation therapy for cervical carcinoma. South Med J 1982; 75: 1195–7.

146 Mazur MT, Hsueh S, Gersell DJ. Metastases to the female genital tract. Cancer 1984; 53: 1978–84.

147 Shepherd JH, Crowther ME. Complications of gynaecological cancer surgery: a review. JR Soc Med 1986; 79: 289–93.

148 Shepherd JH. Cervical cancer: the surgical management of early stage disease. In: Shepherd JH, Monaghan JM eds Clinical Gynaecological Oncology. Oxford: Blackwell, 1985: 63.

149 Averette HE, Nelson JH, NG ABP, Hoskins WJ, Boyce JG. Diagnosis and management of microinvasive (Stage IA) carcinoma of the uterine cervix. Cancer 1976; 38: 414–25.

150 Rutledge FN, Wharton JT, Fletcher GH. Clinical studies with adjunctive surgery and irradiation therapy in the treatment of carcinoma of the cervix. Cancer 1976; 38: 596–602.

151 Fuller AF, Elliott N, Kosloff C, Lewis JL. Lymph node metastases from carcinoma of the cervix, Stage IB and IIA: implications for prognosis and treatment. Gynecol Oncol 1982; 13: 165–74.

152 Million RR, Rutledge F, Fletcher GH. Stage IV carcinoma of the cervix with bladder invasion. Am J Obstet Gynecol 1972; 113: 239–46.

153 Korhonen MO. Adenocarcinoma of the uterine cervix. Prognosis and prognostic significance of histology. Cancer 1984; 53: 1760–3.

154 Rutledge FN, Galakatos AE, Wharton JT, Smith JP. Adenocarcinoma of the uterine cervix. Am J Obstet Gynecol 1975; 122: 236–45.

155 Hill EC, Galante M. Radical surgery in the management of clear cell adenocarcinoma of the cervix and vagina in young women. Am J Obstet Gynecol 1981; 140: 221–6.

156 Heller PB, Barnhill DR, Mayer AR, Fontaine TP, Hoskins WJ, Park RC. Cervical carcinoma found incidentally in a uterus removed for benign indications. Obstet Gynecol 1986; 67: 187–90.

157 Davy M, Bentzen H, Jahren R. Simple hysterectomy in the presence of invasive cervical cancer. Acta Obstet Gynecol Scand 1977; 56: 105–8.

158 Krebs HB, Helmkamp BF, Sevin BU, Poliakoff SR, Nadji M, Averette HE. Recurrent cancer of the cervix following radical hysterectomy and pelvic node dissection. Obstet Gynecol 1982; 59: 422–7.

159 Rutledge F, Seski J. More or less radical surgery. Int J Rad Onc Biol Phys 1979; 5: 1881–4.

160 Thar TL, Million RR, Daly JW. Radiation treatment of carcinoma of the cervix. Semin Oncol 1982; 9: 299–311.

161 Barber HRK. Gynecologic tumors in pregnancy. In: Van Nagell JR, Barber HRK eds, Modern Concepts of Gynecologic Oncology. Boston: John Wright, 1982, 428.

162 Sablinska R, Tarlowska L, Stelmachow J. Invasive carcinoma of the cervix associated with pregnancy: correlation between patient age, advancement of cancer and gestation, and result of treatment. Gynecol Oncol 1977; 5: 363–73.

163 Hacker NF, Berek JS, Lagasse LD, Charles EH, Savage EW, Moore JG. Carcinoma of the cervix associated with pregnancy. Obstet Gynecol 1982; 59: 735–746.

164 Lurain JR, Gallup DG. Management of abnormal Papanicolaou smears in pregnancy. Obstet Gynecol 1979; 53: 484–8.

165 Hannigan EV, Whitehouse HH, Atkinson WD, Becker SN. Cone biopsy during pregnancy. Obstet Gynecol 1982; 60: 450–5.

166 Waldrop GM, Palmer JP. Carcinoma of the cervix associated with pregnancy. Am J Obstet Gynecol 1963; 86: 202–12.

167 Thompson JD, Caputo TA, Franklin EW, Dale E. The surgical management of invasive cancer of the cervix in pregnancy. Am J Obstet Gynecol 1975; 121: 853–63.

168 Funnell JD, Puckett TG, Strebel GF. Kelso JW. Carcinoma of the cervix complicating pregnancy. South Med J 1980; 73: 1308–10.

169 Mikuta JJ, Giuntoli RL, Rubin EL, Mangan CE. The "problem" radical hysterectomy Am J Obstet Gynecol 1977; 128: 119–127.

170 Ulfelder H, Smith CJ, Costello JB. Invasive carcinoma of the cervix during pregnancy. Am J Obstet Gynecol 1967; 98: 424–8.

171 Strauss A. Irradiation of carcinoma of cervix uteri in pregnancy. Am J Roentgenol 1940; 43: 552–66.

172 Guthrie D. Chemotherapy of cervical cancer. Clin Obstet Gynecol 1985 (March); 12: 229–46.

173 Friedlander M, Kaye SB, Sullivan A, Atkinson K, Elliott P, Coppleson M, Houghton R, Solomon J, Green D, Russell P. Cervical carcinoma: a drug-responsive tumour-experience with combined cisplatin, vinblastine, and bleomycin therapy. Gynecol Oncol 1983; 16: 275–81.

174 Coleman RE, Harper PG, Rankin E, Wiltshaw E, Calvert H, Osborne R, Slevin ML, Souhami R, Silverstone AC, Trask CW. A phase two study of Iphosphamide in advanced relapsed carcinoma of the cervix. Presented at 3rd European Conference on Clinical Oncology and Cancer Nursing, Stockholm, Sweden, 1985.

175 Meanwell CA, Blackledge G, Hancock AM, Latief TN, Mould JJ, Spooner D. Phase II study of Iphosphamide in advanced cervical cancer. Presented at 3rd European Conference on Clinical Oncology and Cancer Nursing, Stockholm, Sweden, 1985.

176 Piver MS, Barlow JJ, Vongtama V, Blumenson L. Hydroxyurea: a radiation potentiator in carcinoma of the uterine cervix. Am J Obstet Gynecol 1983; 147: 803–8.

177 The Medical Research Council trial of misonidazole in carcinoma of the uterine cervix. Br J Radiol 1984; 57: 491–9.

178 Potish RA, Twiggs LB, Okagaki T, Prem KA, Adcock LL. Therapeutic implications of the natural history of advanced cervical cancer as defined by pretreatment surgical staging. Cancer 1985; 56: 956–60.

179 Monaghan JM. Surgical management of advanced and recurrent cervical carcinoma: the place of pelvic exenteration. Clin Obstet Gynecol. 1985 (March); 12: 169–82.

180 Keettel WC, Van Voorhis LW, Latourette HB. Management of recurrent carcinoma of the cervix. Am J Obstet Gynecol 1968; 102: 671–9.

181 Barber HRK. Relative prognostic significance of pre-operative and operative findings in pelvic exenteration. Surg Clin Nth Am. 1969 (April); 49: 431–447.

182 Morley GW, Lindenauer SM. Pelvic exenterative therapy for gynecologic malignancy. An analysis of 70 cases. Cancer 1976; 38: 581–6.

183 Ashworth MF, Morton KE, Dewhurst J, Lilford RJ, Bates RG. Vaginoplasty using amnion. Obstet Gynecol 1986; 67: 443–6.

184 Williams EA. Congenital absence of the vagina: a simple operation for its relief. J Obstet Gynaecol Br Comm 1964; 71: 511–2.

185 IARC Working Group of Evaluation of Cervical Cancer Screening Programmes. Screening for squamous cervical cancer: duration of low risk after negative results of cervical cytology and its implication for screening policies. Br Med J 1986; 293: 659–664.

Textbook of Uncommon Cancer
Edited by C.J. Williams, J.G. Krikorian, M.R. Green and D. Raghavan
© 1988 John Wiley & Sons Ltd

Chapter **13**

Malignant Melanoma, Paget's Disease and Sarcoma of the Vulva

Duane E. Townsend

Professor and Vice Chairman, Department of Obstetrics and Gynecology, Director, Gynecologic and Oncologic Services, University of California, Davis, Medical Center, Sacramento, California, USA

INTRODUCTION

Of the three cancers of the vulva to be discussed in this chapter, malignant melanoma is the second most common malignancy of this organ but is the most lethal. Paget's disease is classified as an intraepithelial lesion, although in 20–30% of cases, an invasive adenocarcinoma is present. The sarcomas are comprised of a enormous variety of lesions since they arise from the numerous tissue elements of the vulva.

MALIGNANT MELANOMA

Introduction

Cutaneous malignant melanoma has been increasing rather dramatically over the past two decades with some 22 000 new cases occurring in the United States in 1985 (1). Almost simultaneous with this dramatic increase in incidence has been a remarkable increase in overall 5-year survival. In 1940, less than 40% of patients were alive at 5 years; however, by 1983, the 5-year survival for clinical Stage I disease was 85% (2).

Cutaneous malignant melanoma occurs primarily during the reproductive years. It is extremely rare in childhood, and seldom seen in the elderly except for the lentigo maligna type (3). Occasionally, the lesion is familial. Cutaneous malanoma is divided equally among the sexes. Survival is not equal; women have a better prognosis. Melanoma is six to seven times more common in the white race. It is infrequent in Orientals and blacks. When it occurs in blacks and Orientals, the lesions are primarily on the palms, soles, nailbeds, and mucous membranes. The white population has the disease more commonly on the back and lower legs. The incidence of melanoma is higher in people living closer to the equator, suggesting an ultraviolent etiology. In addition, the death rate is higher in these same individuals. A subset of whites appear to be particularly susceptible to melanoma, i.e. fair-skinned, blue-eyed, blond- or red-haired (3). In addition to solar exposure, there are definite precursor lesions such as junctional nevi.

Classification

In 1967, Clark proposed a new classification of malignant melanoma which was expanded in 1969. The most common, accounting for 70% of melanomas, is called *superficial spreading* (4). This type also has the highest cure rate. It is a lesion which has raised edges and undergoes a lateral growth phase for many years prior to the development of nodules. Histopathologically, the lesion resembles Paget's disease of the breast, i.e. spreading within the epidermis.

The next form is called *nodular* melanoma, which is noted in 15% of cases. It appears to develop de novo as an invasive nodule without lateral spread. It is the most fatal type of melanomas.

Lentigo maligna melanoma, the third type, is found on the sun-exposed surfaces in the elderly. It is a flat, variegated pigmented lesion that grows slowly prior to developing invasive nodules. It has a very high cure rate. This lesion is not found on the vulva.

A fourth type has been called *acral lentiginous* melanoma (5). It is also called the *palmar–plantar–subungual–mucosal* melanoma (6). This tumor is most often seen in blacks and Orientals, infrequently in whites. Histologically, it is similar to that of the lentigo maligna melanoma but is less common. However, this melanoma behaves more aggressively than the lentigo maligna type. It occurs primarily on the palms, soles, nailbeds, and mucous membranes of the oral and nasal cavities, and on the mucocutaneous sites of the genital and anal regions.

There are three major cell types found within malignant melanomas: epithelioid, nevus, and spindle cell. The cell type of the malignancy has little bearing on survival. A neurotropic type is occasionally noted in some melanomas.

Clinical Appearance

Generally, malignant melanomas are dark. The most important factors have to do with the color of the lesin and its border. The single most important factor is thought to be the variegation of color (13). The tumors are not only brown and tan but have various mixtures of blue, red, and white; mixtures of half-tones; and mixtures of browns, tans, and blacks. Color variation is probably related to the location of the melanin within the skin. Inflammation, immune response, and vasodilatation will contribute to a red coloration.. In some instances, the tumors will show a regression with destruction of the melanocyte. Another most common diagnostic feature besides color is the irregularity of the border.

In general, melanomas evolve slowly for a period during which time they are locally invasive and probably do not metastasize. It is during this phase of development that the lesions appear to grow superficially and laterally through the epidermis and dermis prior to penetration and metastases. During the lateral growth phase, melanomas are now most frequently diagnosed and cured by wide local excision.

VULVAR MELANOMA

Incidence

Malignant melanoma of the vulva accounts for 5–10% of all vulvar cancers but is considerably more lethal than the most common, squamous cell carcinoma. The vulva produces 3–5% of all melanomas in women but only accounts for 1–2% of the body surface area (7). There have been over 700 cases of vulvar melanoma reported in the literature. The lesion has not been noted prior to puberty but increases in incidence until the fifth decade of life when it is most common. This is in marked contrast to the cutaneous variety which peaks during the reproductive years. The youngest patient with vulvar melanoma is 14 (7), the oldest being well into her nineties. Prognosis is not linked with age; but some investigators feel that when it does occur in pregnancy, the disease can be extremely virulent (8). A few familial cases have been reported, but they are very uncommon (9). In general, familial melanoma has a high survival rate.

Signs and Symptoms

The most common symptom is pruritus, followed by bleeding, the discovery of a mass, an enlarging mole, and, lastly, burning (8). When a women presents with bleeding, the disease is often advanced, and the prognosis is usually grave. Early detection, as with most cancers, is synonymous with a high chance of cure.

Vulvar melanomas generally will be brown to blue-black, will be flat when they are of the superficial spreading variety, and will be polypoid when they are of the nodular type. Ulceration with bleeding and pain occurs with more advanced lesions. An inflammatory reaction will make a tumor appear red. The lesions can occur anywhere on the vulva, but the most common sites are clitoris and labia minora (8). When lesions do occur in this area, adequate surgical margins are difficult to obtain. Melanomas have been found in association with dystrophies, squamous cell disease, and are sometimes confused with urethral carbuncles, Bartholin gland cysts, and hemangiomas. The various types of melanomas, as mentioned previously, i.e. superficial spreading, nodular, etc., are distributed similar to that of the cutaneous melanomas. The FIGO staging of the vulva is not a reliable index of patient survival for melanomas (10). The thickness of the lesion as well as the invasion into the skin correlate best with the prognosis of vulvar melanoma. When the disease has metastasized or spread to the vagina or to regional lymph nodes, prognosis is dismal (11, 12).

Prognostic Factors

Survival rates from different series of vulvar melanoma vary from as low as 10% (13) to as high as 54% (14). However, 5-year survival rates are misleading in that patients with melanomas have recurred as late as 12 years from initial therapy (15). When the lesions involve the regional lymph nodes, most patients have recurrence and die within 2 to 3 years of therapy, but an occasional long-term survival has been reported (15). When the disease recurs in the treatment field, there have been no reported survivors (14). The significance of lymph node involvement, and its impact upon prognosis are depicted in Table 1.

TABLE 1 VULVAR MELANOMA: INFLUENCE OF POSITIVE NODES ON SURVIVAL (11, 14–25)

	Positive nodes	Negative nodes
Total	99	155
Alive	6	79
Percentage	6	51

Note the 6% survival in the 99 cases with groin node metastases contrasted with 51% 5-year-survivors of those cases where the lymph nodes were found to be disease free.

FIGO staging is depicted in Table 2. Patients with Stage I disease had a 50% 5-year survival, and this dropped to 20% with Stage IV disease. This is in contrast to squamous cell carcinoma (noted in brackets) which has a vastly higher survival for the early stage disease.

In 1967, Clark, attempting to correlate histogenesis and biological behavior, classified malignant melanoma according to the depth of invasion. The Clark classification is divided into five levels:

Level I: All of the malignant cells are above the basement membrane.

Level II: The neoplastic cells have broken through the basement membrane and have extended into the superficial portion of the papillary dermis.

Level III: The malignant cells have extended to the level of the subpapillary vessels but not into the reticular dermis.

TABLE 2 VULVAR MELANOMA: SURVIVAL BY FIGO STAGING (14, 19–23, 26)

	I	II	III	IV
Total	54	18	21	10
Alive	27	8	7	2
Percentage	50 (91.1)[a]	44 (80.9)	35 (48.9)	20 (15.3)

[a] Survival of squamous cell carcinoma of the vulva.

Level IV: The neoplastic cells have extended into the reticular dermis.

Level V: The tumor cells have invaded the subcutaneous fat.

In 1970, Breslow (27) suggested that the thickness, cross-sectional area, and depth of invasion were additional factors that had to be considered in cutaneous melanomas. The Breslow technique measured the thickest portion of the melanoma from the surface of the intact epithelium to the deepest point of invasion. The depth of penetration is then categorized:

Less than 0.76 mm
0.76 to 1.50 mm
1.51 to 2.25 mm
2.26 to 3.0 mm
Greater than 3.0 mm.

Only the more recent articles have attempted to employ these classifications to vulvar cancer.

Chung felt that the Clark system was difficult to apply to the vulva because of a poorly defined papillary dermis as well as the absence of a papillary dermis for the vulvar mucosa (15). He suggested a modification of the Clark scheme by measuring the depth of invasion from the granular layer of the vulvar skin or outer most epithelial of the squamous mucosa. He suggested five levels as did Clark. The Chung modification of the Clark levels is as follows:

Level I: Tumour confined to the epithelium.

Level II: Superficial penetration of tumor into the dermis or lamina propria to a depth of 1 mm or less as measured using a hand micrometer from the granular layer or outermost epithelial layer in the squamous mucosa.

Level III: Penetration between 1 and 2 mm deep into the subepithelial tissues.

Level IV: Invasion beyond 2 mm but not into underlying fat.

Level V: Invasion of melanoma into underlying fat.

In Tables 3, 4, and 5 are given the respective survival rates according to the Clark, Breslow, and Chung methods of classifying vulvar melanomas. Despite the differences in classifying the cancer, it is obvious that the early invasive lesions have a remarkably high survival rate. In Tables 3 and 4, the cutaneous melanoma's survival rate for Stage I disease is given in brackets (2) for each of the Clark and Breslow classifications. Note the significantly higher rates of survival for the cutaneous lesions. This difference in survival is puzzling. It is not due to the type of melanoma found on the vulva, i.e. nodular, superficial spreading, etc., since the various types occur with the same frequency for the cutaneous variety. The cell types of vulvar melanoma are appropriately distributed between epithelioid, nevus, and spindle. However, one problem with comparing the vulvar lesion to the cutaneous melanomas is the difficulty, as noted by Chung, in completely defining comparable layers of the vulva to that of the skin. It may well be that a significant number of vulvar cases should be allocated to higher levels which have poorer survival rates. In addition, part of the difference is probably due to lymph node metastasis which was not always clearly defined in respect to the level of classification of the melanoma. Lastly, adequate surgical margins may be difficult to obtain because of tumor location.

Fewer authors have used the Chung classification. Again, there is a very high survival for the early disease, i.e. levels I and II.

Recently, Phillips (29) following Bagley's (30) classification for cutaneous melanomas suggested that vulvar melanomas be stratified as high, medium, or low risk, depending upon the level of invasion and tumor thickness. The low risk melanomas were those that were less than 0.76 mm in thickness and were at Clark level II or III. Moderate risk melanomas were defined as those less than 0.7 mm in thickness and a level IV, and all melanomas between 0.76 and 1.5 mm of thickness as well as melanomas more than 1.5 mm but level III. The high risk categories are those greater than 1.5 mm of thickness and levels IV and V.

TABLE 3 VULVAR MELANOMA: SURVIVAL BY CLARK LEVELS (4, 16, 18, 21, 22, 25, 28)

	I	II	III	IV	V
Total	4	17	26	23	37
Alive	4	15	16	8	8
Percentage	100 (100)[a]	88 (99)	62 (95)	35 (75)	22 (39)

[a] Survival of Stage I cutaneous melanoma.

TABLE 4 VULVAR MELANOMA: SURVIVAL BY THICKNESS OF LESION (BRESLOW) (14, 15, 17, 18, 21)

	0.76 mm	0.76–1.49 mm	1.50–4.0 mm	4.0+
Total	15	15	38	42
Survival	15	11	21	8
Percentage	100 (99)[a]	73 (94)	55 (78)	19 (42)

[a] Survival of Stage I.

TABLE 5 VULVAR MELANOMA: SURVIVAL OF PATIENTS USING MODIFIED CLARK LEVELS (CHUNG) (15–19, 23)

	I	II	III	IV	V
Total	1	13	12	22	17
Survival	1	11	6	8	7
Percentage	100	85	50	36	41

Using this method, Phillips (29) was able to extract 12 patients with low risk disease from articles by Chung (15), Cleophax (31), and his own series. In the articles reviewed for this chapter, an additional 15 cases with low risk factors were uncovered. It was urged by Phillips that these patients be managed by simple local resection and without the necessity of node dissection, since in all cases the patients are alive and well.

Detection and Evaluation

Any nevus of the vulva should be resected with an adequate margin. If the patient has a large lesion, then a deep wedge biopsy should be taken. There is no evidence to suggest that a deep biopsy of a melanoma will affect prognosis. More importantly, improper diagnosis can lead to inappropriate therapy. Once a diagnosis has been made of malignant melanoma, appropriate pretreatment evaluation must be made. If the patient has an early lesion, i.e. minimal invasion, Chung I or II, or Clark I or II, then wide excision with a 3 cm margin is all that is necessary. A chest x-ray should be sufficient as a baseline. Additional studies are probably unnecessary in this patient since the prognosis is excellent.

With more advanced disease, then a more thorough evaluation must be carried out in order to prepare the patient for appropriate therapy. Evaluation should include a computed tomography (CT) scan, a bone scan, chest x-rays, and appropriate blood studies. If there is disease around the anus, then a barium enema must be performed along with protosigmoidoscopy and/or colonoscopy. A cystoscopic examination is most important, particularly if the disease is near the urethra. The vulva, vagina, and cervix must be carefully scanned with a colposcope to pick out any occult disease or early metastases. The CT scan of the abdomen and pelvis should include careful examination of the liver and retroperitoneal nodes. Lymphangiograms may be of additional benefit. Monoclonal antibody scans are currently under study for cutaneous melanoma. It may be possible with this technology to detect early metastases which would greatly influence therapy. Moreover, attempts are underway to tag the monoclonal antibody with radioactive isotope as well as drugs in order to treat recurrent diseases (32).

Treatment

The single most important step in the management of malignant melanoma is adequate surgical margins. With the cutaneous lesion, it is now suggested that a margin of 3 to 5 cm be obtained. For vulvar melanoma, this is easily performed when the lesions are present on the labia majora, but it is difficult when lesions are on the clitoris or labia minora. Local failure is a problem of inadequate central resection. Physicians are often reluctant to remove portions of the urethra or the vagina in order to obtain an adequate border. The depth of resection is similar for that of squamous cell disease.

Lymphadenectomy

The role of lymphadenectomy for cutaneous melanoma has not been fully resolved. There have been several series (33, 34) which point out that lymphadenectomy done at the time of the initial resection for cutaneous melanoma does not improve survival when compared to those cases when the nodes are taken once they become clinically apparent. However, for vulvar disease, an en bloc resection with removal of the primary lesion and its draining lymph system up to the regional lymph nodes is possible. Morrow (8) and Poderantz (14) argue that the problem of tumor embolization is thus not a consideration in contrast to the cutaneous lesions where en bloc resection is often impossible to perform. Poderantz feels that the recurrence of only one groin lesion in

his large series of cases supports his position. However, it can be argued that in a patient with lymph node metastases, the chance of survival is very dim. Consequently, leaving the lymphadenectomy until the lymph nodes are clinically apparent may have a similar role as that for the cutaneous lesions. Despite this seemingly unresolved issue, the general approach to the melanoma patient is to perform a radical vulvectomy with an en bloc removal of the draining lymphatic system, including the regional nodes. Pelvic lymphadenectomy probably offers nothing for the patient with malignant melanoma even if the inguinal nodes are involved. However, Chung (15) did have one 12-year survivor with positive pelvic nodes who then died of recurrence. His case remains the only one with such a long-term survival. It is not known how long the patient would have survived if the pelvic nodes had not been removed.

The role of exenteration in the woman with malignant melanoma of the vulva is unclear. It has been performed in only two cases (20). In both instances, the patients quickly died of recurrent disease.

Advanced Disease

Patients with advanced or metastatic disease have virtually no chance of survival. Radiation therapy has reduced tumor mass but has not prolonged survival time. In fact, some patients have a more protracted, unpleasant course because of the side effects of radiation. There have been no chemotherapeutic agents or combination of drugs, including immune stimulants, that have been shown to have any significant, beneficial effects with advanced melanomas of the vulva. Perhaps tagged monoclonal antibodies will prove to be of some benefit in these patients.

Summary

It appears at this time that the malignant melanoma of the female genital tract is a more aggressive tumor than other cutaneous melanomas. Fortunately, in contrast to the cutaneous lesion, which is increasing in incidence, there has been no apparent increase in vulvar melanoma. Patients have a poor prognosis primarily due to the advanced stage of the disease at the time of diagnosis. When the malignancy is thin and shows little invasion, the prognosis is excellent, and wide local excision is all that is necessary; even vulvectomy is unnecessary in these patients. With more advanced disease, the standard radical resection of the vulva is employed, although preservation of portions of the vulva could be carried out if adequate margins can otherwise be obtained. Regional node dissection en bloc with the primary tumor is generally recommended. With advanced disease, patient survival is nil.

PAGET'S DISEASE

It has been over 110 years since Paget (35) first described a malignancy of the breast that bears his name. Approximately 25 years later, Dubrewilh (36) described the first case of vulvar involvement with this disease. Since that time, about 200 cases have been reported. This vulvar malignancy is usually classified as an intraepithelial lesion; however, in 20–30% of cases, an invasive adenocarcinoma of the underlying apocrine glands is present (37). The disease has a tendency to recur and is often multifocal. The origin of Paget's disease remains the subject of considerable speculation, although studies suggest that it arises from a pleuripotential cell of the germative cell layer of the epidermis which gives origin to cutaneous appendices as well as mature squamous epithelium (38). Paget's disease of the vulva is associated with malignancies elsewhere in the body, particularly breasts and other organs of the female genital tract (39). When it involves the anus, there is a high association of adenocarcinoma of the rectum.

Symptoms and Gross Appearance

The disease usually begins in the hair-bearing areas of the vulva, genital folds, or perianal region. It will then extend and involve the labia minora and internal structures, including the urethra. Thus, the earliest manifestations of the disease are found in the adenexal areas of the organ. Other extramammary sites include axilla, umbilicus, and external ear canal. Since Paget's disease of the breast is almost always associated with underlying malignancy of the breast, a careful evaluation to exclude an underlying malignancy is important when it occurs in an extramammary site.

Most women with Paget's disease are in the sixth decade of life. Usually, the afflicted individual notes an intermittent pruritic area which gradually becomes more sustained and widespread. In some instances, several areas will be involved simultaneously, but this is the exception. If the patient is examined at this time, reddish smudges are usually present in the area of pruritus. This is often mistaken as a contact dermatitis or an area of monilia, and the patient is usually treated symptomatically with some type of antipruritic agent. Often this relieves the symptoms, and the patient and physician think that nothing serious is present. However, as time passes, the disease continues to develop and the pruritus returns. The reddish smudge becomes more intense, and the area develops a deep, fiery-red base which, if ignored, develops thick white keratin patches with interlacing bridges. When the disease involves the anus, the patients mistakenly believe they have hemorrhoids or anal fissures. Again, delay in physician consultation as well as reluctance for biopsy accounts for the advanced stages of the disease.

To the naked eye, the lesions appear to have fairly well-defined borders, but if magnified with a colposcope, a feathery edge is appreciated. The feathery edge which has a soft, orange-pinkish hue colposcopically will have Paget's cells at its border. In fact, Paget's cells will be found 5 mm beyond the colposcopic border of the lesion. As a consequence, when any therapy is contemplated, adequate surgical margins must be taken in order to lessen the chance of recurrence. If the disease is ignored

even further, the patient will eventually develop areas of adenocarcinoma. These are
fairly easy to detect colposcopically in that they
will form small nodules with atypical vessel
within the large, fiery-red field.

The prevalence of invasive adenocarcinoma
in the apocrine glands in vulvar Paget's disease
varies according to the author. The consensus
is that between 20 and 30% of patients with
vulvar Paget's disease will have an invasive
adenocarcinoma (39, 40–42). This usually
occurs in women who have more advanced
disease.

Histology

The Paget's cell is large and has an abundant
cytoplasm that faintly stains with hematoxylin
and eosin. The nucleus often contains prominent, enlarged nucleolus. Mitotic figures are
rare. Isolated cells are seldom seen, and they
are usually found in groups or nests close to the
basal layer. The cells can be found anyplace,
and their presence in hair follicles, ducts, and
glands is not unremarkable (37). When the
lesions involve the sweat glands, it does not
suggest a glandular origin of the cell. When the
cells are present within the epidermis, they
may eventually slough and may be found by
touch cytology as demonstrated by Masukawa
and Friedrich (43).

Etiology

A number of investigators have attempted to
determine the etiology of the Paget's cell.
Studies of the ultrastructure (44) and biochemical nature of the Paget's cell strongly
support a secretory epithelial cell with a
glandular differentiation. Gunn and Gallager
(45) studied 4 patients topographically with
vulvar Paget's disease and noted 2 cases with
multifocality. They felt the Paget's cell arose in
the epidermis. Woodruff's original hypothesis
that the Paget's cell rose from primitive pleuripotential cells (38) has withstood the test of
time and, in fact, was recently supported in
studies by Mozoujian, who evaluated 7 cases of

extramammary Paget's including those of the
vulva and anal–genital region (46). He used an
immunoperoxidase localization of gross cystic
disease fluid protein (GCDFP-15), a marker of
apocrine epithelium; carcinogenic antigen
(CEA); and keratin proteins. He noted immunoreactivity for GCDFP-15 within the Paget's
cell in 6 of 7 cases including 5 in the vulva and 1
in the axilla. None of the Paget's cell exhibited
immunoreactivity for keratin proteins. Using
normal skin as controls, eccrine glands were
immunoreactive for both keratin and CEA;
whereas GCDFP-15 was localized only to
apocrine ducts and glands. As a consequence,
Mozoujian believes that the Paget's cell probably develops from primitive pleuripotential
cells as suggested by Woodruff.

Treatment

Before therapy is undertaken, it is important to
carefully survey the entire patient for other
malignancies. A mammogram of the breast is
important since occult breast carcinomas are
not uncommon with extramammary Paget's
(47). Malignancies of the other organs of the
female genital tract includes cervix (48), uterus, and vagina (39). Urinary bladder and gall
bladder malignancies have also been found in
association with Paget's disease (48, 49).

With the exclusion of other malignancies,
the therapy of the involved tissue is initiated.
When one uses the colposcope and takes
advantage of its magnification, it is possible to
carefully inspect the topographic surface of the
vulva and pick up additional areas of early
Paget's disease. Also, the borders of the lesions
can be more carefully defined to permit a more
accurate resection of the involved area. Wide
local excision with the naked eye is inadequate
in any situation. A standard vulvectomy is
almost a knee jerk reaction, which is inappropriate. Skinning vulvectomies have been advocated by some individuals (49) but, once again,
normal tissue may be sacrificed for the lack of
careful mapping of involved areas. With a
colposcope, areas of invasive adenocarcinoma
can also be detected.

Stacy et al. (48), in attempting to resolve the problems of high recurrence of Paget's disease when only the unmagnified eye is utilized to treat patients, employed frozen section margins at the time of surgery. Using this technique in 5 of 8 cases, additional margins were necessary. In none of the 8 patients where adequate margins had been obtained on frozen section have recurrences developed over a 3- to 8-year time span. However, additional time must transpire since Paget's disease can develop many years from initial therapy.

Laser vaporization has been used in the treatment of patients. Since Paget's disease can extend down into the glandular structures, the area of vaporization must be at least 3 mm deep in order to achieve disease control. A potential problem with laser is the missing of an occult adenocarcinoma. Consequently, only relatively small areas that have been well sampled should be subjected to this form of therapy. The procedure is performed quite easily as an outpatient; patients are not hospitalized.

Paget's Disease of the Anal–Rectal Area

Involvement of the anal–rectal area deserves special attention. Stacy noted that in his 3 cases of anal–rectal involvement, there was an associated adenocarcinoma in all instances. This is a most important consideration in anyone who has a disease in this area, and a thorough evaluation of the lower bowel in addition to a meticulous inspection of other sites must be performed. The evaluation must include a proctosigmoidoscopy, barium enema, and/or colonoscopy.

Invasive Paget's Disease

There is an occasional instance when the Paget's cell will break off from its intraepithelial location and invade underlying tissues and metastasize. Hart and Millman (50) reported an older woman who had undergone a vulvectomy for Paget's disease and then the disease recurred. The lesion was invading the dermis and lymphatics. She had metastatic disease at the time of repeat therapy. The invasion was of the Paget's cell and not an underlying adenocarcinoma.

Follow Up

Patients with Paget's disease obviously must be carefully followed for a long period of time. The physician must continue to carefully survey the other areas where malignancies can occur, i.e. breasts and other genital sites.

Summary

In summary, Paget's disease remains one of the more fascinating lesions of the vulva being classified as an intraepithelial lesion but associated in a number of instances with a secondary invasive adenocarcinoma. Patients with this disease often present in advanced stages because of failure to diagnose at appropriate time. Therapy does not necessarily require vulvectomy but rather careful mapping and adequate margins. Before therapy is undertaken, the exclusion of cancer in other sites of the body must be meticulously carried out and the exclusion of an associated invasive adenocarcinoma must be performed.

SARCOMA OF THE VULVA

Sarcoma of the vulva is one of the more captivating group of malignancies afflicting this portion of the body. The most common type is leiomyosarcoma (51, 52) with neurofibrosarcoma and rhabdomyosarcoma slightly less frequent.

The number of tumor types is extensive because of the multitude of tissue elements present within the vulva (37). In additon to the previously mentioned sarcomas, the list includes hemangiosarcoma (37) malignant hemangiopericytoma (37), epithelioid sarcoma (53, 54) fibrosarcoma (55), neurogenous sarcoma, malignant mesothelioma, alveolar cell soft part sarcoma (56), embryonal stromal sarcoma, lymphoma (reticulum cell sarcoma), liposarcoma, malignant schwannoma, and angiosarcoma. The total number of sarcomas reported in the literature is about 175.

Signs and Symptoms

Most sarcomas develop on the labia majora, the perineal body or Bartholin's gland area. Generally, a small lump will develop which the patient ignores. The lump gradually increases in size and begins to become uncomfortable particularly with pressure during sexual activity. As the mass enlarges, the pain increases, the clothing becomes very sensitive, and sexual activity becomes impossible. Most sarcomas as they enlarge and invade the local tissues spread hematogenously. However, metastasis to regional lymphatics has been noted. In most cases, the enlarging mass evolves fairly slowly, but when the cells are anaplastic, rapid enlargement is common. Delay in diagnosis is particularly a problem with the sarcomas since the lesions are often subepithelial arising within the deeper tissue elements. Patients have a tendency to ignore these lumps thinking that the mass is probably a result of some type of trauma. Physicians, likewise, often imagine that the mass is nothing more than a sebaceous cyst or some type of benign growth. By the time the tumors are sampled, metastasis may have occurred. When the sarcomas are removed, they often appear encapsulated; however, in many cases, tumor strands will be at the edge of resection.

The age span for all sarcomas is from approximately one month to 70 years with most patients being in the sixth decade of life. The rhabdomyosarcomas usually develop at an earlier age and spread rapidly.

The major problem with the sarcomas is the differential diagnosis. The multitude of different sarcomas that develop results in problems of pathological interpretation. There are a number of benign lesions which are confused with sarcomas, which, if inappropriately diagnosed, will lead to unnecessary radical therapy. Fibromatosis (37) is a lesion which is made up of well-differentiated fibroblasts with so-called pushing margins. The disease can locally recur if inadequately resected but does not metastasize. Pseudosarcomatous fasciitis (57) appears as chronic granulation tissue. It has a mixture of chronic inflammatory cells often within a myxoid mass of fibroblasts. Dermatofibrosarcoma protuberans (58, 59) is a well-differentiated fibrosarcoma that is usually multinodular, basically benign, and the fibroblasts are arranged in a storiform pattern. Again, local recurrence is common if incompletely excised.

The use of the electron microscope has been particularly valuable in determining whether a lesion is benign or malignant (53, 54, 57). In fact, it is urged that anytime a patient is diagnosed as having a sarcoma, an ultrastructural evaluation be performed to assist in therapeutic decisions.

Treatment

The type of therapy depends upon the type of lesion being diagnosed. Leiomyosarcomas, by and large, have been treated by radical resection (51) along with removal of regional lymph nodes. This same treatment holds true for the neurofibrosarcomas and the rhabdomyosarcomas. With the less aggressive lesions such as liposarcoma and low grade fibrosarcomas, wide local resection is all that is necessary. If patients do have a recurrence after initial therapy, a repeat resection is often successful in treating the problem.

Radiation therapy should be tried in those patients who have recurrent disease as it has been beneficial in some cases. DiSaia used chemotherapy in a number of patients and reported surprisingly good success in controlling distant as well as local disease (51).

While most series report a relatively low survival for the sarcomas, late diagnosis of the disease is probably the causal factor. Early diagnosis results in a high cure rate, and if lesions are picked up at a reasonably early stage, the patient's expectation for cure is quite high.

REFERENCES

1 Silverberg E. Cancer Statistics. 1985; 35: 19.

2 Sober AJ et al. Cutaneous melanoma in the-northeastern United States: data from the Melanoma Clinical Cooperative Group. In: Balch CM, Milton G eds Cutaneous Melanoma: Clinical Management and Treatment Results Worldwide. Philadelphia: JB Lippincott: 437.

3 Sober AJ, Rhodes AR, Mihm MC, Fitzpatrick TB. Neoplasms: malignant melanoma. In: Fitzpatrick TB, Eisen AZ, Wolff K, Freedberg IM, Austen KF eds Dermatology in General Medicine. New York: McGraw-Hill: 947–1004.

4 Podratz KC, Gaffey TA, Symmonds RE, Johansen KL, O'Brien PC. Melanoma of the vulva: an update. Gynecol Oncol 1983; 16: 153.

5 Reed RJ. Acrolentiginous melanoma. In: New Concepts in Surgical Pathology of Skin. New York: John Wiley & Sons: 99.

6 Seiji M et al. Malignant melanoma of the palmar–plantar–subungual–mucosal type: clinical and histopathological features. In: Klaus SN ed Pigment Cell, Vol 5. Basel: Karger: 95.

7 Friedman RJ, Kopf AW, Jones WB. Malignant melanoma in association with lichen sclerosus on the vulva of a 14-year-old. Am J Dermatol 1984; 6: 253.

8 Morrow CP. Melanoma of the female genital tract. In: Coppleson M ed Gynecology Oncology: Fundamental Principles and Clinical Practice, Vol 2. New York: Churchill Livingstone: 784–792.

9 Gleicher N, Cohen CJ, Deppe G, Gusberg SB. Familial malignant melanoma of the female genitalia: a case report and review. Obstet Gynecol Rev 1979; 34: 1.

10 Morrow CP, DiSaia PJ. Malignant melanoma of the female genitalia: a clinical analysis. Obstet Gynecol Surv 1976; 31: 233.

11 Morrow CP, Rutledge FN. Melanoma of the vulva. Obstet Gynecol 1972; 39: 745.

12 Morrow CP, Townsend DE. Malignant tumors of the vulva. In: Synopsis of Gynecology Oncology. New York: John Wiley & Sons: 1971: 78–84.

13 Johnson TL, Kumar NB, White CD, Morley GW. Prognostic features of vulvar melanoma: a clinicopathologic analysis. Int J Gynecol Pathol 1986; 5: 110.

14 Poderantz KC, Gaffey TA, Symmonds RE, Johansen KL, O'Brien PC. Melanoma of the vulva: an update. Gynecol Oncol 1983; 16: 153.

15 Chung AF, Woodruff JM, Lewis JL. Malignant melanoma of the vulva. Obstet Gynecol 1975; 45: 638.

16 Bastable JH, Gompel C, Verhest A. Malignant melanoma of the vulva. Diag Gynecol Obstet 1980; 2: 55.

17 Beller U, Demopoulos R, Beckman EM. Vulvovaginal melanoma. J Repro Med 1986; 31: 315.

18 Benda JA, Platz CE, Anderson B. Malignant melanoma of the vulva: a clinical-pathologic review of 16 cases. Int J Gynecol Pathol 1986; 5: 202.

19 Bouma J, Weening JJ, Elders A. Malignant melanoma of the vulva: report of 18 cases. Europ J Obstet Reprod Biol 1982; 13: 237.

20 Edington PT and Monaghan JM. Malignant melanoma of the vulva and vagina. Br J Obstet Gynecol 1980; 87: 422.

21 Jaramillo BA, Ganjei P, Averette HE, Sevin B, Lovecchio JL. Malignant melanoma of the vulva. Obstet Gynecol 1985; 66: 398.

22 Simonsen E, Alm P, Johnsson J.-E, Trope C. The recovery pattern of patients with vulvar melanoma treated by combined surgery and radiation therapy. Ann Chirurgiae et Gynaecol 1982; 71: 334.

23 Warner TFCS, Hafez GR, Buchler DA. Neurotropic melanoma of the vulva. Cancer 1982; 49: 999.

24 Karlen JR, Piver MS, Barlow JJ. Melanoma of the vulva. Obstet Gynecol 1975; 45: 181.

25 Ariel IM. Malignant melanoma of the female genital system: a report of 48 patients and review of the literature. J Surg Oncol 1981; 16: 371.

26 Phillips GL, Twiggs LB, Okagaki T. Vulvar melanoma: a microstaging study. Gynecol Oncol 1982; 14: 80.

27 Breslow A. Thickness, cross-sectional areas and depth of invasion in the prognosis of cutaneous melanoma. Ann Surg 1970; 172: 902.

28 Baltzer J, Kurzl RY, Lohe KJ, Zander J. Melanoma of the vulva. J Repro Med 1986; 31: 825.

29 Phillips GL, Twiggs LB, Okagaki T. Vulvar melanoma: a microstaging study. Gynecol Oncol 1982; 14: 80.

30 Bagley FH, Cody B, Lee A, Legg MD. Changes in clinical presentation in management of malignant melanoma. Cancer 1981; 2: 126.

31 Cleophax JP, Pilleron JD, Durand JC, Lourant M. Le mélanome de la vulve. Gynécologie 1977; 27: 333.

32 Spitler L et al. The therapy of patients with malignant melanoma using a monoclonal anti-melanoma antibody-Ricin a chain immunotoxin. Cancer Res 1987; 47: 1717.

33 Sim FH, Taylor WF, Ivins JC, Pritchard DJ, Soule EH. A prospective randomized study of the efficacy of routine elective lymphadenectomy in management of malignant melanoma. Cancer 1978; 41: 948.

34 Veronesi U et al. Inefficiency of immediate node dissection in stage I melanoma of the limbs. N Engl J Med 1977; 297: 627.

35 Paget J. On disease of the mammary areola, preceding cancer of the mammary gland. St Barth Hosp Rep 1874; 10: 87.

36 Dubrewilh W. Paget's disease of the vulva. Br J Dermatol 1901; 13: 407.

37 Ferenczy A. Pathology of malignant tumors of vulva and vagina. In: Coppleson M ed Gynecology Oncology: Fundamental Principles and Clinical Practice. New York: Churchill Livingstone: 285–338.

38 Woodruff JD. Paget's disease of the vulva: review; report of two cases. Obstet Gynecol 1955; 5: 175.

39 Friedrich Jr EG. Intraepithelial neoplasm of vulva. In: Coppleson M ed Gynecology Oncology: Fundamental Principles and Clinical Practice, Vol 1. New York: Churchill Livingstone: 313–19.

40 Dietel M, Bahnsen J, Stegner HE, Holzel F. Paget's disease of the vulva with underlying apocrine adenocarcinoma and local lymph node invasion. Path Res Pract 1981; 171: 353.

41 James LP, Worsham GF, Hoskins WJ, Belcik R. Apocrine adenocarcinoma of the vulva with associated Paget's disease. Acta Cytol 1983; 28: 178.

42 Pitman GH, McCarthy JG, Perzin KH, Herter FP. Extramammary Paget's disease. Plas Reconst Surg 1982.

43 Masukawa T, Friedrich EG. Cytopathology of Paget's disease of the vulva. Acta Cytol 1978; 22: 476.

44 Stegner HE. Ultrastructure of preneoplastic lesions of the vulva. J Repro Med 1986; 31: 815.

45 Gunn R, Gallager S. Vulvar Paget's disease: A topographic study. Cancer 1980; 46: 590.

46 Mazoujian G, Pinkus GS, Haagensen DE. Extramammary Paget's disease-evidence for an apocrine origin. Am J Surg Pathol 1984; 8: 43.

47 McKee PH, Hertogs KT. Endocervical adenocarcinoma and vulval Paget's disease: a significant association. Br J Dermatol 1980; 103: 443.

48 Stacy D, Burrell MO, Franklin E. Extramammary Paget's disease of the vulva and anus: Use of intraoperative frozen-section margins. Am J Obstet Gynecol 1986; 155: 519.

49 Breen JL, Smith CH, Gregori C. Extramammary Paget's disease. Clin Obst Gyn 1978; 4: 1107.

50 Hart WR, Millman JB. Progression of intraepithelial Paget's disease of the vulva to invasive carcinoma. Cancer 1977; 40: 2333.

51 DiSaia PJ, Rutledge R, Smith JP. Sarcoma of the vulva. Obstet Gynecol 1971; 38: 180.

52 Davos I, Abell MR. Soft tissue sarcoma of the vulva. Gynecol Oncol 1976; 4: 70.

53 Hall DJ, Grimes MM, Goplerud DR. Epithelioid sarcoma of the vulva. Gynecol Oncol 1980; 9: 237.

54 Ulbright TM, Brokaw SA, Stehman FB, Roth LM. Epithelioid sarcoma of the vulva. Cancer 1983; 52: 1462.

55 Hall JSE, Amin UF. Fibrosarcoma of the vulva: Case reports and discussion. Int Surg 1981; 66: 185.

56 Shen J, D'ablaing G, Morrow CP. Alveolar soft part sarcoma of the vulva: Report of first case and review of literature. Gynecol Oncol 1982; 13: 120.

57 Gaffney EF, Bhagirath M, Bryan JA. Nodular fasciitis (pseudosarcomatous fasciitis) of the vulva. Int J Gynecol Pathol 1982; 1: 307.

58 Soltan MH. Dermatofribrosarcoma protuberans of the vulva. Br J Obstet Gynecol 1981; 88: 203.

59 Bock JE, Andreasson B, Thorn A, Holck S. Dermatofibrosarcoma protuberans of the vulva. Gynecol Oncol 1985; 20: 129.

Section **II**

Urological Tumours

Textbook of Uncommon Cancer
Edited by C.J. Williams, J.G. Krikorian, M.R. Green and D. Raghavan
© 1988 John Wiley & Sons Ltd

Chapter **14**

Rare Tumours of the Testis and Paratesticular Tissues

C.R. Hamilton and
A. Horwich
Clinical Academic Unit, Institute of Cancer Research and The Royal Marsden Hospital, Downs Road, Sutton, Surrey, UK

INTRODUCTION

The testes originate embryologically from the posterior abdominal wall. They have both endocrine and reproductive functions, and tumours of the testes and their adnexae (Figure 1) reflect this diversity both of origin and function. The majority of these neoplasms arise from germinal epithelium. Rarely tumours of lymphoid, interstitial or ductal origin arise in the testes and this chapter describes these together with tumours of paratesticular, mesothelial or connective tissues. The subsections of this chapter are as follows:

Non-Hodgkin's lymphoma of the testis.
Gonadal stromal tumours.
Adenocarcinoma of the rete testis.
Paratesticular rhabdomyosarcoma.
Malignant mesothelioma of the tunica vaginalis.

NON-HODGKIN'S LYMPHOMA
OF THE TESTIS

History

The first description of malignant lymphoma of the testis in 1877 is accredited to the French worker Malassez (1). The British surgeon Curling (2) also recognized it as a distinct tumour entity and in a case report published by Hutchinson (1889) (3) many of the notable features of this disease were illustrated in that the patient was elderly, had bilateral tumours and the disease disseminated widely to involve bone and subcutaneous tissues (a feature also of Malassez's original case). Early reports documented particular aspects of these rare tumours to be the age distribution of patients, the pattern of dissemination and the tendency to bilateral involvement. Ficari (4) reviewed the literature from 1877 to 1947; 10/18 cases were over 50 years of age, the skin was involved in 10 cases and the disease was bilateral in 8. More recently, Gowing (1976) (5) reported on 128 cases. Seventy-eight per cent were over 50 years of age, 20% had bilateral testicular involvement, and 62% had died of disseminated disease within 2 years. However, 15/124 treated by orchidectomy survived disease-free for 5 or more years supporting the conclusion that testicular lymphoma occurs as a primary manifestation of non-Hodgkin's lymphoma as well as in the context of disseminated disease.

The prognosis has been considered poor, in keeping with the aggressive histological

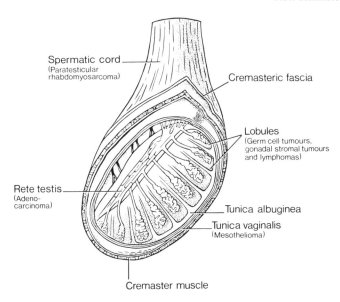

Figure 1 Diagram of testis and spermatic cord indicating sites of tumour origin. Paratesticular rhabdomyosarcoma may arise from connective tissue of the cord or of adjacent structures.

appearance of these tumours. However, the importance both of stage, emphasized by Kiely et al. [6] and the exact histological type [7] are now recognized, as is the high relapse rate in patients with early stage disease, leading to the investigation of systemic therapy even in Stage I disease.

Epidemiology and Aetiology

Testicular tumours are rare, affecting from < 1 to 4.5 per 100000 per year and there are marked racial and geographic variations [8].

The reported incidence is increasing [9] and the vast majority of these tumours arise from germinal epithelium. Non-Hodgkin's lymphoma accounts for approximately 5% of all testicular neoplasms (Table 1). The relative incidence increases with age (Figure 2). In patients over 50 years old lymphomas account for 25–50% of all testicular neoplasms (15). Nearly 80% of the cases reported by the British Testicular Tumour Panel were over 50, contrasting with just three children reported in the same series (5).

Extranodal non-Hodgkin's lymphoma pre-

TABLE 1 INCIDENCE AND AGE DISTRIBUTION OF TESTICULAR LYMPHOMAS

Series	Overall number of testicular tumours	Number with lymphoma	Age distribution
Eckert and Smith (1963) (10)	665	35 (5%)	—
Gowing (1976) (5)	2106	140 (6.5%)	78% over 50 years
Mehrotra et al. (1978) (11)	292	22 (7.5%)	—
Ciatto and Cionini (1978) (12)	280	12 (4%)	—
Read (1981) (13)	1307	51 (4%)	50% over 50 years
Hayes et al. (1983) (14)	220	17 (8%)	—

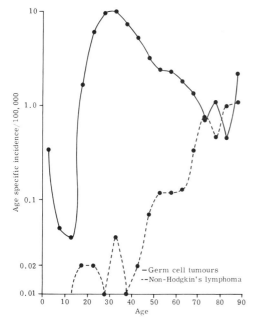

Figure 2 Incidence of germ cell tumours and of lymphomas of the testis by age of presentation. (Data from Thames Cancer Registry.)

senting in the testis is uncommon. The Princess Margaret Hospital, Toronto, was the sole radiation facility serving a population of four million and between January, 1967 and December, 1978, 1934 new patients with non-Hodgkin's lymphoma were referred of whom 16 (0.83%) had a primary testicular presentation (15). Wahal et al. (16) reported on non-Hodgkin's lymphoma in north India, and of 1283 cases, 264 (21%) were extranodal of which 20 (1.5%) presented with a testicular lesion. The aetiology of testicular lymphoma is unknown. Association with maldescent, trauma and familial occurrence, although all described, are probably not of aetiological significance (5).

Pathology and Biology

Testicular lymphoma may present with a very large testicular mass. Kiely et al. (6) recorded one case measuring 16 × 9 cm and weighing 750 g. In the British Testicular Tumour Panel

(BTTP) series (5) the largest tumour measured 13 × 10 × 8 cm and weighed 380 g. The cut surface may appear homogeneous or have yellowish areas of necrosis present and the colour has been variously described as cream, pink, grey or buff. No capsule is present and the lesions have ill-defined edges. Local extension is common.

Gowing (5) gives a full histological description of these tumours and the features that help to distinguish them from seminoma. In this series (5) all the tumours were composed of either poorly differentiated cells of the lymphocytic series or of lymphomas of larger undifferentiated cell type.

The classification most widely applied to testicular lymphoma has been that of Rappaport (17) and using this virtually all reported cases are of diffuse histiocytic or diffuse poorly differentiated lymphocytic type. Other classifications have been used and some have been compared to the Rappaport classification with regard to prognosis. Turner et al. (7) reported on 35 cases of malignant lymphoma of the testis classified both by the Rappaport criteria and the International Working Formulation of non-Hodgkin's lymphoma (18). All the tumours showed a diffuse pattern of growth and 29 were diffuse histiocytic lymphomas. In the Working Formulation 22 of these were of intermediate grade (large cell cleaved, large cell non-cleaved) and 7 high grade (immunoblastic lymphoma). Patients with intermediate grade lymphomas had a significantly better survival than those with high grade tumours and this difference was independent of stage. Jackson and Montessori (19) compared the Rappaport and Lukes and Collins (20) classification of malignant lymphoma and were able to separate the 16 adult cases, all described as diffuse histiocytic lymphomas into three groups using the Lukes and Collins classification (15) and demonstrated a significant trend in prognosis, patients with large cleaved cell lymphoma having the best outlook. Baldetorp et al. (21) analysed 24 patients, classifying the tumours according to the Rappaport and Kiel (22) classifications, and commented that there

TABLE 2 PROGNOSIS OF TESTICULAR LYMPHOMA

Author	Stage[a]	Number	% disease-free survival at 5 years
Gowing (1976) (5)	I–IV	128	12
Sussman et al. (1977) (23)	I–IV	37	20
Jackson and Montessori (1980) (19)	I–IV	194	14.5
Read (1981)[b] (13)	I/IIA	24	40
	IIB/IV	27	0
	I–IV	51	20

[a] Staging according to the Ann Arbor classification (24).
[b] I+IIA — no palpable metastases; IIB–IV — clinically overt metastases.

seemed to be survival advantages for patients with centroblastic/centrocytic lymphomas compared to those with immunoblastic or centroblastic lymphoma.

The prognosis of testicular non-Hodgkin's lymphoma is poor (Table 2). In the British Testicular Tumour Panel series, 62% had died of disseminated lymphoma within 2 years of presentation and only 15 of the 124 patients treated by orchidectomy survived 5 or more years postoperatively. Jackson and Montessori (19) confirmed this low 5-year survival rate by tabulating reported series up to 1977 and found only 28 out of 194 (14.5%) patients surviving disease free for > 5 years. In keeping with the aggressive nature of the disease most patients who succumb to lymphoma do so within the first 2 years, but there are a proportion of deaths that occur later. Sussman et al. (23) noted that of 37 patients, 24 (65%) died of disseminated disease; 71% of these died within the first year post orchidectomy, 17% within the second, 4% within the third, none in the fourth and 8% within the fifth year of follow-up. In all 80% of evaluable patients died of disseminated lymphoma within 5 years.

Undoubtedly survival is related to stage at presentation. Kiely et al. (6) stated that 'The prognosis for lymphoma clinically localised to the testis at the time of original diagnosis is relatively favourable after orchidectomy and radiation therapy to the regional lymph nodes. The previously held belief that life expectancy is poor for men with testicular lymphoma was due to failure in most reports to separate survival of those patients with localised tumour from that of patients with disseminated involvement at the time of orchiectomy.' In their study based on 31 patients, 17 had no evidence of lymphoma elsewhere in the body following orchidectomy. Staging procedures were not extensive, lymphography only occasionally being used. Most patients received postoperative radiotherapy to the regional nodes. Of the 17 patients, 5 survived for more than 5 years and a further 5 patients were alive without evidence of lymphoma with follow-up of 1–3 years.

The Royal Marsden Hospital series (24) demonstrated a significant benefit in lymphoma-free survival for 18 patients with Stage I–II disease compared to 6 patients with Stage III/IV disease, but there was no difference in the probability of lymphoma-free survival between the 10 Stage I and 8 Stage II patients. Turner et al. (7) also noted that increasing Stage correlated with decreasing survival; 8/14 Stage IE patients were alive and well with a mean follow-up of 2.5 years compared to 7/8 Stage IIE patients who died of disseminated lymphoma with survival ranging from 3 to 61 months (mean 27 months). The 2 patients with Stage IV disease both rapidly succumbed in less than 4 months. Buskirk et al. (25), reporting on 17 patients, did note a difference in survival between Stages IEA and IIEA with 73% of the former and 25% of the latter group surviving 2 years. No patient presenting with Stage IV disease survived 2 years. Tepperman et al. (15) analysed 16 patients and found that para-aortic nodal involvement was the strongest adverse prognostic factor. Median survival without this was 57+ months, but if the nodes were involved it was 6 months (p = 0.002). No patient with para-aortic node involvement survived beyond 19 months. Also described were two exceedingly rare cases, one of a primary nodular lymphoma of the testis and one of a mixed seminoma/lymphoma.

These tumours often disseminate widely. In the BTTP series (5) 13 (10%) had clinical evidence of disseminated disease at the time of orchidectomy. In series reported since 1980 the incidence of dissemination at the time of orchidectomy varies from 35 to 70% (13, 15, 21, 24, 25) (Table 3); this apparent increase probably reflects more sophisticated and sensitive staging procedures. The sites of possible metastatic involvement are numerous and reflect both lymphatic and hematogenous spread (Table 3). In the more recent series para-aortic node involvement as the sole extra-

gonadal site of disease occurred in just over one-third of cases. Less common sites of disease at presentation include clinical Stage III disease (9%), skin (7%), bone (5%), bone marrow (3%), liver (3%), upper airways (3%) and central nervous system (2%).

Sites of involvement at relapse are varied (Table 4) but the high incidence of upper airways (15%), central nervous system (10%) and bone involvement (10%) are noteworthy. The aggressive nature of the disease is also reflected in the short time to relapse in patients treated with local or locoregional therapy for early stage disease with most relapses within 2 years. Of the patients in the series shown in Table 3 (excluding Read (13)) with local and locoregional disease, 63% relapsed, and of relapses, 85% did so within 1 year and all within 2 years. In 14 patients with Stage IV disease, survival times ranged from 1 to 29 months (mean 8 months, median 3 months).

Bilateral testicular involvement occurs more

TABLE 3 TESTICULAR LYMPHOMA: STAGE DISTRIBUTION

Author	Number of cases				Stage IV major sites involved
	IE	IIE	IIIE	IV	
Duncan et al. (1980) (24)	10	8	2	4	Skin (3), Lung (1)
Read (1981) (13)		28	6	17	Bone (4), Skin (4), Lung (3), CNS (3), Upper airways (4), Bone marrow (2), Liver (1)
Tepperman et al. (1982) (15)	5	7	1	3	Liver (2)
Buskirk et al. (1982) (25)	11	4	0	2	Bone marrow (2)
Baldetorp et al. (1984) (21)	8	8	3	5	Bone (2), Liver (1), Skin (1)

TABLE 4 TESTICULAR LYMPHOMA: SITES OF RELAPSE

Author	Number of cases	Number relapsing	Major sites of relapse
Duncan et al. (1980) (24)	24	13	Upper aiways (5), Bone (5), Nodal (4), CNS (2)
Read (1981) (13)	51	—	Liver (11), Skin (9), CNS (5), Lung (5), Bone (2)
Tepperman et al. (1982) (15)	16	8	Nodal (4), CNS (3), Lungs (2)
Buskirk et al. (25)	17	11	Upper airways (5), CNS (2), Nodal (2), Mediastinum (2)
Baldetorp et al. (1984) (21)	24	13	Nodal (6), Upper airways (2), other testes (3)

commonly in testicular lymphoma than in any other testicular tumour with an incidence of the order of 20%. This is synchronous in about 5% of cases (5). Duncan (24) commented that patients presenting with bilateral testicular lymphoma usually have advanced disease with only 1/11 patients reported in the medical literature surviving > 2 years following locoregional therapy.

Clinical Features

Enlargement of the testicle is the usual presenting feature. The duration of symptoms in Talerman's series (26) varied from a few weeks to 3 years but was usually less than 6 months. Pain is present in 8–24% of cases and in 402 reported cases there appears to be a right to left preponderance of 1.4:1. The clinical features that may help to differentiate this tumour from the more common germ cell tumours and seminoma are the patient's older age, the tendency to bilateral involvement, lack of association with maldescent, the different pattern of metastatic spread and a lack of non-metastatic manifestation of malignant disease such as gynaecomastia. In the British Testicular Tumour Panel series (5) 78% of lymphoma patients were over 50 years of age and of all testicular tumour patients over 50 years, 26% had lymphoma. Many other authors have commented on this striking difference in age distribution from the more usual testicular tumours. In the series of Eckert and Smith (10) the mean age for lynphoma was 59.8 years compared to 33 years for teratoma and 42.3 years for seminoma.

Investigation and Staging

Patients should be staged according to the Ann Arbor classification (27). Important areas of clinical assessment include the contralateral testis, regional and other lymph node areas, the skin, the neurological system and the upper airways.

The following investigations are recommended: full blood count and differential, erythrocyte sedimentation rate, bone marrow aspirate and trephine biopsy, renal and liver function tests, alpha-fetoprotein and BHCG estimation, chest x-ray, bipedal lymphangiography and/or computerized assisted tomography of the abdomen and cerebro-spinal fluid cytology. Staging laparotomy has been infrequently reported and is not recommended in view of the age and stage distribution of patients and the emphasis on systemic treatment.

Management and Prognosis

Important considerations for appropriate management include the patient's age and general condition, the histological subtype and the stage of the disease.

Surgery. A radical inguinal orchidectomy is the recommended procedure. Historically, this was the only available method of treatment and undoubtedly can result in cure of a minority of patients. In Gowing's series (5) 15/124 patients treated by orchidectomy survived 5 or more years.

Radiotherapy. Abdominal and pelvic lymph node irradiation, e.g. by an inverted-Y field, has a role either as an adjuvant following orchidectomy or to treat overt disease; it has been employed alone and in combination with chemotherapy. The radiotherapy prescription as shown in Table 5 has varied in different institutions with a midplane dose recommendation of between 30 and 40 Gy in 20 fractions over 4 weeks using megavoltage equipment.

With orchidectomy and adjuvant radiotherapy, approximately 50% of Stage I patients and 20% of Stage II patients can be expected to be long-term survivors. Data on abdominal control of disease are scant, but following orchidectomy and radiotherapy abdominal recurrence was only seen as a solitary event in 2 cases and in conjunction with more widespread disease in 3 cases in the collected series of Duncan et al. (24), Tepperman et al. (15) and Buskirk et al (25). In view

TABLE 5 TESTICULAR LYMPHOMA: RADIOTHERAPY RESULTS

Author	Stage	Number of patients	Radiotherapy prescription	Disease-free survival
Duncan et al. (1980) (24)	IE	9	30–40 Gy in 20–24 in 34 days daily fractionation	45% 30% } at 5 years
	IIE	7		
Read (1981)[a] (13)	I/IIA	24	30 Gy in 20 — over 4 weeks	40% 0% } at 5 years
	IIB	4		
Tepperman et al. (1982) (15)	IE	4	25 Gy in 20 over 4 weeks	75% 17% } at 2 years
	IIE	6		
Buskirk et al. (1982) (25)	IE	8	25–40 Gy in 20 over 4 weeks	50% 33% } at 2 years
	IIE	3		

[a] Manchester staging system.

of the high systemic relapse rate consideration should be given to the use of adjuvant chemotherapy in early stage disease, this approach showing some promise in early stage lymphomas at other sites (28).

Chemotherapy. In recent series (13, 15, 24, 25) the survival rate of patients with Stage III and IV disease is very low. Of 35 patients with such extensive disease only one survived for more than 5 years. These results may be improved by the use of modern combination chemotherapy regimens, where high (> 75%) complete response rates have been reported especially by the use of alternating combinations such as M-BACOP (Skarin et al.) (29), PROMACE-MOPP (Fisher et al.) (30) or MACOP-B (Klimo and Connors) (31). However, these aggressive regimens are very toxic in elderly patients and CHOP is a less intensive alternative (McKelvey et al., 1976) (32). Chemotherapy has also been used in Stage I and II disease either alone or in combination with radiotherapy, but with insufficient frequency to make any useful statement.

Recommendations

In view of the high systemic relapse rate for patients with Stage I and Stage II disease we would recommend systemic chemotherapy followed by para-aortic and pelvic lymph node radiotherapy, 40 Gy mid-plane in 23 fractions over $4\frac{1}{2}$ weeks. The choice of chemotherapy would depend on histology of the disease and the age and health of the patient. Six courses of CHOP (32) could be considered appropriate.

Patients with more advanced disease, Stage III or IV should be managed as for advanced lymphoma at other sites (33), choice of chemotherapy again depending on histology, age and general health of the patient. CNS prophylaxis should be considered for those patients with advanced lymphoma of lymphoblastic type.

GONADAL STROMAL TUMOURS (GST)

Introduction

Mostofi et al. (1959) (34) referred to Sertoli and Leydig cell tumours as 'tumours of the specialised gonadal stroma', and suggested a common origin for these cell types. Although they are uncommon, they have attracted attention both because of the age distribution at presentation and because they may be hormonally active.

Leydig cells are named after Franz von Leydig (born 1821), the German anatomist who first described them. They arise embryologically from the posterior urogenital ridge secreting primarily testosterone, but also lesser amounts of oestrogens. They are capable of producing testosterone from cholesterol and secrete just under 10 mg of testosterone per day (35).

Sertoli cells are named after a Milan physiologist, Enrico Sertoli (born 1842) and they form the supporting cells of the seminiferous tubules lying between the germinal cells often with clumps of spermatids buried in their cytoplasm. Sertoli cells have certain features characteristic of hormone producing cells and although apparently unable to generate steroids they may be able to promote their interconversion.

The vast majority of GSTs are benign but about 10% metastasize (36). It is difficult to predict the malignant phenotype from the presenting characteristics. Surgery remains the mainstay of treatment.

Leydig Cell Tumour

Epidemiology and Aetiology

In the British Testicular Tumour Panel series of 2739 testicular tumours, 43 (1.6%) (37) were LCT. Mostofi (38) records a 3% and Ward et al. (39) a 2% incidence. The age of the BTTP series ranged from 21 to 81. Most published cases of LCT have occurred in adult life; childhood cases are rare (40).

Leydig cell hyperplasia may occur with testicular atrophy and although LCTs are reported with maldescent and atrophy, this association is of uncertain significance (37). Constant luteinizing hormone stimulation of the testis in experimental animals can induce both Leydig cell hyperplasia and LCT (41). Kim et al. (1985) (42) reported that only 37 cases of malignant LCT had been described; the average age was nearly 63 years.

Pathology and Biology

These tumours arise within the substance of the testis and are usually well demarcated with a striking yellow brown colour. They can, however, involve the rete testis and spermatic cord and do vary widely in size, the range in the BTTP series being 0.7–10 cm (37).

No seminiferous tubules are seen within the tumour and this helps to differentiate LCT from interstitial cell hyperplasia. The cells may be polygonal or fusiform in shape and usually have a granular cytoplasm in which crystalloids of Reinke may be seen. Mitotic figures can be frequent and do not necessarily imply malignancy (37).

Features of the primary lesion that should arouse suspicion of malignancy include large size (> 5 cm), lack of encapsulation, presence of satellite nodules, areas of necrosis and on microscopy, a very high mitotic index and vascular or lymphatic invasion (37). In the review by Kim et al. (42), 84% of the malignant LCTs were 5 cm or greater in diameter, 74% had an infiltrative margin and 72% lymphatic or vascular invasion.

In tumours behaving in a malignant fashion, metastases are present at diagnosis in about 25% of cases and develop in the remainder usually within 3 years. Recurrence after 5 years can occur but is uncommon (42). The commonest sites of metastases include the regional lymph nodes (68%), liver (45%), lung (45%), and bone (27%) (42).

Clinical Features

Malignant LCT tumours usually present in adult life. In the review by Grem et al. (43) the age range at presentation was 20–82 with a median age of 58 years. Painless testicular enlargement was present in 81%. All patients in this series by definition had metastases, 72% with regional node involvement, 43% with pulmonary metastases, 38% with hepatic metastases and 28% with lung involvement. Gynaecomastia was present in 19%. Metastases were present in 22% at presentation and developed within one year in a further 19%.

Investigations

A full endocrinological assessment of the pituitary/gonadal axis is advised with particular attention to androgen, oestrogen and progesterone production (35). The value of these data is that if elevated titres are noted they can act as a tumour marker. Elevation of urinary ketosteroids were seen in 14/22 patients (64%), of serum and/or urinary androgens in 12/22 patients (54%) and of serum or urinary oestrogens in 11/22 patients (50%) with metastatic Leydig cell tumours (43).

Computed tomography (CT) scanning of the chest and abdomen and/or lymphangiography should also be performed.

Management and Prognosis

Surgery. Inguinal orchidectomy is the treatment of choice for LCT and will cure the majority of patients. Malignancy is often defined in terms of the presence of metastic disease and surgery has been used to resect established regional nodal disease (44, 45) and also solitary pulmonary metastases (46) (this patient alive and disease-free 9 years from presentation and 3 years from resection of pulmonary disease). Cure can be anticipated if the disease is confined to the area resected. Most patients have multiple sites of metastases and surgery is not recommended in these circumstances.

Radiotherapy. This was prescribed for 11/32 patients with malignant LCT reviewed by Grem et al. (43). No objective responses were seen but 2 patients (bone metastases and a retroperitoneal mass) noted reduction in pain. Total radiation dose varied but no response was recorded in patients receiving 48 Gy (47), and 50 Gy (48) respectively as well as those receiving lower doses.

Chemotherapy. This has been presented only in the setting of advanced metastatic disease. Two out of 7 patients treated with *o, p'*-DDD responded, one with a reduction in liver size and falling urinary 17-ketosteroids and another with resolution of pulmonary nodules (43, 49).

Standard chemotherapy regimens incorporating adriamycin and cis-platinum have had no major benefit and more experimental therapy with Ionidamine, which can impair spermatogenesis probably via changes induced in Sertoli cells, although producing symptomatic improvement in 1/2 patients, produced no objective responses (43).

Prognosis is variable with a median survival of 2 years (range 2 months to 17 years). Survival after detection of metastases ranged from 1 month to 9 years with 2/3 patients dying within 2 years. As stated, metastases in the series of Grem et al. (43) were present at diagnosis in 22% and developed within 1 year in a further 19%.

Recommendations

Inguinal orchidectomy is recommended both to establish the diagnosis and to remove the primary lesion. In those patients whose tumours appear benign and whose hormone profile returns to normal post orchidectomy, no further treatment is recommended beyond surveillance. Those patients with histological features suspicious of malignancy should be fully investigated and if no evidence of spread of disease is found it is reasonable to monitor the patients closely, reserving lymphadenectomy for those who relapse either solely in regional nodes or with limited resectable pulmonary disease. Those patients who have disease limited to the regional nodes at presentation should have initially a retroperitoneal lymphadenectomy performed. Radiotherapy and chemotherapy should be reserved for palliation of patients with widespread or unresectable disease.

Sertoli Cell Tumour (SCT)

Epidemiology and Aetiology

In the BTTP series there were 32 SCTs (1.2%) reported (37). At least 7 exhibited malignancy. This figure is in keeping with other large reported series (38). The age of patients ranged from 2 months to 80 years with 7 patients presenting in the first decade of life. Godec (1985) (50) reported the eleventh case of malignant Sertoli cell tumour (excluding the BTTP series patients) and noted that in only 2 cases were children involved. SCT may be found either as pure tumours or in combination with germ cell tumours or other gonadal stromal tumours (36); the aetiology remains obscure.

Pathology and Biology

A full description of these tumours is provided by Symington and Cameron (37). SCTs arise within the testis and in the BTTP series showed considerable variation in size (1–30 cm (37)). They were well demarcated, often cystic and creamy white in colour. Histologically, SCTs usually show evidence of tubule formation and consist of a mixture of epithelial-like and stromal tissue with considerable differences in appearance being noted both within individual tumours and between different tumours. Call–Exner-like bodies are sometimes noted within larger aggregations of cells.

In the BTTP series, 7 cases were malignant. One child had a lymphadenectomy for regional node enlargement and remained disease-free 8 years later (51) and 6 patients died from SCT, 5 within 18 months. The sites of metastatic involvement included regional nodes, liver, lung, bone and brain. In 4/7 cases the tumour invaded either the rete testis, epididymis or spermatic cord and in all cases lymphatic and/or vascular invasion was seen.

The time from presentation to detection of metastases was generally short — 8/11 cases in a recent review (50) developed metastases within 1 year, although long disease-free intervals are occasionally noted.

Clinical Features

SCTs usually present with testicular swelling and 29/32 in the BTTP series did so in this manner (37). They may also be discovered on routine examinations or as an incidental finding either at autopsy or at operation for maldescent (37).

Gabrilove et al. (52) reported on 72 cases of SCT of which 60 were benign. Seventeen cases presented < 1 year of age, and 28 between 20 and 45 years. Malignancy was noted in only one child less than 10 years of age and was predominantly seen in patients over 25 years of age. Gynaecomastia was recorded in 17/72 cases of which it was associated with malignancy in 7. Hormone studies have been infrequent but elevation in serum and urinary oestrogens and testosterones have been reported.

Investigations

A full endocrinological assessment of the pituitary/gonadal axis is advised with particular attention being paid to androgen, oestrogen and progesterone production (35).

CT scanning of the chest and abdomen and lymphangiography should also be performed particularly when the primary tumour exhibits features of malignancy. BHCG, alpha-fetoprotein and placental alkaline phosphatase should also be measured to exclude germ cell tumour.

Management and Prognosis

Surgery. Inguinal orchidectomy is the treatment of choice for SCT and will cure the majority of patients.

Retroperitoneal lymph node dissection has been performed both as a staging/adjuvant (53) procedure and to resect established metastatic disease. The value of the former procedure though not tested in a trial setting, is apparent in case reports in which long-term survivors are reported following resection of both microscopic and macroscopic nodal disease (51, 54). In Godec's series reviewing 11 cases with malignant SCT, 4 had retroperitoneal lymph node dissection for nodal disease and 3 remain disease-free at 5 years, 7 months and 6 months respectively (50).

Radiotherapy. This has also been prescribed as adjuvant treatment to the inguinal nodes and to treat recurrent disease. In general, high radiation doses (> 40 Gy) have been recommended. The efficacy is unknown in an adjuvant setting, but combined with surgery or alone for known metastatic disease 3/5 patients remain alive at 5 years, $2\frac{1}{2}$ years and 7 months after treatment (50).

Chemotherapy. Chemotherapy has been infrequently prescribed for this rare tumour and no documented responses have been recorded.

Recommendations

Inguinal orchidectomy is recommended both to establish the diagnosis and to remove the primary lesion. In those patients whose tumours appear benign and whose hormone profile returns to normal post orchidectomy, no further treatment is recommended. Those patients with histological features suspicious of malignancy should be fully investigated and if no evidence of spread of disease is found it is reasonable to monitor the patients closely, reserving lymphadenectomy for those who relapse either solely in regional nodes or with limited resectable pulmonary disease. Those patients who have disease limited to the regional nodes at presentation should have initially a retroperitoneal lymphadenectomy performed. Radiotherapy should be reserved for palliation of patients with widespread or unresectable disease.

The prognosis is variable in the BTTP series (37) 6/7 with malignant SCT died within 18 months, and 1 after 18 years (histologically confirmed). In the series of Godec (50), 4/11 remain alive, deaths occurring within 2 years in 5/7 that died.

ADENOCARCINOMA OF THE RETE TESTIS (ART)

History

This tumour was first described by Curling (1853) (55). Feek and Hunter (1945) (56) outlined the histological criteria for diagnosis and Schoen and Rush (1959) (57) emphasized

its aggressive nature. More recently Sarma and Weilbaecher (1985) (58) confirmed its rarity reporting the twenty-first case and reviewed the literature indicating that long-term survival post orchidectomy was possible.

Epidemiology and Aetiology

This is a very rare tumour with less than 30 cases reported in the English literature. The age at presentation ranges from 20 to 89 years with a median of 47 and mean of 50 years (58). The aetiology is unknown although some patients have had a history of undescended testis (59), chronic epididymitis (60) or trauma (61).

Pathology and Biology

The rete testis forms part of the collecting system of the testis and tumours arising in the region tend to be located at the hilum. The largest ART measured $10 \times 10 \times 8$ cm and was yellow-grey in colour (60). A full description of these tumours is given by Mostofi and Price (62) who describe the tendency for this tumour to form papillary structures. The differential diagnosis includes seminoma invading the rete testis, adenocarcinoma arising from embryonic remnants and mesothelioma. Also, in cryptorchidism the relative increase or even hyperplasia of the cells of the collecting system can be misinterpreted as ART.

ART is an aggressive tumour both by virtue of local extension and local recurrence after excision and of wide dissemination. In 17 cases recently reviewed with adequate follow-up data, 10 patients developed metastases within 1 year of presentation (58). Sites of metastatic involvement included regional nodes, lung and liver.

Clinical Features

The tumour may arise in either testis and only one bilateral case is recorded. The most common presenting feature is an enlarging scrotal mass which may be tender and can have an associated hydrocele. The primary tumour can infiltrate widely, one case presenting with a scrotal sinus and urethral fistula with involvement of the prostate, trigone and ureteric orifices noted at autopsy (63). ART can also present with symptoms due to either nodal or metastatic disease.

Investigation and Staging

The authors recommend CT scanning of the thorax and abdomen and lymphangiography to assess extent of disease at diagnosis. Chest x-ray and routine haematological and biochemical tests should also be performed as well as serum estimations of alpha-fetoprotein and BhCG, and placental alkaline phosphatase in order to help in the differential diagnosis.

Management and Prognosis

Surgery. A radical inguinal orchidectomy is recommended and as local recurrence has been recorded after scrotal interference (64); this may be considered as indication for hemiscrotectomy.

Only 2 cases are recorded in which a retroperitoneal lymph node dissection was performed and where there is adequate follow-up information (58, 65). In one case the nodes were negative for tumour and in the other a solitary nodal metastasis was removed; both patients remain disease-free at 7 and $3\frac{1}{2}$ years respectively.

Radiotherapy. This has been prescribed to treat extensive local disease at the primary site, following orchidectomy as an adjuvant to the regional lymph nodes, and to treat metastatic disease.

The one patient presenting with extensive local disease and treated with radiotherapy alone (dose not stated) died 40 days from presentation having had no apparent response (63). In the 5 patients receiving adjuvant radiotherapy, one died at 2 months with metastases involving the skin and inguinal nodes and follow-up times were less than 1 year

in the remainder; the impact of radiotherapy in an adjuvant setting remaining unclear (58).

Of 14 patients presenting with or developing metastases, radiotherapy was prescribed in 7. In only one case was comment made about a beneficial response to radiotherapy, the patient remaining symptom-free at 5 months from presentation. Dose response data and information on local control with radiotherapy could not be ascertained (58) although in the report by Whitehead et al., no regression was seen despite an applied dose of 76 Gy using cobalt-60 (66).

Chemotherapy. This has been infrequently used and only in the setting of overt metastatic disease. No responses have been seen to combinations of cyclophosphamide, 5-fluorouracil and actinomycin D (66) or to single agent methotrexate (58).

Recommendations

Patients should have a radical inguinal orchidectomy and a hemiscrotectomy if scrotal violation has occurred. This establishes the diagnosis and should control the primary site. If no evidence of metastases is present on staging then consideration should be given to retroperitoneal lymph node dissection, based on the single case report of a long-term survivor who had a solitary lymph node metastasis resected (65). An alternative policy is one of surveillance with particular attention being paid to the regional lymph nodes reserving surgery for patients relapsing in that site alone.

Patients with metastatic disease limited to the regional nodes should be managed by surgery. Patients with distant metastases should be treated with palliative intent reserving radiotherapy and chemotherapy for specific symptoms. More information is required on the chemotherapy responsiveness of these tumours, especially using combinations that are active in germ cell tumours (67).

The prognosis overall is poor with only 5/17 patients remaining disease-free for periods of 5 months to 7 years (58).

PARATESTICULAR
RHABDOMYOSARCOMA (PTR)

History

Rokitansky is credited with the first case report of rhabdomyosarcoma affecting the spermatic cord (68) and in 1934 a review by Hirsh (69) pointed out that the majority of cases occurred in childhood. Tanimura and Furata (70) reviewed the literature and noted that the majority of patients died with disseminated disease within 1 year and that the overall prognosis was poor. Alexander (71), however, reported 2 long-term survivors who presented in early childhood when aged $2\frac{1}{2}$ years and 3 months and thought that the prognosis of this disease in young children was not necessarily so bad as had been previously claimed. This view was upheld in Gowing's series (68) and by Green (72) when reviewing available data from older surgical cases. The value of chemotherapy in rhabdomyosarcoma was clearly demonstrated in the 1970s and with the advent of effective chemotherapy Olive et al. (73) were able to demonstrate that regional surgery or radiotherapy was unnecessary in lymphogram negative patients managed by orchidectomy and adjuvant chemotherapy thus diminishing potential toxicity from these procedures. At present, attempts are being made to reduce toxicity from chemotherapy in early stage disease and improve chemotherapy for bad risk patients. The role of surgery and radiotherapy are as yet to be redefined.

Epidemiology and Aetiology

The most frequently encountered malignant tumour affecting the soft tissues in childhood is rhabdomyosarcoma. Between 1954 and 1973 2048 cases of malignancy in childhood were recorded by the Manchester University Children's Tumour Registry (CTR), and of these, 85 cases (4%) were rhabdomyosarcoma. Of 150 consecutive cases of soft tissue sarcoma seen by that group, 94 (63%) were rhabdo-myosarcomas (74). The overall incidence in Britain is approximately 4 cases per year per million of the population under 15 years of age (75) and this figure is in keeping with the United States experience reported by Young and Miller (76). Geographic variations in incidence are noted with Sweden having a particularly low incidence of approximately one case per year per million in children (77). A slight male to female preponderance is noted from collected series (72). In the CTR it was 1.5:1 (74). Paratesticular rhabdomyosarcoma represented 4% of the CTR cases and 8% of 573 cases from collected series (72) of rhabdomyosarcoma at all sites.

The aetiology of rhabdomyosarcoma is unknown. The fact that the tumour tends to occur at sites of fusion between the three layers of embryonic tissues and is more frequent in children with other anomalies (78) implicates problems of organ development in the aetiology.

An association with genetically transmitted disease exists, rhabdomyosarcoma occurring more frequently in particular with von Recklinghausen's disease (79). Interestingly, in von Recklinghausen's disease compound tumours consisting of schwannian elements and rhabdomyosarcoma are seen (80). These are sometimes called 'Triton' tumours after the experiments of Locatelli (81) in which implantation of the cut end of the sciatic nerve into Tritons (a small salamander) induced the growth of supernumerary limbs leading to the supposition that endoneural cells may be able to differentiate into muscle. There may also be a higher incidence of breast cancer in relatives (82).

The age incidence of rhabdomysarcoma shows two peaks, an early one around 5 years of age and one later on during adolescence (76). This bimodal distribution in age of presentation is also seen in paratesticular rhabdomyosarcoma (72). In the 22 cases referred to the British Testicular Tumour Panel series (68) a better prognosis was associated with younger age.

Pathology and Biology

PTR usually arises in the spermatic cord but it can compress or invade neighbouring structures such as the epididymis or testes and may be very extensive. The largest lesion in the BTTP series measured $14 \times 12 \times 7$ cm and weighed 980 g (68).

The histological subtype of PTR is embryonal rather than pleomorphic or alveolar and as indicated by Willis (83) arises from primitive embryonic tissue. Research on myocyte development shows that cross striations do not become apparent until the fourteenth week of embryonic life and the absence of such striations does not therefore preclude the diagnosis of rhabdomyosarcoma (84, 85). The usual histological appearance is of a myxoid stroma in association with small dark ovoid or spindle cells with varying degrees of myoblastic differentiation (74). These ovoid cells may show enlargement around an eccentrically placed nucleus producing the so-called 'Tadpole' or 'Tennis racquet' cells. Two histopathological

TABLE 6 CLASSIFICATION OF RHABDOMYOSARCOMA

The Rhabdomyosarcoma Group of the International Society of Paediatric Oncology (SIOP) Classification (86):

1. Embryonal type (293 cases)
   1.1 Dense
       1.1.1 Poorly differentiated   37%
       1.1.2 Well differentiated   14%
   1.2 Loose
       1.2.1 Botryoid   11%
       1.2.2 Non-botryoid   15%
   1.3 Alveolar   23%
2. Adult type (1 case)

Intergroup Rhabdomyosarcoma Classification (IRS) System (87) (581 cases):

1. Embryonal   57%
2. Alveolar   19%
3. Botryoid   6%
4. Pleomorphic   1%
5. Special undifferentiated type 1   4%
6. Special undifferentiated type 2   3%
7. Undifferentiated mesenchymal sarcoma   10%

classifications are shown in Table 6 (86, 87). The prognostic significance of such groupings is not yet clear.

Electron microscopy can help establish the diagnosis (88) by showing actin and myosin filaments. Antibodies to muscle proteins are useful for immunohistological assessments (89), especially to myosin or vimentin (90). These may help differentiate rhabdomyosarcoma from other small round cell tumours such as neuroblastoma, Ewing's sarcoma or lymphoma.

Paratesticular rhabdomyosarcoma may remain localized to the region of the spermatic cord and orchidectomy alone leads to a relapse-free survival of approximately 50% at 2 years with an even better outlook in those under 7 years compared to those over 7 years of age (77% versus 37% recurrence-free survival) (72). PTR is associated with a high incidence of regional lymph node involvement. Raney et al. (91) reported on 20 children with PTR presenting after 1972 one of whom had an abdominal mass at diagnosis. Fifteen of the children had surgical staging and 6 (40%) had node involvement. Not all these patients had lymphography or CT scanning and the incidence of node involvement in more rigorously defined Stage I patients may be lower. In fact 6 patients in the series had a normal lymphogram and on surgical staging 1 (16%) had node involvement. The incidence of node involvement does not vary with age (72).

Haematogenous metastases are uncommon at presentation occurring in less than 5% of patients (72), liver, bone marrow and lung involvement all being reported (72). The most common sites of recurrence after treatment for early stage disease include the retroperitoneal lymph nodes, lung, bone and bone marrow.

Clinical Features

The most common presenting feature is an enlarging painless scrotal mass. Duration of symptoms varied in Johnson's (92) series of 18 patients between 24 hours and 4 months and in 7 cases the tumour was initially unrecognized (hydrocele in 4, hernia in 2, epididymitis in 1). An associated hydrocele may be present (72). Less commonly symptoms are due to metastatic disease, especially in the regional lymph nodes. The presence of a scrotal mass in a child, especially if separate from the testis, should suggest the possibility of rhabdomyosarcoma.

Investigation

The following investigations are recommended: full blood count, differential and erythrocyte sedimentation rate, alpha-fetoprotein and BhCG estimation, renal and liver function tests, chest x-ray, CT scanning of the thorax and abdomen and bipedal lymphangiography.

The UICC published a TNM classification in 1982 (93) for rhabdomyosarcoma which has been widely accepted. Table 7 outlines the categories and clinicians are encouraged to use or at least relate their staging system to that of the UICC to allow comparison of studies. In Table 7 the Intergroup Rhabdomyosarcoma Study classification (94) is also shown.

Management and Prognosis

Surgery. Radical inguinal orchidectomy both confirms the diagnosis and usually completely removes the primary tumour. Prior scrotal violation, e.g. needle biopsy, may be regarded as an indication for hemiscrotectomy. With orchidectomy alone information from collected surgical series (72) suggests an approximately 50% 2 year relapse-free survival rate, this figure being higher in those under 7 years of age compared to those over 7 years of age (77% versus 37%) (72). For example, of 7 cases of PTR reported by Malek et al. (1972) (95) essentially treated by orchidectomy, 3 patients remained disease-free (follow-up of $1\frac{1}{2}$, 3 and 39 years) and 4 patients subsequently developed metastases (all older children).

TABLE 7 STAGING OF RHABDOMYOSARCOMA

TNM	Summary	pTNM	
T1	Confined to organ/tissue	Limited to organ	pT1
T1a	≤5 cm	Excision complete	
T1b	>5 cm		
T2	Involving other organs/tissues Effusion	Invasion beyond organ Excision incomplete	pT2
T2a	≤5 cm	Microscopic residual tumour	pT3a
T2b	≤5 cm	Macroscopic residual tumour	pT3b
T3/4	(Not applicable)	Non-resectable tumour	pT3c
N1	Regional involvement	Nodes completely resected	pN1a
		Nodes incompletely resected	pN1b

Intergroup Rhabdomyosarcoma Study (IRS):
Group I   Localized disease, completely removed, regional nodes not involved
           1.1 Confined to muscle or organ of origin
           1.2 Contiguous involvement with infiltration outside the muscle organ of origin, as through fascial planes
           Inclusion in this group includes both gross impression of complete removal and microscopic confirmation of complete removal
Group II   II.1 Grossly removed tumour with microscopic residual disease; no evidence of gross residual tumour; no evidence of regional node involvement
           II.2 Regional disease, completely removed (no microscopic residual disease)
           II.3 Regional disease with involved nodes, grossly removed, but with evidence of microscopic residual disease
Group IV   Distant metastatic disease present at onset

Arlen et al. (96) also correlated risk of recurrence with older age. Surgery has been used diagnostically to sample retroperitoneal nodes and also as a therapeutic measure with the rationale that PTR more frequently involves regional lymph nodes than rhabdomyosarcoma presenting at other sites and if all involved lymph nodes were to be resected and no other sites of metastatic disease exist, cure could be anticipated.

In the Intergroup Rhabdomyosarcoma Study reported by Raney et al. (91), 12 patients had radical lymphadenectomies and 3 patients lymph node sampling. This information was used as a guide to further management with node negative patients being randomized for adjuvant radiotherapy and node positive patients all receiving radiotherapy. All patients received adjuvant chemotherapy. None of the node negative patients and only one of the node positive patients relapsed (pulmonary metastasis). Five patients who did not undergo surgical staging had no clinical or radiological incidence of disseminated PTR and they also received adjuvant radiotherapy and chemotherapy and none have relapsed.

Surgical confirmation on the accuracy of lymphangiography is scarce. Raney reported on 1/6 (16%) lymphangiogram negative patients having involved nodes at retroperitoneal lymph node dissection and more recently Debruyne et al. (1985) (97) reporting on 7 patients with PTR found 2 with positive lymphangiograms and of the 5 patients with negative lymphangiograms 4 underwent further surgical staging and 2 (50%) were found to have involved lymph nodes.

Surgery also has a role in the management of patients who relapse and, when combined with chemotherapy and radiotherapy, has led to prolonged survival (73).

Radiotherapy. The Intergroup Rhabdomyosarcoma Study (IRS) series examined the role of local radiotherapy in 13 patients with completely excised primaries and no evidence of nodal metastases, randomizing patients to receive or not to receive local radiotherapy, in addition to adjuvant chemotherapy. No patient in either arm developed local recurrence suggesting that radiotherapy to the primary site is not usually indicated but could be considered if scrotal contamination has occurred (91).

Radiotherapy has also been recommended to the regional nodes as an adjuvant in Stage I PTR and also to treat known abdominal or pelvic nodal disease often in conjunction with chemotherapy and surgery. Historical series fail to confirm any advantage on patients managed by orchidectomy and radiotherapy versus orchidectomy alone (72) and radiotherapy to the para-aortic and pelvic lymph nodes in young children will produce growth impairment. In the IRS series (91) all 6 patients with nodal involvement received regional radiotherapy and only one patient relapsed (pulmonary metastases). These 6 patients had all been surgically staged and the authors comment that the good abdominal control of disease may reflect adequacy of node removal rather than control of disease by radiotherapy or chemotherapy. Tefft et al.(1980) (98) addressed the question of regional lymph node irradiation in rhabdomyosarcoma of the genitourinary tract in childhood, reporting on 58 cases. Thirty-eight patients had lymph node sampling of which 15 were positive. Eleven out of 15 patients with positive lymph nodes and 6/23 with negative lymph node sampling received radiotherapy as did 10 patients with no node sampling. The radiation prescription varied up to a maximum of 45 Gy in 5 to 6 weeks. In the entire series only one patient (who received 45 Gy to the regional nodes) failed in regional nodes. Despite the lack of demonstrable benefit either in terms of local control or survival the authors of this paper suggested that regional node irradiation was a wise precaution when nodes were found to be involved by tumour, but that doses should be limited to 35 Gy in 4 weeks.

Radiotherapy in combination with surgery and chemotherapy can result in prolonged survival in patients relapsing in regional lymph nodes (73).

Sequential hemibody radiotherapy (5 Gy to each half with a 6–8 week gap between treatment) in conjunction with chemotherapy and autologous marrow grafting if required has been used for 6 patients with disseminated rhabdomyosarcoma (2 cases were PTR). Five out of 6 have died of disease with a median duration of survival of 30 months and 1 patient remains disease-free at 15 months from diagnosis (99).

Chemotherapy. Rhabdomyosarcoma in childhood responds to single agents but it was the success of combinations (72) that led to chemotherapy having a major role in the management of PTR.

The adjuvant value of chemotherapy in rhabdomyosarcoma in which all disease has been apparently surgically resected was demonstrated by Heyn et al. (100) where 8/15 (53%) of patients treated by surgery and local radiotherapy developed recurrence or metastases versus 3/17 (17.6%) of patients receiving adjuvant chemotherapy (actinomycin D and vincristine). This achieved statistical significance (p = 0.03) and of interest is that of the 11 relapsing patients, 7 have died from disease, 6 in the non chemotherapy arm despite chemotherapy for relapse.

The early studies (91) on the impact of adjuvant chemotherapy on microscopic nodal disease in PTR was often obscured by the routine use of either para-aortic node dissection or abdominal radiotherapy. The study by Olive et al. (73) on 19 children with complete tumour removal and negative lymphangiograms confirms the effectiveness of combination chemotherapy as an adjuvant in this group. Eighteen out of 19 received adjuvant chemotherapy alone with combinations of vincristine, adriamycin, actinomycin D and cyclophosphamide, and of these 18 only one relapsed with spermatic cord and iliac lymph node involvement, and he was successfully salvaged with combined modality treatment and was considered cured 56 months later. The conclusion of the SIOP (Société Internationale d'oncologie Pédiatrique) rhabdomyosar-

coma group was that para-aortic lymphadenectomy was unnecessary in these 'low risk' patients defined by complete surgical resection and negative lymphangiograms and that chemotherapy could probably be reduced to a total duration of 8 months based on their results. Debruyne et al. (97), however, make the point that in their series of 7 patients with PTR those with negative surgical staging were successfully managed with less toxic chemotherapy using vincristine and actinomycin D alone for 11 months and that those with involved nodes could be selected for more aggressive chemotherapy.

Inference regarding the role of chemotherapy in metastatic PTR maybe drawn from studies of rhabdomyosarcoma at other sites. Using vincristine and actinomycin D in conjunction with appropriate surgery and radiotherapy Heyn et al. (100) achieved approximately a 20% 5-year survival in 14 patients with metastatic disease at presentation. The Intergroup Rhabdomyosarcoma Study (101, 102) series tested vincristine and actinomycin D against those two agents plus cyclophosphamide (VAC) and found no survival difference between the two regimens in patients with microscopic residual disease and/or nodal involvement with approximately a 70% relapse-free survival at 5 years. They also compared VAC and VAC plus adriamycin in patients with more advanced disease (gross residual disease/systemic metastases) achieving a response rate of over 80% in each arm with no differences in duration of response or survival being noted. In the report of Maurer et al. (101) from 1977, 423 children had been entered on the Intergroup Rhabdomyosarcoma Study series with 85 with microscopic or regional nodal disease and 151 with gross residual or metastatic disease. Less than 10% of patients with metastatic disease at presentation were alive at 2 years compared to over 60% with gross residual disease post surgery at presentation.

In the Children's Solid Tumour Group study reported by Kingston et al. (1983) (103) the 5-year predicted actuarial survival rate for

TABLE 8 RHABDOMYOSARCOMA—RESULTS OF TREATMENT

Series	Site	Stage	Number of patients	Treatment	% disease-free survival	Median duration of observation
Arlen et al. (1968) (96)	PTR	A11	6	S,R,C	50	3 years
Malek et al. (1971) (95)	PTR	A11	7	S,R	43	3 years
Raney et al. (1978) (91)	PTR	I[a]	13	S,C±R	100	23 months
		II	6	S,R,C	83	16 months
		IV	1	S,R,C	0	—
Olive et al. (1983) (73)	PTR	I[b]	19	C	89	>3 years
		II–IV	13	—	46	—
Debruyne et al. (1985) (97)	PTR	I–IIIE[a]	7	S,R,C	100	27 months
Kingston et al. (1983) (103)	All	All[c]	73	S,R,C	45	5 years[d]
		IV	14	S,R,C	<15	—

[a] IRS staging system.
[b] SIOP staging system.
[c] RMH/Barts staging system.
S=Abdominal surgery; R=radiotherapy; C=chemotherapy.
[d] Actuarial % disease-free survival at 5 years.

children with disease confined to the tissue of origin and no evidence of nodal or metastatic spread was 86% compared to 21% for those with extension outside the tissue of origin. Of the 73 children reported, 14 had distant metastases at presentation and were treated with VAC chemotherapy, surgery being usually confined to biopsy only and radiotherapy being prescribed to bulky disease. Approximately 15% survived 2 years. Results of treatment are shown in Table 8.

Since 1974, 17 cases of PTR have been managed at the Royal Marsden Hospital; 12 had no evidence of dissemination at presentations and 10 of these received adjuvant chemotherapy; 4 of this group relapsed in regional nodes at 14–35 months and 3 were salvaged with further chemotherapy, radiotherapy and surgery and remain disease free 2–10 years from presentation. Three children had regional nodal involvement at presentation and with a combined approach all are disease free at 9 months to 4 years from presentation. Of the two children with widespread metastases 1 died from PTR at 29 months from presentation and the other is disease free 7 years after presenting with hypercalcaemia,

bone marrow infiltration and bone destruction from PTR which was managed with orchidectomy and 2 years of chemotherapy with combinations of vincristine, adriamycin, actinomycin and oral cyclophosphamide.

Management summary. Adjuvant treatment is indicated following primary surgery for clinical Stage I PTR and the most extensive experience has been with 'VAC' chemotherapy. Cure rates are high >85% and it may be that less toxic chemotherapy could be employed particularly in those with negative surgical staging (97). The role of post chemotherapy radiotherapy is not established and we would only recommend it in post pubertal patients since (1) the prognosis in the older patient is not quite so good, (2) there would be a less significant effect on bone growth. An 'inverted Y' field is treated, 40 Gy in 20 fractions over 4 weeks.

Patients presenting with abdominal lymph node involvement should be managed by combined modalities. It is beneficial to use chemotherapy post orchidectomy and use nodal disease as a marker of response. In patients with a complete radiological response an argument for continued chemotherapy alone can be made (86), but the author's preference is to recommend surgical confirmation of response. In those presenting prior to their growth spurt with residual disease post chemotherapy the authors would recommend a surgical approach to the control of intra-abdominal disease. In those post puberty an argument for irradiation can be made and if this is to be combined with excision of previously abnormal nodes our preference would be radiotherapy followed by surgery.

Disseminated PTR should be managed as rhabdomyosarcoma at other sites and although high response rates using combinations of vincristine, cyclophosphamide and adriamycin are seen (102, 103) overall survival is poor (103).

MALIGNANT MESOTHELIOMA OF THE TUNICA VAGINALIS

Introduction

The tunica vaginalis surrounds the testis being formed from the processus vaginalis, which in eSsence is part of the peritoneum that is carried down to the scrotum during the descent of the testis. Malignant medothelioma of the tunica vaginalis (MMTV) is extremely rare and was first described in 1957 (104). Its association with prior asbestos exposure has been emphasized increasingly, 4/6 recently reported cases having such a history (105). Surgery represents the only potentially curative treatment and must be meticulously performed in view of the tendency for local recurrence. Careful appraisal of regional nodes is important as this represents a major pathway of dissemination. In the presence of metastatic disease radiotherapy and chemotherapy are used palliatively with optimal treatment yet to be defined.

Epidemiology and Aetiology

Malignant mesotheliomas can arise from any part of the body where a mesothelial mem-

brane exists; however, tumours of the tunica vaginalis (MMTV) are very rare. Antman et al. (105) reported on 6 cases adding them to the 18 already described in the literature. The age range of these patients was 21–78; the median age, however, was 60 with the majority of patients presenting during or after middle age. Of the 6 cases added to the literature by Antman 4 gave a clear history of prior asbestos exposure which may be of similar relevance in the aetiology of these tumours to that in malignant mesothelioma at other sites (106). Japko et al. (1982) (107) described a case in a 30 year old man who presented with a right scrotal swelling caused by MMTV. A detailed occupational history revealed that for 8 years the patient had worked as a pipe fitter in an oil refinery; his work involved placing asbestos insulation around large pipe-lines which he straddled during the insulation process.

Pathology and Biology

The gross and microscopic appearances of mesothelioma of the tunica vaginalis have been described by Mostofi and Price (108). The tumour usually presents as a hydrocele associated with a scrotal mass. The hydrocele fluid is often clear but can be blood stained and the tumour is seen as a papillary structure standing out from the clear smooth lining of the sac. Great variation in histological appearance occurs but it is often possible to trace continuity between the cells lining the hydrocele and the tumour itself. Mesothelial cells may produce hyaluronic acid but do not produce mucin so that immunohistochemical stains may help distinguish MMTV from metastatic lesions. Mesothelial cells also have distinct ultrastructural features, including abundant microvilli, and electron microscopy can be helpful in diagnosis (109). Regional lymph node involvement has been reported in 3/8 cases undergoing laparotomy and diffuse visceral nodules were seen in a further 2 cases (105). Distant metastases at presentation are rare but are seen on relapse with pulmonary involvement being the most readily apparent. MMTV also tends to recur locally and in the regional lymph nodes (105).

Time from initial therapy to relapse can vary considerably from months to many years. In a series of 24 patients there were 9 recurrences, 3 by 1 year, 5 by 2 years and 7 by 3 years from presentation (105).

Clinical Features

Malignant mesothelioma of the tunica vaginalis presents with a scrotal mass in association with a hydrocele and there may be a history of prior asbestos exposure. The tumour can produce multiple nodules and occasionally malignant mesothelioma of the peritoneum can spread to involve the tunica vaginalis and vice versa.

Investigations and Staging

In view of the propensity to spread to involve abdominal lymph nodes and lung, lymphangiography and CT scanning of the thorax and abdomen is recommended along with routine haematological and biochemical investigations.

Management and Prognosis

Surgery. Surgery is the mainstay of treatment for MMTV and a radical inguinal orchidectomy is the optimal surgical procedure. Transcrotal procedures are associated with local recurrence and where scrotal violation has occurred hemiscrotectomy should be considered. Patients who have radiological evidence of regional lymph node involvement with no evidence of distant metastases, require lymph node dissection, which can be curative—one such patient with histologically confirmed regional node involvement survived 15 years disease-free following such a procedure (110).

Retroperitoneal lymph node dissection as an adjuvant therapy is more controversial. As no other therapy except surgery is curative in MMTV an argument for a retroperitoneal lymph mode dissection at presentation can be

made in a patient with good general health; however, benefit from this treatment depends on the abdominal nodes being the only site of metastases. Of 8 patients undergoing laparotomy 3 were found to have lymph node involvement of whom only 1 survived disease-free. Three patients had negative laparotomies of whom 1 relapsed with groin nodes, 1 at the primary site and 1 remained disease-free. The 2 remaining patients were discovered to have multiple visceral nodules of disease at laparotomy. Sixteen patients did not undergo laparotomy and of these, only 2 relapsed with abdominal disease at 5 and 10 years respectively (105). A reasonable alternative approach would therefore be to monitor patients radiologically, reserving lymphadenectomy for those who relapse only in nodes.

Radiotherapy. This has been prescribed as part of the primary management of MMTV in 5/24 cases reported in the literature (107, 111, 114). The total doses prescribed varied from 25 Gy to 50 Gy and fractionation and overall time were not specified. In 2 of the cases patients were known to have spread of disease at laparotomy with either nodal or visceral deposits. Follow-up times ranged from 1.5 to 36 months and the impact of radiotherapy on survival is not clear.

It has also been used for those patients who develop local recurrence following surgery (105). Of 3 patients with such a complication 1 received radiotherapy (45 Gy total dose over approximately 1 month) following resection of the recurrence and, although he subsequently died from pulmonary metastases, he suffered no further local recurrences.

Radiotherapy can also be prescribed palliatively and occasional short partial responses are recorded (115).

Chemotherapy. A number of agents have been used to treat recurrent or metastatic MMTV. Partial responses were recorded in 3/7 such patients with doxorubicin-containing chemotherapy probably being the most active (105). The similarity between MMTV and malignant mesothelium at other sites would suggest that one may deduce from phase II studies that chemotherapy is largely ineffective although partial responses to high dose cisplatin were seen in 3/24 patients (116).

Recommendations

Radical inguinal orchidectomy and hemiscrotectomy for those patients with previous scrotal violation lead to a high local control rate. In those with no evidence of metastatic disease, patients should be followed clinically with special attention being paid to the primary site and the regional lymph nodes. Patients relapsing in these sites with no evidence of other disease should undergo further surgery and if resection margins are in doubt, consideration may be given to high dose local radio therapy. Similarly, patients presenting with metastatic disease solely involving the regional nodes should undergo radical surgery in an attempt to cure.

Patients relapsing with disseminated disease or who have unresectable disease should be managed palliatively. The efficacy of current chemotherapy is unproven though transient responses have occurred either to doxorubicin alone or in combination with cyclophosphamide and 5-fluorouracil. It is also likely that high doses of radiation would be required to cause tumour regression.

ACKNOWLEDGEMENTS

The authors are indebted to Mrs Julie Butcher for typing the manuscript and would also like to thank the Thames Cancer Registry for the data for Figure 2 and the Department of Medical Art for help with the illustrations.

REFERENCES

1 Malassez M. Lymphadénome du testicule. Bull Soc Anat Paris 1877; 52: 176.
2 Curling TB. In: A Practical Treatise on Diseases of the Testis, 4th edition. London: Churchill: 353.
3 Hutchinson J. Lymphosarcoma of both testes with considerable interval of time. Br Med J 1889; 1: 413.
4 Ficari A. A case of lymphosarcoma with metastases in unusual situations. J Path Bact 1950; 62: 103–11.
5 Gowing NFC. Malignant lymphoma of the testis. In: Pugh RCB ed Pathology of the Testis. London: Blackwell Scientific Publications, 1976: 334–55.
6 Kiely JM, Massey BD, Harrison EG, Utz DC. Lymphoma of the testis. Cancer 1970; 26: 847–52.
7 Turner RR, Colby TV, MacKintosh FR. Testicular lymphomas: a clinicopathologic study of 35 cases. Cancer 1981; 48: 2095–102.
8 Waterhouse J, Muir C, Shanmugaratnam K, Powell J. In: Cancer Incidence in Five Continents, Vol IV. International Agency for Research on Cancer, Lyon.
9 Waterhouse JAH. Epidemiology of testicular tumours. J Soc Med 1985: 3–7.
10 Eckert H, Smith JP. Malignant lymphoma of the testis. Br Med J 1963; ii: 891–4.
11 Mehrotra RML, Wahal KM, Agarwal PK. Testicular lymphoma: A clinicopathologic study of 22 cases. Indian J Pathol Microbiol, 21; 1978: 91–6.
12 Ciatto S, Cionini L. Malignant lymphoma of the testis. Acta Radiol Oncol 1979; 18: 572 6.
13 Read G. Lymphomas of the testis—results of treatment 1960–1977. Clin Radiol 1981; 32: 687–92.
14 Hayes MMM, Sacks MI, King HS. Testicular lymphoma: A retrospective review of 17 cases. S Afr Med J 1983; 64: 1014–16.
15 Tepperman BS, Gospodarowicz MK, Bush RS, Brown TC. Non-Hodgkin's lymphoma of the testis. Radiology 1982; 142: 203–8.
16 Wahal KM, Mehrota R, Agrawal PK. Extra nodal lymphomas in North India. J Indian Med Assoc 80; 1983: 130–2.
17 Rappaport H. Tumors of the hematopoietic system. In: Atlas of Tumor Pathology, Section 3, fasc. 8. Washington, DC: Armed Forces Institute of Pathology, 1966: 91–161.
18 The Non Hodgkin's Lymphoma Pathologic Classification Project. National Cancer Institute Sponsored study of classification of non Hodgkin's lymphomas. Cancer 1982; 49: 2112–35.
19 Jackson SM, Montessori GA. Malignant lymphoma of the testis: Review of 17 cases in British Columbia with survival related to pathological subclassification. J Urol 1980; 123: 881–3.
20 Lukes RJ, Collins RD. Immunological charac-

terisations of human malignant lymphomas. Cancer; 1974: 1488–1503.

21 Baldetorp LA, Brunkrall J, Cavallin-Stahl E, Henrikson H, Holm E, Olsson AM, Akerman M. Malignant lymphoma of the testis Br J Urol 1984: 56: 525–30.

22 Lennert K, Mohri N, Stein H, Kaiserling E. The histopathology of malignant lymphoma. Br J Haematol 1975; 31: Suppl 1193.

23 Sussman EB, Hajdu SI, Lieberman PH, Whitmore WF. Malignant lymphoma of the testis. A clinicopathologic study of 37 cases. J Urol 1977; 118: 1004–7.

24 Duncan PR, Checa F, Gowing NFC, McElwain TJ, Peckham MJ. Extranodal non-Hodgkin's lymphoma presenting in the testicle: A clinical and pathologic study of 24 cases. Cancer 1980; 45: 1578–84.

25 Buskirk SJ, Evans RG, Banks PM, O'Connell MJ, Earle JD. Primary lymphoma of the testis. Int J Radiat Oncol Biol Phys 1982; 8: 1699–1703.

26 Talerman A. Primary malignant lymphoma of the testis. J Urol 1977; 118: 783–6.

27 Carbone PP, Kaplan HS, Musshoff K, Smithers DW, Tubiana M. Report of the committee on Hodgkin's disease staging classification. Cancer Res 1971; 31: 1860–1.

28 Miller TP, Jones SE. Chemotherapy of localised histiocytic lymphoma. Lancet 1979: 358–60.

29 Skarin A, Canellos G, Rosenthal D et al. Therapy of diffuse histiocytic and undifferentiated lymphoma with high dose methotrexate and citrovonum rescue, bleomycin, adriamycin, cyclophosphamide, oncovin and decadron (M-BACOP). Proc Am Soc Clin Oncol 1980; 21: 463.

30 Fisher RI, DeVita VT, Hubbard SM et al. Pro MACE-MOPP combination chemotherapy: Treatment of diffuse lymphomas. Proc Am Soc Clin Oncol 1980; 21: 468.

31 Klimo P, Connorts JM. MACOP-B chemotherapy for the treatment of diffuse large cell lymphoma. Ann Intern Med 1985; 102: 596–602.

32 McKelvey EM, Gottlieb JA, Wilson HE et al. Hydroxyldaunomycin (adriamycin) combination chemotherapy in malignant lymphoma. Cancer 1976; 38: 1484–93.

33 Horwich A, Peckham MJ. 'Bad risk' non Hodgkin's lymphoma. Sem Oncol 1983; 20: 35–55.

34 Mostofi FK, Theiss, EA, Ashley DJB. Tumors of specialized gonadal stroma in human male patients. Cancer 1959; 12: 944–57.

35 Campbell EJM, Dickinson CJ, Slater JDH,

Edwards CRW, Sikora EK. In: Clinical Physiology, 5th edition. Blackwell Scientific Publications 1984: 651–708.

36 Javadpour N. Gonadal stromal tumours of the testis. In: Javadpour N ed Testicular Cancer. 19:383–6.

37 Symington T, Cameron KM. In: Pugh RCB ed Pathology of the Testis. London: Blackwell Scientific Publications, 1976; 259–303.

38 Mostofi FK. Testicular tumours. Cancer 1973; 32: 1186–1201.

39 Ward JA, Krantz S, Mendeloff J, Haltiwanger E. Interstitial cell tumour of the testis: Report of two cases. J Clin endocrinol 1960; 20: 1622–32.

40 Johnstone G. Pre-pubertal gynaecomastia in association with an interstitial cell tumour of the testis. Br J Urol 1967; 39: 211–20.

41 Bonset GM. Malignant tumours of the interstitial cells of the testis in Strong A mice treated with triphenylethylene. J Path Bact 1942; 54: 149–154.

42 Kim I, Young RH, Scully RE. Leydig cell tumours of the testis. Am J Surg Path 19, 9: 177–192.

43 Grem JL, Robins I, Wilson KS, Gilchrist K, Trump DL. Metastatic leydig cell tumor of the testis. Cancer 1986; 58: 2116–19.

44 Lockhart JL, Dalton DL, Vollmer RT, Glenn JF. Nonfunctioning interstitial cell carcinoma of testes. Urology 1976; 8: 392–4.

45 Kippel KF, Jonas U, Hohenfellner R, Walther D. Interstitial cell tumor of testis: a delicate problem. Urology 1979; 14: 79–82.

46 Parker RG. Treatment of apparent solitary pulmonary metastases. J Thorac Cardiovasc Surg 1958; 36: 81–7.

47 Feldman PS, Kovacs K, Horvath E, Adelson GL. Malignant Leydig cell tumor: Clinical, histologic and electron microscopic features. Cancer 1982; 49: 714–21.

48 Davis S, DiMartino NA, Schnieder G. Malignant interstitial cell carcinoma of the testis. Cancer 1981; 47: 425–31.

49 Azer PC, Braunstein GD. Malignant Leydig cell tumor: Objective tumor response to o,p'-DDD. Cancer 1981; 47: 1251–55.

50 Godec CJ. Malignant Sertoli cell tumour of the testicle. J Urol 1985; 16: 185–8.

51 Rosvoll RV, Woodward JR. Malignant Sertoli cell tumor of the testis. Cancer 1968; 22: 8–13.

52 Gabrilove JL, Freiberg EK, Leiter E, Nicolis GL. Feminising and non-feminising Sertoli cell tumours. J Urol 1980; 124: 757–67.

53 Weitzner S, Addridge JE, Lamar Weems W. Sertoli cell tumour of the testis. J Urol 1979; 13: 87–9.

54 Herera LO, Wilks H, Wills JS, Loper GE. Malignant (androblastoma) Sertoli cell tumor of testis. J Urol 1981; 18: 287–90.

55 Curling TB. Observations on cystic disease of the testicle. Medic-Chir Trans 1853; 36: 449.

56 Feek JD, Hunter WC. Papillary carcinoma arising from rete testis. Arch Pathol 1945; 30: 399.

57 Schoen SS, Rush BF. Adenocarcinoma of the rete testis. J Urol 1959; 82: 356–63.

58 Sarma DP, Weillbaecher TG. Adenocarcinoma of the rete testis. J Surg Oncol 1985; 30: 67–71.

59 Dundon C. Carcinoma of the rete testis occurring ten years after orchidopexy. Br J Urol 1952; 24: 58–63.

60 Desberg T, Tanno V. Adenocarcinoma of the rete testis. J Urol 1964; 91: 87–9.

61 Brown NJ. Miscellaneous tumors of mainly epithelial type. The pathology of testicular tumours. Br J Urol (Suppl) 1964; 36: 70–7.

62 Mostofi FK, Price EB. Tumors of the Male Genital System, Washington DC: Armed Forces Institute of Pathology, 1973: 170–3.

63 Roy JB, Boumann WE, Lewis TM, Fahmy A, Pitha J. Adenocarcinoma of rete testis. J Urol 1979; 14: 270–2.

64 Schapira HE, Engel M. Adenocarcinoma of rete testis. NY State J Med 1972; 72: 1283.

65 Winter CC, Puenta E, Lai DY, Sharma HM. Papillary carcinoma of the rete testis. J Urol 1981; 18: 168–70.

66 Whitehead ED, Valensi QJ, Brown JS. Adenocarcinoma of the rete testis J Urol 1972; 107: 992–9.

67 Peckham MJ, Barrett A, Liew, KH, Horwich A, Robinson B, Dobbs HJ, McElwain TJ, Hendry WF. The treatment of metastatic germ-cell testicular tumours with bleomycin, etoposide and cis-platinum (BEP). Br J Cancer 1983; 47: 613–19.

68 Gowing NFC. Paratesticular tumours of connective tissue and muscle. In: Pugh RCB ed Pathology of the Testis. London: Blackwell Scientific Publications, 1976: 317–33.

69 Hirsch EF. Rhabdomyosarcoma of the spermatic cord. Am J Cancer 1934; 20: 398–403.

70 Tanimura H, Furata M. Rhabdomyosarcoma of the spermatic cord. Cancer 1968; 22: 1215–20.

71 Alexander F. Pure Testicular Rhabdomyosarcoma. Br J Cancer 1968; 22: 498–501.

72 Green DM. Diagnosis and Management of Malignant Solid Tumour in Infants and Children. Martinus Nijhoff Publications: 15–90.

73 Olive D, Flamant F, Zucker JM, Voute P, Brunat-Mentigny M, Otten J, Dutou L. Para-

aortic lymphadenectomy is not necessary in the treatment of localised paratesticular rhabdomyosarcoma. Cancer 1984; 54: 1283–7.

74 Marsden HB. In: D'Argio GJ, Evans AE, eds Bone Tumours and Soft Tissue Sarcomas. London: Edward Arnold, 1985: 14–25.

75 Draper GJ, Birch JM, Bithell JF, Kinnier Wilson LM, Leck I, Marsden HB, Morris Jones PH, Stiller CA, Swindell R. Childhood cancer in Britain 1953–1975: Incidence, mortality and survival. Studies in Medical and Population Subjects 1982 No. 37. London: HMSO.

76 Young JL, Miller RW. Incidence of malignant tumours in U.S. children. J Pediatr 1975; 86: 254–8.

77 Ericsson JL-E, Karnstrom L. Mattsson B. Childhood cancer in Sweden. 1958–1974. Acta Paediatr Scand 1978; 67: 425–32.

78 Voute PA, Barrett A. Rhabdomyosarcoma. In: Voute PR, Barrett A. Bloom HJG, Lemele J eds Cancer in Children: Clinical Management, 2nd edition. Springer Verlag, 1986: 316–25.

79 McKeen EA, Bodurtha J, Meadows AT, Douglass EC, Mulvhill JJ. Rhabdomyosarcoma complicating multiple neurofibromatosis. J Pediatr 1978; 93: 992–3.

80 Woodruss JM, Chernik NL, Smith MC, Millett WB, Foote FW Jr. Peripheral nerve tumors with rhabdomyosarcomatous differentiation (malignant Triton: tumors). Cancer 1973; 32: 426.

81 Locatelli P. Formation de Membres Surnuméraires. CR Assoc 20e réunion Turin 1925: 279–82.

82 Li FP, Fraumeni JF. Rhabdomyosarcoma in children: epidemiologic study and identification of a familiar cancer syndrome. J Natl Cancer Inst 1969; 43: 1365–73.

83 Willis RA. In: Pathology of Tumours London: Butterworth, 1948: 589–590.

84 Patton RB, Horn RC Jr. Rhabdomyosarcoma: Clinical and pathological features and comparison with human fetal and embryonal skeletal muscle. Surgery 1962; 52: 572–84.

85 Porterfield JF, Zimmermann LE. Rhabdomyosarcoma of the orbit. A clinico pathological study of 55 cases. Virchows Archiv [A] 1962; 335: 329–44.

86 Flamant F, Rodary CH, Voute PR, Otten J. Primary chemotherapy in the treatment of rhabdomyosarcoma in children: Trial of the International Society of Paediatric Oncology SIOP preliminary results. Radiother Oncol 1985; 3: 187–293.

87 Gaiger AM, Soule EH, Newton WA. Pathology of rhabdomyosarcoma. Experience of the

intergroup rhabdomyosarcoma study 1972–8. Natl Cancer Inst Monogr 1981; 56: 19–27.

88 Mierau GW, Favara BE. Rhabdomyosarcoma in children. Ultrastructural study of 31 cases. Cancer 1980; 46: 2035–40.

89 Toskos M, Howard R, Costa J. Immunohistochemical study of alveolar and embryonal rhabdomyosarcoma Lab Invest 1983; 48: 148–55.

90 Gabbiani G, Kapanci Y, Barazzone P, Franke W. Immunochemical identification of intermediate size filaments in human neoplastic cells. Am J Pathol 1981; 104: 206.

91 Raney RB Jr, Hays DM, Lawrence W Jr, Soule EH. Tefft M, Donaldson MH. Paratesticular rhabdomyosarcoma in childhood. Cancer 1978; 42: 729–36.

92 Johnson DE, McHugh TA, Jaffe N. Paratesticular rhabdomyosarcoma in childhood. J Urol 1982; 128: 1275–6.

93 Spiesse B, Hermanek P, Scheibe O, Wagner G. In: Spiesse B, Hermanek P, Scheibe O, Wagner G eds UICC T.N.M. Atlas: Illustrated Guide to the TNM. pTNM Classification of Malignant Tumours, 2nd edition. Berlin, Heidelberg, New York, Tokyo: Springer, 1982.

94 Mauer HM, Donaldson M, Gehan EA. The intergroup rhabdomyosarcoma study, J Natl Cancer Inst Monogr 1981; 56: 61–8.

95 Malek RS, Utz DC, Farrow GM. Malignant tumours of the spermatic cord. Cancer 1972; 29: 1108–13.

96 Arlen M, Grabstald H, Whitmore WF Jr. Malignant tumours of the spermatic cord Cancer 1969; 23: 525–32.

97 Debruyne FMJ, Bokkerink JPM, de Vries JDM. In: Khoury S, Kuss R, Murphy G, Chatelain C, Karr JP eds Testicular Cancer. Alan R. Liss, 507–517.

98 Tefft M, Hays D, Raney RB Jr, Lawrence W, Soule E, Donaldson MH, Sutow WW, Gehan E. Radiation to regional nodes for rhabdomyosarcoma of the genitourinary tract in children: Is it necessary? Cancer 1980; 45: 3065–8.

99 Munoz LL, Wharam MD, Kaizer H, Beventhal G, Ruymann F. Magna-field irradiation and autologous marrow rescue in the treatment of pediatric solid tumours. Int J Radiat Oncol Biol Phys 1983; 9: 1951–4.

100 Heyn RM, Holland R, Newton WA et al. The role of combined chemotherapy in the treatment of rhabdomyosarcoma in children. Cancer 1974; 34: 2128–42.

101 Maurer HM, Moon T, Donaldson M. The Intergroup Rhabdomyosarcoma Study: A preliminary report. Cancer 1977; 40: 2015–26.

102 Maurer HM. The intergroup rhabdomyosarcoma study: Update, November 1978. Natl Cancer Inst Monogr 1981; 56: 61–8.

103 Kingston JE, McElwain TJ, Malpas JS. Childhood rhabdomyosarcoma: Experience of the Children's Solid Tumour Group. Br J Cancer 1983; 48: 195–207.

104 Barbera V, Rubino M. Papillary mesothelioma of the tunica vaginalis. Cancer 1957; 10: 183–9.

105 Antman K, Cohen S, Dimitrov NV, Green M, Muggia F. Malignant mesothelioma of the tunica vaginalis testis. J Clin Oncol 1984; 2: 447–51.

106 Wagner JC. Asbestos carcinogenesis. Br J Cancer 1975; 32: 258–9.

107 Japko K, Horta AA, Schreiber K, Mitsudo S, Karwa GL, Singh G, Koss LG. Malignant mesothelioma of the tunica vaginalis. Cancer 1982; 49: 119–27.

108 Mostofi FK, Price EB. Tumors of the Male Genital System. Washington DC. Armed Forces Institute of Pathology, 1973: 170–3.

109 Ehya H. Cytology of mesothelioma of the tunica vaginalis metastasis to the lung. Acta Cytol 1985; 29: 79–84.

110 Arlen M, Grabstald H, Whitmore WF. Malignant tumors of the spermatic cord. Cancer 1969; 23: 525–32.

111 Kasdon EJ. Malignant mesothelioma of the tunica vaginalis propria testis: Report of two cases. Cancer 1969; 23: 1144–50.

112 Fishelovitch D, Meiraz Z, Green I. Malignant mesothelioma of the testicular tunica vaginalis. Br J Urol 1975; 47: 208.

113 Tang CK, Gray GD, Keuhnelian JG. Malignant peritoneal mesothelioma in an inguinal hernia sac. Cancer 1976; 37: 1887–90.

114 Eimoto T, Inoue I. Malignant fibrous mesothelioma of the tunica vaginalis: A histologic and ultrastructural study. Cancer 1977; 39: 2059–66.

115 Fligiel Z, Kaneko M. Malignant mesothelioma of the tunica vaginalis propria testis in a patient with asbestos exposure: A case report. Cancer 1976; 37: 1478–84.

116 Mintzer DM, Kelsen D, Frimmer D, Heelan R, Gralla R. Phase II trial of high dose cisplatin in patients with malignant mesothelioma. Cancer Treat Rep 1985; 69: 711–12.

Textbook of Uncommon Cancer
Edited by C.J. Williams, J.G. Krikorian, M.R. Green and D. Raghavan
© 1988 John Wiley & Sons Ltd

Chapter **15**

The Biology and Management of Small Cell Undifferentiated Carcinoma of the Prostate

Margaret E. Jelbart*,
Pamela J. Russell*
Peter Russell† and
Derek Raghavan*‡

* *Urological Cancer Research Unit, † Department of Anatomical Pathology and ‡ Department of Clinical Oncology, Royal Prince Alfred Hospital and University of Sydney, Sydney, Australia*

INTRODUCTION

Little is known about the biology of small cell undifferentiated carcinoma of the prostate (SCUCP). Until recently, there has been no experimental model for the study of this disease, and our current knowledge is based on published data consisting predominantly of case reports. Furthermore, this entity has been recognized only infrequently, and has represented less than 1% of prostatic tumours. In some systems of classification of prostatic neoplasms, SCUCP has not even been described as a separate entity (1). In fact, SCUCP probably occurs with greater frequency than has hitherto been recognized. For example, Sommers (1957) (2) demonstrated in an autopsy study of 109 patients with prostatic carcinoma (without any other malignancies) that 14% had adrenal cortical hyperplasia, which could imply the presence of occult SCUCP with ectopic production of adrenocorticotrophic hormone (ACTH). In the same study, one-third of the 43 cases in which parathyroid tissue was studied had histological evidence of glandular hyperplasia (perhaps implying the presence of raised levels of parathyroid hormone (PTH)).

In view of the rarity of previous experience, it is not possible to be dogmatic about the optimal management of this disease. However, we have attempted to review the available literature, and have drawn upon our experience, as well as adapting some principles from the management of the more common variant of small cell undifferentiated cancer (SCUC) which arises as a bronchogenic tumour.

PATHOLOGY

Approximately half of the cases of SCUCP reported in the literature have been associated with clinical syndromes suggesting ectopic hormone production, directing the pathologist's attention to particular morphological and functional details consistent with neuroendocrine differentiation. For more than 40 years, it has been known that endocrine-paracrine cells (argentaffin- or argyrophil-staining) are present in the normal and hyperplastic prostate gland (3–5). Just as SCUC of the lung has been thought to arise from the so-called bronchial K-cells (6), the histologically similar SCUCP may also derive from this type of cell (7). However, more recent studies have indicated considerable overlap between both pulmonary and prostatic SCUC and the more common epithelial malignancies at both histological and ultrastructural levels (8, 9). Indeed, a significant majority of SCUCP have presented as mixed tumours with a prominent epithelial component, or have emerged during the treatment of prostatic adenocarcinomas. Thus SCUCP and prostatic adenocarcinoma may have a common cell of origin (see below). Further complicating the issue, carcinoid tumours also occur in the prostate, either in isolation or with coexistent adenocarcinoma, and may well form part of a continuum with SCUC as there is substantial histological overlap between the two patterns.

The pathology of SCUCP reflects these considerations and the characteristic morphology is of sheets and nests of uniform cells almost devoid of cell-to-cell orientation. At best, there is some focal suggestion of perivascular or peripheral palisading along the epithelial–stromal interfaces, but more typically, no such arrangement is apparent. Microscopic or larger foci of tumour necrosis are prominent, as is the 'streaming effect' of haematoxyphilic debris. The tumour infiltrates widely and diffusely in a lymphoma-like fashion with poorly circumscribed margins at the advancing edge (Figure 1). Lymphatic and blood vessel permeation are usually evident, and small tumour emboli may be seen at a distance from the infiltrating edge of the carcinoma. The stroma between the tumour islands is immature and fibroblastic. Remnants of normal prostatic tissue may be seen, entrapped or encircled by the carcinoma.

Cytologically, the small uniform cells have

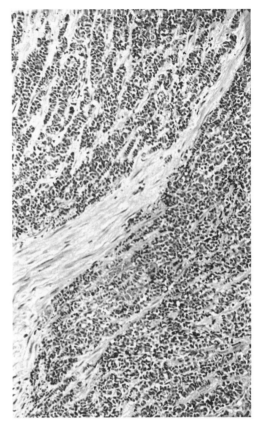

Figure 1 Small cell undifferentiated prostate cancer—note pattern of infiltration.

rounded hyperchromatic nuclei, coarse chromatin and usually inapparent nucleoli. Mitotic figures are numerous, occurring at a rate of five to ten per high power field in most regions. The cytoplasm is scanty and, in many areas, the nuclei appear 'naked' (Figure 2). Mucin stains are negative, while argyrophil granules (Grimelius technique) are variably present. Argentaffin granules are usually not observed (Fontana–Masson method). By the immunoperoxidase technique, the profile of tumour markers (Table 1) includes positive staining for neuroendocrine (non-specific enolase (NSE), bombesin and chromogranin) and various polypeptide hormones (see below), and negative staining for markers of prostatic glandular differentiation (prostate-specific

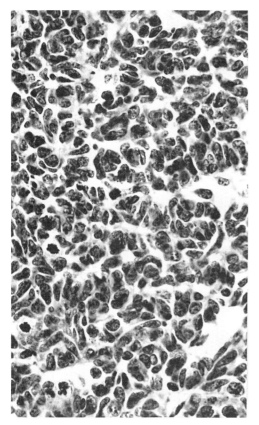

Figure 2 Small cell undifferentiated prostate cancer—note scanty cytoplasm and dominance of nuclei.

antigen (PSA) and prostatic acid phosphatase (PAcP)).

The electron microscopic features of SCUCP are similar to those of SCUC occurring at other sites, and include typical small (140–250 nm), roughly circular neurosecretory dense-core granules (10, 11). Small, well-formed desmosomes have been described in at least one study (11).

Most cases of SCUCP described to date have shown concurrent or antecedent prostatic adenocarcinoma (Table 3). In those tumours with a mixed pattern, the adenocarcinoma has been of the moderately to poorly differentiated microacinar type, with intermingling of tumour elements and transitional areas. We regard identification of an adenocarcinomatous component as an important confirmation

that the tumour has arisen in the prostate, although it is not an absolute requirement for the diagnosis of SCUCP. In many instances, such confirmation has not been possible before autopsy has been performed, and hence the definitive diagnosis of SCUCP has often not been achieved sufficiently early in the clinical course to be of benefit to the patient.

An alternative explanation for the presence of SCUC in the prostatic region is that the lesion represents a metastasis from a bronchogenic tumour (12, 13). With an increasing awareness of the entity of SCUCP, clinicians and pathologists may be able to stage the tumours more appropriately and thus establish the correct diagnosis at an earlier stage.

In those tumours with mixed elements of SCUC and adenocarcinoma, these latter regions have retained their immunoreactivity for PSA and PAcP in large measure (Table 1). It should be borne in mind that, in as many as one-third of prostatic carcinomas, spanning the entire histological spectrum, occasional cells may contain argyrophil granules and will show immuno-staining suggestive of neuroendocrine differentiation (14, 15).

TUMOUR MARKERS AND ECTOPIC HORMONE PRODUCTION

Polypeptide hormones constitute the major biochemical markers of SCUCP, exhibiting features characteristic of the endocrine-paracrine cells described above (so-called amine precursor uptake and decarboxylation or 'APUD' cells). The production of these hormones is associated morphologically with argyrophil staining or, at an ultrastructural level, with the presence of the neurosecretory granules previously discussed. However, the production of these 'ectopic' hormones (Table 2) which can be demonstrated immunohistochemically in tumour tissue or by radioimmunoassay of blood, is not exclusive to SCUCP (16). For example, the production of ACTH, anti-diuretic hormone (ADH) and calcitonin has been reported in patients with non-small cell carcinoma of the lung and with a variety of

TABLE 1 CELLULAR EXPRESSION OF TUMOUR ANTIGENS (IMMUNOHISTOCHEMICAL DEMONSTRATION)

Histological element	Tumour antigen					Reference
	PAcP	PSA	CEA	NSE	EMA	
SCUC ⎱	−	ND	−	ND	ND	
AdCA ⎰	+	ND	+/−	ND	ND	Schron et al. (9)
SCUC ⎱	ND	−	+	+	ND	Ghandur-Mnaymneh et al. (24)
AdCA ⎰	ND	+	−	−	ND	
Carcinoid ⎱						
AdCA ⎰	+[a]	+[a]	ND	ND	ND	Ghali and Garcia (32)
SCUC/carcinoid	ND	+	ND	ND	ND	Almagro (33)
SCUC	−	−	−	−	ND	Bleichner et al. (60)
SCUC	−[b]	−[b]	+[c]	+[d]	ND	Ro et al. (11)
SCUC ⎱	+[e]	+[e]	+[c]	+	ND	
AdCA ⎰	+	+	+[e]	−	ND	Ro et al. (11)
SCUC	−	−	+[f]	+[a]	+	Van Haaften-Day et al. (49)

[a] Variable
[b] 1/9 cases positive.
[c] 5/18 cases positive.
[d] 6/9 cases positive.
[e] 2/9 cases positive.
[f] 4/9 cases positive.
Key: AdCA: adenocarcinoma; ND: not done, PSA, NSE, PAcP, EMA, CEA; see text.

TABLE 2 HORMONES EXPRESSED IN SCUCP

Histology	Hormone	Method		Reference
		RIA	IPX	
Oat cell	ACTH	+	+	Wenk et al. (10)
Undiff ⎱ AdCA ⎰	ACTH	+	ND	Wise et al. (29)
SCUC ⎱	ACTH	ND	+ ⎱	Vuitch and Mendelsohn (21)
AdCA ⎰	ACTH	ND	− ⎰	
SCUC	ACTH	−	ND	Hindson et al. (28)
SCUC	ACTH	−[a]	−[a]	Van Haften-Day et al. (49)
Undiff ⎱ AdCA ⎰	ACTH	+	ND	Holland (61)
Undiff ⎱ AdCA ⎰	ACTH	+	ND	Lovern et al. (62)
Carcinoid ⎱ AdCA ⎰	ACTH	+	+	Ghali and Garcia (32)
Carcinoid ⎱ AdCA ⎰	ACTH	+	+	Capella et al. (14)
SCUC	CRF	+	+	Carey et al. (25)
SCUC	ADH			Sellwood et al. (23)

[a] cf. Jelbart et al. (26).
Key: RIA: radioimmunoassay; IPX: immunoperoxidase; ND: not done; CRF: corticotrophin releasing factor; ADH: anti-diuretic hormone; ACTH: adrenocorticotrophic hormone.
+ = detected; − = not detected.

other tumours. Even in classical adenocarcinoma of the prostate, hypercalcaemia (which may be due to the production of parathyroid hormone (PTH) or a PTH-like substance) has been reported (17–19). Paradoxically, prostate adenocarcinoma may be associated with hypocalcaemia, but it is not known whether this is due to the production of an ectopic hormone.

To date, ACTH appears to be the most common ectopic hormone in SCUCP, either in association with clinically evident Cushing's syndrome or solely on the basis of biochemical, immunohistochemical or endocrinological tests (10, 20–22). ADH has been described in association with 2 cases of primary SCUCP (23, 24) and there has been a case report of a metastatic SCUCP that elaborated corticotrophin (25). In addition, we have demonstrated low levels of bombesin-like immunoreactivity and the production of somatostatin in a cell line derived from a xenografted SCUCP (26), as discussed below.

However, cases of SCUCP have been described in which no ectopic hormone production has been detected (9, 27, 28). Furthermore, in several of the cases in which ectopic hormone production is thought to have occurred, the diagnosis has merely been presumptive, on the basis of biochemical changes (e.g. hypokalaemic alkalosis) or autopsy data (adrenal hyperplasia) (2, 29, 30).

The characteristic markers of prostate cancer, PSA and PAcP, are not usually expressed in foci of SCUCP, although they are often detected immunohistochemically in coexistent regions of adenocarcinoma (Table 1). By contrast, these markers have been demonstrated in both the adenocarcinomatous and carcinoid components of prostatic carcinoid tumours (31–33). In typical adenocarcinoma of the prostate, these markers are more ubiquitous. In a detailed study of 60 prostate cancers graded according to the system of the M.D. Anderson Hospital, all Grade I–III tumours expressed PSA and PAcP, whereas 5% of Grade IV tumours failed to reveal these antigens (34). Heyderman et al. (1984) (35)

showed that 100% of prostate cancers stained positively for PAcP, but demonstrated heterogeneity of expression within individual tumour deposits.

A variety of epithelial and other tumour markers have been reported in cases of SCUCP, although their use appears limited. For example, carcinoembryonic antigen (CEA) has been demonstrated in 25% of prostate cancers (35), but is not a specific marker. Its expression has been correlated with decreasing differentiation of the adenocarcinoma cells (34, 36). As shown in Table 1, CEA is also variably expressed in SCUCP, and may be associated with either, both or neither of the elements of SCUC and adenocarcinoma.

Epithelial membrane antigen (EMA) is expressed in normal prostate cells (37) and is seen focally in up to 80% of prostate adenocarcinomas, although its presence does not correlate with histological grade (34, 35). It is not found on cells of normal endocrine tissue nor in classical neuroendocrine tumours, but has been reported to be expressed by some SCUC of lung (37).

Neurone-specific enolase (NSE), an enzyme of anaerobic glycolysis that is present in neuroendocrine cells, has been extensively reported as a marker of SCUC of the lung. Recently its expression has been found to vary with both the proliferative state and the level of oxygenation of bronchogenic SCUC (38), and we do not regard it as a useful clinical marker for this tumour phenotype. There is discordance of expression of NSE and of the classical prostate markers: In one study, NSE was expressed in 6 of 9 cases of pure SCUCP, none of which stained for PSA or PAcP (11), a pattern also reported by Ghandur-Mnaymneh et al. (1986) (24). Conversely, Ro et al. (1987) (11) described one case of SCUCP which stained for PSA and PAcP but did not express NSE. In mixed tumours, the adenocarcinomatous components did not stain for NSE, whereas 5 of 10 tumours expressed this antigen in regions of SCUC differentiation (11, 24).

In clinical practice, the role of these markers has been restricted predominantly to diagnosis, and in partcular to the more detailed characterization of undifferentiated tumours. In contrast to the serial measurement of blood levels of alpha-fetoprotein and human chorionic gonadotrophin in the management of germ cell and trophoblastic tumours, CEA appears to have little role in the monitoring of the clinical course of SCUCP. The potential role of NSE and EMA has not yet been defined in this context. Although the measurement of ectopic hormones could, in theory, provide an index of the efficacy of treatment of SCUCP, this approach has not been well documented to date. It is not clear whether the presence of these ectopic hormones (or their corresponding clinical syndromes) acts as an adverse prognostic determinant per se, although several of the cases of SCUCP with ectopic hormone production have been characterized by short survival.

DNA CONTENT AND CHROMOSOMAL ANALYSIS

Flow cytometry has been used to measure the DNA content of tumour cells (diploid or aneuploid) and to assess the percentage of cells that are involved in DNA synthesis and cell division. The flow cytometric analysis of prostatic adenocarcinoma has been reviewed by Sandberg (1980) (39). Poorly differentiated prostatic adenocarcinoma is usually aneuploid (40, 41), often in the triploid to tetraploid range. By contrast, well differentiated tumours are predominantly diploid. Approximately two-thirds of moderately differentiated tumours are aneuploid, in the near tetraploid region (41). We are not aware of any detailed studies of the DNA content of SCUCP, other than the information that we have gained from our assessment of a xenografted line (42), as discussed below.

Chromosomal analysis of cell lines derived from prostatic adenocarcinomas has shown them to be mostly triploid or tetraploid, with one showing a pseudodiploid profile (reviewed by Pittman et al., 1987) (42). Direct karyotyping has been recorded for four primary carcinomas and one bone marrow metastasis (43,

44). The most common abnormalities described in these studies included deletions of the long arm of chromosome 10, chromosome 7, structural rearrangements of chromosome 1, and loss or rearrangement of the Y chromosome. These chromosomal alterations did not correlate with the level of histological differentiation of the tumours. Our studies of the xenografted line of SCUCP have revealed a hypodiploid karyotype with several structural alterations, as discussed below.

The cytogenetics of bronchogenic SCUC, which have been studied by direct karyotyping and by the analysis of cell lines established in vitro (45, 46), provide an interesting contrast to the data obtained from studies of typical prostatic adenocarcinoma. Marked chromosomal heterogeneity has been reported in the bronchogenic tumours, with a wide range of consistent abnormalities. These have included deletion of a part of the short arm of chromosome 3, the presence of markers associated with chromosomes 1, 6 and 11 and the detection of minute and double minute chromosomes. Although the chromosome 1 markers were of a variable structure, 6 and 11 frequently took the form of 6q− and 11p+ (46). However, as noted below, there is an interesting similarity of the 1p+ marker chromosome in a model of SCUCP with that shown in a cell line of SCUC of lung (42).

ONCOGENES AND PROSTATE CANCER

The expression of oncogenes, their possible mutation, rearrangement, or amplification in cancer tissue, is the subject of intensive study. To date, no studies of oncogenes have been reported in SCUCP. However, for completeness it is worth noting that preliminary data are available with respect to typical prostatic adenocarcinoma. The *ras* oncogene, which encodes a 21 000—dalton protein (p21), is expressed in prostate cancer tissue, correlating directly with the degree of nuclear anaplasia and inversely with the level of glandular differentiation (47). Large amounts of *ras* and *myc* mRNA have been demonstrated in poorly and moderately differentiated prostatic cancer cell lines (48). It may, however, be possible to distinguish between the levels of differentiation at a molecular level on the basis of expression of the *fos* oncogene (which is associated with rapidly dividing cells). However, further data from the SCUCP xenograft and from lines of bronchogenic SCUC will be required to define the true relationship between SCUCP, prostatic adenocarcinoma and SCUC of lung.

A XENOGRAFT MODEL OF SMALL CELL UNDIFFERENTIATED CARCINOMA OF THE PROSTATE

We have established a xenograft line, designated UCRU-PR-2, from a primary prostatic SCUCP and have characterized it in serial passages in nude mice and in tissue culture (26, 49). Immunohistochemistry has revealed heavy staining for CEA and NSE, and focal areas of expression of EMA. By contrast, PAcP, PSA and ACTH and a range of polypeptide hormones have not been detected by these methods (49). However, radioimmunoassay has revealed the production of ACTH by all tumour fragments tested and by cells in tissue culture (26). Calcitonin was not detected, but bombesin-like immunoreactivity was present in low levels in some samples.

Despite negative immunohistochemistry, the serum of tumour-bearing nude mice contained human PAcP. This difference may reflect the high tumour:host mass ratio in the xenograft model (50). This discrepancy suggests that if clinically relevant and technically feasible, more accurate assessment of hormone and enzyme content of SCUCP may be obtained by methods other than the more convenient immunohistochemistry.

Flow cytometry has shown UCRU-PR-2 to be consistently diploid. The karyotype is hypodiploid with non-random losses of chromosomes 6, 7, 10 and 13, and with structural rearrangements of chromosomes 1 and 2. In addition, three unidentified markers have been detected. Thus, the xenografted SCUCP shows

the deletion of chromosome 10 which is characteristic of prostatic adenocarcinoma and, as previously noted, a similarity of the 1p+ chromosome found in some samples of bronchogenic SCUC.

HISTOGENESIS

The histogenesis of SCUCP is controversial. These tumours are morphologically similar to other tumour types which ectopically secrete hormones and which exhibit the neuroendocrine features of 'APUD' cells. It has been proposed that APUD cells are derived from the neural crest (51) and that this origin is shared by a varitety of 'neuroendocrine' tumours. A neural crest origin is thus postulated for those tumours that produce peptide hormones and which are characterized ultrastructurally by the presence of neurosecretory granules. For SCUCP, this would imply origin from the argentaffin/argyrophil cells that are normally present in the prostate (10, 14, 52). However, there is accumulating evidence that APUD cells in the gastrointestinal and respiratory tracts may not be derived in this fashion, but may have differentiated within the developing endoderm during the course of embryogenesis (53–55).

The major alternative hypothesis to the neural crest origin for SCUCP is that it arises through divergent differentiation within otherwise typical prostatic adenocarcinomas (16, 56). As shown in Table 3, several patients have been reported in whom an initial presentation of adenocarcinoma of the prostate preceded the development of SCUCP (9, 24, 27, 49). In some instances, SCUCP and adenocarcinoma coincide, with clear transition zones evident (9, 24). Similarly areas of transitional overlap have previously been reported between seminoma and teratoma of the testis (57), two tumours originally thought to have separate origins but subsequently shown to derive from a common precursor cell. Thus it is conceivable that SCUCP and adenocarcinoma of the prostate share a common cell of origin, with their respective phenotypes repre-

TABLE 3 SMALL CELL UNDIFFERENTIATED CANCER OF PROSTATE: CLINICAL DETAILS

Age	Pattern of SCUCP	Presence of Adeno CA	Expression of PSA/PAcP	Ectopic hormones	Sites — Local	Bone	Other	Response — Hormone therapy	Chemo-therapy	Sites at autopsy	Series
56	?	Yes	?	+	+	+	–	Yes	NA	B, L, Pr, Sp, N	Wise et al. (1965) (29)
58	Undiff.	Yes	+	+	+	+	Pl effusion Adrenal	Yes	NA	?	Wise et al. (1965) (29)
63	Undiff.	Yes	?	+	+	–	Liver	Yes	NA	Pr, L	Hall (1968) (30)
57	Undiff.	Yes (undiff.)	?	+	+	+	Liver	NA	NA	L, Lu, B	Newmark et al. (1973) (20)
66	Undiff.	Yes	–	+	+	–	Liver	Yes	NA	L, Sp, Gb, N	Lovern et al. (1975) (62)
62	Oat cell	Yes?	–	+	+	–	–	NA	NA	Pr, N, Bl	Wenk et al. (1977) (10)
76	Undiff.	Yes	?	+	+	–	–	NA	NA	Pr	Holland (1978) (61)
77	Carcinoid	Yes	?	?	+	–	–	NA	NA	Pr	Montasser et al. (1979) (63)
77	Carcinoid	No	?	?	+	–	–	NA	NA	Pr	Wasserstein and Goldman (1981) (64)
80	Undiff.	Yes	+	–	+	–	–	Yes	No	Pr, N, B	Schron et al. (1984) (64)
67	Undiff.	Yes	+	–	+	+	Liver	No	?	Pr, B, L, Lu, N, Pe	Schron et al. (1984) (9)
70	Undiff.	Yes	+	+	+	+	–	Yes	?	Pr, N, B, L	Schron et al. (1984) (9)
76	Carcinoid	Yes	+	+	–	–	–	NA	NA	N, Sp, Lu, M, Ad, Pr, L	Ghali and Garcia (1984) (32)
61	Undiff.	No	–	–	+	+	Left SCF Liver	No	Yes	Lu, L, Sp, Ad, M, N, Br	Hindson et al. (1985) (28)
70	Carcinoid	Yes	+	?	+	–	–	NA	NA	Pr, N, B, Lu	Almagro (1985) (33)
73	Oat cell	Yes	–	+	+	+	Liver	NA	NA	Pr, B, N, Pl, Pe, St	Ghandur-Mnaymneh et al. (1986) (24)
60	Undiff.	No	–	–	+	–	Liver	NA	NA	Pr, L, N, Ad	Bleichner et al. (1986) (60)
72	Undiff.	Yes (small acinar)	+	–	+	+	–	Yes	NA	Br, L, Lu, Bl	Van Haaften-Day et al. (1987) (49)

M: marrow; B: bone; Lu: lung; L: liver; BPl: pleura; Pr: prostate; Br: brain; Sp: spleen; Gb: gall bladder; St: stomach; Ad: adrenal; Bl: bladder; Pe: pericardium; PSA: prostate specific antigen; PAcP: prostatic acid phosphatase; SCF: supraclavicular fossa; NA: not applicable. N: nodes.

senting a function of divergent differentiation. Although incomplete, our initial studies of the xenografted SCUCP support this concept: Serial passages exhibit concurrent features of epithelial differentiation (CEA, EMA, PAcP) as well as neuroendocrine function (NSE, neurosecretory granules). Whether the production of polypeptide hormones is attributed to an endodermal or neuroectodermal origin, this index of functional differentiation is most easily explained by origin from a pluripotential stem cell. Whatever the histogenesis, it is clear that SCUCP is often intimately associated with elements of adenocarcinoma. Thus, the formulation of a plan of management, both diagnostic and therapeutic, should take into account the presence of tumour cells with a wide range of potential characteristics—both with respect to histology and expression of tumour markers, as well as sensitivity to hormonal manipulation, radiotherapy or cytotoxic agents. Equally, the management of ordinary adenocarcinoma of the prostate may require modification as it appears likely that SCUCP has previously been under-diagnosed, and may well account for a proportion of 'resistant' prostatic adenocarcinomas.

CLINICAL PRESENTATION

The prospective clinical diagnosis of SCUCP is rarely made, with the majority of cases having been diagnosed either at autopsy or late in the course of the disease. As shown in Table 3, there are many similarities to the presentation of ordinary adenocarcinoma of prostate. Indeed antecedent or concomitant adenocarcinoma is often present. The population of patients consists of males, predominantly in the age range of 60 to 80 years, with features of local and distant involvement. Thus, the presenting symptoms include urinary outflow obstruction, frequency, nocturia, haematuria and occasionally rectal symptoms due to the effects of the enlarged prostate. A common feature is pain due to osseous metastases that distinguishes SCUCP clinically. In the small number of available case reports, there have

been several instances of metastasis to the liver, spleen and lung parenchyma, which are relatively unusual features for prostatic adenocarcinoma.

In approximately half of the reported cases (including some in which a presumptive diagnosis of SCUCP has been made in retrospect), patients have presented with 'endocrine' syndromes, including adrenal hyperfunction, inappropriate ADH production or hypercalcaemia (Table 3). In these instances, biochemical disturbances such as hypokalaemic alkalosis or hyponatraemia have required treatment if recognized in time. In one case, the presenting feature of hypokalaemic alkalosis was an acute psychosis (30).

DIAGNOSIS

Perhaps the most important prerequisite to the correct diagnosis of SCUCP is awareness of the entity. Pathologists may seek to establish the diagnosis histologically, by utilizing special stains or electron microscopy. However, the appropriate clinical investigations, including assay for ectopic hormones, should be performed in patients in whom the diagnosis is suspected clinically: e.g. in patients with unusual presentations, unexplained biochemical abnormalities or unexpected patterns of spread.

A relatively simple approach to investigation can be used. The medical history should elicit symptoms of local and metastatic involvement, and in particular features that would suggest hepatic, splenic or pulmonary deposits. Furthermore, the symptoms of the clinical syndromes associated with ectopic hormone production should be elicited: hyperadrenalism (Cushing's syndrome, hypertension, acne, obesity, etc.); inappropriate ADH production (fluid retention, fluid overload, problems associated with hyponatraemia); hypercalcaemia (constipation, malaise, anorexia, clouded consciousness). It should be noted that patients with ectopic ACTH production may not show classical Cushing's syndrome, and may appear cachexic and pigmented. Furthermore, the physical examination should be directed towards staging the disease (determining the sites of involvement) and assessing the possiblity of ectopic hormone production. Routine biochemical and haematological tests may be augmented by the assay of ACTH, ADH, calcitonin, PTH and bombesin (if possible). These tests should not be carried out in all patients with prostate cancer, but rather in those in whom there is a reasonable clinical suspicion of the presence of SCUCP. PAcP and PSA should also be measured in the blood as they may reflect the presence of a component of adenocarcinoma. In fact, from our xenograft studies, it appears likely that SCUCP itself may release low levels of PAcP (49).

In addition to routine staging of the tumour, including a limited skeletal survey and/or bone scan, computerized axial tomographic (CAT) scanning should be performed to detect abnormalities in the pelvic or retroperitoneal lymph nodes, liver and spleen. A plain chest x-ray should be routine in staging, notwithstanding the rarity of pulmonary metastases in typical prostatic adenocarcinoma, in view of the incidence of this site of metastasis in SCUCP (Table 3).

If all staging tests are negative, suggesting that the tumour is localized to the prostate, we perform a CAT scan of the brain and a bone marrow aspiration biopsy and trephine before defining the plan of management. However, these tests are not routine in the very elderly patient in whom a conservative approach to treatment is proposed.

TREATMENT

In view of the infrequent early diagnosis of this condition, it is not possible to define the 'optimal' management of localized SCUCP. Integral to any approach is definition of the extent of disease, as outlined above. In the situation of SCUCP apparently localized to the prostate, several approaches are possible:

1. radical radiotherapy, in an attempt to achieve local control and perhaps cure;

2. radical prostatectomy, to control the adenocarcinomatous elements and to reduce the bulk of the primary tumour;

3. concurrent or sequential combination cytotoxic chemotherapy, administered to control both local disease and systemic micrometastases in a fashion analogous to that employed for bronchogenic SCUC (58).

The criteria for the use of radical local treatment (radiotherapy or prostatectomy) are more stringent than for pure adenocarcinoma in view of the propensity for SCUCP to metastasize early and widely. With regard to the optimal dose of radical radiotherapy, there is controversy as to whether a lower dose (40–50 Gy over 4–5 weeks) is appropriate (based on the marked radiosensitivity of SCUC of lung), or whether a more conventional, higher dose (60–70 Gy) should be applied, analogous to prostatic adenocarcinoma. We believe that the latter approach should be used in view of the potential for admixture of elements of SCUC and adenocarcinoma in these tumours.

No controlled studies of adjuvant cytotoxic chemotherapy have been carried out in cases of localized SCUCP, and it is not possible to make any recommendations at the present time. In view of the rarity of the disease, it is unlikely that the appropriate studies could be completed. Thus any decision regarding the use of adjuvant cytotoxic chemotherapy should be influenced substantially by considerations such as the age and general fitness of the patient, his attitude to receiving cytotoxics, geographical accessibility, available facilities, etc.

There are only scattered anecdotal reports in the literature referring to patients with established metastatic disease. The cytotoxic agents that are active against bronchogenic SCUC, including cyclophosphamide, vincristine, doxorubicin and etoposide (58), yield objective responses in metastatic SCUCP (28, 59). The use of three- or four-drug combination regimens yields objective response rates of the order of 60–75% in SCUC of the lung (58). No published series of patients with metastatic

SCUCP has been large enough to define an objective response rate; however, it is quite likely that this will be lower than for bronchogenic tumours in view of the heterogeneity of SCUCP with the admixture of elements of adenocarcinoma.

The role of hormonal manipulation should not be forgotten. In several of the cases summarized in Table 3, sustained objective remission was achieved by bilateral orchidectomy or the use of systemic oestrogens. Whether this treatent was effective in tumours composed of dominant elements of adenocarcinoma is not clear; in that situation, it is possible that the treatment selected in favour of elements of SCUC, which predominated at the time of relapse (i.e. hormonal manipulation controlled elements of adenocarcinoma, allowing outgrowth of SCUC).

It should also be emphasized, however, that patients treated by hormonal manipulation for SCUCP should be monitored very closely. Some of the available case reports describe rapid deterioration and death within a few weeks after the institution of hormonal treatment. If a patient with SCUCP fails to respond to hormonal manipulation, we believe that a trial of cytotoxic chemotherapy may be warranted in a attempt to prolong life and to palliate the symptoms of the disease. In the management of prostatic adenocarcinoma, we usually allow a minimum of 2 months before assessing response to hormonal manipulation (unless the patient is rapidly deteriorating). By contrast, the patient wth SCUCP should be reviewed within 2–4 weeks, depending upon the extent and severity of the disease. In a patient receiving systemic oestrogens in whom progressive disease is documented, we would continue the oestrogens at least during a transition period after the introduction of cytotoxics to cover any hormonally sensitive populations of tumour cells (e.g. foci of adenocarcinoma).

PROGNOSIS

To date, the prognosis for SCUCP has been dismal, largely because the diagnosis has been recognized late (or even at autopsy) in the majority of cases. The definition of median survival is complicated by the fact that several of the reported cases have apparently had biphasic tumours with elements of adenocarcinoma and SCUC. Sustained responses to hormonal manipulation may have reflected an initial dominance of adenocarcinoma, whereas the rapid decline after documentation of SCUCP may have reflected a selection process due to the initial treatment, failure to apply the most appropriate treatment for a SCUC, or an altered biological state of the tumour. Although the majority of patients have survived less than 6 months from the time of documentation of SCUC it should be noted that most of them did not receive cytotoxic therapy.

CONCLUSION

The biology of small cell undifferentiated carcinoma of the prostate is poorly understood. Morphologically and functionally it bears a closer resemblance to bronchogenic SCUC than to prostatic adenocarcinoma. However, there is also a substantial overlap with the characteristics of adenocarcinoma, due either to the presence of concurrent elements of this histological subtype or as an inherent biological function of the SCUC cell. Although the histogenesis of SCUCP has not been defined with certainty, we favour the concept of a common stem cell of origin, based on the available data and our own studies of a xenografted tumour line. Future studies of the molecular biology of this interesting tumour may yield important insights into the biology of tumour growth and its interface with the production of a variety of ectopic hormones and tumour antigens. Until these issues are clarified, one of the most important aspects of clinical management remains the need to consider the entity in the differential diagnosis of a prostatic neoplasm.

REFERENCES

1 Mostofi FK, Price EB Jr. Atlas of Tumor Pathology: Tumors of the Male Genital System.

Second series. Fascicle 8. Washington DC: Armed Forces Institute of Pathology, 1973: 177–259.

2 Sommers SC. Endocrine changes with prostatic carcinoma. Cancer 1957; 10: 345–58.

3 Pretl K. Zur Frage der Endokrinie der menschlichen Vorsfeherdruse. Virchows Arch Abt A Path Anat 1944; 312: 392–404.

4 Feyrter, F. Uber das urogenitale Helle-Zellen-System des Menschen. Z Mikrosk-Anat Forsch 1951; 57: 324–344.

5 diSant'Agnese PA, de Mesy Jenkin KL, Churukian CJ, Agarwal MM. Human prostatic endocrine-paracrine (APUD) cells. Arch Pathol Lab Med 1985; 109: 607–12.

6 Bonikos DS, Bensch KG. Endocrine cells of bronchial and bronchiolar epithelium. Am J Med 1977; 63: 765–71.

7 Azzopardi JG, Evans DJ. Argentaffin cells in carcinoma: Differentiation from lipofuscin and melanin in prostatic epithelium. J Pathol 1971; 104: 247–251.

8 Berger CL, Goodwin G, Mendelsohn G et al. Endocrine related biochemistry in the spectrum of human lung carcinoma. J Clin Endocrinol Metab 1981; 53: 422–9.

9 Schron DS, Gipson T, Mendelsohn G. The histogenesis of small cell carcinoma of the prostate. An immunohistochemical study. Cancer 1984; 53: 2478–80.

10 Wenk RE, Bhagavan B, Levy R, Miller D, Weisburger W. Ectopic ACTH, prostatic oat cell carcinoma and marked hypernatremia. Cancer 1977; 40: 773–8.

11 Ro JY, Tetu B, Ayala AG, Ordonez NG. Small cell carcinoma of the prostate. II. Immunohistochemical and electron microscopic studies of 18 cases. Cancer 1987; 59: 977–82.

12 Smedley HM, Brown C, Turner J Ectopic ACTH-producing lung cancer presenting with prostatic metastases. Postgrad Med J 1983; 59: 371–2.

13 Hodge GB, Carson CC. Oat cell carcinoma of lung masquerading as prostatic carcinoma. Urology 1985; 25: 69–70.

14 Capella C, Usellini L, Buffa R, Frigerio B, Solcia E. The endocrine component of prostatic carcinomas, mixed adenocarcinoma–carcinoid tumors, and non-tumor prostate: Histochemical and ultrastructural identification of the endocrine cells. Histopathology 1981; 5: 175–192.

15 Bono AV, Pozzi E. Endocrine-paracrine cells in prostatic carcinoma nad clinical course of the disease. Eruop Urol 1985; 11: 185–8.

16 DeBustros A, Baylin SB. Hormone production by tumours: Biological and clinical aspects. Clin Endocrinol Metab 1985; 14: 221–56.

17 Barkin J, Crassweller PO, Roncari DAK, Onrot J. Hypercalcemia associated with cancer of prostate without bony metastases. Urology 1984; 24: 368–71.

18 Patel S, Rosenthal JT. Hypercalcemia in carcinoma of prostate. Its cure by orchiectomy. Urology 1985; 25: 627–9.

19 Linehan WM, Kish ML, Chen SL, Andriole GL, Santora AC. Human prostate carcinoma causes hypercalcemia in athymic nude mice and produces a factor with parathyroid hormone-like bioactivity. J Urol 1986; 135: 616–20.

20 Newmark SR, Dlhuh RG, Bennett AH. Ectopic adrenocorticotropin syndrome with prostatic carcinoma. Urology 1973; 2: 666–8.

21 Vuitch MF, Mendelsohn G. Relationship of ectopic ACTH production to tumor differentiation. A morphologic and immunohistochemical study of prostatic carcinoma with Cushing's syndrome. Cancer 1982; 47: 296–9.

22 Slater D. Carcinoid tumour of the prostate associated with inappropriate ACTH secretion. Br J Urol 1985; 57: 591–2.

23 Sellwood RA, Spencer J, Azzopardi JG, Wapnick S, Welbourn RB, Kulatilake AE. Inappropriate secretion of antidiuretic hormone by carcinoma of the prostate. Br J Surg 1969; 56: 933–5.

24 Ghandur-Mnaymneh L, Satterfield S, Block NL. Small cell carcinoma of the prostate gland with inappropriate antidiuretic hormone secretion: morphological, immunohistochemical and clinical expressions. J Urol 1986; 135: 1263–66.

25 Carey RM, Varma SK, Drake CR, Thorner MO, Kovacs K, Rivier J, Vale W. Ectopic secretion of corticotropin-releasing factor as a cause of Cushing's syndrome. A clinical, morphologic and biochemical study. N Engl J Med 1984; 311: 13–20.

26 Jelbart ME, Russell PJ, Fullerton M, Funder J, Raghavan D. Ectopic hormone production by a prostatic small cell carcinoma xenograft line. Molec.Cell Endocrinol, 1988; 55: 167–72.

27 Smith CS. Small cell carcinoma of the prostate. J Urol 1985; 133: 371A, abstract 1029.

28 Hindson DA, Knight LL, Ocker JM. Small-cell carcinoma of prostate. Transient complete remission with chemotherapy. Urology 1985; 26: 182–4.

29 Wise HM Jr, Pohl AL, Gazzaniga A, Harrison JH. Hyperadrenocorticism associated with 'reactivated' prostatic carcinoma. Surgery 1965; 57: 655–64.

30 Hall TC. Symptomatic hypokalaemic alkalosis in hyperadrenocorticism secondary to carcinoma of the prostate. Cancer 1968; 21: 190–2.

31 Ansari MA, Pintozzi RL, Choi YS, Ladove RF. Diagnosis of carcinoid-line metastatic prostatic carcinoma by an immunoperoxidase method. Am J Clin Pathol 1981; 76: 94–8.

32 Ghali VS, Garcia RL. Prostatic adenocarcinoma with carcinoidal features producing adrenocorticotropic syndrome. Cancer 1984; 54: 1043–8.

33 Almagro UA. Argyrophilic prostatic carcinoma. Case report with literature review on prostatic carcinoid and "carcinoid-like" prostatic carcinoma. Cancer 1985; 55: 608–14.

34 Ellis DW, Leffers S, Davies JS, Ng ABP. Multiple immunoperoxidase markers in benign hyperplasia and adenocarcinoma of the prostate. Am J Clin Pathol 1984; 81: 279–84.

35 Heyderman E, Brown BM, Richardson TC. Epithelial markers in prostatic, bladder and colorectal cancer. An immunoperoxidase study of epithelial membrane antigen, carcinoembryonic antigen, and prostatic acid phosphatase. J Clin Pathol 1984; 37: 1363–9.

36 Ghazizadeh M, Kagawa S, Izumi K, Maebayash K, Takigawa H, Saidi T, Kawano A, Kurohawa K. Immunohistochemical detection of CEA in benign hyperplasia and adenocarcinoma of the prostate with monoclonal antibody. J Urol 1984; 131: 501–4.

37 Sloane JP, Ormerod MG. Distribution of epithelial membrane antigen in normal and neoplastic tissues and its value in diagnostic tumor pathology. Cancer 1981; 47: 1786–95.

38 Reeve JG, Stewart J, Watson JV, Wulfrank D, Twentyman PR, Bleehen NM. Neuron specific enolase expression in carcinoma of the lung. Br J Cancer 1986; 53: 519–528.

39 Sandberg AA. The prostatic cell: chromosomal and DNA analysis. In Murphy GP ed The Prostatic Cell: Structure and Function Part A. New York: Alan R. Liss, Inc 1980; 75–92.

40 Kjaer TB, Thommesen P, Frederiksen P, Bichel P. DNA content in cells aspirated from carcinoma of the prostate treated with oestrogenic compounds. Urol Res 1979; 7: 249–51.

41 Tribukait B, Esposti PL, Ronstrom L. Tumour ploidy for characterization of prostatic carcinoma: flow cytofluorometric DNA studies using aspiration biopsy material. Scand J Urol Nephrol (Suppl) 1980; 55: 59–64.

42 Pittman S, Russell PJ, Jelbart ME, Wass J, Raghavan D. Flow cytometric and karyotypic analysis of a primary small cell carcinoma of the prostate: A xenografted cell line. Cancer Genet Cytogenet 1987; 26: 165–9.

43 Oshimura M, Sandberg AA. Isochromosome 17 in prostatic cancer. J Urol 1975; 114: 249–50.

44 Atkin NB, Baker MC. Chromosome 10 deletion

45 Whang-Peng J, Bunn PA Jr, Kao-Shan CS et al. A non-random chromosomal abnormality, del 3p (14–23), in human small cell lung cancer (SCCL). Cancer Genet Cytogenet 1982; 6: 119–34.

46 Wurster-Hill DH, Cannizzaro LA, Pettengill OS, Sorenson AD, Cate CC, Maurer LH. Cytogenetics of small cell carcinoma of the lung. Cancer Genet Cytogenet 1984; 13: 303–30.

47 Viola MV, Fromowitz F, Oravez S, Deb S, Finkel G, Lundy J, Hand P, Thor A, Schlom J. Expression of ras oncogene p21 in prostate cancer. N Engl J Med 1986; 314: 133–7.

48 Rijnders AWM, Van der Korput JAGM, van Steenbrugge GJ, Romijn JC, Trapman J. Expression of cellular oncogenes in human prostatic carcinoma cell lines. Biochem Biophys Research Commun 1985; 132: 548–54.

49 Van Haaften-Day C, Raghavan D, Russell P, Wills EJ, Gregory P, Tilley W, Horsfall DJ. Xenografted small cell undifferentiated cancer of prostate: Possible common origin with prostatic adenocarcinoma. The Prostate 1988; 11: 271–9.

50 Raghavan D, Gibbs J, Nogueira-Costa R et al. The interpretation of makrer protein assays: A critical appraisal in clinical studies and on zenograft model. Br J Cancer 1980; 41 Suppl IV: 191–4.

51 Pearse AGE, Pollak JM. Neural crest origin of the endorine polypeptide (APUD) cell of the gastrointestinal cell and pancreas. Gut 1971; 12: 783–788.

52 Kazzas BA Argentaffin and argyrophilic cells in the prostate. J Pathol 1974; 112: 189–93.

53 Andrew A. An experimental investigation into the possible neural crest origin of pancreatic APUD (islet) cells. J Embryol Exp Morphol 1976; 35: 577–93.

54 Fontaine J, LeDouarin NM. Analysis of endoderm formation in the avian blastoderm by the use of quail-chick chimeras: Problem of the neuroectodermal origin of the cells of the APUD series. J Embryol Exp Morphol 1977; 41: 209–222.

55 Sidhu GS. The endodermal origin of digestive and respiratory tract APUD cells. Histopathologic evidence and a review of the literature. Am J Pathol 1979; 96: 5–20.

56 Mendelsohn G, Maksem JA. Divergent differentiation in neoplasms. Pathologic, biologic and clinical considerations. In: Pathology Annual, Part 1, Vol. 21, 1986: 91–119.

57 Raghavan D, Heyderman E, Monaghan P et

al. When is a seminoma not a seminoma? J Clin
Pathol 1981; 34: 123–8.

58 Morstyn G, Ihde DC, Lichter AS et al. Small
cell lung cancer 1973–1983: Early progress and
recent obstacles. Int J Radiat Oncol Biol Phys
1984; 10: 515–39.

59 Raghavan D. (unpublished data)

60 Bleichner JC, Chun B, Klappenbach RS. Pure
small cell carcinoma of the prostate with fatal
liver metastasis. Arch Pathol Lab Med 1986;
110: 1041–44.

61 Holland EA. Prostatic adenocarcinoma with

ectopic ACTH production. Br J Urol 1978; 50:
538–41.

62 Lovern WJ, Farris BL, Wettlaufer JN, Hare S.
Ectopic ACTH production in disseminated
prostatic adenocarcinoma. Urology 1975; 5:
817–20.

63 Montasser AY, Ong MG, Mehta VT. Carcinoid
tumor of the prostate associated with adenocarcinoma. Cancer 1979; 44: 307–10.

64 Wasserstein PW, Goldman RL. Diffuse carcinoid of prostate. Urology 1981; 18: 407–9.

Textbook of Uncommon Cancer
Edited by C.J. Williams, J.G. Krikorian, M.R. Green and D. Raghavan
© 1988 John Wiley & Sons Ltd

Chapter **16**

Adult Wilms' Tumour: A Dilemma

Derek Raghavan*†
Paul Harnett* and
Peter Russell‡
* Department of Clinical Oncology, Royal Prince Alfred
Hospital, Sydney,
† Urological Cancer Research Unit, Royal Prince Alfred
Hospital and University of Sydney, and
‡ Department of Anatomical Pathology, Royal Prince
Alfred Hospital, Sydney, Australia

INTRODUCTION

Wilms' tumour, or nephroblastoma, was first reported as a distinct entiy more than 150 years ago (1, 2). It occurs predominantly as a disease of young children, occurring in about 1 in 13 500 live births (3). It is second in frequency to neuroblastoma among solid abdominal malignancies in young children, and appears to have no sex predominance. The true incidence of this disease in adults is difficult to define as it is combined with renal cell carcinoma in most published statistics. However, it is clear that in all published series the incidence of Wilms' tumour (WT) is substantially less in adults than in children, and adult WT accounts for less than 1% of cases (4–6). An additional problem in determining its incidence has been the histological overlap with other tumours, and several early reports of the disease in adults may, in fact, have represented renal cell carcinomas or sarcomas (7, 8). More than 50 synonyms have been described for this entity (8).

PATHOLOGY AND HISTOGENESIS

WT is usually a solitary lesion occurring in the upper or lower pole of the kidney, and is often very large with a median reported weight greater than 500 grams (9). In 5–10% of cases it occurs bilaterally (10), although it is not clear whether this represents multicentric growth or the phenomenon of metastasis (11). Macroscopically the tumour replaces most of the renal parenchyma, compressing the residuum to one side. The cut surface of the tumour is usually greyish-white, with a rubbery texture. Areas of haemorrhage, necrosis and cyst formation are often present.

WT is thought to arise from pluripotential nephrogenic blastema of mesodermal derivation and can thus produce epithelial and stromal elements (9). Its histology is remarkably variable, differing from one tumour to another and from area to area within individual tumours (9). Three elements are regularly present: epithelial, stromal and blastema-

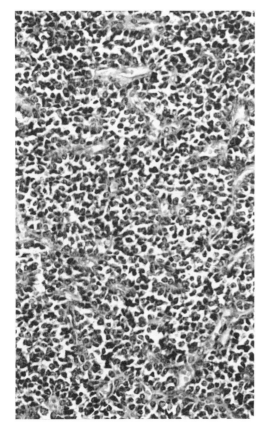

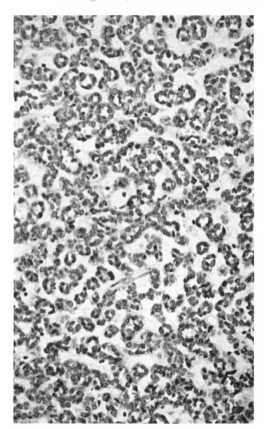

Figure 1 Typical pattern of adult Wilms' tumour with a monotonous population of uniform small cells with scanty cytoplasm and rounded hyperchromatic nuclei. H&E, original magnification: ×225.

Figure 2 Tubular pattern in adult Wilms' tumour. Tubules are formed of the same uniform small cells as are noted in Figure 1. H&E, original magnification: ×225.

tous. The epithelial elements may be obviously glomerular or tubular. The glomerular structures do not contain endothelial or mesangial elements. In some tumours, mesenchymal structures predominate. Sheets of spindle-shaped cells or islands of immature myxoid tissue are interposed by foci of cartilage, fibroblastic connective tissue, skeletal muscle or bone. The less well differentiated elements are often difficult to distinguish from neuroblastoma, being composed of small cells with round hyperchromatic nuclei, scanty cytoplasm and a high mitotic rate.

The diagnosis of adult WT must be based on rigorous histological criteria (Figures 1–3). In particular, confusion with the sarcoma-like

variant of renal cell carcinoma can occur, and the presence of typical elements of renal cell carcinoma (hypernephroma) precludes the diagnosis (7).

In children, the anaplastic or sarcomatous variants of WT constitute the least favourable histological patterns and are independently associated with a worse prognosis with respect to metastasis, efficacy of treatment, relapse and survival (12, 13).

A similar situation appears to apply to the adult patient, although the data are less defined (4–8). The anaplastic variant, in particular, is associated with a hyperdiploid DNA content and a variety of chromosomal rearrangements (14). These cytogenetic abnor-

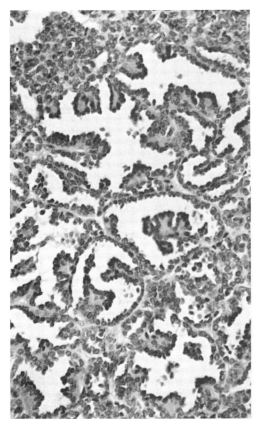

Figure 3 Irregular tufted structures resembling primitive glomeruli. H&E, original magnification: ×225.

malities may well confer an inherent resistance to radiotherapy and chemotherapy.

The tumour tends to invade the renal veins and often will metastasize to the lungs (9). Less commonly, liver and bone metastases will be found (15), and occasional spread to the contralateral kidney has been reported (4). Bone marrow involvement (16), and metastasis to the sigmoid colon, the orbit, the spinal cord and the brain have also been documented infrequently (4). The tumour may spread via the lymphatic channels, affecting regional and distant lymph nodes, or it may spread within the abdominal cavity, invading contiguous or other intraperitoneal organs (4–8).

EXPERIMENTAL MODELS

Several experimental models of WT have been

described (9, 17). The tumour occurs spontaneously in several animal species, including pigs, rats, rabbits, cattle and horses (18). The tumours arising in rats may be of particular significance as a model of adult WT as they characteristically occur at about 8 months of age, i.e. in young adult rats. A spontaneous nephroblastoma that arose in a Furth–Wistar rat has been transplanted in males and females and has been characterized intensively. Histological and ultrastructural studies have shown marked similarity to the human disease (19). Hormonal manipulation has altered the growth rate of the tumour, although the 'take' rates are equivalent in males and females. Tumours have been grown in a variety of sites, including subcutaneous, intramuscular and intrarenal, with host survival being shortest in the latter site. Growth kinetics of cells derived from tumours growing at different sites were the same (20). These tumours have been used as models for radiotherapy and chemotherapy programmes (21).

Experimental WTs have also been induced in rats by chemical carcinogens, such as the plant glycoside cycasin (22) and dimethyl benzanthracene (23); however, it should be noted that renal cell carcinomas can also be induced by these agents.

The intraveneous injection of a strain of avian myeolomatosis virus into newly hatched White Leghorn chickens also produces nephroblastoma in 10% of cases. The tumours resemble the human disease histologically, although they appear not to metastasize. These tumours often have a multifocal origin. Histological and ultrastructural studies have suggested that this tumour originates from blastema tissue present in the post-embryonic kidney (24).

The xenograft model, in which human tumours are transplanted subcutaneously into congenitally athymic nude mice, has also been explored (25). Fogh and colleagues established a cell line, designated SK-NEP-1, from a patient with Wilms' tumour and demonstrated rapid growth characteristics in tissue culture (25). They were also able to initiate a xenograft line in nude mice and studied morphology and karyotype of the tumour. The morphology of WT was maintained in serial passages, and a human karyotype was demonstrated, including a hypodiploid–hyperdiploid complement with a range of abnormalities and chromosomal markers.

CLINICAL PRESENTATION

Several cumulative series of adults with WT have been reported, although there appears to be considerable overlap in the cases cited (4–8). Nevertheless, there is a consistency of features of the adult population presenting with this disease. The mean age of presentation is approximately 30 years, with a similar median figure. The age range of reported cases has been 17 to 80 years, the lower figure representing an arbitrary distinction from the childhood disease. There is an approximately equal sex incidence.

The commonest presentation of WT in the adult is flank or abdominal pain, often accompanied by macroscopical haematuria, the sensation of an abdominal mass or distension, or constitutional features (4–8). These include weight loss, malaise, anorexia, nausea, vomiting, fever and amenorrhea. There have been occasional reports of sciatic pain, testicular pain (26) or scrotal swelling (27) as the presenting features of WT. Nondiagnostic urinary symptoms may be noted, including frequency, nocturia or urinary outflow obstruction.

Up to 25% of patients have metastases at presentation. Pulmonary deposits occur most often, and may either be asymptomatic or may cause dyspnoea or chest pain. Some patients present with bone pain and abdominal pain may reflect hepatic or nodal metastases.

In some instances, patients have been completely asymptomatic, with the tumour having been detected at a routine physical examination. The duration of symptoms, when present, is variable, ranging from a few days to more than 2 years (4–7), largely because of the non-specific nature of the features of early disease.

Physical examination usually reveals a large abdominal mass and local tenderness, often with associated abdominal distension. The patients with advanced disease are often cachexic. Hypertension is a relatively common feature, at least in children (27), and may be due to the production of renin by the tumour (28). A varicocele may be detected in association with the large abdominal mass (29), erroneously suggesting the diagnosis of testicular cancer in younger male patients.

There may be evidence of a malignant pleural effusion (4) or of other less common sites of metastatic disease, such as hepatomegaly or bone tenderness. Occasionally, peripheral lymph nodes are enlarged, and other possible diagnoses must then be excluded, including malignant lymphoma, germ cell tumours, or adenocarcinoma of uncertain primary site.

The specific diagnosis of Wilms' tumour in the adult is often made late as there are no specific features to distinguish it from other renal tumours. As with typical renal cell carcinomas, the primary site is notoriously asymptomatic, contributing to late diagnosis. In fact, in most reported series, approximately 50% of the adults with WT have had Stages 3–5 disease (4–8) (see also Table 1), as compared to only 30% of children (9, 30). By contrast, Kilton et al. (7) reported that more than 60% of adults had localized disease at presentation, on the basis of a highly selected series.

WT occurs in children in association with a wide range of chromosomal abnormalities and unusual clinical syndromes (9, 30). In particular, there is a raised incidence of aniridia, hemihypertrophy and genitourinary abnormalities in these children (9, 30). From the available literature, such syndromes appear to have been documented less often in adults, although it should not be forgotten that the disease is much less common in adult patients, and some of the paediatric syndromes result in early death (thus reducing the likelihood of association in adults).

INVESTIGATION AND STAGING

The approach to the investigation of patients with adult WT depends on whether the diagnosis is anticipated preoperatively (e.g., if a fine needle aspiration biopsy has already been performed on the renal mass) or if the diagnosis has been achieved at nephrectomy. In fact, if the diagnosis of WT is suspected, we believe that fine needle aspiration biopsy may be hazardous as there is a risk of rupturing the tumour and causing intra-abdominal contamination; this, in turn, is associated with a worse prognosis with regard to abdominal recurrence and death (13).

Most commonly a series of tests will have been completed prior to the diagnosis. In the usual clinical setting, an abdominal mass has been investigated prior to the laparotomy. Biochemical screening may have suggested the presence of liver or bone metastases, urinary tract dysfunction, or the presence of hyperuricaemia due to turnover of tumour cells. A full blood count may reveal the anaemia of chronic disease, may show derangements due to marrow infiltration, or may even reflect the production of erythropoietin by the tumour (more commonly associated with renal cell carcinoma).

Plain x-rays of the abdomen may show renal calcification or blunting of the psoas shadow, neither of which allows the distinction between WT and renal cell carcinoma. An intravenous pyelogram will often show distortion of the calyces, sometimes with splaying of the contrast material around the mass. In a small lesion, intrarenal distortion of the calyces may be the only finding. However, none of these changes is specific in the adult patient.

Computerized axial tomographic (CAT) scanning of the abdomen is useful in detecting the extent of intra-abdominal spread and in defining the sites of involvement—regional or mesenteric nodes, liver, contralateral kidney, etc. A CAT scan of the chest may demonstrate mediastinal or lung parenchymal deposits, although a simple chest x-ray constitutes an adequate initial screen for pulmonary metastases.

Arteriography is useful prior to surgery, providing definition of the tumour vasculature and often helping to localize a small primary tumour. Once again, there is no specific pattern associated with WT, and tumours may have reduced, increased or normal vascularity (4, 32, 33).

We have found the gallium scan to be a useful aid to staging, with uptake in both the primary site and, of greater importance, in metastases (34). In the patient who has already undergone radical nephrectomy, a gallium scan may help to define occult metastases. If not previously performed, a postoperative abdominal CAT scan may also provide another parameter of residual disease (for comparison after radiotherapy or chemotherapy) and may reveal involvement not detected at laparotomy.

Cerebral metastases occur uncommonly in adult WT (4–8), and we do not believe that cerebral CAT scanning is routinely indicated in the work-up of such a patient, especially in the absence of symptoms of central nervous system involvement (headache, visual impairment, cerebral dysfunction). In fact, the presence of a cerebral metastasis would not necessarily contraindicate radical surgery for the primary tumour in an attempt to achieve long-term control, although the sequence of treatment could be altered.

Bone marrow biopsy, however, should be performed routinely in any patient who is due to undergo treatment for apparently localized disease. Marrow infiltration is of importance both prognostically and with respect to the choice of optimal management. Furthermore, it may complicate programmes of aggressive combination cytotoxic chemotherapy, especially with regard to marrow recovery.

We stage the disease according to the classification of the US National Wilms' Tumour Study Group (Table 1) (5), although the TNM system is used more widely in Europe.

TABLE 1 STAGING OF ADULT WILMS' TUMOUR (NATIONAL WILMS' TUMOUR STUDY GROUP (5))

Stage	Distribution of disease
1	Tumour limited to the kidney and completely excised; surface of the renal capsule intact; tumour not ruptured before or during removal; no residual tumour beyond margins of resection.
2	Tumour extends beyond kidney, but fully excised; regional extension of tumour and penetration through outer surface of renal capsule into peri-renal soft tissue; vessels outside renal substance are infiltrated or contain tumour thrombus; there may have been *local* spillage of tumour confined to the flank.
3	Incomplete excision, without haematogenous metastases. This stage occurs if one or several of the following conditions are present: a tumour biopsy was taken before or during surgery, tumour rupture before or during surgery; perito-neal metastases, as distinguished from the simple tumour adhesions of Stage 2; invasion of lymph nodes beyond the local regional nodes; complete excision impossible.
4	Haematogenous metastases to lungs, liver, bones, brain, etc.
5	Bilateral renal tumours

TREATMENT

Prior to the introduction of cytotoxic chemo-therapy, the long-term survival of all patients with WT was less than 30% (35, 36). However, since chemotherapy has been used routinely, children with WT have been cured in 60–85% of instances, depending on the histology and stage of the disease. Although uncommon, there are now more than 30 documented cases of adult WT treated in the era of modern chemotherapy (with or without radiotherapy) (Table 2). As can be seen, the results are less impressive than in the paediatric population, although long-term control has been achieved in nearly half of the cases (4–8, 37–40).

There are important problems in the assess-ment of the results of treatment in adult WT, especially when attempting to set them into a historical or chronological context.

1 Definition of the entity. Some (or many) of the cases reported in the medical literature may represent misdiagnosis of renal cell carci-noma or other tumours.

2 Selection bias. There is a tendency for investigators and journal editors to prefer to report 'positive data', and hence there may be a bias in the literature in favour of 'successful' attempts at treatment (41). Although there are many reports of failed treatment, one still cannot assess with certainty whether there is such a bias of reporting.

3 Variation of staging and the phenome-non of 'stage migration'. Since the advent of CAT scanning in the late 1970s, more accurate staging has been possible, and hence the potential for more appropriate selection of treatment for each stage of disease. This, in turn, could have resulted in apparently improved survival figures, rather than being due to improved treatment per se.

4 Selection of patients. It is likely that the distribution and characteristics of patients who receive treatment has changed, with the increasing realization that long-term responses can be achieved by aggressive treatment regi-mens.

5 Improved diagnosis. Pathologists may now recognize the entity of adult WT with a greater frequency and level of confidence, and thus tumours previously diagnosed as renal cell carcinomas may now be considered for aggres-sive treatment; conversely, tumours misdiag-nosed as adult WT may be excluded from such programmes.

6 Inadequate treatment. Many reports have described regimens of treatment, incor-porating chemotherapy in particular, which would currently be regarded as sub-optimal (4, 5, 7, 29, 37, 38) or in which the details of treatment are too scanty to allow adequate assessment of efficacy. Of particular impor-tance is the occurrence of dose reduction,

TABLE 2 THREE-DRUG CHEMOTHERAPY (±RADIOTHERAPY) FOR ADULT WILMS'
TUMOUR

Sex/age		Stage	Radiotherapy administered	Drugs[a]	Salvage regimen	Survival (months)	Series (ref.)
F	36	3	Yes	VAD	?	30[b]	Byrd et al (5)
M	23	4	?	VAC	?	30[b]	Byrd et al. (5)
F	19	4	Yes	VAD	—	36+	Byrd et al. (5)
M	20	1	Yes	VAD	?	24+	Byrd et al. (5)
M	25	4	No	VACB	?	12[b]	Byrd et al. (5)
F	53	4	Yes	VACD	?	12[b]	Byrd et al. (5)
M	63	4	Yes	VAD	?	12[b]	Byrd et al. (5)
?	20	2	Yes	VAD	?	24+	Byrd et al. (5)
F	28	1	Yes	VAD	—	18+	Byrd et al. (5)
?	26	4	No	VAD	?	12[b]	Byrd et al. (5)
F	25	2	Yes	VAC	—	18+	Byrd et al. (5)
F	17	3	Yes	VAC	—	12+	Byrd et al. (5)
F	19	4	Yes	VAD	—	24+	Babaian et al. (4)
M	34	3	Yes	VAD	RT	15[b]	Chung et al.(38)
M	63	4	Yes	VAD	VAC	?[b]	Abadir (37)
M	38	4	No	VAC	?	5[b]	Prat et al. (39)
F	44	3	Yes	VAD	J/VECD/RT	56[b]	Raghavan et al. (34)
F	60	1	No	VAC/VAD	—	30+	Raghavan et al. (34)

[a] Drug regimen not specified in most reports.
[b] Deceased.
Key: A: Actinomycin D; V: vincristine; C: cyclophosphamide; D: doxorubicin; E: etoposide; J: carboplatin;
B: bleomycin.

either with regard to absolute dosage, frequency or duration of administration, which could reduce the likelihood of cure.

7   The phenomenon of data recycling. A
set of data may appear in the medical literature more than once, having been reported initially and then being included in one or more reviews, each of which contributes to an inflated number of cases and a biased distribution of characteristics of patients and results of treatment (42).

Notwithstanding these difficulties, the results achieved in the management of adult WT have some similarities to the paediatric population. The use of surgery, wide field irradiation and combination chemotherapy together appear to yield the best results in each stage of disease. Although a 'state of the art' has not yet been defined, it is appropriate to summarize some of the important issues in the management of adult WT.

Surgery

There are important differences in the role of surgery for the management of WT in children and in adults. In children, there is often a high index of suspicion that a renal or abdominal mass may represent WT, and the surgical approach can be planned accordingly. It has previously been reported that a wide transabdominal approach is the most appropriate for this condition as it allows adequate staging, the delivery of a large abdominal mass without rupture, and the possibility of contralateral renal biopsy. Aron (1974) reported a 67% 2-year survival for patients after a transabdominal incision, compared to a figure of 52% after a flank approach (43).

In the adult, the diagnosis of WT is usually not suspected preoperatively, and thus in most instances, a conventional approach for a renal cell carcinoma has been employed. Tumour spillage is undesirable whatever the histology, and thus adequate exposure must be obtained to allow delivery of the tumour without rupture. In the adult, bilateral WT is a rare phenomenon, and it is thus probably not essential to extend the incision to allow contralateral biopsy nor to use an anterior approach as a secondary procedure.

If the diagnosis of WT is suspected and an anterior approach has been used, the abdominal cavity should be examined carefully for tumour spread, and suspicious areas biopsied (44). Free peritoneal fluid or blood should be collected for cytological examination. Although the details of surgical dissection are beyond the scope of this review, the operation should include adequate sampling of lymph nodes, biopsy of any hepatic lesions, and an aggressive surgical approach to the removal of tumour thrombi from the inferior vena cava (44). It is of particular importance that the tumour be removed en bloc, without transgression of the capsule or rupture of tumour tissue.

If the diagnosis of WT is achieved postoperatively (i.e. from routine histopathological reporting), further surgical management depends, to some extent, upon the nature of the preceding operation. If the tumour has been removed completely and adequate staging achieved, further intervention is usually not warranted. However, if the tumour has merely been biopsied without an attempt at removal, a second laparatomy may be necessary (ideally performed by an experienced surgical oncologist).

In some cases, resection of the tumour is not possible in the first instance. Adequate biopsies must be taken, and the patient should then be treated by chemotherapy and/or radiotherapy. A second-look laparotomy may then be appropriate to ensure removal of the residual tumour mass (45).

Radiotherapy

The role for radiotherapy in the management of WT has been defined in the paediatric population. Prior to the introduction of cytotoxic chemotherapy, radiotherapy was used routinely for preoperative reduction of tumour bulk or for postoperative control of residual disease (35, 36, 46, 47). Although local control was achieved, the majority of patients eventually died of metastatic disease. Preoperative radiotherapy increases the risk of incorrect diagnosis, and has subsequently been shown to have no impact on long-term survival (30).

In children, radical abdominal radiotherapy can cause major abnormalities of skeletal growth and long-term damage to the liver and kidneys (30). In the adult population, growth abnormalities are not a problem, and the liver and remaining kidney can be protected by lead shields. Hussey et al. (48) have demonstrated that doses of irradiation less than 24 Gy, when combined with chemotherapy, are sufficient to achieve local tumour control.

However, as previously noted, the prognosis in adults is worse than in children. Accordingly, although there has been no definitive study of radiation dosage/fractionation, the US National Wilms' Tumour Study Group have recommended a higher dose (45 Gy in 1.8 Gy fractions) of whole abdominal irradiation, with shielding of the kidney and liver to restrict normal tissue damage (5). It must be emphasized, however, that there is a paucity of data regarding the optimal role of radiotherapy in the management of adult WT, and the final decisions should be made in collaboration by the surgeon, the radiotherapist and medical oncologist. Ideally, such patients should be managed according to standard predefined protocols, and the radiation dosage adjusted to the nature of concomitant chemotherapy; thus, it should not be forgotten that doxorubicin can act as a potent radiosensitizer and can induce the phenomenon of 'radiation recall'.

Radiotherapy may also have a role in the management of cerebral metastases or of pulmonary recurrence. In the latter situation, useful palliation of dyspnoea or chest pain can be achieved by whole lung irradiation, although severe radiation-induced pneumonitis can occur at higher doses, especially in the patient treated with doxorubicin (30).

Chemotherapy

The introduction of cytotoxic chemotherapy into the management of WT in children, more than 25 years ago, effected a dramatic improvement in cure rates for all stages of the disease (30, 45, 49–52). Single agent response rates of 20–40% were demonstrated for actinomycin D (49), vincristine (50), several alkylating agents (30, 51) and subsequently doxorubicin (52). Subsequently randomized clinical trials have demonstrated the superiority of two-drug combination regimens over single agents (30, 45) and more recently an added survival benefit from a three-drug combination of vincristine, actinomycin D and doxorubicin (30, 45, 53).

In the management of adult WT, similar response rates have been achieved, although long-term survival figures have been lower (4–8). However, as previously noted, the details of the cytotoxic regimens employed have been scanty in several instances (4, 5) and the doses clearly sub-optimal by current standards in other reports (29, 37, 38). It is even possible that errors in the dosage of actinomycin D cited in some reports (doses in 'milligrams' instead of 'micrograms') may have contributed to the confusion (4, 6). It appears, nevertheless, that the highest chance of cure for adult WT is afforded by a combined modality approach, incorporating radical surgery, whole abdominal irradiation and combination chemotherapy, such as that employed by the National Wilms' Tumour Study Group (5). Several issues remain unresolved, including the optimal combination and dosage of cytotoxics, the most appropriate duration of treatment, and the most effective schedule for the interaction of radiotherapy and chemotherapy.

Another problem that will require further study is the management of the patient with relapsed WT. As previously noted, radiotherapy has been used to palliate the symptoms of the disease. There have also been isolated case reports of sustained remission after salvage chemotherapy for adults with relapsed WT (5,

34, 40). In these instances, the mainstay of treatment has been the use of vincristine, doxorubicin, cyclophosphamide or actinomycin D singly or in combination, sometimes augmented by radiotherapy or the resection of residual tumour nodules. A series of phase II trials have demonstrated activity of etoposide and ifosfamide against relapsed paediatric WT (54, 55).

PROGNOSIS

The prognosis for adult WT is less well defined than in the paediatric population. Although superficially similar with respect to the combinations of treatment modalities employed, important differences in the wide range of reported treatment programmes in timing and dosage make it difficult to estimate the chance of cure or prolonged survival. In addition, it appears that adult WT is characterized by a risk of late relapse and death (5, 34) in contrast to the experience in childhood (30). Thus 2- and 3-year survival figures do not correlate with cure in the adult.

Despite the problems, the National Wilms' Tumour Study Group have estimated an overall survival rate of 54% at 2 years and 24% at 3 years in a series of 31 patients. In their cases with Stage 1–2 disease, the 3-year actuarial survival was 48%, compared with only 11% for patients with metastases at presentation. However, it should be noted that 7 of the patients who died were treated between 1968 and 1970 (prior to the introduction of CAT scanning and aggressive combination chemotherapy regimens).

CONCLUSION

Adult WT remains a tantalizing and difficult problem in management. Extrapolating from the paediatric experience, most patients should anticipate cure. Yet this does not seem to be reflected by the results in the recent medical literature. Pathologists and clinicians must remain vigilant to the possible diagnosis of this entity, especially in patients with poorly differentiated renal cell carcinoma. If the diagnosis has been made, it appears that the greatest chance of long-term survival or cure is afforded by an aggressive approach to management, combining surgery, irradiation and chemotherapy. In view of its rarity, this disease should not be managed by the isolated clinician. Patients should be referred to Cancer Centres with multi-disciplinary clinics with facilities for aggressive treatment, adequate supportive measures and for data collection and involvement in multi-centre clinical trials. Whenever possible, patients should be entered into trials such as the National Wilms' Tumour Study, in order to rationalize treatment and to allow us to learn more about this unusual disease and eventually to achieve the excellent results seen in children with Wilms' tumours.

REFERENCES

1 Rance TF. Cause of fungus haematodes of the kidneys. Med Phys J 1814; 32: 19.
2 Wilms M. Die Mischgeschwulste der Niere. Leipzig: Arthur Georgi, 1899: 1–90.
3 Ehrlich RM, Goodman WE. The surgical treatment of nephroblastoma (Wilms' tumor). Cancer 1973; 32: 1145.
4 Babaian RJ, Skinner DG, Waisman J. Wilms' tumor in the adult patient: Diagnosis, management, and review of the World medical literature. Cancer 1980; 45: 1713.
5 Byrd RL, Evans AE, D'Angio GJ. Adult Wilms tumor: Effect of combined therapy on survival. J Urol 1982; 127: 648.
6 Roth DR, Wright J, Cawood CD Jr, Pranke DW. Nephroblastoma in adults. J Urol 1984; 132: 108.
7 Kilton L, Matthews MJ, Cohen MJ. Adult Wilms tumor: A report of prolonged survival and review of literature. J Urol 1980; 124: 1.
8 Culp O, Hartman FW. Mesoblastic nephroma in adults: A clinico-pathologic study of Wilms' tumor and related renal neoplasms. J Urol 1948; 60: 552.
9 Bennington JL, Beckwith JB. Atlas of Tumor Pathology: Tumors of the Kidney, Renal Pelvis and Ureter, Second series, Fascicle 12. Washington DC; Armed Forces Institute of Pathology, 1975: 31–91.
10 Fay R, Brosman S, Williams DI. Bilateral nephroblastoma. J Urol 1973; 110: 119.
11 Ragab AH, Vietti TJ, Crest W. Bilateral Wilms' tumor: A review. Cancer 1972; 30: 983.
12 Bonadio JF, Storer B, Norkool P, Farewell VT, Beckwith JB, D'Angio GJ. Anaplastic Wilms' tumor: Clinical and pathologic studies. J Clin Oncol 1985; 3: 513–20.
13 Breslow N, Churchill G, Beckwith JB, Fernbach DJ, Otherson HB, Tefft M, D'Angio GJ. Prognosis for Wilms' tumor patients with nonmetastatic disease at diagnosis—results of the second National Wilms' Tumor Study. J Clin Oncol 1985; 3: 521–31.
14 Douglass EC, Look AT, Webber B, Parham D, Wilimas JA, Green AA, Roberson PK. Hyperdiploidy and chromosomal rearrangements define the anaplastic variants of Wilms' tumor. J Clin Oncol 1986; 4: 975.
15 Bond JV, Martin EC. Bone metastases in Wilms' tumour. Clin Radiol 1975; 26: 103.
16 O'Neill P, Pinkel D. Wilms' tumor in bone marrow. J Pediatr 1968; 72: 396.
17 Sufrin G. Experimental models of renal parenchymal neoplasms. In: Chisholm GD, Williams DI eds Scientific Foundations of Urology, 2nd edition, London: Heinemann, 1982: 667–77.
18 Cotchin E. Spontaneous tumours in young animals. Proc R Soc Med 1975; 68: 653.
19 Tomashefsky P, Furth J, Lattimer JK, Tannenbaum M, Priestly J. The Furth–Columbia rat Wilms' Tumor. J Urol 1972; 107: 348.
20 Saroff J, Chu TM, Gaeta JF, Williams P, Murphy GP. Characterisation of a Wilms' tumor model. Invest Urol 1975; 12: 320.
21 Kedar A, McGarry M, Moore R, Williams P, Murphy GP. Effect of post-operative chemotherapy and radiotherapy on the survival of subcutaneously implanted Furth Wilms' tumor. Oncology 1981; 38: 65.
22 Hirono I, Laqueur GL, Spatz M. Transplantability of cycasin-induced tumors in rats with emphasis on nephroblastomas. J Natl Cancer Inst 1968; 40: 1011.
23 Jasmine G, Riopelle JL. Nephroblastomas induced in ovariectomized rats by dimethylbenzanthracene. Cancer Res 1970; 30: 321.
24 Ishiguro H, Beard D, Sommer JR, Heine U, The G, Beard JW. Multiplicity of cell response to the BAI strain A (Myeloblastosis) avian tumor virus. I. Nephroblastoma (Wilms' tumor): Gross and microscopic pathology. J Natl Cancer Inst 1962; 29: 1.
25 Fogh J. Cultivation, characterization, and identification of human tumor cells with emphasis on kidney testis and bladder tumours. Natl Cancer Inst Monogr 1978; 49: 5.
26 Case Records of the Massachusetts General

Hospital. Case 32–1981. N Engl J Med 1981; 305–331.

27 Sukarochana K, Tolentino W, Kiesewetter WB. Wilms' tumor and hypertension. J Pediat Surg 1972, 5: 573.

28 Ganguly A, Gribble J, Tune B et al. Renin-secreting Wilms' tumor with severe hypertension; report of a case and brief review of renin-secreting tumors. Ann. Intern Med 1973; 79: 835.

29 Vorstman B, Rothwell D. Wilms tumor in adult patient. Urology 1982; 20: 628.

30 Green DM, Jaffe N. Wilms' tumor—model of a curable pediatric malignant solid tumor. Cancer Treat Rep 1978; 5: 143.

31 Miller RW, Fraumeni JF Jr, Manning MD. Association of Wilms' tumor with aniridia, hemihypertrophy, and other congenitial malformations. N Engl J Med 1964; 270: 922.

32 Clark RE, Moss AA, de Lorimier AA, Palubinskas AJ. Arteriography of Wilms' tumor. Am J Roentgenol 1971; 113: 476.

33 Farah J, Lofstrom JE. Angiography of Wilms' tumor. Radiology 1968; 90: 775.

34 Raghavan D, Harnett P, Russell P, Korbel EI, Coorey GJ, Green D. Chemotherapy and radiotherapy for adult Wilms' tumour. Submitted for publication.

35 Harvey RM. Wilms' tumor: Evaluation of treatment methods. Radiology 1950; 54: 689,

36 Klapproth HJ. Wilms' tumor: A report of 45 cases and an analysis of 1351 cases reported in the world's literature from 1940–1958. J Urol 1959; 81: 633.

37 Abadir R. Wilms tumors in adults. J Surg Oncol 1981; 16: 175.

38 Chung TS, Reyes CV, Stefani SS. Wilms tumor in adults. Urology 1984; 24: 275.

39 Prat J, Gray GF, Stolley PD, Coleman JW. Wilms' tumor in an adult associated with androgen abuse. JAMA, 1977; 237: 2322.

40 Hagiwara M, Tachibana M, Jitsukawa S, Murai M, Nakazono M, Hata M, Tazaki H. Multimodal treatment of advanced adult Wilms' tumor. J Urol 1982; 127:535.

41 Simes RJ. Publication bias: The case for an international registry of clinical trials. J Clin Oncol 1986; 4: 1529.

42 Hillcoat BL. Data recycling and misreading: Two potential errors in pooled data from small studies. J Clin Oncol 1984; 2: 1047.

43 Aron BS. Wilms' tumor—A clinical study of eighty-one patients. Cancer 1974, 33: 637.

44 Kumar APM, Pratt CB, Coburn TP, Johnson WW. Treatment strategy for nodular renal blastema and nephroblastomatosis associated with Wilms' tumor. J Pediatr Surg 1978; 13: 281'

45 Champion JE, Wilimas J, Kumar APM. The management of Wilms' tumor. In: Spiers ASD ed Chemotherapy and Urological Malignancy. Berlin: Springer Verlag, 1982: 27–43.

46 Abeshouse BS. Management of Wilms' tumor by national survey and review of the literature. J Urol 1957; 77: 792.

47 Scott LS. Wilms' tumour: Its treatment and prognosis. Br Med J 1956; i: 200.

48 Hussey DH, Castro JR, Sullivan MP, Sutow WW. Radiation therapy in management of Wilms' tumor. Radiology 1971; 101: 663.

49 Farber S, D'Angio G, Evans A, Mitus A. Clinical studies of actinomycin D with special reference to Wilms' tumor in children. Ann NY Acad Sci 1969; 89: 421.

50 Sutow WW, Thurman WG, Windmiller J. Vincristine (leurocristine) sulfate in the treatment of children with metastatic Wilms' tumor. Pediatrics 1963; 32: 880.

51 Finklestein JZ, Hittle RE, Hammond GD. Evaluation of a high dose cyclophosphamide regimen in childhood tumors. Cancer 1969; 23: 1239.

52 Tan C, Rosen G, Ghavimi F. Adriamycin (NSC123127) in pediatric malignancies. Cancer Chemother Rep 1975; 6: 259.

53 D'Angio GJ, Evans AE, Breslow N et al. The treatment of Wilms' tumor: Results of the second National Wilms' Tumor Study. Cancer 1981; 47: 2302.

54 Douglass EC, Wilimas JA, Sackey K, Casper J. Nitschke R. Efficacy of combination cisplatin (DDP) and VP–16 in the treatment of recurrent and advanced Wilms' tumor (WT). Proc Am Soc Clin Oncol 1986, 5: 201 (abstract).

55 Demeocq F, Tournade MF, Lemerle J et al: Ifosfamide (IFO) is an active drug in Wilms' tumor (WT). A phase II study of the French Society of Pediatric Oncology Proc Am Soc Clin Oncol 1986, 5: 204 (abstract).

Textbook of Uncommon Cancer
Edited by C.J. Williams, J.G. Krikorian, M.R. Green and D. Raghavan
© 1988 John Wiley & Sons Ltd

Chapter **17**

Primary Adenocarcinoma of the Urinary Bladder and Urachus

Sonny L. Johansson and
Claes R. Anderström
*Department of Pathology and Microbiology and
Eppley Institute for Cancer and Allied Diseases, University
of Nebraska Medical Center, Omaha, Nebraska, USA and
Department of Urology, Kärnsjukhuset, Skövde, Sweden*

INTRODUCTION

Primary adenocarcinoma of the urinary bladder may be of urachal or non-urachal origin. The first case of urachal adenocarcinoma of the bladder was described by Hue and Jacquin in 1863 (1) and the first case of non-urachal adenocarcinoma of the bladder was reported in 1883 by Posner (2) and Sperling (3) who each described one case. This tumor entity was better delineated by Begg (4, 5) who reviewed 18 cases of urachal adenocarcinoma. Since then approximately 300 cases of urachal carcinomas have been reported in the Western and Japanese literature (for review, see references 5 and 7). A recent overview reported on 325 cases of primary non-urachal adenocarcinoma, 208 of which were presented in a total of eight series, the remaining cases appearing as smaller series of patients or case reports (8). Approximately 80% of the cases of non-urachal adenocarcinoma have been published since 1970.

Primary adenocarcinoma of the bladder (including both urachal and non-urachal tumors) is an uncommon tumor and the incidence has been estimated to vary between 0.55 and 3.93% of all bladder tumors. (9–11) (Table 1) Between 1958 and 1973 approximately 13 000 new cases of bladder tumors were reported to the Swedish Cancer Registry (14). One hundred and fifty-seven of these tumors were registered as primary adenocarcinomas of the bladder. However, a careful evaluation of all cases revealed that 45 were erroneously reported or mis-diagnosed (15). Thus, during this 16-year period adenocarcinomas comprised 0.86% of the total number of bladder cancers (14). Twenty-two of these tumors were considered to be urachal, an incidence of 0.17% of all bladder tumors. Based on the figures from Sweden the incidence of urachal carcinoma can be calculated to be approximately one case per 5.8 million inhabitants and the incidence of adenocarcinoma of the bladder proper is about one case per 1.1 million individuals. It appears as if primary adenocarcinomas of the bladder, urachal or non-urachal, are more common in Japan than in Western Europe and the United States (6).

We agree with Begg (16) who suggested that the urachus is a modified part of the urinary

275

TABLE 1   INCIDENCE IN DIFFERENT COUNTRIES OF PRIMARY ADENOCARCINOMA OF THE BLADDER
(URACHAL AND NON-URACHAL) EXPRESSED AS A PERCENTAGE OF ALL BLADDER TUMORS

| Country | Author | Data derived from | Total number of bladder tumors | Number of patients (incidence—%) | |
				Adenocarcinoma of the bladder proper	Adenocarcinoma of the urachus
England	Thomas et al. (12)	United Leicester, Derby and Sheffield Hospitals	5300	25 (0.47)	18 (0.34)
Federal Republic of Germany	Jakse et al. (13)	University of Mainz	715	13 (1.80)	5 (0.70)
Japan	Ichikawa (9)	38 University Hospitals	1018	40 (3.93)	12 (1.18)
Sweden	National Bureau of Health (14)	The Swedish Cancer Registry	13000	90 (0.86)	22 (0.17)
United States	Jacobo et al. (11)	Bladder Tumor Registry	2628	20 (0.76)	6 (0.23)

bladder rather than a separate organ. Embryologically the major hypothesis states that the urachus is of cloacal origin with the upper position of the bladder joining the allantois at the level of the umbilicus. The process that occurs is apparently the following: at birth the apex of the bladder is located 4 cm above the symphysis and as it rapidly descends it pulls the urachus with it. The upper portion of the bladder becomes narrower to form the urachus, and the rest of the bladder takes its adult retropubic position. The final position of the urachus is approximately two-thirds of the distance between the dome of the bladder and the umbilicus. The adult urachus is approximately 5 cm long. The regressive changes generally occurring result in closure of both the cephalad end at the umbilicus and the caudal end at the bladder wall resulting in obliteration also of the middle segment of the urachus, converting it to a solid cord of fibrous tissue. However, dissection between the transversalis fascia and peritoneum within the space of Retzius reveals an urothelial lined canal in 32–70% of individuals in an autopsy series (17). The urothelium in the urachus is structually similar to and differs only slightly from that of the urinary bladder. Focal columnar metaplasia is present in approximately one-third of these cases (17). The configuration of the urachal remnant within the bladder wall varies from that of a uniform narrow tube to

structures showing random microcystic dilatation or irregular lateral pouches. The microscopic remnants in normal non-tumor bearing individuals are of little or no clinical significance but it is important for the urologists and pathologists to be aware of their existence. The rare disorders occurring in the urachus include fistula and cyst formation, infections, with or without concomitant calculus formation, and neoplasia of the urothelial lining or surrounding stroma (12).

ETIOLOGY

There are at least two predisposing factors in the development of primary adenocarcinoma of the bladder, exstrophy of the bladder and schistosomiasis (18). Thus, adenocarcinomas of the bladder are considerably more common in areas of endemic schistosomiasis. Adenocarcinoma is also the most common tumor arising in the exstrophic bladder. Bladder exstrophy occurs in 1:50000 births (19). In a review by Nielsen and Nielsen (20) 81 cases of carcinoma originating in exstrophic bladder were reported. In 75 cases both a clinical and histological description was included and 6 cases only comprised a clinical description. In 68 of the patients the tumor was diagnosed as adenocarcinoma, in 1 case as urothelial carcinoma and the remaining ones were reported to be squamous cell carcinoma or undifferen-

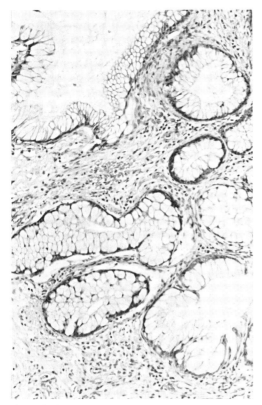

Figure 1 Glandular metaplasia of the urinary bladder (enteric type). H&E, original magnification: ×144.

tiated carcinoma. The tumors are generally diagnosed in the third to sixth decade of life and 60 of 81 cases occurred between 40 and 70 years of age. Only occasional cases occurring in individuals older than 70 years have been reported (21). The bladder mucosa surrounding the tumors in patients with bladder exstrophy generally shows extensive glandular metaplasia and inflammation (Figure 1).

An additional factor which more recently has been associated with the development of adenocarcinoma is the non-functional bladder (3, 22–25). In 1963, Kickham and Keegan (26) described the presence of mucinous epithelium of the bladder of a man who had had a non-functioning bladder for 10 years. In the same year Gordon reported on 2 patients with intestinal metaplasia of the bladder mucosa one of whom had undergone ureterocolic

anastomosis in adolescence (6). At the age of 50 the patient had developed markedly atypical papillary lesions histologically strikingly similar to villous adenoma of the colon. The lesion coexisted with extensive mucinous metaplasia of the urothelium. Silber (24) described 2 patients with non-functioning bladders, Ito and Martin, and Young and Parkhurst each described one patient all of whom developed invasive adenocarcinoma (23, 25). The patients with non-functioning bladder have a small but definite risk of developing bladder cancer and should be followed closely with regard to this possibility. Another minor anterior closing defect of the urinary tract is epispadias. This condition also appears to be associated with increased risk of developing adenocarcinoma. The setting appears to be the same as in patients with bladder exstrophy, namely the tumor develops in a bladder with extensive proliferative cystitis (27, 28). It also raises the question of whether a close follow-up by cystoscopy is indicated for patients with successful epispadias repair.

Based on the fact that the bladder proper and the urachus are so closely related it seems tempting to assume that adenocarcinomas of the urinary bladder and the urachus have the same etiology and pathogenesis. The prevalent theory suggests that adenocarcinoma of the urinary bladder proper develops from urothelium having the potential to undergo metaplasia to mucinous and glandular epithelium (29). The bladder mucosa is exposed to carcinogens and/or chronic irritation which may induce epithelial proliferation with subsequent development of bud-like projections from the bladder epithelium into the lamina propria. These bud-like projections, commonly referred to as von Brunn's nests, can acquire lumina, resulting in cystitis cystica. The urothelial lining of these small cystic structures may develop into columnar epithelium by means of metaplasia resulting in cystitis glandularis (Figure 2). This lesion may proliferate and become neoplastic resulting in an adenocarcinoma of the bladder. This theory is strongly supported by the fact that at birth exstrophic

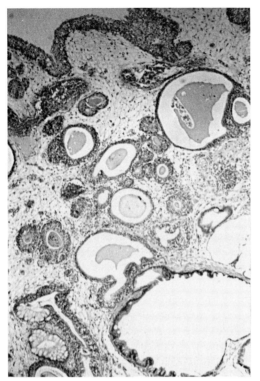

Figure 2 Bladder mucosa showing normal urothelium (top), von Brunn's nest, cystitis cystica and cystitis glandularis (glandular metaplasia) (bottom). H&E, original magnification: ×60.

bladder is lined with normal urothelium. Glandular epithelium develops later as a result of chronic inflammation (30). This theory has been challenged by Engel and Wilkinson in a study of bladder exstrophy since they were able to document the presence of cystitis cystica and glandularis in a patient only 5 days old (22). However, the existence of adenocarcinomas of the renal pelvis and ureter associated with ureteritis and/or pyelitis cystica and glandularis also favors the total potentiality-metaplasia theory (31–34).

The etiology and pathogenesis of urachal carcinomas may be difficult to explain and still remains poorly understood. Thus Schubert et al. (17) carefully examined 122 bladders and found intratubular urachal remnants in 32%, and in one-third of the cases columnar metaplasia was present. Communication between the urachal rest and the bladder lumen was not demonstrated. The authors concluded that even if communication did exist into the urachal lumen, reflux of urine would be unlikely because of the minute diameter and the presence of mucin and other secretions. Consequently it would be difficult to explain the development of urachal carcinoma on the basis of carcinogens present in the urine. Therefore it seems likely that the carcinogenic factors responsible for the development of urachal carcinomas are different from those responsible for adenocarcinomas arising in the renal pelvis, ureter and bladder proper.

MORPHOLOGY

Grossly primary adenocarcinomas may be nodular, papillary, sessile or ulcerative lesions. Thus, cystoscopically the tumors are not clearly different from conventional urothelial carcinomas. Whether urachal or non-urachal the adenocarcinomas can exhibit a number of histological patterns: (1) glandular; (2) colloid (mucinous); (3) papillary; (4) signet ring cell; (5) clear cell (mesonephric); and (6) adenoid cystic carcinoma. In the largest series of adenocarcinomas so far reported half of the 64 cases exhibited pure pattern and the other half was a mixture of two or more patterns (Table 2). The cases included in the study demonstrated adenocarcinomatous features within at least two-thirds of the examined area. Besides the patterns mentioned above, areas of undifferentiated carcinoma, urothelial carcinoma or squamous cell carcinoma were occasionally seen. The tumors with a glandular pattern exhibited anastomosing glands lined by tall columnar epithelium with enteric looking cells (Figure 3). The colloid tumors demonstrated scattered monomorphic cells or aggregates of cells lying in pools of mucin (Figure 4). The papillary adenocarcinomas showed papillary projections generally covered by pseudostratified cylindrical epithelium (Figure 5). These tumors are usually invasive but focally the tumors present as markedly atypical non-invasive papillary tumors which histologically

TABLE 2   CORRELATION BETWEEN HISTOLOGICAL APPEARANCE AND
LOCATION IN 64 CASES OF PRIMARY ADENOCARCINOMA OF THE
BLADDER *(Reproduced with permission from Cancer (15))*

Location of tumor	Histological appearance						
	Glandular ca	Colloid ca	Papillary adenoca	Signet ring cell ca	Clear cell ca	Mixed pattern[a]	Total
Dome	7	5	3	1		13	29
Lateral walls	7	1			1	6	15
Trigone	2		2			9	13
Posterior wall		3				2	5
Other						2	2
Total	16	9	5	1	1	32	64

[a] Mixed tumor pattern includes the 5 main patterns as well as foci of urothelial squamous cell and
adenoid cystic differentiation or undifferentiated carcinoma.
ca: carcinoma; adenoca: adenocarcinoma.

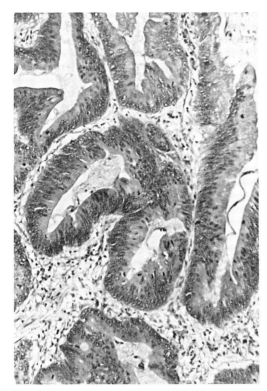

Figure 3 Adenocarcinoma of the urinary bladder, glandular type. Van Gieson, original magnification: ×144. *(Reproduced with permission from Cancer (15).)*

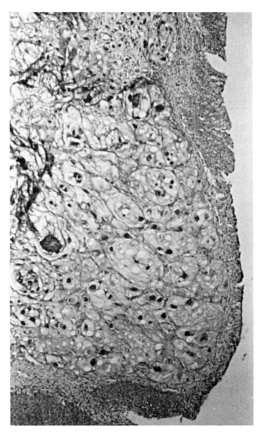

Figure 4 Mucinous adenocarcinoma of the bladder (colloid carcinoma) exhibiting scattered monomorphic cells in a pool of mucin. Note intact covering urothelium. H&E, original magnification: ×60.

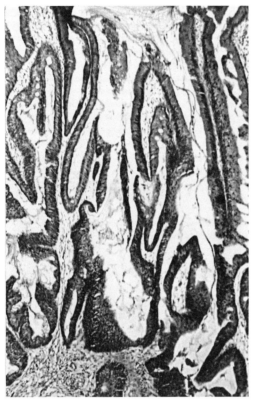

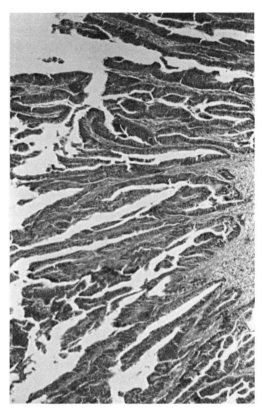

Figure 5 Papillary adenocarcinoma of the urinary bladder comprising papillary projections covered by a
pseudstratified columnar epithelium. PAS, original
magnification: ×60. (*Reproduced with permission
from Cancer (15).*)

Figure 6 Atypical papillary non-invasive bladder
tumor lined with columnar epithelium undistinguishable from atypical villous adenoma. H&E, original
magnification: ×60.

are undistinguishable from villous adenoma
(35–37) (Figure 6). The signet ring cell carcinoma consisted of signet ring cells in clusters or
single cells frequently associated with a marked
fibrosis and thickening of the bladder wall (see
below). The clear cell adenocarcinomas,
which sometimes are referred to by their old
name mesonephric carcinoma, may have a
variety of patterns including tubular, glandular, cystic and papillary structures lined by
cells with a clear cytoplasm or with a hobnail
appearance (Figure 7) (see below). As was
mentioned above, mixtures of more than one
histological pattern are seen in half of the
patients with adenocarcinoma of the bladder
and/or urachus (Figure 8).

Thus, histologically, it is not possible to
differentiate urachal carcinoma from non-

urachal carcinoma. However, it has been
suggested that following criteria should be
fulfilled in order to establish a diagnosis of
urachal carcinoma (38, 39):

1. Tumor located in the dome or anterior wall
   of the bladder.
2. The main bulk of the tumor located in the
   muscle rather than in the lamina propria.
3. Ramifications of the tumor are present
   extending into the bladder walls and with
   extension into the space of Retzius, anterior
   abdominal wall or umbilicus.
4. Urachal remnant present associated with
   tumor.
5. Intact or ulcerated surface epithelium overlying the tumor with a sharp demarcation
   between the tumor and the surface epithe-

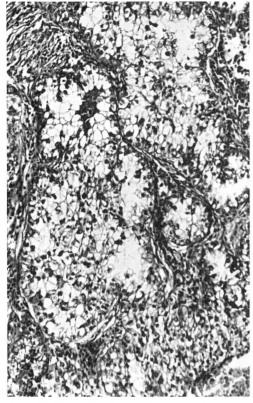

Figure 7 Clear cell adenocarcinoma of the urinary bladder exhibiting a glandular and trabecular pattern. Van Gieson, original magnification: ×144. (*Reproduced with permission from Cancer (15)*.)

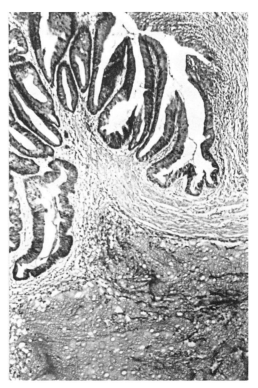

Figure 8 Adenocarcinoma of bladder with papillary (top) and mucinous features (bottom). PAS, original magnification: ×60.

lium that is devoid of glandular and polypoid proliferation such as cystitis glandularis.

However, we agree with Johnson et al. (40) who suggest—that these criteria for inclusion into a urachal carcinoma are too restrictive. Certainly not all urachal tumors need to arise at the dome of the bladder, since Schubert et al. (17) observed urachal remnants in the midline of the vertex in only 54% of their patients and identified remnants in posterior wall in 44% and in the anterior wall in 2%. Due to the fact that inflammation and cystitis cystica go hand in hand, one may occasionally encounter areas of cystitis cystica in bladders with urachal carcinomas. Therefore the presence of proliferative cystitis, such as cystitis cystica or cystitis glandularis, should not exclude a diagnosis of

urachal carcinoma unless a definite transition from cystitis glandularis to malignancy is demonstrated. This also was stated by Ward (41). He described cystitis cystica and glandularis but not intestinal metaplasia bordering an otherwise classic case of urachal carcinoma. The presence of urachal rests in association with a malignancy may aid the pathologist in making the diagnosis of urachal carcinoma, and sometimes the urachus is clearly identifiable grossly in association with a tumor (Figure 9). However, with this exception we have not been able to demonstrate urachal rests in any of our 64 patients nor were Johnson et al. (40) able to. In our own cases the explanation may be that the cases were studied retrospectively and also to some extent related to the extent of the tumors. Therefore the fulfillment of the three following criteria seem more appropriate to designate a bladder carcinoma as a urachal adenocarcinoma: (1) tumor

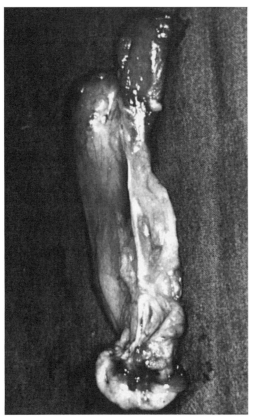

Figure 9 Surgical specimens of a urachal carcinoma operated on with resection of bladder and urachus. (Tumor and bladder bottom; urachus and surrounding tissue top.)

located in the anterior or posterior wall or in the dome of the bladder; (2) presence of sharp demarcation between the tumor and surface epithelium; and (3) exclusion of secondary spread from a primary tumor outside the bladder.

Approximately 90% of the tumors involving the urinary bladder are urothelial carcinomas and a high proportion of these tumors are multiple. In contrast the marked majority of the primary adenocarcinomas of the bladder, whether urachal or not, are solitary lesions. Another major difference between urothelial carcinomas and adenocarcinomas is the location of the tumor since approximately 50% of the latter are located in the dome or the anterior wall of the bladder while less than

10% of conventional urothelial carcinomas are found in this location of the bladder (29). The association of cystitis cystica and cystitis glandularis has been observed in approximately 50% of the cases of adenocarcinoma of the bladder (7, 13, 39, 40, 42). Several cases have described longstanding cystitis glandularis preceding or associated with adenocarcinoma of the bladder (43–47). In some case reports, the progression of cystitis glandularis into adenocarcinoma has prompted some authors to call this a precancerous lesion, but in most cases this does not seem to be justified, especially in view of the fact that mapping studies of urinary bladders have shown that by the age of 60 almost 100% of the population have foci of proliferative cystitis (48, 49).

Like practically all malignant tumors adenocarcinomas of the bladder can be subjected to malignancy grading. We have found that it is practical to apply a 4 grade malignancy scale based on glandular and cellular atypia. Grade I is well differentiated carcinoma; Grade II, moderately differentiated, Grade III, poorly differentiated; and Grade IV, undifferentiated (anaplastic) carcinoma. Thus, the system parallels the WHO grading system used for urothelial tumors (50). Mucinous adenocarcinomas and signet ring cell carcinomas are considered poorly differentiated carcinomas. The grade reported should be based on the area showing the lowest differentiation even if such an area is small.

The non-urachal adenocarcinomas can be staged as conventional urinary bladder tumors. T_A represents non-invasive tumor, T_1 tumor invades the lamina propria, T_2 microscopic involvement of the superficial muscular coat; T_{3A} tumor involving the deep muscle; T_{3B} extends into the perivesical fat; T_{4A} tumors involve the prostate or uterus; and T_{4B} tumors are fixed to the pelvic wall (51). Sheldon and associates (52) suggested the following staging system for urachal carcinoma: Stage I, no invasion beyond the urachal mucosa; Stage II, invasion confined to the urachus; Stage III, local extension into the bladder (IIIA), abdominal wall (IIIB), peritoneum (IIIC), or

TABLE 3   CORRELATION BETWEEN TUMOR LOCATION, GRADE,
           STAGE AND SIZE *(Reproduced with permission from Cancer
           (15))*

			Tumor location		
	Dome	Trigone	Lateral walls	Posterior wall	Other location
Differentiation					
Well	3	1	2	0	0
Moderate	10	3	4	0	0
Poor or anaplastic	16	9	9	5	2
Stage					
Lamina propria	2	1	3	0	0
Muscular wall	7	4	5	1	1
Perivesical growth	11	5	6	0	0
Metastases or local extension					
to other organs	9	3	1	4	1
Estimated size					
<2 cm	7	0	2	0	0
2–5 cm	9	6	7	2	0
>5 cm	13	7	6	3	2

viscera other than the bladder (IIID); and Stage IV, metastases to the regional lymph nodes (IVA), or distant sites (IVB). Adenocarcinoma of the bladder, whether originating in the bladder proper or in the urachus, is generally high stage disease. Sheldon et al. (52) reported that 83% of the patients with urachal carcinoma had at least Stage III disease. In our series of 64 adenocarcinomas only 6 cases had superficial invasion (that is into lamina propria), while 18 had muscular invasion, 22 patients had perivesical growth and 18 patients had extension to other organs or distant metastases (Table 3). The size of the tumors varied considerably: 14% of the tumors were smaller than 2 cm in diameter, 38% measured between 2 and 5 cm, and the remaining 48% were larger than 5 cm (Table 3).

Primary adenocarcinoma of the bladder metastasizes in a similar fashion as conventional urinary bladder carcinoma. In our series of 64 cases, 30 of the patients dying from primary adenocarcinoma of the bladder were subjected to a complete post-morten examination. Pul-

TABLE 4   THE SITE OF TUMOR SPREAD IN 30 AUTOPSIED PATIENTS WITH PRIMARY ADENOCARCINOMA OF THE BLADDER *(Reprinted with permission from Cancer (7))*

	Autopsied (%)
Lungs	40
Liver	37
Skeleton	37
Regional lymph nodes	33
Adrenals	20
Peritoneum	17
Skin	10
Various	17
Locally advanced tumor	43

monary metastases were found in 40% of the cases, liver and skeletal metastases were seen in 37% of the cases, and metastases to regional lymph nodes in 33% of the patients (Table 4). The pattern of metastases is virtually identical to that of high stage urothelial carcinoma (53–55).

Signet Ring Cell Carcinoma

Signet ring cell carcinoma is a rare histological variant of adenocarcinoma of the bladder, and these tumors have frequently been reported separately. The first 2 cases were described in 1955 by Saphir (56). Up to now 37 cases have been reported, 20 of which have occurred in the Chinese or Japanese literature, and the other 17 cases are derived from European and American reports (57–61). Approximately half of the cases originate in the bladder proper; the other half are urachal. However, when reviewing the different case reports we found it very difficult to evaluate if there were only focal areas of signet ring cell carcinoma within the tumor, that is the tumor was of mixed pattern, or if it had a more general signet ring cell appearance. The histological setting of signet

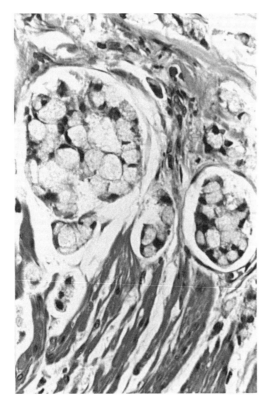

Figure 10 Primary bladder adenocarcinoma, signet ring cell type, invading smooth muscle. Note the vacuolated, mucin filled cells with compressed eccentric nuclei. H&E, original magnification: ×210.

ring cell carcinoma may be that of signet ring cells in a mucinous pool separated by cords of fibrous tissue or diffusely invading signet ring cells associated with a marked scirrhous stroma. The signet ring cells exhibit a mucin filled vacuole filling most of the cell with a slightly curved nucleus located peripherally close to the cell membrane (Figure 10). The mucinous content, which appears clear in routine stains, is strongly periodic acid–Schiff (PAS) and mucicarmine positive. Two cases studied by histochemistry and stained with PAS, mucicarmine, Alcian blue at pH 2.5 and 1.0, high iron diamine and colloid iron, demonstrated the presence of acid sulfomucins which are specific for colonic epithelium (58). The bladder generally has been described as thickened with grayish-white to shaggy reddish-brown color. The resemblance to linitis plastica of the stomach is striking and only occasional cases have been described as sessile, polypoid or fungating. There is a strong male preponderance in the number of reported cases; almost 90% of the patients so far reported have been males. Unlike the other types of adenocarcinoma of the urinary bladder the dominant presenting symptoms were irritative voiding symptoms found in 79% of the patients and hematuria in 64%. Fifty percent of the patients had ureteral obstruction which usually was asymptomatic (60). The prognosis of this variant of bladder adenocarcinoma is extremely poor and the tumor does not seem to respond to either radiation or chemotherapy (60). In our experience, the prognosis is more related to the high stage of these tumors than to the presence of the signet ring cells, which was also suggested by Johnson et al. (40).

Clear Cell Adenocarcinoma

Clear cell adenocarcinoma of the bladder is an even more uncommon variant of primary bladder carcinoma than signet ring cell carcinoma (62). In a recent excellent critical review by Young and Scully (63) concerning clear cell carcimonas of the urinary tract, which also included a review of slides of earlier cases, 6 tumors were reported to originate in the bladder and 13 in the urethra. An additional case has been reported by Hausdorfer et al. (64), and this tumor was diagnosed by urine cytology. The patients were all women aged 35 to 78 years. The majority of the tumors have been papillary although some were sessile. The major differential diagnosis is nephrogenic adenoma; this condition, however, is seen in younger individuals and two-thirds of the patients are males (65). The cells of the clear cell carcinoma have a clear glycogenated cytoplasm with significant nuclear atypia and abundant mitotic figures (Figure 8). Hobnail cells are frequently seen. In contrast the cells of nephrogenic adenoma lack significant atypia, have scanty cytoplasm and exhibit only occasional mitotic figures. The tumor cells of clear cell carcinoma stain positively with mucicarmine, Alcian blue, PAS with diastase and oil red 0 (66, 67).

HISTOCHEMISTRY AND ULTRASTRUCTURAL FEATURES

There are very few studies reporting on the histochemistry of the mucin in adenocarcinoma of the bladder. Tiltman and Maytom (68) examined bladder adenocarcinomas and found the urachal carcinomas contain neutral and sulfated mucopolysaccharides. In contrast, colonic carcinomas and adenocarcinomas of the urinary bladder proper produced sulfated acid mucopolysaccharides such as O-acetylated sialomucins. Identical results were found in the histochemistry studies done by Alroy et al. (69). Similarly, Wells and Anderson (70) demonstrated non-urachal adenocarcinomas to contain O-acetylated sialomucins which are present also in cystitis glandularis. The demonstration of O-acetylated sialic acid by the periodate borohydride/potassium hydroxide PAS (PB/KOH/PAS) technique has been regarded as a unique reaction to the epithelial mucin in the normal terminal ileum and large intestine (71). In a detailed histochemical analysis (20) of a case of adenocarcinoma

originating in the exstropic bladder it was found that the epithelial lining of the non-tumorous bladder mucosa had the appearance of normal colonic epithelium with crypt formation and production of colon specific mucins (O-acetylated sialic mucin). This is in accordance with the results of Culp (72) who studied the mucosa in patients with bladder exstrophy without tumor formation. He found that 73% of the specimens had colonic epithelium. Paneth cells and argyrophil cells are sometimes seen. Although these cells are not a normal constituent of the colonic mucosa, they may be seen in association with chronic inflammation, probably developing through metaplasia of the colonic epithelium due to inflammation (25, 61, 73). Since the urothelium is of cloacal origin and derived from the primitive gut, it is not surprising that the metaplastic glandular epithelium often is of colonic type and adenocarcinomas resembling colonic type are not uncommon.

The study by Alroy et al. (89) is the only major investigation that concerns ultrastructural evaluation of adenocarcinoma of the bladder. They failed to detect any features specific for adenocarcinoma of the bladder and concluded that the appearance was similar to adenocarcinoma cells of other organs. However, they described ultrastructural features such as coexistence of numerous 70F and 100F desmosomes and attenuation of tight junctions and the frequent occurrence of diminished gap junctions and they suggested that this reflected neoplastic transformation and bidirectional differentiation (74).

SYMPTOMS AND CLINICAL INVESTIGATION

The predominant clinical symptoms in patients with urachal adenocarcinomas are gross hematuria and abdominal mass, which are present in 71% and 11% of the patients, respectively (75). Dysuria and frequency have been reported to be present in 10% of the patients and lower abdominal pain in 6%. Mucous in the urine is a rare symptom and

only seen in up to 4% of the patients. Occasionally patients with urachal carcinoma can
present with hematuria despite the absence of a
visible tumor (76), but in almost 90% of the
cases the tumor is endoscopically visible. The
majority of patients with urachal carcinomas
have been reported to be male subjects. Thus
Gazizadeh et al. (75) found 72% of their
patients to be males in a large series of urachal
adenocarcinomas. The mean age was 51 years
for both sexes. Almost 50% of the tumors have
been diagnosed in the fifth and sixth decade
but occasional cases have been reported in
children (77). The majority of cases of non-
urachal carcinomas have also been reported in
men, approximately 70% of them with a mean
age of 60 to 66 years (12, 15). Most of these
patients also present with macroscopic hematuria which is present in 67 to 82% of the cases
(8, 12, 15). Dysuria has been reported in about
25% of the patients (15). The tumor location
in the three largest series of adenocarcinomas
of the bladder (12, 15, 39) which comprised
160 patients, was as follows: (a) dome or
anterior wall in 70 patients (44%); (b) the
lateral wall in 32 patients (20%); (c) the
trigone in 31 cases (19%); and (d) posterior
wall in 13 patients (8%). In the remaining 14
patients the tumor occupied more than one
area of the bladder (9%).

The tumor may appear as a protruding flat,
papillary or polypoid mass, sometimes demonstrating bloody or mucinous discharge from
the area of the urachal orifice (76, 78–80).

Transurethral resection biopsy reveals adenocarcinoma. The histological diagnosis of
adenocarcinoma of the bladder should alert
the physician to the following differential
diagnosis:

1. Metastatic adenocarcinoma.
   A. From distant organs to the bladder.
   B. From direct extension from the prostate,
      colon or female genital tract.
2. Primary adenocarcinoma (non-urachal).
3. Urachal adenocarcinoma.

It is generally not possible to determine the
origin of adenocarcinoma by microscopic

examination. However, in cases of prostatic
carcinoma involving the bladder, immunoperoxidase stain for prostatic specific antigen
(PSA) or prostatic specific acid phosphatase
(PSAP) provides a specificity and sensitivity
that may indicate the diagnosis as a primary
prostatic carcinoma. In a recent publication
Epstein et al. (28) examined 15 primary
bladder adenocarcinomas and 9 tumors with a
mixed glandular and transitional pattern and
found that 3 of 11 tumors in men and 2 of 4
tumors in women showed positivity for PSAP.
Also among the mixed tumors 1 of 5 among
men and 2 of 4 among women showed positively for PSAP while all 24 tumors stained
negatively for PSA. The studies were done with
antisera from several different companies and
it seems as if PSA is more reliable than PSAP in
diagnosing prostatic adenocarcinoma,
although we generally use both in uncertain
cases. In most other cases the diagnosis is
dependent on clinical findings. Further investigation should include radiological examination of the gastrointestinal tract, intravenous
pyelogram, computed tomography of the
abdomen, colonoscopy in selected cases and
careful gynecological examination in females.
When the patients seek medical aid for their
bladder symptoms the adenocarcinoma is unlikely to be metastatic. Direct extension of the
bladder from colonic carcinoma, prostatic
carcinoma and carcinoma of the female genital
tract is not uncommon. Clinically this is
frequently quite apparent. The incidence of
cancer metastatic to the urinary bladder is low
if direct overgrowth from tumors in neighbouring organs is excluded. In a study of 5000
autopsy cases, Klinger (81) found 142 cases of
cancer with metastases to the urinary tract, 33
of which involved the bladder and in 13 of
these cases the bladder was the only genitourinary organ involved. Twenty-seven of the 142
patients had urinary tract symptoms but these
were not symptoms bringing the patient to the
physician. The late symptoms produced by
tumors metastatic to the bladder are due
primarily to invasion of the muscularis of the
bladder or the lamina propria. By the time the

bladder is symptomatic the symptoms from the primary tumor are generally apparent.

Radiology

The radiological findings in adenocarcinoma involving the bladder proper are rather characteristic. Urachal tumors frequently demonstrate a filling defect in the dome and stippled calcification is seen in the bladder dome or in the supravesicular region. The calcification can be seen on conventional radiography and has, when present, been considered almost pathognomonic for urachal carcinoma (82, 83). However, frequently such calcification remains undetected in the plain radiogram. Dystrophic calcification occurs by deposition of calcium salts in degenerating or necrotic tissue and is particularly prevalent in coagulation necrosis (84). It has been reported to occur in many tumors and is frequently seen in renal cell carcinoma. It is the most frequent form of abnormal calcification (85). To distinguish this from that encountered on the surface of bladder tumors occurring within the submucosa of the tumor is important. This type of calcification is seen in approximately 0.5% of bladder tumors (86). Such patterns are easily distinguished by computed tomography. Microscopic dystrophic calcification not detected in the plain radiograph can be clearly delineated by computed tomography (84, 87, 88) which also may delineate tumor involvement of the bladder wall, perivesical or peri-urachal tissue or extension to other organs of importance in surgical planning.

MANAGEMENT AND PROGNOSIS

The diagnosis of a primary adenocarcinoma of the urinary bladder and urachus is justified only after a complete clinical investigation with biopsy and is extremely ominous for the prognosis of the patient. Although various treatment modalities have been used, the prognosis remains poor and the 5-year survival rates reported vary between 6 and 33% (12, 15, 39, 66, 80). The poor prognosis of adeno-

carcinomas of the bladder and urachus has been related to the late appearance of symptoms which is explained by their frequent location in the bladder vault or urachus. Accordingly, Mostofi et al. (39) found urachal adenocarcinomas to present a more unfavourable prognostic outlook for the patient compared to adenocarcinomas of the urinary bladder proper. However, contrary to the report of Mostofi et al. (39), Thomas et al. (12), Malek et al. (10) and Anderström et al. (15) found the prognosis for patients whose tumor was located in the anterior wall, dome or urachus not to be worse than that for patients with adenocarcinomas located in other parts of the bladder. The 5-year survival rate recorded for patients with tumors located in the dome of the bladder was even higher than that of patients with tumors located in other parts of the bladder (10, 12, 15). Furthermore, no correlation between tumor location and tumor stage was present (15). It is quite clear that high stage lesions are frequently seen at diagnosis regardless of tumor location, supporting the assumption of late symptom appearance. Thus, adenocarcinomas seem to be associated with late symptoms whether the tumor is located in the dome or the anterior wall or in other parts of the bladder. In various series 80 to 100% of the tumors have been reported to be invasive (10–12, 15, 34, 66, 80), and the 5-year survival rate has been found to be significantly influenced by tumor stage (Table 5). Thus the 5-year survival rate was 29% when the tumor infiltrated the lamina propria or muscular wall (15) (Table 5). When perivesical growth, or extension to other organs or metastases, were present, the 5-year survival rate declined to 15 and 7%, respectively (15). Thus, tumor stage must be considered to be one of the main predictors for the prognosis of adenocarcinoma of the bladder or urachus, and adequate clinical staging is mandatory before definite treatment is carried out.

Another significant finding necessitating a thorough clinical investigation is the high frequency of metastases which has been reported in patients with adenocarcinomas of

TABLE 5   CORRELATION BETWEEN EXTENT OF TUMOR GROWTH
AND SURVIVAL *(Reprinted with permission from Cancer (15))*

Years	Lamina propria or muscular wall, N=24		Perivesical growth, N=22		Extension to other organs or metastases, N=18	
	Observation time (yrs)	Survival (%)	Observation time (yrs)	Survival (%)	Observation time (yrs)	Survival (%)
0–1	20.33	70	15.09	45	7.43	15
1–2	16.16	58	7.91	21	2.83	7
2–3	11.75	45	4.00	21	2.00	7
3–4	10.50	37	3.50	15	2.00	7
4–5	8.08	29	3.00	15	2.00	7

the bladder or urachus (11, 12, 15, 39, 66, 80). The sites of metastases in adenocarcinomas were found to be similar to that of urothelial bladder tumors. The incidence of pulmonary, liver, osseous and lymph node metastases were found to be 40, 37, 37 and 33% respectively in 30 autopsied patients (15) (Table 4). The metastases in patients with urachal carcinomas as reported by Whitehead and Tessler (80) and Kakizoe et al. (66) seem frequently to involve the lungs, regional lymph nodes, peritoneum and the omentum. The pattern of metastases thus seems to differ somewhat between adenocarcinomas originating in the bladder proper and the urachus.

The very poor outcome in the 37 cases of signet ring cell carcinoma reported so far suggests tumor grade to be of importance for the prognosis of these tumors since signet ring cell carcinomas as well as mucinous adenocarcinomas are considered to be poorly differentiated. However, the majority of adenocarcinomas originating both in the urinary bladder and urachus appear to be poorly differentiated and generally there has not been any significant correlation between the degree of tumor differentiation and survival. Although it has not been possible to demonstrate a significant decrease in survival rate in patients with poorly differentiated tumors compared to patients with moderately well differentiated tumors, the results reported indicate grade to be of some importance for the prognosis (15). How-

TABLE 6   CORRELATION BETWEEN ESTIMATED TUMOR SIZE AND SURVIVAL *(Reproduced with permission from Cancer (15))*

Years	Tumor size <5 cm, N=33		Tumor size>5 cm, N=31	
	Observation time (yrs)	Survival (%)	Observation time (yrs)	Survival (%)
0–1	25.6	62	17.3	29
1–2	19.2	48	7.8	13
2–3	13.8	38	4.0	13
3–4	12.5	33	3.5	10
4–5	10.8	30	2.3	6

ever, tumor stage seems to be more important for the prognosis although poorly differentiated tumors frequently also are deeply infiltrating and have a marked tendency to spread laterally in the lamina propria and muscular coat.

The significance of tumor size was investigated in our series of 64 primary adenocarcinomas of the bladder and urachus (15), and we found that 29 of 31 patients with a tumor diameter exceeding 5 cm died of their tumor (Table 6). In contrast more than 50% of patients with a tumor diameter of less than 2 cm were still alive at the end of the study or died from intercurrent diseases. The data support tumor size as a consideration in tumor evaluation before therapy is administered.

When considering the influence of definite treatment on survival rates the location of tumor recurrence is of importance. Local recurrence following surgical removal is very common both in patients with and without distant metastases (10–12, 15, 34, 66, 80). This is in accordance with histological examination often revealing unexpectedly wide and deep infiltration not suspected clinically. In the evaluation of possible urachal adenocarcinoma tumor position is of importance. As was described by Begg (15), the urachus is located in the space of Retzius. Considered in its widest sense it embraces all the space surrounded by the posterior and upper aspects of the symphysis pubis and the transversalis fascia anteriorly, and behind the bladder as far as its peritoneal reflection and above that by the peritoneum. The lateral boundaries are the umbilical arteries. These structures and the urachus meet above forming the ligamentum commune which reaches the umbilicus. The ligamentum commune consists merely of drawn-out adventitial muscular and elastic tissue although some cellular components from the urachus may remain even in the umbilicus (20). In patients with adenocarcinomas of the bladder and/or urachus it is important not only to remove the primary lesion but also its ramifications and possible extensions. Most patients reported were treated by surgery, and adequate surgical excision of the tumor was considered to be the only method of value.

Mostofi et al. (39), Whitehead and Tessler (80), Thomas and Ward (12), Anderström et al. (15) and Kakizoe et al. (11) found partial bladder resection to result in the highest survival rates. However, in our study (15) careful selection rather than therapeutic effectiveness seemed to have influenced the results. The tumors of the patients treated by partial bladder resection were of smaller size and of lower grade than the tumors of the patients subjected to other treatment modalities but no difference in tumor stage was recorded. Complete removal of the urachus and overlying peritoneum was performed only in a few of the patients. According to the review by Kakizoe et al. (66) the remission time improved when an extended partial bladder resection was performed, and considering the high frequency of local recurrence the minimal surgical procedure to be performed seems to be a partial bladder resection with wide margins within the bladder wall. In conventional urothelial tumors, partial resection of the bladder is rarely performed because of the high incidence of local recurrence and multiple tumors. Primary adenocarcinomas of the bladder differ markedly in that aspect since multiple tumors are very rare and were only found in 3 of our 64 cases (15). In cases with potential urachal tumors, en bloc removal of the soft tissue of the space of Retzius including peritoneum and possibly the transversalis fascia should be carried out. It is important to stress that it is sometimes difficult preoperatively to distinguish between urachal carcinomas and benign urachal cysts and therefore Bourne and May (89) suggested total surgical extirpation of the urachus. However, as pointed out by McGeoy and Lewis (36) the effectiveness of removing a clinically uninvolved umbilicus must be questioned. If the tumor is of limited size and location in the mobile part of the bladder and not extending through the bladder wall or urachus, partial bladder resection or extended partial bladder resection in urachal cases seems to be adequate treatment. In other curatively treated cases we believe, although superiority is not proven, that total cystectomy in bladder cases and extended total cystectomy in urachal cases should be performed, considering the very poor prognosis for these patients, the extremely high incidence of local recurrences and the often unexpectedly wide and deep infiltration found at histological examination. If the chance of complete tumor removal appears to be enhanced by regional lymph node extirpation and extensive resection of the abdominal wall this should be employed in individual cases.

Transurethral resection seems to be adequate curative treatment only in those extremely rare instances where a non-infiltrating adenocarcinoma of the urinary bladder not potentially urachal in origin is present (54). In urachal cases transurethal resection can never be considered efficacious as the deepest part of the tumor can not be removed with certainty.

Radiotherapy has been considered of little value in several reported series (11, 12, 66, 80). However, Mostofi et al. (39) and Thomas et al. (12) have reported occasional cases with long term remission. In contrast, Whitehead and Tessler (80) and Kakizoe et al. (66), in their reviews of urachal adenocarcinomas, found that radiotherapy resulted only in transient remission, and the patients eventually all died of urachal tumor. Systematically administered preoperative radiotherapy and total cystectomy has not been performed but might provide a more favorable prognosis in more advanced cases.

Only in a few cases has chemotherapy been used as adjuvant therapy (7, 47, 75). As yet chemotherapy has not been shown to be effective in the control of the disease. However, as the tumor often is discovered in advanced stages with potentially disseminated disease, chemotherapy needs to be studied further. This could only be achieved in a multicenter national or international study because of the rarity of the tumor. The number of primary adenocarcinomas of the bladder or urachus in the United States will probably not exceed 300 per year based on the incidence figures found in Sweden and on reported cases from the United States.

ACKNOWLEDGMENTS

This work was supported by the Department of Pathology and Microbiology, University of Nebraska Medical Center, Omaha, Nebraska. The authors thank Cheryl Gerharter for excellent secretarial help.

REFERENCES

1 Hue L, Jacquin M. Cancer colloide de la lombille et de paroi abdominale anterieure ayant envahi la vessie. Union Méd de la Sienen-Inf Rouen 1863; 6:418–25.
2 Posner. Ein Fall von Carcinom der Harnblase. Berl. Klin Wochnschr 1883; 392–4.
3 Sperling A. Zur Statistik der Primaren Tumoren der Harnblase. (Thesis.) Berlin: Gustav Schade, 1883.
4 Begg RC. The colloid adenocarcinomata of the bladder vault arising from the epithelium of the urachal canal: with a critical survey of tumours of the urachus. Br J Surg 1931; 18: 422–66.
5 Begg RC. Colloid tumour of the urachus invading the bladder. Br J Surg 1936; 23: 769–72.
6 Gordon A. Intestinal metaplasia of the urinary tract epithelium. J Path Bact 1963; 85: 441–4.
7 Jones WA, Gibbons RP, Correa RJ, Jr Cummings KB, Mason JT. Primary adenocarcinoma of bladder. Urology 1980; 15: 119–22.
8 Peterson RO. Urologic Pathology. Philadelphia: JB Lippincott 1986: 289–90, 354–60.
9 Ichikawa T. Remote results of bladder tumors. Jpn J Urol 1958; 49: 602–10.
10 Malek RS, Rosen JS, Odea MJ. Adenocarcinoma of bladder. Urology 1983; 21: 357–9.
11 Jacobo E, Loening S, Schmidt JD, Culp DA. Primary adenocarcinoma of the bladder: A retrospective study of 20 patients. J Urol 1977; 117: 54–6.
12 Thomas DG, Ward AM, Williams JL. A study of 52 cases of adenocarcinoma of the bladder. Br J Urol 1971; 43: 4–15.
13 Jakse G, Schneider H-M, Jacobi G.H. Urachal signet-ring carcinoma, a rare variant of vesical adenocarcinoma: Incidence and pathological criteria. J Urol 1978; 120: 764–6.
14 National Board of Health and Welfare. The Cancer Registry. Cancer Incidence in Sweden 1958–1973, Stockholm 1971–1979.
15 Anderstrom C, Johansson SL, von-Schultz L. Primary adenocarcinoma of the urinary bladder. A clinicopatholigic and prognostic study. Cancer 1983; 52: 1273–80.
16 Begg RC. The urachus: Its anatomy, histology and development. J Anat 1930; 64: 170–83.
17 Schubert GE, Pavokovic MB, Bethke-Bedurftig BA. Tubular urachal remnants in adult bladders. J Urol 1982; 127: 40–2.
18 Abehouse BS. Exstrophy of the bladder, complicated by adenocarcinoma of the bladder and renal calculi. J Urol 1943; 49: 259–89.
19 Pugh RCB. Lower urinary tract. In: Anderson WAD, Kissane JM eds Vol 1, Chapt 23. Pathology, St Louis: CV Mosby 1977: 980–1.
20 Nielsen K, Nielsen KK. Adenocarcinoma in exstrophy of the bladder the last case in Scandinavia? A case report and review of literature. J Urol 1983; 130: 1180–82.
21 Beynon J, Zwink R, Chow W, Sturdy DE. The

late presentation of adenocarcinoma in bladder exstrophy. Br J Surg 1985; 72: 989.

22 Engel RM, Wilkinson HA. Bladder exstrophy. J Urol 1970; 104: 699–704.

23 Ito TY, Martin DC. Tumors of the bladder in renal transplant patients: report of a case of adenocarcinoma and review of known cases. J Urol 1977; 117: 52–3.

24 Silber SJ. Carcinoma in the bladder left behind. J Urol 1973; 110: 675–7.

25 Young RH, Parkhurst EC. Mucinous adenocarcinomas of bladder. Case associated with extensive intestinal metaplasia of urothelium in patient with nonfunctioning bladder for twelve years. Urology 1984; 24: 192–5.

26 Kickham CJ, Keegan JJ. The bladder 'left behind'. J Urol 1963; 89: 689–91.

27 Altamura MJ, Gonick P, Brooks JJ. Adenocarcinoma of the bladder associated with epispadias: Case report and update. J Urol 1982; 127: 322–4.

28 Epstein JI, Kuhajda FP, Lieberman PH. Prostate-specific acid phosphatase immunoreactivity in adenocarcinomas of the urinary bladder. Hum Pathol 1986; 17: 939–42.

29 Mostofi FK. Potentialities of bladder epithelium. J Urol 1954; 71: 705–14.

30 Formiggini B, Contributo allo studio della mucosa vesicale extrofica. Riforma Med 1920; 36: 352–62.

31 Ackerman LV. Mucinous adenocarcinoma of the pelvis of the kidney. J Urol 1946; 55: 36–45.

32 Blacklock ARE, Geddes JR, Black JW. Mucinous and squamous metaplasia of the renal pelvis. J Urol 1983; 130: 544–5.

33 Brawer MK, Waisman J. Mucinous adenocarcinoma probably arising in the renal pelvis and ureter: A case report. J Urol 1980; 123: 424–5.

34 Ragins AB, Rolnick HC. Mucus producing adenocarcinoma of the renal pelvis. J Urol 1950; 63: 66–78.

35 Assor D. A villous tumor of the bladder. J Urol 1978; 119: 287–8.

36 McGeoy TJ, Lewis CW Jr. Mucinous adenocarcinoma of the urachus. J Urol 1966; 96: 317–19.

37 O'Brien AM, Urbanski SJ. Papillary adenocarcinoma in situ of bladder. J Urol 1985; 134: 544–6.

38 Wheeler JD, Hill WT. Adenocarcinoma involving the urinary bladder. Cancer 1954; 7: 119–35.

39 Mostofi FK, Thompson RV, Dean AL Jr. Mucous adenocarcinoma of the urinary bladder. Cancer 1955; 8: 741–58.

40 Johnson DE, Hodge GB, Fahdi NAD, Ayala AG. Urachal carcinoma. Urology 1985; 26: 218–21.

41 Ward AM. Glandular neoplasia within the urinary tract. The aetiology of adenocarcinoma of the urothelium with a review of the literature. Virchows Arch Abt A Path 1971; 352: 296–311.

42 Kramer SA, Bredael J, Croker BP, Paulson DF, Glenn JF. Primary non-urachal adenocarcinoma of the bladder. J Urol 1979; 121: 278–81.

43 Shaw JL, Gislason GJ, Imbriglia JE. Transition of cystitis glandularis to primary adenocarcinoma of the bladder. J Urol 1958; 79: 815–22.

44 Susmano D, Rubenstein AB, Dakin AR, Lloyd FA. Cystitis glandularis and adenocarcinoma of the bladder. J Urol 1971; 105: 671–4.

45 Edwards PD, Hurm RA, Jaeschke WH. Conversion of cystitis glandularis to adenocarcinoma. J Urol 1972; 108: 568–570.

46 Gyorkey F, Kyung-Whan M, Krisko J, Gyorkey P. The usefulness of electron microscopy in the diagnosis of human tumors. Hum Pathol 1975; 6: 421–41.

47 Lin JI, Yong HS, Tseng CH, Marsidi PS, Choy C, Pilloff B. Diffuse cystitis glandularis associated with adenocarcinomatous change. Urology 1980; 15: 411–15.

48 Ito N, Hirose M, Shirai T, Tsuda H, Nakanishi K, Fukushima S. Lesions of urinary bladder epithelium in 125 autopsy cases. Acta Pathol Jpn 1981; 31: 545–55.

49 Wiener DP, Koss LG, Sablay B, Freed SZ. The prevalence and significance of Brunn's nests, cystitis cystica and squamous metaplasia in normal bladder. J Urol 1979; 122: 317–21.

50 Mostofi FK, Sobin LH, Torloni H. Histological Typing of Urinary Bladder Tumors. Geneva: WHO, 1973.

51 Manual for Staging of Cancer. American Joint Committee of Cancer Editors, 2nd edition, Beahrs OH, Myers MH (eds). Philadelphia: Lippincott 1982: 171–3.

52 Sheldon CA, Clayman GV, Gonzalez R, Williams RD, Fraley EE. Malignant urachal lesions. J Urol 1984; 131: 1–8.

53 Cooling CE. Review of 150 postmortems of carcinoma of the urinary bladder. In: Wallace DM ed Tumours of the Baldder: Neoplastic Disease of Various Sites. Edinburgh: E & S Livingstone, Baltimore: Williams and Wilkins, 1959: 171–86.

54 Fetter TR, Boagev JH, McCuskey B, Seres JL. Carcinoma of the bladder: Site of metastases. J Urol 1959; 81: 746–8.

55 Tabbara WS, Mehio AR. Metastatic patterns of bladder carcinoma. In: Bladder Cancer Part A: Pathology, diagnosis and surgery. New York: Alan Liss, 1984: 145–60.

56 Saphir O. Signet-ring cell carcinoma of the urinary bladder. Am J Pathol 1955; 31: 223–31.

57 Braun EV, Ali M, Fayemi O, Beugard E.

Primary signet-ring cell carcinoma of the urinary bladder: Review of the literature and report of a case. Cancer 1981; 47: 1430–5.

58 Kitamura H, Sumikawa T, Fukuoka H, Kanisawa M. Primary signet-ring cell carcinoma of the urinary bladder: Report of two cases with histochemical studies. Acta Pathol Jpn 1985; 35: 675–86.

59 Alonso-Gorrea M, Mompo-Sanchis JA, Jorda-Cuevas M, Froufe A, Jimenez Cruz JF. Signet ring cell adenocarcinoma of the urachus. Eur Urol 1985; 11: 282–4.

60 Hongyoung C, Lamb S, Pintar K, Jacobs SC. Primary signet-ring cell carcinoma of the urinary bladder. Cancer 1984; 1985–90.

61 Pallesen G. Neoplastic paneth cells in adenocarcinoma of the urinary bladder: A first case report. Cancer 1981; 47: 1834–7.

62 Minervini R, Urbano U, Fiorentini L. Mesonephric adenocarcinoma of bladder. Eur Urol 1984; 10: 141–2.

63 Young RH, Scully RE. Clear cell adenocarcinoma of the bladder and urethra. A report of three cases and review of the literature. Am J Surg Pathol 1985; 9: 816–26.

64 Hausdorfer GS, Chandrasoma P, Pettross BR, Carriere CA. Cytologic diagnosis of mesonephric adenocarcinoma of the urinary bladder. Acta Cytol 1985; 823–6.

65 Young RH, Scully RE. Nephrogenic adenoma. A report of 15 cases, review of the literature, and comparison with clear cell adenocarcinoma of the urinary tract. Am J Surg Pathol 1986; 10: 268–75.

66 Kakizoe T, Matsumoto K, Andoh M, Nishio Y, Kishi K. Adenocarcinoma of urachus. Report of 7 cases and review of literature. Urology 1983; 21: 360–6.

67 Schultz RE, Bloch MJ, Tomaszewski JE, Brooks JJ, Hanno PM. Mesonephric adenocarcinoma of the bladder. J Urol 1984; 132: 263–5.

68 Tiltman AJ, Maytom PAN. Adenocarcinoma of the urinary bladder. Histochemical distinction between urachal and metastatic carcinomas. S Afr Med J 1977; 51: 74–5.

69 Alroy J, Roganovic D, Banner BF, Jacobs JB, Merk FB, Ucci AA, Kwan PWL, Coon JS, Miller AW. Primary adenocarcinomas of the human urinary bladder: Histochemical immunological and ultrastructural studies. Virchows Arch (Pathol Anat) 1981; 393: 165–81.

70 Wells M, Anderson K. Mucin histochemistry of cystitis glandularis and primary adenocarcinoma of the urinary bladder. Arch Pathol Lab Med 1985; 109: 59–61.

71 Culling CFA, Reid PE, Burton JD, Dunn WL. A histological method of differentiating lower gas-trointestinal tract mucins from other mucins in primary or metastatic tumours. J Clin Pathol 1975; 28: 656–8.

72 Culp DA. The histology of the exstrophied bladder. J Urol 1964; 91: 538–48.

73 Satake T, Takeda A, Matsuyama M. Argyrophil cells in the urachal epithelium and urachal adenocarcinoma. Acta Pathol Jpn 1984; 34: 1193–9.

74 Alroy J, Weinstein RS. Unusual cell junction complex in canine mammary gland adenoacanthomas. J Natl Cancer Inst 1976; 56: 667–70.

75 Ghazizadeh M, Yamamoto S, Kurokawa K. Clinical features of urachal carcinoma in Japan: Review of 157 patients. Urol Res 1983; 235–8.

76 Begg RC. Haematuria from an undetected urachal tumour. Lancet 1952; 2: 18–19.

77 Raghavaiah NV, Redy CR. Adenocarcinoma of the bladder in a boy. J Urol 1976; 116: 526–8.

78 Green NW. Gelatinous carcinoma of the bladder. Ann Surg 1915; 42: 501–4.

79 Nadjmi B, Whitehead ED, McKiel CF, Graf EC, Callahan DH. Carcinoma of the urachus: report of 2 cases and review of the literature. J Urol 1968; 100: 738–43.

80 Whitehead ED, Tessler AN. Carcinoma of the urachus. Br J Urol 1971; 43: 468–6.

81 Klinger ME. Secondary tumors of the urinary tract. J Urol 1951; 65: 144–53.

82 Bandler CG, Roen PR. Mucinous adenocarcinoma arising in urachal cyst and involving bladder. J Urol 1950: 64: 504–10.

83 Beck AD, Gaudin HJ, Bonham DG. Carcinoma of the urachus. Br J Urol 1970; 42: 555–62.

84 Nesbitt JA, Walther PJ. Computed tomographic imaging of microscopic dystrophic calcification in urachal adenocarcinoma. Urology 1986; 17: 184–6.

85 McAfee JG, Donner MW. Differential diagnosis of calcification encountered in abdominal radiographs. Am J Med Sci 1962; 243: 609–50.

86 Miller SW, Pfister RC. Calcification in uroepithelial tumors of the bladder. Report of 5 cases and survey of the literature. Am J Roentgenol Radium Ther Nucl Med 1974; 121: 827–31.

87 Cooperman LR. Carcinoma of urachus with extensive abdominal calcification. Urology 1978; 12: 614–16.

88 Lupetin AR. Adenocarcinoma of the urachus: computed tomography diagnosis. J Comput Tomogr 1985; 9: 65–7.

89 Bourne CW, May JE. Urachal remnants: Benign or malignant? J Urol 1977; 118: 743–7.

90 Elem B, Alam SZ. Total intestinal metaplasia with focal adenocarcinoma in a schistosoma-infested defunctioned urinary bladder. Br J Urol 1984; 56: 331–3.

91 Kanokogi M, Uematsu K, Kakudo K, Shimada K, Jkoma F. Mesohephric adenocarcinoma of the urinary bladder: An autopsy case. J Surg Oncol 1983; 22: 118–20.

92 Logothedis CJ, Samuels ML, Ogden C. Chemotherapy for adenocarcinomas of bladder and urachal origin: 5-fluorouracil, doxorubicin and mitomycin C. Urology 1985; 26: 252–5.

93 Makar N. Some observations on pseudoglandular proliferations on the bilharzial bladder. Acta Uniointernationalis Contra Cancrum 1962; 18: 599–607.

94 Miller DC, Gang DL, Gavris V, Alroy J, Ucci AA, Parkhurst EC. Villous adenoma of the bladder: a morphologic or biologic entity? Am J Clin Pathol 1983; 79: 728–31.

95 Nocks BN, Heney NM, Daly JJ. Primary adenocarcinoma of urinary bladder. Urology 1983; 21: 26–9.

96 Spataro RF, Davies RS, McLachlan MSF, Linke CA, Barbaric ZL. Urachal abnormalities in the adult. Radiology 1983; 149: 659–63.

97 Vesth N, Kay L, Nordkild P. Adenocarcinoma in the defunctionalized bladder. Scand J Urol Nephrol 1985; 19: 303–4.

Textbook of Uncommon Cancer
Edited by C.J. Williams, J.G. Krikorian, M.R. Green and D. Raghavan
© 1988 John Wiley & Sons Ltd

Chapter **18**

Urothelial Malignancy of the Upper Tracts

Derek Raghavan,
Peter Russell,
James Wong,
Bruce Pearson and
L. Trevor Malden
Urological Cancer Research Unit, Department of Anatomical Pathology, Department of Urology and Department of Clinical Oncology, Royal Prince Alfred Hospital, Sydney, NSW, Australia

INTRODUCTION

Carcinoma of the upper urothelial tracts is an uncommon malignancy, accounting for less than 10% of urinary tract neoplasia (1–5). Whereas cancer of the bladder constitutes the fifth commonest malignancy in adult males, upper tract tumours occur only once for every 20 to 60 new cases of bladder cancer per year (4, 5). As urothelium lines the entire urinary tract, these tumours may occur synchronously or metachronously in several sites, including the bladder.

Although urothelial malignancy of the upper tracts shares many morphological and functional characteristics with tumours of the bladder, there are important differences which influence diagnosis, treatment and prognosis. We review these factors and present an overview of the management of this disease.

PATHOLOGY

Pathologically, malignant neoplasms occur-ring in the renal pelves and ureters are characterized by two major features. Firstly, they are variants within a limited histological spectrum, based upon transitional cell epithelium and its ability to undergo benign or malignant squamous and glandular metaplasia (Table 1). Although glandular differentiation occurs in approximately one-quarter of transitional cell carcinomas (TCC) of the upper urinary tracts, the term 'adenocarcinoma' is reserved for 'pure' carcinomas of this type. Similarly, squamous elements may be found in about one-fifth of urinary tract transitional cell carcinomas; the term 'squamous cell carcinoma' is best restricted to 'pure' malignant squamous lesions. Undifferentiated carcinomas exhibit no recognizable maturation towards any of these three cell types. Very rarely, other tumour types will be demonstrated, including melanomas, sarcomas or metastases (5, 6).

The second major pathological feature of upper tract tumours is their multifocal origin (noted in up to 50% of cases) (5–8). This

TABLE 1 HISTOLOGICAL CLASSIFICATION OF UPPER TRACT UROTHELIAL TUMOURS

Type	Frequency (%)
Pure transitional cell carcinoma	55
Transitional cell carcinoma with:	
glandular differentiation	20
squamous differentiation	15
glandular and squamous differentiation	5
Adenocarcinoma	3
Squamous cell carcinoma	1
Undifferentiated carcinomas	1

TABLE 2 STAGE AND GRADE OF UPPER TRACT UROTHELIAL TUMOURS[a]

Extent of tumour	Jewett classification	TNM classification
Carcinoma-in-situ	0	T_0
Non-invasive	—	T_a
Invasion of lamina propria	A	T_1
Invasion of superficial muscle	B_1	T_2
Invasion of deep muscle but no penetration through adventia	B_2	T_3
Penetration through adventitia of pelvis, ureter or renal capsule	C,D	T_4 ($N+M0_{-1}$)

[a] Modified from reference 30.
Grade: I: well differentiated; II: moderately differentiated; III: poorly differentiated.

phenomenon is observed in cases of multiple carcinomas in a single renal pelvis, ureter and bladder, where implantation metastases from the most proximal lesion may be a possible explanation. However, multifocal growth is also observed with multiple benign papillomas, which should not implant, and in simultaneous in-situ or infiltrating carcinomas in both kidneys or both ureters, where multicentric autochthonous neoplasia is the only likely explanation.

The gross and histological appearances of individual lesions are determined by which of two major growth patterns is present. From a presumed in-situ or intra-epithelial stage, tumour growth may be papillary or infiltrating. Intra-epithelial TCC is rarely observed in the ureters or renal pelves except in association with (and usually at the margins of) a papillary or infiltrating malignancy. Papillary TCCs make up the majority of epithelial malignancies of the upper urinary tracts (approximately 85%) and, grossly, are soft, sessile, translucent, papillary excrescences, occurring most frequently in the lower portion of the ureters. Larger examples, such as those found in the renal pelves, tend to be partly necrotic and haemorrhagic. Advanced ureteric cancers may be manifested simply as hydronephrosis or may present as a large, infiltrative retroperitoneal mass.

Adenocarcinomas are infrequently reported in the renal pelvis and extremely rarely in the

ureters. They tend to be raised, indurated lesions with a glistening or mucoid cut surface and are associated with dilatation of the pelvicalyceal system due to outflow obstruction. By contrast, squamous carcinomas are usually solid, indurated and ulcerated lesions, which fix the affected renal pelvis or ureter to the surrounding structures by infiltrative growth. They may occur anywhere in the upper urinary tracts.

Standard systems of classification of grade and stage have been established for these tumours, analogous to their vesical counterparts (Table 2). Histologically, the intra-epithelial stage of TCCs may be characterized by cellular atypia and marked nuclear hyperchromatism, an increase in the number of cell layers of the epithelium with only mild cellular changes, or a combination of both. Papillary TCCs show disordered multilayered growth of atypical transitional cells thrown into broad papillary folds which project into the lumen of the affected pelvis or ureter. The papillary or villous processes have a delicate fibrovascular core and may show coalescence of their tips in less well differentiated lesions. A prominent lymphocytic infiltrate is often present in the lamina propria at the base of the

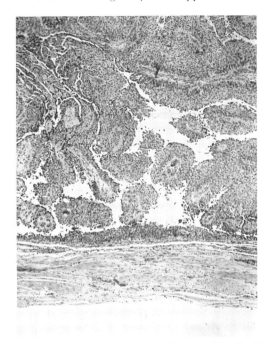

Figure 1 Well differentiated papillary transitional cell carcinoma at the pelvi-ureteric junction. Note the thinness of the pelvic muscularis at the bottom of the figure. H&E, original magnification: ×30. (*Figures 1–3 courtesy of Dr J. Philips, Sydney.*)

TABLE 3 UPPER TRACT TCC: DIFFERENTIATION VERSUS STAGE IN 157 CASES[a]

Stage[b]	Grade[b]		
	Well differentiated	Moderately differentiated	Poorly differentiated
0	18	14	1
A	2	22	11
B	1	13	8
C	0	7	24
D	0	10	26

[a] Data from references 5, 8, 10, 31.
[b] See Table 2 for definitions.

carcinoma. Perhaps the most important difference from bladder cancer is the absence of a substantial layer of muscle surrounding the urothelium and supportive tissue, and hence a reduced barrier to spread (Figure 1).

Infiltrating TCCs are generally moderately or poorly differentiated (Grade. II and III) tumours and show greater cytological anaplasia and mitotic activity. The normally polyhedral transitional cells may show marked spindling, giving rise to a sarcoma-like appearance. This is of particular relevance when there is renal parenchymal involvement as renal cell carcinomas may give rise to a similar pattern and a clear distinction between these two primary sites may not always be possible. There is an inverse correlation between the level of differentiation and the stage of the disease (Table 3).

Squamous cell carcinomas exhibit irregular branching tongues and cords of polyhedral cells projecting in a tentacular fashion into desmoplastic stroma which frequently shows a lymphocytic infiltrate. Tumour cells show a spectrum of differentation from poorly differentiated small cells to large eosinophilic cells with obvious intercellular bridges. Keratin production is also variable and, in the better differentiated examples, keratin pearls may be numerous.

Adenocarcinomas also vary from well differentiated tubulopapillary tumours composed of tall columnar mucus-secreting cells with hyperchromatic basal nuclei, to poorly differentiated solid adenocarcinomas with only occasional attempts at acinus formation. Well differentiated adenocarcinomas must be distinguished from the far more common non-neoplastic pyelitis or ureteritis glandularis. Undifferentiated carcinomas are characterized by solid sheets of uniform small cells (Figure 2) and some are probably analogous to the prostatic small cell carcinomas described in Chapter 15.

Ultrastructurally, transitional cell carcinomas show residua of the native epithelium from which they arise—namely, basal cell attachments to the basal lamina by hemidesmosomes, lateral cell-to-cell attachments (maculae adherentes), and tight junctions at the luminal angles of the surface cells. Characteristic lateral cisternae and intracellular tonofilaments are regularly present.

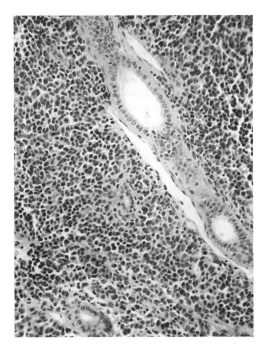

Figure 2 Undifferentiated small cell carcinoma of pelvic origin infiltrating renal medullary tissue. H&E, original magnification: ×150.

EPIDEMIOLOGY

These tumours occur predominantly in the older age groups, especially in the fifth to eighth decades; the mean age at presentation in most reported series is 60–65 years (1–10). In most series, the male to female ratio is approximately equal, in contrast to the male predominance in bladder cancer. The increased prevalence of females probably is due to associated consumption of phenacetin-containing analgesic compounds.

In the first half of this century, a common practice among the lower socio-economic classes, and especially among female factory workers, was the ingestion of excessive quantities of phenacetin-containing analgesic compounds (4, 6, 11). These preparations appear to have yielded transient euphoria, making them an attractive 'opiate' for workers engaged in boring and repetitive tasks. In addition, this practice was habit-forming. In the 1950s and 1960s, it became clear that this social practice was linked to the development of chronic renal failure, on the basis of 'analgesic nephropathy'. It has subsequently been shown that there is a causal relationship between analgesic abuse and the development of urothelial malignancy with lag periods ranging from 4 to more than 40 years (4, 11–13). In our own experience, more than half of the patients presenting with upper tract TCC have a history of analgesic abuse (8).

Cancer of the renal pelvis has also been reported in association with chronic nephropathy in patients in the Balkan states (14), although the exact mechanism is unknown.

Other aetiological associations have been reported, including cigarette smoking (8, 10, 15), industrial exposure (15, 16) and coffee drinking (17). Congenital renal tract anomalies have also been reported in association with upper tract malignancy, although it is not known whether they have a common aetiology (7).

INVESTIGATION

Clinical Presentation

The commonest presenting symptom of upper tract malignancy is macroscopical haematuria, which occurs in more than 70% of patients (1–3, 7–10). Less frequently patients present with flank pain, abdominal pain, weight loss, or urinary symptoms (such as frequency, nocturia, dysuria). Occasionally metabolic or para-neoplastic syndromes are noted (18–23). Up to 10% of patients are asymptomatic, with the tumour being detected at routine medical examination or in the investigation of an intercurrent problem (8, 10).

Physical examination usually reveals the presence of an abdominal mass or tenderness. It is not possible clinically to distinguish between a renal cell carcinoma and a TCC of the renal pelvis. Similarly, the distinction between a large tumour of the ureter and a mass of lymph nodes or a tumour of the gastrointestinal tract can be very difficult. In some instances, the primary tumour will not be obvious, but the patient will have evidence of metastases—most commonly to the regional lymph nodes, bone or liver (1–3, 6–10).

Initial Assessment

A detailed history and physical examination is required to reveal the possible local and systemic effects of the disease. In an academic clinical practice, useful features that should be documented include occupational history, personal habits (analgesic abuse, cigarette intake), ethnic origin, family history and history of prior malignancies.

The initial assessment of such patients should include the evaluation of renal and hepatic function, serum uric acid, serum calcium and a full blood count. Occasionally, the measurement of plasma carcinoembryonic antigen (CEA) or human chorionic gonadotrophin (HCG) may reflect sub-clinical disease, although rarely of clinical value in our experience.

Urine should be examined cytologically for malignant cells, and a sample should also be assessed for bacterial growth. In a patient with a previous history of bladder cancer, persistent haematuria or sterile pyuria may signal an occult tumour of the upper tracts and thus mandates further investigation.

Radiological Studies

Simple screening tests, such as plain radiographs of the abdomen or chest, may be helpful in staging the tumour. The loss of the psoas shadow may reflect a large ureteric tumour or the involvement of regional lymph nodes. Aberrant patterns of calcification may be seen. Occasionally metastatic deposits may be seen in the vertebrae or pelvic bones. Similarly a chest radiograph may reveal metastatic disease, although this is uncommon at presentation.

Intravenous urography commonly shows a fixed, irregular radiolucent filling defect in the renal pelvis or ureter. Calcification may be present in up to 70% of cases. Obstruction with

renal malfunction has been reported in about 30% of renal pelvic lesions and 45% of tumours of the ureter (2, 3, 8, 20, 22). In some instances, the examination will be completely normal, and in other cases there will be failure to visualize the kidney (10).

In association with cystoscopy and examination under anaesthesia, retrograde urography is often useful in defining more clearly the site and size of an upper tract tumour, with a filling defect being present in more than 80% of cases (22). Small volumes of contrast dye, diluted dye or double contrast studies with air/contrast may provide greater resolution. Cytological assessment, brush or basket biopsy, or ureterorenoscopy may be carried out at the same time, providing further information.

Computerized axial tomographic (CAT) scanning can be particularly helpful in determining the nature of a filling defect. CAT scanning may reveal intrusion into the renal pelvis, infiltration of the renal parenchyma or invasion of the perinephric space. Thickening of the wall of the ureter or adjacent involvement may also be seen. The tumour may be staged at the same time, with the assessment of regional and distant lymph nodes, the contralateral kidney, the liver and other potential sites of metastasis.

Renal arteriography may be useful in defining the nature of a filling defect, although its utility varies with the experience of the radiologist (24). We do not routinely recommend this procedure in the evaluation of upper tract tumours because of the 25–40% error rate, its invasiveness and the ready availability of CAT scanning. Although small tumours may not have vascular abnormalities, arteriography can occasionally be helpful preoperatively in defining the vascular anatomy of a large and otherwise ill-defined tumour, and the procedure is used in some centres to help the surgeon to plan the operation.

Radionuclide Scans

Radionuclide bone scans may be of use in determining the presence of osseous metastases as part of an initial staging protocol. Although such metastases are not commonly present at presentation, it is helpful to document their absence when radical surgery is contemplated. We do not believe that an isolated 'hot spot' in a bone scan should preclude surgery. At the very least, histological or radiological confirmation of unequivocal bone metastases would be required. Since the introduction of CAT scanning, we have not used radionuclide liver scanning in the staging of these tumours.

Endoscopic Examination

In view of the potential for field defects and multifocal involvement, cystoscopy, biopsy and examination under anaesthesia are integral to the optimal management of upper tract tumours. In addition to retrograde pyelography, as described above, brushing of the upper tracts may provide tissue for histological and cytological examination (15). Furthermore, catheter lavage and aspiration (barbotage) of the upper tracts may allow measurement of urinary CEA, which affords a relatively sensitive and specific index of upper tract malignancy (Table 4).

The procedures of barbotage may also improve the yield of cells for cytological assessment, although the quality of the preparations may be distorted by the physical disruption of cellular architecture. Although varying with the experience of the cytologist and the procedures used, the overall reported accuracy of urinary cytology in this context ranges from 40 to 70% (26, 27).

TABLE 4 PRELIMINARY EXPERIENCE
WITH URINARY CEA IN
DIAGNOSIS OF UPPER TRACT
TUMOURS[a]

	Urinary CEA (μg/ml)	
Tumour status	<2.5	⩾2.5
Present	1	5
Absent	13	1[b]

[a] Wong et al. in preparation.
[b] Positive bacteriological culture.

The uretero-renoscope can be used to visualize the entire length of ureter and renal pelvis. This also affords the opportunity to perform a biopsy with forceps or a basket. However, this procedure carries a risk of perforation of the upper tracts and must be performed with caution.

Fine Needle Aspiration Biopsy

The technique of fine needle aspiration biopsy (Figure 3) offers a useful alternative to endoscopic examination or retrograde brush biopsy under radiographic control when attempting to obtain a tissue diagnosis. A narrow gauge biopsy needle is introduced percutaneously into the putative tumour mass, controlled either by radiological image intensification or under ultrasound or CAT scan visualization.

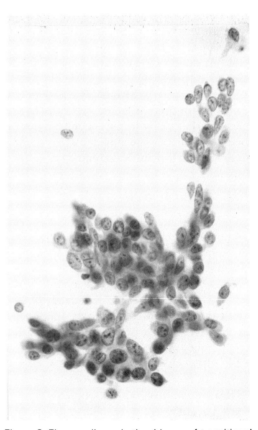

Figure 3 Fine needle aspiration biopsy of transitional cell carcinoma (same lesion as Figure 1). H&E, original magnification: ×300.

An experienced cytopathologist must be available to assess the specimen immediately; if an inadequate specimen has been provided, the procedure can be repeated. There is, however, a theoretical risk of tumour seeding along the needle tract, and the technique should only be applied by experienced staff (28).

TREATMENT

Surgery

Surgical excision is the treatment of choice of upper tract tumours (2, 7, 9, 10, 19). Nephro-ureterectomy is the preferred operation, and it has been shown that subsequent bladder recurrence occurs less often if a cuff of bladder is removed with the lower end of the affected ureter (2, 29, 30). The results of treatment are markedly influenced by the grade of the tumour (Table 5), with well differentiated tumours having a substantially better prognosis (1–3, 9, 10). Similarly low stage tumours have a better outcome than advanced disease (6, 31).

The optimal approach to surgery remains a controversial issue. Conservatism in the surgery of renal pelvic and ureteric tumours has been advocated intermittently for the past 50 years (32, 33). Several techniques have been reported, including partial excision of the renal pelvis, partial nephrectomy, partial ureterectomy and, more recently, percutaneous endoscopic resection of a renal pelvic tumour. These procedures may be carried out in association with radiotherapy. In most reports, conservative surgery has been used in patients with renal failure, poor general medical condition, bilateral tumours or solitary kidneys (30–35).

By contrast, the exponents of radical surgery claim longer survival figures (1, 30) and have suggested that the good results reported after conservative approaches reflect careful selection of patients, failure to report poor results (36) or that they are merely due to the long natural history of the low grade and low stage tumours included in the relevant series.

It should be emphasized, however, that the results of both conservative and radical surgery reflect non-randomized clinical trials, and the differences may be due to many factors. For example, more robust patients may be selected for radical surgery, thus favouring this approach. By contrast, more aggressive surgical approaches may be applied to 'high risk' tumours. Ideally, this issue might be resolved by a randomized multicentre trial. However, in view of the low incidence of these tumours, such a study might not be feasible because of low accrual of patients.

In the absence of unequivocal data, our routine approach for Grade II to III invasive tumours is to perform a nephro-ureterectomy with removal of a cuff of bladder. It is particularly important to monitor such patients regularly for evidence of recurrence in

TABLE 5 GRADE AND STAGE VERSUS PROGNOSIS: % 5-YEAR SURVIVAL

Reference	Stage					Grade		
	0	A	B	C	D	I	II	III
Batata and Grabstaldt (36)	—	90	43	17	0	—	—	—
Bloom et al. (1)	←60→		←28→		0	←56→		16
Booth et al. (7)	←73——→			←31→		73	40	33
Heney et al. (31)	100	95	82	29	0	100	81	29
Williams and Mitchell (2)[a]	←48→		←11——→			36	40	25
Williams and Mitchell (3)[b]	←42→		←15——→			45	10	0

[a] Renal pelvic tumours.
[b] Ureteric tumours.

the contralateral upper tract or bladder. In addition to regular physical examination and endoscopic assessment (with or without retrograde pyelography), we routinely check urinary cytology, and more recently we have commenced an investigational programme of assessment of CEA in urinary samples obtained directly from the upper tracts (Wong et al., in preparation). Additional investigations are performed, depending upon the preference of the clinician: chest radiography, CAT scanning of abdomen and occasionally radionuclide bone scans.

For patients who are poor candidates for aggressive surgery becasue of their general medical condition or the presence of metastases, nephrectomy alone is sometimes performed for tumours of the renal pelvis, accepting the risk of recurrence in the ureteric stump in order to reduce the extent and hazards of operation. Our approach to low grade, low stage tumours has been individualized, and conservative techniques are often employed in patients with chronic renal failure, analgesic nephropathy or solitary kidneys (after prior surgery for cancer or due to chronic infection). It should be emphasized, however, that there is a risk of local tumour seeding after opening the renal pelvis in a conservative technique (37). It has been reported that this risk can be reduced by the use of appropriate packing, suction via a ureteric catheter or irrigation with tumoricidal solutions (37), such as hydrogen peroxide, Milton solution, Betadine solution, 0·25% eusol or nitrofurazone.

It is clear that the selection of cases for conservative treatment is particularly important. It appears that tumours of the renal pelvis have a higher relapse rate than those in the ureter (21, 38) and, as previously noted, grade and stage are important determinants of outcome (1–10).

Radiotherapy

There is relatively limited published information regarding the utility of radiotherapy as the definitive treatment of upper tract tumours

(20, 39–41). A major difficulty has been the inability to deliver tumoricidal doses of irradiation without causing excessive damage to normal tissues, such as the kidneys, bowel or liver. Brady et al. (39) have described a small series of patients with ureteric cancer, treated by radiotherapy as the primary modality. Three of 6 patients survived more than 3 years. Preoperative treatment has also been assessed in a single-arm study of efficacy and toxicity, although long term survival data have not been reported (41). More recently, intraoperative radiotherapy (42) has been used for high grade, high stage upper tract tumours, thus allowing higher doses to be delivered to the tumour while normal tissues are retracted from the field of irradiation. It has also been proposed that postoperative radiotherapy improves the prognosis of patients with ureteric tumours (9, 20, 40), although these series have been uncontrolled.

In general, the role of radiotherapy in the management of upper tract tumours has not been defined. There have been substantial problems in the non-invasive staging of these tumours, and many of the published data antedate the use of CAT scanning for staging or planning of treatment. As noted previously, the rarity of these tumours has made the application of randomized trial design very difficult, and we know of no current studies designed to define the true role of radiotherapy in this context.

Cytotoxic Chemotherapy

Although there is extensive published information regarding the efficacy and toxicity of cytotoxic chemotherapy in the management of urothelial malignancy (43–45), there is a paucity of data relating specifically to tumours of the upper urinary tracts. In general, published studies of cytotoxic chemotherapy for urothelial cancer have incorporated isolated cases of upper tract malignancy, without separating their specific response rates or survival figures. We are not aware of any major studies which have specifically addressed the role of cytotoxic chemotherapy for upper tract tumours. Although one can extrapolate the data available for bladder cancer to some extent, there are two important factors to be considered:

1. Tumours of the upper tracts are often more advanced and widespread at diagnosis due to the reduced investing layers of fat and muscle; hence the response to chemotherapy may be different, perhaps reflecting the results obtained in large volume, metastatic bladder cancer.
2. Upper tract urothelial malignancy is often associated with chronic renal failure (due to antecedent analgesic abuse) and thus drug metabolism may be impaired, altering the profile of toxicity; furthermore, these patients may be generally less fit and less able to adhere to the regimens of cytotoxic therapy.

There is, however, clear evidence that upper tract tumours may respond to cytotoxic chemotherapy (46–48). The drugs that appear to induce objective response in these tumours include cisplatin, methotrexate, doxorubicin and the vinca alkaloids (a similar spectrum to bladder cancer).

Although several reports of the use of combination cytotoxic regimens for urothelial malignancy include patients with upper tract tumours, there is no clear evidence that these combinations produce improved survival compared with the use of single agents (49–51). The recently reported use of the combination of cisplatin, methotrexate and vinblastine (with or without doxorubicin) for urothelial cancer has been of particular interest (52, 53). To date, no response rates or survival figures have been reported for these regimens when applied specifically to upper tract tumours. We have treated two patients with upper tract tumours with the MVAC regimen (53) without achieving objective response, although others have had some success with this regimen in the management of upper tract tumours (Dr C. Sternberg, personal communication). Furthermore, we have treated similar patients with less intensive regimens, such as single

agents or two-drug combinations (50), and have secured long term remissions (8).

Our current practice is to treat patients with upper tract tumours according to protocols established for urothelial tumours that arise in any site. In particular, selected patients are offered treatment according to a randomized multicentre trial in which cisplatin is compared to the MVAC regimen (Dr L. Einhorn, Chairman). Particular attention is required for patients with a prior history of excessive analgesic intake, with meticulous documentation and monitoring of renal function, care with hydration and choice of cytotoxic agents. For patients whose general medical condition is not adequate for treatment with the MVAC regimen, single agent chemotherapy may be used. Not all patients will receive chemotherapy, especially in the context of advanced age, poor medical condition and established hepatic or bone metastases.

PROGNOSIS

The outcome of treatment is influenced to the greatest extent by the grade and stage of the disease (1–10, 19, 22, 31). As shown in Table 5, low grade, low stage tumours are commonly associated with long term survival. A broad range of survival figures has been reported for high grade, advanced stage disease, depending upon the age and fitness of the patients, treatment used and the presence or absence of metastases at first presentation (Table 5). As previously noted, it is not yet clear whether the use of more aggressive combination cytotoxic regimens will influence the long term prognosis of patients with metastatic disease.

SUMMARY

There are many similarities in the biology of cancers of the upper and lower urinary tract, including epidemiology, pathology and some aspects of treatment. However, important differences, such as site of origin, sex incidence, patterns of growth and metastasis and response to treatment, mandate that they be considered as distinct entities. We have assessed some of the important differences between bladder cancer and upper tract tumours, and have reviewed the current approaches in management. The death rate from high grade, high stage upper tract tumours remains high, and further advances in preventative medicine and in the techniques of early diagnosis and management will be required if the majority of patients with this disease are to be cured.

REFERENCES

1 Bloom NA, Vidone RA, Lytton B. Primary carcinoma of the ureter. A report of 102 new cases. Urol 1970; 103: 590–8.
2 Williams CB, Mitchell JP. Carcinoma of the renal pelvis: A review of 43 cases. Br J Urol 1973; 45: 370–6.
3 Williams CB, Mitchell JP. Carcinoma of the ureter: A review of 54 cases. Br J Urol 1973; 45: 377–87.
4 Johansson S, Angervall L, Bengtsson U, Wahlqvist L. Uro-epithelial tumours of the renal pelvis associated with abuse phenacetin-containing analgesics. Cancer 1974; 33: 743–53.
5 Chasko SB, Gray GF, McCarron JP Jr. Urothelial neoplasia of the upper urinary tract. Pathol Ann 1981; 16/2: 127–53.
6 Bennington JL, Beckwith JB. Tumors of the kidney, renal pelvis and ureter. In: Atlas of Tumor Pathology, Fascicle 12, Second Series. Washington DC: Armed Forces Institute of Pathology, 1975.
7 Booth CM, Cameron KM, Pugh RCB. Urothelial carcinoma of the kidney and ureter. Br J Urol 1980; 52: 430–5.
8 Malden LT, Raghavan D, Philips J et al. Urothelial cancer of the upper tracts: A report of 72 cases, including responses to chemotherapy. Submitted for publication.
9 Babaian RJ, Johnson DE. Primary carcinoma of the ureter. J Urol 1980; 123: 357–9.
10 Werth DS, Weigel JW, Mebust WK. Primary neoplasms of the ureter. J Urol 1981; 125: 628–31.
11 McCredie M, Ford JM, Taylor JS, Stewart JS. Analgesics and cancer of the renal pelvis in New South Wales. Cancer 1982; 49: 2617–25.
12 Adam WR, Dawborn JK, Price CG, Ridell J, Story H. Anaplastic transitional cell carcinoma of the renal pelvis in association with analgesic abuse. Med J Aust 1970; 1: 1108–9.
13 Bengtsson U, Johansson S, Angervall L. Malignancies of urinary tract and their relation to analgesic abuse. Kidney Int 1978; 13: 107–13.
14 Petkovic SD. Epidemiology and treatment of renal pelvic and ureteral tumours. J Urol 1975; 114: 858–65.
15 Schmauz R, Cole P. Epidemiology of cancer of the renal pelvis and ureter. J Nat Cancer Inst 1974; 52: 1431–4.
16 McAlpine JB. Papilloma of the renal pelvis in dye workers: Two cases, one of which shows bilateral growth. Br J Surg 1947; 35: 137–40.
17 Armstrong B, Garrod A, Doll R. A retrospective study of renal cancer with special reference to coffee and animal protein consumption. Br J Cancer 1976; 33: 127–36.
18 Bourne HE, Tremblay RE, Ansell JS. Stupor, hypercalcemia and carcinoma of the renal pelvis. N Eng J Med 1964; 271: 1005–6.
19 Wagle DG, Moore RH, Murphy GP. Primary carcinoma of the renal pelvis. Cancer 1974; 33: 1642–8.
20 Batata MA, Whitmore WF Jr, Hilaris BS, Tokita N, Grabstald H. Primary carcinoma of the ureter: A prognostic study. Cancer 1975; 35: 1626–32.
21 Mazeman E. Tumours of the upper urinary tract calcyces, renal pelvis and ureter. Eur Urol 1976; 2: 120–8.
22 Murphy DM, Zincke H, Furlow WL. Management of high grade transitional cell cancer of the upper urinary tract. J Urol 1981; 125: 25–9.
23 Kakizoe T, Fujita J, Murase T et al. Transitional cell carcinoma of the bladder in patients with renal pelvic and ureteral cancer. J Urol 1980; 124: 17–19.
24 Eklund L, Tothlin J. Angiography in carcinoma of the renal pelvis and the ureter. Acta Radiol Diagnost 1976; 17: 676–82.
25 Gill WB, Lu CT, Bibbo M. Retrograde brush biopsy of the ureter and renal pelvis. Urol Clin North Am 1979; 6: 573–86.
26 Sarnacki CT, McCormack LJ, Kiser WS et al. Urinary cytology and the clinical diagnosis of urinary tract malignancy. A clinicopathologic study of 1400 patients. J Urol 1971; 106: 761–4.
27 Zincke H, Aguilo JJ, Farrow GM, Utz DC, Khan AU. Significance of urinary cytology in the early detection of transitional cell cancer of the upper urinary tract. J Urol 1976; 116: 781–3.
28 Gibbons RP, Bush WH, Burnett LL. Needle tract seeding following aspiration of renal cell carcinoma. J Urol 1977; 118: 865–7.
29 Strong DW, Pearse HD. Recurrent urothelial tumours following surgery for transitional cell carcinoma of the upper urinary tract. Cancer 1976; 38: 2178–83.

30 Cummings KB. Nephroureterectomy: Ratio-nale in the management of transitional cell carcinoma of the upper urinary tract. Urol Clin North Am 1980; 7: 569–78.

31 Heney NM, Nocks BN, Daly JJ, Blitzer PH, Parkhurst EC. Prognostic factors in carcinoma of the ureter. J Urol 1981; 125: 632–6.

32 Petkovic SD. A plea for conservative operation for ureteral tumors. J Urol 1972; 107: 220–3.

33 Vest SA. Conservative surgery in certain benign tumors of the ureter. J Urol 1945; 53: 97–121.

34 Petkovic SD. Conservation of the kidney in operations for tumors of the renal pelvis and calcyces: A report of 26 cases. Br J Urol 1972; 44: 1–8.

35 Brown HE, Roumani GK. Conservative surgi-cal management of transitional cell carcinoma of the upper urinary tract. J Urol 1974; 112: 184–7.

36 Batata MA, Grabstald H. Upper urinary tract urothelial tumors. Urol Clin North Am 1976; 3: 70–86.

37 Fraley EE. Cancer of the renal pelvis. In: Skinner DG, DeKernion JB eds Genitourinary Cancer. Philadelphia, London, Toronto, WB Saunders, 1978: 134–49.

38 Zincke H, Neves RJ. Feasibility of conservative surgery for transitional cell cancer of the upper urinary tract. Urol Clin North Am 1984; 11: 717–24.

39 Brady LW, Gislason GH, Faust DS, Kazem I, Antoniades J, Davis JA. Radiotherapy—a valu-able adjunct in the management of carcinoma of the ureter. JAMA, 1968; 206: 2871–4.

40 Holtz F. Papillomas and primary carcinoma of the ureter: Report of 20 cases. J Urol 1962; 88: 380–5.

41 Almgaard LE, Freedman D, Ljungqvist A. Carcinoma of the ureter. Scand J Urol Nephrol 1973; 7: 165–7.

42 Martinez A, Gunderson LL. Intraoperative radiation therapy for bladder cancer. Urol Clin North Am 1984; 11: 693–8.

43 Raghavan D, Pearson B, Duval P et al. Initial intravenous cisplatinum therapy: Improved management for high risk bladder cancer? J Urol 1985; 133: 399–402.

44 Yagoda A. Chemotherapy of metastatic bladder cancer. Cancer 1980; 45: 1879–88.

45 Turner AG, Hendry WF, Williams GB et al. The treatment of advanced bladder cancer with methotrexate. Br J Urol 1977; 49: 673–8.

46 Sternberg JJ, Bracken RB, Handel PB, Johnson DE. Combination chemotherapy (CISCA) for advanced urinary tract carcinoma. JAMA 1977; 238: 2282–7.

47 Voy Eyben F, Mattsson W, Glißberg I, Lind-holm EE. Chemotherapy of advanced transitio-nal cell carcinoma of the renal pelvis: Report of 3 cases treated with vinblastine and chloroethyl-cyclohexyl-nitrosourea. J Urol 1979; 121: 367–8.

48 Kotake T, Usami M, Miki T et al. Combination chemotherapy including adriamycin for advanced transitional cell carcinoma of the urinary tract. Cancer Chemother Pharmacol 1983; 11 (Suppl): 38–42.

49 Soloway MS, Einstein A, Corder MP, Bonney W, Prout GR, Coombs J. A comparison of cisplatin and the combination of cisplatin and cyclophosphamide in advanced urothelial cancer. A National Bladder Cancer Collabora-tive Group A Study. Cancer 1983; 52: 767–72.

50 Hillcoat BL, Raghavan D. A randomised com-parison of cisplatinum (C) versus cisplatinum and methotrexate (C + M) in advanced bladder cancer. Proc Am Soc Clin Oncol 1986; 5: 110 (abstract).

51 Khandekar JD, Elson PJ, DeWys WD, Slayton RE, Harris DT. Comparative activity and toxi-city of cis-diammine dichloroplatinum (DDP) and a combination of doxorubicin, cyclophos-phamide and DDP in disseminated transitional cell carcinoma of the urinary tract. J Clin Oncol 1985; 3: 539–45.

52 Harker WG, Meyers FJ, Freiha FS, Palmer JM, Shortliffe LD, Hannigan JF, McWhirter KM, Torti FM. Cisplatin, methotrexate, and vinblas-tine (CMV): An effective chemotherapy regi-men for metastatic transitional cell carcinoma of the urinary tract. A Northern California Onco-logy Group Study. J Clin Oncol 1985; 3: 1463–70.

53 Sternberg CN, Yagoda A, Scher HI et al. Preliminary results of M-VAC (methotrexate, vinblastine, doxorubicin and cisplatin) for transitional cell carcinoma of the urothelium. J Urol 1985; 133: 403–7.

Section **|||**

Thoracic Tumours

Chapter **19**

Malignant Mesothelioma

James A. Talcott and
Karen H. Antman
*Division of Medicine, Dana Farber Cancer Institute,
Harvard Medical School, Boston, MA, USA*

INTRODUCTION

Although rare (approximately 2200 cases per year in the United States) (1, 2) malignant mesothelioma is important for several reasons. It is widely considered uniformly and rapidly lethal. No consistently effective treatment has yet been developed. More importantly, the tumor is strongly associated with an environmental carcinogen, asbestos, which is widely distributed. Seven to eight million living persons have been exposed to asbestos at work between 1940 and 1970 (3). Large numbers of public and private buildings, including an estimated 10 000 public schools, contain asbestos with potential for aerosolization into the environment (4).

The incidence of mesothelioma rises rapidly with time since first exposure, with a detectable increased incidence beginning about 20 years from first exposure (5–7). While industrial exposure of American workers to asbestos has been markedly reduced in recent years because of statutory and judicial developments (see below), even if all new asbestos exposures can be avoided, a large increase in new cases of mesothelioma is likely. Two recent estimates, based on different techniques, predict 19 000 (8) and 80 000 (9) new cases of asbestos-associated mesothelioma in the 30–50 year period beginning in 1980.

A number of obstacles have hindered the development of effective treatment of mesothelioma. The diagnosis of mesothelioma is difficult to establish. Robertson in 1924 (10) argued that all epithelial pleural tumors represented metastatic growths from other occult primary sites. He postulated that sarcomas, however, could arise de novo from the pleura (10). Klemperer and Rabin in 1931 first proposed a unified concept of primary pleural neoplasms including localized, benign mesothelioma and both epithelioid and sarcomatous variants of diffuse malignant mesothelioma (11). Histologically, the epithelial variant of malignant mesothelioma may differ only subtly from the much more common metastatic adenocarcinomas to the pleura. Consequently, until relatively recently, pathologists were reluctant to diagnose mesothelioma without the opportunity that post-mortem examination provided to sample the tumor extensively, observe the pattern of spread and eliminate other possible primary sites of cancer (12) Winslow and Taylor (13) argued as late as 1960 that diagnostic criteria for malignant mesothelioma should include 'progressive growth of tumor in a characteristic manner, resulting in the death of the patient.' Although electron microscopy and immunohistochemical techniques based on monoclonal antibody technology have substantially improved the ability of pathologists to diagnose mesothelioma (14–16), these techniques are themselves imperfect and not universally available. Diagnostic disagreement among pathologists in putative cases remains common (17, 18) particularly if litigation is involved.

Studies of mesothelioma treatment have been hindered by the tumor's rarity and varied natural history. Single institutions have been unable to accumulate sufficient patients for powerful statistical analysis of outcomes following therapeutic intervention. The natural history of mesothelioma obscures the interpretation of large published therapeutic trials. Because mesotheliomas are generally rapidly lethal, the impact of any treatment producing significant numbers of long-term survivors should be easily recognized. However, a small percentage of patients have survived for long periods (> 2–16 years) in most large published series, including series of patients treated symptomatically (19). Thus the interpretation of reported prolonged survival resulting from treatment is complicated. Selection bias is difficult to avoid in nonrandomized trials. The median survival of patients with the epithelioid variant (13–29 months) is longer than that of those with the sarcomatoid or mixed variants (7–12 months) (20–22). Therefore, comparisons should be made within histologic subtypes.

Nevertheless, significant progress has been made in techniques for obtaining tissue for diagnosis, the use of immunohistochemical techniques and electron microscopy and in clinical staging of the mesotheliomas before and after treatments. Cooperative groups have organized trials to compare treatments in larger number of patients. The legislated reduction of occupational and incidental exposure of individuals to the primary carcinogen, asbestos, although belated and incomplete, suggests that the incidence of malignant mesothelioma may decline in the future.

BENIGN MESOTHELIOMA

Benign, well localized tumors of the serous membranes were distinguished from the diffuse, malignant variety by Klemperer and Rabin (23) who equated localized disease with benign mesothelioma and diffuse disease with malignant mesothelioma. Stout and Murray (24) proposed the mesothelial origin of the localized variety based on cell culture techniques.

Benign and malignant mesotheliomas differ dramatically in their natural history. While localized malignant mesotheliomas have occasionally been diagnosed (25) localized benign tumors demonstrate little, if any, invasive or metastatic potential. Malignant mesothelioma, in contrast, invades locally early in the disease course with direct extension to nearby organs and metastases to distant sites a common preterminal development. Solitary pleural tumors have been variously labelled fibrous, benign or localized mesothelioma, subpleural fibroma, or localized fibroma of the pleura (26). Histologically, benign mesotheliomas resemble fibromas.

The tumor is approximately one-third as common as diffuse malignant mesothelioma (27), and most common in midlife from the fifth to the seventh decades but rare in children. The lack of association with asbestos exposure is reflected in the slight preponderance of women and in symmetrical distribution in the chest. In contrast, malignant mesothelioma has a striking male predominance due to occupational exposure and occurs more frequently in the right chest cavity, perhaps because the lesser deviation of the right main stem bronchus at the carina allows heavier inhaled asbestos exposures on the right.

The solitary fibrous tumor of the pleura presents most commonly as an asymptomatic mass discovered on chest x-ray. Symptoms when they occur are due to local tumor growth, such as cough, chest pain and dyspnea, or systemic complaints such as fever, clubbing, or osteoarthropathy. Large tumors were frequently associated with arthralgias in one series (28). Associated pleural and pericardial effusions may be serosanguineous and may compromise cardiac and pulmonary function (29). Hypoglycemia occurs in approximately 4% of reported cases, more commonly than in malignant mesothelioma (30). Galactorrhea, suggesting abnormal central endocrine regulation, has also been reported (31). Systemic effects usually resolve following resection (28, 32, 33).

While tumors may become enormous, reaching several kilograms, smaller tumors have been reported recently, presumably because of earlier diagnosis (30). Tumors arise most commonly from the visceral pleura and may hang on a vascular stalk. The tumor may extend into the lung directly from the pleura or from pleural rests (28). The tumor is a generally rounded, clearly marginated pleural mass on chest x-ray (34). The differential diagnosis includes primary and secondary malignancies, other benign tumors such as hemangiomas and lipomas, organizing inflammation (pseudotumors), and loculated pleural fluid. Pulmonary sequestration, infarcts, granulomas, hamarto mas, and hydatid cysts may be confused with the intrapulmonary variant. The CT scan most accurately distinguishes a pleural from an intrapulmonary mass. Fluoroscopy may be helpful since the respiratory motion of a mass adherent to the lung is opposite to that of a mass adherent to the chest wall. A cyst may be diagnosed by ultrasound.

Grossly, these tumors are usually rounded, rubbery, firm and well circumscribed and may be pedunculated. The tumor parenchyma is generally grey-white or yellow. Pathologic features associated with malignancy such as hemorrhage, necrosis, and calcification may be prominent in larger tumors. Microscopically, the tumors are composed of elongated cells with oval fusiform nuclei, dark homogeneous cytoplasm and inconspicuous nucleoli. Larger tumors may be highly vascular. An intact layer of mesothelium covers the tumor mass. Predominantly epithelial or mixed tumors are very rare and should suggest malignant mesothelioma (28, 30). Microvilli are absent or primitive on electron microscopy (26). The cell of origin of these tumors is unclear, although the bulk of histochemical studies suggest a submesothelial fibroblast (30). The apparent admixture of fibroblasts and mesothelial elements may result from a common precursor cell capable of differentiation to both surface mesothelium and connective tissue (35).

Natural History and Therapy

The tumor has a benign natural history subject to complete resection and cure although recurrences as late as 17 years have been reported (28, 36). Large tumors may be locally invasive and cause death within 2 years (28, 37, 39). An atypical microscopic appearance in a large tumor may suggest sarcoma, but this should not deter attempted resection for cure. When the primary pathology is ambiguous biopsy of an apparently clinically uninvolved area of pleura may document diffuse mesothelioma.

A tumor of mesothelial origin with a long natural history characterized by multiple recurring peritoneal cysts has recently been described and distinguished from cystic lymphangiomas (40, 42).

EPIDEMIOLOGY

Asbestos

The association of asbestos exposure and the subsequent development of malignant mesothelioma was established by Wagner and associates who observed 47 mesotheliomas in a crocidolite asbestos-mining area in South Africa. Of 33 patients initially described (the remainder were added in an addendum), 32 had a history of asbestos exposure. Of these, 6 were miners, 4 had industrial exposure and the remainder lived near the mines and were only incidentally exposed. The study carefully documented both occupational and indirect exposure, the development of mesothelioma in persons without pulmonary evidence of asbestos-related disease, and the greater than 20-

year delay between exposure and diagnosis (5).

Other etiologic associations have been demonstrated in only a small minority of mesothelioma patients without identified asbestos contact. Mesothelioma in man has been reported after exposure to radiation (43–45), thorium dioxide (Thorotrast) (46, 47), beryllium (22), and perhaps zeolite, a fibrous aluminium silicate (48, 49) although exposure to asbestos may have occurred in the latter case (50).

Mineralogy

'Asbestos' refers to a family of commercially produced silicate fibers whose length:width ratio is generally high and defined as greater than 3. Asbestos occurs in two configurations: the long, straight amphiboles, including crocidolite and amosite, and the serpentines, predominantly chrysotile. Over 90% of asbestos currently used worldwide is chrysotile (51). Crocidolite is the most carcinogenic fiber type, amosite is intermediate and chrysotile is the least potent carcinogen (52–54).

Mechanism of Carcinogenesis

The mechanism of carcinogenesis of asbestos remains obscure. Implicated fiber characteristics include narrow width, which allows greater lung penetration (55), increased length-to-width ratio (56), and chemical stability, which protects the fiber against removal by macrophages or the mucociliary tree (57). In rats, inhaled amphibole fibers accumulate in the lungs, much more than chrysotile fibers, attesting to the greater penetration and stability of amphibole fibers (55). The leaching of magnesium, which stabilizes adjacent strands of chrysotile, may hasten its breakdown in vivo (58). How asbestos reaches the peritoneum is unclear, whether through penetration of swallowed fibers through bowel wall or retrograde flow from the pleural lymphatic space. Only one gastrointestinal mesothelioma occurred in 189 rats with a lifelong diet containing 10%

chrysotile (59). The relative risk of gastrointestinal adenocarcinomas in asbestos workers is about 3 times, far less than that for peritoneal mesothelioma (60, 61).

Malignancies have been induced in mice by chrysotile and anthophyllite, asbestos varieties with a relatively weak association with human cancer (43, 44). Stanton and co-workers (62) found that fibers more than 8 μm in length and less than 1.5 μm in diameter more commonly cause tumors in animals. In addition, they observed that fiberglass, nonsilicon-containing substances such as aluminium oxide, and chrysotile were potent carcinogens in animals. Thus shape, rather than chemical properties, appears to determine the tumorogenicity of asbestos (62). Substances which cause experimental animal tumors could conceivably cause human cancer if the material could reach and remain in contact with the relevant serosal surfaces. Churg and co-workers reported a case in which mesothelioma arose in the pericardium of a patient treated for pericardial effusion with topical application of dust composed of tremolite and anthophyllite asbestos and fiberglass (63). Foreign bodies have induced related sarcomas in experimental systems (64, 65). Interestingly, in the in vivo mouse explant system of Brand and colleagues, neoplastic transformation occurs early after implantation of a foreign body, but transformed cells do not begin proliferating for long periods (66).

Persons at Risk

Wagner's observations of a strong asbestos–mesothelioma association in the South African mining community have been extended to British, European, North American, and Australian industries such as textiles (67), insulation (68) and ship building (69). In the United States the most important occupational exposures are construction trades (7.5 million), automobile maintenance (6.4 million) and shipbuilding and repair (6.1 million, including 4.3 million temporary workers during World War II) (9). An estimated four million Americans have been heavily exposed to asbestos (70). Out of all deaths in asbestos insulation workers followed for several decades 7.7% could be attributed to mesothelioma (6, 71). The relative risk of mesothelioma in insulators in the United States and Canada is 46.0 (72). An increased incidence of asbestos-associated mesothelioma exposure is expected in the next 30–50 years with published estimates of between 19 000 and 80 000 new cases in that interval (8,9).

In a cohort of insulation workers followed for up to 50 years, Selikoff first detected an increase in the incidence of mesothelioma at 15–19 years after the first exposure. The incidence rose steadily to 5.5 per 1000 person-years after first exposure at an interval of 45–50 years (72). Unlike asbestos-associated lung cancers, no difference in smoking rates have been found in asbestos-exposed workers with and without mesothelioma (73). Many patients with asbestos-associated mesothelioma have no evidence of the lung parenchymal and pleural fibrosis characteristic of patients with a heavy asbestos exposure (74).

Beginning with the descriptions of Wagner in 1960, an increased incidence of mesothelioma in residents of neighborhoods surrounding major industrial sites utilizing asbestos (5, 75, 76), have been well documented. In addition, x-ray changes characteristic of asbestos exposure (77, 78) and an increased risk of mesothelioma were found in family contacts of asbestos workers (79). Families have been found in which more than one member developed mesothelioma (80, 81). These are best explained on the basis of common exposures to asbestos presumably from dust brought home on the person of the asbestos worker.

Studies counting asbestos fibers and ferruginous bodies, or 'asbestos bodies' in lung tissue, have demonstrated levels of 100–500 fibers/gram of lung tissue in persons living in major cities. The potential risk of such casual exposures is uncertain (82–84). In a study in rats, mesothelioma could be produced by as little as a single day's exposure to inhaled asbestos (55). Other evidence also suggests the lack of

threshold dose of asbestos for mesothelioma (85). Even if a threshold exposure is necessary for development of mesothelioma, it is useful to assume a linear relationship between dust levels and cancer risk for evaluating changes in dust standards, since individual exposures will vary at a given average or peak dust concentration (7). Documentation of mesothelioma associated with surprisingly small exposures, along wth the 25–40% of patients without recollection of contact with asbestos (86), have raised concern about the risk of mesothelioma in patients with minimal environmental exposures, such as in public buildings with unmaintained asbestos insulation (4). These uncertainties about the risk of low, nonoccupational asbestos exposures have made formulation of public health policy difficult and controversial.

Screening for cancer in asbestos-exposed workers has been examined for cost-effectiveness. Screening for colon cancer, a prevalent malignancy with a relative risk of approximately three in exposed workers, appears worthwhile. Although lung cancer is common, screening may not be useful since therapies are ineffective and diagnostic techniques insensitive (87). No practical means of screening for mesothelioma has been proposed.

Thus, while asbestos-associated mesothelioma remains a striking example of environmental carcinogenesis, much remains incompletely understood. Development of rational measures to protect the public health are hampered by uncertainty about the threshold of asbestos exposure necessary to produce disease. Important co-carcinogens or individual susceptibility may be contributory factors. Estimates of asbestos exposures are imprecise. Cellular and genetic changes involved in malignant transformation and the mechanism by which the shape of the asbestos fiber initiates malignant transformation are as yet unclear.

Legislative Issues

Mesothelioma, like asbestos-associated interstitial lung disease (asbestosis) and bronchogenic carcinoma of the lung, could be reduced substantially by preventing occupational and casual asbestos exposure. In the United States, industrial asbestos exposure is largely controlled by standards set by the Occupational Safety and Health Administration. Approximately 50 000 to 100 000 persons have filed or will file product liability suits against companies which make and use asbestos products to claim damages for asbestos-related diseases.

A brief review of the scientific evidence linking asbestos with serious disease and the American statutory response to this challenge in the last 80 years illustrates the difficulty of controlling by statute a potential cause of serious disease. The history of regulatory legislation in the United States has been reviewed recently (88). Castleman, however, has observed that statutory protections in the industrialized nations do not prevent high levels of exposure to workers in the less developed world, where practices prohibited elsewhere may continue unregulated (89).

One of the first descriptions of disability from asbestos-related disease occurred in 1906. Murray described a 33-year-old man with 14 years of asbestos exposure in a dusty card room (90). All 10 other co-workers with whom he began working had already died. Cooke reported the first case in the medical literature, chronic lung disease in a 33-year-old woman with an 18-year history of asbestos exposure (91). In 1918, a US Labor Department report by Frederick L. Hoffman, vice-president of Prudential Life Insurance Company of New York, stated that asbestos dust 'unquestionably' exposed workers to 'a considerable dust hazard' (92). Little actuarial data existed for asbestos workers in North America since American and Canadian life insurance companies refused to insure them without a large premium surcharge for their expected excess mortality. In 1930 Meriweather reported pulmonary fibrosis in 95 of 363 patients exposed to asbestos dust (93). In response, Great Britain attempted to control asbestos exposures by the Asbestos Industry Regulations of 1931 which regulated handling of raw asbestos but not

asbestos textiles (94). In the United States, the Walsh-Healey Public Contracts Act in 1936 forbade most contractors or suppliers to the Federal Government to allow 'working conditions which are unsanitary or hazardous or dangerous to the health and safety of the employees' (95). Walsh-Healey, however, set no standards until 1942, had minimal provisions for surveillance and but a single enforcement provision, exclusion of the violator from further federal contracts. The likelihood of careful surveillance and strict enforcement fell as the United States prepared for and then fought World War II. Military manufacturing intensified dramatically in 1939 with the onset of war in Europe. In the effort to provide adequate cargo ships despite heavy losses, the number of shipyard workers grew from 177 300 in July, 1940, to a peak of almost two million in 1944. Selikoff has estimated that 4 500 000 workers were employed in shipyards in World War II (6). A committee headed by Dr Philip Drinker surveyed the hazards of the shipyard workplace (96). Minimum health and safety standards for Navy shipyards were promulgated, including segregation of dusty work, requirements for ventilation, respirators and periodic medical examinations for those who worked at any job exposed to asbestos dust (97). A study of pipe insulators, flawed by short and incomplete follow-up, erroneously concluded that pipe insulation posed little hazard of asbestosis (98). The health and safety program of the US Maritime Commission was terminated after World War II.

In 1946, on the basis of field studies in which asbestos fiber concentrations in workplace air samples were measured, the American Conference of Government Industrial Hygienists (ACGIH) recommended a standard of five million asbestos particles per cubic foot of air (99). By 1948, 31 states had adapted similar threshold limit values (TLV) for asbestos. In 1955, Richard Doll reported increased lung cancer rates in asbestos workers (100). In 1960, under the provisions of the Longshoremen and Harbor Workers Compensation Act, the federal government adopted the ACGIH standard for asbestos dust for shipyard work. The same year, Wagner reported an association between asbestos exposure and mesothelioma in South Africa (5).

Seilkoff's study of mortality in asbestos insulation workers presented in 1964 at the Biological Effects of Asbestos Conference in New York, demonstrated the risk to those intermittently handling finished asbestos products (101). In 1968, Harries found asbestosis in workers refitting and repairing ships in British shipyards, demonstrating the risk of removing asbestos (102). In 1969, the United Kingdom replaced the 1931 standards and extended controls to every industrial process producing asbestos dust (103). In the United States, the Clean Air Act of 1970 authorized the Environmental Protection Agency (EPA) to establish American national emission standards for hazardous air pollutants. Asbestos was included among the three substances first named, and emission standards were published in 1973. Temporary standards proposed for allowable asbestos fiber exposures were among the first acts of the Occupational Safety and Health Administration (OSHA). A permanent standard proposed in 1972 was delayed until 1976 while industry objections based on costs and benefits of such a control program were considered.

In 1973, product liability law was applied to asbestos products manufacturers in a suit by an insulation worker who developed asbestosis (104). In 1976, the Consumer Products Safety Commission first banned consumer products containing respirable asbestos. In 1982, under the Toxic Substances Control Act (Tosca), the EPA required identification of asbestos-containing materials in schools and the notification of those exposed.

The future development of asbestos standards is unpredictable, although public awareness of the hazards of asbestos apparently preclude relaxed standards. Future standards should reflect current epidemiological data to define industry-specific or fiber-type-specific standards and to define allowable exposures in public buildings (105). Cooperation among industry, unions, and occupational health researchers can develop work techniques which make stringent standards more practical and effective (106).

Physician's Role in Evaluating Asbestos-associated Diseases

Clinicians considering the diagnosis of asbestos-related disease, including asbestosis, lung cancer, and mesothelioma, should take a careful exposure history and assess disability (107). While the criteria by which disability and judicial product liability awards are made are currently nonuniform, the use of standard disability panels might substantially reduce this variation (105, 108).

The diagnosis of asbestosis is made by documenting characteristic pulmonary fibrosis in the setting of asbestos exposure. Radiologic evidence of characteristic chest x-ray changes, quantified using standard radiographic reference films (109), is usually combined with evidence of restrictive lung disease or diffusion abnormalities on pulmonary function tests and an asbestos exposure history. The importance of asbestos exposure in causing lung cancer is usually determined by weighting the asbestos exposure, smoking history, and other causes of pulmonary disease. Malignant mesothelioma is presumed to be asbestos-caused when diagnosed a suitable interval (> 15 years) after an asbestos exposure of even brief duration (105). The pathologic diagnosis of mesothelioma, however, is often found to be erroneous and thus must be confirmed by an expert pathologist. The physician must inform the patient promptly of the diagnosis of asbestos-related disease and its likely cause, since the patient must apply for compensation before the expiration of the statute of limitations period, which may be as short as 30 days for applications for workers' compensation (107) but is usually 2 years or less from diagnosis.

The detection of future occupational and environmental diseases is unpredictable. Ehrenreich and Selikoff have described the steps comprising such investigations, and recommended mandatory involvement by the medical examiner or forensic pathologist in death related to occupational disease, as opposed to occupational traumatic death (110). However, observations by alert clinicians are essential to identify potential new associations between environmental pathogens and human disease.

CLINICAL MANAGEMENT

Presentation

Mesothelioma is an uncommon tumor in the United States with about 1 case per 100 000 reported in 1975 (2) and an estimated incidence of 2200 total cases for 1985 (54). The tumor tends to occur in the fifth through eighth decades with a median age at diagnosis of between 50 and 60. In most mesothelioma series, a male predominance of 2–5 to 1 is reported (20, 21, 111, 112) reflecting increased occupational exposure. The tumor is rare in childhood (113, 114). Although an asbestos exposure has been reported for some childhood cases the latency period would have to be much shorter than that for adults, implying a different pathogenetic process.

Although the vast majority of mesotheliomas occur in the pleura and the peritoneum, malignant mesothelioma occurs occasionally in other serosal sites, such as the tunica vaginalis testis (115–121), and the pericardium (20, 22, 112, 122). Mesothelioma in the tunica vaginalis may be underdiagnosed (123).

Pleural mesothelioma occurs most frequently in the right chest cavity, possibly because of the less acute angle of the right mainstem bronchus at the carina. Asbestos-related mesotheliomas tend to be in the lower part of the lung, a predilection shared by the fibrosis of asbestosis.

While 80% of all mesotheliomas are pleural, peritoneal mesotheliomas predominate in the most heavily exposed workers (124). Patients with pleural mesothelioma almost always present with chest pain, dyspnea, or both. A larger minority of patients presents with vague sys-

temic complaints of fatigue, weight loss, anorexia, or malaise. Clubbing or pulmonary osteoarthropathy occurs in up to 9% of patients (21), signs associated more frequently with benign localized mesotheliomas and advanced asbestosis (125). In a small fraction, < 5%, mesothelioma is discovered on a routine chest x-ray in an asymptomatic person.

Typically chest pain in mesothelioma tends to be insidious, nonpleuritic and vaguely localized to the chest wall. Sudden chest pain has occurred rarely in association with hemothorax (112). Unfortunately, chest pain usually progresses and responds poorly to palliative radiotherapy. Dyspnea, the presenting symptom in a third to a half of patients (21, 22, 126), is often exertional initially, and usually progressive. Repeated thoracentesis often relieves dyspnea at first, but tumor progression eventually obliterates the pleural space and encases the lung, causing severe unilateral restrictive lung disease.

Patients with peritoneal mesothelioma usually present with abdominal pain, a palpable mass or increased girth. Ascites may be detectable in 30–90% on physical examination (13, 22, 127) and even more frequently by CT scan (128). Tumor associated hypoglycemia, first reported in 1930 in a patient with an intrathoracic fibrosarcomas (129) is associated with pleural and peritoneal mesothelioma as well as variety of other mesenchymal tumors (31, 130).

Mesothelioma is invasive locally, growing along incision scars or thoracentesis entry sites in approximately 5% of cases (20) and forming chest wall and abdominal masses more frequently later (21). Common local complications of pleural mesothelioma include pain, restrictive lung disease, and pericardial invasion with effusion and tamponade. Brachial plexopathy, Horner's syndrome, dysphagia, and superior vena cava syndrome are less common. Although late superficial hepatic invasion is common, symptomatic liver dysfunction is rare. Thromboembolism and other clotting abnormalities occur frequently (20, 112). The median survival is less than 18 months in most large series and less than 12 months for peritoneal mesothelioma (13, 22, 95, 127, 130). There are a few patients in most large series with a 5-year survival following a variety of treatment combinations (20, 22, 111, 112), or symptomatic treatment (19).

A well differentiated papillary mesothelioma seen in younger women is apparently more indolent with 3 of 6 patients surviving 7–29 years in one series (131). Katsube described a syndrome of intraperitoneal cysts of apparent mesothelial origin with prolonged survival accompanied by frequent recurrence (132).

Radiologic Evaluation

Chest x-ray demonstrates most pleural thickening, effusions, and lung nodules. The differential diagnosis of unilateral pleural thickening and effusion includes metastatic cancer, particularly adenocarcinoma which may present with extensive pleural thickening indistinguishable from mesothelioma, a so-called 'pseudomesothelioma' (133). Metastatic malignancies which can cause pleural effusions include carcinomas of lung, breast, pancreas, stomach, ovary, kidney, and bladder, as well as malignant thymona (134). In only about 60% of carcinomas metastatic to the pleura is an effusion present (135). Effusions occur in approximately one-fourth of patients with Hodgkin's and non-Hodgkin's lymphoma and leukemia (136). In one report, pleural masses were found in 31% of chest x-rays in patients with lymphoma in a referral center, but were never the sole expression of the disease (137).

The plain chest film can also demonstrate asbestos-related lung changes especially in the contralateral lung, such as pleural thickening and plaques, calcification, free-flowing effusions and parenchymal fibrosis (125). Parenchymal fibrosis or pleural plaques, which mark asbestos exposure, occur in 20% of patients with pleural and 50% of those with peritoneal mesothelioma (21). Oblique (45°) films have been suggested to improve the evaluation of the pleura (138).

CT scans are the best radiologic technique for staging, preoperative planning, and documenting response to therapy (139, 140). Extending the thoracic scan through the diaphragm to the upper abdomen will occasionally demonstrate extension through the diaphragm as well as hepatic invasion (139). Lung and soft tissue settings allow detection of other pleural and parenchymal abnormalities (136). Radiologic changes associated with asbestos exposure and mesothelioma include the following.

1 Pleural thickening. Patients without malignancy usually manifest a bilateral, fairly uniform process involving the visceral pleura. Like pleural placques (138), these are markers of significant asbestos exposure (141). Most investigators feel pleural disease alone does not cause pulmonary compromise, although this has been disputed (142). An irregularly thickened, nodular pleura is seen in some presentations of mesothelioma (143). Thickened fissures due to a combination of fibrosis, tumor, and associated fluid strongly suggest mesothelioma in patients with extensive pleural changes (133, 144).

2 Plaques. The most common site of asbestos-related change is the pleura, where plaques occur in approximately one-third to one-half of persons surviving > 20 years after a significant asbestos exposure. Plaques are often not diagnosed anti mortem (138, 145). These localized 3–5 mm fibrous thickenings of the parietal pleura are usually multiple and most commonly occur on the inferior posterior and lateral walls adjacent to the fifth to eighth rib. While most pleural plaques are smooth and regular, patients with advanced asbestosis may have large, irregular masses indistinguishable from those seen in mesothelioma and pleural metastatic cancer (144).

Pleural fluid or thickening was seen in 100% of ipsilateral and 86% of contralateral lungs in a CT study (140). A 'shaggy' cardiac border is uncommon (5%) in advanced asbestosis (125). Calcified pleura plaques are not seen until

20 years from first asbestos exposure (68). Histologic calification can be demonstrated in up to 87% of patients with pleural mesothelioma (146). CT scanning is more sensitive than plain films in detecting calcification (133, 140). Calcification may vary widely from single small linear deposits to much larger, irregular shapes and is most commonly seen along the diaphragm (147). The tumor itself is never calcified, although calcified plaques into which the tumor invades may appear to be part of the tumor (144).

3 Pleural effusions. The presence of pleural effusions varies widely in reported series from 30 to 80% of patients with mesothelioma (112, 148, 149). Benign asbestos pleural effusion occurring in 3–5% of workers as early as 3 years after first asbestos exposure is the most common thoracic radiologic abnormality during the first 20 years following exposure (145, 150). The diagnosis of benign effusion is made by excluding mesothelioma, metastatic cancer, and, rarely, tuberculosis. Large and progressive serosanquineous pleura and pericardial effusions can be associated with pathologically and clinically benign mesothelial tumors (29).

4 Parenchymal fibrosis. Asbestos-related fibrosis, or asbestosis, begins at the lung base, the reverse of silicosis which first affects the upper lung fields (125). Changes are graded in severity according to the UICC/Cincinnati classification of the pneumoconiosis. Small linear and nodular densities near the bases are the earliest changes (109, 125). These may progress to the honeycomb pattern of advanced interstitial fibrosis, particularly in the more heavily exposed workers, even after asbestos exposure has ceased. Radiologic findings of asbestosis are observed in the contralateral lung in approximately one-fifth of patients with pleural and one-half of those with peritoneal mesothelioma (148).

5 Lung masses. Direct extension into the lung, usually along interlobular septae, causes detectable intraparenchymal masses in 4–15%

(143, 148, 149). The differential diagnosis of lung nodules includes a large variety of other primary or secondary malignancies and localized benign processes. Advanced asbestosis may sometimes produce large lung nodules. Hilar masses occur in 12–30% of mesothelioma patients on CT scan (140), but are much more common in lung carcinoma.

6 Chest wall. Direct extension through the chest wall with or without rib destruction usually occurs late in mesothelioma, frequently following a track of a prior needle biopsy or open biopsy incision. CT scanning may document the extent of infiltration.

7 Distant metastases. Routine bone, liver, and brain scanning are not recommended, since hematogenous metastases are uncommon at presentation.

Diagnosis

Pleural fluid cytology is diagnostic of mesothelioma in at most 5% of cases (112, 151), although nonspecific malignant cells may be detected by light microscopy (152). Electron microscopic evaluation of pleural fluid specimens may document the mesothelial derivation of the malignant cells. Immediate centrifugation under refrigeration and prompt fixation is required to prevent microstructural distortion (swelling of microvilli and disruption of tonofilaments) (153, 154). Because all cells shed into the pleural or peritoneal cavity are included in the resultant pellet, the entire serosal surface is sampled indirectly. In contrast, pleural needle biopsy is useful only when positive, approximately 15–25% of the time, because of sampling error (21, 111, 112). Open biopsy, which allows nearly complete visualization and repeated directed biopsies, is the definitive diagnostic procedure. Thoroscopy, the placement of flexible fiberoptic instruments into the pleural cavity, is useful in diagnosing early pleural mesothelioma. Laparoscopy is similarly useful in peritoneal mesothelioma (130, 155).

Other potentially efficacious diagnostic techniques in suspected mesothelioma include pulmonary function tests, bronchoscopy, and measurement of pleural fluid hyaluronic acid. Pulmonary function tests may document restrictive lung disease in patients with extensive pleural disease and assess the patient's tolerance of pneumonectomy (125). Obstructive spirometric changes are unrelated to mesothelioma or asbestosis (105). Bronchoscopy, while almost negative in pleural mesothelioma, can help rule out bronchogenic carcinoma, the most common malignancy in smoking asbestos workers. The increased hyaluronic acid content of pleural effusions of mesothelioma was first reported by Meyer and Chafee (156). Others have found the test to be insensitive (126), although Roboz et al. reported increased sensitivity using high performance chromatography (157).

Staging is important in pleural mesothelioma since intensive therapies may be aborted if regional or metastatic disease is discovered. In Grant's series, 6 of 13 patients with clinical Stage I pleural mesothelioma were Stage II by CT scan results, although 2 patients with pericardial involvement on T scan underwent surgery despite the higher stage (140).

In peritoneal mesothelioma CT scanning may demonstrate thickening of the peritoneum and mesentary, ascites, and omental involvement (128). Peritoneal carcinomatosis from ovarian or colon cancer or unknown primary and extranodal non-Hodgkin's lymphoma are also included in the diagnostic differential. Peritoneal carcinomatosis from ovarian cancer usually causes less extensive peritoneal thickening than peritoneal mesothelioma. Although needle biopsy guided by ultrasound or CT scan, laparoscopic biopsy or ascites fluid cytology have been utilized for diagnosis, in most cases laparotomy is required. Although CT assessment of extent of disease may aid evaluation for intensive experimental approaches (155), staging systems for peritoneal mesothelioma are currently of little clinical use (158).

Pathology

Klemperer and Rabin (23) postulated the existence of primary epithelioid and sarcomatoid mesothelial malignancies and equated localized tumors with a benign course and diffuse tumors with aggressive malignancy. This unified concept of mesothelial tumors has gained acceptance relatively recently. So tenuous were antemortem diagnoses and so uniformly lethal the disease that Winslow and Taylor (13) argued that the characteristic clinical progression of the tumor documented at autopsy should be a criterion for definitive diagnosis. Stout and Murry in 1952 used cell culture techniques to propose the mesothelial cell as the cell of origin of localized pleural tumors (24). Despite progress in pathologic techniques initial misdiagnosis is commonly discovered when putative mesothelioma specimens undergo expert review. In a large series the Canadian mesothelioma panel confirmed 50% of the diagnosis, were uncertain in 14% and rejected the diagnosis of mesothelioma in 36%, disagreeing 30% of the time among themselves over putative mesothelioma (17). In Los Angeles, a member of the American Mesothelioma Board accepted only 42 of 162 (26%) ostensible mesothelioma cases (18). Kannerstein and Churg, however, confirmed the diagnosis of mesothelioma in 51% of 82 cases, with another 38% considered 'probable' mesothelioma (159). This degree of diagnostic difficulty requires collaboration between the clinician and the pathologist using clinical information to complement gross and microscopic morphology (154, 160). Information about asbestos exposure should not be used to diagnose mesothelioma, however, given the incomplete association between asbestos exposure and mesothelioma and the medicolegal implications (18).

Gross Morphology

Diffuse malignant mesothelioma grossly presents initially as tiny plaques or nodules on the visceral or parietal pleura which tend to coalesce. Ultimately, dense mats of tissue encase the lung or entrap the bowel. There is local extension into subserosal tissues early with pulmonary invasion frequent along the interlobular septa. Compression of the lung, involvement of the diaphragm and extension into the peritoneal cavity, mediastinum, and contralateral pleura are common complications in advanced disease (161).

Mesothelioma occurs in at least three different subtypes, i.e. epithelial (or tubuloepithelial), sarcomatous (or fibrous) and mixed. The more frequent epithelial subtype has a significantly longer reported median survival, 13–29 months, compared to 7–11 months in the sarcomatoid and mixed variants (20–22). Approximately 50–70% of patients have the epithelial variant, with the remainder equally divided between the mixed and sarcomatous variants in pleural disease (20, 22, 130); a greater preponderance of the epithelial subtype occurs in peritoneal mesotheliomas.

The differential diagnosis of epithelial mesothelioma includes those adenocarcinomas which frequently metastasize to the pleura. These include lung (33% of adenocarcinomas metastatic to the pleura), breast (21%), and stomach (7%) (162) and less frequently, ovary, colon, pancreas, kidney, prostate, and thyroid (135). Ovarian and gastric adenocarcinomas most commonly cause secondary peritoneal cancer.

Sarcomatous mesothelioma may be confused with fibrosarcoma, malignant hemangiopericytomas, malignant schwannoma, and malignant fibrous histiocytoma. Keratin, when present, distinguishes mesothelioma from other sarcomas.

A newly described tumor, focal papillary serous adenocarcinoma of peritoneal origin, is probably derived from extraovarian mullerian mesoderm, and is similar to mesothelioma (131, 161, 163, 164).

Histochemical Approaches

Three histochemical techniques are useful (161).

1 Periodic acid Schiff (PAS)–diastase. Diastase digestion eliminates glycogen, leaving mucopolysaccharides to react with the PAS stain. Mesotheliomas may be PAS positive prior to diastase digestion but become negative following removal of glycogen, while 50% of adenocarcinomas are positive both before and after diastase digestion (164).

2 Hyaluronidase–alcian blue. While one-third to one-half of mesotheliomas are initially positive, mesotheliomas become negative following hyaluronidase digestion while adenocarcinomas remain positive.

3 Mucicarmine. Neutral mucous substances, present in 50% of adenocarcinomas (although rarely in prostate or renal carcinoma), are not found in mesotheliomas.

Immunohistochemical Approaches

Most monoclonal antibody techniques attempt to distinguish epithelioid mesothelioma from adenocarcinoma, rather than the less common sarcomatous mesothelioma from sarcoma. Keratins are a family of 19 polypeptides widely distributed in benign and neoplastic tissue. Optimum keratin binding requires pretreatment with trypsin, apparently to expose the appropriate antigenic sites (165). Epithelioid mesotheliomas (and breast carcinomas) usually stain strongly for keratin proteins, while most other adenocarcinomas stain weakly or not at all (166–168); although some laboratories have had difficulty making this distinction (169, 170). Mesotheliomas often have a characteristic diffuse cytoplasmic staining with a dark perinuclear ring, while peripheral staining characterizes adenocarcinomas (167).

Carcinoembryonic antigen stains most adenocarcinomas strongly but most mesotheliomas weakly or not at all (14). One hundred and twenty-nine of 140 adenocarcinomas in published studies reviewed by Corson (161) were positive, compared to 18 of 182 mesotheliomas. In addition, of those evaluated quantitatively, 42 of 52 adenocarcinomas stained strongly or moderately positive, while 63 of 66 mesotheliomas stained weakly or not at all. Antibodies against human milk globule antigens may distinguish breast and other adenocarcinomas from mesothelioma (170), but a second laboratory was unsuccessful in making the same distinction (171). A specific polyclonal mesothelioma antibody useful in diagnosis (172) has been reported, but the antisera was no longer available after the death of the immunized animals producing it. Attempts to develop monoclonal antibodies to specific mesothelioma antigens continue.

Electron Microscopy

While the ultrastructural detail of electron microscopy may allow identification of the tissue source of an unknown cell type, invasion, the sine qua non of malignancy, must be documented by the light microscope (161).

Epithelial mesotheliomas share with adenocarcinomas the features of epithelial differentiation, including microvilli, desmosomes (tight junctions), tonofilaments, and intracytoplasmic lumina. Sarcomatous mesotheliomas lack these features, resembling fibroblasts.

Epithelial mesotheliomas develop long, thin multiply-branched microvilli. Warhol et al (154) used the length-to-diameter ratio (LDR) to distinguish mesotheliomas from other adenocarcinomas. The LDR may be lower in the primitive, blunted microvilli of mixed or poorly differentiated epithelial mesotheliomas although often these tumors have better differentiated areas with higher LDRs. The LDR usual for mesotheliomas is greater than 10 and for adenocarcinomas less than 10, but there may be substantial overlap between 10 and 15. Breast cancer never has an LDR greater than 10. Ovarian adenocarcinomas of mullerian cell origin and endometrial carcinomas are indistinguishable by LDR from mesotheliomas. Lamellar bodies, which may occur in lung and thyroid adenocarcinomas, and microvilli rootlets, seen in cervical and gastrointestinal adenocarcinomas, never occur in mesothelioma (173).

Keratin tonofilaments, usually seen in perinuclear bundles and in the desmosome complex, tend to be more prominent in epithelioid mesotheliomas than in adenocarcinomas. Increased tonofilaments may distinguish mesothelioma from adenocarcinomas such as ovarian tumors with elevated LDRs (174). Prominent tonofilaments occur commonly in breast and colon adenocarcinomas and in areas of squamous differentiation. Electron microscopy may thus reliably diagnose mesothelioma from properly prepared malignant effusions (153). A characteristic electron microscopy, classic immunohistochemical staining, and characteristic clinical course may result in a highly reliable diagnosis of mesothelioma. Prompt performance of the proper stains and electron microscopy would be less likely for a similar tumor prepared as a pathological unknown (154).

Staging

Extent of pleural mesothelioma, determined by Butchart's staging system (175) and subsequent modifications, is inversely related to survival. Antman (112), for example, found that Stage I tumors resulted in a 16-month median survival compared to 9 months for Stage II. Most importantly, nearly all patients with prolonged survival have had Stage I or limited Stage II disease at diagnosis. It is prudent to confine experimental intensive therapies to these patients. No staging system proposed for peritoneal mesothelioma has so far correlated with survival (158), although minimal estimated tumor mass was required for a recently reported multimodality treatment of peritoneal mesothelioma (155).

Mesothelioma invades locally early with regional extension followed by distant metastasis late in the course. Initial workup for distant metastasis is not indicated unless prompted by symptoms or abnormal local findings. Sites of metastatic mesothelioma include liver, spleen, adrenals, pancreas, kidneys, bowel, thyroid, bone and brain (20, 21, 111). CT scanning often documents unsuspected extent of disease (140). Documenting unsuspected advanced cancer often 'upstages' patients, leaving fewer, better-prognosis patients in early-stage groups than before the staging procedure, a process called 'stage migration. Feinstein labelled the improvement in stage-specific survival brought about by more complete evaluation the 'Will Rogers effect' in his lung cancer study (176). Radioactive agents such as gallium (177) or radiolabelled monoclonal antibodies or new imaging modalities such as nuclear magnetic resonance scanning may permit even more precise tumor imaging and consequently more precise patient comparisons.

Therapy

Multiple strategies must be used to develop and test therapy against a rare and difficult to diagnose tumor such as mesothelioma. Multi-institutional cooperative trials are now underway to increase patient numbers (178). Potential therapies may be screened by in vitro techniques or animal systems, such as the nude mouse tumor-explant system of Chahinian (179). Expert pathologic review of accrued cases is necessary to reduce diagnostic uncertainty as well as careful staging to ensure comparable patients in clinical trials. Histologic subtypes, along with other prognostic factors found to significantly affect survival should be reported (and for randomized trials stratified) to reduce confounding variations in natural history.

While treatments producing long-term survivors should suggest hypotheses for future trials, 'long-term survivors' (> 5 years) must be distinguished from apparently disease-free survivors since about 10% of symptomatically treated or untreated patients have a surprisingly long survival (19, 180). Nevertheless, in carefully designed studies the short natural history of ineffectively treated mesothelioma may allow early appreciation of successful treatments; i.e. in a mesothelioma trial (as opposed to a breast cancer trial), a median

survival of 3 years in a treatment group would likely be meaningful.

Surgery

In its localized, benign form, pleural or peritoneal mesothelioma is amenable to complete excision and cure. However, diffuse mesothelioma is usually extensively infiltrative at diagnosis. Pleural mesothelioma's dismal prognosis has been cited to support conservative recommendations for surgery. Lewis argued that surgery is therapeutically useless in pleural mesothelioma (151) or should be reserved solely for symptom palliation. Gaensler in the published discussion of Lewis' presentation, argued that even surgical biopsy was of no value to patients. However, the poor prognosis has also prompted trials of intensive multimodality in an attempt to extend survival and ultimately, with refinements of useful modalities to attempt cure of patients with mesothelioma. Certainly no effective therapy will ever be identified if no trials are attempted.

Pleural Mesothelioma

Lewis et al. (151) argued against surgery because of difficulty in obtaining adequate surgical margins in such an infiltrative disease, the rapid regrowth of tumor in patients treated with pleurectomy and the high hospital mortality in one study utilizing pleuropneumonectomy (181). An alternative to pleuropneumonectomy in some trials is to combine a limited procedure, parietal pleurectomy, with additional radiotherapy and chemotherapy. McCormack and colleagues (182), reviewing the experience at Memorial-Sloan-Kettering (MSK), reported a 21-month median survival in patients with epithelial pleural mesothelioma treated wth pleurectomy, intrapleural colloidal ^{125}I and a variety of single agent chemotherapy regimens. She compared their more recent results with the median of 16-month survival in their prior study of pleurectomy, external beam irradiation and systemic chemotherapy (183). Potential advantages to pleurectomy over pleuropneumonectomy are reduced surgical morbidity and mortality and preservation of potentially vital pulmonary capacity. Careful patient selection and improved surgical technique with experience has dramatically reduced surgical deaths. The surgical mortality in the MSK experience is 1.5%.

A more radical surgical approach including lung resection was attributed by Butchart to Eiselberg (184). Because dyspnea results from severe intrapulmonary shunting and progressive restriction of the ipsilateral lung, it may be averted by lung resection and diversion of the blood supply to the cointralateral lung (185). Shemin has recently described in detail his technique for pleuropneumonectomy (186). Large series of patients treated by pleuropneumonectomy have been reported by Woern (187), Butchart et al. (181) and DeLaria et al. (185). Woern reported 248 patients, 186 treated with pleurectomy and 62 with a radical procedure including pleuropneumonectomy and resection of involved pericardium and diaphragm. Although he found no survival difference between these groups, the combined 5-year survival of 9% is the best survival in a large series (187).

Butchart reported 29 patients treated with pleuropneumonectomy (181). Two of his patients were alive and without disease at 3.5 and 6 years, although 3 nonsurgically treated patients survived for 3 years as well. He felt that 3/4 of his hospital mortality of 31% could have been prevented with more careful patient selection. In particular, he recommended treating only patients less than 60 years old, with Stage I disease after extensive staging and with the frozen section diagnosis of the epithelial variant of mesothelioma.

DeLaria reported a highly selected group of 11 patients, 9 of whom had the epithelial variant of pleural mesothelioma (185). Two patients were surviving at 2 and 4 years respectively. In contrast to Butchart, he had no hospital mortality.

Peritoneal Mesothelioma

In peritoneal mesothelioma removal of all gross cancer is rarely feasible. Surgery is certainly indicated when appropriate for treatment of complications such as bowel obstruction or for localized and/or slowly recurrent cystic mesothelial tumors (127, 130, 158). Because of anatomical considerations and poor results most persons deny a role for noninvestigational surgery in peritoneal mesothelioma except when localized (158). Nevertheless, multimodality therapy including surgery has produced an apparently extended survival in selected patients with peritoneal mesothelioma (155, 188). An interesting recent paper (155) reported 6 of 6 highly selected patients alive 9–21 months following an intensive regimen of debulking surgery, intraperitoneal chemotherapy, and total abdominal irradiation.

Palliative Surgery

The optimal use of surgery for palliation is unclear. Martini et al. (83) proposed palliative pleurectomy for three indications: (1) uncontrollable pleural effusions; (2) trapped lung; and (3) presence of malignant effusion at thoracotomy. In their series of 106 patients with effusions from a variety of malignancies, all were controlled without significant reaccumulation. Overall perioperative mortality was 10%, with no deaths in 14 patients with mesothelioma. Median survival after surgery was 16 months in all patients. Butchart et al. (189) suggested palliative parietal pleurectomy to control effusions and, in combination with chemotherapy and irradiation, for patients excluded from pleuropneumonectomy. DeLaria et al. (185) felt pleuropneumonectomy offered better palliation since shunting of blood to the ipsilateral lung in patients with advanced local disease impeded respiration. Pleurectomy may prevent or relieve chest pain in some cases. Palliative peritoneovenous shunting of intractable ascites led to pulmonary metastases in one reported case (190). The proper role of palliative surgery, radiotherapy, chemotherapy, and narcotic analgesia in all patients remains to be delineated.

Radiation Therapy

Radiotherapy has been used in mesothelioma with objectives ranging from temporary pain relief to cure. Technological advance, such as modern megavoltage sources, computerized dosimetry techniques and new radiation sources such as electron beam and fast neutron therapy (191) complicates attempts to generalize from past reports to present practice. Differing patient characteristics, diagnostic and staging criteria, type and dosage of radiotherapy, and use of additional therapies may limit generalization of reported results to particular patients or larger trials.

Pleural Mesothelioma

Radiotherapy to the chest is limited by scatter to nearby radiosensitive organs, including lung parenchyma, spinal cord, esophagus, and heart. Modern megavoltage radiation sources have simplified the effective delivery of adequate doses (> 45 Gy) of external beam radiation, although toxicity to the lung and heart limit total doses to approximately 60 Gy (192). Several large unrandomized studies have shown little or no benefit for radiotherapy (112), radiotherapy and chemotherapy versus chemotherapy alone (20, 193) or high-dose radiotherapy versus surgery alone, chemotherapy alone, or no treatment (19). Nevertheless, several case reports (111, 194) and series describe one or more patients with greater than 5-year survival after external beam radiation (19, 195–197).

External beam radiation has been occasionally recommended to palliate chest pain from pleural mesothelioma (12, 195, 198, 199, 200, 202). Nevertheless, the responsiveness of pain to radiotherapy is variable and in most cases, unfortunately, temporary. Gordon et al. (1971) retrospectively found significant pain relief for only 18% of patients receiving 8 to 40

Gy, and 66% for those receiving 40 to 57 Gy. The risk of side effects at high total doses must be balanced against the importance of pain relief and the short life expectancy of patients with chest pain from advanced mesothelioma. Regression of tumor may improve lung function, and although radiation pneumonitis may occur promptly, radiation fibrosis occurs beyond the life expectancy of many patients (203).

Intracavitary treatment with radiactive colloids such as ^{32}P of ^{198}Au could theoretically limit toxicity and treat relatively early mesothelioma where nodules are widely scattered but usually not deeply invasive nor metastatic at diagnosis. However, the beta particles emitted by these agents penetrate at most 2–3 mm, and free flow of suspensions of these agents becomes impractical as progressive mesothelioma obliterates the pleural space, limiting this treatment to early mesothelioma. Brady (202) reported 6 of 6 patients treated with radioactive chromic phosphate alive for at least 12 months.

Peritoneal Mesothelioma

Total radiation dosage to the peritoneal cavity is limited by liver and bowel tolerance to approximately 30 Gy, at which half of patients develop nausea, vomiting, and diarrhea and about 10% bowel obstruction. Renal toxicity occurs at lower doses, requiring the use of blocks. Other infrequent side effects of abdominal radiation include radiation hepatitis, prolonged bone marrow suppression, and radiation enteritis, causing chronic malabsorption (191). Aggresive regimens combining fulldose external beam irradiation and chemotherapy have only recently been reported (155). Chahinian et al. (20) reported short survival and no advantage to patients treated with doxorubicin and radiotherapy compared with patients treated with doxorubicin and 5-azacytidine without radiotherapy. Law reported a dramatic response to radiation in another young woman, alive and well at 4 years (19). Antman et al. (155) reported 6 patients with limited-bulk peritoneal mesothelioma out of a total of 13 patients accrued during the same interval treated with sequential debulking surgery including omentectomy, intraperitoneal doxorubicin and cisplatin, systemic doxorubicin, cyclophosphamide and cisplatin and whole abdominal irradiation to at least 30 Gy. All were alive and disease-free at 9–36 month follow-up. Rogoff et al. (188) reported 12 patients with peritoneal mesothelioma treated at Memorial Hospital in New York. Of 4 patients treated with total abdominal and pelvic irradiation and radioactive colloids, 2 survived 9 and 10 years from diagnosis and another 2 were disease-free at 2 and 10 years. One patient had survived 7 years after biopsy alone.

In summary, the proper role for radiotherapy has not yet been established. No treatment using radiotherapy has yet consistently improved survival. These results suggest that radiotherapy combined with surgery and active chemotherapy treatments may prolong the life of selected patients with mesothelioma. Optimal treatment may vary for specific patient subgroups by site, subtype, extent of disease, and comorbid medical problems, such as chronic pulmonary disease. High-dose irradiation of patients with pleural mesothelioma to palliate chest wall pain, while not always effective, should be tried when chest pain is progressive and unresponsive to narcotic analgesics.

Chemotherapy

The small number of chemotherapy treated mesothelioma patients, infrequent controlled trials, the use of many different drug regimens, and the varied natural history of mesothelioma limit the interpretation of data from clinical drug trials. Animal models, such as Smith's serial transfer of hamster mesothelioma induced by intraperitoneal asbestos (105) and Chahinian's model of human mesothelioma lines transplanted to nude mice (179) may complement human studies. Sequential trials of agents in individual patients (206) offer a

means to individualize therapy rationally and increase information about chemotherapy activity from small numbers of patients, although the development of pleotropic drug resistance and the toxicity of chemotherapy severely limit this approach. Larger cooperative trials are underway (178).

Single Agents

Mintzer et al. (207), using cisplatin 120 mg/m^2 at 4- and then 6-week intervals, obtained 3 partial responses in 25 patients, of whom 4 had measurable disease. Four patients had Grade 3 renal toxicity, and 2 patients stopped treatment for neurotoxicity and for persistent nausea and vomiting. Uncontrolled data in two retrospectively analyzed series suggest significant activity for doxorubicin in mesothelioma (193, 208); but another found a low response rate (209). Sorensen et al. (210) found slow progression in all 30 evaluable untreated ambulatory patients treated in a randomized cross-over trial of doxorubicin 60 mg/m^2 versus cyclophosphamide 1500 mg/m^2. Nine patients had epithelial and 23 sarcomatous or mixed varients of mesothelioma. Harvey et al. treated 11 patients whose mesothelioma progressed during 5-FU therapy with doxorubicin. One partial response of 34 months resulted (211). Six of 9 patients given high-dose methotrexate with vincristine responded by chest x-ray criteria (mostly improving effusions) 3 with complete responses for 11–23 months (212). An early small series suggested activity for single-agent 5-FU (213). Harvey et al., however, gave 20 consecutive patients with pleural or peritoneal mesothelioma 5-FU at two dose levels, observing only a single 24-month partial response (211).

Combination Chemotherapy

Yap et al. (208) retrospectively studied 36 patients with pleural mesothelioma confirmed pathologically at M.D. Anderson over 16 years. The disease stage and histological subtypes were not reported. Of 21 patients given doxorubicin-containing regimens 2 of 10 with measurable disease had partial responses. Six of 15 patients who did not receive doxorubicin responded including 1 of 7 given COMF. Despite the ambiguity of the data, the authors conclude that doxorubicin is useful in mesothelioma (208).

Zidar et al. (214) tested cisplatin and doxorubicin adjusted for myelosuppression and observed responses in 4/6 patients by chest x-ray and abdominal ultrasound. Mischler reported a partial response to doxorubicin with DTIC after progression on doxorubicin alone.

Chahinian found that mitomycin C and cisplatin were synergistic in his model of xenografted human mesothelioma cell lines in nude mice. Of 12 patients with both pleural and peritoneal mesothelioma given these drugs 3 had partial responses and a fourth a complete response of 6 months (215).

Jett and Eagan (216) gave 12 Stage I patients CAMEO chemotherapy (cyclophosphamide 350 mg/m^2, doxorubicin 25 mg/m^2, methotrexate 25, etoposide 80 mg/m^2 × 3 days, vincristine 2 mg). Two had regression, and 2 had prolonged stable disease. One patient with stable disease died at 45 months of congestive heart failure, and another was reported alive and apparently disease-free at 32 months.

Intracavitary chemotherapy for early mesotheliomas confined to one serosal surface is theoretically attractive because, like colloidal beta-particle emitters, the cytotoxic agents are isolated to the tumor-bearing area, promoting normal tissues from toxicity. Very high concentrations of chemotherapy agents in the intracavitary space may facilitate diffusion into cancer cells. The relative effectiveness of intracavitary therapy versus conventional intravenous chemotherapy may depend on the importance of concentration gradient on cell uptake, the tumor thickness and vascularity and whether intracavitary treatments improve access to deeper cell layers in later treatments by killing or rendering permeable outer cell layers. When a significant proportion of the drug is absorbed into the circulation the tumor mass is exposed to both standard capillary levels and much higher serosal surface concentrations.

Dimitrov based the studies of high-dose methotrexate in pleural effusions in mesothelioma patients described above in part on sustained high methotrexate levels observed in 'third-space' fluid collections (212). Sustained exposure to the chemotherapy agent rather than high concentration gradients is the goal of this intracavitary theory. Pfeifle et al. (217) gave intracavitary cisplatin 90 mg/m^2 infusions weekly for 3 weeks to 8 patients resulting in moderate hematologic toxicity and frequent nausea and vomiting. One patient previously treated with doxorubicin had a complete response lasting at least 22 month and 3 other patients had resolution of or significantly decreased ascites or pleural effusions. Complications in one Phase I trial of sequential intraperitoneal cisplatin and doxorubicin included peritonitis in 2 patients, ileus in one, and minimal creatinine elevation (< 2) in another patient. One patient responded completely except for two nodules resected from an apparently sequestered intraperitoneal site at the time of second-look surgery and another had significantly decreased ascites and increased performance status for 18 months (218, 219).

In summary, the most effective treatment of mesothelioma remains to be determined. Individualized therapies should not be presented as 'standard treatment'. Every attempt should be made to include each patient who desires therapy in ongoing research protocols. Combination chemotherapy has not been proven superior to single agents in mesothelioma. Doxorubicin, cyclophosphamide, cisplatin, mitomycin C, and methotrexate appear to have clinical activity in mesothelioma. Optimal treatment may require a combination of surgery, full-dose radiotherapy, intracavitary radiation or chemotherapy, and systemic chemotherapy. Trials of intensive therapy must be targeted at patients with minimal disease to justify therapeutic toxicity with a realistic hope of prolonged survival.

ACKNOWLEDGMENT

We are grateful to Miss Theresa Podedworny for careful preparation of this manuscript.

REFERENCES

1 Hinds MW. Mesothelioma in the United States. Incidence in the 1970's. J Occup Med 1978; 20: 469–71.

2 Young JL, Percy CL, Asire AJ, eds. Surveillance, epidemiology and end results: incidence and mortality data, 1973–1977. Bethesda, Md.: National Institutes of Health, 1981. (Nat Cancer Inst Monograph No 57).

3 Hogan MD, Hoel DG. Estimated cancer risk associated with occupational asbestos exposure. Risk Analysis 1981; 1: 67–76.

4 Spooner CM. Asbestos in schools—a public health problem. N Engl J Med 1979; 301: 782–4.

5 Wagner JC, Sleggs CA, Marchand P. Diffuse pleural mesothelioma and asbestos exposure in the North Western Cape Province. Br J Industr Med 1960; 17: 260–71.

6 Selikoff IJ, Hammond EC, Seidman H. Mortality experience of insulation workers in the United States and Canada, 1943–76. Ann NY Acad Sci 1979; 330: 91–116.

7 Peto J. Dose-response relationships for asbestos-related disease: implications for hygiene standards. Part II. Mortality. Ann NY Acad Sci 1979; 330: 195–203.

8 Walker AM, Loughlin JE, Friedlander ER, Rothman KJ, Dreyer NA. Projections of asbestos-relate disease 1980–2009. J Occup Med 1983; 25: 409–25.

9 Nicholson WJ, Perkel G, Selikoff IJ. Occupational exposure to asbestos: population at risk and projected mortality, 1980–2030. Am J Industr Med 1982; 3: 259–311.

10 Robertson HE. 'Endothelioma" of the pleura. J Cancer Res 1924; 8: 317–75.

11 Klemperer P, Rabin CR. Primary neoplasms of the pleura. A report of five cases. Arch Pathol 1931; 11: 385–412.

12 Saccone A, Coblenz AA. Endothelioma of the pleura. With report of two cases. Amer J Clin Path 1943; 13: 186–207.

13 Winslow DJ, Taylor HB. Malignant peritoneal mesotheliomas. A clinicopathological analysis of 12 fatal cases. Cancer 1960; 13: 127–36.

14 Wang N, Huang S, Gold P. Absence of carcinoembryonic antigen-like material in mesothelioma. Cancer 1979; 44: 937–43.

15 Said JW, Nash G, Tepper G, Banks-Schlegel S. Keratin proteins and carcinoembryonic antigen in lung carcinoma: an immunoperoxidase study of fifty-four cases, with ultrastructural correlations. Hum Pathol 1983; 14: 70–6.

16 Warhol MJ, Hickey WF, Corson JM. Malignant mesothelioma. Ultrastructural distinction from adenocarcinoma. Am J Surg Pathol 1982; 6: 307–14.

17 McDonald AD, Magner D, Eyssen G. Primary malignant mesothelioma tumors in Canada, 1960–1968. A pathological review by the Mesothelioma Panel of the Canadian Tumor Reference Centre. Cancer 1973; 31: 869–76.

18 Wright WE, Sherwin RP, Dickson EA, Bernstein L, Fromm JB, Henderson BE. Malignant mesothelioma: incidence, asbestos exposure, and reclassification of histopathology. Br J Industr Med 1984; 41: 39–45.

19 Law MR, Gregor A, Hodson ME, Bloom HJG, Turner-Warwick M. Malignant mesothelioma of the pleura: a study of 52 treated and 64 untreated patients. Thorax 1984; 39: 255–9.

20 Chahinian AP, Pajak TF, Holland JF, Norton L, Ambinder RM, Mandel EM. Diffuse malignant mesothelioma. Prospective evaluation of 69 patients. Ann Intern Med 1982; 96: 746–55.

21 Elmes PC, Simpson MJC. The clinical aspects of mesothelioma. Q J Med 1976; 45: 427–49.

22 Oels HC, Harrison EG, Carr DT, Bernatz PE. Diffuse malignant mesothelioma of the pleura: a review of 37 cases. Chest 1971; 60: 564–70.

23 Klemperer P, Rabin CR. Primary neoplasms of the pleura. A report of five cases. Arch Pathol 1931; 11: 385–412.

24 Stout AP, Murray MR. Localized pleural mesothelioma. Investigation of its characteristics and histogenesis by the method of tissue culture. Arch Pathol 1942; 34: 951–64.

25 Urschel HC, Paulson DL. Mesotheliomas of the pleura. Ann Thorac Surg 1965; 1:559–74.

26 Briselli MB, Mark EJ, Dickersin GR. Solitary fibrous tumors of the pleura: eight new cases and review of 360 cases in the literature. Cancer 1981; 47: 2678–89.

27 Legha SS, Muggia FM. Pleura mesothelioma: clinical features and therapeutic implications. Ann Intern Med 1977; 87: 613–21.

28 Okike N, Bernatz PE, Woolner LB. Localized mesothelioma of the pleura. Benign and malignant variants. J Thorac Cardiovasc Surg 1978; 75: 363–72.

29 Hansen RM, Caya JG, Clowry LJ, Anderson T. Benign mesothelial proliferation with effusion. Clinicopathological entity that may mimic malignancy. Am J Med 1984; 77: 887 92.

30 Briselli MB, Mark EJ. Solitary fibrous tumors of the pleura and benign extrapleural tumors of mesothelial origin. In: Antman K, Aisner J eds Asbestos Related Malignancy. Orlando, Fl.: Grune & Stratton, 1986.

31 Case Records of the Massachusetts General Hospital (Case 9–1984). N Engl J Med 1984; 310: 580–7.

32 Wierman WH, Clagett OT, McDonald JR. Articular manifestations in pulmonary diseases: an analysis of their occurrence in 1024 cases in which pulmonary resection was performed. JAMA 1954; 155: 1459–63.

33 Benoit HW, Ackerman LV. Solitary pleural mesotheliomas. J Thorac Surg 1953; 25: 346–57.

34 Goodman L. Roentgen of the month: a diagnosable coin lesion. Chest 1976; 70: 405–6.

35 Godwin MC. Diffuse mesotheliomas. With comment on their relation to localized fibrous mesotheliomas. Cancer 1957; 10: 298–319.

36 Utley JR, Parker JC, Hahn RS, Bryant LR, Mobin-Uddin K. Recurrent benign fibrous mesothelioma of the pleura. J Thorac Cardiovasc Surg 1973; 65: 830–4.

37 Stout AP, Himadi GM. Solitary (localized) mesothelioma of the pleura. Ann Surg 1951; 133: 50–64.

38 Wanebo HJ, Martini N, Melamed MR, Hilaris B, Beattie EJ. Pleural mesothelioma. Cancer 1976; 38: 2481–4.

39 Clagett OT, McDonald JR, Schmidt HW. Localized fibrous mesothelioma of the pleura. J Thorac Surg 1952; 24: 213–30.

40 Moore JH, Crum CP, Chandler JG, Feldmen PS. Benign cystic mesothelioma. Cancer 1980; 45: 2395–9.

41 Carpenter HA, Lancaster JR, Lee RA. Multilocular cysts of the peritoneum. Mayo Clin Proc 1982; 57: 634–8.

42 Mennemeyer R, Smith M. Multicystic peritoneal mesothelioma: a report with electron microscopy of a case mimicking intra-abdominal cystic hygroma (lymphangioma). Cancer 1979; 44: 692–8.

43 Stock RJ, Fu YS, Carter JR. Malignant peritoneal mesothelioma following radiation for seminoma of the testis. Cancer 1979; 44: 914–19.

44 Babcock TL, Powell DH, Bothwell RS. Radiation-induced peritoneal mesothelioma. J Surg Oncol 1976; 8: 369–72.

45 Antman KH, Corson JM, Li FP, Greenberger J, Sytkowski A, Henson DE et al. Malignant mesothelioma following radiation exposure. J Clin Oncol 1983; 1: 695–700.

46 Maurer R, Egloff B. Malignant peritoneal

47 Dahlgren S. Effects of locally deposited colloidal thorium dioxide. Ann NY Acad Sci 1967; 145: 786–90.

48 Artvinli M, Baris YI. Malignant mesotheliomas in a small village in the Anatolian region of Turkey: an epidemiological study. J Nat Cancer Inst 1979; 63: 17–22.

49 Lilis R. Fibrous zeolites and endemic mesothelioma in Cappadocia, Turkey. J Occup Med 1981; 23: 548–50.

50 Rohl AN, Langer AM, Moncure G, Selikoff IJ, Fischbein A. Endemic pleural disease associated with exposure to mixed fibrous dust in Turkey. Science 1982; 216: 518–20.

51 Craighead JE, Mossman BT. The pathogenesis of asbestos-associated diseases. N Engl J Med 1982; 306: 1446–55.

52 Wagner JC, Berry G, Pooley FD. Mesotheliomas and asbestos type in asbestos textile workers: a study of lung contents. Br Med J 1982; 285: 603–6.

53 McDonald JC, McDonald AD. Epidemiology of mesothelioma from estimated incidence. Preventive Med 1977; 6: 426–46.

54 McDonald AD, McDonald JC. Epidemiology of malignant mesothelioma. In: Antman K, Aisner J eds Asbestos Related Malignancy. Orlando, Fl.: Grune & Stratton, 1986.

55 Wagner JC, Berry G, Skidmore JW, Timbrell V. The effects of the inhalation of asbestos in rats. Br J Cancer 1974; 29: 252–69.

56 Stanton MF, Layard M, Tegeris A, Miller E, May M, Kent E et al. Carcinogenicity of fibrous glass: pleural response in relation to fiber dimension. J Nat Cancer Inst 1977; 58: 589–603.

57 Lee KP, Barras CE, Griffith FD, Waritz RD. Pulmonary response and transmigration of inorganic fibers by inhalation exposure. Am J Pathol 1981; 102: 314–23.

58 Pooley FD. Minerology of asbestos: the physical and chemical properties of the dusts they form. Semin Oncol 1981; 8: 243–9.

59 Donham KJ, Berg JW, Will LA, Leininger JR. The effects of long-term ingestion of asbestos on the colon of F344 rats. Cancer 1980; 45: 1073–84.

60 Hammond EC, Selikoff IJ, Churg J. Neoplasia among insulation workers in the United States with special reference to intra-abdominal neoplasia. Ann NY Acad Sci 1965; 132: 519–25.

61 Miller AB. Asbestos fibre dust and gastrointestinal malignancies. Review of literature with regard to a cause/effect relationship. J Chronic Dis 1978; 31: 23–33.

mesothelioma after cholangiography with Thorotrast. Cancer 1975; 36: 1381–5.

62 Stanton MF, Wrench C. Mechanisms of mesothelioma induction with asbestos and fibrous glass. J Nat Cancer Inst 1972; 48: 797–821.

63 Churg AM, Warnock ML, Bensch KG. Malignant mesothelioma arising after direct application of asbestos and fibre glass to the pericardium. Am Rev Resp Dis 1978; 118: 419–24.

64 Bischoff F, Bryson G. Carcinogenesis through solid state surfaces. Prog Exp Tumor Res 1964; 5: 85–133.

65 Brand KG. Foreign body induced sarcoma. In: Becker FF ed Cancer. A Comprehensive Treatise Vol 1. New York: Plenum Press, 1975: 485–511.

66 Buoen LC, Brand I, Brand KG. Foreign body tumorogenesis: in vitro isolation and expansion of preneoplastic clonal cell preparations. J Nat Cancer Inst 1975; 55: 721–3.

67 O'Donnell WM, Mann RH, Grosh JL. Asbestos, an extrinsic factor in the pathogenesis of bronchogenic carcinoma and mesothelioma. Cancer 1966; 19: 1143–8.

68 Selikoff IJ. The occurrence of pleural calcification among asbestos insulation workers. Ann NY Acad Sci 1965; 132: 351–67.

69 Selikoff IJ, Lilis R, Nicholson WJ. Asbestos disease in United States shipyards. Ann NY Acad Sci 1979; 330: 295–311.

70 Lemen RA, Dement JM, Wagoner JK. Epidemiology of asbestos-related diseases. Env Health Perspectives 1980; 34: 1–11.

71 Frank AL. Clinical observations following asbestos exposure. Env Health Perspectives 1980; 34: 27–30.

72 Selikoff IJ, Hammon EC, Seidman H. Latency of asbestos disease among insulation workers in the United States and Canada. Cancer 1980; 46: 2736–40.

73 McDonald AD, McDonald JC. Malignant mesothelioma in North America. Cancer 1980; 46: 1650–6.

74 Enticknap JB, Smither WJ. Peritoneal tumors in asbestosis. Br J Industr Med 1964; 21: 20–31.

75 Newhouse ML, Thompson H. Mesothelioma of the pleura and peritoneum following exposure to asbestos in the London area. Br J Industr Med 1965; 22: 261–9.

76 Bohlig H, Dabbert AF, Dalquen P, Hain E, Hinz I. Epidemiology of malignant mesothelioma in Hamburg. A preliminary report. Environmental Res 1970; 3: 365–72.

77 Kilburn KH, Lilis R, Anderson HA, Boylen CT, Einstein HE, Johnson SS et al. Asbestos disease in family contacts of shipyard workers. Am J Pub Health 1985; 75: 615–17.

78 Anderson HA, Lilis R, Daum SM, Fischbein AS, Selikoff IJ. Household-contact asbestos neoplastic risk. Ann NY Acad Sci 1976; 271: 311–23.

79 Vianna NJ, Polan AK. Non-occupational exposure to asbestos and malignant mesothelioma in females. Lancet 1978; i: 1061–3.

80 Risberg B, Nickels J, Wagermark J. Familial clustering of malignant mesothelioma. Cancer 1980; 45: 2422–7.

81 Li EP, Lokich J, Lapey J, Neptune WB, Wilkins EW. Familial mesothelioma after intense asbestos exposure at home. JAMA 1978; 240: 467.

82 Churg AM, Warnock ML. Asbestos and other ferruginous bodies. Their formation and clinical significance. Am J Pathol 1981; 102: 447–56.

83 Churg AM. Fiber counting and analysis in the diagnosis of asbestos-related disease. Hum Pathol 1982; 13: 381–92.

84 Mowe G, Glyseth B, Hartveit F, Skaug V. Fiber concentration in lung tissue of patients with malignant mesothelioma. A case-control study. Cancer 1985; 56: 1089–93.

85 Chen W. Mottet NK. Malignant mesothelioma with minimal asbestos exposure. Hum Pathol 1978; 9: 253–8.

86 Peterson JT, Greenberg SD, Buffler PA. Non-asbestos-related malignant mesothelioma. A review. Cancer 1984; 54: 951–60.

87 McNeil BJ, Eddy DM. The costs and effects of screening for cancer among asbestos-exposed workers. J Chronic Dis 1982; 35: 351–8.

88 Nowinski PA. Chronology of asbestos regulation in the United States work places. In: Antman K, Aisner J eds Asbestos related malignancy. Orlando, Fl.: Grune & Stratton, 1986.

89 Castleman BI. The double standard in industrial hazards. Int J Health Serv 1983; 13: 5–14.

90 Murray HM. Report of the Departmental Committee of Compensation and Industrial Disease, 1906.

91 Cooke WE. Fibrosis of the lungs due to the inhalation of asbestos dust. Br Med J 1924; ii: 147.

92 Hoffman FL. Mortality from respiratory disease in dusty trades. Bulletin 231, Bureau of Labor Standards, US Department of Labor, 1918.

93 Merewether ERA. The occurrence of pulmonary fibrosis and other pulmonary affections in asbestos workers. J Industr Hyg 1930; 12: 198–222, 239–57.

94 Statutory Rules and Orders, 1931. Her Majesty's Stationery Office (1932).

95 Walsh-Healey Public Contracts Act, Public

Law 74–846, 49 Stat 2036, 41 USC 35, et seq. (1936).

96 Drinker P. The health and safety program of the U.S. Maritime Commission JAMA 1943; 121: 822–3.

97 Minimum Requirements of Safety and Industrial Health in Contract Shipyards. Washington, D.C.: United States Government Printing Office, 1943.

98 Fleischer WE, Viles FJ, Gade RL. Drinker P. A health survey covering operations in constructing naval vessels. J Industr Hygiene Toxicol 1946; 28: 9–16.

99 American Conference of Government Industrial Hygienists. Proceedings, April 7–13, 1946: 54–6.

100 Doll R. Mortality from lung cancer in asbestos workers. Br J Industr Med 1955; 12: 81–6.

101 Selikoff IJ, Churg J, Hammond EC. The occurrence of asbestosis among insulation workers in the United States. Ann NY Acad Sci 1965; 132: 139–5.

102 Harries PG. Asbestos hazards in naval dockyards. Ann Occup Hyg 1968; 11: 135–45.

103 Asbestos Regulations, 1969, United Kingdom.

104 Borel v. Fibreboard Paper Products Corp., 493 F.2d 1076 (5th Cir. 1973).

105 Weill H. Asbestos-associated diseases. Science, public policy and litigation. Chest 1983; 84: 601–8.

106 Selikoff IJ. Partnership for prevention—the Insulation Industry Hygiene Research Program. Industr Med 1970; 39: 21–5.

107 Casey TS, Hadler NM. The role of the primary physician in disability determination for Social Security insurance and workers' compensation. Ann Intern Med 1986; 104: 706–10.

108 Richman SI. Why change? A look at the current system of disability determination and workers' compensation for occupational lung disease. Ann Intern Med 1982; 97: 908–14.

109 UICC Committee. UICC/Cincinnati classification of the radiographic appearances of the pneumoconioses. A cooperative study by the UICC committee. Chest 1970; 58: 57–67.

110 Ehrenreich T, Selikoff IJ. Forensic detection and investigation of occupational-environmental disease. Am J Forensic Med Pathol 1980; 1: 325–33.

111 Brenner J, Sordilla PP, Magill GB, Golbey RB. Malignant mesothelioma of the pleura. Review of 123 patients. Cancer 1982; 49: 2431–5.

112 Antman KH, Blum RH, Greenberger JS, Flowerdew GS, Skarin AT, Canellos GP. Multimodality therapy for malignant mesothelioma based on a study of natural history. Am J Med 1980; 68: 356–62.

113 Grundy GW, Miller RW. Malignant mesothelioma in childhood. Report of 13 cases. Cancer 1972; 30: 1216–18.

114 Brenner J, Sordilla PP, Magill GB. Malignant mesothelioma in children: report of seven cases and review of literature. Med Pediatr Oncol 1981; 9: 367–73.

115 Barbera V, Rubino M. Papillary mesothelioma of the tunica vaginalis. Cancer 1957, 10: 183–9.

116 Kasden EJ. Malignant mesothelioma of the tunica vaginalis propria testis. Report of two cases. Cancer 1969; 23: 1144–50.

117 Johnson DE, Fuerst DE, Gallagher HS. Mesothelioma of the tunica vaginalis. South Med J 1973; 66: 1295–7.

118 Fligiel Z, Kaneko M. Malignant mesothelioma of the tunica vaginalis propria testis in a patient with asbestos exposure. A case report. Cancer 1976; 37: 1478–84.

119 Jaffe J, Roth JA, Carter H. Malignant papillary mesothelioma of tunica vaginalis testis. Urology 1978; 11: 647–50.

120 Japco L, Horta AA, Schreiber K, Mitsudo S, Karwa GL, Singh G et al. Malignant mesothelioma of the tunica vaginalis testis: report of the first case with preoperative diagnosis. Cancer 1982; 49: 119–27.

121 Antman K, Cohen S, Dimitrov NV, Green M, Muggia F. Malignant mesothelioma of the tunica vaginalis testis. J Clin Oncol 1984; 2: 447–51.

122 Suzuki Y. Pathology of human malignant mesothelioma. Semin Oncol 1980; 8: 268–82.

123 Eimoto T, Inoue I. Malignant fibrous mesothelioma of the tunica vaginalis. A histologic and ultrastructural study. Cancer 1977; 39: 2059–66.

124 Browne K, Smither WJ. Asbestos-related mesothelioma: factors discriminating between pleural and peritoneal sites. Br J Industr Med 1983; 40: 145–52.

125 Soutar CA, Simon G, Turner-Warwick M. The radiology of asbestos-induced disease of the lungs. Br J Dis Chest 1974; 68: 235–52.

126 Antman KH. Malignant mesothelioma. N Engl J Med 1980; 303: 200–2.

127 Moertel CG. Peritoneal mesothelioma. Gastroenterology 1972; 63: 346–50.

128 Whitley NO, Brenner DE, Antman KH, Grant D, Aisner J. CT of peritoneal mesothelioma: analysis of eight cases. AJR 1982; 138: 531–5.

129 Doege KW. Fibrosarcoma of the mediastinum. Ann Surg 1930; 92: 955–60.

130 Brenner J, Sordilla PP, Magill GB, Golbey RB. Malignant peritoneal mesothelioma. Review of 25 patients. Am J Gastro 1981; 75: 311–13.

131 Foyle A, Al-Jabi M, McCaughey WTE. Papill-

ary peritoneal tumors in women. Am J Surg Pathol 1981; 5: 241–9.

132 Katsube Y, Mukai K, Silverberg SG. Cystic mesothelioma of the peritoneum. A report of five cases and review of the literature. Cancer 1982; 50: 1615–22.

133 Rabinowitz JG, Efremedis SC, Cohen B, Dan S, Efremedis A, Chahinian AP et al. A comparative study of mesothelioma and asbestosis using computed tomography and conventional chest radiography. Radiology 1982; 144: 453–60.

134 Rabin CB, Blackman NS. Bilateral pleural effusion. Its significance in association with a heart of normal size. J Mt Sinai Hosp 1957; 24: 45–53.

135 Meyer PC. Metastatic carcinoma of the pleura. Thorax 1966; 21: 437–43.

136 Whitley NO. Computed tomography and malignant mesothelioma. In: Antman K, Aisner J eds Asbestos Related Malignancy. Orlando, Fl.: Grune & Stratton, 1986.

137 Shuman LS, Libschitz HI. Solid pleural manifestations of lymphoma. AJR 1984; 142: 269–73.

138 Hourihane D, Lessof L, Richardson PC. Hyaline and calcified pleural plaques as an index of exposure to asbestos. A study of radiological and pathological features of 100 cases with a consideration of epidemiology. Br Med J 1966; i: 1069–74.

139 Mirvis S, Dutcher JP, Haney PJ, Whitley NO, Aisner J. CT or malignant pleural mesothelioma. AJR 1983; 140: 665–70.

140 Grant DC, Seltzer SE, Antman KA, Finberg HJ, Koster R. Computed tomography of malignant pleural mesothelioma. J Comp Assist Tomog 1983; 7: 626–32.

141 Sargent EN, Gordonson J, Jacobson G, Birnbaum M, Shaub M. Bilateral pleural thickening: a manifestation of asbestos dust exposure. Am J Roentgenol 1978; 131: 579–85.

142 Britton MG. Asbestos pleural disease. Br J Dis Chest 1982; 76: 1–10.

143 Heller RM, Janower ML, Weber AL. The radiological manifestations of malignant pleural mesothelioma. AJR 1970; 108: 53–9.

144 Kreel L. Computed tomography in mesothelioma. Semin Oncol 1981; 8: 302–12.

145 Epler GR, FitzGerald MX, Gaensler EA. Carrington CB. Asbestos-related disease from household exposure. Respiration 1980; 39: 229–40.

146 Meurman L. Asbestos bodies and pleural plaques in a Finnish series of autopsy cases. Acta Pathol Microbiol Scand (Suppl) 1966; 181: 1–107.

147 Solomon A. The radiology of asbestos-related diseases with special reference to diffuse mesothelioma. Semin Oncol 1981; 8: 290–301.

148 Solomon A. Radiological features of diffuse mesothelioma. Environ Res 1970; 3: 330–8.

149 Wechsler RJ, Rao VM, Steiner RM. The radiology of thoracic malignant mesothelioma. CRC Crit Rev Diag Imag 1984; 20: 283–310

150 Gaensler EA, Kaplan AI. Asbestos pleural effusion. Ann Intern Med 1971; 74: 178–91.

151 Lewis RJ, Sisler GE, Mackenzie JW. Diffuse, mixed malignant pleural mesothelioma. Ann Thorac Surg 1981; 31: 53–60.

152 Herbert A, Gallagher PJ. Pleural biopsy in the diagnosis of malignant mesothelioma. Thorax 1982; 37: 816–21.

153 Kobzik L, Antman KH, Warhol MJ. The distinction of mesothelioma from metastatic adenocarcinoma in effusions by electron microscopy. Acta Cytol 1985; 29: 219–25.

154 Warhol MJ. Electron microscopy in the diagnosis of mesothelioma with routine biopsy, needle biopsy, and fluid cytology. In: Antman K, Aisner J eds Asbestos Related Malignancy. Orlando, Fl.: Grune & Stratton, 1986.

155 Antman KH, Osteen RT, Klegar KL, Amato DA, Pomfret EA, Larson DA et al. Early peritoneal mesothelioma: a treatable malignancy. Lancet 1985; iii: 977–81.

156 Meyer K, Chaffee E. Hyaluronic acid in pleura fluid associated with malignant tumor involving pleura and peritoneum. Proc Soc Exper Biol Med 1939; 42: 797–800.

157 Roboz J, Greaves J, Silides D, Chahinian AP, Holland JF. Hyaluronic acid content of effusions as a diagnostic aid for malignant mesothelioma. Cancer Res 1985; 45: 1850–54.

158 Osteen RT. Surgical treatment of peritoneal mesothelioma. In: Antman K, Aisner J eds Asbestos Related Malignancy. Orlando, Fl.: Grune & Stratton, 1986.

159 Kannerstein M, Churg J. Peritoneal mesothelioma. Hum Pathol 1977; 8: 83–94.

160 Kannerstein M, Churg J, McCaughey WTE. Hill DP. Papillary tumors of the peritoneum in women: mesothelioma or papillary carcinoma. Am J Obstet Gynecol 1977; 127: 306–14.

161 Corson JM. Pathology of malignant mesothelioma. In: Antman K, Aisner J eds Asbestos Related Malignancy. Orlando, Fl.: Grune & Stratton. 1986.

162 Chernow B, Sahn SA. Carcinomatous involvement of the pleura. An analysis of 96 patients. Am J Med 1977; 63: 695–702.

163 Kannerstein M, McCaughey WTE, Churg J, Selikoff IJ. A critique of the criteria for the diagnosis of diffuse malignant mesothelioma. Mt Sinai J Med 1977; 44: 485–94.

164 Kannerstein M, Churg J, Magner D. Histo-

chemistry in the diagnosis of malignant mesothelioma. Ann Clin Lab Sci 1973; 3: 207–11.

165 Pinkus GS, O'Connor EM, Etheridge CL, Corson JM. Optimal immunoreactivity of keratin proteins in formalin-fixed, paraffin-embedded tissue requires preliminary trypsinization. J Histochem Cytochem 1985; 33: 465–73.

166 Schlegel R, Banks-Schlegel S, McLeod JA, Pinkus GS. Immunoperoxidase localization of keratin in human neoplasms. Am J Pathol 1980; 101: 41–50.

167 Corson JM, Pinkus GS. Mesothelioma: profile of keratin proteins and carcinoembryonic antigen. An immunoperoxidase study of 20 cases and comparison with pulmonary adenocarcinomas. Am J Pathol 1982; 108: 80–7.

168 Gibbs AR, Harach R, Wagner JC, Jasani B. Comparison of tumour markers in malignant mesothelioma and pulmonary adenocarcinoma. Thorax 1985; 40: 91–5.

169 Adams VI, Unni KK. Diffuse malignant mesothelioma of pleura: diagnostic criteria based on an autopsy study. Am J Clin Pathol 1984; 82: 15–23.

170 Battifora H, Kopinski MI. Distinction of mesothelioma from adenocarcinoma. An immunohistochemical approach. Cancer 1985; 55: 1679–85.

171 Marshall RJ, Herbert A, Braye SG, Jones DB. Use of antibodies to carcinoembryonic antigen and human milk fat globule to distinguish carcinoma, mesothelioma and reactive mesothelium. J Clin Pathol 1984; 37: 1215–21.

172 Singh G, Whiteside TL, Dekker A. Immunodiagnosis of mesothelioma. Use of antimesothelial cell serum in an indirect immunofluorescence assay. Cancer 1979; 43: 2288–96.

173 Warhol MJ, Corson JM. An ultrastructural comparison of mesotheliomas and adenocarcinomas of the lung and breast. Hum Pathol 1985; 16: 50–5.

174 Warhol MJ, Hunter NJ, Corson JM. An ultrastructural comparison of mesotheliomas and adenocarcinomas of the ovary and endometrium. Int J Gynecol Pathol 1982; 1: 125–34.

175 Butchart EG, Ashcroft T, Barnsley WC, Holden MP. Pleuropneumonectomy in the management of diffuse malignant mesothelioma of the pleura. Experience with 29 patients. Thorax 1976; 31: 15–24.

176 Feinstein AR, Sosin DM, Wells CK. The Will Rogers phenomenon. Stage migration and new diagnostic techniques as a source of misleading statistics for survival in cancer. N Engl J Med 1985; 312: 1604–8.

177 Wolk RB. Gallium-67 scanning in the evaluation of mesothelioma. J Nucl Med 1978; 19: 808–9.

178 Samson M, Baker L, Wasser L, Borden E, Wanebo H. Randomized comparison of cyclophosphamide, DTIC, and Adriamycin (CIA) vs. cyclophosphamide and Adriamycin (CA) in patients with malignant mesothelioma (abstr). Proc Am Soc Clin Oncol 1985; 4: 128.

179 Chahinian AP, Beranek JT, Suzuki Y, Bakesi JG, Wisniewski L, Selikoff IJ et al. Transplantation of human malignant mesothelioma into nude mice. Cancer Res 1980; 40: 181–5.

180 Fischbein A, Suzuki Y, Selikoff IJ, Bekesi JG. Unexpected longevity of a patient with malignant pleural mesothelioma. Cancer 1978; 42: 1999–2004.

181 Butchart EG, Ashcroft T, Barnsley WC, Holden MP. Pleuropneumonectomy in the management of diffuse malignant mesothelioma of the pleural. Experience with 29 patients. Thorax 1976; 31: 15–24.

182 McCormack PM, Nagasaki F, Hilaris BS, Martini N. Surgical treatment of pleural mesothelioma. J Thorac Cardiovasc Surg 1982; 84: 834–42.

183 Martini N, Bains MS, Beattie EJ. Indications for pleurectomy in malignant effusion. Cancer 1975; 35: 734–8.

184 Eiselberg AV. Offizielles Protokoll der Gesellschaft der Artze in Wien. Wien Klin Wochenschr 1922; 35: 509.

185 DeLaria GA, Jensik R, Faber LP, Kittle CF. Surgical management of malignant mesothelioma. Ann Thorac Surg 1978; 26: 375–82.

186 Shemin RJ. Surgical treatment of pleural mesothelioma. In: Antman K, Aisner J eds Asbestos Related Malignancy. Orlando, Fl.: Grune & Stratton, 1986.

187 Woern H. Moeglichkeiten und Ergebnisse der chirurgischen Behandlung des malignen Pleuramesothelioms. Thoraxchirurgie 1974; 22: 391–3.

188 Rogoff EE, Hilaris BS, Huvos AG. Long-term survival in patients with malignant peritoneal mesothelioma treated with irradiation. Cancer 1973; 32: 656–64.

189 Butchart EG, Ashcroft T, Barnsley WC, Holden MP. The role of surgery in diffuse malignant mesothelioma of the pleura. Semin Oncol 1981; 8: 321–8.

190 Nervino HE, Gebhardt FC. Peritoneovenous shunt for intractable malignant ascites. A single case report of metastatic peritoneal mesothelioma implanted via Le Veen shunt. Cancer 1984; 54: 2231–3.

191 Lederman GS, Recht A. Radiation therapy of peritoneal mesotheliomas. In: Antman K,

Aisner J eds Asbestos Related Malignancy. Orlando, Fl.: Grune & Stratton, 1986.

192 Weiss RB, Muggia FM. Working conference on mesothelioma treatment trials. Cancer Res 1979; 39: 3799–800.

193 Vogelzang NJ, Schulz SM, Ianucci AM, Kennedy BJ. Malignant mesothelioma. The University of Minnesota experience. Cancer 1984; 53: 377–83.

194 Porter JM, Cheek JM. Pleural mesothelioma. Review of tumor histogenesis and report of 12 cases. J Thorac Cardiovasc Surg 1968; 55: 882–90.

195 Ratzer ER, Pool JL, Melamed MR. Pleural mesotheliomas. Clinical experience with 37 patients. Am J Roentgenol 1967; 99: 863–80.

196 Dobelbower RR, Strubler KA, Vaisman I. Clinical applications of high energy electron beams: the pancreas, pleura and spine. In: Uppinger A, Bataini JP, Irigaray JM, Chu F eds High Energy Electrons in Radiation Therapy. New York: Springer Verlag, 1980: 91–7.

197 Gordon W, Antman KH, Greenberger JS, Weichselbaum RR, Chaffey JT. Radiation therapy in the management of patients with mesothelioma. Int J Radiation Oncology Biol Phys 1982; 8: 19–25.

198 Schlienger M, Eschwege F, Blache R, Depierre R. Mesotheliomas pleuraux malins. Etude de 39 cas dont 25 autopsies. Bull du Cancer 1969; 56: 265–308.

199 Ehrenhaft JL, Sensenig DM, Lawrence MS. Mesotheliomas of the pleura. J Thorac Cardiovasc Surg. 1960; 40: 393–409.

200 Semb G. Diffuse malignant pleural mesothelioma. A clinicopathological study of 10 fatal cases. Acta Chir Scand 1963; 126: 78–91.

201 Reisner K, Huzly A. Pleurogene Tumoren und Pseudotumoren der Pleura. ROEFO 1967; 106: 775–89, 107: 69–80.

202 Brady LW. Mesothelioma—the role for radiation therapy. Semin Oncol 1981; 8: 329–34.

203 Seydel HG. Radiation therapy for pleural mesothelioma. In: Antman K, Aisner J eds Asbestos Related Malignancy. Orlando, Fl.: Grune & Stratton, 1986.

204 Case Records of the Massachusetts General Hospital (Case 47-1980). N Engl J Med 1980; 303: 1283–91.

205 Smith WE, Hubert DD, Holiat SM, Sobel HJ, Davis S. An experimental model for treatment of mesothelioma. Cancer 1981; 47: 658–63.

206 Guyatt G, Sackett D, Taylor DW, Chong J, Roberts R, Pugsley S. Determining optimal therapy—randomized trials in individual patients. N Engl J Med 1986; 314: 889–92.

207 Mintzer DM, Kelsen D, Frimmer D, Heelan R, Gralla R. Phase II trial of high-dose cisplatin in patients with malignant mesothelioma. Cancer Treat Rep 1985; 69: 711–12.

208 Yap BS, Benjamin RS, Burgess A, Bodey GP. The value of Adriamycin in the treatment of diffuse malignant pleural mesothelioma. Cancer 1978; 42: 1692–6.

209 Lerner HJ, Schoenfeld DA, Martin A, Falkson G, Borden AE. Malignant mesothelioma. The Eastern Cooperative Oncology Group (ECOG) Experience. Cancer 1983; 52: 1981–5.

210 Sorensen PG, Bach F, Bork E, Hansen HH. Randomized trial of doxorubicin versus cyclophosphamide in diffuse malignant pleural mesothelioma. Cancer Treat Rep 1985; 69: 1431–2.

211 Harvey VJ, Slevin ML, Ponder BAJ, Blackshaw AJ, Wrigley PFM. Chemotherapy of diffuse mesothelioma. Phase II trials of single-agent 5-fluorouracil and Adriamycin. Cancer 1984; 54: 961–4.

212 Dimitrov NV, Egner J, Balcueva E, Suhrland LG. High-dose-methotrexate with citrovorum factor and vincristine in the treatment of malignant mesothelioma. Cancer 1982; 50: 1245–7.

213 Gerner RE, Moore GE. Chemotherapy of malignant mesothelioma. Oncology 1974; 30: 152–5.

214 Zidar BL, Pugh RP, Schiffer LM, Raju RN, Vaidya KA, Bloom RL et al. Treatment of six cases of mesothelioma with doxorubicin and cisplatin. Cancer 1983; 52: 1788–91.

215 Chahinian AP, Norton L, Holland JF, Szrajer L, Hart RD. Experimental and clinical activity of mitomycin C and cis-diamminedichloroplatinum in malignant mesothelioma. Cancer Res 1984; 44: 1688–92.

216 Jett JR, Eagan RT. Chemotherapy for malignant mesothelioma: CAMEO. Am J Clin Oncol (CCT) 1982; 5: 429–31.

217 Pfiefle CE, Howell SB, Markman M. Intracavitary cisplatin chemotherapy for mesothelioma. Cancer Treat Rep 1985; 69: 205–7.

218 Antmann KH, Pomfret EA, Aisner J, MacIntyre J, Osteen RT, Greenberger JS. Peritoneal mesothelioma: natural history and response to chemotherapy. J Clin Oncol 1983; 1: 386–91.

219 Antman KH, Osteen RT, Montella D. A phase I trial of intracavitary chemotherapy of doxorubicin (Adriamycin) alternating with cisplatin. In: Howell S ed Intra-arterial and Intracavitary Chemotherapy. Boston: Martinus Nijhoff, 1984: 167–78.

Textbook of Uncommon Cancer
Edited by C.J. Williams, J.G. Krikorian, M.R. Green and D. Raghavan
© 1988 John Wiley & Sons Ltd

Chapter **20**

Primary Sarcomas of the Lung

Mark R. Wick* and
J. Carlos Manivel†
*Assistant Professor of Laboratory Medicine and Pathology and† Instructor in Laboratory Medicine and Pathology, Division of Surgical Pathology, Department of Laboratory Medicine and Pathology, University of Minnesota School of Medicine, Minneapolis, Minnesota, USA

INTRODUCTION

Sarcomas originating in the lung are extraordinarily rare lesions, and account for less than 0.1% of all malignant tumors in this organ (1). Moreover, primary mesenchymal bronchopulmonary malignancies are capable of manifesting a diversity of histopathologic appearances, which are identical to those of secondary sarcomas of the lung, and similar to those of 'metaplastic' lung cancers (2, 3). For these reasons, the diagnosis of primary pulmonary sarcomas is extremely challenging, for both clinicians and pathologists. This chapter will summarize the accumulated data on such neoplasms, and discuss the application of specialized pathologic techniques for their classification. Fibrosarcomas, leiomyosarcomas, malignant hemangiopericytomas, malignant fibrous histiocytomas, angiosarcomas, rhabdomyosarcomas, chondrosarcomas, osteosarcomas, and neurogenic sarcomas of the lung shall be considered, with comments on the differential diagnosis of each of these tumor entities.

DEMOGRAPHIC FEATURES AND CLINICAL HISTORY

Regardless of histologic type, sarcomas of the lung occur in a wide age range; they have been seen in neonatal life, as well as in advanced adulthood (4–7). This fact notwithstanding, most are observed in middle life or in elderly individuals, without a preference for gender (7–12). Caucasians with such tumors are best represented in the literature, although many reports have not specified the racial origins of the patients concerned. Similarly, information on occupations and exposure to potential carcinogenic agents has generally been lacking, and comment cannot be made on these factors.

Symptoms and signs attending pulmonary sarcomas are dependent on the location of the tumors, rather than their histologic types. Peripheral lesions are often asymptomatic, and are found incidentally on chest roentgenograms, or cause chest pain due to extension into the pleura and chest wall. Central neoplasms involving bronchi commonly cause

dyspnea, cough, and hemoptysis; if endobronchial and obtrusive, they may produce endogenous pneumonia (7). Sarcomas which infiltrate or arise in the pulmonary arterial tree
typically serve as the sources of tumor emboli,
mimicking the signs and symptoms of idiopathic venous thromboembolism (9). Those
lesions which manifest extensive intrapulmonary spread may cause alveolar hemorrhage
and respiratory failure (12, 13). Clinical presentation of pulmonary sarcomas by extrathoracic metastasis is virtually unknown.

Aside from the latter point, these features are
identical to those seen in conjunction with
bronchogenic carcinomas (14). However, the
rapidity of symptomatic evolution is usually
greater in carcinoma cases, and patients with
epithelial tumors are older at diagnosis by an
average of two to three decades (15). Furthermore, a history of cigarette smoking is characteristically obtained with carcinomas, but not
sarcomas (7, 14, 15).

RADIOGRAPHIC FEATURES
OF PULMONARY SARCOMAS

The roentgenographic characteristics of sarcomas of the lung are not diagnostic, but may be
suggestive of such tumors (16). Peripheral
lesions are usually larger (greater than 5 cm in
diameter), with rounded borders and a lack of
central cavitation (16–18). Occasional neoplasms display diffuse, multifocal growth
throughout one or both lung fields, simulating
metastatic lesions (12). Central tumors either
present as nondescript hilar densities, or produce obstructive pneumonia, with segmental
or lobar consolidation. Again, all of these
radiographic appearances recapitulate those of
various bronchogenic carcinomas (14).

CLINICAL EVALUATION AND
STAGING

Because of the greater likelihood that a mesenchymal tumor of the lung is metastatic rather
than primary, appropriate radiographic investigations are mandatory before making a diag-

nosis of indigenous pulmonary sarcoma. Those
sites which are most likely to harbor an occult
sarcoma are the uterus, the alimentary tract
(particularly the stomach), and the deep soft
tissues (15). Therefore, depending on the preoperative suspicion that a pulmonary mass is
sarcomatous, barium-contrast studies of the
gastrointestinal tract and computed tomograms of the abdomen and pelvis are in order.
Accordingly, the determination of whether a
lung tumor is epithelial or mesenchymal
becomes extremely important to this initial
evaluation. This is best accomplished by bronchoscopy and transbronchial biopsy of accessible central lesions, or by transthoracic needle
biopsy of peripheral masses. Exfoliative cytologic studies of sputum are seldom rewarding in
cases of pulmonary sarcomas (19, 20).

A formal staging system for sarcomas of the
lung has not yet been devised. However,
tumors which are confined to the lumen of a
bronchus, or which are small and do not
involve the pulmonary arteries or pleura have
a prognosis which is better than that of large,
invasive lesions. Obviously, neoplasms that are
intravascular, have invaded the chest wall, or
have metastasized to distant sites at diagnosis
are clinically advanced, with a correspondingly adverse outlook. The histologic type and
grade of pulmonary sarcomas does not appear
to influence prognosis significantly.

SPECIAL PATHOLOGIC
TECHNIQUES IN THE STUDY
OF SARCOMAS OF THE LUNG

The pathologist is typically confronted with a
poorly differentiated spindle-cell neoplasm, in
cases proving to be primary pulmonary sarcomas. As in the soft tissues, such tumors are often
difficult to classify exactly without the use of
special morphologic techniques. The latter are
basically twofold, and include transmission
electron microscopy, and immunohistochemistry.

Ultrastructural studies are facilitated by
proper fixation of tumor tissue in glutaraldehyde solution, immediately after procurement.

Retrieval of specimens from formalin or paraffin blocks for this purpose yields vastly inferior results. Hence, clinicians should be encouraged to submit fractionated biopsies in suitable fixative, or to contact the surgical pathologist before the biopsy procedure, in order that he or she may be present to supervise the handling of the tissue obtained.

On the other hand, immunocytochemical evaluations may be performed satisfactorily on conventionally processed, formalin-fixed specimens (21, 22). Commercially available antibodies to several tumor-cell determinants are particularly useful in the evaluation of sarcomas; the latter are described briefly in the following sections.

Cytoskeletal Intermediate Filaments

The lineage of differentiation followed by normal and neoplastic tissues is indicated by the type of intermediate filament proteins which they express (23–26). These include five classes; namely, cytokeratin (CK) (27–29), desmin (DES) (27, 30–34), vimentin (VIM) (27, 28, 31–34), neurofilament protein (NFP) (35), and glial fibrillary acidic protein (GFAP) (35, 36). Cytokeratins are a family of polypeptides, ranging in molecular weight from 40000 to 70000 (24, 25, 34). They are seen only in tissues and tumors manifesting epithelial differentiation, and their immunohistologic presence therefore excludes a diagnosis of most sarcomas. In contrast, vimentin is observed primarily in mesenchymal cellular proliferations (27, 28, 31, 33, 34), although some carcinomas also appear to coexpress VIM with CK (37). Desmin is restricted in distribution to myogenous cells, both smooth and striated (24, 27, 28, 30–34). Neurofilament protein and GFAP are detectable only in neuronal-neuroendocrine and glial tissues, respectively (35, 36), and their presence would not be expected in sarcomas.

Special procedures must be applied to the detection of cytokeratins in formalin-fixed tissues, since this mordant appears to 'mask' CK in many cases (38, 39). Proteases, including pepsin, trypsin, and pronase, should be allowed to react with tissue specimens before application of antibodies to CK, to maximize the expression of this intermediate filament protein (38–40). In another vein, we have not encountered any commercial antibodies to VIM which fail to cross-react extensively with CK in formalin-fixed specimens (41). Hence, immunohistologic evaluations for vimentin must always be accompanied by concomitant staining for CK; if the latter is present, reactivity for VIM should be discounted.

Other Filament Proteins

Actin is another cytoplasmic filament protein of particular use in the delineation of sarcomatous differentiation. This determinant is largely restricted in distribution to myogenous cells (42, 43).

Cellular Enzymes

Certain cellular enzymatic proteins are of assistance in determining the cellular nature of spindle-cell tumors of the lung. These include neuron-specific enolase (NSE), which is synthesized by neuroendocrine neoplasms (44), and lysozyme (LYSO), alpha-l-antitrypsin (AAT), alpha-l-antichymotrypsin (AACT), which are typically detectable in fibrohistiocytic tumors (45–47).

Cytoplasmic, Nonfilamentous, Nonenzymatic Proteins

Additional cytoplasmic tumor markers include myoglobin (restricted to striated muscle cells) (48–50), S100 protein (seen in chondrocytes and Schwann cells) (51–53), factor VIII-related antigen (specific for endothelial cells) (54–56), and ferritin (found in fibrohistiocytic cells) (46). These are correspondingly applicable in the identification of rhabdomyosarcoma, chondrosarcoma and neurogenic sarcoma, angiosarcoma, and malignant fibrous histiocytoma, respectively.

Membrane Antigens

Stains for membrane proteins provide significant diagnostic information on epithelial and mesenchymal differentiation. Those of greatest usefulness include epithelial membrane antigen (EMA), which is expressed by most epithelial cells (57, 58); Leu 7, seen in Schwann cells and smooth muscle cells (59, 60); and blood group isoantigens A, B, and H (61–63). The last group of determinants is observed in both epithelial and endothelial tissues (63).

Plant Lectins

Lectins are plant extracts which bind selectively to certain sugar residues, in cell membranes and cytoplasm. The lectin with greatest application to the study of sarcomas is *Ulex europaeus* I agglutinin (UEA), which recognizes endothelial cells in all patients, and epithelial cells in individuals of blood group O (64, 65). When used in conjunction with immunonegativity for epithelial markers such as CK and EMA, *Ulex* may be employed as an indicator of angiosarcomatous and hemangioendotheliomatous differentiation.

Not one of the antigens just listed may be used in isolation, to support or negate a particular diagnosis. Rather, panels of immunostains must be applied to compensate for the nonspecificity of individual reactants. These shall be presented subsequently, in discussions of specific neoplasms.

PATHOLOGIC FINDINGS IN SPECIFIC PULMONARY SARCOMAS

Fibrosarcoma (7, 66–74)

Fibrosarcomas of the lung, of which 71 cases have been documented, may present as either endobronchial or intrapulmonary masses. In the former case, they are soft, tan-grey, and polypoid, and measure up to 2.5 cm in diameter. Foci of hemorrhage and necrosis are frequently seen. The mainstem and lobar bronchi of the right lung are more frequently involved than those of the left. Intrapulmonary tumors are circumscribed, lobulated or nodular masses, which are firm and white-grey. Internal areas of necrosis and hemorrhage are again common, but central cavitation is not observed.

Microscopically, fibrosarcomas are composed of interlacing fascicles of spindle cells, with hyperchromatic, elongated, pointed nuclei. A 'herringbone' pattern of growth is evident in some cases (Figure 1), together with stromal fibrogenesis. The latter feature may be highlighted by trichrome or reticulin stains, but is often absent in poorly differentiated tumors. Cytoplasm is scant and amphophilic, and cell borders are poorly defined. Mitotic activity varies widely, and ranges from one to 30 division figures per ten high-power (× 400) fields (Figure 2). Foci of necrosis are frequently apparent.

Ultrastructurally, fibrosarcomas are comprised of fibroblastic or myofibroblastic cells (75, 76). These manifest irregular nuclear outlines, occasionally prominent nucleoli, and dilated rough endoplasmic reticulum, in addition to usual metabolic cell organelles (Figure 3). Some tumors contain intrareticular collagen fibers, and extracellular collagen fibers are commonly arranged at right angles to cell membranes. Pericellular basal laminar material is seen only in neoplasms with myofibroblastic features, together with cytoplasmic thin filaments and occasional dense bodies. Membrane-associated pinocytosis and subplasmalemmal dense plaques are absent.

Immunohistochemical evaluation demonstrates vimentin-reactivity, but CK and EMA are lacking (31, 57). Occasional tumors with myofibroblastic differentiation may also display actin and desmin, but this is not typical of 'pure' fibrosarcoma (31, 43). Fibrohistiocytic markers such as LYSO, AAT, AACT, and ferritin are not seen in this neoplasm (46); neither are factor VIII-related antigen (FVIIIRAG), myoglobin, S100 protein, Leu 7, blood group isoantigens (BGI), or receptors for UEA (60). Neuron-specific enolase is not

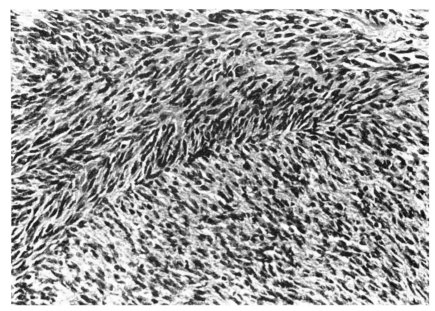

Figure 1   Fibrosarcoma. Spindle-shaped cells grow in a 'herringbone' pattern.

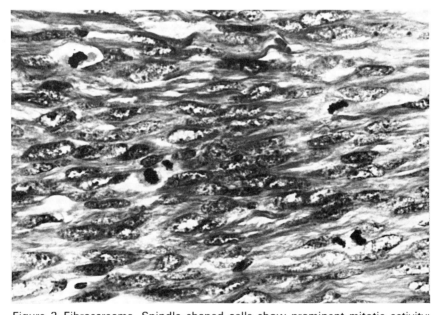

Figure 2   Fibrosarcoma. Spindle-shaped cells show prominent mitotic activity; stromal fibrogenesis is evident.

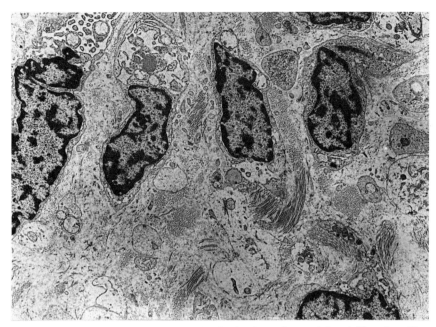

Figure 3 Fibrosarcoma. Elongated cells display irregular nuclei and dilated profiles of rough endoplasmic reticulum intercellular collagen is also seen.

observed in fibrosarcoma, in contrast to its presence in spindle-cell neuroendocrine tumors (carcinoids) (44), which enter into differential diagnosis.

Leiomyosarcoma (7, 15, 18–20, 77–107)

Bronchopulmonary leiomyosarcoma has been described in less than 100 published cases to date. Like fibrosarcoma, it may be seen as an endobronchial or intrapulmonary mass, with virtually identical macroscopic features (Figure 4). Those which are thought to arise from blood vessels in the lung are often intimately adherent to the pulmonary arteries or veins, making resection difficult for the surgeon. Similarly, tumors demonstrating engulfment of major bronchi are hypothesized to take origin from bronchial smooth muscle (15, 101).

Microscopically, leiomyosarcomas are typified by intertwining fascicular growth of spindled tumor cells with dense blunt-ended nuclei, and fibrillar fuchsinophilic cytoplasm, as seen with Masson's trichrome stain. Cell

borders are indistinct, and mitoses again vary widely in number. Fascicles of cells cut in cross section often demonstrate a characteristic perinuclear clear zone within the cytoplasm. Focally, blood vessels may assume a 'staghorn' pattern, like that seen in hemangiopericytoma, and areas of nuclear palisading may also be evident, similar to patterns observed in neural neoplasms (15). Finally, rare leiomyosarcomas of the lung have an epithelioid, polygonal-cell appearance, with distinct cellular borders and more abundant cytoplasm (15). Such lesions are often mistaken for carcinomas.

By electron microscopy, there are five typical findings in the cells of leiomyosarcoma: bundles of cytoplasmic thin filaments, 'dense bodies' associated with such filaments, subplasmalemmal dense plaques, pericellular basal lamina and membrane-associated micropinocytosis (15, 105, 108–110) (Figures 5a and 5b)). Not all of those features are apparent in each case, or in all of the tumor cells in any given lesion. In particular, cytoplasmic actin-like filaments are not especially abundant in

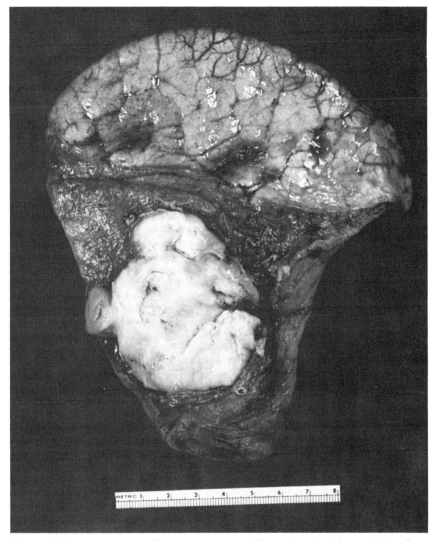

Figure 4 Leiomyosarcoma. Gross appearance. (*Reproduced with permission from Arch Pathol Lab Med 106:510-14, 1982.*)

most pulmonary smooth muscle sarcomas (15). Nevertheless, they are present in sufficient number to make an ultrastructural diagnosis. In the past, one of us (MRW) speculated on the possibility that primary bronchopulmonary leiomyosarcoma might be distinguished from secondary tumors by this characteristic, since the latter often demonstrate marked filamentous development (15).

However, interim study of both types of leiomyosarcoma in the lung has not borne out this hypothesis.

Other fine structural findings which separate leiomyosarcoma from other malignant mesenchymal neoplasms include a tendency for mitochondria to assume polarized positions within tumor cells (15), and the formation of villiform cytoplasmic projections in epithelioid

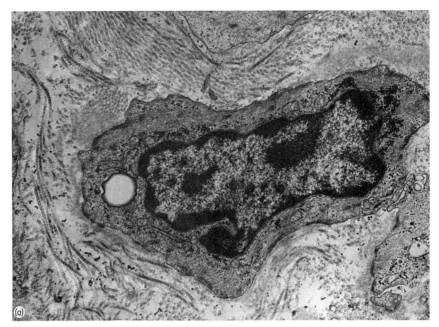

Figure 5a Leiomyosarcoma. Cells are characterized by elongated shape, and numerous cytoplasmic thin filaments.

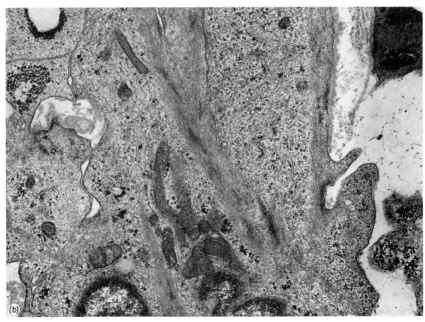

Figure 5b Leiomyosarcoma. Cytoplasmic bundles of thin filaments and associated 'dense bodies'.

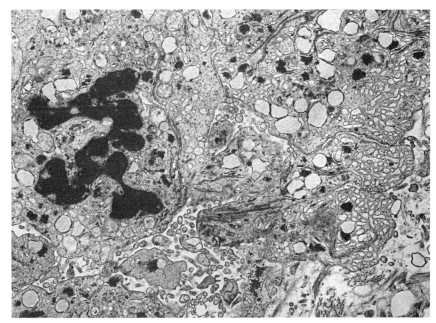

Figure 6 Epithelioid leiomyosarcoma shows numerous villiform cytoplasmic projections. A degenerating cell is present on the left.

lesions (Figure 6). The latter may contain primitive appositional intercellular plaques, but true desmosomes are always absent.

Immunohistologic studies show the regular presence of vimentin and desmin in leiomyosarcomas (26, 31, 60). Actin is also expressed by roughly 60% of cases (43, 60). Leu 7 and S100 protein may be observed in approximately 50% of these neoplasms, in common with the properties of neurogenic sarcomas in soft tissue sites (111). Since neurofibrosarcoma is capable of displaying desmin-reactivity (60, 111), the immunophenotypes of the two tumors overlap significantly. Nevertheless, primary pulmonary neurofibrosarcoma is an entity of questionable existence (7), as discussed below, and our practice is to label any spindle-cell sarcoma of the lung with desmin-, Leu 7-, or S100 protein-positivity as leiomyosarcoma. Of course, this statement is predicated upon concurrent negativity for CK and EMA, inasmuch as these determinants are never apparent in smooth muscle tumors but

typify histologically similar sarcomatoid carcinomas (26, 57). In addition, NSE, LYSO, AAT, AACT, myoglobin, FVIIIRAG, ferritin, BGI, and UEA receptors are absent in leiomyosarcoma (60).

Hemangiopericytoma (16, 112–121)

Thirty-two tumors classified as primary hemangiopericytomas of the lung may be found in the literature. These were seen predominantly in female patients, and were all peripheral intrapulmonary masses with gross appearances like that of leiomyosarcoma.

Microscopically, hemangiopericytoma is comprised of uniform small cells or blunt spindle cells, arranged in solid sheets or around vascular spaces which resemble 'staghorns' (Figure 7). Their nuclear-to-cytoplasmic ratios are high, with oval, hyperchromatic nuclei and scanty amphophilic cytoplasm. Mitoses are extremely variable in frequency, as are foci of necorsis (112).

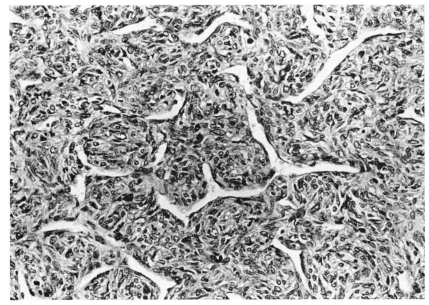

Figure 7 Hemangiopericytoma. Anastomosing vascular channels in a 'staghorn' pattern are surrounded by blunted spindle cells with ill-defined cytoplasm.

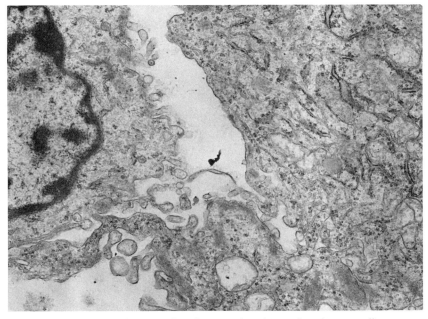

Figure 8 Hemangiopericytoma showing paucity of cytoplasmic organelles; sparse cytoplasmic filaments are present.

By electron microscopy, hemangiopericytoma cells have few distinguishing characteristics (122, 123) (Figure 8). They may contain sparse intermediate cytoplasmic filaments; membrane-associated micropinocytosis and focal pericellular basal lamina may also be apparent. Cytoplasmic dense bodies and subplasmalemmal dense plaques are typically absent, but appositional intercellular junctions may be evident (123).

Similarly, immunocytochemical analysis has shown limited reactivity for most determinants in this neoplasm. Vimentin is detectable in most hemangiopericytomas, and actin is seen in roughly 50%, but desmin, cytokeratin, NSE, EMA, LYSO, AAT, AACT, ferritin, myoglobin, S100 protein, FVIIIRAG, Leu 7, BGI, and receptors for UEA are universally lacking (60).

Malignant Fibrous Histiocytoma (1, 10, 17, 124–129)

Twelve examples of primary malignant fibrous histiocytoma (MFH) of the lung have been documented. All presented as solid, white-tan, peripheral intraparenchymal masses, and varied in size from 1 to 8 cm in greatest dimension. In these and other respects, they were similar in macroscopic character to other pulmonary sarcomas.

Malignant fibrous histiocytoma is microscopically typified by a mixture of spindled and large pleomorphic tumor cells, arranged globally or focally in a mat-like or 'storiform' pattern of growth (Figure 9). Small central intratumoral blood vessels are commonly present at the centers of these storiform structures. The spindle cells are relatively uniform in size, with hyperchromatic or vesicular nuclei and irregular nuclear contours. In isolation, they strongly resemble those observed in fibrosarcoma. However, unlike the latter lesion, pleomorphic giant and polygonal cells also characterize MFH (Figure 10). These elements possess multilobate or multiple nuclei, which may be arranged at the cellular periphery. Cytoplasm is relatively abundant, and may have a 'glassy' homogeneous quality. The tumor stroma is variably fibrous in most cases,

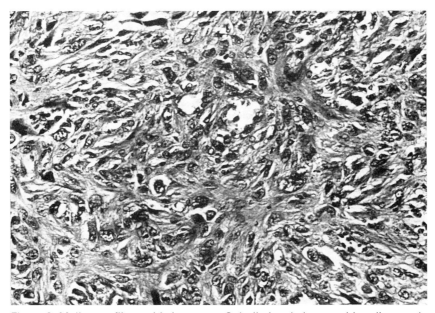

Figure 9   Malignant fibrous histiocytoma. Spindled and pleomorphic cells grow in a 'storiform' pattern.

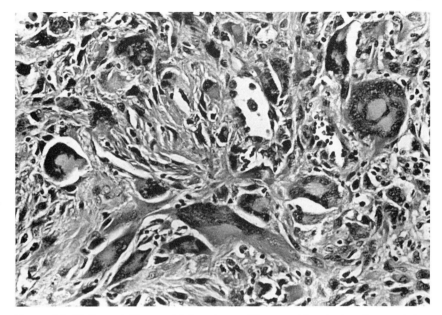

Figure 10 Malignant fibrous histiocytoma. Pleomorphic giant cells are inter-spersed with spindled cells.

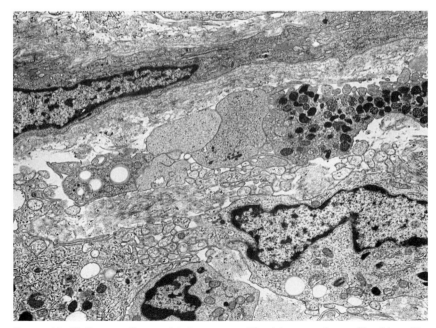

Figure 11 Malignant fibrous histiocytoma. Fibroblast- and myofibroblast-like cells are interspersed with histiocytoid cells that contain numerous lysosomes.

but may also contain areas of myxoid change or acute inflammation. Rarely, matrical osteoid-like material is present. Mitoses range from five to 30 per ten high-power fields (10).

Electron microscopic studies on pulmonary MFH have yielded results identical to those seen in soft tissue tumors of this type (10, 124, 130–133). The neoplastic cells belong to several morphologic classes, which may merge with one another through transitional forms. They include fibroblast- and myofibroblast-like elements (cf. fibrosarcoma, above), and histiocytoid polyglonal and giant cells (Figure 11). The latter display eccentric nuclei with prominent nucleoli, relatively abundant cytoplasm, and ruffled, villiform cell borders. Cellular organelles of note include variably numerous lysosomes, some of which may contain lipid (Figure 12), prominent Golgi complexes, and sparse skeins of intermediate microfilaments. Collagen fibers and amorphous granular material comprise the tumoral matrix. Rare intercellular appositional plaques may be apparent between histiocytoid or myofibroblast-like cells, but true tight junctions are absent.

Those immunoreactants of greatest use in the identification of MFH are vimentin, LYSO, AAT, AACT, and ferritin (26, 45, 46, 134). Of these, vimentin is universally observed, and AACT is next most frequently expressed. As mentioned above, LYSO, AAT, AACT, and ferritin are all 'fibrohistiocytic' markers; however, they may also be produced by anaplastic, pleomorphic carcinomas (which simulate MFH) (60, 135), and it is again important to have negative reactions for CK and EMA in hand before making a diagnosis of malignant fibrous histiocytoma. Desmin and actin are seen in a minority (10–20%) of MFH cases (26, 43), probably as a reflection of myofibroblastic differentiation. Leu 7, NSE, myoglobin, S100 protein, FVIIIRAG, BGI, and receptors for UEA are not present in these tumors (60).

Angiosarcoma (13, 136–138)

Less than 10 well-documented cases of primary

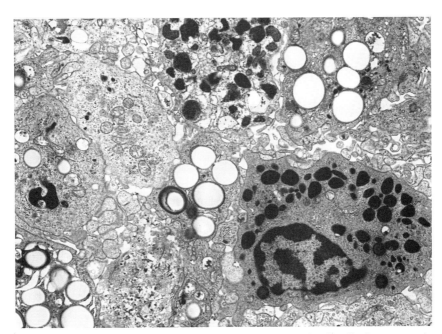

Figure 12 Malignant fibrous histiocytoma. Histiocytoid cells display eccentric nuclei, villiform cytoplasmic borders, and numerous lysosomes.

'classic' angiosarcoma of the lung have been reported. These have usually involved patients in the second and third decades of life, with females predominating, who presented with chest pain and hemorrhagic pleural effusions. Fatal pulmonary hemorrhage has also been documented in conjunction with such neoplasms. Radiographically, angiosarcomas are particularly likely to be confused with metastases, since they assume a multifocal, bilateral, nodular appearance (13).

Grossly, these tumors are soft, hemorrhagic, reddish-blue nodules, which are scattered throughout the lung parenchyma (13). They are found in somewhat greater density in subpleural locations.

Microscopically, classic angiosarcoma has a 'sievelike' appearance, and is composed of interanastomosing vascular channels linked by pump endothelial cells (Figure 13). These cells have a 'hobnail' appearance, in that their hyperchromatic nuclei project into the vascular spaces. Mitotic figures are usually scarce, and cytoplasm is scanty and amphophilic. Foci of hemorrhage, deposition of hemosiderin pigment, and necrosis are common. Occasionally,

areas of papillary growth by the tumor cells may be apparent, as may solid ('dedifferentiated') spindle-cell or epithelioid foci (figure 14). Walls of contiguous bronchioles and preexisting vessels may be infiltrated by these neoplasms. The surrounding lung parenchyma frequently displays organizing pneumonitic changes, as well as hemorrhage and fibrin deposition; peripheral tumor spread along pulmonary lymphatic and venous routes may simulate the appearance of lymphangitic carcinoma.

Ultrastructurally, angiosarcomas manifest polygonal tumor cells which contain moderately abundant microfilaments, as well as Golgi complexes and secondary phagolysosomes. Membrane-associated micropinocytosis is usually prominent, as is pericellular basal lamina (139). Well-developed intercellular junctions are also apparent, into which cytoplasmic microfilaments may insert. Roughly 30% of angiosarcomas contain cells with peculiar rod-like cytoplasmic inclusions, having an internally striated substructure and 'frayed' poles (140) (Figures 15a and 15b). The latter have been termed Weibel–Palade bodies, after

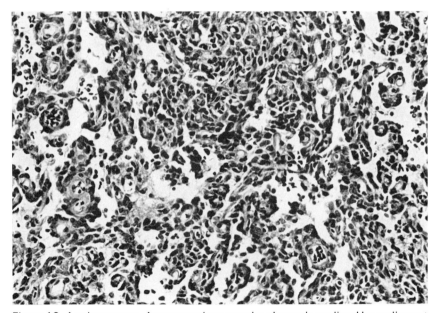

Figure 13 Angiosarcoma. Anastomosing vascular channels are lined by malignant endothelial cells.

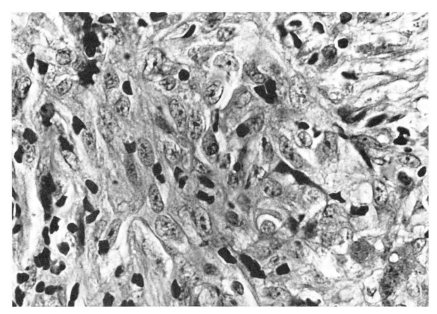

Figure 14 Angiosarcoma. Solid pattern of growth; the cells have an epithelioid appearance.

their describers, and are thought to be specific markers of endothelial differentiation (140, 141).

Factor VIII-related antigen is also restricted to endothelial cells and their neoplasms, but is detectable immunocytochemically in only 30–50% of angiosarcomas (54–56). On the other hand, vimentin is characteristically present in all such tumors (26); BGI and receptors for UEA are seen in approximately 75% of cases (61, 63–65). Since the latter determinants are present in carcinomas as well as vascular tumors (62, 142), negative results for cytokeratin and EMA must accompany the interpretation of UEA- or BGI-positivity as markers for angiosarcoma. Desmin, actin, NSE, LYSO, AAT, AACT, ferritin, myoglobin, S100 protein, and Leu 7 are not found in this lesion (60).

Epithelioid Hemangioendothelioma (So-called 'Intravascular Bronchoalveolar Tumor') (12, 143–154)

Since its initial description over a decade ago,

the enigmatic intravascular bronchoalveolar tumor' (IVBAT) has been further characterized as an endothelial neoplasm of low-grade malignancy, which shares a virtual cellular identity with epithelioid hemangioendotheliomas of the liver and soft tissues (155, 156). Moreover, this lesion demonstrates a marked overlap of its demographic, radiographic, and clinical features which those of angiosarcoma of the lung (12, 13).

In contrast to classic angiosarcoma, however, the tumor nodules of IVBAT are grey-white and solid on gross examination, with a 'chondroid' consistency. Occasionally, they may be centrally calcified. Most are peripheral, multifocal masses, but rare endobronchial examples have been described (12). Individual tumor nodules vary in size from 0.3 to 1.0 cm in diameter.

The microscopic characteristics of the IVBAT are unique among pulmonary neoplasms. This tumor is composed of round to oval nodules with pale, eosinophilic centers and peripheral cellularity (Figure 16). Its advancing edges are confined within alveolar

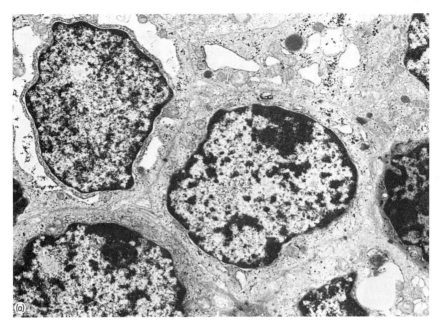

Figure 15a Angiosarcoma. Cells have interdigitating cytoplasmic borders and well-developed intercellular junctions.

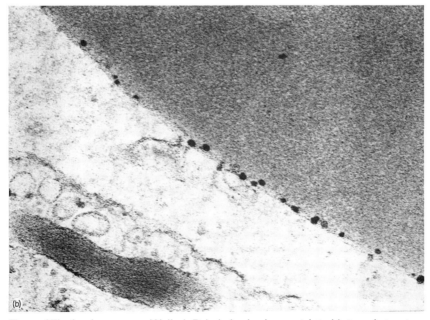

Figure 15b Angiosarcoma. Weibel–Palade body shows striated internal structure and 'frayed' poles.

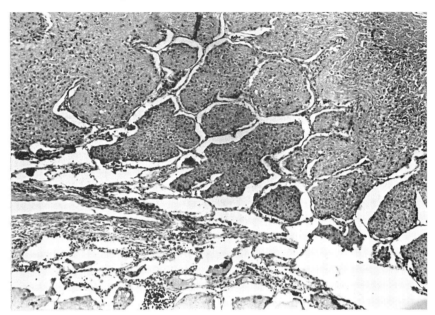

Figure 16 Epithelioid hemangioendothelioma (IVBAT). The tumor is composed of oral nodules. The advancing edges are confined within alveolar spaces.

spaces, with a typical retraction artifact, and have a micropolypoid appearance (Figure 17). Communications between intra-alveolar cell nests are easily seen through the pores of Kohn. Nuclei are round to oval and commonly overlap one another, and cytoplasm is eosinophilic and finely granular, with a 'ground-glass' quality (Figure 18). Mitoses are infrequently observed. Intracytoplasmic vacuoles are often evident in the tumor cells, which, if viable, have well-defined borders. Peripherally, the stroma is myxoid and loose in character, while it centrally assumes a more homogeneous hyaline appearance, and may be dystrophically calcified. The degeneration or necrosis of internal nests of tumor cells, and the just-mentioned stromal qualities yield on overall similarity to cartilaginous lesions; indeed, the IVBAT was initially described as 'primary chondrosarcoma' of the lung (157). In common with classic angiosarcoma, this neoplasm may secondarily infiltrate bronchiolar or pulmonary vascular walls. The surrounding lung parenchyma is normal, without evidence of pneumonitis of fibrosis.

Electron microscopic study of this tumor has demonstrated cellular features which are identical to those of classic angiosarcoma, including the presence of cytoplasmic Weibel–Palade bodies (143, 147, 153, 154). In keeping with its light microscopic appearance, the tumor cells of IVBAT are more closely apposed ultrastructurally than those of angiosarcoma, with more abundant collagenous and amorphous stromal matrix (12).

Correspondingly, the immunocytochemical features of this neoplasm mirror those of angiosarcoma, but reactivity for FVIIIRAG is more common than in the latter neoplasm (approximately 75% of cases) (12, 143, 150, 154). Receptors for UEA are found in nearly every case, and the nonchondroid nature of the IVBAT is confirmed by its uniform S100 protein-negativity (158).

Kaposi's Sarcoma (159–163)

'Classic' or Mediterranean Kaposi's sarcoma usually affects the lung only in the context of disseminated, far-advanced disease, which

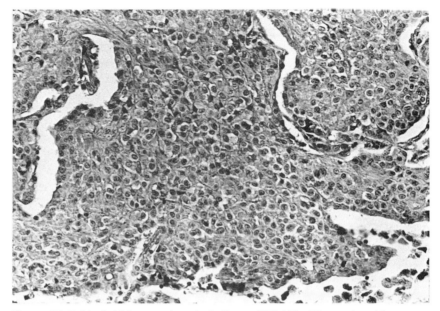

Figure 17 Epithelioid hemangioendothelioma (IVBAT). Micropolypoid appearance of advancing edge.

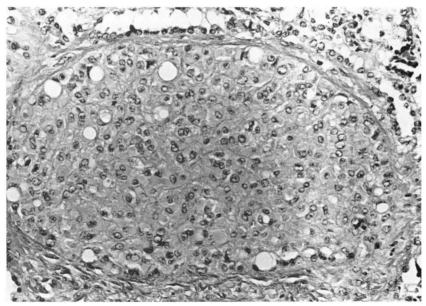

Figure 18 Epithelioid hemangioendothelioma (IVBAT). Tumor cells have finely granular cytoplasm and well-defined margins.

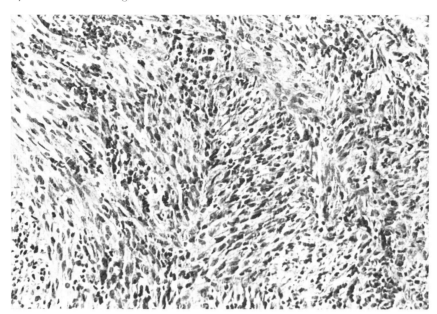

Figure 19 Kaposi's sarcoma. Fascicles of spindle-shaped cells entrap extravasated erythrocytes.

begins in the skin (159, 162). However, patients with the acquired immunodeficiency syndrome (AIDS) may present with pulmonary involvement (manifesting as dyspnea and hemoptysis), in the absence of Kaposi's sarcoma elsewhere (161, 163). Chest radiographs in such cases show only diffuse interstitial infiltrates, without a discrete mass (160). Furthermore, transbronchial or open lung biopsy specimens may display extremely focal abnormalities, necessitating examination of multiple microscopic sections in order to make a diagnosis of this tumor (163).

Histologically, Kaposi's sarcoma is characterized by a combination of telangiectatic vessels and cytologically bland, spindled tumor cells; these tend to be concentrated near pleural surfaces (159, 163). Cell growth occurs in fascicles and sheets, and typically entraps extravasated erythrocytes (Figure 19). Interstitial hemosiderin deposition may also be prominent. Occasional spindle cells contain cytoplasmic cavuoles, or globular, densely eosinophilic inclusions. Mitoses are rare or absent.

Ultrastructural examination of Kaposi's sarcoma discloses varying degrees of endothelial differentiation, as described above. In the spindle cell form of this neoplasm, the tumor cells often express myofibroblast-like features, rather than those of endothelia. The cytoplasmic vacuoles visible at a light microscopic level correspond to ultrastructural lumina, which are unlined by microvilli.

Kaposi's sarcoma is frustratingly difficult to confirm as an endothelial tumor by immunocytochemical means. The angiomatoid form of this lesion expresses FVIIIRAG, BGI, or receptors for UEA; however, spindle-cell Kaposi's sarcoma is reactive only for vimentin in most examples. Rare cases also display desmin or actin, but CK, EMA, NSE, S100 protein, AACT, AAT, LYSO, ferritin, myoglobin, and Leu 7 are universally absent in Kaposi's sarcoma (158).

Rhabdomyosarcoma (11, 164–178)

Rhabdomyosarcoma has accounted for only 25 cases of primary pulmonary sarcoma; in

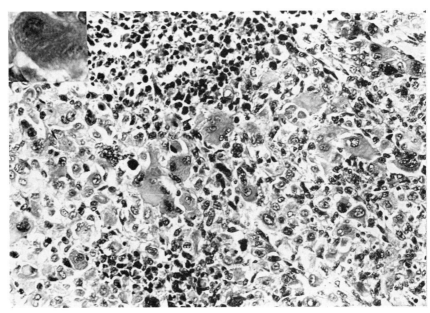

Figure 20 Rhabdomyosarcoma. Cells have abundant, eosinophilic, elongated cytoplasm. Inset: Tumor cell shows cytoplasmic cross-striations.

view of the predominance of pediatric patients with this tumor in other sites, it is somewhat surprising that only 4 examples in the lung have occurred in children (11).

Macroscopically, pulmonary rhabdomyosarcoma has been variously described as a firm, white-grey, intraparenchymal mass, or as a soft, creamy-white tumor, measuring from 8 to 14 cm in diameter. This neoplasm has an apparent tendency to cross lobar septa, and to grossly involve pulmonary veins and bronchi. One lesion was entirely endobronchial, and two in children arose in a congenital adenomatoid malformation (167) and a congenital bronchogenic cyst (166).

Most reported pulmonary rhabdomyosarcomas have been so diagnosed because of the presence of elongaged, 'strap'-like cells with cytoplasmic cross-striations, like those of embryonic myoblasts (Figure 20). These are highlighted by the phosphotungstic acid–hematoxylin stain. Other constituents may include globular cells with refractile, hypereosinophilic cytoplasm, and small, lymphocyte-like elements (Figure 21). Considerable varia-

tin in cell size and shape is commonly evident, and mitoses are abundant. Necrosis and hemorrhage are inconstantly present.

The ultrastructural diagnosis of rhabdomyosarcoma is predicated upon the presence of thick and thin myofilaments within the cytoplasm, which are punctuated by structures resembling the Z-disk of normal sarcomeres (11, 179, 180) (figures 22a and 22b). Glycogen is commonly evident in abundance, and pericellular basal lamina is also apparent (180). Intercellular junctional complexes are absent.

Immunohistochemically, desmin-reactivity is observed in all cell types of this tumor (26, 30, 32), in addition to positivity for vimentin (26). Actin is present in approximately 50% of those tumors comprised of lymphocyte-like elements, while others containing large myoblastic cells almost universally express this determinant (43, 181); NSE may also be detected in this large-cell subpopulation (182). Myoglobin is similarly observed with greatest frequency in differentiated ('pleomorphic') rhabdomyosarcomas, and is a specific marker of striated muscle cells (48–50). Cytokeratin, EMA,

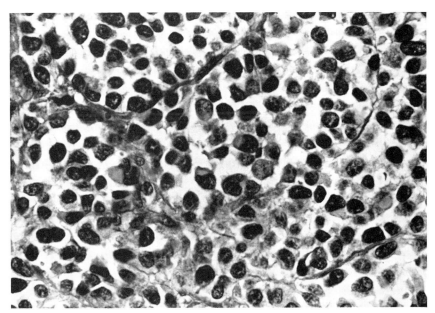

Figure 21 Embryonal rhabdomyosarcoma. Small, lymphocyte-like cells have scanty, densely eosinophilic cytoplasm.

LYSO, AAT, AACT, ferritin, S100 protein, FVIIIRAG, Leu 7, BGI, and receptors for UEA are not observed (60).

The presence of striated muscle tumor in the lung, which lacks rhabdomyocytes in its fully differentiated state (183), may seem problematic histogenetically. We believe that the most reasonable explanation for this phenomenon is that pulmonary rhabdomyosarcomas arise through aberrant, 'divergent' differentiation of neoplastic mesenchymal stem cells in this organ.

Other Intraparenchymal Sarcomas

Sporadic examples of intrapulmonary chondrosarcoma and osteosarcoma have been described (8, 16, 184–190). These have histologic, ultrastructural, and immunohistochemical features like those of primary osseous tumors (191, 192). Chondrosarcomas are microscopically composed of lacunar cells within a myxocartilaginous matrix (Figure 23). These often display a binucleate morphology, with moderate nuclear hyperchromasia.

Tumor cells are commonly arranged in lobules, which may be focally calcified. Mitoses are rare. Ultrastructurally, scalloped cell membranes are evident, with abundant cytoplasmic microfilaments and glycogen pools (191) (Figure 24). Intercellular matrix material is fine granular and abundant. Chondrosarcoma is characterized by vimentin-positivity, as well as reactivity for S100 protein and Leu 7 (60, 192). Cytokeratin, EMA, DES, actin, NSE, LYSO, AAT, AACT, ferritin, myoglobin, FVIIIRAG, BGI, and receptors for UEA are not observed.

Osteosarcomas display polygonal, pleomorphic, or spindled cells, with hyperchromatic nuclei and a moderate amount of amphophilic cytoplasm, which are enmeshed in and refractile, eosinophilic, osteoid matrix (Figure 25). The latter material is extremely variable in quantity and distribution, and must be distinguished from hyalinized collagen. Aside from their production of osteoid, certain examples of this tumor type may be virtually identical to fibrosarcoma or MFH (191). Correspondingly, osteosarcoma cells are often

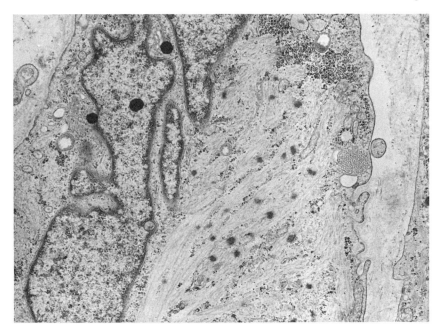

Figure 22a Rhabdomyosarcoma. Focal pericellular basal lamina, glycogen deposits, and cytoplasmic filaments showing sarcomeric differentiation are evident.

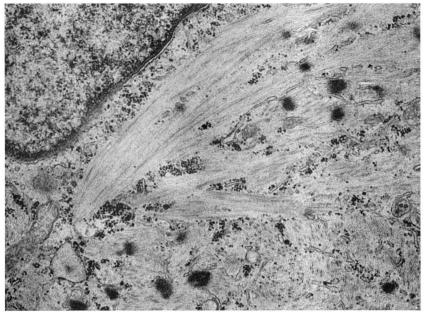

Figure 22b Rhabdomyosarcoma. Sarcomeric differentiation is characterized by thick and thin myofilaments punctuated by densities reminiscent of the Z-disk of normal sarcomeres.

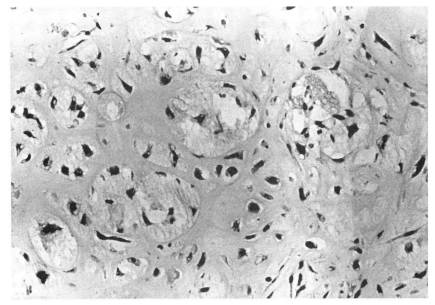

Figure 23 Chondrosarcoma. Tumor cells grow within lacunae surrounded by a myxocartilaginous matrix.

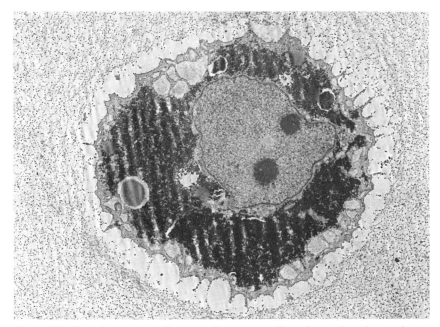

Figure 24 Chondrosarcoma. Tumor cell shows scalloped cytoplasmic membrane and contains abundant glycogen. Intercellular matrix is finely granular.

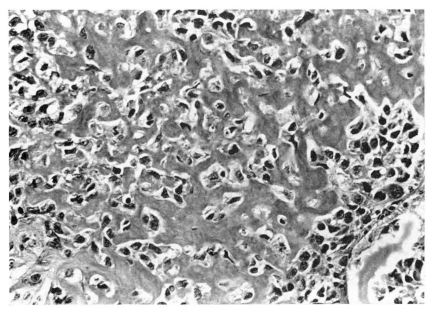

Figure 25 Osteosarcoma. Pleomorphic cells with hyperchromatic nuclei are enmeshed in an osteoid matrix.

indistinguishable ultrastructurally and immu-nohistochemically from those of the latter two neoplasms (60). Hence, the mere presence of verifiable osteoid is sufficient to separate osteo-sarcoma diagnostically from these other tumors.

Isolated examples of primary pulmonary neurofibrosarcoma have been described (193, 194), but illustrative documentation in these cases was suboptimal. One report (194) stated that a spindle-cell mass was focally identical microscopically to neurofibromas of soft tis-sues; however, the patient did not have neuro-fibromatosis, and electron microscopic or immunohistologic data were not provided. True neurofibrosarcomas display elongated, overlapping cytoplasmic processes ultrastruc-turally, which are covered by external basal lamina and may be connected by primitive junctions (195). Vimentin is uniformly expressed by neural neoplasms (26, 60), and S100 protein-reactivity is expected in 60–70% of such tumors (196–198); Leu 7 and desmin may also be observed immunocytochemically

(60, 111). Cytokeratin, EMA, actin, NSE, LYSO, AAT, AACT, ferritin, myoglobin, FVIIIRAG, BGI, and UEA receptors are absent.

Sarcomas of the Pulmonary Arterial Tree (9, 199–241)

Sarcomas of the pulmonary trunk are distinct clinicopathologically from those arising in the bronchi or lung parenchyma; approximately 80 cases have been reported thus far. They typically present with symptoms and signs like those of idiopathic congestive heart failure or venous thromboembolism (203, 218), but are accompanied by dissimilar angiographic or roentgenographic abnormalities in the lung fields (202, 218, 225). The latter include the presence of large, irregular, intravascular fill-ing defects in the pulmonary arteries, with or without a hilar mass (199, 201, 202).

Grossly, pulmonary trunk sarcomas are pre-dominantly confined to the arterial lumen, but often demonstrate transmural invasion into the surrounding lung or mediastinum. They are firm, fleshy, grey-white tumors with internal areas of hemorrhage and necrosis; embolic deposits are commonly present in the pulmonary parenchyma as well.

The microscopic nature of these neoplasms is diverse; several well-documented examples of fibrosarcoma (206, 213), leiomyosarcoma (199, 204, 205, 211), rhabdomyosarcoma (210), malignant fibrous histiocytoma (209, 212), angiosarcoma (236), chondrosarcoma (226), and osteosarcoma (207) have been reported in the pulmonary vasculature. Their histologic features are as described above, in connection with intraparenchymal tumors of these types. In addition, examples labelled as 'fibromyxosarcoma' (237, 238), 'polymorphous sarcoma' (239) and 'mesenchymoma' (240, 241) have been described; most of these cases are culled from the distant literature, and their true histogenesis is considered uncertain. Ultrastructural and immunohistochemical analyses are of similar value in pulmonary artery tumors to that realized in evaluating parenchymal neoplasms of the lung (205, 209–212), and should allow for proper prospective classification of the former lesions in the future.

'Malignant Angioendotheliomatosis'

'Malignant angioendotheliomatosis' is a disorder typified by the intravascular proliferation of uniform, polygonal, cytologically malignant cells; in the past, the latter have been assumed to possess endothelial characteristics, accounting for the nosological designation assigned to this disease (242).

One report of 'angioendotheliomatosis' documented pulmonary arterial involvement, with symptoms and signs like those of thromboembolism, as the presenting manifestation (243). Radiographic investigations disclosed findings consistent with the latter diagnosis, but a lung biopsy revealed the true nature of the process.

The tumor cells in angioendotheliomatosis are loosely arranged within vascular lumina,

including those of the pulmonary arterial system. They contain large vesicular nuclei with prominent nuclei, and scant amphophilic cytoplasm (Figures 26a and 26b). Fibrin-rich thrombi often surround and entrap the proliferating cells.

Ultrastructural examination shows a lack of endothelial characteristics. Rather, the cells in this disorder fail to exhibit junctional complexes, and contain abundant cytoplasmic polyribosomes in the absence of other distinguishing organelles (242). These electron microscopic features are like those of large-cell lymphomas.

Similarly, immunocytochemical studies disclose reactivity for leukocyte common antigen (as described subsequently) on the surfaces of all tumor cells; only those entrapped in fibrin thrombi are reactive for FVIIIRAG, a phenomenon thought to represent passive adsorption of this determinant. The expression of BGI, CK, EMA, DES, actin, NSE, S100 protein, AACT, AAT, LYSO, ferritin, myoglobin, Leu 7, and receptors for UEA is uniformly absent. This constellation of results parallels that seen in lymphoreticular proliferations, leading us to conclude that 'malignant angioendotheliomatosis' is actually an angiotropic malignant lymphoma (242).

DIFFERENTIAL DIAGNOSIS OF PULMONARY SARCOMAS

Metastases

As mentioned earlier in this chapter, the single most important differential diagnostic consideration in cases thought to represent primary sarcomas of the lung is metastatic spread from an extrapulmonary tumor. Special pathologic studies are of no assistance in distinguishing between indigenous and secondary neoplasms, and the clinical characteristics of such lesions also demonstrate considerable overlap. Hence, it is mandatory for the clinicians to initiate appropriate radiographic studies to address this possibility.

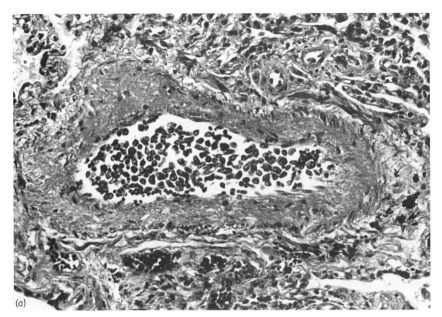

Figure 26a Angiotropic lymphoma ('malignant angioendotheliomatosis'). The lumen of a medium-sized artery contains loosely arranged tumor cells.

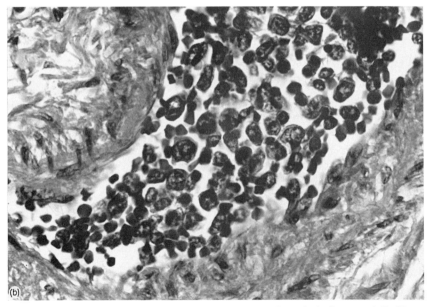

Figure 26b Angiotropic lymphoma ('malignant angioendotheliomatosis'). Neoplastic lymphocytes show pleomorphism, and have large, vesicular nuclei and scanty cytoplasm.

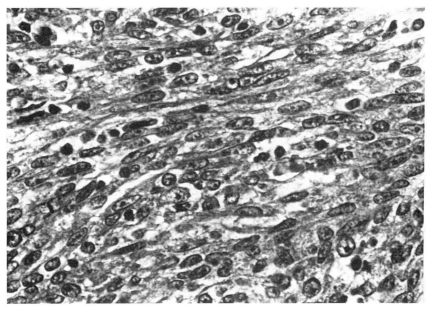

Figure 27 Spindle-cell squamous carcinoma may simulate a sarcomatous neo-plasm.

Sarcomatoid Bronchogenic Carcinoma/Malignant Melanoma

Bronchogenic carcinomas (particularly squamous carcinomas) are capable in rare instances of assuming purely spindle-cell, or pleomorphic and spindle-cell appearances (2, 3, 17, 244) (Figure 27). Moreover, they may also demonstrate confined endobronchial growth (245), a feature which is usually associated with sarcomas. Metastatic or primary malignant melanomas of the lung can mimic the gross and histopathologic features of mesenchymal tumors as well (7, 246) (Figures 28a and 28b). Such neoplasms may be virtually indistinguishable from fibrosarcoma, leiomyosarcoma, or MFH, by conventional pathologic studies (Charter 21).

In these cases, electron microscopy and immunocytochemical analyses are invaluable. Sarcomatoid carcinomas display at-least-focal formation of well-developed intercellular junctions ultrastructurally, and cytoplasmic tonofilaments may also insert into these structures (247) (Figure 29). Melanomas typically contain cytoplasmic premelanosomes (248) (Figures 30a and 30b). None of these findings is present in true sarcomas. Also, CK, or EMA, or both are expected as part of the immunophenotypes of carcinomas, whereas these antigens are lacking in sarcomas (26, 38, 57, 60). Again, we would caution against the omission of these important determinants in immunohistologic evaluations, since others (e.g. AAT, AACT, ferritin) are shared by both epithelial and mesenchymal malignancies (46, 60, 135). Malignant melanoma is reactive for both S100 protein (249) and NSE (250), a combination of results not seen in the sarcomas considered herein.

Carcinosarcoma (17, 251–257)

Carcinosarcoma is defined as a neoplasm manifesting verifiable epithelial and mesenchymal differentiation, within the same mass (17). The most common combinations of such elements in pulmonary tumors include adenocarcinoma or squamous carcinoma, in con-

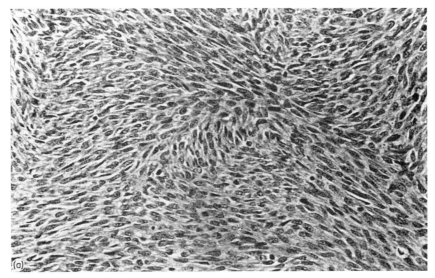

Figure 28a Storiform pattern of growth in a malignant melanoma may simulate a fibrohistiocytic neoplasm.

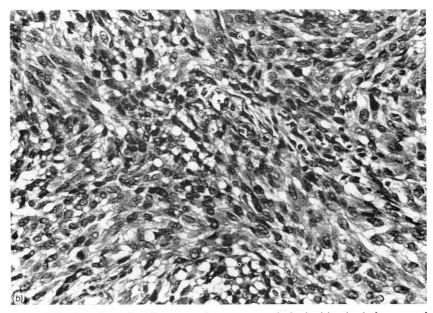

Figure 28b Spindle-cell malignant melanoma can mimic the histologic features of mesenchymal tumors.

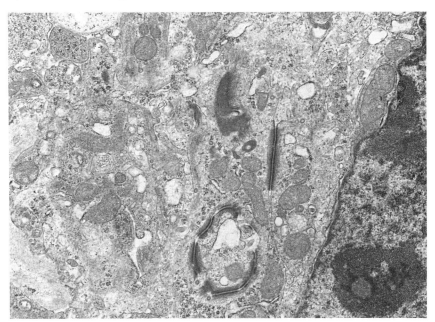

Figure 29 Sarcomatoid squamous carcinoma shows well-developed intercellular junctions and cytoplasmic tonofilaments.

junction with rhabdomyosarcoma, leiomyosarcoma, chondrosarcoma, and osteosarcoma (251–257) (Figures 31 and 31b). Whether or not these neoplasms in fact begin as pure carcinomas and undergo mesenchymal metaplasia is a matter of speculation. However, their clinical behaviours differ sufficiently from pure carcinoma to justify a diagnostic separation between the two (14, 17). Again, ultrastructural and immunocytochemical studies are of great value in delineating the biphasic nature of pulmonary carcinosarcomas. As expected, electron microscopic evidence of two morphologic cell populations is obtained, with one showing epithelial features, and the other displaying an ultrastructural identity to pure sarcomas, as described above (255). Immunohistologic assessment reveals reactivity for CK or EMA in a discrete portion of the mass, accompanied by positive staining for DES, myoglobin, actin, or S100 protein in the sarcomatous components (257).

'Pseudotumors' 'Fibrous Histiocytomas'

Several cases of 'inflammatory pseudotumor' of the lung have been reported, in which certain histopathologic similarities to MFH were evident (17, 258–263) (Figure 32). Other examples of related lesions, particularly in an endobronchial location, have been termed 'fibrous histiocytomas' (264). These masses are in all likelihood not even neoplastic, but instead represent idiosyncratic reactions to injuries. Their cytologic features are bland, without the cellular pleomorphism or nuclear atypia seen in true MFH. In addition, inflammatory cells within and around such lesions are abundant and chronic in nature, unlike the case in most fibrohistiocytic sarcomas. Ultrastructurally and immunohistochemically, 'fibrous histiocytomas' and 'pseudotumors' appear to be myofibroblastic rather than fibrohistiocytic (258, 261–263). Polygonal cells

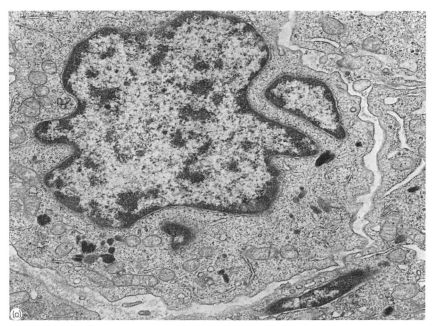

Figure 30a Maligant melanoma shows numerous cytoplasmic premelanosomes.

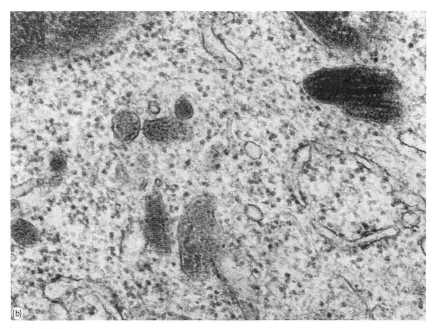

Figure 30b Malignant melanoma. Detail of premelanosomes shows characteristic internal striated structure.

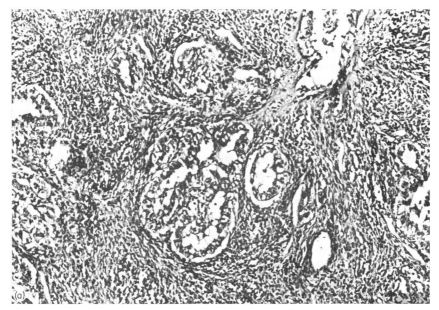

Figure 31a Carcinosarcoma. Adenocarcinomatous elements are surrounded by poorly differentiated sarcomatous cells.

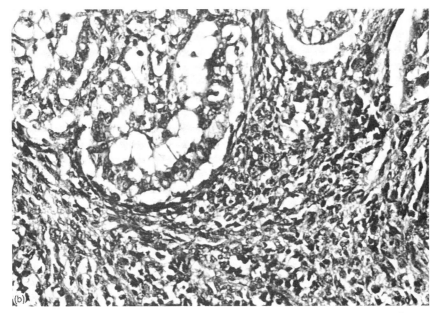

Figure 31b Carcinosarcoma. Glandular structures lined by malignant cells are surrounded by a poorly differentiated sarcomatous stroma.

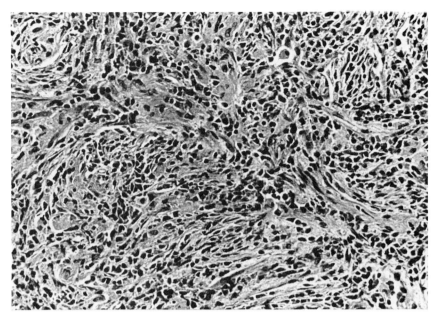

Figure 32 Inflammatory pseudotumor. A 'storiform' pattern of growth is reminiscent of malignant fibrous histiocytoma; however, the cells lack atypia, and a
prominent inflammatory infiltrate is present.

with abundant cytoplasmic lysosomes are not typically apparent by electron microscopy, and immunoreactivity for LYSO, AAT, AACT, and ferritin is lacking (265).

Hemangiomatosis/ Lymphangiomyomatosis

Benign hemangiomatosis and lymphangiomyomatosis may be histologically confused with angiosarcoma and leiomyosarcoma, respectively (266–271). Both are cytologically benign cellular proliferations in the pulmonary interstitium; as their names suggest, hemangiomatosis features a plethora of vascular spaces lined by bland endothelium (Figure 33), and lymphangiomyomatosis is composed of a mixture of banal lymphatic–endothelial and smooth muscular elements (Figure 34). The natural history of both conditions includes substantial morbidity, but this is unlike that associated with neoplastic diseases of the lung. Finally, the mode of clinical presentation of

these disorders is dissimilar to that of pulmonary sarcomas (271).

Chondromas/Leiomyomas

Reports also have been made of benign chondromas and leiomyomas of the lung (272–276). Both of these lesions are typically unassociated with major bronchi, and may be multiple, mimicking metastases radiographically. However, they display exceedingly bland histologic appearances. Nevertheless, since secondary leiomyosarcoma may do so as well, it is worth evaluating the genital tract in women, and the alimentary tract in both sexes, in cases thought to represent leiomyomas of the lung. Chondrosarcoma rarely if ever metastasizes to the lung in the absence of a known extrapulmonary tumor.

Chondromas and leiomyomas of the lung are considered to be hamartomatous lesions (17, 272, 274). The former may constitute part of a triad, including gastric smooth muscle

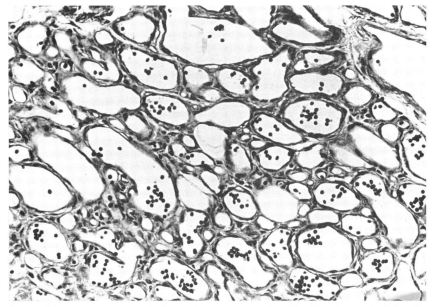

Figure 33 Hemangiomatosis. Vascular spaces are lined by bland endothelial cells.

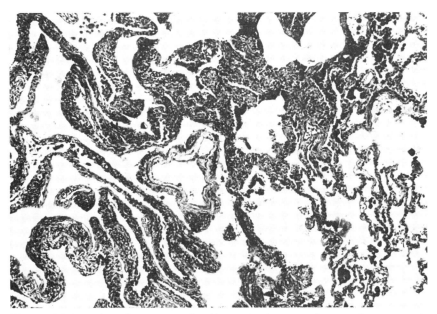

Figure 34 Lymphangiomyomatosis. Hyperplastic smooth muscle surrounds alveolar sacs, vascular structures and bronchioles. Normal lung parenchyma is seen on the right for comparison.

tumors and extra-adrenal paragangliomas, in rare cases (277, 278).

Malignant Lymphoma

This chapter has not considered the characteristics of pulmonary malignant lymphoma, since they are such a specialized group of mesenchymal malignancies, with clinicopathologic features unlike those of 'solid-tumor' sarcomas (279). Rarely, however, malignant lymphoma enters into differential diagnosis with small round-cell sarcomas of the lung, most notably embryonal (lymphocyte-like) rhabdomyosarcoma. The latter manifests reactivity for desmin, actin, or myoglobin (or combinations thereof), while lymphoma lacks all three of these markers (30). Conversely, malignant lymphoma expresses leukocyte-common antigen (a determinant seen in all myeloid and lymphoid cell membranes), whereas rhabdomyosarcoma does not (280). Electron microscopy demonstrates sarcomeric differentiation in rhabdomyosarcoma, but not in lymphoma.

'Atypical Carcinoid' and Small-Cell Neuroendocrine Carcinoma of the Lung

Neuroendocrine carcinomas (NEC; 'atypical carcinoids') of the lung share a potential for spindle-cell growth with sarcomas (Figure 35), and may be endobronchial or intrapulmonary in location, like the latter (281–283). Most NECs are recognizable on conventional microscopy, due to their clustered, organoid cellular growth pattern, and evenly distributed, 'dusty' nuclear chromatin. In questionable cases, ultrastructural study discloses evidence of epithelial differentiation, with intercellular junctional complexes, and cytoplasmic neurosecretory granules (283) (Figure 36). Both of these features are absent in sarcomas. NECs show immunoreactivity for neuron-specific enolase and cytokeratin as well (38, 44).

Small-cell ('oat-cell') neuroendocrine carcinoma is potentially similar in its microscopic appearance to embryonal rhabdomyosarcoma (283, 284) (Figure 37). Small-cell carcinoma is also reactive for NSE and CK, but lacks DES, actin, vimentin, and myoglobin (60). Its ultra-

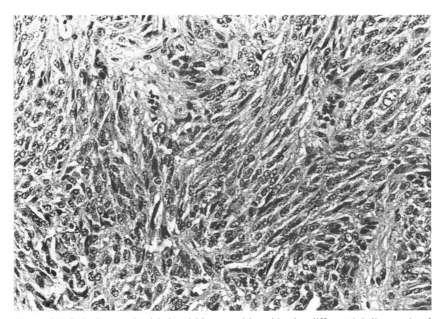

Figure 35 Spindle-carcinoid should be considered in the differential diagnosis of spindle-cell neoplasms of the lung.

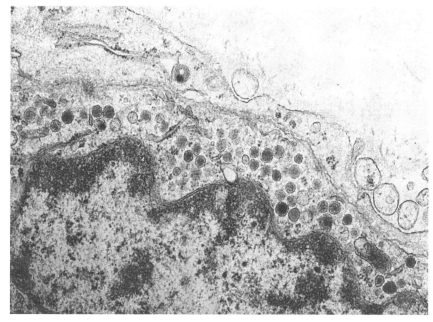

Figure 36 Spindle-carcinoid shows numerous cytoplasmic neurosecretory granules which are membrane-bound and contain a dense core.

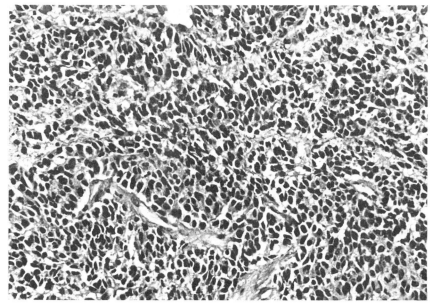

Figure 37 Small-cell (oat-cell) neuroendocrine carcinoma should be considered in the differential diagnosis of small-cell tumors of the lung.

structural attributes are virtually identical to those of NEC (283).

BEHAVIOR AND PROGNOSIS OF PRIMARY PULMONARY SARCOMAS

With isolated exceptions, primary sarcomas of the lung are aggressive tumors, resulting in 60–90% fatality at 5 years' follow-up (7, 9, 10, 12, 13, 15, 285). Endobronchial fibrosarcomas tend to behave more favourably than their intrapulmonary counterparts, but similar comments do not apply to leiomyosarcoma (7). Most tumors cause death by local recurrence and progression, and in general only 30–40% demonstrate extrathoracic metastasis (7, 9, 10, 106). Malignant fibrous histiocytoma of the lung shows a higher metastatic rate, and has a propensity to secondarily involve the brain (10). Seven of 11 patients with this tumor have died. Classic angiosarcoma and pulmonary trunk sarcomas are uniformly fatal (9, 13), probably because of delays in diagnosis and the presence of dissemination upon initial surgery. The IVBAT is an indolent neoplasm with a longer clinical evolution than that of other pulmonary sarcomas. Approximately 35% of patients with this lesion survive beyond 5 years; this may be tantamount to cure, since those who have died have generally done so within 3 years of diagnosis (12). Metastases are seen in a minority of cases, and usually involve the liver; most fatalities with IVBAT are due to progressive intrapulmonary tumor growth. Poor prognostic features of this neoplasm include symptoms at presentation, extensive intravascular or endobronchial spread, and distant metastasis (12).

In the few reported examples of malignant hemangiopericytoma and osteosarcoma of the lung, all patients have died. Other tumor types have insignificant numbers of cases for meaningful comments to be made on their behaviour.

Therapy is currently based on ablative surgery, regardless of histologic tumor type (285). Radiotherapy and chemotherapy have proven to be of little benefit thus far, for any of the sarcomas presented in this chapter.

CLINICAL THERAPEUTIC TRIALS OF POSSIBLE IMPORTANCE TO THE THERAPY OF PRIMARY PULMONARY SARCOMAS

Adjuvant therapeutic protocols that have been specifically designed for primary sarcomas of the lung are currently unavailable. Therefore, one must refer to results obtained in treatment regimens for soft tissue sarcomas of similar histologic types, in order to speculate on the effects of cytotoxic agents on these pulmonary neoplasms. Lopez et al. considered the use of adriamycin and dimethyl triazeno imidazole carboxamide (DTIC) in 40 cases of soft tissue sarcoma (286). Only 10% of patients had complete responses, and 20% underwent partial responses, which were maintained for a median of 28 months. In contrast, however, the median survival of nonresponding patients was 7 months. Those tumors which demonstrated some sensitivity to these drugs included fibrosarcoma and MFH; rhabdomyosarcoma, leiomyosarcoma, and hemangiopericytoma were resistant histotypes. Comparatively more effective protocols may be represented by the combinations of mitomycin C, doxorubicin, and cis-platinum, or cyclophosphamide, vincristine, adriamycin, and dacarbazine, which produced tumor regression in 43% and 48% of cases, respectively, in other reports (287, 288). Fibrosarcomas, leiomyosarcomas, malignant fibrous histiocytomas, angiosarcomas, and rhabdomyosarcomas demonstrated sensitivity to such protocols. It would seem prudent to apply these combination therapies to pulmonary sarcomas, in view of the afore-mentioned poor prognoses of the latter with surgical treatment alone.

Hormonal manipulation represents another potential therapeutic avenue which has not yet been investigated for sarcomas of the lung, particularly leiomyosarcomas. Histologically similar tumors in the uterus behave less aggressively in postmenopausal than in premenopausal women (108), and demonstrate the presence of estrogen receptors (289). These findings suggest that the administration of estrogen-antagonists may have beneficial effects in the treatment of leiomyosarcomas in general.

EXPERIMENTAL WORK WITH IMPLICATIONS FOR THE THERAPY OF PRIMARY PULMONARY SARCOMAS

Immunologic therapeutic approaches to sarcomas in animal models have provided encouraging results. Nomi et al. extracted tumor-specific antigens from methylcholanthrene-induced fibrosarcomas in mice (290). The animals were subsequently inoculated with these determinants after surgical extirpation of the tumors, with concomitant administration of cyclophosphamide. Animals so treated had 70% less metastases, compared to those given cyclophosphamide alone, or no therapy. This regimen appeared to be immunospecific, and did not protect the mice against implantations of another sarcoma type.

In another trial, lymphokine-activated killer lymphocytes were infused intravenously into mice with sarcomas, along with recombinant interleukin-2 (291). This treatment reduced the number of subsequent metastases tenfold, compared to control animals.

Lastly, work being done with tumor antigen-directed monoclonal antibodies may have salutory therapeutic implications. Roth and colleagues studied the binding of several such reagents—B3619, 17-9H3, OST6, OKIa1—to human sarcomas (292). The latter included osteosarcoma, fibrosarcoma, and neurofibrosarcoma. In general, osteosarcomas demonstrated significant avidity for all of these antibodies, followed in order by neurofibrosarcomas and fibrosarcomas. Interestingly, the primary neoplasms showed much greater binding than did their metastases. It is conceivable that directed in vivo immunotherapy (or conjugates of monoclonal antibodies with

cytotoxic agents) may provide effective future treatment modalities for sarcomas of the lung and other sites.

SUMMARY

Primary sarcomas of the lung are rare but aggressive neoplasms. These include fibrosarcoma, leiomyosarcoma, malignant hemangiopericytoma, malignant fibrous histiocytoma, angiosarcoma, epithelioid hemangioendothelioma, rhabdomyosarcoma, pulmonary trunk sarcomas, chondrosarcoma, osteosarcoma, and possibly neurofibrosarcoma. Most of these tumors occur in adult patients, but in age groups generally unlike those associated with bronchogenic carcinomas. Their prognoses are poor, and extirpative surgery is necessary to provide an opportunity for cure. Whether effective adjuvant treatment protocols can be developed to alter this situation remains to be seen.

REFERENCES

1 Paulsen SM, Egeblad K, Christensen J. Malignant fibrous histiocytoma of the lung. Virchows Arch Pathol Anat 1981; 394: 167–76.

2 Love GL, Daroca PJ. Bronchogenic sarcomatoid squamous cell carcinoma with osteoclast-like giant cells. Hum Pathol 1983; 14: 1004–6.

3 Oyasu R, Battifora HA, Buchingham WB. Metaplastic squamous cell carcinoma of bronchus simulating giant cell tumor of bone. Cancer 1977; 39: 119–25.

4 Jimenez JF, Uthman EO, Townsend JW, Gloster ES, Seibert JJ. Primary bronchopulmonary leiomyosarcoma in childhood. Arch Pathol Lab Med 1986; 110: 348–51.

5 Hartman GE, Shochat SJ. Primary pulmonary neoplasms of childhood: a review. Ann Thorac Surg 1983; 36: 108–19.

6 Holinger PH, Slaughter DP, Novak FS. Unusual tumors obstructing the lower respiratory tract of infants and children. Trans Am Acad Ophthalmol Otolaryngol 1950; 54: 223–34.

7 Guccion JG, Rosen SH. Bronchopulmonary leiomyosarcomas and fibrosarcomas: a study of 32 cases and review of the literature. Cancer 1972; 30: 835–47.

8 Sun C-CJ, Krol M, Miller JE. Primary chon-

drosarcoma of the lung. Cancer 1982; 50: 1864–6.

9 Baker PB, Goodwin RA. Pulmonary artery sarcomas. A review and report of a case. Arch Pathol Lab Med 1985; 109: 35–9.

10 Lee JT, Shelburne JD, Linder J. Primary malignant fibrous histiocytoma of the lung. A clinicopathologic and ultrastructural study of five cases. Cancer 1984; 53: 1124–30.

11 Avagnina A, Elsner B, DeMarco L, Bracco AN, Nazar J, Pavlovsky H. Pulmonary rhabdomyosarcoma with isolated small bowel metastasis. A report of a case with immunohistochemical and ultrastructural studies. Cancer 1984; 53: 1948–51.

12 Dail DH, Liebow AA, Gmelich JT, Friedman PJ, Miyai K, Myer W, Patterson SD, Hammar SP. Intravascular, bronchiolar, and alveolar tumor of the lung (IVBAT). An analysis of twenty cases of a peculiar sclerosing endothelial tumor. Cancer 1983; 51: 452–64.

13 Yousem SA: Angiosarcoma presenting in the lung. Arch Pathol Lab Med 1986; 110: 112–15.

14 Israel L, Chahinian A. Lung Cancer: Natural History, Prognosis, and Therapy. New York: Academic Press, 1976.

15 Wick MR, Scheithauer BW, Piehler JM, Pairolero PC. Primary pulmonary leiomyosarcomas. A light and electron microscopic study. Arch Pathol Lab Med 1982; 106: 510–14.

16 Nascimento AG, Unni KK. Sarcomas of the lung. Mayo Clin Proc 1982; 57: 355–9.

17 Carter D, Eggleston JC. Tumors of the Lower Respiratory Tract. In: Atlas of Tumor Pathology, Fascicle 17, Second Series. Washington, DC: Armed Forces Institute of Pathology, 1980.

18 Greene R, McLoud TC, Stark P. Other malignant tumors of the lung. Semin Roentgenol 1977; 12: 225–37.

19 Krumerman MS. Leiomyosarcoma of the lung: primary cytodiagnosis in two consecutive cases. Acta Cytol 1977; 21: 103–6.

20 Sawada K, Fukuma S, Seki Y. Cytologic features of primary leiomyosarcoma of the lung: report of a case diagnosed by bronchial brushing procedure. Acta Cytol 1977; 21: 770–3.

21 Sternberger LA, Hardy PH Jr, Cuculis JJ, Meyer HG. The unlabelled antibody method of immunohistochemistry. Preparation and properties of soluble antigen-antibody complex (horseradish peroxidase-anti-horseradish peroxidase) and its use in the identification of spirochetes. J Histochem Cytochem 1970; 18: 315–33.

22 Hsu S-M, Raine L, Fanger H. Use of avidin-biotin-peroxidase complex (ABC) in immunoperoxidase techniques: a comparison between ABC and unlabelled antibody (PAP) procedures. J Histochem Cytochem 1981; 29: 577–80.

23 Bannasch P, Zerban H, Mayer D. The cytoskeleton in tumor cells. Pathol Res Pract 1982; 175: 196–211.

24 Gown AM, Vogel AM. Monoclonal antibodies to intermediate filaments of human cells. Unique and cross-reacting antibodies. J Cell Biol 1982; 95: 414–24.

25 Virtanen I, Lehto V-P, Lehtonen E, Vartio T, Stenman S. Expression of intermediate filaments in cultured cells. J Cell Sci 1981; 50: 45–63.

26 Miettinen M, Lehto V-P, Badley RA, Virtanen I. Expression of intermediate filaments in soft tissue sarcomas. Int J Cancer 1982; 30: 541–6.

27 Gabbiana G, Kapanci Y, Barrazone P, Franke WW. Immunochemical identification of intermediate-sized filaments in human neoplastic cells. A diagnostic aid for the surgical pathologist. Am J Pathol 1981; 104: 206–16.

28 Ramaekers F, Puts J, Kant A. Differential diagnosis of human carcinomas, sarcomas, and their metastases using antibodies to intermediate filaments. Eur J Cancer Clin Oncol 1982; 18: 1251–7.

29 Tseng SCG, Jarvinen MJ, Nelson WG, Huang JW, Woodcock-Mitchell J, Sun TT. Correlation of specific keratins with different types of epithelial differentiation: monoclonal antibody studies. Cell 1982; 30: 361–72.

30 Altmannsberger M, Weber K, Droste R, Osborn M. Desmin is a specific marker for rhabdomyosarcomas of human and rat origin. Am J Pathol 1985; 118: 85–95.

31 Denk H, Krepler R, Artlieb U, Gabbiani G, Rungger-Brandle E, Leoncini P, Franke WW. Proteins of intermediate filaments: an immunohistochemical and biochemical approach to the classification of soft tissue tumors. Am J Pathol 1983; 110: 193–208.

32 Miettinen M, Lehto V-P, Badley RA, Virtanen I. Alveolar rhabdomyosarcoma: demonstration of the muscle type of intermediate filament protein, desmin, as a diagnostic aid. Am J Pathol 1982; 108: 246–51.

33 Gown AM, Vogel AM. Monoclonal antibodies to human intermediate filament proteins. III. Analysis of tumors. Am J Clin Pathol 1985; 84: 413–24.

34 Osborn M, Weber K. Tumor diagnosis by intermediate filament typing: a novel tool for surgical pathology. Lab Invest 1983; 48: 372–394.

35 Trojanowski JQ, Lee VMY, Schlaepfer WW. An immunohistochemical study of human central and peripheral nervous system tumors, using monoclonal antibodies against neurofilaments and glial filaments. Hum Pathol 1984; 15: 248–57.

36 Velasco ME, Dahl D, Roessman U, Gambetti P. Immunohistochemical localization of glial fibrillary acidic protein in human glial neoplasms. Cancer 1980; 45: 484–94.

37 Herman CJ, Moesker O, Kant A, Huysmans A, Vooijs GP, Ramaekers FCS. Is renal (Grawitz) tumor a carcinosarcoma? Evidence from analysis of intermediate filament types. Virchows Arch Cell Pathol 1983; 44: 73–83.

38 Battifora HA. Recent progress in the immunohistochemistry of solid tumors. Sem Diagn Pathol 1984; 1: 251–71.

39 Sheibani K, Tubbs RR. Enzyme histochemistry: technical aspects. Sem Diagn Pathol 1984; 1: 235–50.

40 Pinkus GS, O'Connor EM, Etheridge CL. Optimal immunoreactivity of keratin proteins in formalin-fixed, paraffin-embedded tissue requires preliminary trypsinization. An immunoperoxidase study of various tumors using polyclonal and monoclonal antibodies. J Histochem Cytochem 1985; 33: 465–61.

41 Erlandson RA. Diagnostic immunohistochemistry: an interim evaluation. Am J Surg Pathol 1984; 8: 615–24.

42 Bussolati G, Gugliotta P, Fulcheri E. Immunochemistry of actin in normal and neoplastic tissues. In: DeLellis RA ed Advanced in Immunochemistry. Masson Monogr Diagn Pathol 1984; 7: 325–41.

43 Mukai K, Schollmeyer J, Rosai J. Immunohistochemical localization of actin. Applications in surgical pathology. Am J Surg Pathol 1981; 5: 91–7.

44 Carlei F, Polak JM. Antibodies to neuron-specific enolase for the delineation of the entire diffuse neuroendocrine system in health and disease. Sem Diagn Pathol 1984; 1: 59–70.

45 DuBoulay CEH. Demonstration of a alpha-l-antitrypsin and alpha-l-antichymotrypsin in the fibrous histiocytomas using immunoperoxidase techniques. Am J Surg Pathol 1982; 6: 559–64.

46 Kindblom L-G, Jacobsen GK, Jacobsen M. Immunohistochemical investigations of tumors of supposed fibroblastic-histiocytic origin. Hum Pathol 1982; 13: 834–40.

47 Meister P, Nathrath W. Immunohistochemical characterization of histiocytic tumors. Diagn Histopathol 1981; 4: 79–87.

48 Brooks JJ. Immunohistochemistry of soft tissue tumors: myoglobin as a tumor marker for rhabdomyosarcoma. Cancer 1982; 50: 1757–63.

49 Corson JM, Pinkus GS. Intracellular myoglobin—a specific marker for skeletal muscle differentiation in soft tissue sarcomas. An immunoperoxidase study. Am J Pathol 1981; 103: 384–9.

50 Mukai K, Rosai J, Hallaway BE. Localization of myoglobin in normal and neoplastic human skeletal muscle cells using an immunoperoxidase method. Am J Surg Pathol 1979; 3: 373–6.

51 Nakajima T, Watanabe S, Sato Y, Kameya T, Hirota T, Shimosato Y. An immunoperoxidase study of S100 protein distribution in normal and neoplastic tissues. Am J Surg Pathol 1982; 6: 715–27.

52 Kahn HJ, Marks A, Thom H, Baumal R. Role of antibody to S100 protein in diagnostic pathology. Am J Clin Pathol 1983; 79: 341–7.

53 Steffansson K, Wollman R, Jerkovic M. S100 protein in soft tissue tumors derived from Schwann cells and melanocytes. Am J Pathol 1982; 106: 261–8.

54 Burgdorf WHC, Mukai K, Rosai J. Immunohistochemical identification of factor VIII-related antigen in endothelial cells of cutaneous lesions of alleged vascular nature. Am J Clin Pathol 1981; 75: 167–71.

55 Guarda LA, Ordóñez NG, Smith JL, Hanssen G: Immunoperoxidase localization of factor VIII in angiosarcoma. Arch Pathol Lab Med 1982; 106: 515–19.

56 Mukai K, Rosai J, Factor VIII-related antigen: an endothelial marker. In DeLellis RA ed Diagnostic Immunohistochemistry. New York: Masson, 1984: 253–61.

57 Pinkus GS, Kurtin PJ. Epithelial membrane antigen—a diagnostic discriminant in surgical pathology: immunohistochemical profile in epithelial, mesenchymal, and hematopoietic neoplasms using paraffin sections and monoclonal antibodies. Hum Pathol 1985; 16: 929–40.

58 Sloane JP, Ormerod MG. Distribution of epithelial membrane antigen in normal and neoplastic tissues and its value in diagnostic pathology. Cancer 1981; 47: 1786–95.

59 Tuthill RJ, Tubbs RR. A study of anti-Leu 7 staining of Schwann cells and neural-crest derived tumours (abstract). Lab Invest 1984; 50: 62A.

60 Wick MR, Abenoza P, Manivel JC. Immunohistochemical findings in tumors of the head and neck. In Gnepp DR ed Pathology of the Head and Neck. London: Churchill Livingstone (in press).

61 Feigl W, Denk H, Davidovits A, Holzner JH. Blood group isoantigens in human benign and malignant vascular tumors. Virchows Arch Pathol Anat 1976; 370: 323–32.

62 Gupta YN, Gupta S, Singh IJ, Khanna NN, Agarwal MK. Epithelial isoantigens A, B, and H in oral carcinomas. Ear Nose Throat J 1985; 64: 51–4.

63 Weistein RS, Coon J, Alrony J, Davidsohn I. Tissue-associated blood group antigens in human tumors. In: DeLellis RA ed Diagnostic Immunohistochemistry. New York: 1981: 239–53.

64 Ordóñez NG, Batsakis JG. Comparison of *Ulex europaeus* I lectin with factor VIII-related antigen in vascular lesions. Arch Pathol Lab Med 1984; 108: 129–32.

65 Miettinen M, Holthöfer H, Lehto V-P, Miettinen A, Virtanen I. *Ulex europaeus* I lectin as a marker for tumors derived from endothelial cells. Am J Clin Pathol 1983; 79: 32–6.

66 Carswell J Jr, Kraeft NH. Fibrosarcoma of the bronchus. Report of a case diagnosed by bronchoscopy and treated by pneumonectomy. J Thorac Surg 1950; 19: 117–22.

67 DeMatteis A, Angeletti CA. Primary fibrosarcoma of the lung. Pathol Microbiol 1964; 27: 129–34.

68 Holinger PH, Johnston KC, Gossweiler N, Hirsch EC. Primary fibrosarcoma of the bronchus. Dis Chest 1960; 37: 137–43.

69 McEachern CG, Sullivan RW, Arata JE, Griest WD, Smith RB. Fibrosarcoma of the bronchus. J Thorac Surg 1955; 29: 368–72.

70 Robb D: A case of neonatal fibrosarcoma of lung. Br J Surg 1958; 46: 173–4.

71 Storey CF. Fibrosarcoma of the bronchus. Report of three cases diagnosed by bronchoscopy and treated by resection. J Thorac Surg 1952; 24: 16–33.

72 Strimel WH Jr, Hansell JR, Bindie R. Primary pulmonary fibrosarcoma. Report of two cases. J Germantown Hosp 1962; 3: 63–72.

73 Temple LJ, Aligazakis C. Fibrosarcoma of bronchus treated by pneumonectomy. Br Med J 1954; ii: 1463–4.

74 Black H. Fibrosarcoma of the bronchus. J Thorac Surg 1950; 19: 123–34.

75 Stembridge VA, Luibel FJ, Ashworth CT. Soft tissue sarcomas: electron microscopic approach to histogenetic classification. South Med J 1964; 57: 772–9.

76 Van Haelst UJGM. General considerations on electron microscopy of tumors of soft tissues. In Fenoglio CM, Wolff M eds Progress in Surgical Pathology, Vol 2. New York: Masson: 1980, 225–57.

77 Agnos JW, Starkey GWB. Primary leiomyosarcoma and leiomyoma of the lung. Review of the literature and report of two cases of leiomyosarcoma. N Engl J Med 1958; 258: 12–16.

78 Brindley GV Jr. Primary malignant tumors of the lung other than bronchogenic carcinoma. Ann Surg 1959; 149: 936–48.

79 Fadhli HA, Harrison AW, Shaddock SH. Primary pulmonary leiomyosarcoma. Review of the literature and report of one new case. Dis Chest 1965; 48: 431–3.

80 Glennie JS, Harvey P, Jewsbury P. Two cases of leiomyosarcoma of the lung. Thorax 1959; 14: 327–32.

81 Guillan RA, Wilen CJW, Zelman S. Primary leiomyosarcoma of the lung. Dis Chest 1969; 56: 452–4.

82 Havard CWH. Hanbury WJ. Leiomyosarcoma of lung. Lancet 1960; ii: 902–4.

83 Hewlett TH, McCarty JE. Pulmonary leiomyosarcoma. Arch Surg 1958; 76: 81–6.

84 Hicks HG. Bronchogenic leiomyosarcoma. Case report with necropsy findings. Dis Chest 1957; 32: 338–40.

85 Johnson EK, Mangiardi JL, Jacobs JB. Primary leiomyosarcoma of the lung treated by pneumonectomy. Surgery 1952; 32: 1010–13.

86 Killingsworth WP, McReynolds GS, Harrison AW. Pulmonary leiomyosarcoma in a child. J Pediatr 1953; 42: 466–70.

87 Mason MK, Azeem PS. Primary leiomyosarcomata of lung. Thorax 1965; 20: 13–17.

88 McNamara JJ, Paulson DL, Kingsley WB, Salinas-Izaquirre SF, Urschel HC Jr. Primary leiomyosarcoma of the lung. J Thorac Cardiovasc Surg 1969; 57: 635–41.

89 Merritt JW, Parker KR. Intrathoracic leiomyosarcoma. Can Med Assoc J 1957; 77: 1031–3.

90 Mylius EA, Aakhus T. Primary pulmonary leiomyosarcoma. Acta Pathol Microbiol Scand 1961; 148 (Suppl): 149–60.

91 Ochsner A, Ochsner S. Pneumonectomy for leiomyosarcoma. Patient well 21 years later. J Thorac Surg 1958; 35: 768–70.

92 Randall WS, Blades B. Primary bronchogenic leiomyosarcoma. Arch Pathol Lab Med 1946; 42: 543–8.

93 Rosen A, Christensen AH, Jamplis RW. Primary leiomyosarcoma of the lung. Case report. Dis Chest 1964; 45: 425–7.

94 Rosenberg D, Medlar E, Douglass R: Concurrent primary leiomyosarcoma and carcinoma of the bronchus. J Thorac Surg 1955; 30: 44–8.

95 Shaw RR, Paulson DL, Kee JL, Lovett VF. Primary pulmonary leiomyosarcomas. J Thorac Cardiovasc Surg 1961; 41: 430–6.

96 Sherman RS, Malone BH. A roentgen study of muscle tumors primary in the lung. Radiology 1950; 54: 507–15.

97 Tocker AM, DeHaan C, Stofer BE. Primary pulmonary leiomyosarcoma. Dis Chest 1957; 31: 328–34.

98 Watson WL, Anlyan AJ. Primary leiomyosarcoma of the lung. Cancer 1954; 7: 250–8.

99 Watson WL, Anlyan AJ. Primary leiomyosarcoma: a clinical evaluation of six cases. In: Watson WL ed Lung Cancer: A Study of 5000 Memorial Hospital Cases. St Louis: CV Mosby, 1968, 428–41.

100 Yacoubian H, Connolly JE, Wylie RH: Leiomyosarcoma of the lung. Ann Surg 1958; 147: 116–23.

101 Morgan PGM, Ball J. Pulmonary leiomyosarcomas. Br J Dis Chest 1980; 74: 245–252.

102 Carlson DH, Hanelin J. Leiomyosarcoma of the thorax. J Can Assoc Radiol 1978; 29: 221–4.

103 Dowell AR. Primary pulmonary leiomyosarcoma: report of two cases and review of the literature. Ann Thorac Surg 1974; 17: 384–94.

104 Ownby D, Lyon G, Spock A. Primary leiomyosarcoma of the lung in childhood. Am J Dis Child 1976; 130: 1132–3.

105 Pritchett PS, Fu Y-S, Kay S. Unusual ultrastructural features of a leiomyosarcoma of the lung Am J Clin Pathol 1975; 63: 901–8.

106 Cameron EWJ: Primary sarcoma of the lung. Thorax 1975; 30: 516–20.

107 Wang NS, Seemayer ThA, Ahmed MN, Morin J. Pulmonary leiomyosarcoma associated with an arteriovenous fistula. Arch Pathol Lab Med 1974; 98: 100–5.

108 Böcker W, Strecker H. Electron microscopy of uterine leiomyosarcomas. Virchows Arch Pathol Anat 1975; 367: 59–71.

109 Nevalainen TJ, Linna JI. Ultrastructure of gastric leiomyosarcoma. Virchows Arch Pathol Anat 1978; 379: 25–33.

110 Knapp RH, Wick MR, Goellner JR. Leiomyoblastomas and their relationship to other smooth muscle tumors of the gastrointestinal tract: an electron microscopic study. Am J Surg Pathol 1984; 8: 449–61.

111 Swanson PE, Manivel JC, Wick MR. Immunoreactivity for Leu 7 in neurofibrosarcoma and other spindle-cell sarcomas of soft tissue. Submitted to Am J Pathol.

112 Enzinger FM, Smith BH. Hemangiopericytoma. An analysis of 106 cases. Hum Pathol 1976; 7: 61–82.

113 Braham J, Sarova-Pinchas I, Pauzner YM, Braf Z. Hemangiopericytoma of the lung with metastasis to the brain. Case report. Israel Med J 1962; 21: 47–50.

114 McCormack LJ, Gallivan WF: Hemangiopericytoma. Cancer 1954; 7: 595–601.

115 McCormack LJ, McIsaac WM, Ragde H, Groves LK, Effler DB: "Functioning" pulmonary neoplasms: I. The carcinoid tumor; II. The hemangiopericytoma. Cleve Clin Q 1961; 28: 145–56.

116 Ochsner S, DeCamp PT: Hemangiopericytoma of the lung. Am Rev Tuberc 1958; 77: 496–500.

117 Wellington JL, Neuman HW: Primary hemangiopericytoma of the lung. Can Med Assoc J 1963; 88: 1295–7.

118 Viswanathan R, Sriramachari S. Pulmonary hemangiopericytoma. Ind J Chest Dis Allied Sci 1981; 23: 104–6.

119 Van Assendelft AHW, Strengell-Usanov L, Kastarinen S. Pulmonary hemangiopericytoma with multiple metastases. Eur J Respir Dis 1984; 65: 380–3.

120 Meade JB, Whitwell F, Bickford BJ, Waddington JKB. Primary hemangiopericytoma of lung. Thorax 1974; 29: 1–15.

121 Alt B, Huffer WE, Belchis DA. A vascular lesion with smooth muscle differentiation presenting as a coin lesion in the lung: glomus tumor versus hemangiopericytoma. Am J Clin Pathol 1983; 80: 765–71.

122 Murad TM, Von Haam E, Murthy MSN. Ultrastructure of a hemangiopericytoma and a glomus tumor. Cancer 1968; 22: 1239–49.

123 Morales AR, Fine G, Pardo V, Horn RC Jr. The ultrastructure of smooth muscle tumors with a consideration of the possible relationship of glomangiomas, hemangiopericytomas, and cardiac myxomas. Pathol Annu 1975; 10: 65–92.

124 Bedrossian CWM, Veroni R, Unger KM, Solman J. Pulmonary malignant fibrous histiocytoma. Chest 1979; 75: 186–9.

125 Kern WH, Hughes RK, Mand BW, Harley DP. Malignant fibrous histiocytoma of the lung. Cancer 1979; 44: 1793–1801.

126 Sajjad SM, Begin LR, Dail DH, Lukeman JM. Fibrous histiocytoma of lung—a clinicopathological study of two cases. Histopathology 1981; 5: 325–34.

127 Larsen K, Vejlsted H, Hariri J. Primary malignant fibrous histiocytoma of the lung. A case report. Scand J Thorac Cardiovasc Surg 1984; 18: 89–91.

128 Chowdhury LN, Swerdlow MA, Jao W, Kathpalia S, Desser RK. Postirradiation malignant fibrous histiocytoma of the lung. Demonst-

ration of alpha-l-antitrypsinlike material in neoplastic cells. Am J Clin Pathol 1980; 74: 820–6.

129 Mills SE, Breyer RH, Johnston FR, Hudspeth AS, Marshall RB, Choplin RH, Cordell AR, Myers RT. Malignant fibrous histiocytoma of the mediastinum and lung. A report of three cases. J Thorac Cardiovasc Surg 1982; 84: 367–72.

130 Limacher J, Delage C, Legace R. Malignant fibrous histiocytoma: clinicopathologic and ultrastructural study of 12 cases. Am J Surg Pathol 1978; 2: 265–74.

131 Taxy JB, Battifora HA. Malignant fibrous histiocytoma: an electron microscopic study. Cancer 1977; 40: 254–67.

132 Harris M. The ultrastructure of benign and malignant fibrous histiocytomas. Histopathology 1980; 4: 29–44.

133 Weiss LM, Warhol MJ. Ultrastructural distinctions between adult pleomorphic rhabdomyosarcomas, pleomorphic liposarcomas, and pleomorphic malignant fibrous histiocytomas. Hum Pathol 1984; 15: 1025–33.

134 Meister P, Konrad EA, Nathrath W, Eder M. Malignant fibrous histiocytoma: histological patterns and cell types. Pathol Res Pract 1980; 168: 193–212.

135 Silva FG, Taylor WE, Burns DK. Demonstration of alpha-l-antitrypsin in yet another neoplasm (letter to the editor). Hum Pathol 1984; 15: 494.

136 Press P. Hemangioendothelio-sarcoma à localization pulmonaire. Poumon Coeur 1958; 14: 930–45.

137 Tralka GA, Katz S. Hemangioendothelioma of the lung. Am Rev Resp Dis 1963; 87: 107–14.

138 Kayser K, Bauer M, Luellig H, Berberich H, Schaaf S. Long-term development of a primary lung sarcoma, probably lymphangiosarcoma—a case report. Thorac Cardiovasc Surg 1984; 32: 178–81.

139 Rosai J, Sumner HW, Kostianovsky M, Perez-Mesa C. Angiosarcoma of the skin: a clinicopathologic and fine structural study. Hum Pathol 1976; 7: 83–109.

140 Carstens PHB. The Weibel-Palade body in the diagnosis of endothelial tumors. Ultrastruct Pathol 1981; 2: 315–25.

141 Weibel ER, Palade GE. New cytoplasmic components in arterial endothelia. J Cell Biol 1964; 23: 101–112.

142 Limas C, Lange P, Fraley EE, Vessella RL. A, B, H antigens in transitional cell tumors of the urinary bladder. Correlation with the clinical course. Cancer 1979; 44: 2099–107.

143 Corrin B, Harrison WJ, Wright DH. The so-called intravascular bronchioloalveolar tumour of lung (low grade sclerosing angiosarcoma): presentation with extrapulmonary deposits. Diagn Histopathol 1983; 6: 229–37.

144 Corrin B, Manners B, Millard M, Weaver L. Histogenesis of the so-called "intravascular bronchioloalveolar tumour." J Pathol 1979; 128: 163–7.

145 Echevarria RA: Angiogenic nature of "intravascular bronchioloalveolar tumor." Arch Pathol Lab Med 1981; 105: 627–8.

146 Ferrer-Roca O: Intravascular and sclerosing bronchioalveolar tumor. Am J Surg Pathol 1980; 4: 375–81.

147 Reynes A, Capron F, Baglin JY, Leclerc P, Prudent J, Rochemaure J. Etude ultrastructurale et histochimique de la "tumeur bronchiolo-alvéolaire sclérosante et intravasculaire" de Dail et Liebow. Revue Franc Maladies Resp 1981; 9: 279.

148 Sherman JL, Rykwalder PJ, Tashkin DP. Intravascular bronchioalveolar tumor. Am Rev Resp Dis 1981; 123: 468–70.

149 Weldon-Linne CM, Victor TA, Christ ML, Fry WA. Angiogenic nature of the "intravascular bronchioloalveolar tumor" of the lung. Arch Pathol Lab Med 1981; 105: 174–9.

150 Weldon-Linne CM, Victor TA, Christ ML. Immunohistochemical identification of factor VIII-related antigen in the intravascular bronchioloalveolar tumor of the lung. Arch Pathol Lab Med 1981; 105: 628–9.

151 Emery RW, Fox AL, Raab DE. Intravascular bronchioloalveolar tumour. Thorax 1982; 37: 472–3.

152 Marsh K, Kenyon WE, Earis JE, Pearson MG. Intravascular bronchioloalveolar tumour. Thorax 1982; 37: 474–5.

153 Azumi N, Churg A. Intravascular and sclerosing bronchioloalveolar tumor. A pulmonary sarcoma of probable vascular origin. Am J Surg Pathol 1981; 5: 587–96.

154 Bhagavan BS, Dorfman HD, Murthy MSN, Eggleston JC. Intravascular bronchioloalveolar tumor (IVBAT). A low-grade sclerosing epithelioid angiosarcoma of lung. Am J Surg Pathol 1982; 6: 41–52.

155 Ishak KG, Sesterhenn IA, Goodman ZD, Rabin L, Stromeyer FW. Epithelioid hemangioendothelioma of the liver: a clinicopathologic and followup study of 32 cases. Hum Pathol 1984; 15: 839–52.

156 Weiss SW, Enzinger FM. Epithelioid hemangioendothelioma. A vascular tumor often mistaken for a carcinoma. Cancer 1982; 50: 970–81.

157 Smith EAC, Cohen RV, Peale AR. Primary chondrosarcoma of the lung. Ann Intern Med 1960; 53: 838–46.

158 Wick MR. Unpublished observations, 1984.

159 Loring WE, Wolman SR: Idiopathic multiple hemorrhagic sarcoma of lung (Kaposi's sarcoma). NY State J Med 1965; 65: 668–77.

160 Misra DP, Sunderrajan EV, Hurst DJ. Japosi's sarcoma of the lung: radiography and pathology. Thorax 1982; 37: 155–65.

161 Epstein DM, Gefter WB, Conard K. Lung disease in homosexual men. Radiology 1982; 143: 7–22.

162 Dantzig PI, Richardson D, Rayhanzadeh S. Thoracic involvement of non-African Kaposi's sarcoma. chest 1974; 66: 522–31.

163 Nash G, Fligiel S. Kaposi's sarcoma presenting as pulmonary disease in the acquired immuno-deficiency syndrome: diagnosis by lung biopsy. Hum Pathol 1984; 15: 999–1001.

164 Lee SH, Reganchary SS, Paramesh J: Primary pulmonary rhabdomyosarcoma: a case report and review of the literature. Hum Pathol 1981; 12: 92–6.

165 Thomas WJ, Koening HM, Ellwanger FR, Lightsey AL. Primary pulmonary rhabdomyosarcoma in childhood. Am J Dis Child 1981; 135: 469–71.

166 Krous HF, Sexauer ChL. Embryonal rhabdomyosarcoma arising within a congenital bronchogenic cyst in a child. J Pediatr Surg 1981; 16: 506–8.

167 Ueda K, Gruppo R, Unger F, Martin L, Bove K. Rhabdomyosarcoma of lung arising in congenital cystic malformation. Cancer 1977; 40: 383–8.

168 Bariffi F, DelBono M, Natali P. Su di un caso rabdomiosarcoma primitive del polmone. Clin Tisiol Univ Napoli 1967; 22: 123–45.

169 Bignardi P. Su un caso di rabdomiosarcoma del polmone. Clinica (Bologna) 1960; 20: 367–77.

170 Conquest HF, Thornton JL, Massie JR, Coxe JW. Primary pulmonary rhabdomyosarcoma. Report of three cases and literature review. Ann Surg 1965; 161: 688–92.

171 Drennan JM, McCormack RJM. Primary rhabdomyosarcoma of the lung. J Pathol Bacteriol 1960; 79: 147–7.

172 Fallon G, Schiller M, Kilman JW. Primary rhabdomyosarcoma of the bronchus. Ann Thorac Surg 1971; 12: 650–4.

173 Forbes GB. Rhabdomyosarcoma of bronchus. J Pathol Bacteriol 1955; 70: 427–31.

174 Gordon LZ, Boss H. Primary rhabdomyosarcoma of lung. Report of a case. Cancer 1955; 8: 588–91.

175 Grouls V, Helpap B. Das Rhabdomyosarkom der Lungen. Thoraxchirurgie 1976; 24: 94–7.

176 Kostelecky A, Stolz J. Lungerhabdomyosarkom. Zbl Chir 1956; 81: 473–80.

177 McDonald S Jr, Heather JC. Neoplastic invasion of the pulmonary veins and left auricle. J Pathol Bacteriol 1939; 48: 533–43.

178 Maschio C. Rhabdomiosarcoma del polmone. Riv Anat Patol Oncol 1956; 11: 1161–80.

179 LaValle-Bundtzen J, Norback DH. The ultrastructure of poorly-differentiated rhabdomyosarcoma: a case report and literature review. Hum Pathol 1982; 13: 301–13.

180 Erlandson RA. Diagnostic Transmission Electron Microscopy of Human Tumors. New York: Masson, 1981.

181 De Jong ASH, van Kessel-van Vark M, Albus-Lutter ChE, Raamsdonk W, Voute PA. Skeletal muscle actin as a tumor marker in the diagnosis of rhabdomyosarcoma in childhood. Am J Surg Pathol 1985; 9: 467–74.

182 Tsokos M, Linnoila RI, Chandra RS, Triche TJ. Neuron-specific enolase in the diagnosis of neuroblastoma and other small round cell tumors in children. Hum Pathol 1984; 15: 575–84.

183 Aterman K, Patel S. Striated muscle in the lung. Am J Anat 1970; 128: 341–9.

184 Morgan HD, Salama FD. Primary chondrosarcoma of the lung. J Thorac Cardiovasc Surg 1972; 64: 465–9.

185 Daniels AC, George H, Strans FH. Primary chondrosarcoma of the tracheobronchial tree. Report of a unique case, and brief review. Arch Pathol Lab Med 1967; 84: 615–21.

186 Greenspan EB. Primary osteoid chondrosarcoma of the lung: report of a case. Am J Cancer 1933; 18: 603–9.

187 Lowell LM, Tuby JG. Primary chondrosarcoma of the lung. J Thorac Surg 1946; 68: 476–90.

188 Bini G: Osservazioni anatomiche et istopatologiche sopra particolari forme di tumori polmonari maligni di nataura mesenchimale. Patologica 1942; 34: 77–88.

189 Nosanchuk JS, Weatherbee L. Primary osteogenic sarcoma in lung: report of a case. J Thorac Cardiovasc Surg 1969; 58: 242–7.

190 Reingold IM, Amromin GD. Extraosseous osteosarcoma of the lung. Cancer 1971; 28: 491–8.

191 Spjut HJ, Dorfman HD, Fechner RE, Ackerman LV. Tumors of Bone and Cartilage. In: Atlas of Tumor Pathology, Fascicle 5, Second Series, Washington DC: Armed Forces Institute of Pathology, 1971.

192 Nakamura Y, Becker LE, Marks A. S100

protein in tumors of cartilage and bone. An immunohistochemical study. Cancer 1983; 52: 1820–4.

193 Bartley TD, Arean VM. Intrapulmonary neurogenic tumors. J Thorac Cardiovasc Surg 1965; 50: 114–23.

194 Roviaro G, Montorsi M, Varoli F, Binda R, Cecchetto A. Primary pulmonary tumours of neurogenic origin. Thorax 1983; 38: 942–5.

195 Erlandson RA, Woodruff JM. Peripheral nerve sheath tumors: an electron microscopic study of 43 cases. Cancer 1982; 49: 273–87.

196 Weiss SW, Langloss JM, Enzinger FM. Value of S100 protein in the diagnosis of soft tissue tumors with particular reference to benign and malignant Schwann cell tumors. Lab Invest 1983; 49: 299–308.

197 Daimaru Y, Hashimoto H, Enjoji M. Malignant peripheral nerve sheath tumors (malignant Schwannomas): an immunohistochemical study of 29 cases. Am J Surg Pathol 1985; 9: 434–44.

198 Matsunou H, Shimoda T, Kakimoto S, Yamashita H, Ishikawa E, Mukai M. Histopathologic and immunohistochemical study of malignant tumors of peripheral nerve sheath (malignant Schwannoma). Cancer 1985; 56: 2269–79.

199 Pain JA, Sayer RE. Primary leiomyosarcoma of the pulmonary artery. Eur J Respir Dis 1984; 65: 139–43.

200 Wackers FJ, van der Schoot JB, Hampe JF: Sarcoma of the pulmonary trunk associated with hemorrhagic tendency. A case report and review of the literature. Cancer 1969; 23: 339–51.

201 Moffat RE, Chang CH, Slaven JE. Roentgen considerations in primary pulmonary artery sarcoma. Radiology 1972; 104: 283–8.

202 Killebrew E, Gerbode F. Leiomyosarcoma of the pulmonary artery diagnosed preoperatively by angiocardiography. J Thorac Cardiovasc Surg 1976; 71: 469–71.

203 Myerson PJ, Myerson DA, Katz R, Lawson JP. Gallium imaging in pulmonary artery sarcoma mimicking pulmonary embolism. Case report. J Nucl Med 1976; 17: 893–5.

204 Shoenfeld Y, Avidor I, Liban E, Levy MJ, Pinkhas J. Primary leiomyosarcoma of the pulmonary artery. Respiration 1981; 41: 208–13.

205 Henrichs KJ, Wenisch HJC, Hofman W, Klein F. Leiomyosarcoma of the pulmonary artery. Virchows Arch Pathol Anat 1979; 383: 207–16.

206 Elphinstone RH, Spector RG. Sarcoma of the pulmonary artery. Thorax 1959; 14: 333–40.

207 McConnell TH. Bony and cartilaginous tumors of the heart and great vessels: report of an osteosarcoma of the pulmonary artery. Cancer 1970; 25: 611–7.

208 Durgin B, Ingleby H. Primary sarcoma of the pulmonary artery. Clinics 1946; 5: 182–9.

209 Paulsen SM, Egeblad K. Sarcoma of the pulmonary artery. A light and electron microscopic study. J Submicroscop Cytol 1983; 15: 811–21.

210 Bleisch VR, Kraus FT. Polypoid sarcoma of the pulmonary trunk. Cancer 1980; 46: 314–24.

211 Hayata T, Sato E. Primary leiomyosarcoma arising in the trunk of the pulmonary artery. Acta Pathol Jpn 1977; 27: 137–44.

212 Hopwood D, McNeill G. Spindle-cell sarcoma of the pulmonary trunk: a case report with histochemistry and electron microscopy. J Pathol 1979; 128: 71–7.

213 Wolf PL, Dickenman RC, Langston JD: Fibrosarcoma of the pulmonary artery, masquerading as a pheochromocytoma. Am J Clin Pathol 1960; 34: 146–53.

214 Jacques JE, Barclay R. The solid sarcomatous pulmonary artery. Br J Dis Chest 1960; 54: 217–20.

215 Ali MY, Lee GS. Sarcoma of the pulmonary artery. Cancer 1964; 17: 1220–4.

216 Friedman HM, Smith CK. Leiomyosarcoma of the pulmonary artery. JAMA 1968; 203: 809.

217 Sethi GK, Slaven JE, Kepes JJ: Primary sarcoma of the pulmonary artery. J Thorac Cardiovasc Surg 1972; 63: 587–93.

218 Altman NH, Shelley WM. Primary intimal sarcoma of the pulmonary artery. Johns Hopkins Med J 1973; 133: 214–22.

219 Hayes WL, Farha SJ, Brown RL. Primary leiomyosarcoma of the pulmonary artery. Am J Cardiol 1974; 34: 615–17.

220 Thijs LG, Kroon TAJ, van Leeuwen TM. Leiomyosarcoma of the pulmonary trunk associated with pericardial effusion. Thorax 1974; 29: 490–4.

221 Rao NG, Krishnaswami S, Cherian G. Sarcoma of the pulmonary artery with metastases to pancreas and adrenal glands. Chest 1974; 66: 459–62.

222 Magilligan DJ, Ryan GF, Salisnjiak MM. Pulmonary artery sarcoma. NY State J Med 1976; 76: 977–9.

223 Olsson HE, Spitzer RM, Erston WF. Primary and secondary pulmonary artery neoplasia mimicking acute pulmonary embolism. Radiology 1976; 118: 49–53.

224 Murthy MSN, Mechstroth CV, Merkle BH. Primary intimal sarcoma of pulmonary valve and trunk with osteogenic sarcomatous ele-

ments. Arch Pathol Lab Med 1976; 100: 649–51.

225 Schmookler BM, Marsh HB, Roberts WC. Primary sarcoma of the pulmonary trunk and/or right or left main pulmonary artery. A rare cause of obstruction of right ventricular outflow. Am J Med 1977; 63: 263–72.

226 Hohbach C, Mall W. Chondrosarcoma of the pulmonary artery. Beitr Pathol 1977; 160: 298–307.

227 Fredericka DN, Hart NJ, Cook SA. Primary sarcoma of the pulmonary artery. Cleve Clin Q 1980; 47: 115–18.

228 Fer MF, Greco FA, Haile KL. Unusual survival after pulmonary artery sarcoma. South Med J 1981; 74: 624–6.

229 Hynes JK, Smith HC, Holmes DR. Preoperative angiographic diagnosis of primary sarcoma of the pulmonary artery. Circulation 1982; 66: 672–4.

230 Wright EC, Wellons HA, Martin RP. Primary pulmonary artery sarcoma diagnosed noninvasively by two-dimensional echocardiography. Circulation 1983; 67: 459–62.

231 Salazar GH, Roth JA, Burns WA. Sarcomas of the pulmonary artery. Am Soc Clin Pathol Check Sample Series (Anat Pathol AP83–10) 1983; 11: 1–5.

232 Chomette G, Auriol M, Delsol M. Sarcome primitif de l'artère pulmonaire à type d'hemangioendotheliosarcome. Ann Anat Pathol 1978; 23: 161–70.

233 Klein F, Zeidler D, Henrichs KJ. Primares spindelzellsarkom der Pulmonalarterie. Onkologic 1979; 2: 209–11.

234 Mizutani T, Morimoto Y, Okada Y. An operative case of primary pulmonary artery sarcoma. Kyobu Geka 1979; 32: 930–6.

235 Barth J, Lehman H, Thermann M. Rhabdomyosarkom der arteria pulmonalis. ROFO 1982; 136: 669–72.

236 Dannheimer IPL, Venter CP. Haemangiosarcoma of the pulmonary valve presenting as a pulmonary stenosis. S Afr Med J 1978; 54: 873–6.

237 Haythorn SR, Ray WB, Wolff RA. Primary fibromyxosarcoma of the heart and pulmonary artery. Am J Pathol 1941; 17: 261–71.

238 Green JR, Crevasse LE, Shanklin DR. Fibromyxosarcoma of the pulmonary artery associated with syncope, intractable heart failure, polycythemia, and thrombocytopenia. Am J Cardiol 1964; 13: 547–52.

239 Martin WC, Tuohy EL, Will C. Primary tumor of the heart (entrance to the pulmonary artery). Am Heart J 1939; 17: 728–34.

240 Hagstrom L. Malignant mesenchymoma in pulmonary artery and right ventricle. Acta Pathol Microbiol Scand 1961; 51: 87–94.

241 Munk J, Griffel B, Kogan J. Primary mesenchymoma of the pulmonary artery: radiological features. Br J Radiol 1965; 38: 104–11.

242 Wick MR, Mills SE, Scheithauer BW, Cooper PH, Davitz MA, Parkinson K: Reassessment of "malignant angioendotheliomatosis:" evidence in favor of its reclassification as intravascular lymphomatosis. Am J Surg Pathol 1986; 10: 112–23.

243 Sy WM, Nissen AW. Radionuclide studies in hemangioendotheliomatosis: case report. J Nucl Med 1975; 16: 915–17.

244 Lichtiger B, Mackay B, Tessmer CF. Spindle cell variant of squamous carcinoma. Cancer 1970; 26: 1311–20.

245 Dulmet-Brender E, Jaubert F, Huchon G. Exophytic endobronchial epidermoid carcinoma. Cancer 1986; 57: 1358–64.

246 Carstens PHB, Kuhns JG, Ghazi C. Primary malignant melanomas of the lung and adrenal. Hum Pathol 1984; 15: 910–14.

247 Battifora HA. Spindle-cell carcinoma: ultrastructural evidence of squamous origin and collagen production by the tumor cells. Cancer 1976; 37: 2275–82.

248 Mazur MT, Katzenstein AA. Metastatic melanoma: the spectrum of ultrastructural morphology. Ultrastruct Pathol 1980; 1: 337–56.

249 Springall DR, Gu J, Cocchia D, Michetti F, Levene A, Levene MM, Marangos PJ, Bloom SR, Polak JM. The value of S100 immunostaining as a diagnostic tool in human malignant melanomas. Virchows Arch Pathol Anat 1983; 400: 331–44.

250 Dhillon AP, Rode J, Leathem A. Neurone-specific enolase: an aid to the diagnosis of melanoma and neuroblastoma. Histopathology 1982; 6: 81–92.

251 Kakos GS, Williams TE, Assor D. Pulmonary carcinosarcoma: etiologic, therapeutic, and prognostic considerations. J Thorac Cardiovasc Surg 1971; 61: 777–83.

252 Sarma DP, Deshotels SJ Jr: Carcinosarcoma of the lung. J Surg Oncol 1982; 19: 216–8.

253 Wright ES, Pike E, Couves CM. Unusual tumors of the lung. J Surg Oncol 1984; 24: 23–9.

254 Gabriel JB, Ibanez I, Kondlapoodi P, Chauhan PM, Hagstrom JWC. Carcinosarcoma of the lung with spindle-cell epithelial component: report of a case. J Surg Oncol 1984; 25: 116–18.

255 Zimmerman KG, Sobonoya RE, Payne CM.

Histochemical and ultrastructural features of an unusual pulmonary carcinosarcoma. Hum Pathol 1981; 12: 1046–51.

256 Razzuk MA, Urschel MC, Race GJ. Carcinosarcoma of the lung. Report of two cases and review of the literature. J Thorac Cardiovasc Surg 1971; 61: 541–7.

257 Huszar M, Herczeg E, Lieberman Y, Geiger B: Distinctive immunofluorescent labeling of epithelial and mesenchymal elements of carcinosarcoma with antibodies specific for different intermediate filaments. Hum Pathol 1984; 15: 532–8.

258 Chen HP, Lee SS, Berardi RS. Inflammatory pseudotumor of the lung. Ultrastructural and light microscopic study of a myxomatous variant. Cancer 1984; 54: 861–5.

259 Titus JL, Harrison EG, Clagett OT, Anderson MW, Knaff L. Xanthomatous and inflammatory pseudotumors of the lung. Cancer 1962; 15: 522–38.

260 Dublier LD, Bryant LR, Danielson GK. Histiocytoma (fibrous xanthoma) of the lung. Am J Surg 1968; 115: 420–6.

261 Berardi RS, Lee SS, Chen HP, Stines GJ. Inflammatory pseudotumors of the lung. Surg Gynecol Obstet 1982; 156: 89–96.

262 Wentworth P, Lynch MJ, Fallis JC, Turner JAP, Lowden JA, Conen PE. Xanthomatous pseudotumor of lung: a case report with electron microscope and lipid studies. Cancer 1968; 22: 345–55.

263 Kuzela DC. Ultrastructural study of a postinflammatory "tumor" of the lung. Cancer 1975; 36: 149–55.

264 Lund C, Sorenson M, Axelsen F, Larsen K. Pulmonary histiocytomas. Eur J Respir Dis 1983; 64: 141–9.

265 Dehner LP. Personal communication, 1986.

266 Powell V: Pulmonary telangiectasis. Thorax 1958; 13: 321–6.

267 Wagenvoort CA, Beetstra A, Spijker J. Capillary haemangiomatosis of the lungs. Histopathology 1978; 2: 401–5.

268 Joliat G, Stalder H, Kapanci Y. Lymphangiomyomatosis: a clinicoanatomical entity. Cancer 1973; 31: 455–61.

269 Banner AS, Carrington CB, Emory WB. Efficacy of oophorectomy in lymphangioleiomyomatosis and benign metastasizing leiomyoma. N Engl J Med 1981; 305: 204–9.

270 Sobonya RE, Quan SF, Fleishman JS: Pulmonary lymphangioleiomyomatosis: quantitative analysis of lesions producing airflow limitation. Hum Pathol 1985; 16: 1122–8.

271 Corring B, Liebow AA. Pulmonary lymphangiomyomatosis. Am J Pathol 1975; 79: 348–82.

272 Butler C, Kleinerman J. Pulmonary hamartoma. Arch Pathol Lab Med 1969; 88: 584–92.

273 McDonald JR, Harrington SW, Clagett OT. Hamartoma (often called chondroma) of the lung. J Thorac Surg 1945; 14: 128–43.

274 Burkhardt A, Otto HF, Kaukel E. Multiple pulmonary (hamartomatous?) leiomyomas. Light and electron microscopic study. Virchows Arch Pathol Anat 1981; 394: 133–41.

275 Silverman JF, Kay S. Multiple pulmonary leiomyomatous hamartomas. Report of a case with ultrastructure examination. Cancer 1976; 38: 1199–1204.

276 Taylor TL, Miller DR. Leiomyoma of the bronchus. J Thorac Cardiovasc Surg 1969; 57: 284–8.

277 Carney JA. The triad of gastric epithelioid leiomyosarcoma, functioning extra-adrenal paraganglioma, and pulmonary chondroma. Cancer 1979; 43: 374–82.

278 Wick MR, Ruebner BH, Carney JA. Gastric tumors in patients with pulmonary chondroma or extra-adrenal paraganglioma: an ultrastructural study. Arch Pathol Lab Med 1981; 105: 527–31.

279 Herbert A, Wright DH, Isaacson PG, Smith JL. Primary malignant lymphoma of the lung: histopathologic and immunologic evaluation of nine cases. Hum Pathol 1984; 15: 415–22.

280 Kurtin PJ, Pinkus GS. Leukocyte common antigen—a diagnostic discriminant between hematopoietic and nonhematopoietic neoplasms in paraffin sections using monoclonal antibodies. Correlation with immunologic studies and ultrastructural localization. Hum Pathol 1985; 16: 353–65.

281 Ranchod M, Levine GD. Spindle-cell carcinoid tumors of the lung. A clinicopathologic study of 35 cases. Am J Surg Pathol 1980; 4: 315–31.

282 Mills SE, Cooper PH, Walker AN, Kron IL. Atypical carcinoid tumors of the lung: a clinicopathologic study of 17 cases. Am J Surg Pathol 1982; 6: 643–54.

283 Fisher ER, Palekar A, Paulson JD. Comparative histopathologic, histochemical, electron microscopic, and tissue culture studies of bronchial carcinoids and oat-cell carcinomas of lung. Am J Clin Pathol 1978; 69: 165–72.

284 Carter D. Small-cell carcinoma of the lung. Am J Surg Pathol 1983; 7: 787–95.

285 Gebauer C. The postoperative prognosis of primary pulmonary sarcomas. Scand J Thorac Cardiovasc Surg 1982; 16: 91–7.

286 Lopez M, DiLauro L, Papaldo P, Perno C-F. Alternating combination chemotherapy of

advanced soft tissue sarcomas in adults. Am J Clin Oncol 1984; 7: 539–42.

287 Bui NB, Chauvergne J, Hocke C, Durand M, Brunet R, Coindre J-M. Analysis of a series of sixty soft tissue sarcomas in adults treated with a cyclophosphamide-vincristine-adriamycin-dacarbazine (CYVADIC) combination. Cancer Chemother Pharmacol 1985; 15: 82–5.

288 Edmonson JH, Long HJ, Richardson RL, Creagan ET, Green SJ. Phase II study of a combination of mitomycin, doxorubicin, and cisplatin in advanced sarcomas. Cancer Chemother Pharmacol 1985; 15: 181–2.

289 Cramer SF, Meyer JS, Kraner JF. Metastasizing leiomyoma of the uterus: S-phase fraction, estrogen receptors, and ultrastructure. Cancer 1980; 45: 932–7.

290 Nomi S, Pellis NR, Kahan BD. Retardation of postsurgical metastases with the use of extracted tumor-specific transplantation antigens and cyclophosphamide. J Nat Cancer Inst 1984; 73: 943–50.

291 Mulé JJ, Shu S, Rosenberg SA: The antitumor efficacy of lymphokine-activated killer cells and recombinant interleukin-2 in vivo. J Immunol 1985; 135: 646–52.

292 Roth JA, Restrepo C, Scuderi P, Baldwin RW, Reichert CM, Hosoi S. Analysis of antigenic expression by primary and autologous metastatic human sarcomas using murine monoclonal antibodies. Cancer Res 1984; 44: 5320–5.

Textbook of Uncommon Cancer
Edited by C.J. Williams, J.G. Krikorian, M.R. Green and D. Raghavan
© 1988 John Wiley & Sons Ltd

Chapter **21**

Primary Malignant Melanoma of the Lung

Amanda Herbert

Consultant Histopathologist, Department of Histopathology, Southampton General Hospital, Tremona Road, SO9 4XY, UK

INTRODUCTION

It is exceptional for malignant melanoma to arise at any site except the skin, eye, juxtacutaneous mucous membranes and, much less often, leptomeninges, all of which are sites normally populated by melanocytes which migrate from the neural crest during fetal life. There are, however, rare instances of primary melanoma arising in many visceral sites including the larynx, trachea, bronchus, oesophagus, gall bladder, rectum, cervix, ovary, vagina, and adrenal glands (1). Although melanocytes have occasionally been found in some of these sites, they have never been demonstrated, or systematically searched for, in the trachea or bronchial tree.

It has been particularly difficult to establish with certainty the existence of primary melanomas in the lung because it is such a common site for metastases. Furthermore, solitary metastases, particularly from ocular melanoma, may arise in the lung many years after the primary tumour was excised (2). The survival following resection of solitary metastatic pulmonary tumours can be surprisingly good, and comparable with that of primary tumours (3). Melanoma is further complicated by the fact that primary cutaneous melanomas

can regress, while still giving rise to metastases (4).

In spite of the wide array of information tending to oppose the acceptance of primary melanoma of lung, there are no less than 18 pulmonary melanomas in the English literature reported as probable primaries at that site (Tables 1 and 2). Although not all of these tumours can be accepted with certainty as true primaries, the evidence overwhelmingly suggests that the lower respiratory tract is an unusual but well established site for the origin of malignant melanoma.

It is important to identify those reported cases which are acceptable as primary tumours, so that the clinical and pathological features can be analysed and recognized during life in order to achieve appropriate treatment and management.

REVIEW OF THE LITERATURE

Lung Melanoma

A case report of 2 patients, in whom multiple melanotic pulmonary tumours were found at necropsy, is often referred to as the earliest record of primary melanoma arising in the

TABLE 1   CLINICAL DETAILS OF CASES OF PRIMARY MELANOMA OF THE LUNG

Reference	Year	Age	Sex	Presentation	Duration	Smoking history	Operation	Other treatment	Other melanomas	Outcome after surgery
Todd (5)	1888	60	M	haemoptysis	1 month	—	none	symptomatic	—	—
		55	M	haemoptysis		—	none	symptomatic	—	—
Funkel and Torrey (6)	1916	40	F	haemoptysis; haemothorax	16 months	—	none	symptomatic	—	—
Carlucci and Schleussner (7)	1942	48	F	chest pain	3 months	smoker	R pneumonectomy	none	none	died postoperatively
Allen and Spitz (8)	1953	49	F			—	resection	—	MM hard palate 6 years before	alive at 2 years
Hsu et al. (9)	1962	20	M	haemoptysis; chest pain	6 months	—	R pneumonectomy	none	numerous moles L leg and foot	died at 2 years with metastases
Salm (10)	1963	45	M	haemoptysis; pneumonia		—	L pneumonectomy	none	none	died at 6 months with metastases
Reed and Kent (2)	1964	71	M	asymptomatic; shadow on routine chest x-ray		no data	LL lobectomy	none	none	alive at 11 years
Reid and Mehta (11)	1966	60	F	chest pain	10 weeks	20/day 5 years	R pneumonectomy	none	none	alive at 10 years
Jensen and Egedorf (13)	1967	61	F	haemoptysis;	6 months	—	segmentectomy LUL	none	none	died at 6 months with metastases
Allen and Drash (14)	1968	40	F	tiredness;		—	RL lobectomy	none	none	alive
Taboada et al. (15)	1972	56	M	asymptomatic; shadow on routine chest x-ray	5 months	non-smoker	LL pneumonectomy wedge resection pneumonectomy	none	none	died at 3 months with metastases
		40	M	asymptomatic; shadow on routine chest x-ray		—	L pneumonectomy	none	none	alive at 3 years
Adebonojo et al. (16)	1979	55	F	haemoptysis; fever;		—	RU lobectomy	adjuvant chemotherapy radiotherapy	benign mole shoulder (biopsied)	alive at 3 years
Robertson et al. (17)	1980	70	F	dyspnoea;	12 months	10/day to age of 50	none	none	none	died at 9 weeks (no surgery)
Gephardt (18)	1981	47	M	died acute pneumonia PH adenoca in lymph node of unknown origin		heavy smoker	none	none	none	PM diagnosis (no surgery)
Carstens et al. (19)	1984	29	F	asymptomatic; shadow on routine chest x-ray		—	RU lobectomy	none	benign naevus biopsied 3 years before	died at 1 month with metastases
Herbert (20)	1987	37	M	haemoptsis;	6 weeks	15/day 25 years	none	vincristine, radiotherapy	none	died within year (no surgery)

TABLE 2 HISTOPATHOLOGY OF PRIMARY MELANOMAS OF THE LUNG

Reference	Specimen	Location	Size	Relation to bronchus	Junctional activity	Metastasis	Post mortem
Todd (5) 1	PM	both lungs—multiple	hens eggs	—		—	limited
2	PM	right lung multiple	—	—		—	limited
Funkel and Torrey (6)	PM	LUL/hilum	—	—		within the lung	limited
Carlucci and Schleusser (7)	R lung	RML, RLL, and hilum	5 cm	tumour in RML, RLL, bronchi and hilar nodes ? site of origin	none		no
Allen and Spitz (8)	Resection	—	—	in bronchus	yes, in squamous and ciliated epithelium	Previous MM	alive at 3 years
Hsu et al. (9)	R lung	RML and anterior RUL	6 cm	origin in UL bronchus	none	died with recurrence	no
Salm (10)	L lung bronchus	2 cm	polypoid tumour	yes, in squamous in bronchus	widespread metaplasia	yes metastases	
Reed and Kent (2)	LLL	'central'	3.5 cm	not related to bronchus	none	none	alive at 10 years
Reid and Mehta (11)	R lung	medical RLL	4.5 cm	intraluminal growth	none	none	alive at 11 years
Jensen and Egedorf (13)	LUL apical segments	uncertain	4 cm	infiltration of lung and bronchus	none	recurrence and metastases	yes
Allen and Dash (14)	RLL	apical lower	5 cm	dome-like projection into bronchus	yes, in ciliated epithelium	none	alive
Taboada et al. (15)	LLL	base	4 cm	no relation to bronchus	none	recurrences in lung and scar	yes
	L lung	LUL	?	overgrowth of bronchus	none	none	alive at 3 years
Adebonojo et al. (15)	R lung	hilum and all lobes	10 cm	arising from R main bronchus infiltrating carina	yes, in ciliated epithelium	hilar mode metastases	alive at 3 years
Robertson et al (16)	PM	hilum and RML	?	R main and RML bronchus	none	died with metastases	yes
Gephardt et al. (18)	PM	RUL	?	polypoid tumour in left main bronchus	none	MM in hilar LN PH adeno in LN	limited
Carstens et al. (19)	RUL	central	4 cm	parabronchial	yes, in squamous epithelium	metastases of unknown origin	yes
Herbert (20)	LUL	central	?	extruding from bronchus	yes, in ciliated epithelium	died with metastases	no

lung (15). In fact this paper includes no discussion about the origin of these tumours, and most subsequent authors consider that the tumours in both these patients could well have been metastatic. Kunkel and Torrey report the case of a young woman with an extensive pulmonary malignant melanoma which was considered to have arisen as a primary growth in the chest (6). Although the diagnosis was made at necropsy, alternative sites of origin were not excluded. Carlucci and Schleussner report another case, unproven by necropsy, in which a possible primary malignant melanoma was surgically resected (7).

In a large series including 337 primary melanomas, Allen and Spitz include a case which they consider to be a primary melanoma of lung (18). These authors state that no melanoma, except the malignant blue naevus, can be regarded with certainty as a primary tumour unless junctional activity can be demonstrated in the overlying epithelium. They describe criteria for differentiating junctional activity from intra-epithelial spread of metastatic melanoma and consider that this histological evidence alone is sufficient to establish the primary nature of a melanoma. The case presented in this series as a primary lung tumour shows junctional activity in squamous and ciliated epithelium, but occurred 6 years after a malignant melanoma had been resected from the hard palate. Subsequent authors, in attempting to establish with certainty the existence of primary melanomas of lung, have been forced to exclude the evidence of cases such as this. This does not alter the fact that Allen and Spitz may have been right in regarding their case as arising as a second primary in the bronchial mucosa. A further case is reported in 1962 by Hsu et al. in which the clinical evidence suggests that a resected pulmonary melanoma may be a primary tumour but there is insufficient histological or follow-up evidence to be certain (9).

The first well documented case, which not only fulfils the histological criteria laid down by Allen and Spitz but also excludes an alternative site of origin both by clinical and subsequent full necropsy examination, was reported by Salm in 1963 (10). This is generally regarded by subsequent authors as the first acceptable example of this condition. In the following years there has been a steady flow of individual case reports suggesting that the condition is less rare than originally believed.

Reed and Kent report 2 cases, one of which concerned the surgical resection of a malignant melanoma in the lung of a 71 year old man who was alive 10 years later without clinical evidence of an alternative primary site or of metastatic disease (2). These authors do not mention histological criteria for establishing the primary nature of the tumour, and themselves regard the site of origin as uncertain. They compare this case with another in which a 66 year old man was alive and well 3 years after resection of a solitary pulmonary metastasis resulting from an intra-ocular melanoma removed 31 years earlier.

Reid and Mehta present 2 cases considered to be primary malignant melanomas arising in the bronchus and trachea respectively (11). The first case resulted from the re-classification, during an extensive review of the pathology of lung cancer, of a lung tumour originally described as large cell anaplastic carcinoma (12). This case, although undoubtedly a malignant melanoma, does not show histological evidence of being a primary tumour. The authors state that there was no clinical evidence of an alternative primary site: there are no necropsy data because the patient was alive and free of disease when the report was written, 11 years after pneumonectomy. The second case is a tracheal tumour, in which there is evidence of junctional activity as well as intraepithelial spread of melanoma cells, which was resected from a man who died postoperatively. Necropsy did not reveal any metastases or an alternative primary site.

Jensen and Egedorf report a case, with necropsy and clinical data to suggest that the tumour was primary, but little histological evidence for this. These authors propose clinical criteria, in addition to histological and pathological ones, to establish the primary nature of these tumours (13).

Allen and Drash report a further case with junctional activity in ciliated epithelium and stress the need to observe the histological criteria for diagnosing the tumour as primary (14). An alternative primary site is excluded by clinical history and the survival time after surgical resection is not stated. Two cases are reported by Taboada et al., one with and one without autopsy confirmation (15). In the only recorded case of a primary melanoma of lung occurring in a black woman, Adebonojo makes the point that surgical treatment was delayed by the initial assumption that the lesion was metastatic (16). Removal of two benign naevi preceded pneumonectomy. Two more case reports, including necropsy data, describe melanomas which appear likely to have arisen in the lung (17, 18).

A recent case report provides histological evidence that the tumours are primary as well as full necropsy and clinical data to exclude an alternative primary site (19). The present author has reported a case, illustrated below, in which histological evidence of primary neoplasia allowed a diagnosis to be made on bronchial biopsy and cytology (20).

Tracheal and Tracheo-bronchial Melanoma

The second patient described by Reid and Mehta provided convincing histological clinical and necropsy evidence for the origin of melanoma in the trachea (11). Mori et al. describe the surgical resection of an early tracheal melanoma (21). There are 2 case reports of multiple tracheo-bronchial malignant melanomas with histological appearances to suggest that they might be primary (22, 23). These tracheal tumours will be included in the discussion of the evidence for regarding melanomas as primary, but have not been included in the Tables 1 and 2 which have been confined to pulmonary malignant melanomas of lung, as reported in the English language literature.

Pleural Melanomaa

There is a single case report of a malignant melanoma arising in the pleura (24). In view of the different histogenesis of mesothelium, this case will not be discussed further.

CASE REPORT OF A PRIMARY MELANOMA OF LUNG (20)

The rarity of this type of lung tumour is reflected by the fact that only one case has been reported in 15 years among the surgical specimens received from the Wessex Regional Cardiothoracic Surgical Unit, during which time there have been approximately 200–250 pulmonary resections per year.

A 37 year old Caucasian man was referred from Jersey for investigation of a 6-week history of haemoptysis. He had smoked 15 cigarettes per day for 25 years but had recently given this up. Chest radiographs showed a shadow, estimated size 6 × 3 cm, situated at the left hilum and extending into the anterior segment of the upper lobe. Tomograms and computed tomography (CT) scanning suggested dilatation of bronchi by mucus distal to an intra-bronchial neoplasm. Bronchoscopy revealed a dark brown/black coloured tumour extruding at the origin of the anterior and apico-posterior segmental bronchi of the upper lobe.

Biopsy of this lesion showed a close-packed spindle-celled invasive tumour with obvious dusky pigmentation which was confirmed to be melanin by Masson–Fontana staining (Figures 1 and 2). The broncial epithelium overlying and adjacent to the tumour, and also the mucous gland ducts in the sub-mucosa, showed the presence of scattered intra-epithelial melanocytes with similar cytological appearance to free infiltrating cells in the underlying tissue (Figure 3). These cells had granular melanin in their cytolplasm. Melanin was also present between the ciliated bronchial cells and within their cytoplasm, particularly under the luminal surface (Figures 4 and 5).

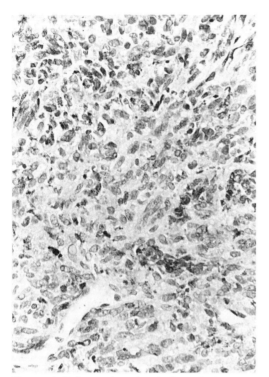

Figure 1 Polygonal and spindle-celled malignant melanoma. H&E.

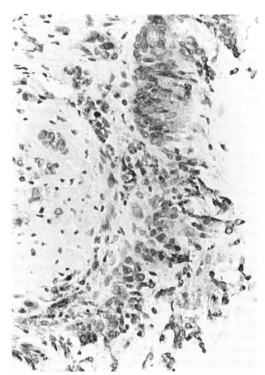

Figure 3 Atypical melanocytes in ciliated bronchial epithelium and infiltrating beneath the epithelium. H&E.

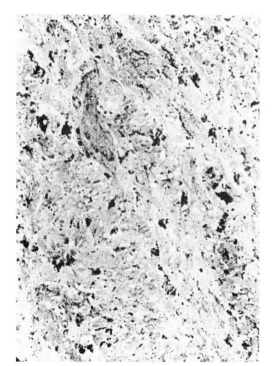

Figure 2 Pigment in tumour confirmed to be melanin. Masson–Fontana.

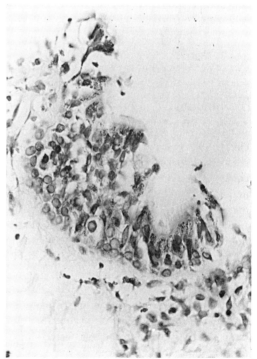

Figure 4 Atypical melanocytes in bronchial epithelium and granular pigment within ciliated cells. H&E.

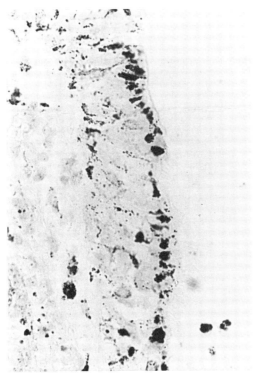

Figure 5   Melanin demonstrated in intra-epithelial melanocytes and within the cytoplasm of
ciliated cells. Masson–Fontana.

The appearance was interpreted as malignant melanoma with junctional activity, and secondary uptake of melanin by ciliated cells. This was evidence of primary neoplasia, and suggested the possibility of an origin in a pre-existing lentigo.

Bronchial brush cytology also showed non-cohesive pigmented malignant melanoma cells and bronchial epithelial cells containing pigment.

A full clinical history and examination did not provide any evidence of an alternative primary site. The bronchial neoplasm was assessed as operable, but resection was not carried out in view of the demonstration of metastases in vertebrae, ribs and liver by CT scanning. He remained well for a few months during which time he received radiotherapy and vincristine. Just over 4 months after bronchoscopy, he was re-admitted with signs

of cerebral metastases and died shortly after-wards. There is no record of a post-mortem.

The diagnosis in this case rests on clinical and histological evidence, both of which suggest that this was a primary neoplasm in the bronchus.

HISTOGENESIS OF MALIGNANT MELANOMA

Before assessing the likelihood of individual tumours being primary growths in the lung, or describing the clinical and pathological features of this group of tumours, it is necessary to consider the development of malignant melanoma in general, the origin of melanocytes and the development melanoma at other mucosal sites.

The Development of Malignant Melanoma

The majority of cutaneous malignant melanomas arise from the neoplastic proliferation of pre-existing melanocytes within the epithelium (25). The nests of neoplastic melanocytes in the lower part of the epidermis are referred to as junctional activity. This can be seen in previously normal skin, the epidermal component of a pre-existing benign naevus or a lentigo (an area of pigmentation, with hyperplasia of melanocytes), and in all these instances the process of neoplasia is the same. It is very rare for malignant change to occur in a blue naevus or in the dermal component of a benign compound or intra-dermal naevus (26).

The classification of cutaneous malignant melanoma into three main types with the addition of acro-lentiginous malignant melanoma as a fourth (25, 27), is still widely used although there has been recent controversy about its clinical and biological significance (28–30).

(a) Malignant melanoma arising in lentigo maligna. Lentigo maligna, otherwise known as Hutchinson's melanotic freckle, is a variegated

pigmented lesion with atypical hyperplastic melanocytes in the basal layer of the epidermis associated with solar degenerative changes in the skin. It is not in itself malignant. Malignant melanoma arising in lentigo maligna occurs at a mean age of 70 years and is twice as common in women.

(b) Malignant melanoma of superficial spreading type. This is the commonest type and is characterized by an intra-epidermal radial growth phase whch precedes and later accompanies the vertical growth phase (dermal invasion). It is commoner in women and occurs at a mean age of 45 years.

(c) Nodular melanoma. This is the least common, carries the worst prognosis, is commoner in men and occurs at a mean age of 50 years. It is characterized by dermal invasion from the outset.

(d) Acro-lentiginous melanoma. This includes sub-ungual melanoma and those arising on the palms and soles. It has a radial growth phase similar to that of lentigo maligna. This type of melanoma is the only one seen with any frequency in black people and occurs equally in men and women.

It used to be considered that malignant melanoma arising in lentigo maligna had a better prognosis than the other types (26, 27). It is now agreed that the prognosis is related to the depth of invasion of the vertical growth phase which is biologically different from the radial growth phase (30).

The Origin of Melanocytes

During the earlier part of this century there was debate and controversy about the origin of the melanocyte, although it was generally agreed that this was the cell of origin for malignant melanoma. The disagreement was between those who held the opinion that

melanocytes were derived from the transformation of basal epidermal cells (31: Allen 1949) and those who believed that the melanocyte was a specific type of cell (32, 33). This was finally confirmed by the experimental work of Rawles and other workers who demonstrated that melanocytes migrate from the neural crest during embryonic life and populate the skin, uveal tract, meninges and ectodermal mucous membranes (34).

Mucosal Malignant Melanoma

The majority of mucosal malignant melanomas, which account for less than 5% of all melanomas, arise in juxta-cutaneous mucosa, such as the ano-rectum, nasal and oral cavity, all of which are ectodermal in origin. Although some of these arise de novo, either as melanoma of superficial spreading type or nodular melanoma, many of those in the mouth, and also vagina, arise in pigmented plaques histologically analogous to lentigo maligna, but with a greater malignant potential (26, 35). Oral and nasal melanomas are commoner in black and oriental races and are related to ectopic pigmentation at these sites (36, 37). Similarly leptomeningeal melanoma is associated with pre-existing pigmentation (27).

The development of malignant melanoma below the level of the oropharynx or above the anorectum is exceptionally rare, which is not surprising in view of the endodermal origin of this epithelium. Melanocytes are not normally found below the level of the oropharnx (38). Genuine primary malignant melanomas have rarely been described in the larynx (39), oesophagus (40), gall bladder (41) and rectum (42) as well as in the lower respiratory tract and pleura. They have also been described in the adrenal (19), ovary, vagina and cervix (1). In an increasing number of these sites, including the larynx, vagina and oesophagus, melanocytes have been demonstrated in a small proportion of individuals in the absence of melanoma and usually in the absence of overt pigmentation (43–45).

The Histogenesis of Malignant Melanoma of Lung

The laryngo-tracheal bud grows caudally as a ventral diverticulum from the foregut, below the pharynx and just proximal to the liver diverticulum, before differentiation of the intervening oesophagus and stomach (46). This process starts at the third week of fetal life and at the fourth week the trachea divides into the two main bronchi. Between the fourth and twelfth weeks the bronchi divide into lobar and segmental branches, at this stage remaining as direct branches of the primary bronchus. It is during this time that migration of neural crest cells occurs. The neural crest develops cranio-caudally and in the human fetus it is present throughout its length by the fourth week after ovulation. Melanocytes are not observed in the fetal dermis until the eighth week, appearing first in the head region. It is during the fourth to eighth week that migration is believed to occur through the embryonic mesenchyme (47). It seems possible that melanocytes could occasionally populate bronchial and other mucosal epithelium during this period of migration.

Reid and Mehta considered that the association of junctional activity with squamous metaplasia in tracheal and bronchial melanomas could be considered to provide evidence for their origin from melanocytic metaplasia of epithelial cells, supporting earlier views of Allen and Spitz that melanomas were epithelial in origin (8, 11). Although it is now recognized that para-endocrine cells of the APUD series arise from local endodermal cells rather than from cells migrating from the neural crest, which is supported by the frequent finding of neurosecretory granules in tumour cells from all types of bronchogenic carcinomas (48), there is no evidence for melanocytic differentiation in any form of carcinoma. Peripheral nerve tumours may show melanocytic differentiation (49), but this group of tumours do not overlap with the spectrum of differentiation seen in either carcinomas or sarcomas.

All the evidence of the embryological development of melanocytes and the biological behaviour of cutaneous melanomas supports the view of Becker (33) that 'cutaneous melanoblasts are distinct from palisade epidermal basal cells. They undergo benign neoplasia to produce pigmented nevus and malignant neoplasia to produce melanoma.' When malignant melanomas do arise in the lung and other unusual sites it seems highly probable that they arise by a similar mechanism to that so clearly described in the skin. It is the aetiological factors which must be different, as with acro-lentiginous and juxta-mucosal melanoma, in that exposure to sunlight is not involved.

EVIDENCE FOR A PRIMARY ORIGIN OF MELANOMA IN THE LOWER RESPIRATORY TRACT

It is evident from the published cases of primary melanoma of lung that different authors use different criteria for establishing the primary nature of the lesions they describe, not all of which are present in any individual case. The evidence can be divided into three broad categories based on histopathological, clinical and necropsy findings.

Histological Evidence

As described by Allen and Spitz and agreed by subsequent authors, the presence of junctional activity, manifest by nests of malignant melanocytes in the epithelium overlying and adjacent to a melanoma, is evidence that it is primary at that site (8, 27, 50). This evidence may be lost in large tumours or when there is ulceration of the overlying mucosa. In the skin, junctional activity must be distinguished from the occasional 'epidermotropic' metastases which invade the epidermis and may simulate primary neoplasia (27). Unlike true junctional activity in a primary melanoma, this does not spread into epithelium adjacent to the tumour which should occur to some extent in a primary melanoma, even a nodular one (27, 51).

Furthermore, these epidermotropic metastases occur as multiple deposits and not as solitary neoplasms.

Junctional activity is mentioned as evidence for primary growth of the melanoma in 6 out of the 15 published cases of pulmonary melanoma in which the history is recorded (8, 10, 14, 16, 19, 20).

Junctional activity is also described in 2 solitary tracheal and 2 multiple tracheo-bronchial melanomas (11, 20–22). The latter 2 reports describe very similar multiple areas of junctional activity with and without invasion. Verweij et al. (22) can find no other source of primary growth and interpret their case as one of multifocal primary tracheo-bronchial melanoma. Rosenberg et al. (23) suggest that the lesions in their case may represent metastases implanted during repeated bronchocopies carried out to fulgurate and control bleeding in a bronchial melanoma, itself a probable metastasis from a facial melanoma. The histological appearance of these multiple tumours would be difficult to distinguish from a mucosal equivalent of epidermotrophic metastases. In two of the solitary melanomas, one pulmonary and one tracheal, malignant cells are seen directly infiltrating the ciliated epithelium overlying the tumour. This is interpreted as direct spread in one case and as evidence for primary neoplasia in the other (11, 14). It must be recognized that junctional activity in ciliated epithelium is less accurately documented and may not always be the exact counterpart of that seen in the skin (22).

In spite of these reservations about the significance of intra-epithelial melanoma cells, there is some convincing evidence of true junctional activity among the published cases, particularly in those reported by Salm, and Allen and Drash (10, 14).

Salm illustrates nests of melanoma cells infiltrating ciliated epithelium and also pagetoid spread within foci of squamous metaplasia adjacent to the tumour base (10). Allen and Drash illustrate a transition between normal ciliated epithelium through epithelium containing basal atypical melanoytes to an area

adjacent to the main tumour mass where the basal melanoma cells are dropping off into nests below the epithelium (14). The appearance in both tumours of a pigmented 'flare' around a largely amelanotic tumour is difficult to reconcile with anything but a primary tumour.

The atypical melanocytes in the adjacent mucosa of the case described by Allen and Drash are very similar to those illustrated in Figure 3 and resemble lentigo maligna rather than superficial spreading melanoma (20). Similar observations have been made about the pigmented flares around other forms of primary mucosal and also acro-lentiginous melanomas, suggesting a comparable histogenesis (26).

Allen and Spitz and Carstens et al. describe and illustrate junctional activity in squamous and/or ciliated epithelium (8, 19) Adebonojo et al. describe but do not illustrate junctional ativity in ciliated epithelium (16). These descriptons and illustrations provide histological evidence for the existence of this entity.

The gross appearance of the tumour is often an important factor in deciding whether a lung tumour is primary or secondary. Metastases are typically well circumscribed lesions situated in the pulmonary parenchyma: lack of bronchial involvement would mitigate against a primary origin. Polypoid intra-bronchial tumours, as described in the majority of published cases of primary melanomas of lung, would be consistent with a primary tumour. Thus the finding of several circumscribed tumours, not related to bronchi and resected on different occasions, raises some doubt in the first case reported by Taboada et al., although an alternative site of origin was not found at necropsy (15). This should better be regarded as pulmonary melanoma of unknown origin, and not as a proven bronchial primary.

In summary, primary melanomas are likely to be intra-bronchial rather than in the pulmonary parenchyma itself, although it may not be possible to establish the bronchial origin if the tumour is large. Junctional activity adjacent to the main tumour mass is strong evidence that it is a primary tumour. It must be interpreted with caution in ciliated epithelium, particularly in multiple lesions or where the infiltration is directly overlying the tumour.

Clinical Evidence

In order to establish that a mucosal melanoma is primary, a full history and examination is required to exclude an alternative primary site. In the published cases, 2 patients had benign naevi resected either as an unrelated previous operation or in order to exclude malignancy (16, 19). The histology in both cases was reviewed as benign. It seems highly unlikely that either of these lesions was misinterpreted, since they were both assessed in the light of the subsequent pulmonary malignant melanoma. In one case report, naevi were described on the lower leg and dorsum of the same foot. These were not biopsied, so that an element of doubt remains (9).

The possibility of multiple primary tumours is raised by the case reported by Allen and Spitz (8). Using their criteria, 3.6% of 337 primary melanomas were multiple. This is higher that most series, which range between 1.3 and 2.3% (52, 53). Although cases without evidence of a previous primary melanoma are required to establish the existence of primary melanoma at a particular site, in an individual case the possiblity of a second primary must be recognized if there is histopathological evidence to suggest that it is primary. This could well be important for patient management and treatment.

Clinical examination to exclude a conventional primary site should include examination of the skin, eyes, nasal and oral cavities, anal canal and genitalia. As well as pigmented and amelanotic lesions and excision scars, it is necessary to be aware of the clinical appearance of regression of a malignant melanoma which is well documented although rare (4, 27). These often look inflamed and hypopigmented and do not return to completely normal skin. There is usually, but not always, a history of a pre-existing melanotic lesion and

metastases are often found in the lymph nodes draining the site. It is possible that such lesions could be missed and be associated with unexplained metastases (54).

Long clinical follow-up after surgical resection is evidence in favour of the lesion being primary rather than metastatic, although the overall survival following surgical resection of solitary pulmonary metastases in general is surprisingly good. For solitary metastases from all sites Moersch and Clagett, and Wilkins et al. report 5-year survivals approaching 30% (3, 55). However, the survival figures for resection of the solitary metastatic melanoma among these cases is not so good: in a survey of 254 cases reported in the literature at that time, Wilkins et al. found no examples of malignant melanoma among the 5-year survivors (55). Reed and Kent report 3-year survival following resection of a single pulmonary metastasis considered to have arisen from an ocular melanoma removed 31 years before (2).

In summary, the diagnosis of primary malignant melanoma of lung requires a full clinical history and examination to exclude the current existence, previous resection or regression of a cutaneous, ocular or juxta-cutaneous melanoma. In the absence of evidence of an alternative primary site, survival beyond 5 years after pulmonary resection is strong clinical evidence in favour of the tumour being primary.

Necropsy Evidence

A full necropsy to exclude alternative sites of origin, such as leptomeninges, nasal cavity, oropharynx, is clearly required to establish with certainty that a particular lung melanoma is primary. Thus Salm gave the first convincing evidence for the existence of this condition as an entity (10). Five of the published cases provide full necropsy data to support the primary nature of the melanoma (10, 13, 15, 17, 19). As with clinical examination, it is necessary to recognize the appearance of regressed melanomas as well as active ones, and to look for cutaneous scars and localizing lymph node metastases.

Certain problems remain, even at necropsy. Thus it is possible that small primaries could be missed, or the site of origin remain obscure. The necropsy in the case reported by Gephardt et al., for example, provided no explanation for the metastatic adenocarcinoma seen in a cervical lymph node biopsy 8 years before the patient presented with a pulmonary melanoma (18). In large series of melanomas there is usually a small group of about 4% with metastases from an unknown primary site (25, 54). There is no comment as to whether any of these patients had necropsies.

With greater acceptance of the lung as a primary site for malignant melanoma the diagnosis is likely to be made more often during life. This is clearly of great value in the management and treatment of patients. Necropsy remains essential for confirmation in order to avoid the overdiagnosis which is likely to occur for a relatively 'optimistic' form of pulmonary involvement by melanoma.

Assessment of Validity of Published Reports

It is impossible to access the validity of some of the individual cases with any degree of certainty, but they have been roughly categorized as 2 'proven', 8 'near proven', 4 'probable' and 4 'improbable' cases as analysed below.

There are 2 published cases which can be described as 'proven' with full histological, clinical and necropsy evidence of having arisen as primary tumours in the lung (10, 19).

There are a further 4 in which the diagnosis seems reasonably certain in that the pathology was consistent with a primary tumour and either long term survival or full necropsy supported this diagnosis (2, 11, 13, 17). The similar histopathological and clinical findings, with rather shorter follow-up, suggest that the second case reported by Taboada et al. and that reported by Adebonojo et al. should be regarded as almost equally probable as should the case reported by Gephardt, with the negative, albeit limited necropsy (15, 16, 28). In spite of the lack of prolonged follow-up or

necropsy, the histopathological appearance of the case reported by Allen and Drash almost certainly represents a primary tumour (14). These 8 cases have been categorized as 'near proven'.

Although reservations have been expressed about the lack of follow-up or necropsy in some of the cases (7, 9), and the 'second' primary reported by Allen and Spitz (8) these cases provide considerable evidence to suggest that they may be primary. The limited histological material available in the case illustrated in Figures 1–5 and the lack of necropsy data leave this case in a similar category of 'probable' (20). Four cases have been assessed as probably metastatic or insufficiently documented (5, 6, 16: case 1).

CLINICAL AND PATHOLOGICAL FEATURES OF 14 PRIMARY MELANOMAS OF LUNG

An analysis of the clinical and pathological features of the 14 'proven', 'near proven' and 'probable' cases should give some useful information on this rare condition.

The case histories of these 14 patients indicate that the mode of presentation is similar to that of primary bronchogenic carcinoma (Table 1). Haemoptysis is the commonest single symptom, followed by chest pain. Three patients were asymptomatic, and found to have shadows on a routine chest x-ray.

In this small number of patients there is a preponderance of females (57%) which is similar to the slight excess of women usually noted for malignant melanoma (25, 27) and the reverse of the male preponderance which is still seen in bronchogenic carcinoma. The ratio of males:females with lung cancer is falling, but was still 6:1 in 1969, the approximate midpoint of the published cases of primary melanoma of lung (46).

Of the 5 cases in which there is a comment about cigarette smoking all were smokers. (One non-smoker is mentioned in the 'improbable' group.) The average age of the patients, which is similar for males and females, is 48 years which is comparable to the expected age for nodular and superficial spreading malignant melanoma (25).

Only 2 of the patients received adjuvant chemotherapy and radiotherapy, so that the effects of this cannot be assessed.

Most of the tumours were polypoid, intraluminal or had infiltrated the bronchial wall (2, 15). Histologically, most were described as pleomorphic/polygonal or spindle-celled tumours. One tumour, which lacked junctional activity, was described as looking similar to a malignant blue naevus (17). They were predominantly pigmented, except for the ones reported by Salm (10) and Allen and Drash (14) which were partially or largely amelanotic, with a pigmented 'flare' around the tumour. This may reflect the fact that amelanotic melanomas in the lung are highly likely to be interpreted as anaplastic carcinomas (12).

There is an impression from these cases that prolonged survival following surgery might be more frequent than would be expected, particularly in view of the size of some of these tumours. The average recorded size is 4.9 cm which is well above the usual size of a resected cutaneous melanoma. In view of this, these pulmonary tumours can only be compared with the worst prognostic group of malignant melanomas, categorized by Clark et al. as level V (25). Of the 12 patients with surgically resected primary malignant melanomas 60% were alive and disease free after an average of 5 years compared with 12% of patients with Level V malignant melanomas after an average of 3.6 years (25). These figures do indicate a somewhat better survival for this rare form of melanoma.

SUMMARY

Eighteen published cases of primary melanoma of the lung have been reviewed, one of which has been illustrated. The evidence suggests that the majority are acceptable as primary tumours. Certain intriguing questions remain to be answered before the histogenesis of this tumour can be explained. Is it possible that melanomas of the lung might arise in premalignant lentigos in the bronchus? Would a systemic search reveal melanocytes in the bronchi of normal individuals? Is the apparent connection with cigarette smoking genuine or coincidental? It is not possible to answer these questions from a retrospective study, but they are more likely to be answered with greater acceptance of the existence of this site for the origin of malignant melanoma so that larger numbers of cases can be analysed.

REFERENCES

1 DasGupta TK, Brasfield RD, Paglia MA. Primary melanomas at unusual sites. Surg Gynecol Obstet 1969; 128: 841–8.

2 Reed RJ, Kent EM. Solitary pulmonary melanomas. J Thorac Cardiovasc Surg 1964; 48: 226–31.

3 Moersch RN, Clagett OT. Pulmonary resection for metastatic tumors of the lungs. Surgery 1961; 50: 579–85.

4 Smith JL, Stehlin JS Jr. Spontaneous regression of primary malignant melanoma with regional metastases. Cancer 1965; 18: 1399–415.

5 Todd FW. Two cases of melanotic tumours in the lungs. JAMA 1888; 11: 53–4.

6 Funkel OF, Torrey E. Report of a case of primary melanotic sarcoma of lung presenting difficulties in differentiating from tuberculosis. NY J Med 1926; 16: 198–201.

7 Carlucci GA, Schleussner RC. Primary (?) melanoma of the lung. A case report. J Thorac Surg 1941–2; 11: 643–9.

8 Allen AC, Spitz S. Malignant melanoma. A clinicopathological analysis of the criteria for diagnosis and prognosis. Cancer 1953; 6: 1–45.

9 Hsu C-W, Wu S-C, Ch'en C-S. Melanoma of the lung. Chin Med J 1962; 81: 263–6.

10 Salm R. A primary malignant melanoma of the bronchus. J Pathol Bacteriol 1963; 85: 121–6.

11 Reid JD, Mehta VT. Melanoma of the lower respiratory tract. Cancer 1966; 19: 627–31.

12 Reid JD, Carr AH. The validity and value of histological and cytological classifications of lung cancer. Cancer 1961; 14: 673–98.

13 Jensen OA, Egedorf J. Primary malignant melanoma of the lung. Scand J Resp Dis 1967; 48: 127–35.

14 Allen MS Jr, Drash EC. Primary melanoma of the lung. Cancer 1968; 21: 154–9.

15 Taboada CF, McMurray JD, Jordan RA, Sey-

bold WD. Primary melanoma of the lung. Chest 1972; 62: 629–31.

16 Adebonojo SA, Grillo IA, Durodola JI. Primary malignant melanoma of the bronchus. J Natl Med Assoc 1979; 71: 579–81.

17 Robertson AJ, Sinclair DJM, Sutton PP, Guthrie W. Primary melanocarcinoma of the lower respiratory tract. Thorax 1980; 35: 158–9.

18 Gephardt GN. Malignant melanoma of the bronchus. Hum Pathol 1981; 12: 671–3.

19 Carstens PHB, Kuhns JG, Ghazi C. Primary malignant melanomas of the lung and adrenal. Hum Pathol 1984; 15: 910–14.

20 Herbert A. Primary malignant melanoma of lung diagnosed by bronchial biopsy. A case report (submitted for publication).

21 Mori K, Cho H, Som M. Primary 'flat' melanoma of the trachea. J Pathol Bacteriol 1977; 121: 101–5.

22 Verweij J, Breed WPM, Jansveld CAF. Primary tracheo-bronchial melanoma. Neth J Med 1982; 25: 163–6.

23 Rosenberg LM, Polanco GB, Blank S. Multiple tracheobronchial melanomas with 10-year survival. JAMA 1965; 192: 717–19.

24 Smith S, Opipari MI. Primary pleural melanoma. A first reported case and literature review. J Thorac Cardiovasc Surg 1978; 75: 827–31.

25 Clark WH Jr, From L, Bernardino EA, Mihm MC. The histogenesis and biologic behavior of primary human malignant melanomas of the skin. Cancer Res 1969; 29: 705–27.

26 Clark WH Jr, Ainsworth AM, Bernardino EA, Yang C-H, Mihm MC, Reed RJ. The developmental biology of primary human malignant melanomas. Sem Oncol 1975; 2: 83–103.

27 McGovern VJ. Melanoma. Histological Diagnosis and Prognosis. Biopsy Interpretation Series. New York: Raven Press, 1983.

28 Ackerman AB, David KM. A unifying concept of malignant melanoma. Hum Pathol 1986; 17: 438–40.

29 Flotte TJ, Mihm MC Jr. The art versus the science of dermatopathology. Hum Pathol 1986; 17: 441–2.

30 Clark WH Jr, Elder DE, Van Horn M. The biologic forms of malignant melanoma. Hum Pathol 1986; 17: 443–50.

31 Allen AC. A reorientation of the histogenesis and clinical significance of cutaneous nevi and melanomas. Cancer 1949; 2: 28–56.

32 Masson P. My conception of cellular nevi. Cancer 1951; 4: 9–38.

33 Becker SW. Microscopic analysis of normal melanoblasts, nevus cells and melanoma cells. In: Gordon M ed Pigment Cell Growth. Pro-

ceedings of the Third Conference on the Biology of Normal and Atypical Pigment Cell Growth. New York: Academic Press, 1953: 109–19.

34 Rawles ME. Origin of the mammalian pigment cell and its role in the pigmentation of hair. In: Gordon M ed Pigment Cell Growth. Proceedings of the Third Conference on the Biology of Normal and Atypical Pigment Cell Growth. New York: Academic Press, 1953: 1–15.

35 Takagi M, Ishikawa G, Mori W. Primary malignant melanoma of the oral cavity in Japan with special reference to mucosal melanosis. Cancer 1974; 34: 358–70.

36 Broomhall C, Lewis MG. Malignant melanoma of the oral cavity in Ugandan Africans. Br J Surg 1967; 54: 581–4.

37 Lewis MG, Martin JAM. Malignant melanoma of the nasal cavity of Ugandan Africans. Relationship of ectopic pigmentation. Cancer 1967; 20: 1699–705.

38 Becker SW. Melanin pigmentation. A systematic study of the pigment of the human skin and upper mucous membranes, with special consideration of pigmented dendritic cells. Arch Dermatol Syph 1927; 16: 259–90.

39 Welsh LW, Welsh JJ. Malignant melanoma of the larynx. Laryngoscope 1961; 71: 185–91.

40 Pomeranz AA, Garlock JH. Primary melanocarcinoma of the esophagus. Ann Surg 1955; 142: 296–301.

41 Walsh TS. Primary melanoma of the gallbladder with cervical metastasis and fourteen and a half year survival. Cancer 1956; 9: 518–22.

42 Mason JK, Helwig EB. Ano-rectal melanoma. Cancer 1966; 19: 39–50.

43 Pesce C, Toncini C. Melanin pigmentation of the larynx. Acta Otolaryngol 1983; 96: 189–92.

44 de la Pava S, Nigogosyan G, Pickren JW, Cabrera A. Melanosis of the esophagus. Cancer 1963; 16: 48–50.

45 Nigogosyan G, de la Pava S, Pickren JW. Melanoblasts in vaginal mucosa. Origin for primary malignant melanoma. Cancer 1964; 17: 912–13.

46 Spencer H. Pathology of the Lung, 4th edition. Oxford: Pergamon Press, 1985: 1–16; 837–932.

47 Zimmermann AA, Becker SW. Precursors of epidermal melanocytes in the negro fetus. In: Gordon M ed Pigment Cell Growth. Proceedings of the Third Conference on the Biology of Normal and Atypical Pigment Cell Growth. New York: Academic Press, 1953: 159–81.

48 Carter D, Eggleston JC. Tumors of the Lower Respiratory Tract. Washington DC: Armed Forces Institute of Pathology, 1979.

49 Enzinger FM, Weiss SW. Soft Tissue Tumors. St Louis: CV Mosby, 1983: 580–675.

50 Lever WF, Schaumburg-Lever G. Histopatho-
    logy of the Skin, 6th edition. Philadelphia: JB
    Lippincott, 1983; 681–725.
51 Kornberg R, Harris M, Ackerman AB. Epider-
    motropically metastatic malignant melanoma:
    differentiating malignant melanoma to the epi-
    dermis from malignant melanoma primary in
    the epidermis. Arch Dermatol 1976; 114: 67–9.
52 Pack GT, Scharnagal IM, Hillyer RA. Multiple
    primary melanoma. A report of 16 cases. Cancer
    1952; 5: 1110–15.
53 McLeod R, Davis NC, Herron JJ, Caldwell RA,
    Little JH, Quinn RL. A retrospective survey of
    498 patients with malignant melanoma. Surg
    Gynecol Obstet 1968; 126: 99–108.
54 Das Gupta TK, Bowden L, Berg JW. Malignant
    melanoma of unknown primary origin. Surg
    Gynecol Obstet 1963; 117: 341–5.
55 Wilkins EW, Burke JF, Head JM. The surgical
    management of metastatic neoplasms in the
    lung. J Thorac Cardiovasc Surg 1961; 42: 298–
    309.

Textbook of Uncommon Cancer
Edited by C.J. Williams, J.G. Krikorian, M.R. Green and D. Raghavan
© 1988 John Wiley & Sons Ltd

Chapter **22**

Bronchial Gland Tumours ('Bronchial Adenomas')

R. Stuart-Harris* and
B.C. McCaughan†
* *Medical Oncology Unit, Department of Medicine, West-mead Hospital, Sydney and*
† *Department of Cardiothoracic Surgery, Royal Prince Alfred Hospital, Sydney, Australia*

INTRODUCTION

Bronchial adenomas were first documented in 1831 (1) and are rare tumours, comprising only about 1% of all primary bronchial tumours (2). However, they account for 8–10% of all bronchial tumours excised (3). They are derived from the epithelium, ducts and glands of the bronchial tree and are more appropriately referred to as bronchial gland tumours. Initially, it was assumed that they were benign tumours, hence the name adenoma ascribed to them in 1882 (4). However, it is now recognized that these tumours represent a wide spectrum of malignant potential. They are usually indolent malignant tumours with long natural histories, although truly benign and frankly malignant forms are not infrequent.

Bronchial gland tumours include the bronchial carcinoid, bronchial adenoid cystic carcinoma (cylindroma), bronchial mucoepidermoid carcinoma, mucous gland cyst adenoma and mixed tumours (salivary gland type). Mucous gland cyst adenomas are very rare indeed (13 cases reported) and are benign, while mixed tumours of salivary gland type are

even rarer (2 cases reported) (3). Neither of these tumours will be described further and the discussion will be limited to the three common tumours of the group, namely: bronchial carcinoid, bronchial adenoid cystic carcinoma and bronchial mucoepidermoid tumours. Bronchial carcinoids account for 90% of these tumours, adenoid cystic carcinoma 8% and mucoepidermoid tumours 2% (5). They occur with similar frequency in males and females, although a slight predominance of females has been noted (3, 6). The median age at presentation is in the fifth decade, although reported ages range from 4 to 82 years (3, 6, 7). However, it should be remembered that the onset of symptoms may antedate detection of the tumour by up to 20 years or more, reflecting their long natural history.

BRONCHIAL CARCINOIDS

Bronchial carcinoids are by far the most commonly encountered tumour of the so-called 'bronchial adenoma' group. However, they should no longer be classified as bronchial adenomas, but rather belong to the neuroendocrine group of tumours, the amine precursor uptake decarboxylase (APUD) tumours and appear to share with small cell carcinoma of the lung a common neuroectodermal stem cell. This has given rise to the concept, as described by DeCaro et al. (8), of the histogenetic spectrum of pulmonary APUD tumours, ranging from the typical well differentiated carcinoid to the undifferentiated small cell carcinoma of the lung. The cell origin for these tumours remains controversial although many favour the Kulchitsky cell of the respiratory epithelium (9). Although usually characterized by a slow growth pattern and a low incidence of metastatic disease, bronchial carcinoids on occasion behave as an aggressive malignant tumour (6).

Clinical Features

There are no known aetiological factors in the causation of bronchial carcinoids. Females slightly outnumber males but not significantly so (6). Patients with these tumours present most commonly in the fifth and sixth decades of life although there is a wide age range (6).

Unlike patients with bronchogenic carcinoma those with centrally located bronchial carcinoids may have respiratory symptoms for many years prior to diagnosis. Common symptoms are those of haemoptysis, dyspnoea and recurrent or persistent pneumonitis. Recent large series report an increasingly greater number of patients being asymptomatic with an abnormality detected on routine chest x-ray (6). These patients usually have a peripherally located tumour.

Less than 5% of patients with a primary bronchial carcinoma present with metastatic disease and of these a rare presentation is that of the carcinoid syndrome. The diagnosis of the carcinoid syndrome is suspected by the characteristic episodic cutaneous flushing and confirmed by a markedly elevated level of urinary 5-hydroxyindoleacetic acid (5-HIAA). Ricci et al. reviewed the literature (10) and found that 2–7% of patients with a primary bronchial carcinoma developed the carcinoid syn-

drome (6, 11, 12). Almost invariably hepatic metastases were present. Todd et al. (11) and Okike et al. (12) have reported patients in whom a bronchial carcinoid produced the carcinoid syndrome in the absence of metastases and following resection the syndrome disappeared. Even in the presence of metastases the most effective management of the carcinoid syndrome is the resection of all tumour bearing tissue wherever possible.

Pathology

Macroscopically, bronchial carcinoids are usually well encapsulated tumours without evidence of invasion into surrounding structures. Bronchoscopically they often have a glistening vascular appearance. When sectioned they characteristically have a tan colouring and may be lobulated.

Light microscopy defines two histological groups of bronchial carcinoid, the typical and atypical carcinoid, as described in the detailed reports from the Mayo Clinic (12, 13). The typical carcinoid has regular polyhedral cells arranged frequently in cords, trabecular and ribbon-like patterns. Although the diagnosis is usually suspected on routine staining techniques, histological confirmation may require argyrophilic stains or electron microscopy to define the characteristic neurosecretory granules. Rarely are mitoses seen in the typical carcinoid.

By comparison the atypical carcinoid may demonstrate one or more of the following features: increased mitotic activity, tumour necrosis, cellular pleomorphism, or increased cellularity and disorganization of the architecture (13).

Lymphatic involvement has been found in 10–20% of bronchial carcinoids (2, 6, 11–17). Although more commonly associated with atypical carcinoids lymphatic involvement will be found in 5–10% of typical carcinoids when a systematic lymph node dissection is routinely performed (6). Long term disease-free survival beyond 10 years following complete resection of the primary tumour and involved lymph nodes has been reported by many authors (6, 11–13, 15, 17). Recurrence following such resections is usually associated with an atypical histological appearance.

Haematogenous spread of a primary bronchial carcinoid is an infrequent occurrence. Hepatic, cerebral and bony metastases are the most common when distant spread occurs and as described previously may give rise to the carcinoid syndrome.

Investigation and Staging

As for the more common forms of bronchogenic carcinoma, the appropriate management of patients with a primary bronchial carcinoid requires an accurate anatomical and pathological diagnosis. By comparison, however, detailed staging procedures have far less importance in the management of patients with primary bronchial carcinoid compared with those with bronchogenic carcinoma. This relates to the good prognosis of carcinoid tumours even in the presence of lymphatic involvement or a cytological positive pleural effusion (6).

Accurate definition of the bronchial extent of these tumours when located centrally is of critical importance in planning surgical resection especially if bronchoplastic procedures are contemplated. Endobronchial tumours accessible to bronchoscopic biopsy will yield pathological confirmation of these tumours in almost all cases (6). However, there has been a reluctance to biopsy such tumours because of the risk of haemorrhage. Nevertheless, in most series significant haemorrhage has not been a major problem (2, 6, 11, 12, 14–17) although haemorrhage necessitating emergency pulmonary resection has been reported (18). Whilst the rigid bronchoscope should always be available when biopsing such tumours, endobronchial biopsy using the flexible fibreoptic bronchoscope presents no real risk of major haemorrhage. When bronchoscopically accessible the tumour should be biopsied because of the low yield from cytological examination of bronchial brushings and wash-

ings even in the presence of endobronchial disease (6). The presence of malignant cells may be identified on cytological examination but the differentiation between carcinoid, small cell carcinoma, or undifferentiated non-small cell bronchogenic carcinoma may not be possible and biopsy may still be necessary. This same constraint applies to fine needle aspiration of peripheral carcinoids. Not infrequently patients with a peripherally located carcinoid are diagnosed as small cell carcinoma of the lung following cytological evaluation of a fine needle aspirate. The correct diagnosis may only be reached after chemotherapy has failed to alter the radiological appearance of the mass and thoracotomy is performed. Peripheral small cell carcinomas are sufficiently rare that all such tumours, in the absence of significant mediastinal lymphadenopathy on computerized tomography, should be considered bronchial carcinoids until proven otherwise.

Staging procedures in these tumours should be limited. In the absence of symptoms of distant metastases routine cerebral, hepatic or bone scanning is not indicated. Mediastinoscopy, a technique often used to determine inoperability in non-small cell lung cancer, is not indicated in patients with a known bronchial carcinoid. The presence of mediastinal lymph node involvement should not per se preclude resection.

Preoperative assessment of cardiopulmonary reserve rarely requires the detailed testing performed in those patients with bronchogenic carcinoma. Patients with carcinoid tumours are frequently non-smokers and younger compared with those patients with primary bronchogenic carcinoma. However, when evaluating patients requiring resection for tumours located in the distal trachea or main stem bronchi assessment of pulmonary function is indicated.

Treatment and Prognosis

Resection remains the only effective treatment modality of primary bronchial carcinoids.

Controversy exists, however, as to the extent of resection necessary to obtain the most favourable results. Endobronchial resection whether used alone or in combination with transbronchoscopic implantation of radioactive sources invariably leads to local recurrence (6, 14, 15, 17, 19, 20) and on occasion distant metastases and even the carcinoid syndrome (6, 10). Endobronchial resection may give a misleading impression because of the very nature of these slowly growing tumours and it is only if the patients are followed long term that the inadequacy of this treatment is appreciated. This must be considered with the increasing use of laser techniques for endobronchial disease. Endobronchial resection, regardless of the technique employed, is an inappropriate first line therapy for patients with a primary bronchial carcinoid other than in those patients in whom medical contraindications prohibit thoracotomy. On the other hand, however, endobronchial treatment especially with the newer laser techniques may have a role in the management of recurrent inoperable tumours.

All patients without medical contraindication to thoracotomy and in whom the disease is limited to one hemithorax should undergo thoracotomy. The demonstration of free pleural fluid or mediastinal lymphadenopathy on computerized axial tomography does not preclude operation. The relative merits of bronchoplastic procedures and conservative resections, as opposed to conventional pulmonary resections, remains controversial. Some have believed that the malignant potential of these tumours has been exaggerated and that lung preserving procedures can be employed in the majority of cases (22, 23). However, it is only when large numbers of patients are reviewed and followed for at least 10 years that it is possible to accurately assess the success of treatment in these tumours which inherently have a slow pattern of growth and late metastases. McCaughan (6) reported recurrences presenting from 20 to 108 months following pulmonary resection for carcinoid (median duration 66 months).

In reviewing 181 patients at the Mayo Clinic, Okike et al. (19) detailed only 19 patients in whom a bronchoplastic procedure was performed. In all of these patients the histology was that of a 'typical' carcinoid, there were no lymphatic metastases and the tumours were small (mean 1.5 mm). At Memorial Sloan Kettering Cancer Center conservative procedures were used selectively for those patients in whom preoperative pulmonary function assessment precluded conventional resection for malignant disease (6). Pulmonary lobectomy was the most commonly performed resection in this series (55% of resections). Sleeve resection or segmentectomy or wedge resection was performed in only 10% of patients, again in patients with small tumours and no lymphatic metastases. Regardless of the extent of resection performed, systematic mediastinal lymph node dissection should routinely be performed, both for staging purposes and effective tumour management.

The actuarial disease-free survival in the Memorial series for bronchial carcinoids was 92% at 5 years and 77% at 10 years (6). The relative roles of tumour size, lymphatic metastases and the histological features of the tumour in influencing the chance of recurrence are difficult to determine. Larger tumours more commonly are atypical carcinoids and have a higher incidence of lymphatic involvement. The most important determinant of survival appears to be the histology (6, 8, 13, 15, 24, 25). Following resection of atypical carcinoids the 5- and 10-year survival percentages are 69% and 52%, compared with 100% and 87% for typical carcinoids (6). These results from the Memorial series reflect those reported from other institutions. It is against these results that any large series of conservative resections must be compared. Unfortunately such a series is not currently available and bronchoplastic and lung conserving operations, whilst appearing an attractive proposition, should be reserved for selected patients with either small typical carcinoids without evidence of lymphatic involvement or in those patients with impaired pulmonary function.

BRONCHIAL ADENOID CYSTIC CARCINOMA

Adenoid cystic carcinoma of the salivary glands was first described by Robin and Laboullens in 1853 (26). However, it is more difficult to date the first report of adenoid cystic carcinoma arising in the bronchial tree. Although one of the first descriptions is attributed to Hamperl in 1937 (27) the first description was probably by Heschl some 60 years earlier (28). Nevertheless, bronchial adenoid cystic carcinoma is now well established as a distinct clinicopathological entity. The original term cylindroma was coined by Billroth in 1859 (29) when describing an orbital growth arising from the lacrimal gland. It should be abandoned in favour of the widely accepted term adenoid cystic carcinoma suggested by Reid in 1952 (30). Clinically, bronchial adenoid cystic carcinoma is a more aggressive tumour than either bronchial carcinoid or bronchial mucoepidermoid tumours, and thus assumes relative importance. Despite this, and also the fact that it is more common than mucoepidermoid carcinoma, it has been the subject of less detailed review in the literature than either of these other two tumours.

Clinical Features

Although bronchial adenoid cystic carcinoma accounts for only 0.1–0.2% of all primary pulmonary neoplasms, it accounts for around 10% of all bronchial adenomas (3, 32). It arises in larger airways, most frequently in the trachea where it comprises one-third of all primary tracheal tumours (33–36). Indeed, only squamous cell carcinoma is more common in this site (35). It has a predilection for the upper third of the trachea, in contradistinction to most other tracheal carcinomas, which usually arise in the lower third (37). As for other tumours included under the category of bronchial adenoma, the incidence in males and females is approximately equal with a peak incidence of presentation in the fifth decade. Adenoid cystic carcinoma is not associated with smoking or other known carcinogens (38) and exhibits no distinct racial predilection (39). The aetiology remains obscure.

Due to their frequent site in the upper trachea, these tumours often present with upper airways obstruction and thus wheezing or apparent late onset asthma, dyspnoea (especially when recumbent), stridor and hoarseness may be prominent symptoms (34, 39, 40). However, when the tumour arises in the trachea it may present relatively late as 75% of the trachea must be occluded before symptoms develop (41). Less frequently haemoptysis, recurrent pneumonitis, pain, weight loss and malaise may be noted.

Pathology

Adenoid cystic carcinoma may be found in numerous sites including the salivary glands (42), lacrimal glands (43), palate (44), maxillary sinus (45), eustachian tubes (46), external auditory canal (47), cervix (48), breasts (49), sweat glands (50), and oesophagus (51), as well as in the bronchial tree.

Macroscopically the tumours are greyish-white or pink in colour and annular or polypoid in appearance. When cut the cells exude mucus. The tumour often extends vertically and horizontally into the cartilaginous wall of the trachea (37), and is usually covered by intact epithelium.

Histologically and ultrastructurally, bronchial adenoid cystic carcinoma is identical with its commoner salivary gland counterparts (34, 52). Thus the tumour is characterized by the growth of cells in long solid cylinders (53). On microscopy, the tumour is classically composed of small, uniform, darkly staining tumour cells arranged in cords, sheets or nests with fenestrations producing a cribriform pattern (37). The centres of the cells often appear canalized giving rise to tubular spaces or cyst-like structures (34, 53). As described earlier, there may be a cylindromatous appearance (54), with cells clustered around a lumen filled with faintly fibrillar material (34). Characteristically, perineural and intraneural infiltration is observed (55). Histochemically, acid phosphatase is found in the tumour cells, although no other common intracellular enzymes have been found (56).

Overall the tumour is a moderately well differentiated, non-encapsulated adenocarcinoma exhibiting aggressive local invasion, which may render complete excision impossible and lead to frequent local recurrence (39). It invades along tissue planes and perineural sheaths and into bones, especially the spine (39). Later, lymphatic spread occurs (53). More distant metastases are rare but have been reported to the lung, brain, liver, bone, skin and kidney (39, 53).

The investigation and management of patients with bronchial adenoid cystic carcinoma is discussed in common with mucoepidermoid carcinoma in the following section.

MUCOEPIDERMOID TUMOURS

Mucoepidermoid tumours arising in the salivary glands were established as a distinct clinicopathological entity in 1945 (57). Mucoepidermoid tumours arising in the bronchial tree were first reported in 1952 (58). Initially, mucoepidermoid tumours of the bronchus were thought to be relatively benign tumours, and were included under the category of bronchial adenoma together with bronchial carcinoid and bronchial adenoid cystic carcinoma (59). When Reichle and Rosemond reviewed 29 patients with bronchial mucoepidermoid tumour (60), they suggested that mucoepidermoid tumours were low grade malignancies characterized by local invasion of the bronchial wall. Although case reports suggested that occasional variants behaved in a more aggressive fashion (59, 61), it was not until 1971 that it was recognized fully that bronchial mucoepidermoid tumours may be high grade malignancies (62). It is now appreciated that these tumours form a spectrum of histological appearances and clinical behaviour ranging from benign tumours through to high grade malignancies. Although

the majority of mucoepidermoid tumours are benign, some are highly malignant and for these tumours the separate term of mucoepidermoid carcinoma should be reserved.

Clinical Features

These tumours are rare comprising only about 2% of all bronchial adenomas. The report from the Memorial Hospital (62) noted only 12 such cases when 5500 patients with lung cancer were reviewed. Other authors (63) noted that only 80 cases had been reported by 1979 and estimated that mucoepidermoid carcinoma would occur less than five times for every 1000 primary bronchial neoplasms. As for other tumours included under the heading of bronchial adenoma, bronchial mucoepidermoid tumours occur in both sexes with a peak incidence in middle to late life. However, reported series indicate a slight male to female predominance (63) and presentation in children has been reported (65-67). No specific aetiological factors have been identified. Although one report (62) noted that the majority of patients were cigarette smokers, there are insufficient data to establish cigarette smoking as a causative factor.

The presenting symptoms of bronchial mucoepidermoid tumours are consequent upon the site of the tumour and the rapidity of its growth. Mucoepidermoid tumours most frequently arise in the proximal bronchi and symptoms of recurrent respiratory infection secondary to endobronchial obstruction are frequent. Cough and haemoptysis have also been frequently reported. As with other tumours of the bronchial adenoma group the discovery of these tumours is sometimes incidental. The duration of symptoms reflects the biological nature of the tumour. The duration of symptoms for high grade tumours is probably less than one year (62), whereas for low grade tumours it can be many years (60).

Pathology

Mucoepidermoid tumours of the bronchus are

believed to arise from the submucosal bronchial gland duct (7) or possibly from the bronchial epithelium itself (8). Phylogenetically, the mucous glands of the bronchi are similar to those of the salivary glands. Hence, the observation that mucoepidermoid tumours of the bronchus are identical histologically to those of the salivary glands is only to be expected (61). Mucoepidermoid tumours usually arise in the proximal bronchi, although two reports have documented a treacheal site of origin (68, 69). Only rarely does the tumour arise in a lobar bronchus (70). Macroscopically they are usually well circumscribed, non-encapsulated, lobulated tumours projecting into the bronchial lumen and covered by normal bronchial mucosa. When the tumour is sectioned numerous mucous filled cysts are apparent. Microscopically bronchial mucoepidermoid tumours consist of a admixture of mucous cells resembling squamous cells and basal cells with swollen cytoplasm and well demarcated cellular boundaries are seen. Although the relative proportions of different cell types vary between specimens and often within the same specimen, elements of epidermoid carcinoma usually predominate. The tumours are positive for mucicarmine, PAS and Alcian blue stains. Mitotic activity and hyperchromatism may be seen rarely.

Mucoepidermoid tumours of the salivary glands are divided into low, intermediate and highly malignant types on the basis of histological appearances and clinical features (71). A sub-division of bronchial mucoepidermoid tumours into low grade and high grade variants has been suggested (63, 72), and in general, clinical behaviour reflects the pathological grading (59, 73, 74). However, patients with a tumour that has a low grade histological appearance have been reported in whom the clinical behaviour is more like that of a high grade lesion (75). The low grade variant is characterized by local invasion and rarely, if ever, metastases. Patients with metastatic disease are more likely to have a tumour which appears as a high grade malignancy on histological examination. Metastases to regional

lymph nodes have been described with later distant metastases to bone, liver, brain, skin (62) and adrenals (76).

Investigations and Staging

Bronchial adenoid cystic carcinomas and mucoepidermoid tumours are most frequently located centrally and hence freely accessible to bronchoscopic biopsy. Excessive haemorrhage has not proved to be a problem with fibreoptic bronchoscopic biopsy. Biopsy will provide the tissue diagnosis in almost all cases and will differentiate mucoepidermoid tumours into high and low grade types which is of importance in planning therapy.

The local extent of tumour must be accurately assessed in planning any definitive resection. This involves endoscopic assessment by the operating surgeon and high resolution computerized tomographic examination to evaluate the extent of extraluminal tumour. However, extensive submucosal and perineural spread may well still conceal the true extent of tumour (73).

In the absence of clinical features suggesting distant metastases, routine staging procedures involving organ imaging are not indicated. Similarly, mediastinoscopy does not form part of the routine preoperative investigation for patients with adenoid cystic carcinoma or mucoepidermoid tumours. Assessment of the patient's pulmonary status is required in older patients with centrally placed tumours in whom pneumonetomy or bronchoplastic procedures are contemplated.

Management and Prognosis

Despite small numbers in all series there is little doubt that complete surgical resection with microscopic clearance of tumour provides the best chance of long term disease-free survival (73, 74). The extent of resection is dependent upon the site and extent of the tumour. The frequent location of adenoid cystic carcinomas in the trachea may demand major tracheal and carinal resection and reconstruction (77). This represents on occasion a technical challenge to thoracic surgeon and aneasthetist alike.

Proximal main stem bronchial tumours frequently require pneumonectomy because of the extensive local invasion so frequently demonstrated by adenoid cystic carcinomas and mucoepidermoid carcinoma. There has been increasing interest in bronchoplastic procedures (70, 78, 79) in these proximally located tumours in order to preserve pulmonary function. There have been only small numbers reported and these comprise selected patients, particularly those with low grade mucoepidermoid tumours. Frozen section examination is required when such resections are performed to ensure microscopic clearance of tumour. When this is achieved such procedures may result in long term disease-free survival.

Routine lymph node dissection should be performed when resecting adenoid cystic carcinomas and mucoepidermoid carcinomas. Even in the presence of extensive lymph node involvement long term survival without evidence of recurrence has been reported following complete surgical resection (73).

When surgical resection is not an option either because of the patient's general medical condition or the extent of disease, radiotherapy with or without endoscopic removal of the tumour has been used (73, 74). The long term results have usually been unsatisfactory with local tumour recurrence. On some occasions endoscopic removal is required as an emergency procedure because of life-threatening tracheal obstruction by tumour (73). There has been increasing interest in newer laser techniques in this regard and these require further assessment. The role of photodynamic therapy using the argon dye laser in these tumours also remains to be evaluated. These later techniques may well have a role in the locally recurrent tumour following prior surgery and/or radiation.

The rarity of these two tumours precludes analysis of survival as detailed for bronchial carcinoids. The prognosis appears to be most dependent upon being able to achieve a complete macroscopic and microscopic clearance of all tumour. When this is achieved long term disease-free survival can be expected. In its absence local recurrence is the rule. The histological grade in mucoepidermoid tumours is of prognostic importance. Low grade tumours can usually be completely excised whilst high grade lesions frequently demonstrate extensive local invasion, lymph node metastases and even evidence of distant spread.

NON-SURGICAL MANAGEMENT

Because the behaviour of these tumours is usually indolent, most patients present with localized disease and are cured by surgery. Hence, experience with non-surgical management has been very limited even for bronchial carcinoid, the commonest of these tumours. Even when non-surgical management with radiotherapy or chemotherapy has been employed, the rarity of these tumours has restricted experience to mere case reports. Nevertheless, the results of non-surgical management are summarized below.

Bronchial Carcinoid

Although one report (80) describes a favourable response to radical irradiation in 3 patients, most other authors describe bronchial carcinoid as a relatively radioresistant tumour, similar to its more frequent counterpart, the gastrointestinal carcinoid. Thus, irradiation should probably be regarded as palliative and not curative for this tumour, but may be of benefit for those patients in whom resection is not possible. The role of irradiation as an adjuvant form of therapy following resection is entirely unknown.

For carcinoid tumours as a group, the limited data that are available suggest that doxorubicin, 5 (5-fluorouracil) FU, dacarbazine (DTIC), actinomycin D, streptozotocin and alkylating agents all may have activity (81). However, it is noteworthy that even the most extensive single agent experience (with doxorubicin) encompassed a total of only 33 patients. Overall, single agents appear disappointing as response rates are usually less than 20%. Combination chemotherapy appears to offer little advantage as response rates are little higher. The largest series of combination chemotherapy was a randomized comparison of 5-FU plus streptozotocin versus cyclophosphamide and streptozotocin (82). The response rate for the 5-FU combination was 44% and for the cyclophosphamide arm 37%. Although it is tempting to assume that bronchial carcinoids might respond similarly, the overall response rate for carcinoids of bronchial origin was only 2/17 (12%), suggesting that they may be less drug sensitive.

Overall, therefore, chemotherapy for bronchial carcinoid appears disappointing, but responses with single agents or combination chemotherapy have been observed occasionally. At present, there are insufficient data to be able to recommend the use of particular cytotoxic drugs, and chemotherapy should be regarded as investigational. Ideally, such treatment should form part of a multicentre clinical trial for patients with symptomatic metastatic disease.

Adenoid Cystic and Mucoepidermoid Carcinoma

As for bronchial carcinoid, radiotherapy or other forms of non-surgical management for these tumours is usually reserved for patients in whom complete resection is not possible or for those with recurrent disease. Bronchial adenoid cystic carcinoma was assumed to be relatively radioresistant, but it is now clear that radical radiotherapy may induce tumour regression (73–85). Some authors (86) advocate postoperative radiotherapy when tumour is close to the resection margins, when there is local lymphatic spread, or perineural invasion. Preoperative radiotherapy has also been used (84).

There are few reports of the use of chemotherapy for adenoid cystic carcinoma, despite the fact that, compared with the other tumours, it is more aggressive and more than 50% of patients may develop distant metastases eventually (87). For example, one series collected 242 patients over a 25-year period (88). However, of a total of 218 patients treated, only 2 received chemotherapy. A further series describes a total of 65 patients receiving chemotherapy (89). Although the numbers of patients in the various treatment subgroups were small, cisplatin, 5-FU, and doxorubicin alone or in combination appeared promising. Thus, adenoid cystic carcinoma should be regarded as a potentially drug responsive tumour and, if chemotherapy is contemplated, these agents should be considered.

The role of radiotherapy in the treatment of bronchial mucoepidermoid carcinoma, remains to be defined. Mucoepidermoid tumours of salivary gland origin are, generally, relatively insensitive to radiation (89). However, little is known about the radiosensitivity of low-grade or high-grade mucoepidermoid tumours of bronchial origin.

Information on the role of chemotherapy in the management of mucoepidermoid is also scant. Although methotrexate, 5-FU, cisplatin, and bleomycin have all been used and occasional responses seen (90), there are insufficient data to be able to recommend any of these agents with confidence.

REFERENCES

Bronchial Carcinoids

1 Laennec RTH. Traité de L'Ausultation Médiate et des Maladies des Poumons et du Coeur, 3rd edition. Paris: Chaud, 1831: 250.
2 Burcharth F, Axelsson C. Bronchial adenomas. Thorax 1972; 27: 442–9.
3 Paulson DL, Ginsberg RJ. Bronchial adenoma. In: Shields TW ed. General Thoracic Surgery, 2nd edition. Philadelphia: Lea and Febiger, 1983: 712–28.
4 Muller H. Zur Entstehungsgeschichte der Bronchialerweiterungen. Inaug. Diss. Univ. Halle. Ermsleben a.H., A. Busch 15, 1882: 1–36.
5 Spencer H. Rare pulmonary tumours. In: Pathology of the Lung, 4th edition, Vol 2. Oxford: Pergamon Press, 1985: 933–1020.

6 McCaughan BC, Martini N, Bains MS. Bronchial carcinoids. J Thorac Cardiovasc Surg 1985; 89: 8–17.

7 Attar S, Miller JE, Hankins J, Thompson BW, Suter CM, Kleger PJ, McLaughlin JS. Bronchial Adenoma: A Review of 51 Patients. Ann Thorac Surg 1985; 40: 126–32.

8 DeCaro LF, Paladugu R, Benfield JR, Lovisatti L, Pak H, Teplitz RL. Typical and atypical carcinoids within the pulmonary APUD tumor spectrum. J Thorac Cardiovasc Surg 1983; 86: 528–36. .

9 Bensch KG, Corrin B, Parients R, Spencer H. Oat-cell carcinoma of the lung. Its origin and relationship to bronchial carcinoid. Cancer 1968; 22: 1163–72.

10 Ricci C, Patrassi N, Massa R, Mineo C, Benedetti-Valentini F Jr. Carcinoid syndrome in bronchial adenoma. Am J Surg 1973; 126: 671–7.

11 Todd TR, Cooper JD, Weissberg D, Delarue NC, Pearson FG. Bronchial carcinoid tumors. J Thorac Cardiovasc Surg 1980; 79: 532–6.

12 Okike N, Bernatz PE, Woolner LB. Carcinoid tumors of the lung. Ann Thorac Surg 1976; 22: 271–7.

13 Arrigoni MG, Woolner LB, Bernatz PE. Atypical carcinoid tumors of the lung. J Thorac Cardiovasc Surg 1972; 64: 413–21.

14 Tollis GA, Fry WA, Head L, Shields TW. Bronchial adenomas. Surg Gynecol Obstet 1972; 134: 605–10.

15 Lawson RM, Ramanathan L, Hurley G, Hinson KW, Lennox SC. Bronchial adenoma. Review of an 18 year experience at the Brompton Hospital. Thorax 1976; 31: 245–52.

16 Smith RA. Bronchial carcinoid tumours. Thorax 1969; 24: 43–50.

17 Markel SF, Abell MR, Haight C, French AJ. Neoplasms of the bronchus commonly designated as adenomas. Cancer 1964; 17: 590–608.

18 Mark JBD. Discussion of Todd et al. (11).

19 Okike N, Bernatz PE, Payne WS, Woolner LB, Leonard PF. Bronchoplastic procedures in the treatment of carcinoid tumors of the tracheobronchial tree. J Thorac Cardiovasc Surg 1978; 76: 281–91.

20 Baldwin JN, Grimes OF. Bronchial adenomas. Surg Gynecol Obstet 1967; 124: 813–18.

21 Jensik RJ, Faber LP, Brown CM, Kittle CF. Bronchoplastic and conservative resectional procedures for bronchial adenoma. J Thorac Cardiovasc Surg 1974; 68: 556–65.

22 Spencer FC. Discussion of Jensik et al. (21).

23 Weisel W. Discussion of Jensik et al. (21).

24 Wilkins EW Jr, Grillo HC, Moncure AC, Scannel JG. Changing times in surgical management

25 Faber LP. Discussion of DeCaro et al. (8).

Adenoid Cystic Carcinoma

26 Price JC, Percarpio B, Murphy PW, Henderson RL. Recurrent adenoid cystic carcinoma of the trachea: intraluminal radiotherapy. Otolaryngol Head Neck Surg 1979; 87: 614–23.

27 Hamperl H. Uber Gutartige Bronchialtumoren (Cylindrome und Carcinoide). Virchows Arch Path Anat 1937; 300: 46–88.

28 Heschl R. Ueber ein Cylindrom der Lunge. Wien Med Wehnschr 1877; 17: 385–90.

29 Billroth T. Beobachtungen uber Geschwulste der Speicheldrusen. Arch Path Anat 1859; 17: 357–75.

30 Reid JD. Adenoid cystic carcinoma (cylindroma) of the bronchial tree. Cancer 1952; 5: 685–94.

31 Payne SW, Ellis FH, Woolner LB, Moersch HJ. The surgical treatment of cylindroma (adenoid cystic carcinoma) and mucoepidermoid tumors of the bronchus. J Thorac Cardiovasc Surg 1959; 38: 709–26.

32 Paulson DL, Ginsberg RJ. Bronchial adenoma. In: Shields TW, ed General Thoracic Surgery, 2nd edition. Philadelphia: Lea and Febiger, 1983: 712–28.

33 Richardson JD, Grover FL, Trinkle JK. Adenoid cystic carcinoma of the trachea. Response to cobalt-60. J Thorac Cardiovasc Surg 1973; 66: 311–14.

34 Hajdu SI, Huvos AG, Goodner JT, Foote FW, Beattie EJ. Carcinoma of the Trachea. Clinicopathological Study of 41 Cases. Cancer 1970; 25: 1448–56.

35 Houston HE, Payne WS, Harrison EG, Olsen AM. Primary Cancers of the Trachea. Arch Surg 1969; 99: 132–40.

36 Markel SF, Abell MR. Adenocystic Basal Cell Carcinoma of the Trachea. J Thorac Cardiovasc Surg 1964; 48: 211–25.

37 Mark EJ. Pathology of tracheal neoplasms. In: Choi NC, Grillo HC ed. Thoracic Oncology. New York: Raven Press, 1983.

38 Carter D, Eggleston JC. Adenoid Cystic Carcinoma. In: Tumors of the Lower Respiratory Tract, Second Series, Fascicle 17. Washington DC: Armed Forces Institute of Pathology, 1980: 199–202.

39 Cleveland RH, Nice CM, Ziskind J. Primary adenoid cystic carcinoma (cylindroma) of the trachea. Radiology 1977; 122: 597–600.

40 Grillo HC. Tracheal tumors: diagnosis and

management. In: Choi NC, Grillo HC ed Thoracic Oncology. Raven Press, 1983: 271–8.

41 Belsey R. Resection and reconstruction of the intrathoracic trachea. Br J Surg 1950; 38: 200–5.

42 Thackray AC, Lucas RB. Tumors of the major salivary glands. In: Atlas of Tumor Pathology, Armed Forces Institute of Pathology, Second Series, Fascicle 10. Washington, DC: Armed Forces Institute of Pathology 1974; 91–9.

43 Gamel JW, Font RL. Adenoid cystic carcinoma of the lachrimal gland: the clinical significance of a basaloid histologic pattern. Hum Pathol 1982; 13: 219–25.

44 Eneroth CM, Hjertman L, Moberger G. Adenoid cystic carcinoma of the palate. Acta Otolaryngol 1968; 66: 248–60.

45 Dodd GD, Jing BS. Radiographic findings in adenoid cystic carcinoma of the head and neck. Ann Otol Rhinol Laryngol 1972; 81: 591–8.

46 Sanderson JN, Silva JS. Multiple thoracic nodules in a young asymptomatic woman. Chest, 1973; 63: 1019–20.

47 Sodagar R. Adenoid cystic carcinoma of the external auditory canal. Eye Ear Nose Throat Mon. 1972; 51: 341–2.

48 Ryden SE, Silberman EM, Goltman RT. Adenoid cystic carcinoma of the cervix presenting as a primary pulmonary neoplasm. Am J Obstet Gynecol 1974; 120: 846–7.

49 Laff HI, Neubuerger KT. Bronchial adenoma with metastasis. Arch Otolaryngol 1944; 40: 487–93.

50 Donahue JK, Weichert RF, Ochsner JL. Bronchial adenoma. Ann Surg 1968; 167: 873–85.

51 Nelms DC, Lura MA. Primary adenocystic carcinoma (cylindromatous carcinoma) of the esophagus. Cancer 1972; 29: 440–3.

52 Hoshino M, Yamamoto I. Ultrastructure of adenoid cystic carcinoma. Cancer 1970; 25: 186–98.

53 Spencer H. In: Pathology of the Lung, 4th edition, Vol. 2. Oxford: Pergamon Press, 1985: 968–9.

54 Eby LS, Johnson DS, Baker HW. Adenoid cystic carcinoma of the head and neck. Cancer 1972; 29: 160–8.

55 Wilkins EW, Darling RC, Soutter L, Sniffen RC. A continuing clinical survey of adenomas of the trachea and bronchus in a general hospital. J Thorac Cardiovasc Surg 1963; 46: 279–91.

56 Willighagen RG, van der Heul RO, van Eijssel TG. Enzyme histochemistry of human lung tumours. J Pathol Bacterol 1963; 85: 279–90.

Mucoepidermoid Tumours

57 Stewart FW, Foote FW, Becker WF. Mucoepidermoid Tumors of the Salivary Glands. Ann Surg 1945; 122: 824–4.

58 Smetana HF, Quoted by Liebow AA. Tumors of the lower respiratory tract. In: Atlas of Tumor Pathology, National Council, Section V, Fascicle 17. Washington DC: Armed Forces Institute of Pathology, 1952: 45.

59 Dowling EA, Miller RE, Johnson IM, Cliier FCD. Mucoepidermoid tumors of the bronchi. Surgery 1962; 52: 600–9.

60 Reichle FA, Rosemond GP. Mucoepidermoid tumors of the bronchus. J Thorac Cardiovasc Surg 1966; 51: 443–8.

61 Ozlu C, Christopherson WM, Allen JD. Mucoepidermoid tumors of the bronchus. J Thorac Cardiovasc Surg 1961; 42: 24–31.

62 Turnbull AD, Huvos AG, Goodner JT, Foote FW. Mucoepidermoid tumors of bronchial glands. Cancer 1971; 28: 539–44.

63 Klacsmann PG, Olson JL, Eggleston JC. Mucoepidermoid carcinoma of the bronchus. An electron microscopic study of the low grade and high grade variants. Cancer 1979; 43: 1720–33.

64 Sniffen RC, Soutter L, Robbins LL. Mucoepidermoid tumours of the bronchus arising from surface epithelium. Am J Pathol 1958; 34: 671–83.

65 Lack EE, Harris GBC, Eraklis AJ, Vawter GF. Primary bronchial tumors in childhood. A clinicopathological study of six cases. Cancer 1983; 51: 492–7.

66 Seo IS, Warren J, Mirkin D, Weisman SJ, Grosfeld JL. Mucoepidermoid carcinoma of the bronchus in a 4-year-old child. Cancer 1984; 53: 1600–4.

67 McDougall JC, Gorenstein A, Unni K, O'Connell EJ. Carcinoid and mucoepidermoid carcinoma of the bronchus. Ann Otol 1980; 89: 425–7.

68 Larson RE, Woolner LB, Payne WS. Iucoepidermoid Tumor of the Trachea. Report of a Case. J Thorac Cardiovasc Surg 1965; 50: 131–7.

69 Trentini GP, Palmieri B. Mucoepidermoid tumor of the trachea. Chest 1970; 62: 336–8.

70 Breyer RH, Dainauskas JR, Jensik RJ, Faber LP. Mucoepidermoid carcinoma of the trachea and bronchus: The case for conservative resection. Ann Thorac Surg 1980; 29: 197–204.

71 Healey WV, Perzin KH, Smith L. Mucoepidermoid Carcinoma of Salivary Gland Origin. A Classification, Clinical-Pathological Correlation, and Results of Treatment. Cancer 1970; 26: 368–88.

72 Carter D, Eggleston JC. Tumors of the Lower Respiratory Tract, Fascicle 17, Second Series,

Washington DC: Armed Forces Institute of Pathology, 1980: 193–8.

73 Conlan AA, Payne WS, Woolner LB, Sanderson DR. Adenoid cystic carcinoma (cylindroma) and mucoepidermoid carcinoma of the bronchus; factors affecting survival. J Thorac Cardiovasc Surg 1978; 76: 369–77.

74 Leonardi HK, Jung-Legg Y, Legg MA, Neptune WB. Tracheobronchial mucoepidermoid carcinoma: Clinicopathological features and results of treatment. J Thorac Cardiovasc Surg 1978; 76: 431–8.

75 Barsky SH, Martin SE, Matthews M, Gazdar A, Costa JC. 'Low Grade' Mucoepidermoid Carcinoma of the Bronchus with 'High Grade' Biological Behaviour. Cancer 1983; 51: 1505–9.

76 Lifschultz BD, Vanecko R, Hidvegi DF. Mucoepidermoid tumors of the bronchus. Ill Med J 1982; 161: 335–9.

77 Grillo HC. Tracheal tumours: diagnosis and management. In: Choi NC, Grillo HC ed Thoracic Oncology, New York: Raven Press, 1983: 271–8.

78 Lowe JE, Bridgman AH, Sabiston DC. The role of bronchoplastic procedures in the management of benign and malignant pulmonary lesions. J Thorac Cardiovasc Surg 1982; 83: 2272–84.

79 Frist WH, Mathisen DJ, Hilgenberg AD, Grillow HC. Bronchial sleeve resection with and without pulmonary resection. J Thorac Cardiovasc Surg 1987; 93: 350–7.

Non-surgical Management

80 Baldwin JN, Grimes OF. Bronchial adenomas. Surg Gynecol Obstet 1967; 124: 813–8.

82 Moertel CG. Treatment of the carcinoid tumor and the malignant carcinoid syndrome. J Clin Oncol 1983; 1: 727–40.

82 Moertel CG, Hanley JA. Combination chemotherapy trials for metastatic carcinoid tumor and the malignant carcinoid syndrome. Cancer Clin Trials 1979; 2: 327–34.

83 Price JC, Percapio B, Murphy PW, Henderson RL. Recurrent adenoid cystic carcinoma of the trachea: intraluminal radiotherapy. Otolaryngol Head Neck Surg 1979; 87: 614–23.

84 Pearson FG, Thompson DW, Weissberg D, Simpson WJK, Kergin FG. Adenoid cystic carcinoma of the trachea. Ann Thorac Surg 1974; 18: 16–29.

85 Cleveland RH, Nice CM, Ziskind J. Primary adenoid cystic carcinoma (cylindroma) of the trachea. Radiology 1977; 122: 597–600.

86 Grillo HC. Management of tracheal tumors. Am J Surg 1982; 143: 697–700.

87 Matsuba HM, Simpson JR, Mauney M, Thawley SE. Adenoid cystic salivary gland carcinoma: a clinicopathologic correlation. Head Neck Surg 1986; 8: 200–4.

88 Spiro RH, Huvos AG, Strong EW. Adenoid cystic carcinoma of salivary gland origin: a clinicopathologic study of 242 cases. Am J Surg 1974; 128: 512–20.

89 Jakobsson PA, Eneroth CM. Variations in radiosensitivity of various types of malignant salivary-gland tumour. Acta Otolaryng 1970; suppl 263: 186–8.

90 Kaplan MJ, Johns ME, Cantrell RW. Chemotherapy for salivary gland cancer. Otolaryngol Head Neck Surg 1986; 95: 165–70.

Textbook of Uncommon Cancer
Edited by C.J. Williams, J.G. Krikorian, M.R. Green and D. Raghavan
© 1988 John Wiley & Sons Ltd

Chapter **23**

Unusual Tumours of the Mediastinum

Peter Harper* and
Bruce Addis†
*Consultant Medical Oncologist, Guy's Hospital, London
and † Consultant Histopathologist and Honorary Senior
Lecturer, Brompton Hospital and Cardiothoracic Institute,
London, UK

ANATOMICAL CONSIDERATIONS

The boundaries of the mediastinum are well defined: the thoracic inlet lies superiorly, the diaphragm inferiorly, the vertebral column posteriorly and the sternum and pleural reflections anteriorly and antero-laterally. Within these anatomical boundaries the mediastinum is traditionally sub-divided into compartments, each 'space' being associated with particular tumours. Not surprisingly these sub-divisions vary from author to author, but we prefer a simple partition into only three areas: the antero-superior, posterior, and middle mediastinal divisions (1, 2). The contents of each dictate the position of the tumours that occur (1–4). These are set out in Table 1.

The antero-superior compartment of the mediastinum is bounded inferiorly by the diaphragm, anteriorly by the sternum and posteriorly by the vertebral column down to the thoracic vertebra, and below this level by the anterior pericardium. The middle compartment of the mediastinum is bounded inferiorly by the anterior pericardium and posteriorly by the oesophagus, and extends down to the diaphragm. The posterior mediastinum lies between the vertebral column and posterior pericardium.

Modern imaging techniques enable radiologists to localize tumours precisely within these clear anatomical landmarks, thereby narrowing the differential diagnosis. Treatment and prognosis, however, depend on an exact histological diagnosis and this requires close cooperation between surgeon and pathologist enabling maximum information to be obtained from biopsy material (see below).

In this chapter emphasis is given to those primary tumours of the mediastinum which most often provide diagnostic and therapeutic problems. Shortage of space precludes inclusion of mediastinal cysts; and tumours of the heart require more detailed discussion than could be provided here. We have also omitted perhaps the most common cause of a mediastinal mass, metastatic carcinoma involving mediastinal lymph nodes: this is a familiar clinical situation and should be considered in the differential diagnosis of any lesion in this area.

411

TABLE 1 THE LOCATION OF MEDIASTINAL TUMOURS[a]

SUPERIOR

Thyroid and parathyroid tumours and hyperplasias

POSTERIOR	MIDDLE	ANTERIOR

Neurogenic tumours:
  neurofibroma
  schwannoma
  malignant nerve
    sheath tumour
  neuroblastoma
  ganglioneuroblastoma
 	
  ganglioneuroma
  paraganglioma
Enteric cysts
	Bronchogenic
	and
	pericardial
	cysts
		Thymic cysts and tumours:
		  thymoma
		  thymic carcinoma
		  carcinoid
		  germ cell tumours
		  lymphomas
		  thymolipoma
		  sarcoma
		Paraganglioma
		Haemangioma
		Lymphangioma

	Lymphadenopathy Mediastinal fibrosis	

[a] From Addis (6).

THE ANTERIOR MEDIASTINUM

Mullen and Richardson have reviewed anterior mediastinal tumours in children and adults (3). In a collective series of 702 adults, thymic lesions accounted for 47% of the tumours recorded, lymphomas 23%, endocrine tumours 16%, and germ cell tumours 15%. In 179 children, the most frequently seen anterior mediastinal tumour was lymphoma (45%), with germ cell tumours accounting for 24%, thymic lesions 17% and mesenchymal tumours 15% (3). Tumours of intrathoracic thyroid and parathyroid glands, mediastinal germ cell tumours and neuroblastoma are well covered in the general literature or other chapters in this book and are not included here.

Signs and Symptoms of Anterior Mediastinal Tumours

Two-thirds of patients will present with specific symptoms, the remaining one-third of tumours being discovered on a routine chest x-ray. The most common symptoms are chest pain, cough and dyspnoea, caused by compression or invasion of adjacent structures. Other less common symptoms include haemoptysis, dysphagia, hoarseness, Horner's syndrome, vena caval obstruction, arrythmias, fever, weakness and weight loss (3, 5).

Obtaining a Biopsy

There can be nothing more frustrating to the practising oncologist than an unclear histological report, where the diagnosis ranges from metastatic undifferentiated carcinoma to a tumour of unknown origin or nature. This is particularly prevalent when tumours of the mediastinum are considered. An adequate, well handled initial biopsy must be obtained (6). Due to the anatomical considerations described above, obtaining a second biopsy can be very traumatic and should be unnecessary.

Immunohistochemistry and electron microscopy now play important roles in tumour diagnosis and formalin fixation is no longer ideal. The intact unfixed specimen should be delivered to the laboratory without delay with as much accurate clinical information as obtainable. This enables the pathologist to make imprints from the cut surface of the fresh tissue for cytological examination, to freeze tissue for immunohistochemistry and, in cases of malignant lymphoma, for gene rearrangement studies. Tissues for electron microscopy should be fixed immediately in glutaraldehyde and the remainder of the specimen can then be fixed in formalin. Cytological diagnosis of mediastinal tumours by fine needle aspiration requires considerable expertise but the technique is growing in popularity (7).

TUMOURS OF THYMIC EPITHELIUM

Tumours of thymic epithelium are now divided into two groups: the few tumours showing unequivocal histological and cytolo-gical evidence of malignancy are classified as thymic carcinomas and the remaining tumours, whatever their clinical behaviour, form the much larger group of thymomas (6, 8, 9).

Thymomas

Thymomas are the most frequent tumours of the anterior mediastinum. They have an equal sex incidence and occur over a wide age range. Rare cases have been reported in children (10, 11) but the majority present in the fifth and sixth decades. Very rarely there is a familial tendency (8).

In a post-mortem study, Bell et al. found that 98% of all thymus glands lie between the manubrium sterni and the xiphisternum (12). Most thymomas therefore occur in the anterior

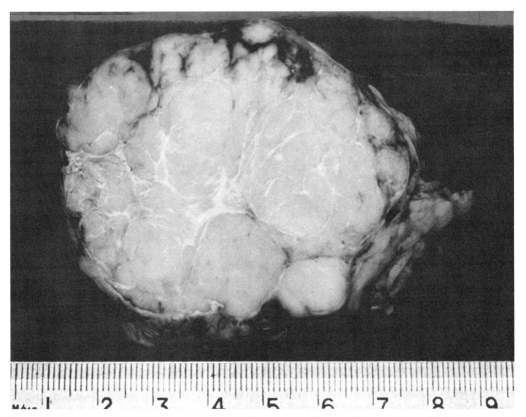

Figure 1. An encapsulated thymoma showing the characteristic nodular pattern with irregular septa of connective tissue.

or superior mediastinum: 75% are found in the anterior mediastinum, immediately above and anterior to the pericardium; approximately 15% occupy both the anterior and superior compartments and 6% are primarily within the superior mediastinum. The remaining 4% develop in the neck in thymic tissue that has failed to descend (9). Isolated examples have been recorded in the middle and posterior mediastinum, and even within lung parenchyma.

Gross pathology. The majority of thymomas are completely or partially encapsulated and the cut surface of a typical tumour shows bulging nodules of soft, cream or light tan-coloured tissue separated by white septa (Figure 1). This nodularity may be lost in some invasive tumours leaving a more uniform cut surface. Cysts may be present in the tumour or in the surrounding compressed normal thymus.

Microscopic appearances. A wide variety of histological appearances is seen, the two main variables being cell morphology and the ratio of epithelial cells to lymphoid cells (6, 9). Epithelial cell nuclei are typically oval with a diameter three to five times that of a lymphocyte, delicate chromatin and a single nucleolus. The cytoplasm is usually pale staining and cell boundaries are indistinct (Figure 2).

Variable numbers of lymphocytes lie between the epithelial cells. The lymphoid population in thymomas is not neoplastic and, as in the normal thymus, consists of T lymphocytes in various stages of maturation. Lymphocytes vary in size and mitoses may be frequent. A high lymphocyte turnover rate may be associated with a population of mononuclear phagocytes containing nuclear debris, giving the tumour a 'starry-sky' pattern. Viable lymphocytes may be present within the cytoplasm of epithelial cells, a phenomenon known as emperipolesis, and these cells may be the

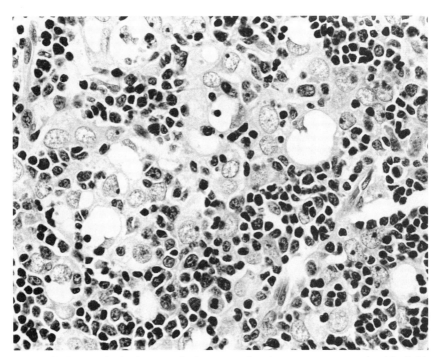

Figure 2. The typical microscopic features of a thymoma are seen in this field, which shows large, pale-staining epithelial cells mixed with a population of lymphocytes (thymocytes).

neoplastic equivalent of the nurse cells of the normal thymus.

Another frequent feature is the presence of perivascular spaces, lying between the capillary basement membrane and the epithelial basement membrane of the tumour cells. These may be widely dilated, even to the extent of forming macroscopic cysts. They contain lymphocytes, plasma cells and mast cells and may be obliterated by structureless hyaline material.

Many thymomas contain spindle cell areas, often merging with the connective tissue of the septa. Some tumours consist purely of spindle cells with elongated nuclei and attenuated cytoplasm, forming closely interlacing bundles of whorls (Figure 3). The lymphocyte population is almost invariably sparse and perivascular spaces are not conspicuous. If spindle cell and typical epithelial areas coexist, lymphocytes tend to infiltrate epithelial areas selectively. Usually epithelial cells are dispersed among the lymphocytes and, if the lymphocyte population predominates, as in the normal thymic cortex, they may not be obvious in routine sections. Often they are more easily seen at the periphery of tumour nodules or around perivascular spaces and, in some tumours, epithelial cell groups and lymphocytes appear separate. In these circumstances epithelial cells seem to lose their dendritic form and show distinct cell outlines. Hofmann et al. have called this variant the 'epidermoid' type of thymoma (13).

In about 20% of tumours tubular or tubulocystic structures, lined by flattened or cuboidal epithelium, are present. True glandular structures, lined by ciliated or mucus-secreting epithelium, are infrequent.

Hassall's corpuscles, usually poorly formed, are present in about 20% of tumours: Rosai and Levine used the term medullary differentiation to describe areas in lymphocyte-rich thymomas where the lymphocytes are more sparsely distributed and rudimentary Hassall's corpuscles can be found (9).

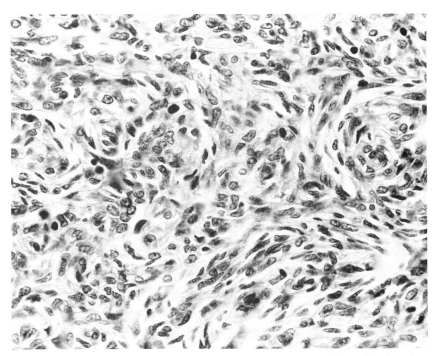

Figure 3 A spindle cell thymoma showing a whorled pattern. Note that lymphocytes are usually sparse in this type of tumour.

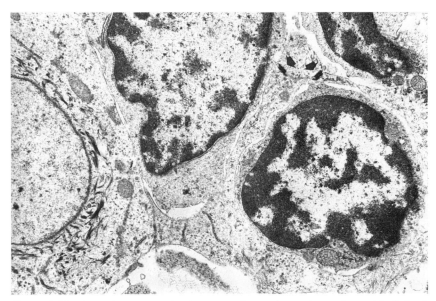

Figure 4 Electron microscopy of a thymoma shows the nucleus of an epithelial cell with long cell processes surrounding lymphocytes. The processes are joined by desmosomes (arrows top right) and bundles of tonofilaments are present in the epithelial cell cytoplasm.

At the ultrastructural level thymic epithelial cell nuclei can be distinguished from lymphocyte nuclei by their larger size, fine diffuse nuclear chromatin and conspicuous nucleoli. The cytoplasmic boundaries and complex interdigitating cell processes are distinct and form a network around the lymphocytes. Bundles of cytoplasmic filaments are usually conspicuous and converge on cell junctions. The latter are of desmosomal type and are usually numerous (Figure 4) (14).

Immunohistochemical features. Like all epithelia, thymic epithelium expresses keratin intermediate filaments and this is of great value in making the distinction between thymoma and malignant lymphoma, especially when only a small biopsy is available (6, 15, 16). Reactivity depends largely on the antibody used: antibodies to low molecular weight keratins give most uniform staining whereas antibodies to higher molecular weight keratins pick out more heavily keratinized cells and

rudimentary Hassall's corpuscles in areas of medullary differentiation (16).

Normal thymic epithelium expresses HLA DR antigens but the distribution varies according to the antibody used (16–21). Loss of reactivity in tumours has been noted by several workers (16, 17, 20). The Leu 7 (HNK-1) antigen is present on normal thymic epithelium and has a very variable expression in tumours (16, 17, 21). There is some evidence that it is more strongly expressed in invasive thymomas (16).

The majority of the lymphocytes in thymomas are immature T cells with a cortical phenotype (17, 21, 22) expressing OKT6 and/or OKT9. Chilosi et al. (18) found foci of mature lymphocytes and Müller-Hermelink et al. (21) have subdivided thymomas into cortical, medullary and mixed types, using the presence of mature T lymphocytes with helper or suppressor phenotype, to help assess medullary differentiation. The validity of this classification and its significance from the standpoint of tumour behaviour has yet to be confirmed.

Malignancy in Thymomas

It is only comparatively recently that there has been more or less general agreement about the use of the term thymoma. Thanks largely to the work of Rosai and Levine previous complex classifications have been discarded and the term has been restricted to tumours of thymic epithelium (9). Even more recently the separate category of thymic carcinoma has emerged. The inclusion of such tumours in earlier series of thymomas undoubtedly blurred the assessment of malignancy (23). Arriagada et al. recently used the term thymic carcinoma to include all invasive or metastatic thymic epithelial tumours whatever their histological appearances, thereby further confusing the situation. In their multicentre retrospective review of 56 macroscopically invasive thymic tumours, microscopic signs of invasion were observed in 68% of cases and nuclear abnormalities were present in 33% of cases (24). We believe that the term thymic carcinoma should be reserved for tumours showing unequivoval histological evidence of malignancy (see below) (25, 26). However, we have seen examples of otherwise unremarkable thymomas which contained foci of apparent malignant transformation.

Rosenberg in a masterly review of the subject (27) comments that benign thymoma has been defined as a tumour that is well encapsulated and does not invade adjacent mediastinal structures; 50–65% of thymomas fit this definition. He considers that the distinction between 'benign' and 'malignant' thymomas is artificial and should be discarded. All thymomas are *potentially* invasive and therefore should be considered as malignant (25).

If tumours with frankly malignant histological appearances are excluded, most authors are agreed that microscopic criteria are of less value in indicating malignant potential than macroscopic invasion. However, several recent series have indicated that tumours with a small lymphocyte population (predominantly epithelial thymomas) are more likely to pursue an aggressive course (3, 16, 28–30). In the absence of macroscopic evidence of invasion, microscopic appearances suggesting capsular invasion are unreliable due to capsular irregularities and should not be used to assess prognosis (16).

Apart from local invasion of the capsule and adjacent structures, including lung, pericardium and myocardium, thymomas tend to spread by seeding to serosal surfaces, occasionally producing large pleural masses. Distant metastasis is rare (9) but spread to lymph nodes, liver, bone, kidney, spleen, central nervous system and peripheral nerves is recorded (31–33). Widespread metastases may occur without local invasion (34). Only 12 examples of metastasizing thymoma were found in the literature by Guillan et al. in 1971 (35); however, over the last two decades an increasing number of cases have been recorded (35–37).

Staging of thymoma. Tumour stage is determined by the extent of invasion at operation. Stage I disease is represented by intracapsular growth with an intact capsule, and may be referred to as benign thymoma. Stage II disease is indicated by growth into surrounding organs, particularly mediastinal fat, pleura or pericardium. Stage III disease represents the addition of intrathoracic metastases. Stage IV lesions have extrathoracic metastases (9).

Associated Disease

Thymomas may be associated with major abnormalities of the immune system. In the Mayo Clinic review 71% of 601 patients with thymoma suffered from 493 other diseases suspected of being associated with the tumour. Of these cases, 423 involved disorders of immunity (38). (See Table 2.)

In their very careful review extending from 1832 to December 1970 the authors have succinctly set out their reasons for inferring that thymoma together with certain diseases creates a 'syndrome' rather than a 'spectrum' of coincidental diseases. In the total of 423 cases of disease related to disorders of immu-

TABLE 2 ABNORMAL IMMUNE DISEASES, ENDOCRINE
ABNORMALITIES AND SEVERE INFECTIONS
ASSOCIATED WITH THYMOMAS. A REVIEW OF
601 CASE HISTORIES[a]

Disease	Combined percentage	
Immune disorder		
Myasthenia gravis	44	
Cytopenias	21	Total patients
Other cancers	17	with one or more
Hypogammaglobulinaemia	6	of this group:
Polymyositis	5	423/601 (89%)
Systemic lupus erythematosus	2	
Rheumatoid arthritis		
Thyroiditis		
Sjögren syndrome		
Chronic ulcerative colitis		
Pernicious anaemia		
Raynaud disease		
Regional enteritis		
Rheumatic endocarditis		
Sarcoid		
Dermatomyositis		
Scleroderma		
Takayasu syndrome		
Endocrine disorders	*17*	
Cushing syndrome	11	Total patients
Hyperthyroidism	3	with one or more
Addison's disease	1	of this group
Pan hypopituitarism	1	20/601 (4%)
Severe infections, etc.	6	Total patients 30/601 (6%)

[a] From Souadjian et al. (38).

nity they included myasthenia gravis (44%), cytopenias (21%), cancer (17%), hypogammaglobulinaemia (6%), polymyositis (5%), and systemic lupus erythematosus (2%). To these can be added case reports of Eaton–Lambert syndrome, Di George syndrome, pemphigus, scleroderma, polyneuritis, polyarthropathy, myotonic dystrophy, regional ileitis and the nephrotic syndrome (38).

Myasthenia gravis. Myasthenia gravis is an acquired autoimmune disorder associated with acetylcholine receptor deficiency at the motor end plate. The quantity of acetylcholine released is normal but the lack of available receptors to bind it reduces the amplitude of the end plate potential. Symptoms therefore are abnormal weakness and fatigability on exertion. A proposed classification of myasthenia gravis is related to presence of absence of thymoma and age of onset.

1. Myasthenia gravis with thymoma: the disease is usually severe and the anticholinesterase receptor antibody level is high. There is no association with either sex of HLA antigen.

2. No thymoma, onset before age 40: the anticholinesterase receptor antibody level is intermediate. There is a female preponderance and an increase associated with HLA-A1, HLA-B8 and HLA-DRw3 antigens (HLA-B12 in Japan).

3. No thymoma, onset after age 40: the anti-cholinesterase receptor antibody level tends to be low. There is a male preponderance and an increased association with HLA-A3, HLA-B7 and HLA-DRw2 antigens.

Muscle antibodies are found in 90%, 5% and 45% respectively in the three types (39–42).

The incidence of myasthenia gravis in published series of thymomas is between 15 and 59%. This variation, it is suggested, is accounted for by referral pattern and the overall figure is approximately 30% (9, 30). In contrast, patients presenting with myasthenia gravis have a much lower incidence of thymoma (8.5–15%), though some 75–85% of such patients overall will have some pathological change in the thymus gland, usually a form of thymic lymphoid follicular hyperplasia (30, 43). Bernatz et al. demonstrated clearly that the most consistent association was not found in the thymoma itself but in the surrounding non-neoplastic thymus: namely, the presence of lymphoid follicles with germinal centres identical to those seen in most patients with myasthenia gravis without thymoma. In their series this was present in 53% of patients with myasthenia gravis and in none of those without (30). In the series of Rosai and Levine the figures were 50% and 5% respectively (9).

The presenting type of myasthenia gravis in patients with thymoma is indistinguishable from that seen in patients without thymoma, although Perlo et al. noted that particularly acute forms of the disease are more common in those with tumours (44). Thymomas associated with myasthenia gravis present in younger individuals than non-myasthenic associated tumours (42), which are more frequently diagnosed in the fourth to sixth decades. The effect of thymectomy on myasthenic symptoms differs according to the underlying pathology: in patients with a thymoma improvement in muscle strength is only found in some 25% of patients, whereas improvement may occur in some 40–60% of patients undergoing thymectomy who do *not*

have an underlying thymoma. Several authors have therefore commented that the main reason for surgery in patients with myasthenia gravis *and* a thymoma is removal of the tumour itself rather than a beneficial effect on the myasthenia gravis (30, 41, 44–46). If surgery is contemplated it should be complete, that is a full anterior mediastinal clearance to avoid the possibility of leaving behind residual islets of thymic tissue. The postoperative management of the patient's respiratory problems following such major surgery is of great importance (41).

Childhood thymoma and myasthenia gravis. Thymomas are exceedingly rare in the first 20 years of life and there were thought to be no associated cases of myasthenia gravis. A recent report describes 2 cases presenting without clinical evidence of myasthenia gravis before thoracotomy, who developed florid myasthenia gravis after thoracotomy for removal of an anterior mediastinal mass later documented to be a thymoma. Their extensive review of the literature revealed 5 other instances (47).

Treatment of myasthenia gravis. Myasthenia gravis should be treated with standard medical treatment consisting of anti-cholinesterase drugs. Some patients may show great improvement after receiving immunosuppressive drugs such as corticosteroids and azathioprine (48).

Red cell hypoplasia. In this condition there is anaemia associated with an almost total absence of red cell precursors in the bone marrow (49). In two-thirds of the cases the abnormality is confined to the red cell series but in approximately one-third of cases there is a concurrent depression of platelets or leukocytes (50). The original reviews estimate that over half the patients with red cell aplasia have an underlying thymoma and that about 5% overall of all thymomas are accompanied by this abnormality (51). Of patients with red cell hypoplasia, 96% are 40 years or older at the time of diagnosis and females predominate slightly.

Histologically if an underlying thymoma is present it is almost invariably of the pure spindle cell type. The incidence of encapsulation and of a benign clinical course is the same as for thymomas in general. Thymectomy will result in remission of the disease in from 25 to 35% of cases (51, 52) and in those who do benefit remission of the erythroid hypoplasia may be prolonged (9, 53).

Hypogammaglobulinaemia. Souadjian et al., in their review of 598 patients in the literature with thymoma, found that hypogammaglobulinaemia was reported in approximately 6% (38). The first description of the association had been made by Good in 1954 (54). The features are repeated infection, diarrhoea and lymphadenopathy. Resection of an underlying thymoma does not alter this aspect of the disease (9).

Management of Thymoma

On a plain chest x-ray the typical thymoma is a mass extending laterally from the main mediastinal shadow into either lung field, the outline being round or oval and often lobulated. In patients with myasthenia gravis, where the tumours may be smaller, a lateral or an oblique view reveals a tumour that is not apparent in the antero-posterior views (55).

Computed tomographic scanning (CT) provides additional information to the standard chest x-ray. Within the spectrum of thymic lesions, although thymoma is the most common diagnosis, the differential diagnosis must include thymic cysts, thymolipomas, thymic carcinoids, and thymic lymphomas. Distinguishingly between malignant and benign thymic lesions is difficult, both radiographically and microscopically. A series of papers have reviewed this situation (4, 56–61).

CT scanning allows excellent definition of the margins of a thymoma. Keen and Libshitz determined the additional information that could be obtained using CT in addition to the standard chest radiograph (57). In their series of 24 patients they found that CT gave additional information in 14 and altered treatment in 2 cases. The presence or absence of invasion into adjacent structures was predicted in 16 of

17 patients in whom CT and surgical correlations could be made (57). Brown et al. in a review of the value of computed tomography in myasthenia gravis could not differentiate thymomas from non-thymomatous masses or thymic hyperplasia from normal glands (62). The presence of local invasion is such an important prognostic factor that we believe CT scanning to be imperative in all patients suspected of having thymoma before a definitive treatment strategy is planned for any patient.

Radioisotope scanning using ^{75}Se-selenomethionine proved positive in 6 of 11 patients with thymoma (63). Its clinical usefulness, in addition to the information available from CT scanning, remains to be determined.

Surgery. For the encapsulated thymoma, complete surgical resection should be curative. In the series of 181 patients reported from the Mayo Clinic who had operations for thymoma between 1941 and 1969, Bernatz et al. showed that the survival curve for patients with non-invasive tumours and no evidence of myasthenia gravis was the same as that for the general population once 4 years had elapsed after surgery (64). The tumour should be removed in its entirety without breach of the capsule. Fechner demonstrated that less than 2% of such cases should recur (65).

In a review of 169 patients with surgically treated thymoma recorded at a single institution over a period of 28 years, Maggi et al. reported a local relapse rate of 3.8% in non-invasive cases and an overall survival of 85% at 5 years (66). In their series the presence of myasthenia gravis was not correlated with a shorter survival, which conflicts with earlier reports (64, 67).

Surgery for malignant (invasive) thymomas. The role of surgery in invasive thymoma remains unclear. This surely reflects the proportion of patients in each series who could undergo complete resection. The majority of series which contain any substantial numbers of patients from a single centre have been collected over many decades and imaging techniques, surgical techniques and supportive care has changed considerably during this time. Sub-analysis of any series therefore has to take account of degree of resection (complete, partial or biopsy alone), the use of radiotherapy, and in some instances the use of chemotherapy. These variables, together with the presence or absence of associated diseases, particularly myasthenia gravis, makes such analysis very difficult. Survival rates do in fact vary from 23% to 54% at 5 years (30, 36, 66, 68).

In the series of Maggi et al. 59 cases (36%) were invasive. A complete resection was possible in just over half (58%) of these invasive cases. Survival at 5 years was 80% for those achieving this complete resection, compared to 59% and 45% respectively for those who had a sub-total resection or biopsy alone (66). Cohen et al. (68), reviewing a series of 23 malignant thymomas treated over a period of 35 years, also found that complete surgical excision offered the best chance of long term survival and there appeared to be no benefit from postoperative radiotherapy in these cases, confirming the views of Sawyer and Foster (69). Many other series, however, continue to recommend postoperative irradiation (36, 42, 70–72).

Significantly, Cohen et al. found no difference in survival between the group of patients receiving irradiation following partial excision of most of their tumour and the group receiving irradiation following only biopsy of the lesion. This observation suggests that there is no value in so called 'de-bulking' procedures, where complete resection cannot be attained (68).

Radiotherapy. In *non-invasive* (benign) thymoma the treatment of choice is complete surgical excision and given the very low rate of local recurrence (2–4%) there is no place for adjuvant radiotherapy. In encapsulated tumours where incomplete surgical excision is attained there is no clear guidance. Many series would recommend radiotherapy in this situation and each case must be judged on its merits. However, given the very slow growth rate of these tumours in the absence of myasthenia gravis or other related immune or endocrine dysfunction, a policy of no treatment and careful follow-up could be justified.

In *invasive thymoma*, support for radiotherapy used in conjunction with complete or incomplete surgical excision comes from a number of sources (36, 37, 39, 45, 46, 73–77) and though radiotherapy is rarely curative there are several well documented long term survivals (see above) (30, 46, 67, 75–78). Certainly irradiation may lead to good local control after incomplete resection (24, 36, 75, 77); however, the results of radiotherapy are poor in cases of late recurrence after surgery (79).

Radiotherapy techniques have varied greatly from series to series and dose has varied from 3000 to 6000 rads. Cohen, in a retrospective analysis, found no survival benefit with irradiation when complete resection was attainable. He also found no survival advantage in patients receiving irradiation following partial excision of most of their tumour when compared with the group receiving irradiation following only biopsy of the lesion. This suggested that there was no value in 'de-bulking procedures' and that the irradiation was of value in gaining local control of thymoma (68). Arriagada et al. had similar findings and agreed that irradiation seemed to decrease the rate of local recurrence in these invasive tumours. Their local recurrence rate was 34% at 2 years and overall survival 46% at 5 years. They did make some recommendations concerning radiotherapy technique: suggesting that the volume to be treated should include the supraclavicular lymph nodes and recommending rather high doses of 4500–5000 rads following complete resection and 5000–5500 rads when resection was incomplete, stressing that great care be taken to limit the dose to the spinal cord to below 4500 rads. Although they perceived that there was a risk involved in such doses they considered it justified (80).

Complications of mediastinal irradiation, including constrictive pericarditis, pericardial effusion with tamponade, coronary artery fibrosis, pneumonitis, pulmonary fibrosis and hypothyroidism are all well known. The use of multiple portals, shrinking fields and lung shielding with sub-carinal blocks may all help to reduce these complications (81). Even moderate doses of radiotherapy may produce pneumonitis (82).

In our opinion, radiotherapy should be given to all cases of invasive thymoma where inadequate clearance had been attained. It is possible that a moderately effective chemotherapeutic regimen could now be developed and future treatments should be interpreted in conjunction with this (see below).

Chemotherapy. The poor prognosis of incompletely resected invasive thymoma, with surgery and radiotherapy as the primary modalities of treatment, makes the development of an effective chemotherapeutic regimen important. To date the results of chemotherapy are interesting but not exciting. Nevertheless, there may be a few promising pointers.

Hu and Levine have recently reported on a single case of treatment with prednisolone and reviewed the chemotherapy literature (83). Their interest was aroused by the prompt and marked regression of mediastinal and pulmonary nodular disease to treatment with prednisolone 60 mgs every day, in a man who had previously been treated with five drugs and low dose irradiation to the mediastinal mass. Including their own case they found 14 patients in the literature where treatment with corticosteroids had resulted in 12 responses (86%), the longest of which lasted 36 months (84–91).

Single agent chemotherapy has been reported in a total of 26 cases and seven drugs, the largest single series being our own using single agent ifosfamide in 8 consecutive patients (92). Cisplatin has been used in 5 cases, complete remission being attained in 3 and partial remission in 2 others (93–97). No response was attained in 2 patients treated with vincristine (98). Doxorubicin achieved 2 partial remissions in 2 patients (99, 100). Chlorambucil and nitrogen mustard achieved

TABLE 3 COMBINATION CHEMOTHERAPY IN THYMOMAS: CISPLATIN-CONTAINING REGIMENS[a]

Regimen	No. of patients	Response (duration)	Reference
BAPP	5	2/5+ PR (4, 12 months) 3/5 SD (4+, 6, 14 months)	37
CP, P	1	CR (4 months)	37
BAPP	9[b]	1 CR, 5 PR	105
AP	1	CR (9+ months)	106
	2	CR (4+, 20+ months)	107
PAC	1	CR (12 months)	108
PAC+VCR	11	4/11 CR (5, 8+, 29+ months) 6/11 PR/ (5+, 6, 9, 12, 16+, 22 months)	109
Total no. of patients	25	10/25 CR, 11/25 PR	

[a] After: Hu and Levine (83).
PR: partial response; SD: stable disease; CR: complete response; PD: progressive disease.
[b] Includes previous 5 patients in Kotsilimbas et al.
BAPP=bleomycin, Adriamycin, cisplatin, prednisone.
CP,P=cisplatin, prednisone.
PAC=cisplatin, Adriamycin, cyclophosphamide.
PACVCR=cisplatin, Adriamycin, cyclosphosphamide+vincristine.

TABLE 4 COMBINATION CHEMOTHERAPY IN THYMOMAS: NON-PLATINUM
CONTAINING REGIMENS[a]

Regimen	No. of patients	Response (duration)	Reference
COPP[b]	5	4/5 PR	110
CVCP	9	(12,33+, 34+ months) 4/9 CR, 1/9 PR (31+, 33+, 41+, 62+ months) 3/9 SD, 1 PD	111
CHOP	2	2/2 PD	74
MVPV	2	2 PR (3 week, 3 months)	98
CA	1	1 CR (13+ months)	111

[a] From Hu and Levine (83).
[b] Radiation therapy included
PR: partial response; SD: stable disease; CR: complete response; PD: progressive disease.
COPP =cyclophosphamide, vincristine, procarbazine, prednisone.
CVCP =CCNU, vincristine, cyclophosphamide, prednisone.
CHOP=cyclophosphamide, adriamycin, prednisone.
MVPV=nitrogen mustard, vincristine, procarbazine, vinblastine.
CA=cyclophosphamide, adriamycin.

no response in 3 patients (101). Maytansine has been tested in 4 patients and achieved 2 brief partial remissions (102, 103). Ifosfamide in our group has achieved a complete remission in 5 of 8 patients (63%) and 2 patients had stabilization of disease. The dose used by us was 1.5 g/m^2 daily for 5 successive days every 3 weeks with mesna to prevent urothelial toxicity (92). The complete remissions have proved durable in 5 of the patients with a follow-up ranging from 6 months to 2 years. Details of combination chemotherapy are given in Tables 3 and 4.

Ten of 25 patients treated with platinum containing chemotherapy achieved a complete remission and 11 of 25 partial remissions. The median duration of these responses is 12 months (37, 104–108). The major non-platinum containing regimens include standard COPP, which Evans et al. reported as showing 4 out of 5 partial remissions, including 2 which continued for 33 and 34 months respectively (109). Daugaard, using CVCP, achieved 4 out of 9 complete remissions lasting from 31 to 62 months (74, 109–111) (Table 5).

Combination chemotherapy is to a certain extent encouraging but there is no clear regimen that has been identified. Single agent cis-

platinum, steroids and the alkylating agents show some promise but such treatment will have to be confined in research protocols to cases where there is no other identified treatment. Ifosfamide could well be useful in combination.

The enticing possibility of in some way reducing the bulk of very large tumours with chemotherapy, thus allowing the possibility of surgery or adequate radiotherapy to be delivered to a smaller tumour volume, is one we should aim for: however, we must remain alert to the possibility of increased toxicity (112).

Prognosis. For non-invasive thymomas 5-year survival may be as high as 83% and 10-year survival has been reported at 65%. For invasive thymomas 5-year survival may be as low as 25% (30), though recent series have achieved approximately 50% (66). Older series have certainly shown that the most important and only consistent factor affecting prognosis is the presence of invasion or metastases. Myasthenia gravis, when associated with an invasive thymoma, was previously thought to have a dismal prognosis, but this may be somewhat better than we first thought (66).

TABLE 5 IMMUNOHISTOCHEMISTRY IN THE DIAGNOSIS OF ANTERIOR MEDIASTINAL TUMOURS

Cytokeratin negative tumours		
Malignant lymphoma	Seminona	Paraganglioma

Confirm by:
Leukocyte common
  Antigen
B and T cell Markers
Surface immunoglobulins
Leu-M1 (Hodgkin's)
	Confirm by:
	Placental alkaline
	  phosphatase
		Confirm by:
		Neurone-specific
		  enolase
		PGP 9.5 (chief cells)
		
		S-100 (supporting cells)

Cytokeratin positive tumours				
Thymoma	Germ cell tumours (often mixed)			
Thymic carcinoma	Carcinoid	Embryonal carcinoma	Yolk sac Choriocarcinoma	carcinoma

Some tumours
HLA-DR and
Leu-7 positive
	Confirm by:
	Neurone-specific
	  enolase
	PGP 9.5
	Specific
	  peptides
	  (e.g. ACTH)
		Confirm by:
		Human Placental
		lactogen
			Confirm by:
			Alpha-fetoprotein
				Confirm by:
				Human Chorionic
				  gonadotrophin

Thymic Carcinomas

Thymic carcinomas form a heterogeneous group of rare tumours. This includes tumours which share many features with typical thymomas but show clear features of malignancy, such as large hyperchromatic nuclei, frequent mitoses and necrosis (Figure 5). The thymic origin may be indicated by fribrous septa, perivascular spaces and a lymphocyte population, which is usually sparse. Several rare variants have been described by Snover et al. (25) and Wick et al. (26). They include squamous cell carcinoma, lymphoepithelioma-like carcinoma, spindle cell carcinoma, sarcomatoid carcinoma, basaloid carcinoma, clear cell carcinoma, small cell undifferentiated carcinoma, mucoepidermoid carcinoma and adenoid cystic carcinoma.

Some examples of squamous cell carcinoma may be cystic and Leong et al. have described an example apparently arising within a benign cyst (113).

The microscopic appearances of lymphoepithelioma-like squamous cell carcinoma are identical to those of poorly differentiated nasopharyngeal carcinoma and this similarity has been further emphasized by a report of its association with Epstein–Barr virus infection (114). Electron microscopy and immunohistochemistry may be necessary to make the distinction from malignant lymphoma (see Table 5).

Clear cell carcinoma of the thymus is regarded as a distinct entity by Wolfe et al. and they stress those features that enable it to be differentiated from metastatic clear cell carcinoma from other sites and mediastinal seminoma (115).

Small cell carcinoma of the thymus resembled its much more common pulmonary counterpart and electron microscopy reveals small numbers of neurosecretory granules. The concept that this tumour is an undifferentiated neuroendocrine carcinoma is supported by an example showing transition from a better

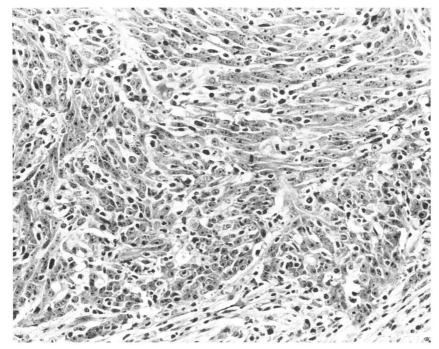

Figure 5 A thymic carcinoma in which the epithelial cells have large prominent nucleoli, a coarse chromatin pattern and frequent mitoses. In this field they appear spindle-shaped and the scattered lymphocytes give a clue to the thymic origin.

differentiated carcinoid to an undifferentiated small cell tumour (116). However, the existence of mixed small cell–squamous cell variants implies an endodermal origin (25).

None of these histological variants is peculiar to the thymus and the possibility that the mediastinal tumour is metastatic must be excluded. The presence of a well circumscribed mediastinal mass and the absence of detectable tumour elsewhere are clearly important.

Primary Thymic Carcinoid Tumours

Since the thymus is of endodermal origin, the presence of endocrine cells, similar to those found in the respiratory and gastrointestinal tracts, is not unexpected. They have proved difficult to demonstrate by traditional staining techniques but recently their presence was shown by Rhode et al. (117) using the general neuroendocrine marker PGP 9.5. Rosai and

his colleagues believe these cells to be the origin of the tumours that they first described in 1972 (118, 119). Wick et al. have reported on 15 cases, 8 of which had been followed up for more than 5 years at the time of publication, and reviewed the pathological and clinical features (120).

Pathology and biology. Thymic carcinoids occur over a wide age range but are most frequent in middle age, the mean age from the two largest series being 48 years (119, 120). There is a strong male predominance. They may be asymptomatic, discovered only by routine chest radiography, or they may cause compression of mediastinal structures. They often reach a considerable size and, although they may appear well circumscribed, infiltration of surrounding structures makes surgical removal difficult (120). The cut surface is uniformly pinkish-tan in colour and they lack

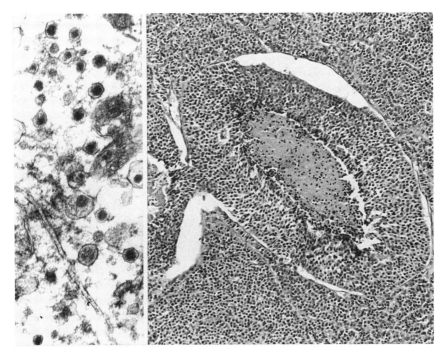

Figure 6 A thymic carcinoid tumour. In many areas of this tumour the characteristic carcinoid pattern was lacking. This field shows a very typical type of necrosis, in which the cells surrounding the necrotic focus separate from the surrounding tumour. Numerous dense core secretory granules are seen by electron microscopy (inset).

the clear encapsulation or white fibrous septa usually seen in thymomas. Minute foci and necrosis or calcification may be visible together with areas of haemorrhage.

In general, the histological features resemble those of carcinoid tumours elsewhere, although different areas of the same tumour may vary. Typically, cells are uniform in size with moderate pale or granular eosinophilic cytoplasm, finely dispersed nuclear chromatin and single inconspicuous nuclei. They form ribbons or cords in a richly vascular stroma. In more cellular areas the pattern is less obvious and cells may form sheets with few diagnostic features (Figure 6). Several unusual variants are described and are particularly likely to be confused with thymic epithelial tumours. These include spindle cell tumours (121), tumours showing rosette formation or a cribriform pattern and those with a sclerotic fibrous stroma (116). Cytoplasmic pigment is occasionally present and may be either lipofuscin (120) or melanin (122).

Rosai et al. have listed the clinical, light microscopic and ultrastructural features that help to distinguish between thymoma and thymic carcinoid (119). At the light microscopic level thymic carcinoids lack fibrous septa, a lymphocyte population and perivascular spaces. Electron microscopy demonstrates numerous dense core neurosecretory granules (Figure 6).

In contrast to bronchopulmonary carcinoids, of which only about 10% have atypical features, the majority of thymic carcinoids are histologically atypical, showing nuclear pleomorphism, significant numbers of mitoses and areas of necrosis. The latter are often characteristic, with a small central focus of necrosis in the centre of a round or oval cellular aggregate separated from the surrounding cells by an artefactual fissure-like space (Figure 6)(119).

The clinical behaviour of thymic carcinoids correlates with the atypical histological features: local recurrence is likely, even after a long interval (119, 120, 123). Metastases frequently involve mediastinal nodes and widespread distant metastasis, including osteosclerotic bone deposits, is not unusual. In the Mayo Clinic series, 11 of 15 patients developed metastases (120).

If endocrine tumours of the thymus, or more correctly tumours of the thymus showing endocrine differentiation, show a spectrum of malignancy comparable to that seen in bronchopulmonary endocrine tumours, it might be expected that a poorly differentiated variant, comparable to small cell carcinoma of the lung, may occasionally occur. Such tumours occur at a younger age than their lung counterparts and it has been suggested that they may have a somewhat better prognosis (119, 124). They are discussed with thymic carcinomas.

Marino and Müller-Hermelink classify thymic carcinoids and small cell carcinomas as neuroectodermal carcinomas (125). Tumours showing a combination of endocrine and epithelial features are well described in the lung and gastrointestinal tract. Wick et al. (116) mention 2 cases of thymic carcinoma with ultrastructural features of carcinoid tumours and the lesion illustrated in Figure 7 is a possible example of dual differentiation. Parts of the tumour showed a microcystic pattern formed by cells with epithelial features and perivascular spaces were frequent. Typical neurosecretory granules were present in small numbers.

Immunohistochemistry has an important role to play in the diagnosis of carcinoid tumours. Like thymomas, they consistently express intermediate filaments of keratin type, provided that the antibody used reacts with keratins of low molecular weight. The report by Miettinen et al. of neurofilaments in a thymic carcinoid may indicate that co-expression of intermediate filament types is a feature but further studies are required (126).

Antibodies of value in recognizing endocrine tumours are anti-neurone-specific enolase (NSE), and PGP 9.5 (117, 127).

In an immunohistochemical study of 12 thymic carcinoids, Wick and Scheitauer demonstrated ACTH in 4 tumours, 3 of which had presented with Cushing's syndrome (116). Somatostatin was present in 6 cases and none stained for calcitonin, VIP, insulin, glucagon or gastrin. In contrast to 'typical' bronchopulmonary carcinoids, where immunoreactive serotonin is usually demonstrable, only one thymic tumour contained serotonin. The tendency for thymic carcinoids to produce ACTH is shared by more aggressive bronchopulmonary neuroendocrine tumours, atypical carcinoids and small cell carcinomas (128) and this correlates with their clinical behaviour. Swinborne-Sheldrake et al. demonstrated ACTH in 3 thymic carcinoids and calcitonin in one tumour in which stromal amyloid was present (129).

Clinical features. Thymic carcinoids *are not* associated with the typical carcinoid syndrome of flushing, diarrhoea and asthma. There have been cases of Cushing's syndrome (130) and there is also an association with the multiple endocrine neoplasia (MEN) syndromes, both type 1 (pituitary, parathyroid and pancreatic islet cell tumours) and type 2 (Sipple syndrome—phaeochromocytoma, medullary thyroid carcinoma and, in some cases, parathyroid hyperplasia).

Salyer et al. in a complete review of the literature up to 1976 provided an extensive pathological and clinical review of 3 cases of their own, 10 additional cases from the literature that they considered proved and 4 cases that they thought likely. They confirmed the male prominance and lack of association with myasthenia gravis or red cell hypoplasia. Thymic carcinoids appeared to be more aggressive tumours than thymomas with local invasion and frequent metastases: however, their review indicated that the clinical course was usually protracted (123). Subsequently, it became apparent that these tumours are far more

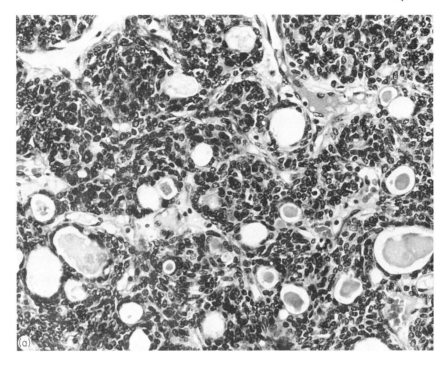

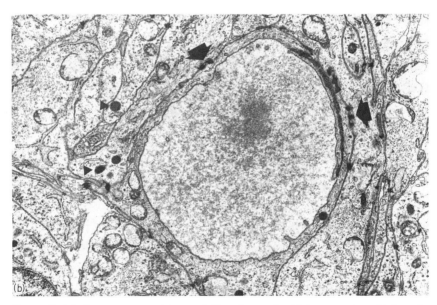

Figure 7 (a) A very unusual type of thymic carcinoid tumour, in which cells surround gland-like spaces. (b) Ultrastructurally they show prominent epithelial features and only scattered neurosecretory granules (arrowheads). The lumen is surrounded by long cell processes with numerous desmosomes (arrows) and occasional microvilli.

malignant than first thought and 5-year survival is only 15% for all treatment methods (3,
131).

Aggressive surgery is the treatment of choice
even if this means sacrificing adjacent normal
tissue. Radiotherapy and chemotherapy have
to date proved ineffective in altering the
progress of the disease though occasional
patients may have had some benefit.

Thymolipoma and Thymic Sarcoma

Rosai and Levine have reviewed the available
literature on thymolipoma (9) and Rosai was
also co-author of a single case of sarcoma of the
thymic stroma with features of a liposarcoma
(131).

Thymolipomas are rare, benign lesions that
account for 2–9% of all thymic tumours. They
may occur at any age but are most frequent in
young adults, with a mean age of 22 years.
They can grow to a large size and a quarter of
the cases reviewed by Rosai and Levine
weighed over 2 kg: the largest tumour on
record weighed over 16 kg (9). Associated
diseases include myasthenia gravis (132), thyr-
otoxicosis, aplastic anaemia and Hodgkin's
disease (133).

These tumours retain the original lobated
form of the thymus and are encapsulated.
Macroscopically, they resemble lipomas but
thin strands of white tissue separate the adipose
tissue. Microscopically, there is a close resemblance to normal thymus with preservation of
normal thymic cortex and medulla in the
strands of thymic tissue. Thymolipomas
appear to be formed by overgrowth of hyperplasia of thymus and associated adipose tissue
but the cause is unknown.

Sarcomas of the thymus are excessively rare.
A single case of rhabdoid sarcoma has been
described under the heading of malignant
histiocytoma (134). The thymic liposarcoma
described above, which occurred in a 39 year
old woman, was found on a routine chest
radiograph (131). Microscopically, it was a
pleomorphic liposarcoma intimately mixed
with histologically normal thymic tissue. It was

resected and she was given postoperative
radiotherapy (4600 rads). Thirty-one years
later a compression fracture of the fifth thoracic vertebra occurred and was thought to be
due to a metastasis. She was given further
radiotherapy. The final outcome was not
known at the time of publication, although the
authors did comment on a further case that
had come to their attention.

Malignant Lymphomas of the Thymus

Hodgkin's disease is limited to the mediastinum in less than 5% of patients and in about a
quarter of these it is confined to the thymus.
The remainder have involvement of mediastinal lymph nodes alone or involvement of both
thymus and lymph nodes. The histological
appearances lead to the earlier terms 'granulomatous thymitis' or 'granulomatous thymoma'
and are those of nodular sclerosing Hodgkin's
disease (6). It is important to note that the
persistence of the mediastinal mass following
therapy may be due to a residual cyst (135–
137). Treatment is entirely conventional with
radiotherapy or radiotherapy and chemotherapy (138). Hodgkin's disease is discussed
further in the section on mediastinal lymphadenopathy.

In children and adolescents, non-Hodgkin's
lymphoma involves the mediastinum in up to
one-third of all cases. Of these, the majority are
of lymphoblastic type and are of T cell origin,
sharing markers with cortical thymocytes.
Their distinctive clinical characteristics
include a tendency to occur in adolescent
males and early dissemination to bone marrow
and the central nervous system. Selective infiltration of the thymus results in an anterior
mediastinal mass, the so-called Sternberg sarcoma (139).

Large cell lymphoma with sclerosis is a
comparatively recently recognized form of
mediastinal lymphoma and there is some evidence that it arises within the thymus (6, 140–
144). It usually presents in the third or fourth
decade and some series indicate a female
predominance (144). Patients frequently pre-

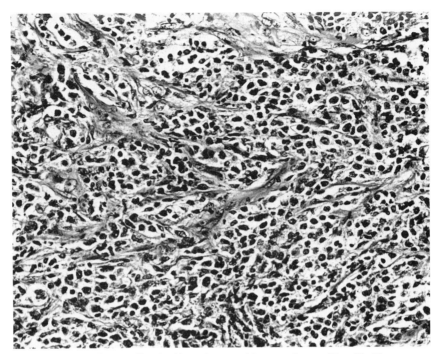

Figure 8 Sclerosing mediastinal lymphoma of large cell type (B cell). The groups of malignant lymphoid cells are separated by fine bands of connective tissue. Such tumours may be mistakenly diagnosed as epithelial in origin or as mediastinal seminomas.

sent with superior vena caval obstruction or symptoms due to infiltration of lung or chest wall and most have a bulky anterior mediastinal tumour.

The characteristic histological feature, which is present to some extent in most of these tumours, is a tendency for tumour cells to be packeted or compartmentalized by a network of narrow connective tissue septa (Figure 8). Tumour cells are large and have the features of a high-grade lymphoma, with prominent nucleoli and a high mitotic rate. Nuclei are frequently folded or lobated and may mimic the Reed–Sternberg cells of Hodgkin's disease. Most cases in which immunohistochemical studies have been undertaken show B cell lineage. Scattered among the neoplastic cells is a population of non-neoplastic T lymphocytes.

Recognition of this type of lymphoma is often far from straightforward, especially when only a small amount of tissue is available. In addition to Hodgkin's disease, the differential diagnosis includes thymoma, thymic carcinoma, carcinoid and seminoma. Immunohistochemistry is helpful and the panel of antibodies should include cytokeratin, leukocyte common antigen, specific B and T cell markers, kappa and lambda light chains and Leu M1 (a useful marker for Reed–Sternberg cells). The absence of cytoplasmic glycogen may help make the distinction from seminoma. Lymph nodes may be involved but spread is characteristically extranodal, the most frequently involved organs being kidney, liver, thyroid, ovary, pancreas and gastrointestinal tract.

Treatment is on conventional lines with chemotherapy, radiotherapy or both. Perrone et al. found that good prognostic signs included marked tumour sclerosis and a good response to initial therapy (144). Conversely, a poor prognosis was likely in patients who were aged

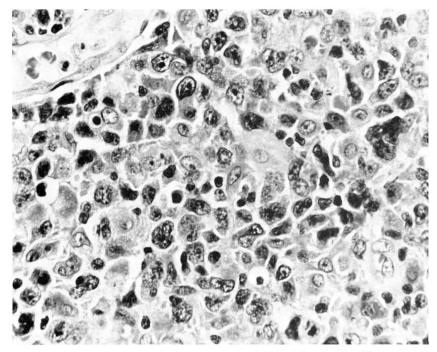

Figure 9 Another example of large cell mediastinal lymphoma (B cell), occurring in a 12 year old child. In this case no sclerosis was apparent and the cells showed a marked degree of pleomorphism.

25 or less at the time of diagnosis, those who had extrathoracic disease at presentation and those whose response to initial therapy was incomplete. Surgical de-bulking of the tumour and the type of initial treatment seemed to have little effect on the outcome.

We have seen a small number of cases of high-grade, non-Hodgkin's mediastinal lymphoma of large cell type occurring in children. All were of B cell type but lacked the typical sclerosis seen in older patients (Figure 9). Similar tumours are probably included in the series of mediastinal non-lymphoblastic lymphoma in children reported by Bunin and her colleagues (145). Treatment in their series was not uniform but resulted in complete remission in 92% of which 74% remained disease-free for 13 to 65 months.

An example of true histiocytic lymphoma of the thymus is reported by Szporn et al. who also demonstrated the distribution of histiocytes in the normal gland (146).

Kubonishi et al. have described a very unusual case of granulocytic sarcoma, presenting as a tumour in the antero-superior mediastinum in a 23 year old male (147). Eight months later the patient developed the blood and bone marrow pictures of acute promyelocytic leukaemia.

Histiocytosis X of the Thymus

Siegal et al. presented detailed pathology and follow-up of 4 cases. All the patients were children, their age at diagnosis ranging from 2 months to 8 years (148). In 2 cases the disease seemed restricted to the thymus and in the other 2 there was extrathymic involvement. Three additional cases were reviewed. Primary treatment was surgical, with complete excision in 2 and partial excision in 2. Two cases received postoperative radiotherapy, one chemotherapy and no information was available on the fourth. All were alive and well with a follow-up of 4 to 14 years. The histological features were characteristic with an infiltrate of Langerhans cells and variable numbers of eosinophils, fibrosis and residual thymic tissue.

Soft Tissue Tumours of the Mediastinum

Mesenchymal tumours of the mediastinum are rare and since the extensive review by Pachter and Lattes in 1963 (149), additions to the literature have consisted mainly of single case reports. The majority arise from adipose tissue or blood vessels.

Tumours of Adipose Tissue

Most intrathoracic lipomas occur in adults and are asymptomatic. They appear to arise in the cardio-phrenic angle and mould themselves around mediastinal structures as they enlarge. Seventy-five per cent arise anteriorly and closely resemble a pericardial cyst on x-ray.

Primary liposarcomas of the mediastinum tend to arise in the posterior mediastinum where they can be confused with neurogenic tumours. Fifty-one cases had been recorded until 1981. Schweitzer and Aguam reviewed the first 50 cases (150, 151) and tabulated all known cases and the various systems of classification of liposarcomas. Their conclusions were that the tumours might occur in any age group, although the average age was 45 years with two-thirds of these patients older than 40 years at presentation. There was an equal sex incidence in their series. The predominant presenting symptoms were respiratory distress, chest pain or a feeling of pressure, cough and weight loss. Seventy-six per cent of patients underwent surgical exploration. Certainly irradiation did cause major remissions in a number of patients, but in their review Friedman and Egan surmised that to arrest the growth of liposarcoma with irradiation they had to administer approximately 9000 rads over a period of 30 to 50 days (152). The treatment of choice for these tumours was clearly that of complete surgical resection.

Survival data were available in 76% of cases. Within this group median survival was 40 months although some patients survived for an extraordinary number of years before dying of the disease. Castleberry, in a general review of childhood liposarcoma, recorded 4 cases of mediastinal tumours (153).

Tumours of Vascular Origin

Benign haemangiomas and lymphangiomas both occur in the anterior mediastinum. Haemangiomas may be of capillary or cavernous type. Most lymphangiomas contain large cystic spaces and are similar to the more common cystic hygroma of the neck, which occurs in childhood and may extend into the mediastinum. Angiomas often attain a large size before causing symptoms and in children respiratory distress may occur either due to rapid enlargement or if haemorrhage occurs into the lesion or into the pleural space (154–157).

In the series of Pachter and Lattes, haemangiopericytomas formed a significant group of tumours (154). Most pathologists now make this diagnosis with caution as many other tumours, including thymomas and pleural fibromas, can mimic the histological appearances. In true haemangiopericytomas the normal histological criteria of malignancy do not correlate well with behaviour. Capsular invasion and infiltration of surrounding structures are more reliable prognostic indicators (154, 158).

An example of mediastinal angiosarcoma is described by Gibbs et al. (159) who stress the value of immunohistochemical staining for factor VIII-related antigen in the diagnosis of malignant endothelial tumours.

Tumours of Muscle Origin (149, 160)

Smooth muscle tumours are extremely rare in the mediastinum and in the series of Rasaretnam and Panabokke there were 7 benign and 2 malignant tumours (160). Leiomyosarcomas may originate in the wall of the pulmonary artery, superior vena cava or even in bronchial cysts. Sunderrajan reports on a case presenting as a superior vena caval syndrome (161). Death usually results from regional extension and metastases, but survival following resection has been reported (160, 161).

There is only a single report of a benign mediastinal rhabdomyoma (162), but primary mediastinal rhabdomyosarcoma is well recognized. The Intergroup Rhabdomyosarcoma Study Committee, in analysing their data, found 10 of 646 patients to have primary mediastinal disease, 8 of whom were male (161). Mediastinal rhabdomyosarcomas tended to occur in older children and were more likely to be of undifferentiated histological type than similar tumours in most other primary sites. All 10 patients were treated on protocol with chemotherapy and radiotherapy with surgical resection if possible (161). The only long term survivor achieved gross resection of disease (162). In the series of 17 patients with intrathoracic disease (including the 10 with mediastinal disease discussed above), 2 who achieved gross surgical clearance were long term survivors, and only 1 of 10 unresected cases survived longer than 2 years (162).

Fibrosarcoma and Malignant Fibrous Histiocytoma

Pachter and Lattes recognized a number of cases of fibrosarcoma of the mediastinum (149). It is possible that at least some of their tumours would now be classified as malignant fibrous histiocytoma and there have been several recent examples. In the case reported by Chen et al. erosion of the thoracic aorta resulted in false aneurysm formation and fatal intrapulmomary haemorrhage (163). Posterior mediastinal tumours were also reported by Natsuaki et al. (164) and Mills et al. (165) one of whose patients had an excellent response to radiotherapy. Poon et al. recorded a case of inflammatory fibrous histiocytoma of the mediastinum in which combination chemotherapy produced remission, sustained for 2 years at the time of publication (166).

Mixed Connective Tissue Tumours and Undifferentiated Sarcomas

Mixed connective tissue tumours (mesenchymomas) have been described in the mediastinum. Most are lipomas, liposarcomas or rhabdomyosarcomas with areas of chondroid or osseous metaplasia (149). Dehner et al. encountered foci of neoplastic cartilage in 2 of 3 malignant mesenchymal tumours of the anterior mediastinum in children. All 3 tumours consisted predominantly of small spindle cells and the term 'thymoblastoma' was tentatively suggested (167). We have seen 2 similar cases in young people: neither contained cartilage and there were no diagnostic ultrastructural features. However, there is no good evidence that such lesions are of thymic origin.

Mediastinal Fibrosis (Sclerosing Mediastinitis)

Though it is not a true neoplasm, mediastinal fibrosis produces similar symptoms and, in small biopsies, the distinction from nodular sclerosing Hodgkin's disease and spindle cell neoplasms may be difficult. The process is one of fibroblast proliferation with deposition of densely collagenized connective tissue and compression of mediastinal structures (168, 169). Inflammatory cells are also a characteristic feature in active areas. In most cases the aetiology is unknown and the thoracic disease may be part of a multifocal process which includes retroperitoneal fibrosis, Riedel's thyroiditis, sclerosing cholangitis, orbital pseudotumour and constrictive pericarditis (170, 171). The drug methysergide is a known cause and some cases may represent an exaggerated reaction to tuberculous or fungal infection (172).

The disease affects all age groups and both sexes but is seen most often in young women. Superior vena caval compression is a frequent feature of mediastinal fibrosis though a rare cause of superior vena caval obstruction overall, accounting for only 1–2% of this syndrome.

There can be involvement of pulmonary vessels, bronchi and even the coronary arteries. The condition is rarely life-threatening but the quality of life in these patients is poor. The results of conservative treatment have been disappointing but with the development of materials specifically designed as venous grafts, and the improved patency rates now reported with autogenous vein grafts, the role of surgery should be reconsidered. This has recently been reviewed (173). Three of 5 cases had major relief of symptoms for many years.

Mediastinal Lymphadenopathy and Other Disorders

A large number of inflammatory and neoplastic diseases can cause enlargement of mediastinal lymph nodes. Some involve mediastinal nodes alone and therefore present as a mediastinal mass, whereas others produce mediastinal lymph node enlargement as part of a generalized lymphadenopathy. Some of the former are discussed here.

Malignant Lymphoma

Malignant lymphoma is one of the commonest causes of a mediastinal mass, accounting for some 44% of cases in the surgical series reported by Wychulis et al. (4). Nevertheless, lymphomas presenting solely as a mediastinal mass are very much less common.

Hodgkin's disease limited to intrathoracic sites occurred in only 44 of the 1470 patients treated over a 20-year period at Stanford (174). Johnson et al. reporting this series found mediastinal nodes to be involved in forty (91%). The predominant subtype is nodular sclerosing and no cause for this particular relationship has yet been put forward (174, 175). Mediastinal Hodgkin's disease may be very bulky indeed and in this situation tumour size is related to duration of remission (138, 174, 175); patients with tumours greater than one-third of chest diameter do significantly less well than those with smaller tumours. For such bulky tumours combination chemotherapy

and radiotherapy have been recommended (138, 174, 175).

In non-Hodgkin's lymphoma, involvement of mediastinal or hilar nodes occurs in 15 to 25% of patients, most often at a late stage when tumour is widely disseminated. Between 9 and 12% of patients have disease apparently confined to the mediastinum at the time of presentation (176, 177). Many of these are lymphoblastic or large cell lymphoma originating in the thymus and these have been discussed.

The remaining tumours are of nodal origin and may be of B cell type, including plasmacytomas, or of post-thymic T cell origin. The treatment and prognosis of a patient with primary mediastinal non-Hodgkin's lymphoma is unclear, both because of the small numbers of patients treated (176, 177) and the lack of uniformity in their treatment. Tumours are characterized by rapid growth and early dissemination and there is a short median survival time in the group of 13 months. Because of this early dissemination, even in clinically localized lesions, and the poor response in 3 such patients initially treated with local radiation therapy, Lichtenstein has suggested the use of combination chemotherapy (176).

Angiofollicular Lymph Node Hyperplasia (Castleman's Disease)

Castleman and his co-workers first described this entity in 1954 as a localized tumour-like mass found in the mediastinum, characterized histologically by 'hyperplasia of lymphoid follicles' (178). In most cases the mass appears to involve lymph node groups and presents as a large asymptomatic localized mass in the mediastinum. Thymic involvement is rare (179). In 1972, Keller et al published an extensive review in which they divided the disease into two histological subtypes, hyaline-vascular, comprising 91% of cases, and plasma cell, representing 9% of cases (180).

In the hyaline-vascular variant the closely packed abnormal follicles consist of layers of small lymphoid cells with hyaline intercellular material. The vascular component consists of a network of small thick-walled vessels, many of which penetrate the follicles. Follicles are more typically reactive in the plasma cell variant and are separated by numerous plasma cells.

The hyaline-vascular type typically produces effects only from its size and position, whereas the plasma cell type is accompanied by a multitude of a systemic effects including fever, anaemia, abnormal liver function tests, renal disease, skin rashes, hypergamma-globulinaemia, the nephrotic syndrome, myasthenia gravis and peripheral neuropathy (179, 180).

The clinical differences between the two types are reflected in quite different outcomes. The hyaline-vascular subtype is a localized, tumour-like, self-limiting process, curable with local therapy. Surgery is the treatment of choice though on occasions radiotherapy may be required. The plasma cell subtype is a systemic disease with a more aggressive course associated with infectious complications and a risk of development of other malignancies (181). The nature of the disease and the relationship between the two types, if any, continues to perplex: in a recent editorial Frizzera found more questions than answers (181).

THE POSTERIOR MEDIASTINUM

Strictly speaking, the posterior mediastinum is the space between the posterior border of the pericardium and the anterior aspect of the vertebral column, but by convention it also includes the paravertebral gutters. Many of the tumours arising in this compartment are of neural origin: in one large series 20% of all mediastinal tumours were neurogenic and they were encountered as frequently as thymomas (4). The remaining lesions found in the posterior mediastinum are oesophageal and enteric cysts, foramen of Morgagni hernias and lymphomas.

Tumours of Neural Origin

Neurogenic tumours in the mediastinum include benign and malignant nerve sheath tumours, arising from peripheral nerves, together with less common tumours of the autonomic nervous system, comprising neuroblastomas, ganglioneuroblastomas, ganglioneuromas and paragangliomas. Patients with nerve sheath tumours may have other features of neurofibromatosis.

Neurogenic tumours of the mediastinum have been reviewed by Akwari and colleagues (182). Among 706 collected cases of mediastinal neurogenic tumours they found 69 (9.8%) with extensions through an intervertebral foramen so that the composite tumour was dumbbell shaped. Histologically two-thirds were of nerve sheath origin and one-third of sympathetic origin, with only 2% arising from paraganglion cells. If the diagnosis of these tumours is made prior to thoracotomy then the initial surgery should be a laminectomy with resection of the intravertebral tumour. If the thoracic extension is small then this can be removed at the same time: if it is larger a separate thoracotomy is required.

Nerve Sheath Tumours (Chapters 29 and 31)

In adults, benign nerve sheath tumours form 75% of posterior mediastinal tumours and they accounted for 39 of the 55 intrathoracic neural tumours in the series of Davidson et al. (183). They are slow growing and often asymptomatic lesions which are usually discovered between the ages of 20 and 40 years. Radiologically, the appearances are of a sharply circumscribed round or oval shadow in the paravertebral gutter and bony erosion can occur with both benign and malignant variants. Early surgical exploration and resection is a universally accepted policy because of doubts about the diagnosis, increasing size of the tumour and the possibility of malignancy. Where this is achieved there are few residual problems.

As Davidson and his colleagues stated (183),

the pathologist's difficulties are perhaps greater than those of the surgeon, for whom the distinction between neurofibroma and neurilemmoma is of relatively little importance.

Two distinct types of benign nerve sheath tumour are recognized, but long-standing lesions may be difficult to categorize because of extensive fibrosis. Neurilemmomas (schwannomas) are of Schwann cell origin and characteristically have two components combined in varying proportions: Antoni-A tissue consists of interlacing bundles of closely packed spindle cells, often with nuclear palisading, and Antoni-B tissue is loose myxoid connective tissue. They are encapsulated and nerve fibres run through the capsule rather than through the tumour. In contrast, neurofibromas have no true capsule and nerve fibres are scattered throughout the tumours. Cells include perineural and endoneural fibroblasts as well as Schwann cells and these appear as scattered spindle cells in a loose stroma. Patients with neurofibromatosis may develop plexiform neurofibromas, which appear as elongated irregular swellings along the course of peripheral or autonomic nerves.

Most malignant nerve sheath tumours (neurofibrosarcomas, malignant schwannomas) occur in patients with neurofibromatosis, often arising from pre-existing neurofibromas. Rapid growth in such a lesion should therefore alert one to the possibility of malignant change. This tends to occur in relatively young patients, usually between 20 and 30 years. In patients without neurofibromatosis malignant nerve sheath tumours occur a decade or so later. Unlike benign nerve sheath tumours, which are virtually confined to the paravertebral area, malignant tumours may also arise in other mediastinal sites and it may be difficult, especially with large tumours, to identify the origin.

For the pathologist, the distinction between malignant nerve sheath tumours and other spindle cell sarcomas, particularly malignant fibrous histiocytoma and fibrosarcoma, may be difficult, especially if the patient lacks the stigmata of neurofibromatosis. A useful immunohistochemical marker for Schwann cells is S-100 protein. Ultrastructurally, nerve sheath tumours characteristically show long cell processes with deposition of basement membrane material between cells.

Tumours of the autonomic nervous system (183, 184) (Chapter 29)

Tumours arising in the posterior mediastinum from autonomic ganglia show a complete spectrum of differentiation from malignant undifferentiated tumours of sympathetic precursor cells (neuroblasts) to benign tumours of fully differentiated ganglion cells.

Neuroblastoma has been fully discussed in standard textbooks. Although the adrenal medulla is the most common primary site, about 16% present in the mediastinum (185). In the series of Wychulis et al. (1971) there were 8 neuroblastomas amongst 212 neurogenic mediastinal tumours (4). They are usually large at the time of presentation and the histological appearances vary from undifferentiated tumours, consisting of sheets of uniform small dark cells with scanty cytoplasm, to better differentiated tumours, in which the cells form rosettes with a central tangle of neural processes. Recent advances in immunohistochemistry have helped in the diagnosis of neuroblastoma: staining for neuron specific enolase is positive (6, 186) and specific monoclonal antibodies for neuroblastoma are described (187).

The basic treatment of neuroblastoma has changed little in the past decade. A localized tumour is curable in a high proportion of patients with combination chemotherapy. Infants have therapeutic advantages compared to children older than 1 year. Disseminated neuroblastoma continues to be a largely fatal disease (188). New treatment modalities developed over the last 8 years, including the use of cis-platinum and the podophyllotoxins VP16-213 and VM26, the possibility of cleaning up bone marrow with monoclonal antibodies and autologous bone marrow transplantation are all contributing to improved results (188–191). Mediastinal tumours may have a better prognosis than adrenal tumours and share a tendency to spontaneous regression or maturation.

Ganglioneuroblastomas are tumours in which the cells show a range of maturation from primitive neuroblasts to fully differentiated ganglion cells (192). Two histological patterns are described; the composite type, in which foci of pure neuroblastoma are present with mature ganglion cells, and the diffuse type, in which undifferentiated and differentiating neuroblastoma cells are intimately mixed with immature bizarre ganglion cells in a fibrillary stroma.

The prognosis for this group is far better than for either neuroblastomas ot intra-abdominal ganglioneuroblastomas. Adams and Hochholzer reviewed 80 cases and demonstrated a 5-year actuarial survival of 88% (192). Prognosis was related to histological pattern, age and extent of disease at diagnosis. Tumours most likely to metastasize were those with a composite pattern and a predominantly neuroblastomatous cell type. Stage 1 tumours were curable by simple excision, Stage 2 tumours treated with surgery and radiation responded as favourably as those that received adjuvant chemotherapy. Late recurrences were not easily treatable. They found on review that these posterior mediastinal tumours were a remarkably homogeneous group. They were encapsulated, grew silently to a relatively large size and were biochemically inactive. Their accessibility to a lateral thoracic approach made total or sub-total excision possible in more than half the cases. Standard treatment for the Stage 1 tumour should be complete surgical excision to de-bulk the mass and to permit accurate staging and diagnosis. Adjuvant radiotherapy in Stage 1 disease should be considered for patients over 12 years old, for tumours of the composite pattern and for incomplete excision. In patients with initially elevated catecholamine metabolites which do not fall to normal after surgery, prognosis is poor and further treatment is necessary.

Ganglioneuromas are benign tumours which are relatively common in the posterior mediastinum, forming about 30% of the neurogenic tumours in the series of Whychulis et al. (4). They are uncommon under the age of 3 years but about half of the patients are younger than 20 years. Most are asymptomatic and chest radiography reveals a large, characteristically poorly defined tumour. These are often adherent to adjacent structures and this makes surgical removal difficult. Grossly they appear soft with a white or yellow surface. Calcification is frequent and they may undergo cystic degeneration. Histologically they resemble normal sympathetic ganglia, consisting of bundles of nerve fibres with ganglion cells scattered singly or in clusters. Every tumour should be thoroughly sampled to exclude foci of less mature cells.

Paragangliomas (Chapters 29 and 36)

Paragangliomas form less than 1% of primary mediastinal tumours (193) and occur either in the anterior mediastinum or, less commonly, in the paravertebral region.

Branchiomeric paragangliomas (chemodectomas) of the anterior mediastinum arise from paraglanglia associated with the arteries and nerves of the branchial arches. These include the aorticopulmonary paraganglia, distributed between the bifurcation of the pulmonary artery and the aortic arch in the area limited by the right pulmonary artery and the ductus arteriosus, and pulmonary paraganglia, within the adventitia of the pulmonary arteries (194). Tumours arising in this area are often attached to the pericardium. Paraganglia associated with the segmental ganglia of the sympathetic chain give rise to paravertebral paragangliomas. Glenner and Grimley recommended that the term phaeochromocytoma be limited to paragangliomas arising in the adrenal medulla (194).

Whereas a high proportion of adrenal tumours secrete catecholamines, few anterior mediastinal tumours are functioning. Aorticosympathetic tumours occupy an intermediate

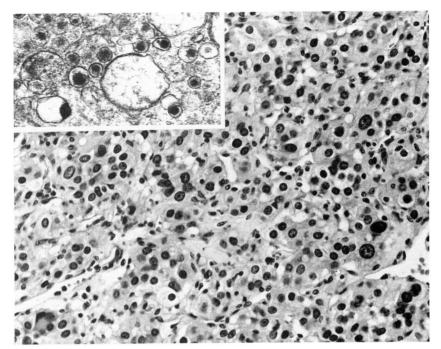

Figure 10 Mediastinal paraganglioma. This tumour arose in relation to a pulmonary artery in the anterior mediastinum. Note the characteristic balls of cells
separated by a capillary network and the degree of variation in nuclear size.
Numerous dense core granules are seen by electron microscopy (inset).

position (195). An association between functioning mediastinal paraganglioma and carotid body tumours has recently been described
(196).

Paragangliomas, whatever their location,
appear as well circumscribed, pinkish-tan coloured or haemorrhagic lesions with a spongy
consistency. Microscopically, they consist of
nests or balls of cells ('Zellballen') surrounded
by a rich network of thin-walled sinusoidal
blood vessels (Figure 10). The cell nests consist
of chief cells, which are large with round or
oval nuclei and abundant clear or eosinophilic
granular cytoplasm, and the less conspicuous
supporting or sustentacular cells, which lie
around the periphery of the cell nests. The
chief cells show argyrophilia and electron
microscopy reveals numerous neurosecretory
granules (Figure 10). Immunohistochemistry
may be necessary to make the distinction
between paraganglioma and carcinoid

tumour: both stain with antibodies to neurone-
specific anolase (NSE) but chief cells do not
express cytokeratins and the supporting cells,
which are of Schwann cell origin, stain for
S-100 protein The usual histological indicators
of malignancy are considered unreliable and
their behaviour is difficult to predict. Late
recurrence is frequent and about 10% metastasize via the blood stream to lungs and bone.

In a review of 36 documented cases by Lack
et al., half the patients were asymptomatic and
the mass was discovered on routine chest
radiography (197). Those with symptoms
complained of hoarseness, dysphagia, chest
pain or discomfort, cough and, in one instance,
haemoptysis. The superior vena caval syndrome was present in 3 cases. Complete surgical resection was achieved in 52%.

Olsen and Salyer (198) later tabulated all
forty cases in the literature and again stressed
that the best therapy is complete surgical

excision, though this was not without its risks. They found that there was a high incidence of aggressive tumour growth in the mediastinum with resultant important morbidity or death in 16 of the 35 cases. Nineteen patients only were alive and well at the time of their review.

Localization of these mediastinal paragangliomas may prove easier in the future due to the development of two-recent techniques: ^{131}I-*meta*-iodobenzylguanidine (^{131}I-*m*IBG) scintigraphy and two dimensional echocardiography (199, 200). ^{131}I-*m*-IBG is a new radiopharmaceutical technique that has proved to be useful in the localization of catecholamine-producing tumours, neuroblastomas and carcinoid tumours. It is taken up and concentrated in adrenergic vesicles (201). Cueto-Garcia et al. described a two-dimensional echocardiographic detection of such a tumour which defined its anatomical relationship to other vascular structures (199).

Paragangliomas, arising in the costo-vertebral sulcus, from residual extra-adrenal chromaffin tissue related to the sympathetic chain, are far less common and occur in a somewhat younger age group. About half of the tumours are functional, producing symptoms due to noradrenaline release (202). Here also, ^{131}I-*m*IBG may offer very interesting treatment potential (200).

Chemotherapy for malignant paraganglioma is unproven but there has been an interesting case report in which carboplatin caused major regression in a patient with tumour metastatic to lung and liver, who had failed to respond to previous therapy (203).

MISCELLANEOUS RARE TUMOUR-LIKE LESIONS OF THE MEDIASTINUM

Occasionally, extramedullary haemopoiesis presents as a large solitary mediastinal mass, usually located along the paravertebral gutter. The primary disease is likely to be hereditary spherocytosis or thalassaemia (204). Even if the diagnosis is considered, it is unlikely that

surgical intervention and confirmatory biopsy can be avoided.

Amyloid disease occasionally presents as a mediastinal tumour by causing massive enlargement of mediastinal lymph nodes. Associated conditions include multiple myeloma (205) and primary bronchopulmonary amyloid (206, 207).

SUMMARY

Careful attention to the situation of a mediastinal tumour will be of great help in limiting the differential diagnosis. Imaging, with plain x-rays, computed tomography and isotope scans, also helps the clinician to form an opinion regarding the most likely origin of the lesion. However, a tissue diagnosis is essential and an adequate biopsy must be obtained: since many mediastinal tumours are quite necrotic a sizable sample should be taken whenever possible. In addition to light microscopy, the newer pathological techniques have much to contribute and in most cases treatment can be based on accurate diagnosis.

ACKNOWLEDGEMENTS

We wish to thank Anne Dewar for the electron photomicrographs.

REFERENCES

1 Burkell CC, Cross JM, Kent HP et al. Mass lesions of the mediastinum. Curr Prob Surg, June 1969.
2 Hammon JW, Sabiston DC. The mediastinum: In Ellis HE, Goldsmith HS eds Thoracic Surgery Haggerstown MD: Harper and Row, 1978.
3 Mullen B, Richardson JD. Primary anterior mediastinal tumours in children and adults. Ann Thorac Surg 1986; 42: 338–45.
4 Wychulis AR, Payne WS, Clagett OT, Woolner. Surgical treatment of mediastinal tumours: A 40 year experience. J Thorac Cardiovasc Surg 1971; 62: 379–91.
5 Silverman NA, Sabiston DC. Primary tumours and cysts of the mediastinum. Curr Probl Cancer. 1977; 2: 1.

6 Addis BJ; The pathology of mediiastinal tumours. In: Hoogstraten B Tumours of the Lung. Mediastinum, Pleura and Clear Wall. Berlin; Springer Verlag. (In press).

7 Tao L-G, Pearson FG, Cooper JD et al. Cytopathology of thymoma. Acta Cytol 1984; 28: 165–70.

8 Wick MR, Sheithauer BW, Dines DE. Thymic Neoplasia in Two Male Siblings. Mayo Clin Proc 1982; 57: 653–6.

9 Rosai J, Levine JD. Tumours of the Thymus. Atlas of Tumour Pathology, Second Series, Fascicle 13. Washington, DC: Armed Forces Institute of Pathology, 1976.

10 Deshpande GN, Fisher JE, Juitt TC, Freeman AL. Malignant thymoma in an eight month old boy. J Surg Oncol 1981; 18: 61–6.

11 King RM, Telander Rl, Smithson WA, Banks PM, Han MT. Primary mediastinal tumours in children. J Paed Surg 1982; 17: 512–20.

12 Bell RH, Knapp BI, Anson BJ et al. Form, size, blood supply and relations of the adult thymus. Q Bull Northwest Univ Med Sch 1954; 28: 156.

13 Hoffman W, Möller P, Manke H.G. Otto HF. Thymoma: a clinicopathologic study of 98 cases with special reference to three unusual cases. Path Res Pract 1985; 179: 337–53.

14 Pascoe HR, Miner MS. An ultra structural study of nine thymomas. Cancer 1976; 37: 317–26.

15 Battifora H, Sun TT, Bahu RM, Rao S. The use of antikeratin antiserum as a diagnostic tool: thymoma versus lymphoma. Hum Pathol 1980; 11: 635–41.

16 Ring N, Addis BJ. Thymoma, an integrated clinicopathological and immunohistochemical study. J Pathol 1986; 149: 327–37.

17 Chan WC, Zaarari JS, Tabei S, Bibb M, Brynes Rk. Thymoma: an immunohistochemical study. Am J Clin Pathol 1984; 82: 160–6.

18 Chilosi M, Iannucci AM, Pizzolo G., Menestrine F, Fiore-Donati L, Jonossy L. Immunohistochemical analysis if thymoma. Evidence for the medullary origin of epithelial cells. Am J Surg Pathol 1984; 8: 309–18.

19 van der Kwast TH, van Vliet E, Chisten E, van Ewijk W, van der Heul RO. An immunohistologic study of the epithelial and lymphoid components of six thymomas. Hum Pathol 1985; 16: 1001–8.

20 Savino V, Berrih S, Dardenne M. Thymic epithelial antigen acquired during autogeny and defined by the anti-p[19] monoclonal antibody, is lost in thymomas. Lab Invest 1984; 51: 292–6.

21 Müller-Hermelink HK, Marino M, Palestro G. Pathology of thymic epithelial tumors. In: Müller-Hermalink HK ed. The Human Thymus Berlin: Springer-Verlag, 1986.

22 Mokhtor N, Hsu SM, Lad RP, Haynes BF. Jaffe ES. Thymoma: lymphoid and epithelial components mirror the phenotype of the normal thymus. Hum Pathol 1984; 15: 378–84.

23 Jain & Frable WJ. Thymoma: analysis of benign and malignant criteria. J Thorac Cardiovasc. Surg 1974; 67: 310–21.

24 Arriagada R, Bretel JJ, Caillaud JM, Garreta L, Guerin RA, Laugier A, Le Chevalier T, Shlienger M: Invasive carcinoma of the thymus. A multicenter retrospective review of 56 cases. Eur J Cancer Clin Oncol 1984; 20: 69–74.

25 Snover DC, Levine JD, Rosai J. Thymic carcinoma; 5 distinctive histological variants. Am J Surg Pathol 1982; 6: 451–70.

26 Vick MR, Scheithauer BW, Weiland LH, Bernatz PE. Primary thymic carcinomas. Am J Surg Pathol 1982; 6: 613–30.

27 Rosenberg JC. Neoplasms of the mediastinum. In: DeVita VT Jr, Hellman S, Rosenburg SA eds Cancer, Principles and Practice of Oncology. Ohiladelphia: B Lippincott, 1986: 599–620.

28 Masaoka A, Mandon Y, Nakahara K, Tanioka T. Follow up study of thymomas with special reference to their clinical stages. Cancer 1981; 48: 2485–92.

29 Verley JM, Hollman KH. Thymoma—A comparative study of clinical stages, histological features and survival in 200 cases. Cancer 1985; 55: 1074–86.

30 Bernatz PE. Harrison EG. Claggett OT. Thymoma: A clinico pathologic study. J Thorac Cardiovasc Surg 1961; 42: 424–44.

31 Fornasiero A, Daniele O, Sperandio P, Morandi P, Fosser VP, Cartei G, Fiorentino MV. Chemotherapy of invasive or metastatic thymoma: Report of 11 cases. Cancer Treat Rep 1984; 68: 1205–10.

32 Ibrahim NB, Briggs JC, Jeyasingham K, Owen JR. Metastasing thymoma. Thorax 1982: 37: 771–3.

33 Vick MR, Nichols WC, Ingle JN, Bruckman JE, Okazaki H. Malignant lymphocytic thymoma with central and peripheral nervous system metastases. Cancer 1981; 47: 2036–43.

34 Yoshido A, Shigematsu T, Mori H, Yoshida H, Fukunishi R. Non-invasive thymoma with widespread blood-borne metastases. Virchows Arch A (Pathol Anat) 1981; 390: 121–6.

35 Guillan RA, Zelman S, Smalley RL, Inglesias PA. Malignant thymoma associated with myasthenia gravis and evidence of extra-thoracic metastasis. Cancer 1971; 27: 823–30.

36 Batata MA, Martini N, Huvos AG, Aguilar RI, Beattie EJ. Thymomas—Clinicopathologic features, therapy and prognosis. Cancer 1974; 34: 389–96.

37 Chahinian AP, Bhardwaj S, Meyer RJ, Jaffrey IS, Kirschner PA, Holland FJ. Treatment of invasive or metastatic cancer; report of eleven cases. Cancer 1981; 47: 1752–61.

38 Souadjian JV, Enriquez P, Silverstein MN, Pepin J-M. The spectrum of diseases associated with thymoma: coincidence or syndrome? Arch Intern Med 1974; 134: 374–9.

39 Burgh NP, Gatzinsky P, Larsson S et al. Tumours of the thymus region. Ann Thorac Surg 1978; 25: 91.

40 Engel AJ, Myasthenia gravis and myasthenic syndromes. Ann Neurol 1984; 16: 519–25.

41 Drachman DB. Myasthenia gravis. Engl J Med 1978; 298: 136–46.

42 Wilkins EW, Edmonds LH, Castleman B. Cases of thymoma at the Massachusetts General Hospital J Thorac Cardiovasc Surg 1966; 52: 313–22.

43 Alpert LI, Osserman KE, Osserman RS, Caerk A. Studies in myasthenia gravis: effects of thymectomy. Results of 185 patients. 1941–1969. Am J Med 1971; 50: 465–74.

44 Perlo Vp, Schwarb RB, Castleman B. Myasthenia gravis and thymoma. In: Brain WR, Norris FH eds The Remote Effects of Cancer on The Nervous System; the Proceedings of a Symposium, Chapter 7 New York and London: Grune and Stratton, 1965: 55–6.

45 Lattes R. Thymoma and other tumours of the thymus. An analysis of 107 cases. Cancer 1962; 15: 1224–60.

46 Gerein AN, Srivastava SP, Burgess J. Thymoma—A 10 year review. Am J Surg 1978; 136: 49.

47 Furman WL, Buckley PG, Green AA, Stokes DC, Chien LT. Thymoma and myasthenia gravis in a four year old child. Cancer 1985; 56: 2703–6.

48 Dractman DB, Shellita J, Khadekar JD, McKever WP et al. Invasive thymoma responsive to oral cortico steroids. Cancer Treat Rep 1978; 62: 1397.

49 Rowland AS. The syndrome of benign thymoma and primary aregenerative anemia; an analysis of forty-three cases. Am J Med Sci 1964; 247: 719–31.

50 Burrows S, Carrol R. Thymoma associated with pancytopenia. Arch Pathol 1971; 92: 465–8.

51 Goldstein J, MacKay JR. Human Thymus, St Louis: Warren H Green, 1969: 319–37.

52 Zenk JV, Todd EP, Dillon M, De Simone P, Utley JR. The role of thymectomy in red cell aplasia. Ann Thorac Surg 1979; 28: 257.

53 Kaung DT, Cech RF, Peterson RE. Benign thymoma and erythroid hypoplasia; thirteen year 'cure' following thymectomy, Cancer 1968; 22: 445–50.

54 Good RA. Agammaglobulinaemia; a provocative experiment of nature. Bull Inv Minn Hosp 1954; 26: 1–19.

55 Seybold WD, McDonald JR, Clagett OT, Good CA. Tumours of the thymus. J Thorac Cardiovasc Surg 1950; 20: 195–214.

56 Kreel L. Radiology of the thymus. Proc R Soc Med 1973; 66: 157–8.

57 Keen SJ, Libshitz. Thymic lesions experience with computed tomography in 24 patients. Cancer 1987; 59: 1520–3.

58 Brown LR, Muhm JR, Grey JE. Radiographic Detection of Thymoma, AJR 1980; 134: 1181–8.

59 Moore AV, Korobkin M, Olanow WE Al. Age-related changes in the thymus gland; CT—pathologic correlation. Am J Radiol 1983; 141: 241–6.

60 Zerhouni EA, Scott WW, Baker RR, Wharam D, Siegelman SS. Invasive thymomas; diagnosis and an evaluation by computed tomography. J Comp Assist Temog. 1982; 6: 92–100.

61 Scatarige JC, Fishman EK, Zerhouni EA, Seigelman SS. Trans-diaphragmatic extension of invasive thymoma. Am J Radiol 1985; 144: 31–6.

62 Brown LR, Muhm JR, Sheedy FF, Unni KK, Bernatz PE, Hermann RC. The value of computed tomography in myasthenia gravis. Am J Radiol 1983; 140: 31.

63 Masaokoka A, Kyo S. [75]Selenomethionine scintiography in mediastinal diseases. J Thorac Cardiovasc Surg 1978; 75: 419–24.

64 Bernatz PE, Khonsari S, Harrison EG, Tailor WF. Thymomas: factors influencing survival. Surg Clin North Am 1973; 53: 885–92.

65 Fechner RE. Recurrence of non-invasive thymomas: report of four cases and review of literature. Cancer 1969; 23: 1423–7.

66 Maggi G, Giaccone G, Donadio M, Ciuffreda L, Dalesio O, Leria G, Trifiletti G, Casadio C, Palestro G, Mancuso M, Calciti A. Thymomas. A review of 169 cases with particular reference to the results of surgical treatment. Cancer 1986; 58: 765–76.

67 Salyer WR, Eggleston JC. Thymoma: A clinical and pathological study of 65 cases. Cancer 1976; 37: 229–49.

68 Cohen DJ, Ronnigen LV, Graber M, Deshong JL, Jaffin J, Burge JR, Zajtchuk R. J Thorac Cardiovasc Surg 1984; 87: 301–37.

69 Sawyer JL, Foster JH, Surgical treatment of thymomas. Arch Surg 1968; 96: 814–17.

70 Kilman JW, Klassen KP. Thymoma. Am J Surg 1971; 121: 710–11.

71 Cohn LH, Grimmes OF. Surgical management of thymic neoplasms. Surg Gynecol. Obstet 1970; 12: 206–15.

72 Braitman H, Herrmann C, Mulder Dj. Surgery for thymic tumours. Arch Surg 1971; 103: 14–16.

73 Hara N, Yoshida T, Furukawa T, Inokuchi K. Thymoma clinico-pathologic features, therapy and prognosis. Japanese J Surg 1980; 10: 232–7.

74 Applequist P, Kostainen S, Franssila K, Mattila S, Grohn P. Treatment and prognosis of thymoma; a review of 25 cases. J Surg Oncol 1982; 20: 265–8.

75 Marks RD, Wallis KM, Pettit HS. Radiation therapy control of 9 patients with malignant thymoma. Cancer 1978; 41: 117–19.

76 Penn CRH, Hope-Stone HF. The role of radiotherapy in the management of malignant thymoma. Br J Surg 1976; 59: 533–9.

77 Ariaratnam LS, Kalnicki S, Mincer F, Botstein C. The management of malignant thymoma with radiation therapy. Int J Radiat Oncol Biol Phys 1979; 5: 77–80.

78 Legg MA, Brady J. Pathology and clinical behaviours of thymomas. A survey of 51 cases. Cancer 1965; 18: 1131–44.

79 Le-Golvan DP, Abell MR. Thymomas. Cancer 1977; 39: 2142–7.

80 Arriagada R, Gerrard-Marchant R, Tubiana M, Amiel JL, Hajj L. Radiation therapy in the management of malignant thymic tumours. Acta Radiol Oncol 1981; 20: 167–72.

81 Carmel RJ, Caplan HS. Mantle Irradiation in Hodgkin's disease. Cancer 1976; 37: 2813–25.

82 Braun SR, do Pico A, Olson CE, Caldwell W. Low dose radiation pneumonitis. Cancer 1975; 35: 1322–4.

83 Hu E, Levine J. Chemotherapy of malignant thymoma. Case report and review of the literature. Cancer 1986; 57: 1101–4.

84 Soffer LJ, Gabrilove JL. Wolff BS. Effect of ACTH on thymic masses. J Clin Endocrinol Metab 1952; 12: 690–6.

85 Platzer RF. Ovalocytosis associated with malignant thymoma. NY State J Med 1970; 70: 430–2.

86 Skeggs DBL. Complications associated with the radiotherapy of thymic tumours. Proc R Soc Med 1973; 66: 155–7.

87 Green JD, Forman WH. Response of thymoma to steroids. Chest 1974; 65: 114–16.

88 Haussen S, Nibbelink D, Hackett E, Vic NA, Cape CA. Effect of adreno cortico-steroid therapy of myasthenia gravis on associated malignant thymomas. (Abstract) Neurology 1975; 25: 347.

89 Posner J, Howieson J, Cvitkovic E. Disappearing spinal cord compression. Oncolytic effect of gluco corticoids and other chemotherapeutic agents on epidural metastases. Ann Neurol 1977; 2: 409–13.

90 Shellito J, Khandikar JD, McKeever WP, Vick NA. Invasive thymoma repsonse to oral cortico-steroids. Cancer Treat Rep 1978; 62: 1397–400.

91 Almog C, Pick A, Weisberg D, Herczeg E. Regression of malignant thymoma with metastasis after treatment with adrenocorticosteroids. Isr J Med Sci 1978; 14: 476–80.

92 Rankin EM, Harper PG, Bryant B, Dussek K, Rowland CG. Ifosfamide: a highly active agent for the treatment of malignant thymoma cancer (in press).

93 Talley RW, O'Bryan RM, Gutterman J, Brownlee RW, McCredie KB. Clinical evaluation of toxic effects of CDDP. (NSC-119875); Phase I clinical study. Cancer Chemother Rep 1973; 57: 465–71.

94 Coccini G, Boni C, Cumo A. Long lasting response to cisplatinum in recurrent malignant thymoma; case report. Cancer 1982; 49: 1985–7.

95 Shetty MR, Aurora RK. Invasive thymoma treated with cis-platinum. Cancer Treat Rep. 1981; 65: 531.

96 Needles B, Kemeny N, Urmacher C. Malignant thymoma; renal metastases responding to cisplatin. Cancer 1981; 48: 223–6.

97 Levin L, Sealy R, Barron J. Syndrome of inappropriate anti-diuretic hormone secretion following cis-platinum in a patient with malignant thymoma. Cancer 1982; 50: 2279–82.

98 Stolinsky DC. Hum GJ. Jacobs EM, Solomon J, Bateman JR. Clinical trial of weekly doses of vinblastine combined with vincristine in malignant lymphoma and other neoplasms. Cancer Chemother Rep 1973; 57: 477–84.

99 Boston B. Chemotherapy of invasive thymoma. Cancer 1976; 38: 49–52.

100 Bonadonna G, Monfardini S, Delena M et al. Phase I and preliminary phase II evaluation of adriamycin. Cancer Res. 1970; 30: 2572–82.

101 Effler DB, McCormack LJ. Thymic neoplasms. J Thorac Cardiovasc Surg 1956; 31: 60–82.

102 Chahinian AP, Nogeire C, Ohnuma T et al. Phase I study of weekly maytansine, given by IV bolus of 24-hour infusion. Cancer Treat Rep 1979; 63: 1953–60.

103 Jaffrey IS, Denefrio JM, Chahinian P. Re-

sponse to Maytansine in a patient with malignant thymoma. Cancer Treat Rep 1980; 64: 193–4.

104 Chahinian AP, Holland JF, Bhardwaj S. Chemotherapy for malignant lymphoma. Ann Intern Med 1983; 99: 136.

105 Mitrov PS, Bergmann L, Tuengerthal S. Induktion einer kompletten Remission mit Adriamycin und Cis-Platin bei einem, invasiv wachsenden Thymom. Dtsch Med Wochenschr 1982; 44: 1667.

106 Klippstein TH, Mitroc PS, Kochendorfer K, Bergmann L. High dose adriamycin and cis-platinum in advanced soft tissue sarcomas and invasive thymomas. Cancer Chemother Pharmacol 1984; 13: 78–81.

107 Campbell MG, Pollard R, Al-Sarraf M. A complete response in metastatic malignant thymoma to cis-platinum, doxorubicin and cyclophosphamide. Cancer 1981; 98: 1315–17.

108 Fornasiero A, Daniele O, Sperandio P, Morandi P. Chemotherapy of invasive or metastatic thymoma; report of 11 cases. Cancer Treat Rep 1984; 68: 1205–10.

109 Evans WK, Thompson DJ, Simpson WJ, Feld R, Phillips MJ. Combination chemotherapy in invasive thymoma, role of COPP. Cancer 1980; 46: 1523–7.

110 Daugaard G, Hanson HH, Rorth M. Combination chemotherapy for malignant thymomas. Ann Intern. Med. 1983; 99: 189–90.

111 Butler WM, Diehl LF, Taylor HG, Weltz MD. Metastatic thymoma with myasthenia gravis. Cancer 1982; 50: 419–22.

112 Trask CW, Joannidies T, Harper PG et al. Radiation inducing lung fibrosis after treatment of small cell carcinoma of the lung, with very high dose cyclophosphamide. Cancer 1985; 55: 57–60.

113 Leong A S-Y, Brown JH. Maignant transformation in a thymic cyst. Am J Surg Pathol 1984; 8: 471–5.

114 Leyvraz S, Henle W, Chaninian AP, Perlmann C. Klein G, Gordon RE, Rosenblum M, Holland JF. Association of Epstein-Barr virus with thymic carcinoma. N Engl J Mid 1985; 312: 1296–9.

115 Wolfe JT, Wick MR, Banks PM, Scheitauer BW. Clear cell carcinoma of the thymus. Mayo Clin Proc 1983; 58: 365–70.

116 Wick MR, Scheitauer BW. Thymic carcinoid. A histologic, immunohistochemical and ultrastructural study of 12 cases. Cancer 1984; 53: 475–84.

117 Rhode J, Dhillon AP, Thompson RJ, Craig R, Leatham A. Neurodocrine cells in thymus and thymic carcinoid. J Pathol 1986; 148: 105A.

118 Rosai J, Higa E. Mediastinal endocrine neoplasm of probable thymic origin related to carcinoid tumour. Clinico pathologic study of 8 cases. Cancer 1972; 29: 1061–74.

119 Rosai J, Levine G, Weber WR, Higa E. Carcinoid tumours and oat cell carcinomas of the thymus. Pathol Annu 1976; 11: 201–26.

120 Wick MR, Carney JA, Bernatz PE, Brown LR. Primary mediastinal carcinoid tumors. Am J Surg Pathol 1982; 6: 195–205.

121 Levine GD, Rosai J. A spindle cell variant of thymic carcinoid tumour. Arch Pathol Lab Med 1976; 100: 293–300.

122 Ho FCS, Ho JCI. Pigmented carcinoid tumour of the thymus. Histopathology 1977; 1: 363–9.

123 Salyer WR, Salyer DC, Egglestone JC. Carcinoid tumours of the thymus. Cancer 1976; 37: 1958–73.

124 Wick MR. Oat cell carcinoma of the thymus. Cancer 1982; 49: 1652–7.

125 Marino M, Müller-Hermerlink HK. Thymoma and thymic carcinoma. Virchows Arch (Pathol Anat) 1985; 407: 119–49.

126 Miettinen M. Partanen S, Lehto V-P, Virtanen I. Mediastinal tumours: ultrastructural and immunohistochemical evaluation of intermediate filaments as diagnostic aids.

127 Wick MR. Neurone specific enolase. In Neuroendocrine tumours of the thymus, bronchus and skin. Am J Clin Pathol 1983; 79: 703–7.

128 Gould VE, Linnoilu RI, Memdi VA, Warren WH. Neuroendocrine cells and neuroendocrine neoplasms of the lung. Pathol Annu 1983; 18: 287–330.

129 Swinborne-Sheldrake K, Gray GF, Glick AD. Thymic epithelial neoplasms. South Med J 1985; 78: 790–800.

130 Huntrakoon M, Lin F, Heitz Pu, Tomita T. Thymic carcinoid tumour with Cushing's syndrome. Arch Pathol Lab Med 1984; 108: 551–4.

131 Havlieck F, Rosai J. A sarcoma of thymic stroma with features of liposarcoma. Am J Clin Pathol 1984; 82: 217–24.

132 Oho HF, Lachen Meyer L, Janzen RWC, Gurtler KF, Fischer K. Thymolipoma in association with myasthenia gravis. Cancer 1982; 50: 1623–28.

133 Pillai R, Yeoh N, Addis B, Peckham M, Goldstraw P. Thymolipoma in association with Hodgkin's disease. J Thorac. cardiovasc Surg. 1985; 90: 306–8.

134 Lemos LB, Hamondi AB. Malignant thymic tumour in an infant (malignant histiocytoma). Arch Pathol Lab Med 1978; 102: 85–9.

135 Keller A, Castleman B. Hodgkin's disease of the thymus gland. Cancer 1974; 133: 1615–23.

136 Lindford KK, Meyer JE, Dedrick CG, Hassell LA, Harris NL. Thymic cysts in mediastinal Hodgkin's disease. Radiology 1985; 156: 37–44.

137 Kim HC, Nosher J, Haas A, Sweeney W, Lewis R. Cystic degeneration of thymic Hodgkin's Disease following radiation therapy. Cancer 1985; 55: 354–6.

138 Kaplan HS, Hodgkin's Disease. Cambridge, Ma: Harvard University Press, 1980.

139 Smith JL, Clein GP, Barker CR, Collins RD. Characterisation of malignant mediastinal lymphoid neoplasm as thymic in origin (Sternberg sarcoma as T-cell disease). Lancet 1973; i: 74.

140 Yousem SA, Weiss LM, Warnke RA. Primary mediastinal non-Hodgkin's lymphomas; a morphologic and immunologic study of nineteen cases. Am J Clin Pathol 1985; 83: 676–80.

141 Waldron JA, Dohring EJ, Farber LR. Primary large cell lymphomas of the mediastinum; an analysis of twenty cases. Sem Diagn Pathol 1985; 2: 281–95.

142 Addis BJ, Isaacson PG. Large cell lymphoma of the mediastinum; a B-cell tumour of probable thymic origin. Histopathology, 1986; 10: 379–90.

143 Menestrina F, Chilosi M, Bonetti F, Lestani M, Scarpa A, Novelli P, Doglioni C, Todeschini G, Ambrosetti A, Fiore-Donati L. Mediastinal large-cell lymphoma of B-type with sclerosis; histopathological and immunohistochemical study of eight cases. Histopathology 1986; 10: 589–600.

144 Perrone T, Frizzera G, Rosai J. Mediastinal diffuse large-cell lymphoma with sclerosis. Am J Surg Pathol 1986; 10: 176–91.

145 Bunin NJ, Hvizdala E, Link M, Callihan TR, Hutsu HO, Wharam M, Warnke RA, Berrard CW, Murphy SB. Mediastinal nonlymphoblastic lymphomas in children: a clinicopathologic study. J Clin Oncol 1986; 4: 154–9.

146 Szporn AH, Dikman S, Jagirdar J. True histiocytic lymphoma of the thymus. Am J Clin Pathol 1984; 82: 734–7.

147 Kubonishi I, Ohtsuki Y, Machida K-I, Agatsuma Y, Tokuoka H, Iwata K, Miyoshi I. Granulocytic sarcoma presenting as a mediastinal tumour. Am J Clin Pathol 1984; 82: 730–4.

148 Siegal GP, Dehner LP., Rosai J. Histiocytosis-X (Langerhans' cell granulomatosis) of the thymus. Am J Surg Pathol 1985; 9: 117–24.

149 Pachter MR, Lattes R. Mesenchymal tumours of the mediastinum. I. Tumours of fibrous tissue, adipose tissue, smooth muscle and striated muscle. Cancer 1963; 16: 74–94.

150 Schweitzer DL, Aguam AS. Primary liposarcoma of the mediastinum. Report of a case and review of the literature. J Thorac Cardiovasc Surg 1977; 74: 83–97.

151 Prohn P, Winter J, Ulatowski L. Liposarcoma of the mediastinum—case report and review of the literature. Thorac Cardiovasc Surg 1981; 29: 119–21.

152 Friedman M, Egan JW. Effect of irradiation on liposarcomas. Acta Radiol Stockh 1960; 54: 225.

153 Castleberry RP, Kelly DR, Wilson ER, Cain WS, Salter MR. Childhood liposarcoma. Cancer 1984; 54: 579–84.

154 Pachter MR, Lattes R. Mesenchymal tumours of the mediastinum. II. Tumours of blood vascular origin. Cancer 1963; 16: 95–107.

155 Azizkhan RG, Dudgeon, BL Buck JR, Colombani PM, Yaster M, Nichols D, Civin C, Kramer SS, Haller JA. Life-threatening airway obstruction as a complication to the management of mediastinal masses in children. J Pedatr Surg 1985; 20: 816–22.

156 Pachter MR, Lattes R. Mesenchymal tumours of the mediastinum. III. Tumours of lymph vascular origin. Cancer 1963; 16: 108–17.

157 Sumner TE, Bolberg FM, Kaiser PE, Shaffner LB. Mediastinal cystic hygroma in children. Pediat. Radiol 1981; 11: 160–2.

158 Kelley MJ, Mannes EJ, Rabin CE. Mediastinal masses of vascular origin. A review. J Thorac Cardiovasc Surg 1978; 76: 559–572.

159 Gibbs AR, Johnson NF, Giddings JC, Powell DEB, Jasani B. Primary angiosarcoma of the mediastinum. Hum Pathol 1984; 15: 687–91.

160 Rasaretnam R, Panabokke RG. Leiomyosarcoma of the mediastinum. Br J Dis Chest 1975; 69: 63–9.

161 Sunderrajan EV, Nuger AM, Rosenholtz MJ, Maltby JD. Leiomyosarcoma in the mediastinum presenting as a superior vena cava syndrome. Cancer 1984; 53: 2553–6.

162 Crist WM, Raney RB, Newton W, Lawrence W, Teffte M, Foulkes MA. Intrathoracic soft tissue sarcomas in children. Cancer 1982; 50: 598–604.

163 Chen W, Chan CW, Mok CK. Malignant fibrous histiocytoma of the mediastinum. Cancer 1982; 50: 797–800.

164 Natsuaki M, Yoshikawa Y, Itoh T, Minato N, Yamada H. Xanthogranulomatous malignant fibrous histiocytoma arising from posterior mediastinum. Thorax 1986; 41: 322–3.

165 Mills SA, Brayer RH, Johnston FR. Hudspeth S, Marshall RB, Choplin RH, Cordell R, Myers RT. Malignant fibrous histiocytoma of the mediastinum and lung. A report of three

cases. J Thorac Cardiovasc Surg 1982; 84: 367–72.

166 Poon MC, Durant JR, Logard MJ, Chang-Poon VY. Inflammatory fibrous histiocytoma: an important variant of malignant fibrous histicytoma highly responsive to chemotherapy. An Intern Med 1982; 97: 858–63.

167 Dehner LP, Franciosi RA, Drake RM, Favara BE. Malignant mesenchymar tumors of the anterior medinstinum-lung: a clinicopathological and ultrastructural study. Lab Invest 1978; 38: 384.

168 Kittredge RD, Nash AD. The many facets of sclerosing fibrosis. AJR 1974; 122: 288–98.

169 Light AM. Idiopathic fibrosis of the mediastinum. A discussion of three cases and review of the literature. J Clin Pathol 1978; 31: 78–88.

170 Comings DE, Skubi KB, van Eyes J, Motulsky AG. Familial multifocal fibrosclerosis. Ann Intern Med 1967; 66: 884–92.

171 Hanly PC, Shub C, Lie JT. Constrictive pericarditis associated with combined retroperitoneal and mediastinal fibrosis. Mayo Clin Proc 1984; 59: 300–4.

172 Weider S, Rabinowitz JG. Fibrous mediastinitis: a late manifestation of mediastinal histoplasmosis. Radiology 1977; 125: 305–12.

173 Mitchell IM, Saunders NR, Maher O, Lennox SC, Walker DR. Surgical treatment of idiopathic mediastinal fibrosis: report of five cases. Thorax 1986; 41: 210–14.

174 Johnson DW, Hoppe RT, Cox RS et al. Hodgkin's disease limited to intra-thoracic sites. Cancer 1983; 52: 8.

175 Mouch P, Goodman K, Hellman S. The significance of mediastinal involvement in early stage Hodgkin's disease. Cancer 1978; 42: 1039.

176 Lichtenstein AK, Levine A, Taylor CR, Boswell B, Rossman S, Feinstein DI, Lukes RJ. Primary mediastinal lymphoma in adults. Am J Med 1980; 68: 509–14.

177 Levitt LJ, Aisenberg AL, Harris NL, Linggood RM, Poppema S. Primary non-Hodgkin's lymphoma of the mediastinum. Cancer 1982; 50: 2486–92.

178 Castleman B, Iverson L, Menendez VP. Localised mediastinal lymph node hyperplasia resembling thymoma. Cancer 1956; 9: 822–30.

179 Karcher DS, Pearson CE, Butler WM, Hurwitz MA, Cassell PF. Giant lymph node hyperplasia involving the thymus with associated nephrotic syndrome and myelofibrosis. Am J Clin Pathol 1982; 77: 100–4.

180 Keller AR, Holchholzer L, Castleman B. Hyaline-vascular and plasma-cell types of giant lymph node hyperplasia of the mediastinum and other locations. Cancer 1972; 29: 670–83.

181 Frizzera G. Castleman's disease: more questions than answers. Hum Pathol. 1985; 16: 202–5.

182 Akwari OE, Spencer Payne W, Onoforio BM, Dines DE, Muhm JR. Mayo Clin Proc 1978; 53: 353–8.

183 Davidson KG, Walbaum PR, McCormack RJM. Intrathoracic neural tumours. Thorax 1978; 22: 359–67.

184 Enzinger FM, Weiss SW. Soft Tissue Tumours. St Louis, Illinois: CV Mosby, 1983.

185 Variend S. Small cell tumours in childhood. J Pathol 1985; 145: 1–26.

186 Dhillon AP, Rhode J, Leathern A. Neurone-specific enolase: an aid to the diagnosis of melanoma and neuroblastoma. Histopathology 1982; 6: 81–92.

187 Kemshead JT, Goldman A, Fritschy J, Malpas JS, Pritchard J. Use of panels of monoclonal antibodies in the differential diagnosis of neuroblastoma. Lancet 1983; i: 12–14.

188 Simone JV. Editorial. The treatment of neuroblastoma. J Clin Oncol 1984; 2: 717–18.

189 Rosen E, Cassady JR, Frantz CN, Kretschmar C, Levey R, Sallan SE. Neuroblastoma: the joint centre for radiation therapy/Danar-Farber Cancer Institute/Children's Hospital experience. J Clin Oncol 1984; 2: 719–32.

190 Kretschmar CF, Frantz CN, Rosen EM et al. Improved prognosis for infants with stage four neuroblastoma. J Clin Oncol 1984; 2: 799–803.

191 Shafford EZ, Rogers DW, Pritchard J. Advanced neuroblastoma; improved response using a multi-agent regimen (OPEC) including sequential cystatin and VM-26. J Clin Oncol 1984; 2: 742–7.

192 Adams SA, Hochholzer L. Ganglioneuroblastoma of the posterior mediastinum. A clinicopathologic review of eighty cases. Cancer 1981; 47: 373–81.

193 Benjamin SP, McCormack LJ, Effler DB, Groves LK. Primary tumours of the mediastinum. Chest 1972; 62: 297–303.

194 Glenner GG, Grimley PM. Tumours of the extra-adrenal paraganglion system (including chemoreceptors). Atlas of Tumour Pathology, Second Series, Fascicle 9. Washington DC. Armed Forces Institute of Pathology, 1974.

195 Ogawa J, Inoue H, Koide S, Kawada S, Shotitsu A, Hata J. Functioning paraganglioma in the posterior mediastinum. Ann Thorac Surg 1982; 33: 507–10.

196 Dunn GD, Brown MJ, Sapsford RN, Mansfield AO, Hemingway AP, Sever PS, Allison D.

Functioning middle mediastinal paragang-lioma associated with intercarotid paragang-liomas. Lancet 1986; i: 1061–4.

197 Lack EE, Stillinger RA, Colvin DB, Groves RM, Burnette DG. Aortico-pulmonary para-ganglioma. Report of a case with ultrastructur-al study and review of the literature. Cancer 1979; 43: 269–78.

198 Olsen JL, Salyer WR. Mediastinal paragang-liomas (aortic body tumour): a report of four cases and a review of the literature. Cancer 1978; 41: 2405–12.

199 Cueto-Garcia L, Shub C, Sheps SG, Puga FJ. Two-dimensional echocardiographic defection of mediastinal phaeochromocytoma. Chest 1987; 6: 834–6.

200 Editorial. Iodobenzylguanidine for location and treatment of pheochromocytoma. Lancet 1984; ii: 905–7.

201 Sheps SG, Brown ML. The localisation of mediastinal paraglangiolmas (pheochromocy-toma). Chest 1987; 6: 807–9.

202 Nigan BK. Intrathoracic chemodectoma with noradrenalin secretion. Thorax 1981; 36: 66–8.

203 Cairnduff F, Smith IE. Carboplatin chemo-therapy for malignant paraganglioma. Lancet 1986; ii: 982 (letter).

204 Verani R, Olson J, Moake JL. Intra-thoracic extra medullary haematopoiesis. Report of case in a patient with sickle cell disease—beta-thalassaemia. Am J Clin Pathol 1980; 73: 133–8.

205 Antoniutto G, Falconieri G, Manconi R. Mas-sive enlargement of mediastinal lymph nodes in a patient with multiple myeloma. Thorax 1983; 38: 151–2.

206 Thompson PJ, Jewkes J, Corrin B, Citron KM. Primary bronchopulmonary amyloid tumour with massive hilar lymphadenopathy. Thorax 1983; 38: 152–4.

207 Shaw P, Grossman R, Fernandes BJ. Nodular mediastinal amyliodosis. Hum Pathol 1984; 15: 1183–5.

Section **IV**

Gastrointestinal Tumours

Textbook of Uncommon Cancer
Edited by C.J. Williams, J.G. Krikorian, M.R. Green and D. Raghavan
© 1988 John Wiley & Sons Ltd

Chapter **24**

Uncommon Cancers of the Esophagus

J.C. Rosenberg

*Hutzel Hospital Surgical Unit, Wayne State University,
Detroit, Michigan, USA*

INTRODUCTION

Greater than 90% of esophageal malignancies are squamous cell carcinomas. They predominate in number over all other esophageal neoplasms, benign or malignant (1). Only the latter will be considered in this chapter and since only uncommon cancers will be discussed, squamous cell carcinomas do not qualify for inclusion. However, there are variants of this neoplasm which are sufficiently infrequent to merit mention in the context of this chapter. Those that will be discussed are the spindle cell carcinoma and its variants, the pseudosarcoma and carcinosarcoma. Infrequently encountered associations of squamous cell carcinoma with lesions such as achalasia and diverticula of the esophagus will also be discussed.

Second in frequency to squamous cell carcinomas are primary adenocarcinomas of the esophagus. Close to 7% of patients with carcinoman of the esophagus will have this diagnosis (2). Most of them will have an underlying Barrett's esophagus. This relationship will be treated extensively.

Other cancers of epithelial origin which will be described are the adenoid cystic carcinomas (cylindromas), mucoepidermoid carcinomas (adenocanthomas), carcinoids and the undifferentiated small cell or oat cell carcinomas. The cancers of nonepithelial origin which will be considered are the leiomyosarcomas, other cancers of mesodermal origin and the malignant melanomas.

VARIANTS OF SQUAMOUS CELL CARCINOMA OF THE ESOPHAGUS

Spindle Cell Carcinoma

This manifestation of squamous cell carcinoma is characterized histopathologically by spindle-shaped cells resembling fibroblasts. It is a poorly differentiated squamous cell carcinoma which can be confused with a sarcoma. The spindle cells, however, have been studied by electron microscopy and have been shown to contain numerous tonofibrils and occasional well-developed desmosomes (3). Desmosomes are characteristically found at the intercellular junction of epithelial cells. Tonofibrils radiate from them and contribute to the 'stiffness' or cytoskeleton of this cell type. However, except for their large size and irregular shape, the spindle cells also resemble actively synthesizing fibroblasts and are closely associated with collagen fibrils. Battifora believes that the spindle cells orginate from mesenchymal metaplasia of squamous cells and that collagen is produced by these metaplastic cells (3). Similar tumors in the skin have shown a gradual transition of the spindle cells to typical squa-mous cells. This view has received support from others (4).

Pseudosarcoma and Carcinosarcoma

Several observers argue that these two designa-tions refer to the same lesion and should be referred to as polypoid carcinomas of the esophagus (5–7). The rationale for this desig-nation resides in the fact that they do indeed have the gross appearance of a polypoid lesion. Adenocarcinomas, inflammatory granulomas, smooth muscle tumors and melanomas may also present as polypoid lesions. In the case of pseudosaromas/carcinosarcomas, the barium esophagram will usually reveal a large poly-poid mass in the middle or lower third of the esophagus. The esophagus is usually distended at the site of the tumour but the degree of esophageal obstruction is considerably less than one would expect from the size of the mass.

Histopathologically, they appear to be spin-dle cell carcinomas which present a varying picture all the way from nests of squamous cells (which may or may not appear malignant) in a spindle cell stroma (referred to as pseudosar-coma), to an intimate mixture of carcinoma-tous and sarcomatous appearing cells growing together as a single tumor (carcinosarcoma). Although it is convincingly argued that these malignancies most likely arise from two differ-ent cell lines, carcinomatous and sarcomatous, which comingle (7) (sometimes referred to as a 'collision' tumor) we regard them as highly undifferentiated squamous cell carcinomas of the spindle cell type.

The majority of carcinosarcomas do not invade very deeply into the underlying tissue. The carcinomatous elements are limited and may be found only at the base of the polypoid mass. Metastases from these tumors are usually sarcomatous in appearance.

According to those authors who make a distinction between carcinosarcomas and pseudosarcomas, the latter differ from the former in that the seemingly sarcomatous

tissue is considered nonmalignant since metas-tases do not occur. However, the distinction between pseudosarcoma and carcinosarcoma is admittedly difficult even to those who believe the two lesions are separate entities. The subsequent course of the patient may often prove the pseudosarcoma to metastasize and demonstrate both sarcomatous and carcino-matous elements in the secondary lesions (5, 7).

Of the combined total of about 80 cases of carcinosarcoma and pseudosarcoma of the esophagus found in the literature, most occurred in men over 50 years of age. The longest survivor was a patient who lived for 6 years after surgical resection of the tumor (7). Turnbull et al. reported 2 of 5 patients alive and free of disease 10 years after a pseudosar-coma was resected. Two of the 5 patients died with metastatic disease (8). This tumor was encountered once in 5000 cases of squamous cell carcinoma in one series (9).

Radical esophagectomy is recommended for cure which is thought to be more readily attained with this variant of esophageal cancer than with the ordinary squamous cell carci-noma (10, 11). A recent publication from Beijing of 4 patients with carcinosarcoma reported them all well 3 to 19 years after radical excision and esophagogastrostomy (12).

Verrucous and Varicoid Carcinomas of the Esophagus

These lesions are variants of fungating squa-mous cell carcinomas (7, 13). They may be confused with esophageal varices when an esophagram is obtained, which is their dis-tinguishing feature.

Infrequently Encountered Associations of Squamous Cell Carcinoma of Esophagus

Tylosis

In a classic summary of this obscure condition, Howel-Evans described this disease which is characterized by changes of the skin of the palms and soles (hyperkeratosis palmaris et plantaris) and papillomas of the esophagus (14). The syndrome occurs as the result of an autosomal dominant gene. Seventy percent of patients with tylosis will develop squamous cell carcinoma of the esophagus.

Achalasia

Approximately 5% of all patients with achalasia have been reported to develop squamous cell carcinomas of the esophagus. The cancers are located in the middle third and lower third in equal frequency (15, 16). It has been reported to occur after the achalasia has been present for 20 years or longer. In some instances the cancer has been thought to be the cause of the achalasia (17). Rarely, an adenocarcinoma may be found in the dilated esophagus (18). Joske and Benedict suspected that the obstructive process somehow led to the squamous cell carcinoma (19). More recent literature continues to implicate retention esophagitis as a premalignant condition (21) The esophagitis is thought to arise from stagnating retained food in the megaesophagus. The advent of fiberoptics for flexible endoscopes and the attendant increased frequency of esophagoscopy should result in an increase in the frequency of reports of squamous cell cancer in patients with achalasia. It is hoped that this will result in the discovery of early lesions and hopefully produce better survival rates (21).

Treatment of the cancer is as for any squamous cell carcinoma. The use of postoperative chemo-radiation therapy rather than preoperatively has had reasonable results in our hands (22). Patients with this unusual association do as poorly as the patients with esophageal cancer (23).

Esophageal Diverticula

Isolated case reports constitute the basis of this uncommon association of conditions. Up to 1976, 35 cases were collected from the literature. Two-thirds of the cancers occurred in pharyngoesophageal diverticula and the remainder of the epiphrenic level. Epithelial cysts of the esophagus do not apparently share this proclivity to develop cancers (24). Only 0.4% of 1249 patients with a pharyngoesophageal diverticulum had an associated squamous cell carcinoma (15). Although it is recommended to treat these cancers as one would any other squamous cell carcinoma, in the aforementioned series, diverticulectomy alone was curative in the absence of full-thickness penetration, nodal metastasis or extension to the line of resection.

Plummer–Vinson (Paterson–Kelly) Syndrome

Sideropenic anemia, glossitis and esophagitis are associated with a 10% incidence of pharyngeal or esophageal cancer. The latter are usually located in the upper esophagus. The syndrome, and thus the cancers, are more frequent in women than men. Nutritional deficiencies have been postulated as etiologic factors (1). The syndrome is apparently less often seen than when it was first described over 65 years ago (26). When strictures are present dysplastic changes and in situ carcinoma can be found at the site of the narrowed esophagus (27).

Lye Stricture

Squamous cell carcinomas have been reported to occur in esophageal strictures secondary to lye ingestion. The cancer occurs at the site of the stricture which is frequently located at the level of the tracheal bifurcation (28). The duration between the detection of the carcinoma and the ingestion of lye varies between 30 and 45 years. The similarity of this lesion to squamous cell carcinomas occurring in chronic draining sinus tracts and chronic skin ulcers suggests a common etiologic mechanism. Like squamous cell carcinomas in these lesions, the carcinoma occurring in a strictured esophagus secondary to caustic injury appears to be less aggressive than the usual forms of squamous cell carcinoma. It has a slightly higher resectability rate than other forms of squamous cell carcinoma (40% vs 30%) and may have a better prognosis. Resection of the extensively strictured esophagus which has to be bypassed is a formidable procedure. The mortality under this condition may be higher than the risk of developing cancer in the excluded esophagus. Since the exact risk is not known, resection of the excluded esophagus is not advised.

ADENOCARCINOMA OF THE ESOPHAGUS

The literature on adenocarcinoma of the esophagus is difficult to summarize since so many authors include gastric lesions which invade the esophagus in their reports. The rationale for doing so is that, irrespective of whether the esophagogastric cancer originates in the esophagus or the stomach, the prognosis and treatment are the same. This may be true for the advanced lesion but as diagnostic technics such as esophagogastroscopy improve, earlier lesions are found and a distinction can be made betweeen primary adenocarcinoma of the esophagus and those which involve it as a result of direct extension from the stomach. Detection of the less advanced lesion may be accompanied by a better understanding of the factors which are responsible for the emergence of these cancers and, hopefully, a better approach to their cure. It is our view that this progression of events is currently taking place with respect to the adenocarcinoma arising in a columnar lined esophagus. Although there are certainly some adenocarcinomas that arise from the sparse glandular elements in the esophagus, the majority of esophageal adenocarcinomas appear to arise from this metaplastic tissue.

Until recently, many authorities doubted the existence of primary adenocarcinoma of the esophagus because it was so rare (29). The Mayo Clinic reported 19 patients with this diagnosis who constituted 3.3% of the 1312

patients with cancer of the esophagus or cardia seen from 1946 to 1963. Turnbull et al. found an incidence of 2.3% among 1918 patients with esophageal cancer seen from 1926 to 1968 at the Memorial Hospital for Cancer in New York (8). In a more recent series of 163 patients with esophageal cancer between 1975 and 1982, 6.7% had a primary adenocarcinoma of the esophagus (2). This figure is close to the one reported from Denmark where 6.9% of the esophageal carcinomas were found to be of the glandular type (30).

Histogenesis of Primary Adenocarcinoma of the Esophagus

The Superficial and Deep Glands of the Esophagus

These are mucus secreting cells which are indistinguishable in appearance from the cardiac glands of the stomach. Secretions from the superficial glands located within the mucosa enter the lumen of the esophagus through ducts lined by a single layer of mucous cells. The deep esophageal glands are located in the submucosa. The terminal portion of the ducts from these glands is lined with squamous cells. The deep esophageal glands are thought to give rise to the mucoepidermoid carcinomas which are occasionally found in the esophagus (7).

Congenital Persistence of the Columnar Lined Esophagus

During early embryonic life, the esophagus is a tube of stratified columnar cells which develops a lumen and then becomes lined with ciliated columnar cells. During the fourteenth week of embryonic life, squamous cells appear in the middle third of the esophagus. They spread craniad and caudad gradually lining the entire lumen of the esophagus by the seventh month of gestation. If this process is arrested during fetal life, segments of the esophagus could remain lined with grandular epithelium rather than squamous epithelium.

Another possible explanation for the congenital presence of small patches of fundic gastric mucosa in the esophagus is that they represent heterotopic deposits of displaced embryonic tissue such as one occasionally sees in a Meckel diverticulum (7).

Columnar Lined Esophagus Resulting from Glandular Mucosa Replacing the Squamous Cell Mucosa under the Influence of Reflux Esophagitis (Barrett's Esophagus)

This is the explanation which is currently the accepted one but it was not appreciated when Barrett first drew attention to the columnar lined lower esophagus in 1950. He originally attributed the phenomenon to a *congenitally* short esophagus. He discarded the possibility that the shortened esophagus was acquired as a result of, 'reflux esophagitis', a term he coined. By 1957 he changes his views on the subject and postulated that the lower esophagus lined by columnar epithelium was most probably, '. . . the result of a failure of the embryonic lining of the gullet to achieve normal maturity', i.e. that it was of congenital origin (31).

As early as 1953, Allison and Johnstone pointed out the relationship between a hiatal hernia, reflux esophagitis and the columnar lined esophagus but did not appreciate the possibility that the reflux esophagitis was responsible for the appearance of the columnar epithelum. Indeed, it was thought that the 'gastric mucosa' in the esophagus contributed to the esophagitis. It is of further interest that one of the 7 patients reported by Allison and Johnstone had an adenocarcinoma in the glandular ('gastric') lining of the esophagus (32).

Barrett's explanation of the presence of a columnar lined lower esophagus held sway for the next 20 years and the lesion is still commonly known as a 'Barrett's esophagus', i.e. a columnar lined esophagus.

Allison continued to accumulate an extensive experience with peptic esophagitis, recognizing that there was incompetence of the esophagogastric spincter mechanism resulting in reflux. However, he focused on the anatomic abnormality (the hiatal hernia) rather than on the physiologic one and concentrated on repairing the hernia. He did not recognize that doing so did not suffice to correct the reflux. By 1970, he still considered the columnar lined esophagus to be a failure of complete development but did recognize that it was liable to malignant degeneration (33). Others began to suspect that reflux esophagitis could be responsible for the presence of the columnar epithelium as early as 1960. Adler's outstanding studies published in 1963 gave great credibility to this explanation—one which was subsequently substantiated and is now widely held (34, 35). It was also at this time that Nissen described his operation, the fundoplication, which effectively prevented reflux esophagitis and has become the standard operation for this condition (36).

Adenocarcinoma in Barrett's Esophagus

Etiologic and Pathologic Considerations

The emphasis placed on Barrett's esophagus in this chapter stems from the fact that 59 to 86% of adenocarcinomas of the esophagus arise in a Barrett's esophagus. It is thus possible that common factors are involved in the causation of both lesions (37). The constituents of the refluxed material which are responsible for the conversion of the squamous epithelium to columnar epithelum are not known. It is difficult to reproduce the lesion in experimental animals (38). Since it has been observed in 9 of 17 patients who had total gastrectomy with esophagojejunostomy one might assume that the alkaline small bowel contents may be crucial in its pathogenesis (39).

Several possibilities exist to explain the replacement of the squamous cell lining by the glandular epithelium (1). Epithelial cells from the stomach may grow up into an esophagus denuded of its mucosa (2). Submucosal esophageal glands or the cardiac glands in the lamina propria may proliferate and cover the denuded luminal surface of the esophagus (3). The squamous cell epithelium may undergo metaplasia under the influence of the esophagitis. The last possibility has been the generally accepted one. However, as indicated above it must not be forgotten that there is a possibility that the columnar lined esophagus can be of congenital origin. Ransom et al. considered the 'extended' form of Barrett's esophagus (extending to 30 cm, or above, from the incisors) to be of congenital origin and to have a greater tendency to undergo malignant degeneration. This group made up half of the 34 patients whom they studied (40).

The microscopic changes which characterize a Barrett's esophagus have been carefully studied by both light and electron microscopy and by immunohistochemical technics (41–43). The mucosa can assume one of three forms. There is usually an admixture of them in any given patient. The gastric-type epithelium tends to be located distally. This type of tissue resembles the mucosa seen in the fundus of the stomach and contains parietal and chief cells. It has an atrophic appearance and the functional status of the acid and pepsinogen secreting cells is unclear. Located proximally in the columnar lined esophagus is intestinal-type epithelium with villi lined by columnar and goblet cells. The changes in this type of mucosa closely resemble the process of 'intestinalization' that one sees in the stomach of patients with atrophic gastritis. Unlike normal intestinal absorptive cells, the columnar cells of this specialized epithelium contain glycoprotein secretory granules, usually lack brush borders and do not absorb lipids. Paneth and neuroendocrine cells can also be found in this tissue. The third type of epithelial cells seen in a Barrett's esophagus are cardiac-type glands which tend to be found between the gastric-type and the proximal intestinal-type.

Barrett's esophagus has been found in 8 to 20% of patients who undergo esophagoscopy for evaluation of esophagitis. The frequency rises to 44% when a stricture complicates the esophagitis (35). The percentage of patients with Barrett's esophagus who subsequently develop adenocarcinoma ranges from 0 to 46.5% (37). Very little is known about the factors responsible for the malignant degeneration of this tissue. However, the finding of a progression of changes from dysplasia to in situ neoplasia to invasive malignancy is consistent with the concept that metaplasia is the process which accounts for the presence of the columnar epithelium in the esophagus. The component of the Barrett's mucosa most often associated with the malignancy is the intestinal-type which is characterized by large numbers of goblet cells. Detailed studies of the adenocarconomas in Barrett's esophagus reveal multiple cell types including keratin-producing cells (44). These investigations support the view that adenocarcinomas, like the Barrett's esophagus itself, are examples of multidirectional differentiation.

Another feature of the adenocarcinoma worthy of mention is that multiple foci of malignancy are often present. There could be genetic components to both the occurrence of Barrett's esophagus and the adenocarcinoma arising from it since these lesions are rarely seen in blacks whereas squamous cell carcinoma is far more common in blacks than in whites (2, 35, 37). Since cigarette smoking and alcohol ingestion are thought to be related to the etiology of squamous cell carcinoma, investigators have looked for this relationship in patients with adenocarcinoma in a Barrett's esophagus. Some reports suggest such a relationship; others do not (37).

Clinical Features

Patients with adenocarcinoma that developed in a Barrett's esophagus are usually white men in the fifth and sixth decades of life with past histories of esophagitis, hiatal hernias and strictures who often smoke and may have a heavy alcohol intake. The higher frequency of cancer of the esophagus of all cell types in men is well established. Skinner et al. found that the male:female ratio among patients with Barrett's esophagus was 2:1. When adenocarcinoma complicated the columnar lined esophagus, the ratio increased to 9:1 (45). Patients with reflux esophagitis secondary to scleroderma and those with reflux caused by cardiomyotomy for achalasia may also be at risk. Peptic ulcer disease and extraesophageal tumors are other conditions frequently associated with Barrett's esophagus.

The absence of a past history of Barrett's esophagus among patients found to have an adenocarcinoma in a columnar lined esophagus is significant. This is a reflection of the difficulty in recognizing the existence of the abnormally located epithelium in the esophagus. Its appearance on endoscopy is not strikingly different from that of squamous cell epithelium and radiologic differentiation is unreliable. Pertechnate scintigraphy has been recommended for the diagnosis of Barrett's esophagus but this radionuclide will only be concentrated by the columnar epithelium when it is of the gastric-type (46).

Barrett's mucosa may be granular with a salmon-pink color or have the velvety appearance of gastric mucosa. Biopsies must be taken to verify the diagnosis. Close surveillance of patients with reflux esophagitis and Barrett's esophagus may result in the detection of adenocarcinomas before they become extensive. Once they cause symptoms they are usually far advanced and have the same poor prognosis as squamous cell carcinomas.

Treatment

Patients with Barrett's esophagus who do not have dysplastic or neoplastic alterations in the columnar lined esophagus may benefit from fundoplication since some patients have experienced regression or stabilization of this process when the reflux of gastric contents was prevented (45, 47).

When patients show evidence of in situ or invasive malignancy in a Barrett's esophagus, esophagectomy followed by adjuvant chemotherapy of the type utilized for gastric adenocarcinoma is recommended (37).

Dysplastic changes present within the Bar-

rett's mucosa present a difficult therapeutic problem. One is less enthusiastic about recommending radical surgery under these circumstances. However, evidence strongly indicates that dysplastic changes are the first stages of invasive carcinoma. This is especially true of 'high-grade' dysplasia which is considered a morphologic marker and precursor of adenocarcinoma (35, 48). Patients with this form of dysplasia are candidates for esophagectomy (37, 45).

The type of esophagectomy required is an extensive one; more extensive than can be performed using the Ivor Lewis approach (1). The columnar mucosa can extend quite high in the esophagus. By utilizing an operation which places the esophagogastric or esophagocolic anastomosis in the neck, one can be more confident that all of the involved mucosa has been removed. A modification of the technic described by McKeown is recommended (49).

The prognosis of patients with adenocarcinoma in a Barrett's esophagus depends upon the pathologic stage of the tumor. The staging system proposed in Table 1 is similar to Duke's system of staging colon carcinoma and may more accurately predict the patient's prognosis and the carcinoma's progression than the TNM system. However, there has not been sufficient material available yet to prove this hypothesis. A recently reported series of 32

TABLE I STAGING OF ADENOCARCINOMA
INVOLVING BARRETT'S ESOPHAGUS

Stage I: Carcinoma limited to the mucosa (including in situ carcinoma) not extending beyond the muscularis mucosa with negative nodes.

Stage II: Carcinoma limited to the esophageal wall but not extending to the adventitia with negative nodes.

Stage III: Any of the above with involved regional lymph nodes or full-thickness wall penetration of the tumor to the adventitia, without invasion of adjacent organs.

Stage IV: Carcinoma invading adjacent organs or with distant metastases.

patients with this cancer revealed a 14.5% survival rate for 5 years.

Adenoid Cystic Carcinoma (Cylindroma)

These tumors show histologic features which are identical with those found in the salivary glands but they act more aggressively and carry a poorer prognosis than the relatively indolent salivary gland cylindromas (7). Epstein et al. studied 6 cases of esophageal adenoid cystic carcinomas and concluded that they were distinct morphologically as well as clinically from the adenoid cystic carcinomas of salivary gland origin (50). These tumors have the typical cystic or cribriform configuration of the tumor cells with some areas of solid or basaloid patterns. In the esophagus, the latter pattern predominates, the cells are more pleomorphic and the overlying squamous mucosa contains focal areas of dysplasia and in situ carcinoma.

Based on a review of the 29 patients with this lesion who are reported in the literature up to 1984, Epstein et al. found that 76% of the tumors occur in males during their sixth decade in contrast to the salivary gland cylindromas which predominate in females in the fourth and fifth decades of life (50). The cancer's aggressive behavior is reflected in the 9-month median survival following diagnosis. It is suggested that these lesions be resected as one would a squamous cell carcinoma of the esophagus (51). Recently, a combination of radiation therapy and cisplatin, cyclophosphamide, vincristine and doxorubicin produced a complete response in a patient with metastases to the lung from an esophageal adenoid cystic carcinoma. The 44 cases culled from the literature up to 1986, confirmed the poor prognosis of these cancers. Thus, further exploration of this form of combination chemotherapy would have some merit (52).

Mucoepidermoid Carcinoma (Adenoacanthoma) of the Esophagus

This tumor is an adenocarcinoma which con-
tains squamous elements. The relative proportion of the two components varies both within and among these cancers. Ming suggests that when the tumor is a well-differentiated adenocarcinoma, some cells undergo squamous metaplasia and can be seen to be surrounded by the unaffected glandular cells (7). These lesions are typically referred to as adenoacanthomas. They may arise from aberrant gastric epithelium. However, there are mucoepidermoid cancers of the esophagus which are thought to arise from the deep mucous glands of the esophagus. They are similar to those found in the salivary glands. In 1978, Woodard et al. could only collect 8 cases of this esophageal lesion, attesting to its rarity (53). Esophageal mucoepidermoid carcinomas are characterized by small groups of mucous cells scattered among large groups of squamous cells. These are very aggressive malignancies and are most often found at the lower end of the esophagus although the tumor reported by Turnbull et al. was located in the upper thoracic esophagus (8). Resection failed to cure this patient and the poor prognosis was comparable to those patients with mucoepidermoid cancers arising from the bronchial glands.

CANCERS OF NEUROENDOCRINE ORIGIN

Primary Oat Cell Carcinoma of the Esophagus

Various names are given to this cancer which is similar in appearance and behaviour to its counterpart in the lung. It is also referred to as a small cell carcinoma, a small cell undifferentiated carcinoma and an apudoma (amine precursor uptake and decarboxylation tumor). A total of 88 cases of this lesion were recently collected from the literature (54). The tumors are thought to be of neuroectodermal origin since most investigators find them to be argyrophilic and on electron microscopy the cells contain neurosecretory granules (55). Immunohistochemical studies have also revealed the presence of ACTH and calcitonin within some of the tumors that have been studied for their capacity to synthesize polypeptide hormones (56). Evidence of Cushing's disease was not present in the patient found to have ACTH in the tumour. However, other patients have been reported with paraneoplastic syndromes such as inappropriate anti-diuretic hormone secretion and hypercalcemia (57).

Because these tumors occasionally also have areas of squamous cell carcinoma within them, and even less often adenocarcinomatous elements, earlier authors had doubts as to the true origin of this malignancy. The accumulated evidence, however, leaves little doubt as to the true nature of this malignancy, i.e. that it is of neuroectodermal origin (58).

Like squamous cell carcinomas, the majority of oat cell carcinomas are equally located in the middle and lower thirds of the esophagus. Men are more frequently involved (3:2) and the tumor is most common in the 50–70 age group (54, 57).

The limited experience with oat cell carcinoma of the esophagus has been dismal. All patients reported have died with disseminated disease. The overall survival is 4.7 months; the longest survival is 24 months (54). Treatment has consisted of resection, radiation and chemotherapy (54, 56, 59). Combination chemotherapy used for patients with oat cell cancer of the lung has provided dramatic (albeit temporary) response with this tumor when it occurs in the esophagus (59, 60).

Carcinoid Tumors of the Esophagus

Further evidence of the neuroendocrine basis of oat cell cancers is the rare carcinoid tumor which is presumed to arise from the same cell type but which is a far less aggressive tumor. Resection of the esophagus is effective therapy (61, 62).

PRIMARY MALIGNANT MELANOMA OF THE ESOPHAGUS

It might be argued that this cancer should be included among those in the previous section since the cells of origin in this malignancy are derived from neural crest tissue, as are apudomas and carcinoids. A recent review of the world literature encompassed 110 patients with this infrequently encountered lesion of the esophagus (63). The tumor is often polypoid and lymphatic and hematologic metastases are common, resulting in a 5-year survival of 4%. Resection is the treatment recommended and has resulted in a 10-year survival in one patient. Average survival, however, is only 13.4 months. Patients with secondary involvement of the esophagus with melanoma outnumber the patients with primary melanoma of the esophagus.

ESOPHAGEAL SARCOMAS

Leiomyosarcoma of the Esophagus

This is the most common malignant nonepithelial tumor in the esophagus. Nonetheless, Choh et al. could only find 44 patients in the English literature with leiomyosarcoma of the esophagus (64). Polypoid lesions which are well differentiated respond best to surgical therapy. Radical excision may at times not be necessary in these extreme instances. Overall, however, the prognosis of patients with this rare cancer is poor. Resection has resulted in several 5 year survivors.

Rhabdomyosarcoma of the Esophagus

These sarcomas, derived from striated rather than smooth muscle, are extremely rare. Resection can result in long-term survival (65).

CHORIOCARCINOMA OF THE ESOPHAGUS

Three cases of this lesion were summarized in 1979 (66). The diagnosis appeared to be easily made by brush biopsy since the characteristic cyto- and syncytotrophoblastic cells can be readily identified.

PRIMARY LYMPHOMA OF THE ESOPHAGUS

Non-Hodgkin's and Hodgkin's lymphoma arising in the esophagus has been reported (67, 68). The radiographic appearance is characterized by a diffuse nodularity as a result of lymphomatous infiltration of the mucosa. This tumor is being seen increasingly in immunocompromised patients (69).

SECONDARY ESOPHAGEAL MALIGNANCIES

The esophagus is not a frequent site of metastatic disease. As indicated above, metastatic malignant melanomas involve the esophagus more frequently than primary melanomas do. Lymphoma involving the esophagus as part of diffuse disseminated disease has also been reported. Direct extension from a lung tumor is perhaps the most frequently seen form of involvement of the esophagus by a malignancy arising in another organ. Microscopic foci of tumor are seen at autopsy in 3 to 4% of patients dying of cancer and in 9% of women dying of breast cancer. The relative frequency of involvement of the esophagus by metastatic breast cancer has resulted in the recognition of the syndrome of postmastectomy dysphagia (72, 73). Fifty-eight cases of esophageal involvement in the course of breast cancer have been reported in the literature. Radiotherapy and chemotherapy may be beneficial in those instances (73). Since the lesion often causes dysphagia by extrinsic compression, care must be taken during esophagoscopy that the esophagus is not perforated (72). Biopsy by exploration of the neck or posterior mediastinum or by needle aspiration using computerized axial tomography can provide tissue for a definitive diagnosis. These lesions can simulate primary esophageal cancers. Other sites of cancer that have been reported to give rise to metastases to the esophagus are the kidneys, pancreas, cervix and bladder (71).

REFERENCES

1 Rosenberg JC, Roth J, Lichter AS, Kelsen DP. Cancer of the Esophagus. In: DeVita V, Hellman S, Rosenberg SA eds Principles and Practices of Oncology, 2nd edition Philadelphia: JB Lippincott 1985: 621–53.
2 Steiger Z, Wilson RF, Leichman L, Busuito MJ, Rosenberg JC. Primary adenocarcinoma of the esophagus. J Surg Oncol 1987 in press.
3 Battifora H. Spindle cell carcinoma: Ultrastructural evidence of squamous origin and collagen production by the tumor cells. Cancer 1976; 37: 2275.
4 Agha FP, Keren DF. Spindle-cell squamous carcinoma of the esophagus: A tumor with biphasic morphology. AJR 1985; 145: 541.
5 Osamura RY, Shinamura K, Hata J, Tramaoki N, Watonabe K, Kubota M, Yamazaki S, Mitomi K. Polypoid carcinoma of the esophagus: A unifying term for "carcinosarcoma" and pseudosarcoma. Am J Surg Pathol 1978; 2: 201.
6 Matsusaka T, Watanabe H, Enjoji H. Pseudosarcoma and carcinosarcoma of the esophagus. Cancer 1976; 37: 1546.
7 Ming SC. Tumors of the esophagus and stomach. In: Atlas of Tumor Pathology, Second Series, Fascicle 7. Washington DC: Armed Forces Institute of Pathology.
8 Turnbull AD, Rosen P, Goodner JT, Beattie EJ. Primary malignant tumors of the esophagus other than typical epidermoid carcinoma. Ann Thorac Surg 1973; 15: 463.
9 Fennell WM, Perold JI. Pseudosarcoma of the esophagus: A case report, S Afr Med J 1977; 52: 37.
10 Postlethwait RW, Wechsler AS, Shelburne JD. Pseudosarcoma of the esophagus. Ann Thorac Surg 1975; 19: 198.
11 DeMeester TR, Skinner DB. Polypoid sarcomas of the esophagus: A rare but potentially curable neoplasm. Ann Thorac Surg 1975; 20: 405.
12 Xu LT, Sun CF, Wu LH, Chang ZR, Liu TH. Clinical and pathological characteristics of carcinosarcoma of the esophagus: Report of 4 cases. Ann Thorac Surg 1984; 37: 197.
13 Yates CW, LeVine MA, Jensen KM. Varicoid carcinoma of the esophagus. Radiology 1977; 122: 605.
14 Howel-Evans W, McConnell RB, Clarke CA, Shepard PM. Carcinoma of the esophagus with keratosis palmaris et plantaris (tylosis): A study of two families. Q J Med 1958; 27: 413.

15 Lortat-Jacob JL, Richard CA, Fekete F, Testart J. Cardiospasm and esophageal carcinoma: Report of 24 cases. Surgery 1969; 66: 969.

16 Just-Viera GO, Haight C. Achalasia and carcinoma of the esophagus. Surg Gynecol Obstet 1969; 128: 1081.

17 Rock LA, Latham PS, Hankins JR, Narsallah SM. Achalasia associated with squamous cell carcinoma of the esophagus: A case report. Am J Gastroenterol 1985, 80: 526.

18 Sigurgeirsson B, Johannson KB, Haroarson S, Onundarson PT, Thorgeirsson G. Acute thoracic inlet obstruction in achalasia with adenoid cystic and squamous cell carcinoma. Ann Thorac Surg 1985; 40: 516.

19 Joske RA, Benedict EB. The role of benign esophageal obstruction in the development of carcinoma of the esophagus. Gastroenterology 1959; 36: 749.

20 Hankins JR, McLaughlin JS. The association of carcinoma of the esophagus with achalasia. J Thorac Cardiovasc Surg 1975; 69: 355.

21 Lamb RK, Edwards CH, Pattison CW, Matthews HR. Squamous carcinoma in situ of the esophagus in a patient with achalasia. Thorax 1985; 40: 795.

22 Rosenberg JC, Franklin R, Steiger Z. Squamous cell carcinoma of the thoracic esophagus: An interdisciplinary approach. Current Problems in Cancer 1981; 5: 1.

23 Wychulis AR, Woolam GL, Andersen HA, Ellis FH. Achalasia and carcinoma of the esophagus. JAMA 1971; 215: 1638.

24 McGregor DH, Mills G, Boudet RA. Intramural squamous cell carcinoma of the esophagus. Cancer 1976; 37: 1556.

25 Huang B, Unni KK, Payne WS. Long term survival following diverticulectomy for cancer in pharyngoesophageal (Zeuker's) diverticulum. Ann Thorac Surg 1984; 38: 207.

26 Ahlbom HE. Simple achlorhydric anaemia, Plummer-Vinson syndrome, and carcinoma of the mouth, pharynx and oesophagus in women: Observations at Radiumhemmet, Stockholm. Br Med J 1936; ii: 331.

27 Entwistle CC, Jacobs A. Histological findings in the Paterson-Kelly syndrome. J Clin Pathol 1965; 18: 408.

28 Hopkins RA, Postlethwaite RW. Caustic burns and carcinoma of the esophagus. Ann Surg 1981; 194: 146.

29 Raphael HA, Ellis HF, Dockerty MB. Primary adenocarcinoma of the esophagus: 18-year review and review of literature. Ann Surg 1966; 164: 785.

30 Cederquist C, Nielsen J, Berthelsen A, Hansen HS. Adenocarcinoma of the esophagus. Acta Chir Scand 1980; 146: 411.

31 Barrett N. The lower esophagus lined by columnar epithelium. Surgery 1957; 41: 881.

32 Allison PR, Johnstone AS. The oesophagus lined with gastric mucous membrane. Thorax 1953; 8: 87.

33 Allison PR. Peptic oesophagitis and oesophageal stricture. Lancet 1970; ii: 199.

34 Adler RH. The lower esophagus lined by columnar epithelium: Its association with hiatal hernia, ulcer, stricture and tumor. J Thorac Cardiovasc Surg 1963; 45: 13.

35 Spechler SJ, Goyel RK. Barrett's esophagus. New Engl J Med 1986; 315: 362.

36 Nissen R. Eine einfache Operation zur beinflussung der Refluxoesophagitis. Schweiz Med Wochenschr 1956; 86: 590.

37 Rosenberg JC, Budev H, Edwards RC, Singal S, Steiger Z, Sundareson AS. Analysis of adenocarcinoma in Barrett's esophagus utilizing a staging system. Cancer 1985; 55: 1353.

38 Bremner CG, Lynch VP, Ellis FH. Barrett's esophagus: congenital or acquired? An experimental study of esophageal mucosal regeneration in the dog. Surgery 1970; 68: 309.

39 Hamilton SR, Yardley JG. Regeneration of cardiac type mucosa and acquisition of Barrett mucosa after estophagogastrostomy. Gastroenterology 1977; 72: 669.

40 Ranson JM, Patel GK, Clift SA, Womble NE, Read RD. Extended and limited types of Barrett's esophagus in the adult. Ann Thorac Surg 1982; 33: 19.

41 Paull A, Trier JS, Dalton D, Camp RC, Loeb P, Goyel RK. The histologic spectrum of Barrett's esophagus. New Engl J Med 1976; 295: 476.

42 Berenson MM, Herbst JJ, Freston JW. Enzyme and ultrastructural characteristics of esophageal columnar epithelium. Digest Dis 1975; 19: 895

43 Jass JR. Mucin histochemistry of the columnar epithelium of the oesophagus: A retrospective study. J Clin Pathol 1981; 34: 866.

44 Banner BF, Memoli VA, Warren WH, Gould VE. Carcinoma with multidirectional differentiation arising in Barrett's esophagus. Ultrastruct Pathol 1983; 4: 205.

45 Skinner DB, Walther BC, Riddell RH, Schmidt H, Lascone C, DeMeester TR. Barrett's esophagus: Comparison of benign and malignant cases. Surgery 1983; 198: 554.

46 Mangla JC. Barrett's esophagus: An old entity rediscovered. J Clin Gastroenterol 1981; 3: 347.

47 Brand DL, Ylvisaker JT, Gelfand M, Pope CE. Regression of columnar esophageal (Barrett's) epithelium after anti-reflux surgery. New Engl J Med 1980; 302: 844.

48 Lee RG. Dysplasia in Barrett's esophagus: Clinicopathologic study of 6 patients. Am J Surg Pathol 1985; 9: 845.

49 McKeown KC. Total three-stage oesophagectomy for cancer of the oesophagus. Br J Surg 1976; 63: 259.

50 Epstein NI, Sears VL, Tucker RS, Egan JW. Carcinoma of the esophagus with adenoid cystic differentiation. Cancer 1984; 53: 1131.

51 Pourzand A, Freant L, Levin R, Peabody J, Absolon K. Primary adenoid cystic carcinoma of the esophagus: Report of a case and review of the literature. J Thorac Cardiovasc Surg 1975; 69: 785.

52 Petersson SR. Adenoid cystic carcinoma of the esophagus: Complete response to combination chemotherapy. Cancer 1986; 57: 1464.

53 Woodard BA, Shelburne JD, Vollmer RT, Postlethwait RW. Mucoepidermoid carcinoma of the esophagus: A case report. Hum Pathol 1978; 9: 352.

54 Sabnathan S, Graham GP, Salama FD. Primary oat cell carcinoma of the esophagus. Thorax 1986; 41: 318.

55 Imai T, Sannoke Y, Okano H. Oat cell carcinoma (APUDOMA) of the esophagus: A case report. Cancer 1978; 41: 358.

56 Johnson FE, Clawson MC, Bashiti HM, Silverberg AB, Brown GO. Small cell undifferentiated carcinoma of the esophagus. Cancer 1984; 53: 1746.

57 Doherty MA, McIntyre M, Arnott SJ. Oat cell carcinoma of the esophagus: A report of six British patients with a review of the literature. Int J Radiat Oncol Biol Phys 1984; 10: 147.

58 Reyes CV, Chejfec G, Jao W, Gould VE. Neuroendocrine tumors of the esophagus. Ultrastruct Pathol 1980; 1: 367.

59 Kelsen DP, Weston E, Kurty R, Cvitkvoic E, Lieberman P, Golbey RB. Small cell carcinoma of the esophagus: Treatment by chemotherapy alone. Cancer 1980; 45: 1558.

60 Rosenthal SN, Lemkin JA. Multiple small cell carcinomas of the esophagus. Cancer 1983; 51: 1944.

61 Rankin R, Nirodi NS, Browne MK. Carcinoid tumor of the esophagus: Report of a case. Scott Med J 1980; 25: 245.

62 Siegel A, Swartz A. Malignant carcinoid of oesophagus. Histopathology 1986; 10: 761.

63 Chalkiadokis G, Wihlm JM, Morand G, Weil-Bousson M, Witz JP. Primary malignant melanoma of the esophagus. Ann Thorac Surg 1985; 39: 472.

64 Choh JH, Khazei AH, Ihm HJ. Leiomyosarcoma of the esophagus: Report of a case and review of the literature. J Surg Oncol 1986; 32: 223.

65 Wobbes T, Rinsma SG, Holla AT, Rietberg M, Leezenberg JA, Collenteur JC. Rhabdomyosarcoma of the esophagus. Arch Chir Neerl 1975; 27: 69.

66 Trillo AA, Accettulo LM, Yecter TL. Choriocarcinoma of the esophagus: Histologic and cytologic findings. A case report. Acta Cytol 1979; 23: 69.

67 Matsuura H, Saito R, Nakajing S, Yoshihara W, Enomoto T. Non-Hodgkins lymphoma of the esophagus. Am J Gastroenterol 1985; 80: 941.

68 Agha FP, Schnitzer B. Esophageal involvement in lymphoma. Am J Gastroenterol 1985; 80: 412.

69 Gedgaudos-McClees RK, Maglinte DD. Lymphomatous esophageal nodules: The difficulty in radiological differential diagnosis. Am J Gastroenterol 1985; 80: 529.

70 Marshall ME. Gastrointestinal metastasis from carcinoma of the breast. J Ken Med Assoc 1973; 81: 154.

71 Anderson MF, Harrell GS. Secondary esophageal tumors. Am J Radiol 1980; 135: 1243.

72 Laforet EG, Kondi ES. Postmastectomy dysphagia. Am J Surg 1171; 121: 368.

73 Boccardo F, Merlano M, Canobbio L, Rosso R, Aste H. Esophageal involvement in breast cancer: Report of six cases. Tumori 1982; 68: 149.

74 Dulchavsky S, Rosenberg JC. Metastases to the esophagus as the presenting manifestation of secondary malignant disease. Ann Thorac Surg 1987 (submitted for publication).

Textbook of Uncommon Cancer
Edited by C.J. Williams, J.G. Krikorian, M.R. Green and D. Raghavan

Chapter **25**

Rare Gastric Tumours

T.S. Ganesan and M. Slevin

ICRF Department of Medical Oncology, St Bartholomew's Hospital, London, UK

INTRODUCTION

The chapter reviews rare tumours of the stomach, but does not cover lymphomas and extramedullary plasmacytomas as they are covered comprehensively in reviews of haematological malignancies. Sarcomas, which comprise 3% of gastric tumours, carcinoid tumours, adenosquamous carcinoma, carcinosarcoma and neurogenic tumours of the stomach in that order of incidence are primarily dealt with in this review. Current research on the pathogenesis is focused mostly on sarcomas and carcinoid tumours. Surgery is still the mainstay of management in all these tumours. Radiotherapy has little role in the management while the role of chemotherapy particularly in carcinoid tumours is being explored at various centres. In general, they are not easy to differentiate from the more common adenocarcinomas clinically and the diagnosis is usually made on biopsy or at operation. The histogenesis of some of these tumours in particular the sarcomas, and neurogenic tumours is not resolved fully. This review encompasses the incidence, aetiology, pathogenesis, clinical features and management of these tumours.

SARCOMAS

Next to adenocarcinoma of the stomach, mesenchymal cell tumours or sarcomas are the commonest neoplasms accounting for 1–3% of gastric tumours. Traditionally most of these have implicated the malignant smooth muscle cell. Histologically these have been difficult to classify since the first description in 1960 (1). Under the recent WHO classification, the term epithelioid or cellular leiomyomas were to include the older 'leiomyoblastomas' (2). Leiomyosarcoma is the malignant version of the former. Appelman and Helwig in their excellent review of this difficult subject established the different clinical, biological and histological characteristics of these tumours (3–5).

Pathologically, leiomyomas and leiomyosarcoma are almost exclusively seen in the stomach, when compared to the rest of the gastrointestinal tract. On gross morphology both types of tumours are large and lobular and occasionally appearing as discrete nodules. Benign tumours are smaller and in one series all malignant tumours were above 6 cm in diameter (4). The malignant tumours are commonly seen in the body of the stomach and less often in the antrum, fundus and cardia. However, benign tumours almost always arise in the body of the stomach. Usually tumours are well circumscribed and appear to be grossly encapsulated. They occur as intramural masses that expand the gastric wall. They can be endogastric, exogastric or dumb-bell shaped. The mucosa overlying the tumour is often ulcerated. Degenerative changes such as hyalinization, haemorrhage and necrosis are common. The anterior wall of the stomach is more commonly involved in benign tumours as opposed to the posterior wall in malignant tumours.

Microscopically benign leiomyomas can be differentiated into a cellular and an epithelioid variant. The predominant cells seen in the former are spindle cells, with well defined borders, clear or eosinophilic cytoplasm and dark staining nucleus, which are arranged loosely. In the epithelioid variety the cells are more plump and round with clear cytoplasm. Often there is a mixture of the two cell types. Palisading and a whorling arrangement of cells are seen as is a strong reticulum fibre pattern. Vessels are also seen usually as capillaries in the tumour. The tumours involve the muscularis propria and submucosa. Pseudocapsule formation is observed, though not by fibrous tissue but by hyalinized bundles of smooth muscle. Mitotic figures are rarely seen in the benign tumours though up to five per 50 high power fields (HPFs) have been reported (4).

Leiomyosarcomas in contrast are made up of similar, round or epithelioid and spindle cells which are closely packed and much smaller in size. The reticulum fibre pattern is indistinct. The nulei are hyperchromatic and there are more mitotic figures usually over five per 50 HPFs. There is a tendency to form alveolar clusters or whorls. Two further varieties based on the differentiation of the cell type can be recognized. Benign leiomyoma can also be seen existing with the more malignant variety if adequate sections of the tumour are performed.

Metastases are uncommon in the benign tumour though it has been recorded (3). In contrast both local and distant metastases are observed with leiomyosarcoma. Locally peritoneum and retroperitoneal organs are the most frequent sites. Haemotogenous spread is more common than lymphatic spread, liver and lungs being common sites. Depending on the accuracy and duration of follow-up, 55%

of patients with well differentiated leiomyosarcomas and 75% of the poorly differentiated variety, show metastatic behaviour (3, 4). This obviously is a major feature in predicting the malignant nature of the neoplasm. Once metastases are documented survival is poor though it can take a long time for them to manifest after removal of the primary tumour.

The nature of the cell causing the tumour has been in doubt, and only by recent ultra-structural studies has it been shown to be myogenic (6, 7). It seems to be composed of cells that seem capable of partial differentiation towards a smooth muscle cell. The basic cell is poorly differentiated. It is occasionally difficult to differentiate leiomyoma from less common varieties of stroma tumour namely the glomus tumour, pericytoma and angioma. However, in a review of over 231 cases (3) no case of haemangiopericytoma could be documented. In a more recent study by Masur and Clark, however, analysis of 28 cases by electron microscopy and immunostaining for the S-100 protein suggests a neural origin for the tumours, previously diagnosed as leiomyomas or leiomyosarcomas except in 2 cases (8).

Leiomyomas are more often seen in the sixth decade as opposed to leiomyosarcomas in the fifth decade. It has been observed at all ages and males have a greater incidence of the tumour. A small minority of cases occur as part of a syndrome in younger people in association with a functioning extra-adrenal paraglanglioma and pulmonary chondroma (9). Two cases have been reported following radiotherapy of the stomach for peptic ulcer (10).

Clinically symptoms are predominantly of upper gastrointestinal haemorrhage. This manifests as either haematemesis or malaena and occurs in about 50% of patients with both benign and malignant varieties of the tumour. Anorexia, nausea and vomiting and generalized abdominal pain or less commonly epigastric pain are observed. Weight loss is more often seen with malignant tumours. A palpable mass is occasionally observed. It is interesting though that up to one-third of patients can be asymptomatic and the tumour detected incidentally. Recurrent or massive upper gastrointestinal haemorrhage in a patient without any other symptom should lead one to suspect a leiomyoma in contrast to the more common carcinoma or peptic ulcer (11, 12).

The differentiation between leiomyoma and leiomyosarcoma is difficult and a combination of clinical and pathological features is necessary. Weight loss and abdominal pain indicate a more malignant tumour. Tumours arising in the cardia and fundus and on the posterior gastric wall are malignant. Size of the tumour, extent of mucosal invasion, histological features and presence of mitotic figures aid in diagnosing malignancy (Table 1).

Endoscopy and a barium meal are usually enough when combined with a biopsy to give a definite diagnosis. x-Ray appearances are characteristic with a large filling defect often with a central ulcer. Laparotomy defines the extent of local invasion and metastases.

Management has been mainly surgical. The exact surgical procedure to be performed is not yet uniformally accepted. In the largest series published (3, 11) local resection seemed to be as good as a subtotal or a total gastrectomy. With respect to the benign tumours out of 65 patients followed up to at least 5 years there was only one patient with metastases (3). In contrast in leiomyosarcomas, metastases were observed in up to 76% on follow-up. In general epithelioid leiomyosarcomas did better and median survival was 5 years. In these patients extent of surgical resection did not seem to alter the prognosis. No definite role for chemotherapy or radiotherapy has been delineated in this tumour. The overall prognosis with leiomyoma is excellent with all patients being cured after local excision. However, in leiomyosarcoma though surgery is potentially curative, once metastases are observed survival is poor.

CARCINOID TUMOURS OF THE STOMACH

Carcinoid tumours have been described in all parts of the gastrointestinal tract with the exception of the oesophagus. Sanders and

TABLE 1 DIFFERENTIATION BETWEEN LEIOMYOMA AND LEIOMYOSARCOMA

	Leiomyoma	Leiomyosarcoma
Age	sixth decade	fifth decade
M:F	2.4:1	2.7:1
Symptoms:	gastrointestinal haemorrhage abdominal pain asymptomatic	weight loss gastrointestinal haemorrhage abdominal pain
Tumour:		
Size	<6–7 cm	>6–7 cm

Location	body of stomach	more common in the
		   body of the stomach but seen in cardia,
		   fundus and antrum

Wall	commonly anterior	commonly posterior
Extent	submucosa and mucosa	extends up to serosa
Metastases	rare	common
Histology:		
Cell type	large epithelial or spindle cells loosely arranged well differentiated <5 mitotic figures per 50 high power fields	small epithelial or spindle cells packed closely well differentiated/poorly differentiated >5 mitotic figures per 50 high power fields
Survival	good	poor

Axtell (13) in their review of gastrointestinal carcinoids estimated the incidence of gastric carcinoids at 3.4% while Godwin's series (14) estimated the incidence at 2%. Askanazy was the first to recognize them and reported it in 1923 (15). Later with the description of the carcinoid syndrome in the 1950s, it was noted that gastric carcinoids were rarely associated with the classical syndrome (4). Carcinoid syndrome has been observed in only 5 out of 86 patients in a review by Sanders and Axtel (13), and Hajdu et al. (16) observed it in one out of 10 patients. Gastric tumours rarely synthesize serotonin and they normally lack the enzyme histidine carboxylase. This biochemical difference also accounts for the fact that few are argentaffin positive.

Grossly the tumours appear as single or multiple submucosal growths and are generally small, firm and well circumscribed. The mucosa is usually intact but occasionally may be ulcerated. Microscopically carcinoid tumours are composed of small uniform cells that are polygonal or cuboidal. They form nests, clusters, cords and strands within the submucosa. The cells contain granules within the cytoplasm which give a positive argentaffin reaction. It is because of their origin from gastrointestinal endocrine cells that they are called apudomas. They are classified as orthoendocrine apudomas producing hormones similar to those of cells of origin. The overall histological appearance is benign though most pathologists now believe that all tumours are potentially malignant. This has been studied in great detail after the initial reports of carcinoid tumours as being benign.

Hajdu et al. demonstrated the relationship of the depth of invasion of tumour into the submucosa and the predilection for metastases (16). The size of the tumour is also important as tumours less than 1 cm rarely metastasize. It is a slowly growing tumour and local metastases to lymph nodes and liver are the common sites. Bone is a frequent site too, and the reaction is often that of an osteoblastic lesion. Local and distant metastases were found in 55% at the time of diagnosis in Godwin's series

(14) and in 28% in Sander's series (13). Hajdu et al. reported 5 out of 10 gastric carcinoids with metastases (16).

An association between atrophic gastritis and enterochromaffin like (ECL) cells has been recognized (17). Some of the factors that increase the risk of adenocarcinomas may also affect ECL cells in the stomach. Spontaneous gastric carcinoids develop only in humans and in an African rodent, *Praomys natalensis*, which also develops spontaneous adenocarcinomas (18). In Wistar rats both tumours have been induced by N-methyl-N' nitro-nitrosoguanidine given orally (19). Occasionally carcinoids are seen following gastro-jejunostomy postulating a role for gastrin (20). Pernicious anaemia has been associated with carcinoid tumours as with adenocarcinomas. It has been suggested that a combination of increased nitrosamines and gastritis in this situation may lead to carcinoid tumour (21). In a review by Moses et al. (17) it was found that 47 out of 66 cases of multiple gastric carcinoids and 14 out of 93 cases of solitary carcinoid tumour had pernicious anaemia. This has been confirmed by Carney et al, in a review of 30 patients at the Mayo Clinic: in 15 patients with multiple carcinoids 75% had pernicious anaemia (22). It is, therefore, reasonable to conclude that along with a threefold increase of stomach carcinoma in patients with pernicious anaemia there is a higher frequency of carcinoid tumours.

Clinically the symptoms of carcinoid are not different from gastric cancer. Epigastric pain is the most frequent symptom followed by malaena, haematemesis, weight loss, anaemia, nausea and vomiting. When these symptoms are associated with attacks of flushing and diarrhoea, a diagnosis of gastric carcinoid should be entertained. In the absence of the latter the diagnosis is usually made at laparotomy. Liver metastasis are observed at a later stage and the liver is often palpable, being hard and nodular.

The usual investigations performed to reach a correct diagnosis are endoscopy and a barium meal. It is difficult to differentiate from cancer in a routine barium meal. 5-Hydrox-yindole-acetic acid (5-HIAA) excretion in the urine is a useful confirmatory test though seldom elevated in gasteric carcinoids.

Treatment is usually surgical, with wide excision of the tumour if malignant. For multiple carcinoids subtotal gastrectomy may be necessary. Removal of the primary even though metastases exist, causes regression of metastases and decrease in symptoms of the syndrome. Solitary liver metastases can be removed surgically and Moertel documented 5 such patients treated at the Mayo Clinic (23). Murray Lyon et al. treated 3 patients with hepatic artery ligation and observed relief of symptoms (14). Further Moertel treated 11 such patients at the Mayo Clinic, and noticed a prompt fall in HIAA and relief of symptoms although of a short duration. The prognosis is generally good with surgical excision of the primary tumour in the absence of metastases. In patients with frank metastases and the carcinoid syndrome with 5-HIAA levels > 150 mg/24 hours a trial of chemotherapy is war-ranted. However, as these tumours are indo-lent the decision to give a patient cytotoxic chemotherapy has to be made carefully in each patient. The general principles of management with chemotherapy are the same as with other metastatic carcinoid tumour. Drugs which are active as single agents include 5-fluorouracil (5-FU) streptozotocin, doxorubicin and DTIC. Combination chemotherapy has been difficult to evaluate and conduct because of the rarity of the disease and the indolent nature of the tumour. Various trials are in progress to assess particular combination regimens. In a review of the treatment of carcinoid tumours no combination was superior and none signifi-cantly increased the overall survival (23).

Hormonal therapy to antogonize the princi-pal effects of the mediators of the carcinoid syndrome is possible. Mild gastrointestinal symptoms can be managed by diphenoxylate or codeine. Serotonin antagonists like cypro-heptadine and methysergide have been useful (23). Parachlorophenylalanine which is an inhibitor of tryptophan 5-hydroxylase is a

useful agent at doses of 2–4 g/24 hours, though not without side effects. Somatostatin can be given only through the intravenous route and may be useful in carcinoid crisis. Human leucocyte interferon has been tried in carcinoid syndrome with marked symptomatic relief and reductions in 5-HIAA excretoin (23).

The prognosis for carcinoid tumour of the stomach is generally good if the disease is localized and the 5-year survival is around 90%. Patients with regional extension of the disease had a 23% 5-year survival. Distant metastases, size of tumour, presence of carci-noid syndrome indicate poor survival and patients are usually dead in under 2 years. However, judicious management of these tumours in a specialist centre can considerbaly improve the quality of life.

SQUAMOUS CELL CARCINOMA OF THE STOMACH

Pure squamous cell carcinoma or adenosqua-mous (adenoacanthoma) carcinoma is a rare disease. By definition the tumour should arise below the cardia as it is difficult to exclude oesophageal lesions. Squamous cell carcino-mas comprise only a small fraction of gastric carcinomas, approximately 0.04–0.7% (26). There is a male predilection with the ratio being 4:1. The neoplasm is only seen in adults and occurs with greater frequency during the sixth decade of life.

The majority of the tumours arise in the pyloric region followed by the body of the stomach. The tumours are exophytic in character, protruding within the lumen of the stomach and often attaining considerable size (27). Microscopically the features of squamous cell carcinoma are to be found. The cells exhibit keratin pearl formation and intercellu-lar bridges.

Considerable discussion has taken place in the literature pertaining to the histogenesis of these tumours. As squamous cellular epithe-lium is not normally found in gastric mucosa certain explanations are possible. Ectopic squamous cell nests in the stomach and squamous metaplasia of glandular epithelium are logical theories. Other explanations are squamous differentiation of adenocarcinoma as has been observed in basal cell carcinoma. Further, the existence of a totipotential gastric cell has been raised as well as an origin from endothelial cells of blood vessels (26, 27).

The frequency of pure squamous cell carcinoma and adenosquamous carcinoma is about equal as reported by Boswell and Helwig (28).

Clinically epigastric pain, nausea, indigestion and an epigastric mass are common features. There is no difference clinically between adenocarcinoma and squamous cell carcinoma. Diagnosis is usually established by radiography and confirmed by gastroscopy.

Treatment is surgical and consists of total or subtotal gastrectomy. Excision is usually possible, because the tumour is often confined to the stomach. The reported 5-year survival is poor at 4–14% and not different from adenocarcinoma (29, 30). Only 5 out of 18 patients presented in the literature were noted to have metastases at the time of publication; however, in the series of Boswell and Helwig (28) all the 12 patients were dead of metastases if adequate follow-up time was provided and death occurred within a median of 7 months from diagnosis.

CARCINOSARCOMA

Carcinosarcoma is a rare malignant neoplasm of the stomach consisting of both epithelial and mesenchymal elements in the same tumour. It is commonly seen in the uterus though cases have been reported in other organs including the stomach. The latter is rare and Queckenstedt in 1904 was the first to report such a case (31). There have been 23 additional cases reported, 16 of the have been from Japan (32). Saphir and Vass in 1938 reviewed the literature and discussed in detail the existence of carcinosarcoma as an entity (33). There has been no change in the incidence of carcinosarcoma in various organs since 1938 (32).

Because carcinoma of the stomach is a common cancer in Japan, carcinosarcoma has also received more attention there (32). Pathologically it has to be differentiated from collision tumour and coexisting carcinoma and sarcoma. Meyer in 1919 and Fould in 1946 classified the tumour by the following histological features (34, 35):

1. Collision tumour: the two components originate in different areas of the stomach and grow together to form a single tumour.
2. Combination tumour: the two components develop simultaneously due to the same aetiological factor, or one precedes the other and there is admixture without any relation between parenchyma and stroma.
3. Composition tumour: the malignancy of the two components develops simultaneously, but the relationship between parenchyma and stroma is maintained.

However, collision tumour is differentiated from true carcinosarcoma (2 and 3) (36, 37). In a review of the 23 reported cases of carcinosarcoma of the stomach at least 7 were of the 'collision' type. Grossly Kitamura (38) divided them into three types depending on their development: (a) general thickening of the gastric wall; (b) chief development beyond serosa; (c) intragastric and polypoid or ulcer like.

In pathological diagnosis the following complicating factors need to be considered carefully: (i) variation and marked anaplasia of carcinoma cells; (ii) large amounts of connective tissue produced in response to chronic inflammation; (iii) invasion of a benign connective tissue tumour by a carcinoma; (iv) invasion of sarcoma by normal or metaplastic epithelial structures (33).

In large carcinomas sarcoma-like proliferation is often observed and can be differentiated by special stains.

The pathogenesis of the tumour has interested several people. Carcinosarcoma in general has been observed after irradiation to organs (39–41). Virchow and Herxheimer believed that a primary carcinoma would stimulate excessive growth of stroma and that carcinosarcoma might result when the proliferation of the latter reached the stage of malignancy (42, 43). Experimental studies by Ehrlich and Apolant showed that the transplanted carcinoma in the mouse could change its histological appearance to carcinosarcoma and eventually to sarcoma (44).

Clinically this tumour affects a younger age group than carcinoma. It is more frequent in male patients and has a propensity for the pyloric region. The symptoms are identical to that of stomach carcinoma and a correct diagnosis is only made at operation or autopsy. Metastasis has been reported in up to 20% at diagnosis and more frequently is of the carcinomatous element.

Management has been essentially surgical which includes partial to total gastrectomy. However, the mortality has been 100% as eventually all patients to date have died of the tumour.

NEUROGENIC TUMOURS OF THE STOMACH (Chapter 29)

Following Verocay's introduction of the word neurinoma (45), with reference to neoplasms arising from Schwann cells, Stout (46) and later Ransom and Kay (47) classified them into neurilemmoma (benign) and neurogenic sarcoma. It is the former which is seen commonly in the stomach and there were 35 patients in Stout's series. In a review of the literature the percentage of neurogenic tumours varies from 2.5% to 10% of all benign gastric tumours. However, until recently histological features of these tumours were not clear cut and it is possible that many leiomyomas were inadvertently classified as neurogenic tumours. Ransom and Kay believed abdominal forms of neurilemmoma usually occur in the stomach and retroperitoneal tissue. The association with von Recklinghausen's disease is often observed.

Neurilemmomas arise from Schwann cells as most believe or contrarily from the endoneurium. The tumours are submucosal, intramural or subserous and variable in size. They are usually well encapsulated and ulcerated over the mucosa. They often grow to a huge size in view of their slow growing nature. Rutten's series (48) describes the varying nature of these tumours with illustrative cases.

Histologically there are two well defined types.

1. The tumour is arranged in an orderly manner with regular fasciculi of the delicate fibrillae, arranged in whorls. There is a regular arrangement of the cell nuclei called the 'palisade' effect which is not pathognomonic. Occasionally tumour cells form syncytium which stains with silver and resembles the Schwann cells.

2. The tumour lacks the regular character in this type. The tissue is more undifferentiated, and shows a reticular structure interspersed with small fluid filled crevices. These so-called microcysts are regarded as degenerative forms. The nuclei are elongated and oval. Tendency to necrosis, absence of the capsule, loss of the palisade structure and frequent mitoses are signs which suggest a malignant nature of the neoplasm.

Malignant degeneration of neurogenic tumours is of the order of 15%. The benign or malignant nature of the neoplasm is difficult to establish only on histological grounds. Melanocytic schwannomas in various locations have been documented. Burns et al. (49) reported one such tumour in the stomach which was resected. Malignant non-chromaffin paraganglioma of the stomach has also been reported (50).

Clinically the symptoms depend on the growth, type and localization of the tumour. Epigastric pain, malaena or haematemesis, palpable mass are some of the features. Recurrent gastric haemorrhages with prolonged asymptomatic intervals are seen in up to 36% of cases (51). Subserous tumours are associated with a tendency to undergo torsion or suppuration. Malignant degeneration is a real and frequent complication.

Diagnosis is confirmed by a barium meal and endoscopy. Usually it is a smooth encapsulated tumour. Occasionally if ulcerated it is difficult to differentate from gastric carcinoma.

Treatment is normally surgical consisting of excision allowing an adequate margin.

ACKNOWLEDGEMENTS

This work was supported by the Imperial Cancer Research Fund. We are grateful to Dr P.F.M. Wrigley and Dr A.J. Stansfeld for critical comments. Our thanks to Claire Adams who typed the manuscript.

REFERENCES

Sarcomas

1 Martin JF, Basin P, Feroldi J, Cabanne F. Tumeurs myoides intra-murales de l'estomac—considérations microscopiques à propos de 6 cas. Ann Anat Pathol (Paris) 1960; 5: 484–97.
2 Enzinger FM, Lattes R, Torloni H. Histological typing of soft tissue tumours. International histological classification of tumours no 3. Geneva: World Health Organization, 1969.
3 Appelman HD, Helwig EB. Sarcomas of the stomach. Am J Clin Pathol 1977; 61: 2–10.
4 Appelman HD, Helwig EB. Gastric epithelioid leiomyoma and leiomyosarcoma (leiomyoblastoma). Cancer 1976; 38: 708–28.
5 Appelmann HD, Helwig EB. Cellular leiomyomas of the stomach in 49 patients. Arch Pathol Lab Med 1977; 101; 373–7.
6 Cornog JL. The ultrastructure of leiomyoblastoma: with comments on the light microscopic morphology. Arch Pathol 1969; 87: 404–10.
7 Salazar H, Totten RS. Leiomyoblastoma of the stomach—an ultrastructural study. Cancer 1970; 25: 176–85.
8 Masur MT, Clark HB. Gastric stromal tumours. Am J Surg Pathol 1983; 7: 507–19.
9 Carney JA. The triad of gastric epithelioid leiomyosarcoma, functioning extra-adrenal paraganglioma, and pulmonary chondroma. Cancer 1979; 43: 374–82.
10 Lieber MR, Winans CS, Griem ML, Moosa R, Elner VM, Franklin WA. Sarcomas arising after radiotherapy for peptic ulcer disease. Dig Dis Sci 1985; 30: 593–9.
11 Schiu NH, Farr GH, Papachristou DN, Hajdu SI. Myosarcomas of the stomach: Natural history, prognostic factors and management. Cancer 1982; 49: 177–87.
12 Stout AP. Bizarre smooth muscle tumours of the stomach. Cancer 1962; 15: 400–9.

Carcinoid Tumours of the Stomach

13 Sanders RJ, Axtell HK. Carcinoids of the gastro-intestinal tract. Surg Gynecol Obstet 1964; 119: 369–80.
14 Godwin JD. Carcinoid tumours. Cancer 1975; 36: 560–9.
15 Askanazy M. Zur Pathogenese der Magenkrebse und über ihren gelegentlichen Ursprund aus angeborenem epithelian Keimen in der Magenwand. Deutsche Med Wehnsehr 1923; 1: 49–53.
16 Hajdu SI, Winawer SJ, Laird Myers WP. Carcinoid tumors. Am J Clin Pathol 1974; 61: 521–8.
17 Moses RE, Frank BR, Leavitt M, Miller R. The syndrome of type A chronic atrophic gastritis, pernicious anaemia and multiple gastric carcinoids. J Clin Gastroenterol 1986; 8(1): 61–5.
18 Randeria JD. Gastric carcinoids and adenocarcinoma in the untreated and the chemically treated mastomys of the Y and Z strains. Abst Proc XIIth Int Cancer Cong. Buenos Aires, 1978.
19 Tahara E, Ito K, Nakagami K et al. Induction of carcinoids in the glandular stomach of rats by N-methyl-N-nitro-N-nitro-soguanidine. J Cancer Res Clin Oncol 1981; 100: 1–12.
20 Bordi C, Senatore S, Missale G. Gastric carcinoid following gastrojejunostomy. Am J Dig Dis 1976; 21: 667–71.
21 Wilander E. Achylia and the development of gastric carcinoid. Virchows Arch (Pathol Anat) 1981; 394: 151–60.
22 Carney JA, Vay L, Go W et al. The syndrome of gastric argyrophil carcinoid tumors and nonantral gastric atrophy. Ann Intern Med 1983; 99: 761–3
23 Moertel CG. Treatment of the carcinoid tumour and the malignant carcinoid syndrome. J Clin Oncol 1983; 11: 727.
24 Murray Lyon IM, Parsons VA, Blendis LM, Dawson JL, Rake MO, Laws JW, Williams R. Treatment of secondary hepatic tumours by ligation of the hepatic artery and infusion of cytotoxic drugs. Lancet 1970; ii: 172.
25 Engstrom PF, Lavin PT, Moerytel CG, Folsch E, Douglas HO Jr. Streptozotocin plus fluorouracil versus doxorubicin therapy for metastatic carcinoid tumour. J Clin Oncol 1984; 2: 1255.

Squamous Cell Carcinoma of the Stomach

26 Straus R, Heschel S, Fortmann DJ. Primary adenosquamous carcinoma of the stomach. Cancer 1969; 21: 985–95.
27 Rioux A, Masse SR. Pure squamous cell carcinoma of the stomach. Can J Surg 1979; 22: 238–9.
28 Boswell JT, Helwig EB. Squamous cell carcinoma and adenocanthoma of the stomach a clinicopathological study. Cancer 1965; 18: 181.
29 Altschuler JH, Shaha JA. Squamous cell carcinoma of the stomach. Cancer 1966; 19: 831–8.
30 Antoniades J ed. Uncommon Malignant Tumours. 1982: 10.

Carcinosarcoma

31 Queckenstedt H. Ueber Karzinosarkome. Leipzig, 1904. Cited by Saphir O and Vass A (33).
32 Tanimura H, Furuta M. Carcinosarcoma of the stomach. Am J Surg 1967; 113: 702–9.
33 Saphir O, Vass A. Carcinosarcoma. Am J Cancer 1938; 33: 331.
34 Meyer R. Beitrag zur Verstanding über die Namengebung in der Geschwulstlehre. Zentralbl Allg Path 1919; 30: 291.
35 Fould L. Carcinosarcoma. Am J Cancer 1940; 39: 1.
36 Stout AP, Humphreys GH, Rottenberg LA. A case of carcinosarcoma of the esophagus. AJR 1949; 61: 461.
37 Bergmann M, Ackerman LV, Kemler RL. Carcinosarcoma of the lung. Review of the literature and report of two cases treated by pneumonectomy. Cancer 1951; 4: 919.
38 Kitamura S. Study on carcinosarcoma of stomach. Gann 1950; 41: 15.
39 Hill RP, Miller FN. Combined mesenchymal sarcoma and carcinoma (carcinosarcoma) of the uterus. Cancer 1951; 4: 803.
40 Butcher HR Jr, Seaman WB, Eckert C, Saltzstein S. An assessment of radical mastectomy and postoperative irradiation therapy in the treatment of mammary cancer. Cancer 1964; 17: 480.
41 Knezevic-Zvac J. Carcinoma sarcoma uteri after radiotherapy of carcinoma colli. Med Arkh 1960; 14: 45.
42 Virchow R. Die krankhaften Geschwulste, Vol 2, Berlin: A Hirschwald, 1864–1865.
43 Herxheimer G. Der Carcinoma sarcomatodes nebst Beschreibung eines einschlagigen Tumors des Oesophagus. Beitr Path Anat 1908; 44: 150.
44 Ehrlich P, Apolant H. Zur Kenntnis der Sarkomentwicklung bei Carcinomtransplantationen. Zentralbl Allg Path 1906; 17: 513.

Neurogenic Tumours of the Stomach

45 Verocay J. Beitr Path Anat 1910; 70: 1.
46 Stout AP. Am J Cancer 1935; 24: 751.
47 Ransom HK, Kay EB. Ann Surg 1940; 112: 700.
48 Rutten APM. Neurogenic tumours of the stomach. Br J Surg 1965; 52: 920–5.
49 Burns DK, Silva FG, Forde KA, Mount PM, Brent Clark H. Primary melanocytic schwannoma of the stomach. Cancer 1983; 52: 1432–41.
50 Westbrook KC, Bridger WM, Williams GD. Malignant nonchromaffin paraganglioma of the stomach. Am J Surg 1972; 124: 407–9.
51 Palmer ED. Medicine 1951; 30: 81.

Chapter **26**

Uncommon Pancreatic Tumors

Monty S. Metcalfe* and
John S. Macdonald†

* University of Kentucky Medical Center, Veterans Administration Hospital, Lexington, Kentucky and † Lucille Parker Markey Cancer Center, University of Kentucky Medical Center, Lexington, Kentucky, USA

INTRODUCTION

Cancer of the pancreas is responsible for approximately 25 000 cancer deaths per year in the United States. The incidence if 10/100 000 in the general population. After age 30, in both men and women and in every population, rates increase with age in a log-linear fashion. The incidence in the eighth decade is 40 times that in the fourth decade. There appears to be a trend of steadily increasing incidence of this tumor, although because of problems of classification and ascertainment, it is by no means clear that the increase is real rather than apparent (1).

Numerous epidemiologic studies have looked for etiologic factors in pancreatic cancer. It has been felt that there is an increased incidence in patients with diabetes (2–7) and chronic pancreatitis (8–10); however, there are no studies that would suggest a causal relationship. One rare entity that does seem to carry an increased risk of pancreatic cancer is hereditary pancreatitis (11). Other factors that have been investigated include coffee (10, 12), radiation exposure (13–17), asbestos exposure (18–20), diet (21–23), and tobacco (24–30). Except for tobacco, there is little if any reason to suspect any of these as

having a major role in the etiology of pancreatic cancer.

The degree of this tumor's lethality is reflected by the fact that while it is the seventh most common cancer, it is the fourth most common cause of cancer deaths in the United States. The overall survival at one year is 10% and 2% at 5 years (31). The reasons for the grim prognosis are many, but can be distilled into three major causes: (1) late diagnosis due to the non-specific, vague complaints which may not arouse suspicion at a time when an early diagnosis and surgical cure are possible; (2) the relatively ineffective therapy for advanced disease; and (3) the fact that surgery is only capable of curing 15% of resectable patients.

A detailed pathological classification of pancreatic malignancies would serve no clinical purpose if all of the separate entities possessed a similar prognosis. Fortunately it has become apparent that this is not the case, at least for a small minority of pancreatic malignancies (32). A classification of pancreatic malignancies is suggested in Table 1. Basically this divides pancreatic tumors into those of the exocrine and those of the endocrine pancreas. The tumors of the endocrine pancreas are those of islet cell origin such as the insulinoma,

TABLE 1 CLASSIFICATION OF PANCREATIC
MALIGNANCIES

Tumors of presumed ductal origin
   Duct cell adenocarcinoma
   Giant cell carcinoma
      Giant cell carcinoma (epulis–osteoid type)
   Adenosquamous carcinoma
   Microcystadenocarcinoma
   Mucinous adenocarcinoma
   Cystadenocarcinoma
Tumors of presumed acinar origin
   Acinar cell carcinoma
Tumors of mixed acinar, ductal, and islet cell origin
Tumors of uncertain origin
   Pancreatoblastoma
   Oncocytic carcinoma
   Papillary and cystic, solid, solid and papillary tumor
   Small cell carcinoma
Lymphomas
Sarcomas
Islet cell tumors
   Insulinomas
   Glucagonomas
   Somatistatinomas
   Vipomas
   Carcinoid

---

glucagonoma, etc. The exocrine pancreatic tumors are represented by tumors of presumed ductal cell origin (33, 34), of which the majority are the common ductal adenocarcinoma. Also included are less common variants such as the squamous cell carcinoma, giant cell carcinoma and the cystadenocarcinoma. Other uncommon tumors of the exocrine pancreas include acinar cell carcinoma, lymphomas, and sarcomas.

BACKGROUND

In this review the common ductal adenocarcinoma will not be dealt with in detail except to serve as a baseline for comparison for the less common tumors. The ductal adenocarcinoma accounts for approximately 75–90% of all pancreatic malignancies (32, 35–37). There is an overall male to female predominance of 1.5–2:1, although the ratio approaches unity with advancing age. There appears to be an increased incidence in blacks (1). The tumor occurs in all age groups but is rare before the age of 25 (31), most patients being in the 50–70 age range. Approximately 70% of ductal adenocarcinomas occur in the head of the pancreas, with 20% occurring in the body and 10% in the tail of the gland (35–37). The vast majority of patients present with at least regional metastatic disease, if not widespread disease. The most common sites of metastasis include: regional lymph nodes in 18–25%, liver in 21–80%, peritoneum in 11–23%, lungs in 7–28%, and abdominal carcinomatosis in 25% (38). Presenting signs and symptoms are of a non-specific nature, including weight loss and pain in over 70%; jaundice is present in 80% of patients with tumors of the head, of the gland, but is uncommon in tumors of the body and tail. Other presenting symptoms may include anorexia, nausea, vomiting, weakness, and constipation. All of these are non-specific, but are present in at least 25% of patients. Common presenting signs are jaundice and hepatomegaly in over 80% of patients with tumors of the head of the gland, while tumors of the body and tail more often present with hepatomegaly, and abdominal mass or ascites. The current recommended diagnostic work up for a patient thought to have a possible pancreatic tumor would include an ultrasound followed by a computed tomography (CT) scan (depending on the results of the ultrasound). If an abnormality is detected, endoscopic retrograde cholangiopancreatography (ERCP) with cytology is recommended if available. If a lesion is identified that appears to be localized and potentially resectable an angiographic examination should be obtained preoperatively. If a patient has obvious metastatic disease at presentation, then diagnostic evaluation should be limited to establishing a tissue diagnosis from the most available site. This may include fine needle biopsy of the pancreas (31, 39).

Morphologically these tumors present as ill-defined, indurated masses gray-white or gray in color on cut section. Microscopically they are composed of different sized duct-like structures, with an abundant stromal reaction. They vary from well to very poorly differentiated. Mucin stains are usually positive (10).

Due to the nature of the presenting complaints, very few patients are able to be approached surgically with curative intent. Only 15% of patients who are initially considered to have localized disease after non-invasive work up are found to be resectable with curative intent. In addition the operative mortality at various institutions for surgical intervention can be considerable for a Whipple procedure or a total pancreatectomy. Given the entire group of patients resected for cure, only 10% survive for 5 years, the prognosis for ampullary tumors being somewhat better due to their earlier presentation from obstructive jaundice (39). Age per se has little effect on outcome with younger patients doing as poorly as the more elderly (41). Radiation and chemotherapy have made only slight impact on survival of patients with metastatic disease, although the use of combined modality therapy in locally advanced disease may hold promise. The benefit of these modalities in the adjuvant setting has yet to be established (42).

UNUSUAL TUMORS OF THE EXOCRINE PANCREAS

Cystadenocarcinomas represent 1–1.5% of pancreatic cancers (32, 35). There are no known epidemiologic or etiologic factors that would separate this tumor from the ductal adenocarcinoma. Pathologically these tumors tend to be large, ranging in size from 2 to 30 cm in diameter, with mean diameters reported of 10.1–10.5 cm in separate series (43, 44). Grossly these tumors tend to be round, they may be lobulated or smooth, and usually are well encapsulated, although occasionally tumor is found to break the surface. One-half to two-thirds of these cysts are multilocular. The cyst walls range from 1 to 20 mm in thickness, and tend to be fibrous. Not uncommonly the cyst wall contains prominent vessels and calcifications are not unusual. The cysts tend to be filled with fluid which may be mucoid or gelatinous. Microscopically the cysts are lined by columnar cells with papillary formation. It would appear that the majority of cases are found to have coexisting areas of benign appearing epithelium. This raises the question whether or not the benign cystadenoma may give rise to its malignant counterpart (45, 46). Most authors agree that the mucinous cystadenomas and cystadenocarcinomas are of ductal cell origin (44, 47), while the serous cystadenomas are felt to be of acinar origin with little malignant potential. The confirmation of the malignant nature of a cystadenomatous lesion is based on (1) local invasion, (2) involvement of regional nodes, (3) cyst wall invasion, and (4) histologic dedifferentiation. Most of these tumors tend to be of low bioloic grade as evidenced by 11/21 tumors graded as Broders' Grade I and 9/21 as Grade II lesions in one series (46).

Clinically these tumors have been reported in patients with a wide age range from 23 to 77 years. The mean age is 50–60, the median age is 48 (44). There would appear to be a slight female predominance, although not to the degree reported in the benign cystadenoma where the ratio is reported to be 4.6:1–9:1 (43,

45). The cystadenocarcinoma is remarkable for its long duration of symptoms prior to diagnosis, averaging 22 months in one report (48). The most common presenting signs and symptoms are abdominal pain, which tends to be more common in the left upper quadrant. Jaundice is remarkable for its absence (45). Although jaundice has been reported to occur from mucinous obstruction of the biliary tree without direct compression by tumor (49). The clinical history is also remarkable for the absence, as a rule, of alcohol abuse, trauma, cholelithiasis, drug abuse or prior pancreatitis (44, 46, 48). Diagnostically a high index of suspicion must be maintained due to the absence of the above conditions, the long duration of symptoms and the vagueness of the complaints. The plain abdominal films are reported to show a mass effect in 50–67% of cases, with calcifications being noted in 10% (45). Routine barium upper gastrointestinal series are positive in 50–95% of cases, the most common abnormalities being either indentation of the lesser curvature of the stomach or C-loop deformities of the duodenum (43). As most of the literature dealing with these tumors antedates widespread use of ultrasonography or CT scanning, the exact value of these procedures cannot be stated based on the available literature. However, based on their utility in the diagnostic evaluation of the common ductal adenocarcinoma, one would presume that they would be the diagnostic procedure of choice currently. It has been reported that the sunburst calcifications typical of these lesions are best appreciated with CT scanning (50). Once a cystic lesion of the pancreas has been demonstrated, the differential diagnosis must include the benign cystadenoma, cystadenocarcinoma and the more common pseudocyst. Due to the frequent coexistence of benign areas in the malignant cystadenocarcinoma, needle biopsies are felt to be inadequate to rule out the possibility of malignancy. The risk of seeding the biopsy tract has also been raised as an objection to this procedure, although the exact incidence of this complication is not known (43). If the diagno-

sis is in doubt, exploration should be undertaken. At the time of surgery approximately 50% of patients will be found to have localized disease without evidence of metastatic disease. Twenty to 25% of patients will be found to have either liver, nodal, or peritoneal spread at the time of exploration. In contrast to the more common ductal adenocarcinoma, curative resection may be attempted even in the presence of local nodal involvement or direct local extension to adjacent organs (43). The surgical procedure of choice is in part dictated by the location of the lesion, which is slightly more common in the body and tail than in the head of the gland. Therefore distal pancreatectomy as well as 'cystectomy' with a rim of normal tissue have been the most common operations performed. Whipple procedures and total pancreatectomies have also been performed. Due to the small number of reported cases the preferred operation cannot be clearly determined. Survival in patients who are able to undergo a total excision is markedly better than in the ductal adenocarcinoma (35). Reported 5-year survival rates range from 38 to 68% with 23% 10-year survivors in one series (43, 48). In addition, patients who have a subtotal resection still have a mean survival of 30 months from diagnosis to death, reinforcing the apparent more 'benign' course of this tumor type (44). Reports of the use of chemotherapy and radiotherapy are too few to draw meaningful conclusions.

Adenosquamous carcinoma, also known as adenocanthoma, has been reported to represent from 3.8% (32) to as much as 11% (51) of all pancreatic tumors. Most series report 3–4%. There appears to be a male to female ratio of approximately 3:1 (35). Due to the extremely small number of cases, it is difficult to define any specific epidemiologic or etiologic association. It has been suggested that there may be an association with chronic pancreatitis (52); this needs further substantiation. It has also been suggested that there may be an association with prior radiation exposure, with a relatively long latency prior to the appearance of the tumor, similar to radiation induced thyroid disease (36). The validity of this theory must also await further reports.

Pathologically these tumors exist as mixtures of squamous and adenocarcinomatous elements (53). Pure squamous cell carcinomas are very rare. Virtually all tumors show areas of transition from adenocarcinoma to areas of squamous metaplasia to areas of frank squamous cell carcinoma. As these tumors are felt to be of ductal origin, this implies that the adenocarcinoma cells are able to undergo metaplastic changes into squamous forms (51, 53, 54). It should be noted that some authors have found small areas of squamous carcinoma in a high proportion of carefully sectioned tumors originally felt to be pure ductal adenocarcinoma. Little is mentioned in regard to the gross appearance and size, 4–10 cm diameters (51, 53, 55), of these tumors that would allow differentiation from the more common ductal adenocarcinoma.

Clinically there are no apparent unique features of these tumors. The diagnostic evaluation and management of these tumors is little different from the ductal adenocarcinoma. One feature of note is the unique angiographic appearance of these tumors. They are reported to have marked hypervascularity with an obvious tumor blush. This is said to distinguish the adenosquamous carcinoma, as well as the cystadenocarcinoma and angiosarcoma from the common ductal carcinoma (56). Unfortunately the prognosis of the adenosquamous carcinoma is also similar, if not worse than the common ductal cancer. The mean survival in one series was reported to be 9 months from the onset of symptoms. In another series 0/18 survived for one year (33). On a more optimistic note a series of patients with gastrointestinal squamous cell tumors of various primary sites, were treated with single agent chemotherapy with bleomycin. There were only two pancreatic tumors in this small series, but one-half responded with a complete regression of disease (57). The duration of response and survival are not mentioned. This may give hope that therapeutic programs such as those directed toward squamous cell carcinoma of the anus (58, 59) and esophagus (60, 61) might be effective in pancreatic squamous cell cancers as well. Due to the uncommon nature of this tumor it will be very difficult to accumulate a series to test this hypothesis.

Acinar cell carcinoma has been reported to represent 1–13.4% of all pancreatic tumors (32, 62), with most series reporting 1–2% (32, 35). There is a male predominance. There are again no proven unique epidemiologic or etiologic features of this tumor compared to the ductal adenocarcinoma. It is of interest to note that acinar cell neoplasms can be induced in rats by the carcinogenic agent, azaserine (63). To date no definite agents have been linked to human acinar cell tumors. Grossly they tend to be large tumors, ranging from 2 to 15 cm in diameter. They are lobulated, soft and fleshy in consistency, usually yellowish in color with obvious zones of necrosis and hemorrhage on gross sectioning. Microscopically these tumors appear as an acinar arrangement of regular round or columnar cells with basally situated nuclei with a deeply eosinophilic cytoplasm and occasional zymogen granules. Mitotic figures are usually sparse (64). These tumors may bear a slight resemblance to an islet cell tumor or small cell carcinoma. By electron microscopy the cytoplasm is shown to contain abundant rough endoplasmic reticulum and numerous mitochondria. Electron dense zymogen granules are also usually apparent (64). It is not uncommon to have tumors of mixed ductal and acinar composition, 4/11 in one series (64).

Clinically these tumors occur in all age groups, and are thought to have a slightly younger mean age than the common ductal adenocarcinoma (35, 64), although tumors have been reported in children on rare occasions. Acinar cell tumors are located more commonly in the tail of the gland than in the head. Common presentations include complaints of pain, weight loss, and/or an abdominal mass. Jaundice is uncommon reflecting this tumor's usual location. A unique syndrome occurring in elderly patients, predominantly males, has been described in association with acinar cell carcinoma (66–68). Clinical features include malaise, eosinophilia, nodular skin lesions, and polyarthritis. Microscopically the skin nodules reveal fat necrosis (66). The skin lesions first appear on the lower extremities, but later appear on the upper extremities on the chest and abdomen and scalp (67). This wide distribution helps to differentiate these lesions from erythema nodosum with which they may be confused clinically (67). The arthritis involves both small and large joints. There is pain with motion, but little swelling, erythema or warmth of the affected joints. Fat necrosis has been seen in or about the articular tissue (67). An eosinophilia ranging from 15 to 21% was reported in 10/14 patients in one series (67). It is postulated that high circulating levels of pancreatic lipase are responsible for the fat necrosis (67). It is not unusual for these patients to present with obvious metastatic disease and an occult primary tumor. Thrombotic non-bacterial endocarditis occurred in 3/11 patients in one series which suggests a possible high incidence in this tumor (64). Diagnostically and therapeutically these tumors do not differ from the ductal adenocarcinoma. There are reports of markedly elevated carcinoembryonic antigen (CEA) levels being found in patients with acinar cell carcinoma (69), but it is not clear that this is a unique feature of this particular histology of pancreatic malignancy (70). Mean survival from diagnosis is reported to range from 4.3 to 6.5 months which is not significantly different from the common ductal tumor (35, 64).

Pleomorphic adenocarcinoma, also known as the giant cell carcinoma or sarcomatoid carcinoma, represents 2.1–12.8% of pancreatic malignancies (38). This tumor is not unique in any known epidemiologic fashion. The exact cell of origin is debated with some favoring a true mesenchymal origin consistent with its sarcomatous appearance, an acinar cell origin based on a report in which electron microscopy was suggestive of this (71), or most widely accepted an origin from ductal cells (72–74). Clinically there is a slight male to female predominance (75). The mean age is 67 (76),

the median age is 65 (75). There is a reported pronounced tendency for these tumors to occur in the body and tail (35, 74, 75, 77) although in one series there was an equal distribution between head, body, and tail.

Their presentation resembles that of other tumors occurring in similar locations in the pancreas. Abdominal pain, weight loss, anorexia, and left upper quadrant mass are all common presenting complaints. Ascites may occur (75). Jaundice is uncommon as one would expect. Most patients are found to have widely metastatic disease at the time of diagnosis. Local–regional disease and distant hematogenous spread are both common. Common sites of spread include liver, lungs, and regional nodes; of interest in one series was a significant incidence of spread to mediastinal and hilar nodes which is unusual for common ductal carcioma (75). These tumors also tend to be locally invasive (74).

Pathologically these tumors tend to be large, mean of 8.9 cm in diameter with a range of 4.5–18 cm (76). Areas of gross hemorrhage and necrosis are common. Microscopically they tend to grow in a loose sarcomatoid pattern with mono- and multinuclear giant cells. The giant cells themselves are large pleomorphic cells, with vacuolated nulei with prominent nucleoli and coarse chromatin and eosinophilic cytoplasm. The giant cells are interspersed in a background of malignant tumor cells with a spindle cell configuration. There are fibrous septae of reticulin fibers around the tumor cells (76).

Cytophagocytosis of red blood cells (RBCs) by the tumor cells is common, as is cannibalism of tumor cells by the malignant giant cells. Care must be taken to differentiate this tumor from melanoma, choriocarcinoma, sarcoma, hepatocellular carcinoma, angiosarcoma, and liposarcoma (75, 76, 78).

There would appear to be nothing unusual about the diagnostic or therapeutic approach to this tumor type. Mean survival from diagnosis is usually 3–4 months (75, 77), although occasional long term survivors have been reported. There is a question whether these long term survivors may represent a subgroup of the giant cell carcinoma in that the giant cells are of a morphologically different variety than in the more common form. The giant cells in this subgroup resemble osteoclasts and therefore this subgroup has been referred to as the epulis–osteoid type of giant cell carcinoma (35, 79). Whether this represents a unique subtype with a better prognosis still awaits confirmation (40).

Microadenocarcinoma represents 1–3% of pancreatic tumors (35). The mean age in one small series was 39.7 years (40). These tumors tend to be large, with a median diameter of 14 cm. The head and tail of the pancreas have both been reported as the more common site (35, 40). Microscopically small glands of more uniform and small size than in the usual ductal cancer are present. These glandular structures are centered in sheets of tumor cells. The nuclei of the cells are uniform and of intermediate size. The cytoplasm is scant and pale staining. Mucin stains are positive. There is more necrosis and less fibrosis than is seen with ductal adenocarcinoma (35). Care must be taken to distinguish this tumor from carcinoid tumor. Clinically these patients present with disseminated disease and the prognosis is grim with a mean survival of 2–11.2 months (35, 40).

Mucinous and colloid adenocarcinoma represents approximately 2% of pancreatic malignancies (35). This is a marked male predominance. The median age is similar to the more common ductal tumor. A history of chronic pancreatitis and ethanol abuse is commonly obtained in these patients, although there is no proof of a causal relationship. These tumors tend to present with a large, soft mass in the head of the pancreas. Grossly they have a mucoid or gelatinous appearance. Microscopically there are large cystic spaces filled with mucin, and lined by tall columnar, non-papillary glandular epithelium. Frequently nests of tumor cells are found floating in lakes of mucin (35). The median survival has been reported to be 9–11 months (35); in one series 3/5 were alive at one year, but none at 5 years. It has been suggested that this tumor may have a slightly better prognosis than the common ductal adenocarcinoma, but this would not appear to be significantly better.

The papillary and cystic carcinoma also known as the *solid and papillary carcinoma*, is rare; the exact incidence is unknown but is probably about 1% of pancreatic tumors. It is most common in young females, mean age of 24 in one series (80), and may be more common in blacks. Patients most commonly present with complaints of an abdominal mass with or without pain, most often in the left upper quadrant. The mass may have been present for a prolonged period, in one case greater than 2 years. The most common location is reported to be in the head of the gland.

Grossly these tumors are large, mean 10 cm in one series (80). They are encapsulated by fibrous tissue (81) and obviously hemorrhagic on cut section. Microscopically solid and cystic areas with hemorrhage are noted. Sheets of cells surround thin walled vessels containing intact RBCs. Other areas show a distinct papillary configuration. Nuclei are round with inconspicuous nucleoli, and the chromatin is finely dispersed (35). Cholesterol granulomas are common. Tumors have been reported to stain positive for alpha$_1$-antitrypsin (81). PAS positive material has also been noted in the cystic space (81). Electron microscopy reveals abundant mitochondria. There are reports of pre-zymogen granules (82) although others report the absence of zymogen granules and dense core neurosecretory granules. Therefore the exact cell of origin is debated; some feel this is an acinar cell tumor (81, 82), while others feel that it arises from the smallest ducts.

This tumor has a clearly better prognosis than the common ductal adenocarcinoma, even when metastatic disease is found. Exact survival figures are not available but most series report most, if not all, patients alive and free of disease after simple resection (80, 83). Radical pancreatectomy is not felt to be necessary by most authors. Deaths due to metastatic disease have been reported, however. There is one report of a patient with locally advanced unresectable disease treated with 4000 rads with some tumor regression; at the time of publication the patient was reported to be doing well with evidence of disease regressing by CT scan (84). It should be noted that the patient still had residual disease after radiation and the long term outcome of this case is not reported. The exact role that radiation may play in this tumor is therefore unclear, but might be considered in a case with palliative intent.

Extrapulmonary small cell carcinoma accounts for 1% of pancreatic cancers based on two large series. There were 5/485 and 7/508 small cell cancers reported in these large series of pancreatic malignancy (35, 85). There would appear to be a male predominance. The age range in one series was 42–73 with a mean of 60 (85). Most patients presented with jaundice and weight loss. Four of the 5 cases were located in the head of the gland. The mean diameter of the tumors was 4.2 cm. Grossly the cancer was firm, gray-white, with areas of necrosis and hemorrhage. Local and regional disease was extensive (85). Metastatic disease was noted in regional and distant nodes, liver, and lungs. Microscopically the tumor consisted of sheets and nests of small, round cells with markedly hyperchromatic nuclei and poorly defined cytoplasm. A scant fibrous stroma was also noted. Mitotic activity is prominent.

Clinically these patients have done very poorly with all patients reported dead within 2 months in one series (85). More recently there is a report of 2 patients treated with combination chemotherapy with one of these achieving a pathologic complete remission documented by laparotomy (86). Certainly in view of the advances in the therapy of pulmonary small cell carcinoma, it is not unreasonable to approach pancreatic small cell cancer in a similar manner. The use of combination chemotherapy should be the basic approach, supplemented by radiation or surgery should the clinical situation indicate (87). Interestingly there are at least 2 reported cases of ectopic hormone production by a pancreatic small cell tumor. One was shown to produce ACTH, the other produced an unidentified substance that was felt to be the cause of the patient's hypercalcemia (88, 89). Several authors warn that the presence of a lung primary must always be considered, as the vast majority of patients with a pancreatic mass that proves to be small cell will have metastatic tumor from a lung primary site (87, 90).

Pancreatoblastoma is a very uncommon pancreatic malignancy representing less than 1% of pancreatic cancers (35). It presents in a very young population, age range 15 months to 13 years in one series (91). Patients present with an abdominal mass and discomfort. Grossly these tumors present as encapsulated masses, most commonly in the head of the pancreas (92). They tend to be of large size, some reported to be greater than 10 cm in diameter (52, 91). Microscopically there are small cells with scant cytoplasm; these cells occur in sheets, but with focal glandular arrangements present. Mucin stains are positive in the glandular lumina. Mixed with the small cells are larger, deeply eosinophilic cells with zymogen granules present in the cytoplasm. Irregular nests of well differentiated epidermoid cells without keratinization are also present. The exact cellular origin of these tumors is arguable (91-5). Clinically patients are reported to do well after surgical removal although the follow-up in most cases has been short.

Oncocytic carcinoma is very rare, representing less than 1% of pancreatic malignancies. Cases have been too few to state with certainty age or sex trends. Presenting signs and symptoms are usually related to an enlarging mass, with or without abdominal pain. Grossly the tumors are usually large, diameters of 7–12.5 cm being reported (40, 96). They may be more common in the tail of the gland. The cut surface is yellow-white with focal hemorrhage (96). The tumor is composed of solid sheets of cells with abundant granular, eosinophilic cytoplasm. The nuclei are large and irregular in size and shape. The chromatin pattern is coarse and nuclei are prominent. Fine bands of fibrous tissue are present. Rare glandular structures may be seen (96). Remarkable features by electron microscopy include abundant mitochondria and a scarcity of other cytoplasmic organelles. Also notable from their absence is the lack of zymogen and neurosecretory granules (96). The clinical course of this tumor is marked by malignant behavior as evidenced by local splenic invasion, perineural invasion and peripancreatic nodal involvement. The prognosis cannot be compared to the more common ductal cancer due to the lack of cases.

Stage I lymphomas of the pancreas must be extremely uncommon. However, pancreatic involvement by intraabdominal lymphoma is probably not terribly rare (97, 99). Most lymphomas involving the pancreas would appear to be large cell or small, cleaved cell tumors. When dealing with a possible pancreatic lymphoma, the problem of differentiation from an anaplastic carcinoma must be kept in mind, and adequate tissue obtained. The use of needle biopsies in these instances may well be unrewarding (100). Therapy should be based on stage and histology as with other lymphomas.

True sarcomas clearly originating in and localized to the pancreas are rare. Certainly pancreatic involvement with retroperitoneal sarcomas occurs. It is difficult in reviewing old case reports to be sure of the exact histologic diagnosis (101, 102). As with lymphomas, it is important to realize that the distinction of sarcoma from lymphoma and anaplastic carcinoma may be very difficult even with adequate tissue, therefore the same tenet in regard to utility of needle biopsy in lymphoma is equally applicable here.

Mixed cell tumors of the pancreas have been reported (103, 104). Combinations of acinar, ductal and islet cell differentiation, including at least one case of trilineage differentiation, occur. This is not totally unexpected as experimental embryologic studies have provided evidence for differentiation of endocrine cells within the endodermal epithelium (105–107). Cases have been too few to make accurate statements about clinical associations or behavior, although reported cases have shown

malignant behavior with infiltrative growth, perineural invasion, nodal and distant metastases (103, 104).

ENDOCRINE TUMORS OF THE PANCREAS

The pancreas has two functions, an exocrine function and an endocrine function. The previously discussed neoplasms of the pancreas have all arisen from one or another of the cellular components of the exocrine pancreas. Tumors of the endocrine pancreas will be described in this section of this chapter. The tumors of the endocrine pancreas fall into two groups: (1) the islet cell tumors, and (2) carcinoid tumors. As a general entity, endocrine neoplasms of the pancreas have been of great interest to pathologists, oncologists, and endocrinologists because of their unique clinical and pathologic features and the protean clinical manifestations that can result from the biologically active materials secreted by these neoplasms.

Islet cell tumors represent the most common endocrine neoplasms of the pancreas. The vast majority of these tumors must remain asymptomatic since there is a marked difference in prevalence of islet cell tumors in autopsy series versus clinical series. Rates as high as 1500/100 000 incidence have been reported in autopsy series whereas the clinical incidence of islet cell neoplasia is approximately 1/100 000 population (108 109). The pathology of islet cell tumors depends not only upon the light microscopic identification of neoplasia of islet cells, but also upon sophisticated staining and/or other techniques to define what particular hormone or hormones the neoplasms produce. The classic Grimelius silver stain (110) was one of the early approaches to defining a tumor as a pancreatic endocrine tumor. Now, however, electron microscopy, which is capable of defining the morphology of granules within the islet cells, and imunohistochemistry, which may stain for particular polypeptides produced by endocrine tumors, are also very helpful techniques. In poorly differentiated tumors histo-

TABLE 2 PANCREATIC ISLET CELL TUMORS

Cell type (immunohistochemical staining)	Product	Syndrome
A	Glucagon	Glucagonoma
B	Insulin	Insulinoma
D	Gastrin, somatostatin	Zollinger–Ellison syndrome, somatostatinoma
D_1	VIP	Pancreatic cholera
PP	Pancreatic polypeptide	No clearly defined syndrome

chemical staining for neuron-specific enolase is now considered to be a simple and specific technique for detecting neuroendocrine tissue. Since islet cells are of neuroendocrine origin, this approach can be useful in defining these neoplasms. Table 2 defines the islet cell neoplasms by the polypeptides produced by these tumors and the clinical syndromes that may be associated with them. Occasionally more than one product may be secreted in patients with islet cell tumors.

Islet cell tumors generally occur sporadically. The etiology of these malignancies is unknown. However, there are familiar syndromes in which neuroendocrine tumors occur. Wermer (111) and Sipple (112) describe two inherited syndromes of multiple neuroendocrine neoplasia of which clinicians must be aware. In Wermer's syndrome or multiple endocrine neoplasia (MEN type 1) patients may have tumors of the pituitary gland, thyroid gland, and pancreas most commonly islet cell tumours. In Sipple's syndrome (MEN type 2) patients present with parathyroid tumors, pheochromocytomas and medullary carcinoma of the thyroid, but uncommonly have pancreatic tumors. The importance of these inherited neuroendocrine tumor syndromes concerns screening for the detection of families at risk for neuroendocrine neoplasms. Patients with islet cell neoplasm should be questioned in regard to any familial history and if that is present family members should be evaluated for the possible presence a MEN syndrome.

Islet Cell Tumor Syndromes

Zollinger–Ellison syndrome (113) results from the secretion of gastrin by an islet cell tumor containing delta granules. The typical patient presents with a symptom complex marked by recurrent gastric ulceration due to hypersection of gastrin and resultant gastric acid production (114). Occasionally patients will also have a syndrome of diarrhea which is secondary to rapid intestinal transit time (115). The Zollinger–Ellison syndrome may also be a manifestation of the MEN-1 syndrome.

Diagnosis of a Zollinger–Ellison syndrome (ZES) depends upon documenting elevations in gastric acid output and fasting serum gastrin levels. A fasting serum gastrin level of greater than 1000 p/ml is considered diagnostic of ZES (116). In patients suspected of this syndrome with less elevated serum gastrin levels, a secretion stimulation test may be performed. If the serum gastrin increases to greater than 200 p/ml over baseline after administration of secretin this is strong evidence for the existence of the ZES. Although the vast majority of patients with ZES will have islet cell tumors of the pancreas, occasionally the syndrome is produced by extrapancreatic tumors typically in the duodenal wall (115). CT scanning and ultrasonography will occasionally demonstrate a mass in the pancreas and also may demonstrate liver metastases. Frequently, however, the primary site of a Zollinger–Ellison tumor will not be demonstrated before surgery (116). Newer techniques including portal venous sampling for gastrin and intraoperative ultrasonography of the pancreas to detect small tumors are being explored (116). The assessment of whether the islet cell tumor is benign of malignant frequently can only be made at the time of surgery. Approximately 25% of patients with ZES have malignant tumors. The malignancy or benignity of an islet cell tumor is not defined by histopathology but rather by the presence or absence of local invasion and/or metastases.

The treatment of ZES entails antitumor therapy and therapy aimed at the inhibition of the physiologic effect of gastrin. In the past before the advent of potent H_2 histamine receptor blockers, total gastrectomy was a frequent therapeutic approach to patients with ZES (118). Obviously with the removal of the end organ affected by hypersecretion of gastric acid, symptoms could be relieved. Now with the use of H_2 blockers including cimetidine and rantidine, inhibition of gastric acid secretion secondary to gastrin can be achieved pharmacologically (116). Frequently the doses required to effectively suppress gastric acid secretion in ZES are considerably higher than the standard dosages of H_2 blockers. Effective antitumor therapy (118) can be carried out by resection of the tumor mass secreting gastrin and by the use of partial cytoreduction with surgery and cytotoxic chemotherapy. Since the chemotherapy for all islet cell tumors is similar, this will be discussed at the end of this section.

Insulinomas. These are the most common islet cell tumors and are neoplasms of beta cells. The syndrome of insulinoma depends upon demonstration of hypoglycemia with inappropriately elevated plasma levels of immunoreactive insulin (119). Fasting hypoglycemia with elevation of serum plasma insulin levels particularly if 'big' insulin (pro insulin) is elevated makes a diagnosis of insulinoma highly likely. Occasionally patients will have hypoglycemia and elevated insulin levels secondary to the surreptitious self-administration of insulin. If this is suspected, the plasma may be assayed for anti-insulin antibodies which develop when porcine or beef insulin is injected (118). Insulinomas are almost always benign and resection of the primary tumor will effectively manage this syndrome.

Glucagonoma. Islet cell tumors containing alpha granules may produce glucagon (118). The physiologic effect of glucagon is to increase serum glucose levels by stimulating gluconeogenesis and glycogenolysis in the liver. In patients with glucagonoma the hypersecretion of glucagon results in carbohydrate intolerance and hyperglycemia. The hyperglycemia is usually mild. In addition to metabolic abnormalities these patients may also present with a characteristic dermatitis termed necrolytic migratory erythemia (120). Other features including weight loss, anemia, diarrhea and hypoaminoacidemia have also been noted (121, 122). It should be emphasized that glucagonomas are very rare tumors. On presentation, this tumor is usually malignant with most patients having metastatic disease to the liver (118, 123). The diagnosis of glucagonoma depends upon demonstrating that a patient with hyperglycemia and the other clinical manifestation of this syndrome has grossly elevated plasma glucagon levels. In many instances glucagon levels are in excess of 2000 pg/ml (118, 123).

Somatostatinoma. Somatostatinoma, another extremely rare islet cell tumor, was originally described in 1977 (124). Less than 30 patients have been described in the world literature with somatostatinoma. Somatostatin producing tumors contain delta granules and are associated with mild diabetes, steatorrhea and cholelithiasis (125). Elevated somatostatin may be measured by radioimmunoassay in the serum of these patients. The overall natural history of this disease is unknown although most patients have malignant disease with metastases to the liver (125). It is thus likely that patients will have a natural history similar to that seen with the Zollinger–Ellison syndrome where most patients have hepatic metastases at the time of diagnosis. There is little information available for the treatment of this syndrome. Certainly surgical resection of the tumor should be attempted if technically feasible and non-surgical approaches such as chemotherapy may have some beneficial effect.

Vipoma. This tumor is responsible for the watery diarrhea, hypokalemia and achlorhydria (WDHA) syndrome (118). Another name for this condition is the pancreatic cholera syndrome. Although profuse diarrhea may be seen with the Zollinger–Ellison syndrome, those patients all have increased gastric acid production and thus do not exhibit achlorhydria. In the past there has been a debate in the literature in regard to the particular hormone responsible for the WDHA syndrome. Now there is general agreement that vasoactive intestinal peptide (VIP) is the major polypeptide producing this syndrome (125). Strong presumptive evidence for causation by VIP has been developed from studies in which normal volunteers have been given VIP infusions and the syndrome has been reproduced (126). The clinical manifestations of this disease are characterized by profuse watery diarrhea and hypokalemia. A characteristic of the WDHA syndrome is that diarrhea persists even when all oral intake is stopped. The hypokalemia is presumably on the basis of potassium loss in diarrheal stools. The great majority of patients with vipoma present with metastatic disease to the liver. Antitumor therapy (surgery and chemotherapy) is similar to that for other islet cell tumors.

Pancreatic polypeptide producing islet cell tumors. Recently patients have been described with islet cell tumors that produce only pancreatic polypeptide (PP) (127). One such patient had an associated WDHA syndrome and in others the only manifestation was malignant islet cell tumor with hepatomegaly and concomitant elevation of serum levels of pancreatic peptide (118). Other hormones measured including insulin, glucagon, somatostatin, VIP, and gastrin were low as was

urinary excretion of 5-hydroxyindole-acetic acid (5-HIAA). This islet cell tumor may have a significant relationship with the MEN-1 syndrome. In screening 12 family members in the MEN-1 families, three were found to have elevated serum levels of pancreatic polypeptide and on evaluation were found to have pancreatic tumors. Removal of these tumors resulted in normalization of the pancreatic polypeptide levels (128).

Treatment of islet cell tumors. In a patient with hormonally active islet cell tumor the aim of surgical intervention is to remove as much tumor mass as possible (118). Vigorous attempts should be made to achieve preoperative localization of the tumor. Such attempts would include localization of the tumor within the pancreas by use of CT scan, ultrasound, arteriography, and selective venous sampling for the localization of polypeptide producing tissue. Once the tumor is localized in the body and tail of the pancreas and if it is greater than 1 cm in size, a distal pancreatectomy may be performed. If the tumor is less than 1 cm in diameter or if it is located in the head of the pancreas enucleation of the tumor mass may be performed.

In patients with metastatic disease to the liver having significant symptoms from polypeptide production one should consider surgical resection of functioning metastases. Other approaches that may be useful are embolization of metastases via the hepatic artery and rarely heptic radiation therapy (129, 130). The reason that partial resection is a viable alternative in islet cell tumors is a result of the natural history of these tumors. Growth of islet cell neoplasms may be very slow and the patient's major morbidity may be related to the hormonal products being produced by the tumor. Thus partial resection may give patients long periods of significant remission from the morbidity of their disease (118).

Medical management of islet cell tumors. In patients with Zolinger–Ellison syndrome high doses H_2 blockers, either cimetidine or ranitidine, can relieve all symptoms of gastrinoma (117). In patients with insulinoma not treatable by resection, diazoxide (131) may effectively prevent hypoglycemic crises.

There is evidence now that a somatostatin analogue may be useful in the treatment of islet cell tumors (132). The hormone somatostatin is able to decrease peptide release from islet cell tumors. However, the normal plasma half-life of somatostatin is very short so that aside from approaches using continuous infusion, therapy of islet cell tumors would be impractical. Recently (132) a long acting somatostatin analogue (SMS-201-995) has been evaluated in patients with islet cell malignancies who are ill with symptoms from the polypeptides being produced by the tumor. Beneficial effects (132) have been seen in patients with vipomas and with ZES following the use of somatostatin analogue. There is also some evidence that somatostatin analogue may result in tumor regression. Further evaluation of this approach is necessary to define its full role in the management of islet cell tumors.

The chemotherapy of islet cell tumors. A characteristic of all islet cell tumors is the relative indolence of their progression. When compared to other malignant tumors of the gastrointestinal tract such as the common adenocarcinoma of stomach, pancreas, and colon, metastatic islet cell carcinoma is a very slowly progressive disease. For this reason, the patients are considered candidates for cytotoxic chemotherapy only when they have failed other procedures such as surgery, radiation, and anti-hormonal therapies (133). Because these patients may then have a poor performance status and be quite ill, they may be relatively poor candidates in whom to expect response to chemotherapy. The major drug that has been shown to be useful in islet cell tumors is the naturally occurring methyl nitrosourea streptozotocin. This drug is known to have a toxic effect on the pancreatic beta cells in animals and was thought therefore to be a drug likely to have benefit for humans with insulinoma (134). Clinical trials with streptozotocin used alone showed an approximate 30–40% response rate in metastatic islet cell carcinomas (135). The combinations of streptozotocin and 5-FU have also been shown to be beneficial with combinations of 5-FU plus straptozotocin producing response in 50–60% of patients (136).

Currently the Eastern Cooperative Oncology Group is comparing 5-FU plus streptozotocin to doxorubicin plus streptozotocin and a third arm of chlorozotocin alone. The results of this study are not available at present. However, it is clear that streptozotocin combinations appear to be the most appropriate chemotherapeutic approaches for islet cell carcinomas. In the future, attempts will be made to refine these so that toxicity will be decreased with the maintenance of excellent chemotherapeutic affect.

Carcinoid Tumors

Carcinoid tumors, as do islet cell tumors, develop from neuroectodermal tissue and may also be associated with other endocrine tumors in the MEN-1 and MEN-2 syndromes (137). Fully 85% of these tumors occur in three organ sites: the rectum and sigmoid, appendix and small bowel. The pancreatic carcinoids are rare and represent less than 5% of the total carcinoid tumors reported. The carcinoids are of interest because they may be associated with a syndrome characterized by diarrhea and flushing and thought to be due to production of a wide variety of biologically active compounds by the tumors. Compounds that have been associated with carcinoid tumors include histamine, bradykinin, serotonin and prostaglandins (138). Carcinoids from the gastrointestinal tract that metastasize almost always metastasize first to the liver. Pancreatic carcinoid tumors metastasizing to the liver will almost always be associated with an elevation of urinary 5-HIAA. Symptoms due to the carcinoid syndrome such as diarrhea, flushing, retroperitoneal or endomyocardial fibrosis are relatively uncommon. In one series of 209 patients with documented carcinoid tumors only 14 or 6.7% had evidence of carcinoid syndrome (139). Even in patients with liver metastases, less than 50% will evidence the carcinoid syndrome. With the rarity of primary pancreatic carcinoid tumors and the infrequent occurrence of carcinoid syndrome, it can be seen that a pancreatic tumor producing the carcinoid syndrome would be a distinctly rare event.

The treatment of carcinoid tumors is similar to the therapy of islet neoplasms since patients may need pharmacologic therapy to antagonize the physiologic effects of biologically active substances produced from these tumors along with cytoreductive therapy (surgery, radiation, chemotherapy). A variety of approaches including adrenergic blocking agents, kinin antagonists, serotonin synthesis inhibitors, histamine receptor antagonists and peripheral serotonin antagonists have been used to treat symptoms of carcinoid syndrome (140). However, most of the time, the diarrhea and/or flushing can be treated with simple symptomatic therapy. In patients with florid carcinoid syndrome or in patients who develop a marked exacerbation of their carcinoid syndrome, long-acting somatostatin analogue have recently been used. Investigators at the Mayo Clinic (140) have reported complete amelioration of carcinoid syndrome in 22 of 25 patients refractory to other therapeutic measures. In 18 of 25 cases there was a greater than 50% reduction in urinary 5-HIAA. There was also some suggestion that somatostatin analogue may produce objective tumor regression in some patients with metastatic carcinoid tumors. Further studies will be required to define the full spectrum of activity of somatostatin analogues in the carcinoid tumor.

The chemotherapy of carcinoid tumors is similar to that of islet cell tumors. Single agents including doxorubicin, 5-FU, and DTIC have activity in 15–25% of patients (138). 5-FU plus streptozotocin has been compared to cyclophosphamide and streptozotocin in this disease by the Eastern Cooperative Oncology Group study (141); 33% of the patients receiv-

ing 5-FU plus streptozotocin and 27% receiving cyclophosphamide combined with streptozotocin responded. These results indicate that the chemotherapy of carcinoid syndrome is not as effective as the chemotherapy of islet cell tumors. Thus new approaches to therapy such as somatostatin analogue perhaps combined with chemotherapy need exploration.

The surgical management of patients with carcinoid tumor is of great importance since this approach may be curative. It is unlikely that a patient wth a primary carcinoid of the pancreas will present to a physician at a time when his tumor is still localized. However, if such is the case, appropriate resection should be curative. In patients with metastatic carcinoid, the basic principles for surgical management are similar to those discussed with islet cell tumors. Carcinoid tumors are like islet cell neoplasms, very indolent malignant processes. Therefore, partial cytoreduction by surgery such as resection of hepatic tumors or the removal of intra-abdominal metastases may give the patient excellent, relatively long term palliation. One should consider the use of non-curative, but cytoreductive surgical procedures as palliative approaches for patients with carcinoid tumors who are significantly symptomatic with either bulk disease or carcinoid syndrome not controllable by medical means. There is good evidence that carcinoid tumor patients who have resection of bulk disease may attain palliation from symptoms and be given months or in many cases years of remission (138). Other approaches such as hepatic artery ligation for metastatic liver disease also should be considered as a palliative. In the Mayo Clinic experience 18 of 25 patients developed significant remission of symptoms from this procedure (138).

REFERENCES

1 Mack TM. Pancreas. In: Schottenfeld D, Graumeni JF ed Cancer Epidemiology and Prevention. WB Saunders, 1982: 638–67.
2 Marble A. Diabetes and Cancer. N Engl J Med 1934; 211: 339–49.
3 Ellinger F, Landsmana H. Frequency and

course of cancer in diabetics. NY St J Med 1944; 44: 259–65.

4 Bell ET. Carcinoma of the pancreas. Am J Pathol 1957; 33: 499–523.

5 Cohen GF. Early diagnosis of pancreatic neoplasms in diabetics. Lancet 1965; ii: 1267–1474.

6 Bauer FW, Robbins SL. An autopsy study of cancer patients. JAMA 1972; 221: 1471–4.

7 Kessler II. Cancer Mortality Among Diabetics. J Nat Cancer Inst 1970; 44: 673–86.

8 Burch GE, Ansari A. Chronic alcoholism and carcinoma of the pancreas. Arch Intern Med 1968; 122: 273–5.

9 Wynder EL. A case control study of cancer of the pancreas. Cancer 1973; 31: 641–8.

10 Lin RS, Kessler II. A multifactorial model for pancreatic cancer in man. JAMA 245: 147–52.

11 Kattwinkel J, Loepy A, DiSant'Agnese PA. Hereditary pancreatitis: three new kindreds and a critical review of the literature. Pediatrics 1973; 51: 55–69.

12 MacMahon B, Yen S, Trichopoulos D. Coffee and cancer of the pancreas. N Engl J Med 1981; 304: 630–3.

13 Tavassoli FA, Lynch RG. Occult adenocarcinoma of the pancreas in a 17-year-old patient with immunosuppressed leukemia. Gastroenterology 1974; 66: 1054–7.

14 Jablon S, Kato H. Studies of the mortality of A-bomb survivors, 5 radiation dose and mortality, 1950–1970. Rad Res 1972; 50: 649–98.

15 Matanoski GM, Seltser R, Sartwell PE. The current mortality rates of radiologists and other physicians specialists: specific causes of death. Am J Epidemiol 1975; 101: 199–210.

16 Hutchinson GB. Late neoplastic changes following medical irradiation. Cancer 1976; 37: 1102–10.

17 Court-Brown WM, Doll R. Mortality from cancer and other causes after radiotherapy for ankylosing spondylitis. Br Med J 1965; ii: 1327–32.

18 Levy BS, Sigurdson E, Mandel J. Investigating possible effects of asbestos in city water: surveillance of gastrointestinal cancer incidence in Duluth, Minnesota. Am J Epidemiol 1976; 103: 362–8.

19 Kanarek MS. Asbestos in drinking water and cancer incidence in the San Francisco Bay area. Am J Epidemiol 1980; 112: 54–72.

20 Selikoff IJ, Seidman H. Cancer of the pancreas among asbestos insulation workers. Cancer 1981; 1469–73.

21 Bjelke E. Epidemiologic studies of cancer of the stomach, colon, and rectum; with special emphasis on the role of diet. Scand J Gastroenterol 1974; 9: 1–53.

22 Kark JD. Serum vitamin A (retinal) and cancer incidence in Evans County, Georgia. J Nat Cancer Inst 1981; 66: 7–16.

23 Wald N. Low serum vitamin A and subsequent risk of cancer. Lancet 1980; ii: 813–15.

24 Kahn HA. The Dorn study of smoking and mortality among U.S. veterans: report on eight and one-half years of observation. Nat Cancer Inst Monogr 1966; 19: 1–125.

25 Hammond EC. Smoking in relation to the death rates of one million men and women. Nat Cancer Inst Monogr 1966; 127–204.

26 Weir JM, Dunn JE. Smoking and Mortality: A Prospective Study. Cancer 1970; 25: 105–12.

27 Best EWR. A Canadian Study of Smoking and Health. Ottawa, Canada. Dept Natl Health and Welfare; 1966.

28 Cederlof R. The Relationship of Smoking and Some Social covariables to Mortality and Cancer Morbidity. Stockholm, The Karolinska Institute 1975.

29 Doll R, Peto R. Mortality in relation to smoking: 20 Years Observations on Male British Doctors. Br Med J 1976; 2: 1525–36.

30 Hirayama T. Prospective studies on cancer epidemiology based on census population in Japan. In: Nieburgs HE ed Prevention and Detection of Cancer, Vol 1, Etiology. Marcel Dekker, 1978: 1139–48.

31 Moossa AR, Lewis MH, Bowie JD. Clinical features and diagnosis of pancreatic cancer. In: Moossa AR ed Tumors of the Pancreas. Williams and Wilkins 1980; 429–42.

32 Morohoshi KT, Held G, Kloppel G. Exocrine pancreatic tumours and their histological classification. A study based on 167 autopsy and 97 surgical cases. Histopathology 1983; 6: 645–61.

33 Cubilla AL, Fitzgerald PJ. Morphological patterns of primary nonendocrine human pancreas carcinoma. Cancer Res 1975; 35: 2234–48.

34 Chen J, Baithun SI, Ramsay MA. Histogenesis of pancreatic carcinomas: a study based on 248 cases. J Pathol 1985; 146: 65–76.

35 Cubilla AL, Fitzgerald PJ. Cancer of the pancreas (nonendocrine): a suggested morphologic classification. Sem Oncol 1979; 6: 285–97.

36 Cubilla AL, Fitzgerald PJ. Classification of pancreatic cancer (nonendocrine). Mayo Clin Proc 1979; 54: 449–58.

37 Cubilla AL, Fitzgerald PJ. Surgical pathology of tumors of the exocrine pancreas. In: Moossa AR ed Tumors of the Pancreas. Williams and Wilkins, 1980: 159–93.

38 Kloppel G. Pancreatic, Nonendocrine Tumours. In: Kloppel G, Heitz PU ed Pancreatic Pathology. Churchill Livingstone, 1984; 79–113.

39 Moossa AR. Pancreatic Cancer: Approach to diagnosis, selection for surgery and choice of operation. Cancer 1982; 50: 2689–98.

40 Chen J, Baithun SI. Morphological study of 391 cases of exocrine pancreatic tumours with special reference to the classification of exocrine pancreatic carcinoma. J Pathol 1985; 146: 65–76.

41 Jochimsen PR, Pearlman NW, Lawton RL. Course and treatment results of young patients with carcinoma of the pancreas. Surg Gynecol Obstet 1977; 144: 32–4.

42 O'Connell MJ. Current status of chemotherapy for advanced pancreatic and gastric cancer. J Clin Oncol 1985; 3: 1032–9.

43 Hodinson DJ, ReMine WH, Weiland LH. A clinicopathologic study of 21 cases of pancreatic cystadenocarcinoma. Ann Surg 1978; 188: 679–84.

44 Compagno J, Oertel JE. Mucinous cystic neoplasms of the pancreas with overt and latent malignancy (cystadenocarcinoma and cystadenoma). Am J Clin Pathol 1978; 69: 573–80.

45 Becker WF, Welsh RA, Pratt HS. Cystadenoma and cystadenocarcinoma of the pancreas. Ann Surg 1965; 161: 845–63.

46 Cullen PK, ReMine WH, Dahlin DC. A clinicopathological study of cystadenocarcinoma of the pancreas. Surg Gynecol Obstet 1963; 117: 189–95.

47 Setia U, Bhatia G. Pancreatic cystadenocarcinoma associated with strongyloides. Am J Med 1984; 77: 173–5.

48 Warren KW, Hardy KJ. Cystadenocarcinoma of the pancreas. Surg Gynecol Obstet 1968; 127: 734–6.

49 Ito Y, Blackstone MO, Frank PH, Skinner DB. Mucinous biliary obstruction associated with a cystic adenocarcinoma of the pancreas. Gastroenterology 1977; 73: 1410–12.

50 Mullens JE, Barr JR, Barron PT. Cystadenoma and cystadenocarcinoma of the pancreas. Can J Surg 1983; 26: 529–31.

51 Ishikawa O, Matsui Y, Aoki I, Iwanaga T, Terasawa T, Wasa A. Adeno-squamous carcinoma of the pancreas. Cancer 1980; 46: 1192–6.

52 Horie A, Yano Y, Kotto Y, Miwa A. Morphogenesis of pancreatoblastoma, infantile carcinoma of the pancreas. Cancer 1977; 39: 247–54.

53 Cihak RW, Kawashima T, Steer A. Adenocanthoma (adenosquamous carcinoma) of the pancreas. Cancer 1971; 29: 1133–40.

54 Cubilla AL, Fitzgerald PJ. Morphological lesions associated with human primary invasive nonendocrine pancreas Cancer Res 1976; 36: 2690–8.

55 Wilozynski SP, Valente PT, Atkinson BF. Cytodiagnosis of Adenosquamous Carcinoma of the Pancreas. Acta Cytol 1984; 28; 733–6.

56 Sprayregen S, Schoenbaum SW, Messinger NH. Angiographic features of squamous cell carcinoma of the pancreas. J Can Assoc Rad 1975; 26: 122–4.

57 Ravry M, Moertel CG, Schutt AJ, Hahn RG, Reitemeier RJ. Treatment of advanced squamous cell carcinoma of the gastrointestinal tract with bleomycin. Cancer Chemo Rep 1973; 57: 493–5.

58 Leichman L, Nigro N, Vaitkevicius VK, Considine B. Cancer of the Anal Canal. Am J Med 1985; 78: 211–15.

59 Nigyro ND, Seydel HG, Considine B, Vaitkevcius VK, Leichman LII, Kinzie J. Combined pre-operative radiation and chemotherapy for squamous cell carcinoma of the anal canal. Cancer 1983; 51: 1826–9.

60 Franklin R, Steiger Z, Vaishampayan G, Asfaw I, Rosenberger J, Loh J, Hoschner J, Miller P. Combined modality therapy for esophageal squamous cell carcinoma. Cancer 1983; 51: 1062–71.

61 Leichman L, Steiger Z, Seydel HG, Dindugru A, Kinzie J, Toben S, MacKenzie G, Shell J. Pre-operative chemotherapy and radiation therapy for patients with cancer of the esophagus: a potentially curative approach. J Clin Oncol 1984; 2: 75–9.

62 Miller JR, Baggenstoss AH, Comfort MW. Carcinoma of the pancreas. Cancer 1951; 4: 233–41.

63 Longnecker DS, Curphey TJ. Adenocarcinoma of the pancreas in azaserine treated rats. Cancer Res 1975; 35: 2249–58.

64 Webb JN. Acinar cell neoplasms of the exocrine pancreas. J Clin Pathol 1977; 30: 103–12.

65 Mah PT, Loo DC, Tock EPC. Pancreatic acinar cell carcinoma in childhood. Am J Dis Child 1974; 128: 101–4.

66 MacMahon HE, Brown PA, Shen EM. Acinar cell carcinoma of the pancreas with subcutaneous fat necrosis. Gastroenterology 1965; 49: 555–9.

67 Mullin GT, Caperton EM, Crespin SR, Williams RC. Arthritis and skin lesions resembling erythema nodosum in pancreatic disease. Ann Intern Med 1968; 68: 75–87.

68 Burns WA, Mathews MJ, Hamosh M, Vander Weide G, Blum R, Johnson FB. Lipase-secreting acinar cell carcinoma of the pancreas with polyarthropathy. Cancer 1974; 33: 1002–9.

69 Horie Y, Gomyoda M, Koshimoto Y, Ueki J,

Ikeda F, Murawaki Y, Kawamura M, Hirayama C. Plasma carcinoembryonic antigen and acinar cell carcinoma of the pancreas. Cancer 1984; 53: 1137–42.

70 Tracey KJ, O'Brien MJ, Williams LF, Klibaner M, George PK, Saravis CA, Zamcheck N. Signet ring carcinoma of the pancreas, a rare variant with very high CEA values. Dig Dis Sci 1984; 29: 573–6.

71 Rosai J. Carcinoma of the pancreas simulating giant cell tumor of bone. Cancer 1968; 22: 333–44.

72 Pour RM. Induction of unusual pancreatic neoplasms with morphologic similarity to human tumors, and evidence of their ductal/ductular origin. Cancer 1985; 55: 2411–16.

73 Robinson L, Damjenow I, Brezina P. Multinucleated giant cell neoplasm of pancreas. Arch Pathol Lab Med 1977; 101: 590–3.

74 Alguacil-Garcia A, Weiland LH. The histologic spectrum, prognosis, and histiogenesis of the sarcomatoid carcinoma of the pancreas. Cancer 1977; 39: 1181–9.

75 Tschang TP, Garza-Garza R, Kissane JM. Pleomorphic carcinoma of the Pancreas. Cancer 1977; 39: 2114–26.

76 Guillan RA, McMahon J. Pleomorphic adenocarcinoma of the pancreas. Am J Gastroenterol 1973; 60: 379–86.

77 Guillan RA. Pleomorphic adenocarcinoma of the pancreas. Cancer 1968; 21: 1072–9.

78 Freund U. Pleomorphic giant cell tumor of the pancreas. Isr J Med Sci 1973; 9: 84–8.

79 Kay S, Harrison JM. Unusual pleomorphic carcinoma of the pancreas featuring production of osteoid. Cancer 1969; 23: 1158–62.

80 Compagno J, Oertel JE, Kremzar M. Solid and papillary epithelial neoplasms of the pancreas, probably of small duct origin: a clinipathologic study of 52 cases. Lab Invest 1979; 40: 248–9.

81 Kloppel G, Morohoshi T, John HD, Oehmichen W, Opitz K, Angelkort A, Lietz H, Ruckert K. Solid and cystic acinar cell tumour of the pancreas. Virchows Arch (Pathol Anat) 1981; 392: 171–83.

82 Bombi JA, Mills A, Badal JM, Piulachs J, Estape J, Cardesa A. Papillary-cystic neoplasm of the pancreas. Cancer 1984; 54: 780–4.

83 Kuo TT, Su IJ, Chien CH. Solid and papillary neoplasm of the pancreas. Cancer 1984; 54: 1469–74.

84 Fried P, Cooper J, Balthazar E, Fazzini E, Newall J. A role for radiotherapy in the treatment of solid and papillary neoplasms of the pancreas. Cancer 1985; 56: 2783–5.

85 Reyes CV, Wang T. Undifferentiated small cell carcinomas of the pancreas. Cancer 1981; 47: 2500–2.

86 Fer MF, Levenson RM, Cohen MH. Extrapulmonary small cell carcinoma. In: Greco FA, Oldham RK, Bunn PA ed Small Cell Lung Cancer. Grune and Stratton, 1981: 301–25.

87 Richardson RL, Weiland LH. Undifferentiated small cell carcinomas in extrapulmonary sites. Sem Oncol 1982; 9: 484–96.

88 Hobbs RD, Stewart AF, Ravin ND, Carter D. Hypercalcemia in small cell carcinoma of the pancreas. Cancer 1984; 53: 1552–4.

89 Corrin B, Gilby ED, Jones NF, Patrick J. Oat cell carcinoma of the pancreas with ectopic ACTH secretion. Cancer 1973; 31: 1523–7.

90 Ibrahim NBN, Briggs JC, Corbidhley C.M. Extrapulmonary oat cell carcinoma. Cancer 1984; 54: 1645–61.

91 Buchino JJ, Castello FM, Nagaraj HS. Pancreatoblastoma. Cancer 1984; 53: 963–9.

92 Taxy JB. Adenocarcinoma of the pancreas in childhood. Cancer 1976; 37: 1508–18.

93 Hamoudi AB, Misugi K, Grosfeld JL, Reiner CB. Papillary epithelial neoplasm of pancreas in a child. Cancer 1970; 26: 1126–34.

94 Frable WJ, Still WJS, Kay S. Carcinoma of the pancreas. Infantile type. Cancer 1971; 27: 667–73.

95 Grosfeld JL, Clatworthy HW, Hamoudi AB. Pancreatic malignancy in children. Arch Surg 1970; 101: 370–5.

96 Huntrakoon M. Oncocytic carcinoma of the pancreas. Cancer 1983; 51: 332–6.

97 Gray GM, Rosenberg SA, Cooper AD, Gregory PB, Stein DT, Herzenberg H. Lymphomas involving the gastrointestinal tract. Gastroenterology 1982; 82: 152–3.

98 Wasldron JA, Magnifico M, Duray PH, Cadman EC. Retroperitoneal mass presentations of B-immunoblastic sarcoma. Cancer 1985; 56: 1733–41.

99 Rosenfelt F, Rosenberg SA. Diffuse histiocytic lymphoma presenting with gastrointestinal tract lesions. Cancer 1980; 45: 2188–93.

100 Ackerman NB, Aust JC, Bredenberg CE, Hanson VA, Rogers LS. Problems in differentiating between pancreatic lymphoma and anaplastic carcinoma and their management. Ann Surg 1976; 184: 705–8.

101 Neibling HA. Primary Sarcoma of the Pancreas. Am Surg 1968; 34: 690–3.

102 Brooke WS, Maxwell JG. Primary sarcoma of the pancreas. Am J Surg 1966; 112: 657–61.

103 Schron DS, Mendelsohn G. Pancreatic carcinoma with duct, endocrine, an acinar differentiation. Cancer 1984; 54: 1766–70.

104 Reid JD, Yuh SL, Petrelli M, Jaffe R. Ductu-

loinsular tumors of the pancreas. Cancer 1982; 49: 908–15.

105 Andrew A. An experimental investigation into the possible neural crest origin of pancreatic APUD (islet cells). J Embryol Exp Morphol 1976; 35: 577–93.

106 Fontaine J, DeDovarin NM. Analysis of endoderm formation in avian blastoderm by the use of quail chick chimeras: problem of the neuroecto-origin of the cells of APUD series. J Embryol Exp Morphol 1977; 41: 209–22.

107 Nicolesco S, Popescu-Miclosani S, Coste C, Valica M. Morphological significance of association of epithelial cords and duct-like structures in certain tumors of the pancreatic islets. Endocrinology 1978; 16: 227–30.

108 Schein PS, De Lellis RA, Kahn CR. Islet cell tumors. Current concepts and management. Ann Intern Med 1973; 79: 239–57.

109 Moldow RE, Connelly RR. Epidemiology of pancreatic cancer in Connecticut. Gastroenterology 1978; 55: 667–86.

110 Grimelius L. A silver nitrate stain for alpha2 cells in human pancreatic islets. Acta Soc Med Upsallen 1968; 73: 243.

111 Wermer P. Genetic aspects of adenomatosis of endocrine glands. Am J Med 1954; 16: 363–71.

112 Sipple JH. The association of pheochromocytoma with carcinoma of the thyroid gland. Am J Med 1961; 31: 163–8.

113 Zollinger RM, Ellison EH. Primary peptic ulcerations of the jejunum associated with islet cell tumors of the pancreas. Ann Surg 1955; 142: 709.

114 Jensen RT. Zollinger-Ellison Syndrome: Current concepts and management. Ann Intern Med 1983; 98: 5–78.

115 Regan PT, Malagelada JR. A reappraisal of clinical, roentgenographic and endoscopic features of the Zolinger-Ellison syndrome. Mayo Clin Proc 1978; 53: 19–23.

116 McCarthy DM, Jensen RT. Zollinger-Ellison syndrome—current issues. In: Cohen S, Soloway RD eds Hormone-Producing Tumors of the Gastrointestinal Tract. New York: Churchill Livingstone, 1985: 25–55.

117 McGuigan JE, Wolfe MM. Secretin injection test in the diagnosis of gastrinoma. Gastroenterology 1980; 789: 1324.

118 Brennan MF, Macdonald JS. Cancer of the endocrine system. In: DeVita VT, Hellman S, Rosenberg SH eds Cancer Principles and Practice of Oncology Philadelphia: JB Lippincott, 1985; 1179–241.

119 Stefanini P, Carboni M, Petrassi N. Beta islet cell tumors of the pancreas. Results of a study on 1067 cases. Surgery 1974; 75: 597–609.

129 Becker WS, Kahn D, Rothman S. Cutaneous manifestations of internal malignant tumors. Arch Derm Syph 1972; 45: 1069.

121 Malinson CN, Bloom SR, Warin AP. A glucagonoma syndrome. Lancet 1974; ii: 1–5.

122 Holst JJ. Glucagon-producing tumors. In: Cohen S, Soloway RD eds Hormone-producing Tumors of the Gastrointestinal Tract. Churchill Livingstone, 1985; 57–84.

123 Leichter SB. Clinical and metabolic aspects of glucagnoma. Medicine 1980; 59: 100.

124 Ganda OP, Weir GC, Soeldner JS. Somatostatinoma: a somatostatin-containing tumor of the endocrine pancreas. N Engl J Med 1977; 296: 963–98.

125 Boden G, Shimoyama R. Somatostatinoma. In: Cohen S, Soloway RD eds Hormone-producing Tumors of the Gastrointestinal Tract. New York: Churchill Livingstone, 1985: 85–99.

126 Kane MG, O'Dorisio TM, Krejs GL. Intravenous VIP infusion causes secretory diarrhea in man. N Engl J Med 1983; 309: 1501–6.

127 Glasser B, Vinik AI. Clinical findings in patients with malignant tumors secreting pancreatic polypeptide (PP). Clin Res 1979; 27: 627a.

128 Friesen SR, Kimmel JR, Tomita T. Pancreatic polypeptide as a screening marker for pancreatic polypeptide apudomas in multiple endocrinopathies. Am J Surg 1980; 139: 61–72.

129 Clouse ME, Lee RGL, Duszlak EJ. Hepatic artery embolization for metastatic endocrine-secreting tumors of the pancreas. Gastroenterology 1983; 85: 1183–6.

130 Tochner ZA, Kinsella TJ, Glatstein E. Hepatic irradiation in the management of metastatic hormone-secreting tumors. Cancer 1985; 56: 20–24.

131 Bleecker JJ, Chowdhury F, Goldner MG. Thiazide therapy in hypoglycemia of metastatic insulinoma. Clin Res 1964; 12: 456.

132 Kvols L, Schutt A, Buck M. Treatment of metastatic islet cell carcinomas with a long acting somatostatin analogue. Proc Smer Soc Clin Oncol 1986; 5: 85.

133 Haller DG. Chemotherapeutic management of endocrine-producing tumors of the gastrointestinal tract. In: Cohen S, Soloway RD eds Hormone-producing Tumors of the Gastrointestinal Tract. New York: Churchill Livingstone, 1985: 129–37.

134 Murray-Lyon IM, Eddleston ALWF, Williams R. Treatment of multiple hormone producing malignant islet cell tumors with streptozotocin. Lancet 1968; ii: 895.

135 Broder LE, Carter SK. Results of therapy with

Streptozotocin in 52 Patients. Ann Intern Med 1973; 79: 108–18.

136 Moertel CG, Hanley JA, Johnson LA. Streptozotocin alone compared with streptozotocin plus fluorouracil in the treatment of advanced islet cell carcinoma. N Engl J Med 1980; 303: 1189.

137 O'Dorisio TM, Vinik AL. Pancreatic polypeptide and mixed polypeptide-producing tumors of the gastrointestinal tract. In: Cohen S, Soloway RD eds Hormone-Producing Tumors of the Gastrointestinal Tract. New York: Churchill Livingstone, 1985: 117–28.

138 Moertel CG. Treatment of the carcinoid and the malignant carcinoid syndrome. J Clin Oncol 1983; 1: 727–40.

139 Moertel CG. Small intestine. In: Holland JF, Free E eds Cancer Medicine, Philadelphia: Lea and Febiger, 1973: 1574–84.

140 Kvols LK, Moertel CG, O'Connell MJ et al. Treatment of the malignant carcinoid syndrome: evaluation of a long-acting somatostatin analogue. New Engl J Med 1986; 315: 663–704.

141 Moertel CG, Hanley JA. Combination chemotherapy trials in metastatic carcinoid tumor and the malignant carcinoid syndrome. Clin Cancer Trials 1979; 2: 327–34.

Textbook of Uncommon Cancer
Edited by C.J. Williams, J.G. Krikorian, M.R. Green and D. Raghavan
© 1988 John Wiley & Sons Ltd

Chapter **27**

Uncommon Tumours of the Hepatobiliary System

G.H. Millward-Sadler* and Ralph Wright†

Consultant Pathologist and Senior Lecturer, University of Southampton Medical School, Southampton and † Professor of Medicine and Honorary Consultant Physician, University of Southampton Medical School, Southampton, UK

INTRODUCTION

Tumours of the hepatobiliary system may show striking differences in pathology and clinical presentation, depending on age, race and geography. Hepatocellular carcinoma (HCC) is one of the commonest neoplasm world-wide but is rare in Western society. There are, however, unusual variants both in their clinical manifestation and pathology: only these will be described in the present chapter.

Neoplasms of childhood differ greatly from those in adults. Primary tumours dominate the picture in children, whereas in adults the majority of tumours are metastatic. Primary, malignant liver tumours are also rare, except for hepatocellular carcinomas.

The ease of production of liver tumours in experimental animals facilitates investigation of aetiological and surgical problems. Improved diagnostic aids and operative techniques encourage surgical approach to resection of the tumours and liver transplantation for primary neoplasms of the liver is becoming feasible.

The classification of primary liver malignant tumours is set out in Table 1 with those

especially likely to develop in childhood being indicated. Childhood liver tumours have recently been comprehensively reviewed (1). An American study showed that carcinomas comprised 90% of primary hepatic neoplasms seen in a 36-year period in adults (2).

The clinical presentation of tumours of the liver and those of the biliary tract will differ. Malignant hepatic tumours usually present with right upper quadrant pain, malaise, weight loss and fever, but may have characteristic syndromes due, for example, to the secretion of tumour products, such as in the carcinoid syndrome. The rapidity of onset and clinical course may also vary depending on the type of tumour. Tumours of the biliary tree usually present with obstructive jaundice, but the presentation and clinical course may also differ depending on the site of obstruction.

CLINICAL FEATURES OF PRIMARY LIVER CELL CANCER

The clinical features of these unusual liver cell cancers do not differ significantly from that seen more commonly with primary HCC except where indicated below.

TABLE 1 CLASSIFICATION OF PRIMARY
MALIGNANT LIVER TUMOUR

Epithelial:

Liver:	Hepatocellular carcinoma
	Hepatoblastoma[a]
Gallbladder and	Carcinoma,
cystic duct:	miscellaneous
Biliary tree:	Cholangiocarcinoma of:
	cystic duct
	intrahepatic
	Bifurcation
	common bile duct
	periampullary
Miscellaneous:	Carcinoid tumour
	Squamous carcinoma

Mesodermal:

Liver:	Angiosarcoma
	Epithelioid haemangioendothelioma
	Malignant mesenchymoma[a]
	Undifferentiated (embryonal) sarcoma[a]
Biliary tree:	Embryonal rhabdomyosarcoma[a]
Miscellaneous:	Leiomyosarcoma
	MFH
	Fibrosarcoma in AIDS

Mixed:

	Combined carcinoma
	Malignant mixed hepatic tumour[a]
	Carcinosarcoma

[a] Childhood tumours.

They usually present with right upper quadrant pain, rapidly enlarging hepatomegaly, malaise and weight loss. Occasionally there is the development of portal hypertension with variceal bleeding or the Budd–Chiari syndrome as a result of the extension of the tumour into the hepatic veins, or thrombosis of these veins. Ascites and oedema may also be present.

The diagnosis is based on the clinical features and the demonstration of intrahepatic tumour by abdominal ultrasound or computed tomography (CT scan), or angiography. The most essential feature in diagnosis is liver biopsy which may have to be done under ultrasound guidance. A rapid diagnosis can be made by cytological examination of a dab preparation of the fresh tissue, or examination after cytospin of the fluid into which the biopsy has been taken.

HEPATOCELLULAR CARCINOMA (HCC) UNUSUAL VARIANTS

Extrahepatic Manifestations of HCC

These may be grouped as endocrine manifestations, metabolic changes and haematological syndromes and have been reviewed by Margolis and Homey (3), and Cochrane and Williams (4).

Endocrine manifestations include erythrocytosis, hypercalcaemia, sexual changes and hyperthyroidism. The erythrocytosis may be due to production of erythropoietin or its substrate by tumour cells, or to decreased inactivation of erythropoietin by the diseased liver. Hypercalcaemia may be due to multiple skeletal metastases or to production of parathyroid hormone like substances by the tumour. Sexual precocity and gynaecomastia are due to production by the tumour of gonadorophin and somatotrophin like hormones, and hyperthyroidism has been described (5).

Metabolic changes include hypoglycaemia, due either to increased glucose utilization by the tumour or to decreased glucose production by the diseased liver. Hyperlipidaemia, possibly due to uncontrolled cholesterogenesis by tumour cells has been described as well as macroglobulinaemia and porphyria.

Haematological syndromes include dysfibrinogenaemia (6), possibly due to release of an antifibrinolytic substance, and dysproptinaemias such as raised levels of cryofibrinogen, haptoglobin or caeruloplasmin (4).

Pedunculated Carcinoma (Figure 1)

Occasionally HCC protudes from the capsular surface as a pedunculated growth with little invasion into the liver (7). These pedunculated varieties are thought to arise from accessory lobes of liver and even from ectopic liver tissue (8). To confirm an origin from such a source it is necessary to demonstrate non-neoplastic liver at the site. Because of its pedunculated nature and minimal invasion of the liver, these

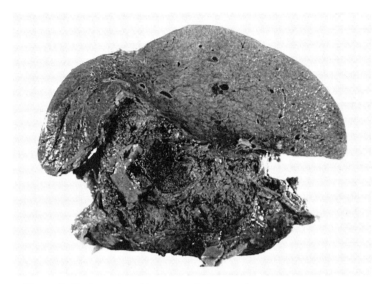

Figure 1 Pedunculated hepatocellular carcinoma: coronal slice of liver with a large massive tumour arising from the inferior surface of the liver. There is minimal invasion of the liver but resection was impossible because of involvement of porta hepatis.

tumours are especially amenable to surgical resection and have a relatively good prognosis. There are no histological differences from other examples of HCC.

Fibrolamellar Carcinoma

This distinctive variant of HCC is found in young non-cirrhotic patients, usually female, and grows slowly as a single mass which can often be resected. It is characterized by large, polygonal cells with abundant deeply eosinophilic cytoplasm and large vesicular nuclei, each with a prominent eosinophilic nucleolus (9, 10). The cells are arranged in trabeculae separated by delicate lamellae of parallel bundles of collagen which blend and merge to form broad swathes of fibrous tissue (Figure 2). A characteristic set of tumour markers, namely carcinoembryonic antigen, alpha$_1$-antitrypsin and fibrinogen, is demonstrable within tumour cells and helps to define the tumour (11).

Sclerosing Carcinoma

These tumours arise as solitary masses in non-

cirrhotic liver, are grey-white in appearance and firm in texture. Macroscopically it is virtually impossible to differentiate these tumours from cholangiocarcinomas. Sclerosing HCC is associated with hypercalcaemia (12).

HEPATOBLASTOMA

These tumours (sometimes called embryonal hepatic tumours) occur in the first 2 years of life, but have been recorded in adult life (1, 13–16). They also arise prenatally (17). The tumour is thought to arise from primitive hepatic blastoma capable of differentiating into malignant epithelial and mesenchymal elements (14).

Clinical Features

There is a slight male preponderance and familial cases sometimes occur. Presentation is with abdominal swelling and hepatomegaly, but anorexia, diarrhoea and vomiting may occur. Rupture of the tumour can present as an acute abdominal emergency with a haemoperitoneum. There is no association with cirrhosis

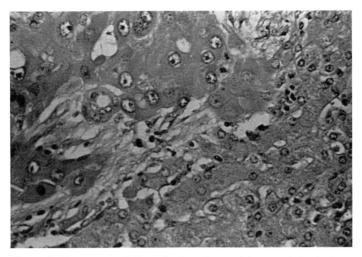

Figure 2 Tumour top left at the interface with non-cirrhotic liver
bottom right. Tumour cells have abundant cytoplasm, large vesicular nuclei and prominent nucleoli. The fibrous tissue at the interface
is of tumour origin with collagen bundles in parallel arrays. H&E,
original magnification: ×400.

(18). Rarely, a thrombocytosis may be present in the peripheral blood (19). A variety of conditions and congenital abnormalities has been described in patients with hepatoblastoma (18–20). These include hemi-hypertrophy, renal abnormalities, osteoporosis and precocious virilization in males. Raised serum levels of alpha-fetoprotein (AFP) are consistently present and a cell line from a hepatoblastoma has been established that secretes AFP in quantity (21).

Pathology

The tumour mass is usually single, but occasionally multiple nodules are seen. The tumour is usually situated in the right lobe and may vary in size from 6 to 17 cm in diameter, with a soft consistency in two-thirds of cases (13). Two types of hepatoblastoma have been identified by Ishak and Glunz (18), the epithelial and the mixed types, but a rare anaplastic mucoid variant also occurs (22, 23). The mixed type of hepatoblastoma occurs more often in females.

Epithelial Type

This has a rather uniform cut surface. Histolo-

gically there are different proportions of fetal and embryonal cells (Figure 3). Fetal hepatocytes resemble small hepatocytes, may contain fat and glycogen, can secrete bile, and are arranged in cords separated by sinusoids. Areas showing a macro-trabecular pattern have been described (24). Embryonal cells are primitive, small, dark, blast-like cells, with a tendency to form rosettes and imperfect acinar structures. They often form and surround small vascular lakes. Mitotic activity is more frequent. Foci of even smaller, darker, more undifferentiated cells resembling neuroblastoma can sometimes be found within these embryonal areas. Rarely in occasional tumours, foci of squamous differentiation and even melanin pigmentation occur.

Foci of haematopoiesis are consistently found in the sinusoids between the fetal liver cells, but are rare in the embryonal areas and are not seen in the non-neoplastic liver.

Mixed Type

Macroscopically this is a lobulated tumour of variegated colouring (tan, haemorrhagic or greenish-grey) which may contain foci of calci-

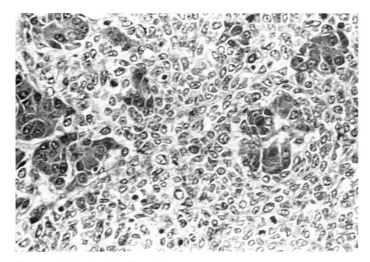

Figure 3 Small islands of large tumour cells resembling fetal hepatocytes are embedded in a background of smaller tumour cells with scanty cytoplasm resembling embryonal hepatocytes. H&E, original magnification: ×250.

fication. Histologically the epithelial elements are the same but mixed with elements of a primitive mesenchymal stroma containing foci of osteoid, cartilage or striated muscle.

Between one-quarter and one half of all hepatoblastomas are in the mixed category; the proportion rises with the degree of care used to examine the tumour (1).

Anaplastic Type

The anaplastic hepatoblastoma is a variant in which the small undifferentiated cells, sometimes found as small foci in the embryonal areas of a more typical tumour, predominate. Small foci of typical epithelial tumour cells can usually be found (23). Abundant stromal mucin production has been recorded in this subtype (22).

Teratoid Hepatoblastoma

A variant showing teratoid features has recently been described (25).

Differential Diagnosis

This is limited. The mixed type is similar to,

and sometimes confused with, the malignant hepatic mixed tumour which contains a well differentiated hepatocellular carcinomatous element amongst its components. The anaplastic variant has to be distinguished both from neuroblastoma, and undifferentiated (embryonal) sarcomas.

Prognosis

This is directly related to the feasibility of complete surgical resection: recurrence following resection usually occurs within 3 years but may not happen until after 5 years. Successful resections have been recorded (13, 26). If untreated they are uniformly fatal, metastasizing to abdominal lymph nodes, lungs and brain. Adverse histological prognostic features (1, 23, 24) relate to the degree of anaplasia in the tumour, but an increased embryonal cell component is associated with a higher risk of recurrence following resection. A dominant fetal cell pattern is associated with the best chance of recurrence-free survival but tumours with a macro-trabecular component in these 'fetal' zones do badly.

Treatment

Treatment must be aimed at achieving surgical resection where feasible: anecdotal evidence suggests this may be faciliated by aggressive chemotherapy even in otherwise seemingly inoperable cases (27). Even if chemotherapy fails to achieve this, survival can be increased (29).

CARCINOMA OF THE GALLBLADDER

This disease of elderly ladies almost invariably occurs in association with gallstones (28). Despite this only a small proportion of patients with gallstones develop carcinoma so that other aetiological factors must be involved though these have not been defined. Although often thought of as a rare condition a number of studies have stressed the frequency of the tumour (29–31). The tumour has been found in 0.2% of all gallbladder operations in Sweden (32). In the United States it is more common in Caucasians than Negroes and is particularly high in American Indians in the south west of America (33). The female to male ratio is 3:1 and the peak age instance is 70–75 years of age, though it has been described in young patients (31). The disease is usually well advanced by the time of diagnosis—especially in the patient presenting with obstructive jaundice (34). Occasionally the gallbladder carcinoma can be diagnosed preoperatively by ultrasound examination, CT scanning or endoscopic retrograde cholangiopancreatography (ERCP) when tissue may be obtained for a cytological diagnosis (35). Occasionally early and even in situ examples may be found incidentally in gallbladders removed because of gallstones. When such in situ carcinoma involves Aschoff–Rokitansky sinuses, invasive carcinoma will be mimicked. The early carcinomas are found in the fundus and may be seen as a mucosal plaque or as a papillary excrescence. The papillary tumours, though rare (36), can be multifocal and may extend to involve or obstruct the cystic duct (37). The

gallbladder, if not completely replaced by tumour, almost always shows evidence of preceding chronic cholecystitis associated with the presence of gallstones and there may be the dystrophic calcification of a 'porcelain gallbladder'. It is estimated that a radiologically demonstrable porcelain gallbladder has a 20% chance of harbouring a carcinoma (38, 39). Most commonly the carcinoma has extensively replaced the gallbladder wall and direct invasion of the liver from the gallbladder bed has occurred. A firm grey/white mass of tumour is then produced centred on the site of the gallbladder. Lymphatic permeation by tumour also occurs and can result in blockage of the cystic duct as well as metastases to lymph nodes in the free edge of the lesser omentum.

While the diagnosis at laparatomy may be obvious, it is not possible to distinguish microscopically between adenocarcinomas arising from the gallbladder and the rest of the biliary tree. The majority are well differentiated desmoplastic adenocarcinomas, a few are mucinous adenocarcinomas and a small proportion are less well differentiated or anaplastic. Squamous carcinoma of the gallbladder occurs in approximately 5% of cases, with squamous differentiation identifiable in another 5% of the adenocarcinomas. These latter tumours are best referred to as adenosquamous carcinoma.

Treatment

Since most tumours have already infiltrated the liver or porta hepatis at the time of operation, it is usually only feasible to confirm the diagosis by taking a biopsy; sometimes a palliative bypass is possible.

When the carcinoma is found incidentally at operation or on subsequent microscopic examination of the gallbladder (40) the prognosis is much better. In this series, 11 of the 32 patients had cancer confined to the mucosa and sub-mucosa with a 5-year survival of 63.6%. When full thickness involvement of the gallbladder wall was present the patients were all dead within $2\frac{1}{2}$ years.

Early diagnosis is facilitated by frozen section examination of suspicious areas at the time of cholecystectomy for gallstones. The value of radical excision of the gallbladder bed and part of the liver is controversial; the whole subject has been reviewed by Blumgart and Imrie (35). There have been some reports of a modest prolongation of survival after adjunctive therapy (41), but it is doubtful whether chemotherapy or radiotherapy, or a combination of both produces any marked improvement.

OTHER MALIGNANT TUMOURS OF THE GALLBLADDER

Melanoma can occur in the gallbladder and may be either primary (42, 43) or secondary. Melanoma is the most common metastatic tumour to the gallbladder.

Oat cell carcinoma may arise from the gallbladder and has a very bad prognosis. In one series all patients were dead within one year of diagnosis (44).

Carcinosarcomas and a variety of monomorphic sarcomas are even rarer primary tumours of the gallbladder but have been described (45, 46).

CARCINOMA OF THE CYSTIC DUCT

This is a very rare lesion which is often indistinguishable from cancer arising in the bile ducts or the adjacent gallbladder. Nishimura et al (47) have reviewed 25 cases and recommend radical excision with a hepaticojejunostomy.

CHOLANGIOCARCINOMA

Carcinomas of the biliary tree can be subdivided into those arising within the liver—the intrahepatic cholangiocarcinomas and cholangiolocellular carcinomas, and those arising from the extrahepatic biliary tree. Intrahepatic cholangiocarcinomas (Figure 4) are less often seen than hepatocellular carcinomas. An American study reported that 75% of primary liver carcinomas were hepatocellular (48) while in a Natal series only 7% of 442 hepatic neoplasms were cholangiocarcinomas (49). Cholangiocarcinomas are distributed fairly uniformly in the world, unlike HCC (50), occur most frequently in the sixth decade, and have no male predominance (51).

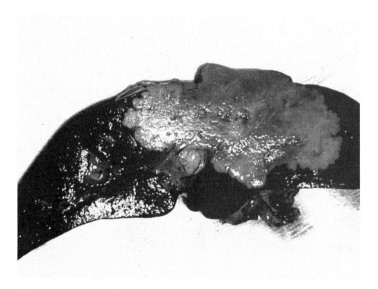

Figure 4 Coronal slice of non-cirrhotic liver showing a large single pale sharply defined and hard mass of cholangiocarcinoma.

Aetiology

Aetiological factors of importance can be divided into infections/infestations, drugs/toxins, predisposing diseases and congenital anomalies.

Infections and Infestations

Most examples of cholangiocarcinoma arising in association with infections and infestations relate to the liver flukes *Clonorchis sinensis* (52) and *Opisthorchis viverrini* (53). In the Far East the liver fluke (*C. sinensis*) resides in bile ducts and releases ova into the hepatic parenchyma, causing suppurative cholangitis and hepatic scarring. Amongst 38 cases of clonorchiasis in Hong Kong, 10 had HCC, 7 had intrahepatic cholangiocarcinoma, one had carcinoma of the common bile duct and one had lymphoma (52). Extrahepatic biliary carcinoma in typhoid carriers is six times more frequent than in matched controls (54).

Extrinsic Carcinogens

Dried and salted fish, which is the vehicle of transmission for infestations with *O. viverrini* (53), is also a potential source of nitrosamine and aflatoxin ingestion. Other potential extrinsic carcinogens include anabolic steroids (55) and thorium dioxide (56). In the 120 reported liver tumours caused by Thorotrast, cholangiocarcinoma was present in one-third of the cases—the same percentage as angiosarcoma (56).

Congenital Anomalies

Sporadically cholangiocarcinoma arises in a congenital anomaly of the biliary tree but no large series has been collected. Congenital intrahepatic dilatation of the bile ducts (57, 58), biliary microhamartomas (von Meyenburg complexes) (59), and biliary atresia (60) have all been recorded. Malignant change has also been found in a biliary cystadenoma (61).

Predisposing Diseases

Carcinoma in bile ducts is a rare, well recognized complication of chronic ulcerative colitis (62) and primary sclerosing cholangitis (63). The extrahepatic system is most frequently the primary site but origin from intrahepatic bile ducts has also been recorded.

Cirrhosis is less often present in cholangiocarcinoma than in HCC (2, 50, 52, 64) and a relationship to hepatitis B virus (HBV) infection has not been demonstrated. The role of gallstones in the aetiology of extrahepatic biliary carcinoma is not proven.

Clinical Features

Tumours at the hilum of the liver usually present as problems in the differential diagnosis of obstructive jaundice, whereas cholangiocarcinomas present with abdominal pain, anorexia and jaundice. In both groups jaundice is a more frequent initial symptom than in HCC (51) but otherwise the clinical features are similar. Alpha-fetoprotein (AFP) is not produced by these tumours (50). Clinically cholangiocarcinoma may be suspected when both an elevated AFP and a bruit are absent.

Cholangiocarcinoma of the bile duct can be classified by its location into the upper third which includes the common hepatic duct and the confluence of the hepatic duct; the middle third between the cystic duct and upper border of the duodenum; and the lower third between the upper border of the duodenum and the ampulla of Vater. The latter is generally referred to as periampullary carcinoma. The clinical features, diagnosis and treatment will differ.

Bile Duct Cancer at the Hilum of the Liver

Adenocarcinoma of the hepatic ducts at its bifurcation within the portal hepatis, otherwise known as the Klatskin tumour (65), and of the major intrahepatic bile ducts (66) differs from tumours elsewhere in the biliary tree. It has been reviewed by Blumgart and Imrie (35).

The tumour is slow growing and presents with the features of obstructive jaundice.

In early reports it was proposed that tubal drainage should be undertaken, rather than resection, and that the prognosis was relatively good. More recently, because of the advent of more accurate diagnosis with ultrasonography, percutaneous transphepatic cholangiography (PTC) and ERCP, accurate localization of the hilar cholangiocarcinoma (Figure 5) has been more readily achieved and has altered management. Fine needle aspiration cytology can be carried out under radiological control. Preoperative cholangiography and angiography give an excellent guide to the extent of the tumour and help determine whether or not resection can be readily carried out (35, 67).

Diagnostic difficulty may be experienced in disinguishing intrahepatic bile duct carcinoma or carcinoma at the hilum from sclerosing cholangitis, particularly as both conditions can be associated with ulcerative colitis. Cytological examination may be necessary to make this distinction. The surgical approach to treatment of these tumours has been fully reviewed by Blumgart and Imrie (35). They strongly advocate primary resection, contrary to earlier approaches, though the number of patients in which this can be undertaken is limited. Alternatives include some form of bypass surgery, intubation through the tumour, a transhepatic endoprosthesis and a U-tube technique (68). Following bypass surgery, radiation (69) or chemotherapy (70) may be used as an adjunctive therapy. The prognosis is poor with a 50% survival at one year and virtually none surviving at 5 years (71).

Tumours of the Common Bile Duct and Ampulla

Tumours of the middle and lower third of the bile duct (periampullary tumours) have similar presentation. They usually present with colestatic jaundice, dark urine, pale stools and pruritus as well as weight loss. The gallbladder is often enlarged and palpable (Courvoisier's sign) but may not be dilated if there has been preceding cholecystitis, particularly in association with gallstones.

The liver may be enlarged and tender and if spread has occurred outside of the biliary tree to the peritoneum ascites may be present. Liver function tests show a raised alkaline phosphatase in most cases, moderate elevation of the transaminases, marked elevation of the bilirubin and prolongation of the prothrombin time which is correctable by vitamin K. A raised AFP is present in less than 20% of cases and hepatitis B surface antigen and anti-mitochondrial antibody are usually negative.

Haematobilia may occur and bleeding is particularly common with ampullary carcinomas when the jaundice may be intermittent and the stools mixed with blood. This, combined with the steatorrhoea, gives the stools a

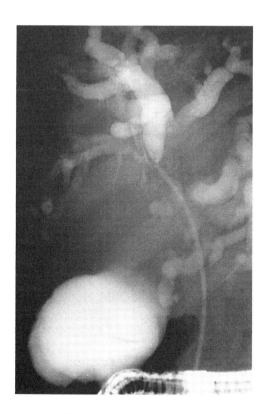

Figure 5 ERCP of hilar cholangiocarcinoma with dilated intrahepatic bile ducts.

characteristic silvery appearance which is, however, rare.

It is essential to establish preoperatively the site of the tumour to facilitate surgery. This can be done by ultrasound which shows dilatation of the ducts with or without dilatation of the gallbladder and sometimes a characteristic narrowing at the site of obstruction. Computed tomography may give information about spread of the lesion beyond the bile ducts.

The most useful investigations for localizing the site of the tumour are PTC or preferably ERCP (Figure 6). ERCP has the advantage of permitting aspiration of material for cytology or for direct biopsy of the tumour.

Direct surgical resection of the tumour with the aim of cure has been undertaken and has been reviewed by Braasch (72), Pitt et al. (73),

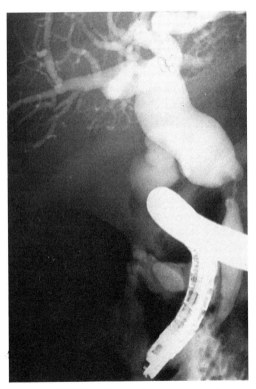

Figure 6 ERCP of cholangiocarcinoma of common bile duct with shouldered stricture clearly demonstrated.

Blumgart and Imrie (35) but the results are poor.

Palliation and relief of the obstruction may be achieved by introducing a stent through the tumour at ERCP, by transhepatic biliary drainage, or by surgical bypass.

The use of radiation and chemotherapy has been reviewed by Pilepich (69) and Andrews and Smith (70) but these have little influence on survival.

Pathology

Macroscopic Appearances

Cholangiocarcinomas have a fibrous stroma giving a firm white appearance (Figure 4). The tumour may be massive, nodular or diffuse in type. The edges of the tumour are less well defined than in HCC, and show an infiltrating pattern of growth. Necrosis, bile-staining, haemorrhage and vascular invasion are less common than in HCC. Most cholangiocarcinomas arise peripherally but the hilar cholangiocarcinoma in the porta hepatis presents as obstructive jaundice at an early stage (74).

Microscopic Appearances

Histologically, cholangiocarcinomas are usually well differentiated sclerosing adenocarcinomas, with a well marked acinar pattern and a desmoplastic stroma (Figure 7). They may be mucin-producing but necer secrete bile. A few exhibit a papillary pattern and some are anaplastic. In biopsy material it may be difficult to distinguish these tumours from metastatic adenocarcinomas, especially those arising in the pancreas or the extrahepatic biliary tree, or from sclerosing acinar forms of HCC. When the tumour first invades blood vessels, the vascular baement membrane is used and cyst-like spaces are created rather than solid intravascular tumour nodules (2). Extensive invasion of larger vessels is not seen. Rarely an adenosquamous carcinoma arises in the extrahepatic biliary tree (75).

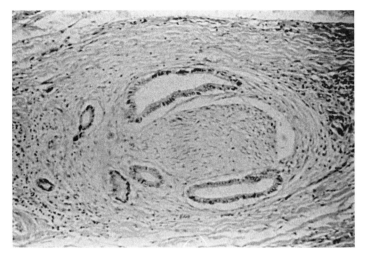

Figure 7 A nerve in the centre of the figure is surrounded by well differentiated desmoplastic adenocarcinoma of the biliary tree. Such perineural invasion can be the most definitive feature of malignancy in some well differentiated examples. H&E, original magnification: ×160.

OTHER PRIMARY CANCERS OF LIVER AND BILIARY TREE COMBINED CARCINOMAS

These carcinomas contain both hepatocellular carcinoma and cholangiocarcinoma. A recent survery of 24 cases divided these tumours itno three subgroups: types I, II and III. Type I tumours are collision tumours where hepatocellular carcinomas and cholangiocarcinomas simultaneously coexist. Type II are true combined tumours with the two histological parts mixed and can be seen to merge with each other. Type III have a fibrolamellar appearance but the glands secrete mucin (76).

Cholangiolocellular Carcinoma

A cholangiolocellular carcinoma derived from cholangioles has been described by Steiner and Higginson (77). This carcinoma resembles and is difficult to distinguish from cholangiocarcinoma but has small acini lined by uniform cuboidal-cells in a sclerotic stroma, rather than the flattened and pleomorphic malignant aci-

nar cells of the cholangiocarcinoma. There is some uncertainty about this rare entity, as it is also difficult to distinguish from sclerosing HCC. Peters (78) observed that all three types of sclerosing carcinoma—sclerosing HCC, cholangiocarcinoma and cholangiolocellular carcinoma have an association with hypercalcaemia.

Biliary Cystadenocarcinoma

A rare biliary cystadenocarcinoma has been described (79). It is claimed that this arises from a cystadenoma (61) or a congenital cyst (80).

Carcinoid Tumour

This is most commonly present as metastatic tumour within the liver (81) and is very rare as a primary hepatic tumour when it is thought to originate from scattered argentaffin cells present in gallbladder and bile duct epithelium (2) including the ampulla of Vater (82). It may produce a carcinoid syndrome. Hypoglycaemia has also been a recorded association (83). Recently carcinoid differentiation has been described with a primary hepatocellular carcinoma (84). Other apudomas that secrete other neuroendocrine hormones such as pancreatic polypeptide (85) occasionally arise from intrahepatic bile duct epithelium.

Squamous Carcinoma

This rare entity usually arises in the wall of a simple liver cyst (2, 86, 87), but has also been recorded in association with hepatolithiasis.

ANGIOSARCOMA

Aetiology

Angiosarcoma of the liver is a rare tumour which has specific and interesting aetiological associations. The tumour has been associated with cirrhosis (88), arsenic ingestion (89) and thorium dioxide (Thorotrast) administration (90-93). The early reports of this tumour mostly come from wine producing countries in Europe where arsenic was used by vineyard workers in insecticide sprays and dusts (89).

Thorotrast was widely used in several countries as an x-ray imaging medium and angiosarcoma is one of the more common tumours that can develop several years after initial exposure (90, 92, 94). Angiosarcoma has more recently been reported in males working with the polymerization of vinyl chloride, particularly those handling the monomer (95-97). The period of exposure ranged from 4 to 28 years. Oestrogens (98, 99) and androgenic anabolic steroids (100) have also been implicated as possible causes of this tumour.

Clinical Features

Symptoms are usually non-specific, and include malaise, anorexia, weight loss and right upper quadrant pain. Jaundice and abdominal swelling from ascites are late features. Hepatomegaly and splenomegaly are present on initial examination. The patients may have anaemia, and micro-angiopathic haemolysis has been recorded (88, 101).

Pathology

Macroscopically, the tumour is composed of greyish-white or haemorrhagic nodules

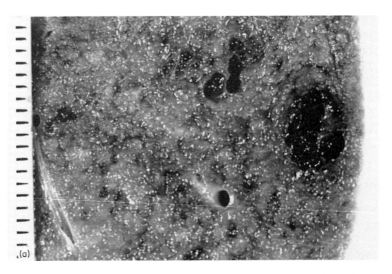

Figure 8a High power macroscopic detail of liver containing black nodules of an angiosarcoma. The largest nodule is 7 mm in diameter.

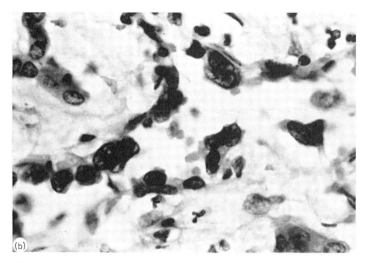

Figure 8b Angiosarcoma: large hyperchromatic pleomorphic tumour nuclei with scanty cytoplasm are forming a vascular channel. H&E, original magnification: ×600.

(Figure 8a). It spreads to the lungs, to the nodes of the porta hepatis and occasionally to the spleen (97). Involvement of the bone marrow and peritoneal surfaces has also been recorded (88). Rupture of a superficial nodule in the liver may result in haemoperitoneum.

Histologically there are plump, pleomorphic spindle cells with a clearly malignant appearance which form solid nodules of tumour and vascular channels (Figure 8b). Their endothelial derivation can be confirmed by an immunoperoxidase technique demonstrating factor VIII-related antigen in the cells, although this antigen is usually only focally present. At the edges of the tumour the cells invade and extend along the hepatic sinusoids. In the deeper parts of the tumour, the dilated vascular channel resemble blood lakes, and islands of residual hepatic parenchyma appear to float in these lakes. Extramedullary haematopoiesis is a regular feature of the tumour sinusoids (1, 88, 97).

Course and Prognosis

The tumour is rapidly progressive and patient

survival time is short, being usually less than one year after presentation (88, 102).

EPITHELIOID HAEMANGIOENDOTHELIOMA

This is a rare variant of a hepatic angiosarcoma (103–105). It arises most commonly in middle age, but no adult age is exempt. It affects women twice as commonly as men and a relationship to oral contraceptive use has been suggested (105). The majority of patients present with upper abdominal pain and weight loss, but jaundice and haemoperitoneum have also been recorded. The tumour nodules are usually multiple, firm and white. Histologically two cell types are present—dendritic cells with mucin-negative intracytoplasmic lumina, and large plump epithelioid cells. Immunoperoxidase studies for factor VIII-related antigen are positive. The tumour shows intravascular and intrasinusoidal growth with secondary stromal sclerosis and calcification. The tumour is very slow growing, with 25% of patients surviving 5 years even with inoperable tumours, but extrahepatic metastases eventually occur.

OTHER PRIMARY SARCOMAS

Malignant Mesenchymoma

The malignant mesenchymoma is rare and is found only in children. It grows rapidly but does not metastasize. On gross inspection it varies in colour from greyish-white to reddish-purple. Histologically, there is undifferentiated mesenchymal tissue often associated with extramedullary haematopiesis, differentiated smooth or striated muscle fibres and fibroblastic and myxoid connective tissue. Any of the spindle cell elements may be sarcomatous, and muscle cells may appear as giant myoblasts, sometimes with cross-striations. Osteoid tissue and bone are not seen in this tumour.

Embryonal Rhabdomyosarcoma

The embryonal rhabdomyosarcoma (sarcoma botryoides) is a rare tumour found at several potential sites including the extrahepatic biliary tree. It arises in childhood, most frequently in girls (106), but rarely it occurs in adults at this site. The tumour protrudes into the lumen of the biliary tree in a polypoid manner and is covered by an intact layer of non-neoplastic biliary epithelium. The small mesenchymal tumour cells are increased in number in sub-epithelial zones producing the 'cambian' layer: only rarely is full differentiation towards muscle with the formation of cross-striations seen. The tumour usually presents with obstructive jaundice. It is frequently inoperable and so has been associated with poor survival. Prolonged survival can occur with modern chemotherapeutic regimens and in some instances resections can be subsequently performed.

Monomorphic Sarcomas

Monomorphic sarcomas (15) are rare and usually occur in elderly subjects. A predominance of myoblasts in some tumours classes them as hepatic rhabdomyosarcomas or leio-myosarcomas, while in other cases a fibrosarco-matous pattern is evident. Sarcomas arising in the ligamentum teres have been seen in younger patients and are more accessible to resection (107). Leiomyosarcomas arising in the liver occur in adults of middle age (15) and have a worse prognosis than those in the ligamentum teres.

Malignant fibrous histiocytoma occurs on rare occasions (108–111). Fibrosarcoma has been described in an African child with AIDS (112).

Undifferentiated (Embryonal) Sarcomas

The majority of undifferentiated (embryonal) sarcomas of the liver, occur in the 6 to 15 years age group. Amongst 31 cases only 13% were older than 16 years. Isolated examples are seen in adults up to the age of 80 years (personal observations). These cases present as an abdominal mass and/or abdominal pain, and the average survival is less than one year (113, 114). This rare sarcoma is a large, single globular tumour showing areas of necrosis, haemorrhage and gelatinous degeneration (Figure 9a). A pseudocapsule demarcates the tumour. The main component is undifferentiated sarcomatous tissue, with stellate or spindle cells packed in fascicles or lying loosely in a myxoid stroma (Figure 9b). Characteristically there are single or small groups of large polygonal cells which contain PAS-positive and diastase-resistant globules in their cytoplasm. These globules stain intensely for $alpha_1$-antitrypsin using immunochemical techniques. At the edges of the mass, degenerating dilated bile ducts and islands of hepatocytes are seen, giving a resemblance to the mesenchymal hamartoma, of which this may be the malginant counterpart.

Malignant Hepatic Mixed Tumour

These tumours generally develop during childhood but are exceedingly rare. They characteristically contain a mixture of mesenchymal and epithelial elements. The epithelial compo-

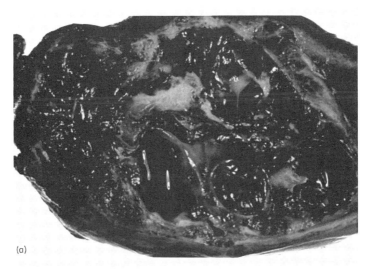

(a)

Figure 9a Embryonal sarcoma showing many large areas of cystic and mucoid degeneration and irregular white nodules of solid tumour.

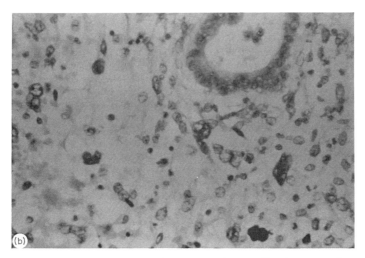

(b)

Figure 9b Loosely textured mononuclear cells, incorporating several tumour giant cells with bizarre hyperchromatic nuclei, have entrapped a dilated bile duct at the edge of the tumour. H&E, original magnification: ×250.

nent is a well differentiated hepatocellular, squamous or papillary carcinoma. The mesenchyme is usually poorly differentiated, although foci of osteoid or bone may be present. Malignant hepatic mixed tumours with a hepatocellular carcinomatous element but a benign mesenchyme (such as osteoid or bone) have sometimes been called 'liver cell carcinomas of childhood'. This term is not preferred (2). Differentiation from other tumours is made on histological and ultrastructural grounds (49).

Carcinosarcoma

Mixed tumours are occasionally encountered
which contain both hepatocellular carcinoma
and sarcomatous elements intimately mixed
(2), and some may in fact be separate malignancies; in others both elements are present in
metastases (2). These rare tumours must be
distinguished, where possible, from spindle-cell
variants of hepatocellular carcinoma and from
malignant hepatic mixed tumours of childhood.

REFERENCES

1 Weinberg AG, Finegold MJ. Primary hepatic
   tumours of childhood. Hum Pathol 1983; 14:
   512–37.
2 Edmondson HA. Tumours of the liver and
   intrahepatic bile ducts. In: Atlas of Tumour
   Pathology, Section VII, Fascicle 25. Washington DC. Armed Forces Institute of Pathology, 1958.
3 Margolis S, Homey C. Systemic manifestations
   of hepatoma. Medicine (Baltimore) 1972; 51:
   381–91.
4 Cochrane AMG, Williams R. Humoral effects
   of hepatocellular carcinoma. In: Okuda K,
   Peters RL eds Hepatocellular Carcinoma.
   London: John Wiley & Sons, 1976: 333–52.
5 Helzberg JH, McPhee MS, Zarling EJ, Lukert
   BP. Hepatocellular carcinoma: an unusual
   course with hyperthyroidism and inappropriate thyroid-stimulating hormone production. Gastroenterology 1985; 88: 181–4.
6 Gralnick HR, Givelber H, Abrams E. Dysfibri-
   nogenemia   associated   with   hepatoma;
   increased carbohydrate content of the fibrinogen molecule. Engl J Med 1978; 299: 221–6.
7 Horie Y, Katoh S, Yoshida H et al. Pedunculated hepatocellular carcinoma. Report of
   three cases and review of literature. Cancer
   1983; 51: 746–51.
8 Lieberman MK. Cirrhosis in ectopic liver
   tissue. Arch Pathol 1966; 82: 443–6.
9 Craig JR, Peters RL, Edmondson HA, Omata
   M. Fibrolamellar carcinoma of the liver: a
   tumour of adolescents and young adults with
   distinctive clinico-pathologic features. Cancer
   1980; 40: 372–9.
10 Wong LK, Link DP, Frey CF, et al. Fibrolamellar hepatocarcinoma; radiology, management and pathology. AJR 1982; 139; 172–5.
11 Teitelbaum DH, Tuttle S, Carey LC, Klausen
   KP. Fibrolamellar carcinoma of the liver.
   Review of three cases and the presentation of a

characteristic set of tumour markers defining
this tumour. Ann Surg 1985; 202: 36–41.
12 Omata M, Peters RL, Tatter D. Sclerosing
   hepatic carcinoma: relationship to hypercalcaemia. Liver 1981; 1: 50–5.
13 Baggenstoss AH. The pathology of tumours of
   the liver in infancy and childhood. In: Pack
   GT, Islami AH eds Tumours of the Liver,
   London: William Heinemann, 1970: 240–58.
14 Honan RP, Haqqani MT. (1980) Mixed hepatoblastoma in the adult: case report and review
   of the literature. J Clin Pathol 1980; 33; 1058–
   63.
15 Ishak KG. (1976) Mesenchymal tumours of
   the liver. In: Okuda K, Peters RL eds Hepatocellular Carcinoma. London: John Wiley &
   Sons, 1976; 247–307.
16 Meyer P, Li Volsi VA, Cornog JL. Hepatoblastoma associated with an oral contraceptive.
   Lancet 1974; ii: 1387.
17 Benjamin E, Landon M, Marsden HB. Hepatoblastoma as a cause of intra-uterine foetal
   death. Case report. Br J. Obstet. Gynaecol
   1981; 88: 329–32.
18 Ishak KG, Glunz PR. (1967) Hepatoblastoma
   and hepatocarcinoma in infancy and childhood. Cancer 1967; 20: 396–422.
19 Napoli VM, Campbell WG. Heptoblastoma in
   infant sister and brother. Cancer 1977; 39:
   2647–50.
20 Beach R, Betts P, Radford M, Millward-Sadler
   GH. Production of human chorionic gonadotrophin by a hepatoblastoma resulting in precocious puberty. J Clin Pathol 1984; 37: 734–7.
21 Hata Y, Uchino J, Sato K et al. Establishment
   of an experimental model of human hepatoblastoma. Cancer 1982; 50: 97–101.
22 Joshi VV, Kaur P, Ryan B et al. Mucoid
   anaplastic hepatoblastoma. A case report.
   Cancer 1984; 54: 2035–9.
23 Lack EE, Neave C, Vawter GF. Hepatoblastoma: a clinical and pathological study of 54
   cases. Am J Surg Pathol 1982; 6: 693–705.
24 Gonzales-Crussi F, Upton MP, Maurer MS.
   Hepatoblastoma: attempt at characterisation
   of histologic subtypes. Am J Surg Pathol 1982;
   6: 599–612.
25 Manivel C, Wick MR, Abenoza P, Dehner LP.
   Teratoid Hepatoblastoma: a nosological
   dilemma of solid embryonic neoplasms of childhood. Cancer 1986; 57: 2168–74.
26 Exelby PR, Filler RM, Grosfeld JL. (1974)
   Liver tumours in children in the particular
   reference to hepatoblastoma and hepatocellular carcinoma. American Academy of Paediatrics. Surgical Section Survey. J Pediatr Surg
   10, 329–37.

27 Andreassy RJ, Brennan LP, Siegel MM. et al. Preoperative chemotherapy for hepatoblastoma in children: report of six cases. J Pediatr Surg 1980; 15: 517.

28 Parkash OM. On the relationship of cholelithiasis to carcinoma of the gallbladder and on the sec dependency of the carcinoma of the bile ducts. Digestion 1975; 12: 129.

29 Chandler JG, Fletcher WS. A clinical study of primary carcinoma of the gall bladder. Surg Gynecol Obstet 1963; 117: 297–300.

30 Cooke L, Avery-Jones F, Keich MK. Carcinoma of the gallbladder. A statistical study. Lancet 1953; ii: 585–7.

31 Hamrick RE Jr, Liner FJ, Hastings PR, Cohn I. Jr. (1982) Primary carcinoma of the gallbladder. Ann Surg 195: 270–3.

32 Warren KW, Choe DS, Plaza J, Relihan M. Results of radical resection for periampullary cancer. Ann Surg 1975; 181: 534–40.

33 Diehl AK. Epidemiology of gallbladder cancer: a synthesis of recent data. J Nat Cancer Inst 1980; 65: 1209–14.

34 Fahim RB, McDonald JR, Richards JC, Ferris DO. Carcinoma of the gallbladder: a study of its modes of spread. Ann Surg 1982; 156: 114–22.

35 Blumgart LH, Imrie CW. (1985) Tumours of the extrahepatic biliary tree and pancreas. In: Wright R, Millward-Sadler, GH, Alberti KGMM, Karran SJ eds Liver and Biliary Disease. Eastbourne: Baillière Tindall, 1985: 1495–522.

36 Vaittinen E. Carcinoma of the gallbladder: A study of 390 cases diagnosed in Finland 1953–1967. Ann Chir Gynaecol (Suppl) 1970; 168: 7–81.

37 Appleman RM, Morlock CG, Dahlin DC, Adson MA. Long term survival in carcinoma of the gallbladder. Surg Gynecol Obstet 1963; 117: 459–64.

38 Piehler JM, Crichlow RW. Primary carcinoma of the gallbladder. Surg Gynecol Obstet 1978; 147: 929–42.

39 Polk HC Jr. Carcinoma and the calcified gallbladder. Gastroenterology 1966; 50: 582–5.

40 Bergdahl L. Gallbaldder carcinoma first diagnosed at microscopic examination of gallbladders removed for presumed benign disease. Ann Surg 1980; 191: 19–22.

41 Treadwell TA, Hardin WJ. Primary carcinoma of the gallbladder: the role of adjunctive therapy in its treatment. Am J Surg 1976; 132: 703–6.

42 Naguib SE, Aterman K. Presumed primary malignant melanoma of the liver. Am J Dermatopathol 1984; 6 (Suppl.): 231–43.

43 Mills SE, Cooper PH. Malignant melanoma of the digestive system. In: Sommers SC, Rosen PP. eds Pathology Annual, Part 2, Vol 18. Norwalk, Connecticut; Appleton-Century-Crofts, 1–26.

44 Albores-Saavedra J, Soriano J, Larraze-Hernandez O, Aguirre J, Henson DE. Oat cell carcinoma of the gallbladder. Hum Pathol 1984; 15: 639–46.

45 Willen R, Willen H. Primary sarcoma of the gallbladder. A light and electronmicroscopical study. Virchows Arch. (Pathol Anat) 1982; 396: 91–102.

46 Born MW, Ramey WG, Ryan SF, Gorden PE. Carcinosarcoma and carcinoma of the gallbladder. Cancer 1984; 53: 2171–7.

47 Nishimura A, Mayama S, Nakano K et al. Carcinoma of the cystic duct: case report. Japanese Surg 1975; 5: 109–17.

48 Edmondson H, Peters RL. Liver. In: Anderson WAD, Kissane JM eds Pathology. St Louis: Mosby, 1977: 1321–428.

49 Schonland MM, Millward-Sadler GH, Wright DH, Wright R. Hepatic tumours. In: Wright R, Millward-Sadler GH, Alberti KGMM, Karren SJ eds Liver and Biliary Disease. Eastbourne: Baillière Tindall, 1985: 1137–84.

50 Anthony P. Primary carcinoma of the liver. Coll Surg Engl 1976; 15: 517.

51 Okuda K, Kubo Y, Okazaki N et al. Clinical aspects of intrahepatic bile duct carcinoma including hilar carcinoma. A study of 57 autopsy proven cases. Cancer 1977; 39: 232–46.

52 Purtilo DT. Clonorchiasis and hepatic neoplasms. Trop Geograph 1976; 28: 21–27.

53 Flavell DJ. Liver fluke infection as an aetiological factor in bile duct carcinoma of man. Trans Soc Trop Med Hyg 1981; 75: 814–24.

54 Welton JC, Marr JS, Friedman SM. Association between hepatobiliary cancer and typhoid carrier state. Lancet 1979; i: 791–4.

55 Stromeyer FW, Smith DH, Ishak KG. (1979) Anabolic steroid therapy and intrahepatic cholangiocarcinoma.

56 Battifora HA. (1976) Thorotrast and tumours of the liver. In: Okuda K, Peters RL eds Hepatocellular Carcinoma. New York: John Wiley & Sons, 1976: 83–94.

57 Chen KT. Adenocarcinoma of the liver. Association with congenital hepatic fibrosis and Caroli's disease. Arch Pathol Lab Med 1981; 105: 294–5.

58 Gallagher PJ, Mills RR, Mitchison MJ. Congenital dilatation of the intrahepatic bile ducts with cholangiocarcinoma. J Clin Pathol 1972; 25: 804–8.

59 Cruickshank AH, Sparshott SM. Malignancies in natural and experimental hepatic cysts: experiments with aflatoxin in rats and the malignant transformation of cysts in human livers. J Pathol 1971: 104; 185–90.

60 Kulkarni PB, Beatty EC. Cholangiocarcinoma associated with biliary atresia. Am J Dis Child 1977; 131: 442.

61 Iemoto Y, Kondo Y, Fukamachi S. Biliary cystadenocarcinoma with peritoneal carcinomatosis. Cancer 1981; 48: 1664–7.

62 Ritchie JK, Allan RN, Macartney J et al. Biliary tract carcinoma associated with ulcerative colitis. Q J Med 1974; 43: 263.

63 Chapman RWG, Arborgh BAM, Rhodes JM et al. Primary sclerosing cholangitis: a review of its clinical features. Gut 1980; 21: 870.

64 Shikata T. Primary liver carcinoma and liver cirrhosis. In Okuda K, Peters RL eds Hepatocellular Carcinoma. New York: John Wiley & Sons, 1976: 53–71.

65 Klatskin G. Adenocarcinoma of the hepatic duct at its bifurcation within the porta hepatis. Am J Med 1965; 38: 241–56.

66 Altemeier WA, Gall EA, Zinninger MM, Hoxworth PI. Sclerosing carcinoma of the major intrahepatic bile ducts. Arch Surg 1957; 75: 450–60.

67 Voyles CR, Bowley NB, Allison DJ et al. Carcinoma of the proximal extrahepatic biliary tree. Radiological assessment and therapeutic alternatives. Ann Surg 1983; 197: 188–94.

68 Terblanche K. Carcinoma of the proximal extrahepatic biliary tree—definitive and palliative treatment. Surg Annu 1979; 11: 249–65.

69 Pilepich MV. Radiation in carcinoma of the extrahepatic bile duct. In: Wanebo HJ ed Hepatic and Biliary Cancer. New York and Basel: Marcel Dekker, 1987: 417–27.

70 Andrews WG. Smith FP. Chemotherapy for cholangiocarcinoma and gallbladder cancer. In: Wanebo HJ ed Hepatic and Biliary Cancer. New York and Basel: Marcel Dekker, 1987: 453–7.

71 Tomkins RK, Thomas D, Wile A, & Longmire WP Jr. (1981) Prognostic factors in bile duct carcinoma. Analysis of 96 cases. Ann Surg 194, 447–57.

72 Braasch JW. Surgical resection of cancer of the midduct and distal common bile duct: the Lahey Clinic experience. In: Wanebo HJ ed Hepatic and Biliary Cancer. New York and Basel: Marcel Dekker, 1987: 357–75.

73 Pitt HA, Roslyn JJ, Tompkins RK. Surgical resection of bile duct cancer: The UCLA experience. In: Wanebo HJ ed Hepatic and

Biliary Cancer. New York and Basel: Marcel Dekker, 1987: 339–55.

74 Whelton MJ, Petrelli M, George P et al. Carcinoma at the junction of the main hepatic ducts. Q J Med 1987; 38: 211–30.

75 Landsberg L, Khodadadi J, Goldstein J. Adenosquamous carcinoma of the common bile duct. J Surg Oncol 1986; 33: 109–11.

76 Goodman ZD, Ishak KG, Langloss JM et al. Combined hepatocellular-cholangiocarcinoma. A histological and immunohistochemical study. Cancer 1985; 55: 124–35.

77 Steiner PE, Higginson J. Cholangiolo-cellular carcinoma of the liver. Cancer 1959; 12: 753–9.

78 Peters RL. Pathology of hepatocellular carcinoma. In: Okuda K, Peters RL eds Hepatocellular Carcinoma. London: John Wiley & Sons, 1976: 107–69.

79 Ishak KG, Willis GW, Cummins SD, Bullock AA. Biliary Cystadenoma and cystadenocarcinoma. Report of 14 cases and review of the literature. Cancer 1977; 38: 322–38.

80 Devine P, Ucci AA. Biliary cystadenocarcinoma arising in a congenital cyst. Hum Pathol 1985; 16: 92–4.

81 Hodgson HJF, Maton PN. Carcinoid and neuroendocrine tumours of the liver. In: Williams R, Johnson PJ eds Liver Tumours. London and Philadelphia: Baillière Tindall, 1987: 35–61.

82 Boissonas A, Buttin S, Khalifa P et al. Tumeur carcinoidienne vatero-duodénale et neurofibromatose de Recklinghausen. Ann Méd Interne (Paris) 1985; 136: 46–8.

83 Ali M, Fayeuci AO, Braub EV. Malignant apudoma of the liver with symptomatic intractable hypoglycaemia. Cancer 1978; 42: 686–92.

84 Barsky SH, Linnoila I, Triche TJ, Costa J. Hepatocellular carcinoma with carcinoid features. Hum Pathol 1984; 15: 892–4.

85 Warner T, Seo ISD, Madura JA, Polak JM, Pearse AGE. PP-Producing apudoma of the liver. Cancer 1980; 46: 1146–51.

86 Bloustein PA, Silverberg SG. Squamous cell carcinoma originating in an hepatic cyst. Cancer 1976; 38: 2002.

87 Song E, Kew MC, Grieve T et al. Primary squamous cell carcinoma of the liver occurring in association with hepatolithiasis. Cancer 1984; 53: 542–6.

88 Pollard SM, Millward-Sadler GH. Malignant haemangioendothelioma involving the liver. J Clin Pathol 1974; 27: 214–21.

89 Regelson W, Kim U, Ospina J, Holland JF. (1968) Haemangioendothelial sarcoma of liver

from chronic arsenic intoxication by Fowler's solution. Cancer 1968; 21: 514–22.

90 Baxter PJ, Langlands AO, Anthony PP et al. Angiosarcoma of the liver: a marker tumour for the late effects of Thorotrast in Great Britain. Br J Cancer 1980; 41: 446–53.

91 Tesluk H, Nordin WA. Haemangioendothelioma of the liver following thorium dioxide administration. Arch Pathol 1955; 60: 493–501.

92 Vianna NJ. Tumours in patients with angiosarcoma of the liver. Ann Intern Med 1981; 95: 185–6.

93 Visfeldt J, Poulsen H. (1972) On the histopathology of liver and liver tumours in thorium-dioxide patients. Acta Pathol Microbiol Scand, Section A: Pathology, 1972; 80: 97–108.

94 Kojiro M et al. Thorium dioxide-related angiosarcoma of the liver: pathomorphologic study of 29 autopsy cases. Arch Pathol Lab Med 1985; 109: 853–7.

95 Creech JL, Johnson MN. (1974) Angiosarcoma of liver in the manufacture of polyvinyl chloride. J Occupational Med 1974; 16: 150–1.

96 Duck BW. Vinyl chloride carcinogenesis. Br J Cancer 1975; 32: 260.

97 Makk L, Delmore F, Creech JL, Ogden LL, Fadell EH, Songster CL, Clanton J, Johnson MN, Christopherson WM. Clinical and morphological features of hepatic angiosarcoma in vinyl chloride workers. Cancer 1976; 37: 149–63.

98 Hoch-Ligeti, C. Angiosarcoma of the liver associated with diethylstilboestrol. JAMA 1978; 240: 1510–11.

99 Monroe FS, Riddell RH, Siegler M, Baker AL. Hepatic angiosarcoma. Possible relationship to long-term oral contraceptive ingestion. 1981.

100 Falk H, Thomas LB, Popper H, Ishak KG. Hepatic angiosarcoma associated with androgenic–anabolic steroids. Lancet 1979; ii: 1120–3.

101 Alpert LI, Benisch B. Hemangioendothelioma of the liver associated with microangiopathic hemolytic anemia. Am J Med 1970; 48: 624–8.

102 Baker H. de C., Pagett GE, Dawson J. Haemangioendothelioma (Kupffer cell sarcoma) of the liver. J Pathol Bacteriol 1965; 72: 173–182.

103 Ishak KG, Sesterhenn IA, Goodman ZD et al. Epithelioid haemangioendothelioma of the liver. A clinicopathologic and follow-up study of 32 cases. Hum Pathol 1984; 15: 839–52.

104 Eckstein RP. Epithelioid haemangioendothelioma of the liver: report of two cases histologically mimicking veno-occlusive disease. Pathology 1986; 18: 459–62.

105 Dean PJ, Haggitt RC, O'Hara CJ. Malignant epithelioid haemangioendothelioma of the liver in young women: relationship to oral contraceptive use. Am J Surg Pathol 1985; 9: 695–704.

106 Ruymann FB, Raney RB Jr, Crist WM et al. (1985) Rhabdomyosarcoma of the biliary tree in childhood: a report from the Intergroup Rhabdomyosarcoma Study.

107 Tomaszewski MM, Kuenster JT, Hartman K et al. Leiomyosarcoma of the ligamentum teres of liver: case report. Paediatr. Pathol 1986; 5: 147–56.

108 Dehner LP. Malignant fibrous histiocytoma arising in the liver. Arch Pathol Lab Med 1986; 110: 773–4.

109 Conran RM, Stocker JT. Malignant fibrous histiocytoma of the liver: a case report. Am J Gastroenterol 1985; 80: 813–15.

110 Alberti-Flor JJ, O'Hara MF, Weaver F et al. Malignant fibrous histiocytoma of the liver. Gastroenterology 1985; 89: 890–3.

111 Fukayama M, Koike M. Malignant fibrous histiocytoma arising in the liver. Arch Pathol Lab Med 1986; 110: 203–6.

112 Ninane J, Moulin D, Latinne D et al. AIDS in two African children—one with fibrosarcoma of the liver. Eur J Paediatr 1985; 144: 385–90.

113 Stocker JT, Ishak KG. Undifferentiated (embryonal) sarcoma of the liver: a report of 31 cases. Cancer 1978; 42: 336–48.

114 Forbes A, Portmann B, Johnson P, Williams R. Hepatic sarcomas in adults: a review of 25 cases. Gut 1987; 28: 668–74.

Textbook of Uncommon Cancer
Edited by C.J. Williams, J.G. Krikorian, M.R. Green and D. Raghavan
© 1988 John Wiley & Sons Ltd

Chapter **28**

Unusual Tumours of the Colon, Rectum and Anus

Irving Taylor

Department of Surgery, University of Southampton, South-ampton, UK

COLORECTAL TUMOURS

Colorectal adenocarcinoma is now the second commonest malignancy in the Western world with approximately 20 000 new cases per annum in the UK alone. Other malignant tumours in this region are extremely rare and in general can only be distinguished from adenocarcinoma on the basis of histological examination. Some of these rare tumours produce rather unusual appearances on endos-copy as well as on barium studies which might raise a suspicion in the mind of the clinician but, in general, management will only be affected by the final histological report.

Leiomyosarcoma

Smooth muscle malignant tumours have been recognized in both the rectum and colon. It is possible that they arise from benign leiomyo-mas, which occur more frequently. Rectal leiomyosarcomas are more frequent than col-onic ones. Only 29 colonic and approximately 100 rectal leiomyosarcomas had been reported in the literature (1, 2).

Clinical Factors

The tumours have been described in both male and females, the majority being over 50 years of age. Rectal tumours are usually large and bulky and the patient has a sensation of a mass in the rectum. Bleeding, constipation and symptoms of obstruction may all be present (3).

In one series (4) 4 of 5 patients with colonic leiomyosarcoma exhibited lower abdominal pain, change in bowel habit, rectal bleeding and weight loss. Colonic tumours can occasio-nally grow to enormous sizes with few symp-toms. Rarely the finding of an abdominal mass may be the presenting symptom.

Diagnosis

This is based on rectal examination, endoscopy (either sigmoidoscopy or colonoscopy) and by barium enema examination. Usually a barium enema shows a projecting or constricting lesion which is not readily distinguishable from a carcinoma (Figure 1). Occasionally endo-scopic biopsy may confirm the diagnosis but more often the biopsy is insufficient for defini-tive histological confirmation. If the mucosa overlying the tumour appears intact this should arouse the suspicion that the lesion is not a typical carcinoma (5).

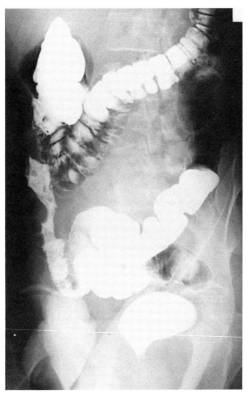

Figure 1 Barium enema appearance of a leiomyosarcoma in the ascending colon.

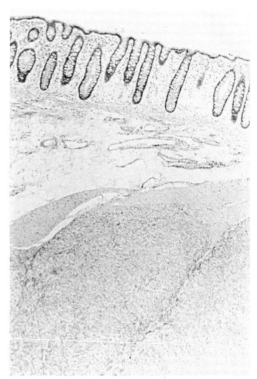

Figure 2 Histological appearance of leiomyosarcoma of the colon (original magnification: ×40).
The normal large bowel mucosa overlies a large
rounded mass of smooth muscle tumour cells. In
this instance the tumour arises from the muscularis propria, but frequently it arises from the
muscularis mucosa.

Histology

There is great variation in the histological
characteristics of leiomyosarcoma. Some are
well differentiated lesions composed of spindle-
shaped cells, others are more immature
plumper cells of varying size and shape with
deeply staining oval nuclei. Mitosis is usually
common and bizarre giant cells can occasionally be recognized (4).

The overlying mucosa is usually intact
(Figure 2). Spread is commonly local, often
along the submucosal plane. Frequently, however, invasion into perirectal or ischiorectal fat
occurs as well as into the mesocolon.

Blood stream spread is also recognized with
liver and lung metastases (6). It is generally
considered that lymph node involvement does
not occur.

Treatment

Surgery. Surgical excision is the single most
important therapy. Often this is performed on
the assumption that an adenocarcinoma is
present. Accordingly for rectal lesions which
are large and low (less than 6 cm from the anal
verge) abdominoperineal excision is performed. For more proximal lesions a restora-
tive procedure, anterior resection, is usually
undertaken. Occasionally local excision of
leiomyosarcoma of the rectum has been performed on the basis of possible benign muscle
tumour. However, the incidence of local recurrence following this procedure is very high
indeed.

For colonic lesions standard resections are

carried out, e.g. right hemicolectomy, transverse colectomy or left hemicolectomy.

It would appear that the most satisfactory treatment for rectal leiomyosarcoma is radical removal by abdominoperineal excision with emphasis on wide ablation of the rectum itself rather than on extensive removal of lymphatics, which are seldom involved (5). However, the results are not good. In one small series of rectal lesions 5 of 11 patients died with disease within 5 years of resection (4).

Radiotherapy. Radiotherapy should perhaps be retained for selected patients who develop significant symptoms from local recurrence.

Chemotherapy. Although some sarcomas will respond well to single agent or combination chemotherapy, there is little evidence that such treatment can prolong survival. Adjuvant chemotherapy is being tested in soft tissue sarcomas though there is too little experience in large bowel leiomyosarcomas to allow any useful conclusions to be drawn. Few randomized studies of such treatment at other sites have been reported; in that of Omura et al. (7) adjuvant Adriamycin showed no benefit when used in uterine sarcomas.

Carcinoid Tumours

Malignant carcinoid tumours can occur anywhere along the gastrointestinal tract. They are thought to arise from the Kulchitsky cells of the crypts of Zieberkuhn. They are of endodermal origin and show basophil granules which have an affinity for silver stains—hence the alternative name of argentaffinoma (8, 9).

Clinical Features

Carcinoids in the colon and rectum are rare, much less frequently encountered that in either the small bowel or appendix (Table 1). It usually presents as a single growth which forms a small nodular thickening in the mucosa and submucosa and is often asymptomatic. As it enlarges it produces a sessile or occasionally

TABLE 1 DISTRIBUTION OF CARCINOID TUMOURS[a]

Organ	Proportion of all carcinoids (%)	Range (%)
Appendix	41.6	35–45
Small bowel	26.9	20–33
Rectum and sigmoid	17.1	12–24
Lung and bronchi	9.3	4–14
Oesophagus and stomach	2.3	2–3
Ovary	1.5	0.3–0.9
Biliary tract	0.21	0.1–0.3

[a] From Macdonald JS. Carcinoid tumours. In: DeVita VT, Hellman S, Rosenberg SA eds Cancer: Principles and Practice of Oncology. Philadelphia: Lippincott, 1982: 1019–24.

pendiculated polyp which may ulcerate the mucosa. They have been described in all age ranges between 30 and 80 (8).

When small and polypoid (less than 2 cm in diameter) they tend not to produce any symptoms. Large tumours in the rectum can result in bleeding (especially if mucosal ulceration occurs) and constipation. Colonic carcinoids only produce symptoms when much larger and result in invasion of the serosal surface or beyond (8, 10).

It is extremely rare for carcinoids of the large bowel and rectum to produce the carcinoid syndrome. This is true even in unquestionably malignant tumours which have produced liver metastases. Accordingly the syndrome will not be further discussed in this review.

The diagnosis should be considered when small, firm submucosal nodules are palpated on rectal examination. Lesions of more than 1 cm have frequently metastasized to lymph nodes (90%) and to distant sites (60%) at the time of presentation. In contrast Hadju et al. (11) found no evidence of either local or distant metastases in 20 patients with superficial invasive tumours.

Endoscopy

Rectal carcinoids often appear as yellowish lesions. Large tumours can appear ulcerative

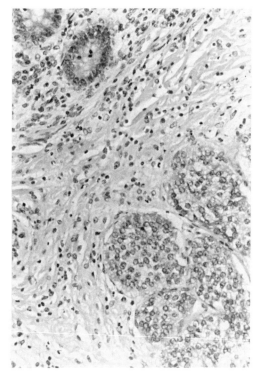

Figure 3 Histological appearance of carcinoid of the colon (original magnification: ×200). The base of mucosal crypts are seen top left. Nests of small polygonal cells are present in the submucosa. Specific silver stains, such as Grimelius, can confirm the identity of this tumour.

and if so this usually indicates deeper invasion. Biopsy should be fairly deep in order to obtain a positive diagnosis. Histologically they have the typical appearance of carcinoid tumours (Figure 3).

Treatment

In the case of small lesions biopsy removal is considered adequate if complete excision can be assured. These are usually well differentiated lesions. For larger lesions in the rectum, certainly if less than 2 cm in diameter, wide local excision is possible often by the anal route.

In one series of 40 patients followed up for over 20 years, with tumours less than 1 cm, all had local excision (10) and none of the patients died of their carcinoid tumour.

However, if there is evidence from the biopsy specimen or following excision that extension of the carcinoid into or beyond the muscle coat of the rectum is present, or if the tumour is greater than 2 cm in diameter, then local excision is unlikely to be adequate (8, 12, 13). In these cases wide excision, including anterior rectosigmoid resection or abdominoperineal resection is required if any improvement in survival is to be achieved.

Other Therapies

Too few cases of carcinoid of the large bowel have been treated with radiotherapy or chemotherapy for any meaningful conclusions to be drawn. In carcinoid of the small bowel, radiotherapy has generally been ineffective and chemotherapy (5-FU, streptozotocin, cyclophosphamide, methotrexate, doxorubicin) of limited palliative value (14). The risk of a carcinoid crisis should, however, be borne in mind, especially in those rare patients who have severe symptoms. Response to chemotherapy is more common in foregut carcinoids and in one series the survival for patients receiving chemotherapy for colonic carcinoid was particularly poor (Table 2). Recently, human leukocyte interferon has been shown to have activity in carcinoid tumours, though

TABLE 2 RESPONSE AND SURVIVAL AFTER CHEMOTHERAPY FOR CARCOID TUMOURS: EFFECT OF ANATOMICAL SITE[a]

Site of primary	Response Rate (%)	Median Survival (months)
Small bowel	41	29.3
Pancreas	42	21.6
Lung	12	14.9
Colon	—	10.1
Unknown	17	8.0

[a] From Moertel CG, Hanley HA. Combination chemotherapy trial for metastatic carcinoid tumour and malignant carcinoid syndrome. Cancer Clin Trials 1979; 2: 327–31.

most responses were biochemical (15). In general, however, the outlook is good with a 5-year survival rate of 13%.

ANORECTAL TUMOURS

Young et al. (17), reporting on data for the Surveillance, Epidemiology and End Results (SEER) programme of the National Cancer Institute, found an age adjusted incidence for anorectal tumours of 0.6 per 100 000 population/year.

Basal Cell Carcinoma

The anal skin is very rarely the site of a basal cell carcinoma. In one review from St Mark's Hospital only 10 cases occurred in over 4000 colorectal tumours treated between 1928 and 1956 (18).

Clinical Features

The tumours are usually on the anal verge or lower anal canal. These have distinct rolled edges with a central shallow ulcer. It rarely if ever invades deeper or adjacent tissues and does not metastasize.

The patients usually complain of pain or irritation related to 'piles'. The inguinal lymph nodes are not involved but may be enlarged due to associated anal sepsis.

Histology

The tumour consists of typical sheets of basophilic staining cells containing large blue nuclei and minimal cytoplasm. It arises from the basal cells of the malpighian layer of the skin.

Treatment

The most effective therapy is adequate surgical excision. This is almost invariably curative. Primary excision is usually possible if the tumour is small. If the tumour is larger, then partial closure leaving the rest of the wound to heal by granulation is adequate. Radiotherapy can be used if surgery is contra-indicated (65).

Squamous (Epidermoid) Carcinoma of the Anal Region

This uncommon tumour accounts for about 2% of all tumours of the large bowel. A variety of different tumours are seen in the anal region as its embryological development is complex (see section on cloacogenic carcinoma, below). However, about 30% are keratinizing tumours, though Stearns and Quan have suggested that all pathological variants of epidermoid carcinoma should be considered together when discussing treatment (19).

Tumours of the anal region predominate in males (sex ratio 3:1), whereas tumours of the anal canal are more common in women (sex ratio 2:1) (20). Conditions causing chronic irritation of the anal canal or perianal region appear to be associated with the disease (20–26). Because of the frequency of benign anorectal disease and the rarity of anal carcinoma it is hard to establish a causal relationship, though the association of mucinous adenocarcinoma with chronic anal fistula is the strongest (27), with over 130 cases of this association reported in the literature. There also seems to be a relationship between male homosexuality and anal cancer (28) and multiparity in women (29).

Although the anal canal is short (up to 3 cm), its anatomy is complex (Figure 4 and 5). Though transitional epithelium is found at the pectinate line, modified squamous epithelium may extend up to the area of the anal glands so that squamous carcinomas may arise within the rectum (30, 31). Tumours (mucoepidermoid) of the anal glands at the base of the columns of Morgagni have been described (32). Below the pectinate line modified squamous epithelium continues down to the anal verge where stratified squamous epithelium takes over.

In an analysis of the presenting site in 189 cases of squamous carcinoma the majority were found to be adjacent to the pectinate line

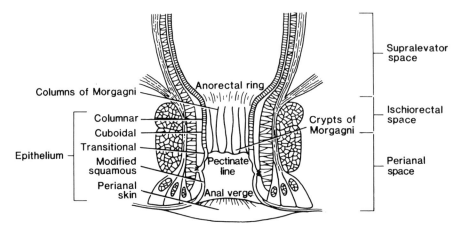

Figure 4 Schematic representation of the anatomy of the anorectal region.

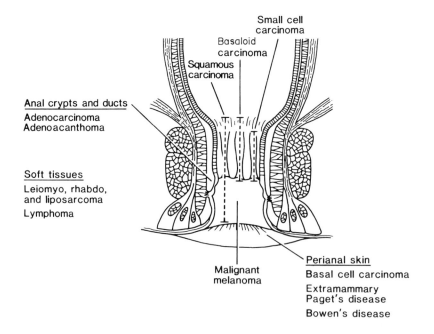

Figure 5 Anatomical sites of uncommon tumours of the anorectal region.

(Figure 6) (33). Local spread, often longitudinal, occurs by invasion into perianal tissues; it is analogous to the longitudinal spread seen in oesophageal carcinoma (34). Vaginal invasion is common (30%) as are metastases to the prostate, urethra, bladder and sacrum (34). The direction of lymphatic spread appears to be related to the tumour site but may be altered with obstruction (21). Sugarbaker et al. (36) in a review, presented data from four studies; tumours of the anal margin were found to have mesenteric nodes in 14 of 53 cases (26%) compared with 86 of 200 (43%) of anal canal tumours. Sterns and Quan (19) found

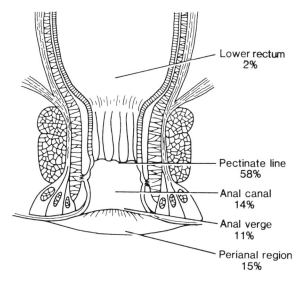

Figure 6 Proportion of anorectal tumours by anatomical
site (33).

groin metastases in 44 of 109 patients (40%), pelvic lymph node metastases in 15 of 45 patients (33%); the incidence of spread did not appear to be related to the anatomical position of the primary tumour. Liver (3%) and lung (3%) metastases appear to have been a relatively uncommon presenting feature in two large collected series (9, 37).

Presentation and Staging

Rectal bleeding is the commonest symptom being reported in 27% to over 60% of series (38). This often simulates the pattern of bleeding seen in benign anorectal conditions. About 40% of patients have anorectal discomfort or pain, often aggravated by defecation. Other less common symptoms are change in bowel habit, awareness of an anal mass, tenesmus, pruritus and discharge. Because its symptoms mimic those of benign conditions, diagnosis is often delayed. Early biopsy of suspicious lesions is recommended as carcinoma will be found occasionally.

The TNM staging system (UICC) and TNM checklist for anal tumours are shown in Tables 3 and 4. Other staging systems have

been proposed by Richards et al. (39) and Paradis et al. (40) (Table 5). In the large recent Mayo Clinic series (41) a modification of the ABC system was used: B was modified to B_1 invasion into the internal sphincter, B_2 invasion into the external sphincter and B_3 invasion into adjacent pelvic tissues.

Histology

The WHO (42) divide anal carcinomas into (1) squamous cell carcinoma, (2) cloacogenic carcinoma, (3) mucoepidermoid carcinoma, (4) adenocarcinoma, (5) undifferentiated carcinomas. There are no special features differentiating squamous carcinoma of the anus from those at other sites. These tumours may form a continuum with cloacogenic tumours.

Treatment

Surgery has been the primary therapy for squamous tumours in the anorectal region. Many report combining results for squamous tumours with those of non-keratinizing varieties. The extent of surgery depends on the location and degree of spread of the tumour.

TABLE 3 ANAL CANAL AND ANAL ORIFICE: TNM PRE-TREATMENT CLINICAL CLASSIFICATION AND POST-SURGICAL CLASSIFICATION (UICC, 1980)

The classification applies only to carcinoma.

Minimum Requirements for Assessment:
T – Clinical examination; radiography and endoscopy.
N – Clinical examination and radiography.
M – Clinical examination and radiography.

Anatomical Sites:
Two anatomical sites are identified: Anal Canal ICD-O T-154.2, and Anal Orifice ICD-O T-173.5

ANAL CANAL
T –   Primary Tumour

Tis   Pre-invasive carcinoma (carcinoma in situ).
T0   No evidence of primary tumour.
T1   Tumour occupying not more than one third of the circumference or length of the canal and not infiltrating the external sphincter muscle.
T2   Tumour occupying more than one third of the circumference or length of the anal canal or tumour infiltrating the external sphincter muscle.
T3   Tumour with extension to rectum or skin but not to other neighbouring structures.
T4   Tumour with extension to other neighbouring structures.
TX   The minimum requirements to assess the primary tumour can not be met.

N –   Regional Lymph Nodes

The regional lymph nodes for the Anal Canal are the peri-rectal nodes and the nodes distal to the origin of the inferior mesenteric artery.
N0   No evidence of regional lymph node involvement.
N1   Evidence of involvement of regional lymph nodes.
NX   The minimum requirements to assess the regional lymph nodes can not be met.

ANAL ORIFICE
T –   Primary Tumour

Tis   Pre-invasive carcinoma (carcinoma in situ).
T0   No evidence of primary tumour
T1   Tumour 2 cm or less in its greatest dimension strictly superficial or exophytic.
T2   Tumour more than 2 cm by not more than 5 cm in it greatest dimension or tumour with minimal infiltration of the dermis.
T3   Tumour more than 5 cm in its greatest dimension or tumour with deep infiltration of the dermis.
T4   Tumour with extension to muscle, bone, etc.
TX   The minimum requirements to assess the primary tumour can not be met.

N –   Regional Lymph Nodes

The regional lymph nodes for the Anal Orifice are the inguinal nodes.

N0   No evidence of regional lymph node involvement.
N1   Evidence of involvement of movable unilateral regional lymph nodes.
N2   Evidence of involvement of movable bilateral regional lymph nodes.
N3   Evidence of involvement of fixed regional lymph nodes.
NX   The minimum requirements to assess the regional lymph nodes can not be met.

ANAL CANAL AND ANAL ORIFICE
M –   Distant Metastases

M0   No evidence of distant metastases.
M1   Evidence of distant metastases (specify, using recommended abbreviations).
MX   The minimum requirements to assess the presence of distant metastases can not be met.

POST-SURGICAL HISTOPATHOLOGICAL CLASSIFICATION (p.TNM)
pT – Primary Tumour
The pT categories correspond to the T categories.

pN – Regional Lymph Nodes
The pN categories to the N categories.

pM – Distant Metastases
The pM categories correspond to the M categories.

Histopathological Grading (G): Record as G1—High degree of differentiation, G2—Medium, G3—Low or Undifferentiated, GX—Not assessed.

Additional Descriptors; For recurrent cases, add prefix r. For cases having other treatment before surgery, add prefix y.

STAGE-GROUPING
No stage grouping is at present recommended.

TABLE 4 STAGING CHECKLIST (UICC, 1980)

ANAL ORIFICE   ANAL CANAL

PRE-TREATMENT CLINICAL CLASSIFICATION (TNM)
→ Please check one or more items in each section as applicable.

Site and Extent of Tumour	PRIMARY TUMOUR		→If not assessed check TX ☐	Category
Site: Anal Canal ☐ Anal Orifice ☐	Pre-invasive carcinoma (carcinoma in situ)		☐	Tis
Size in greatest dimension . . cm	No evidence of primary tumour		☐	T0
	Anal Canal	≤ 1/3 anal canal ☐ · Ext. sphincter not infiltrated ☐		T1
		> 1/3 anal canal ☐ · Ext. sphincter infiltrated ☐		T2
		Extension only to: Skin ☐ · Rectum ☐		T3
		Extension to other neighbouring structures ☐		T4
	Anal Orifice	2 cm or less ☐ · Strictly superficial or exophytic ☐		T1
		> 2 to 5 cm ☐ · Minimal infiltration of dermis ☐		T2
		More than 5 cm ☐ · Deep infiltration of dermis ☐		T3
		Extension to muscle, bone, etc. ☐		T4
	REGIONAL LYMPH NODES	→If not assessed check NX ☐		Category
	Anal Canal	No evidence of involvement ☐		N0
		Evidence of involvement ☐		N1
	Anal Orifice	No evidence of involvement ☐		N0
		Evidence of involvement · Movable · Unilateral ☐		N1
		· · Bilateral ☐		N2
Regional lymph nodes Histologically: negative ☐ positive ☐		· Fixed nodes ☐		N3
	DISTANT METASTASES	→ If not assessed check MX ☐		Category
Histological diagnosis:	No evidence of distant metastases		☐	M0
	Evident of distant metastases (specify)		☐	M1
. . . . Grade:	Category: pT pN pM Stage: G			
			Date	

POST-SURGICAL HISTOPATHOLOGICAL CLASSIFICATION (p. TNM)
→ Please check one or more items in each section as applicable.

Site and Extent of Tumour	PRIMARY TUMOUR		→ If not assessed, check pTX ☐	Category
Site: Anal Canal Anal Orifice ☐	Pre-invasive carcinoma (carcinoma in situ)		☐	pTis
Size in greatest dimension . . cm	No evidence of primary tumour		☐	pT0
	Anal Canal	≤ 1/3 anal canal ☐ · Ext. sphincter not infiltrated ☐		pT1
		> 1/3 anal canal ☐ · Ext. sphincter infiltrated ☐		pT2
		Extension only to: Skin ☐		pT3
		Extension to other neighbouring structures ☐		pT4
	Anal Orifice	2 cm or less ☐ · Strictly superficial or exophytic ☐		pT1
		> 2 to 5 cm ☐ · Minimal infiltration of dermis ☐		pT2
		More than 5 cm ☐ · Deep infiltration of dermis ☐		pT3
		Extension to muscle, bone, etc. ☐		pT4
	REGIONAL LYMPH NODES	→ If not assessed check pNX ☐		Category
	Anal Canal	No evidence of invasion ☐		pN0
		Evidence of invasion ☐		pN1
	Anal Orifice	No evidence of invasion ☐		pN0
		Evidence of invasion · Movable · Unilateral ☐		pN1
		· · Bilateral ☐		pN2
Regional lymph nodes: Histologically: negative ☐ positive ☐		· Fixed nodes ☐		pN3
	DISTANT METASTASES	→ If not assessed, check pMX ☐		Category
Histological diagnosis.	No evidence of distant metastases		☐	pM0
	Evidence of distant metastasis (specify)		☐	pM1
. . . . Grade:	Category: pT pN pM Stage: G			

TABLE 5 ALTERNATIVE STAGING SYSTEMS FOR SQUAMOUS CARCINOMA
OF THE ANAL CANAL

ABC Classification (39)[a]
A: Tumour confined to anal mucosa and submucosa
B: Invasion into extra-anal tissues without regional lymph node involvement
C: Metastasis into regional lymph nodes

Roswell Park Memorial Institute Classification (40)
0: Carcinoma in situ
I: Sphincter muscle not involved
II: Sphincter muscle involved
III: Regional metastasis
A—perirectal nodes only
B—inguinal modes
IV: Distant metastasis

[a] See text for Mayo Clinic modification (41).

The Mayo Clinic recommend local excision only for anal canal tumours of less than 2 cm below the dentate line (41). Abdominoperineal resection is recommended for less favourable anal canal tumours, some workers also advocating pelvic lymph node dissection in selected patients (19, 33, 40, 43). Total pelvic exenteration may be considered if the bladder or urethra is involved (44). In women excision of the perianal tissues may need to be wide, including the posterior portion of the vaginal wall (33).

Excision of the involved pelvic nodes has been commonly recommended in the past, though the outcome is very poor despite this; in collected series, only 11 of 67 (16%) patients presenting with inguinal node metastases survived 5 years (36). In contrast, 36 of 70 patients (51%) developing inguinal node metastases after initial therapy survived 5 years; for this reason Sugarbaker et al. (36) recommended a watch and wait policy in patients who are pelvic node negative at presentation. The importance of stage at presentation is shown clearly in the Mayo Clinic (41) review of their experience in 188 cases of squamous and cloacogenic carcinomas (Figure 7).

Radiotherapy

These tumours are generally as radiosensitive

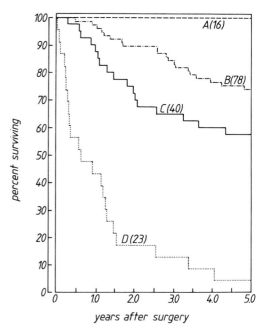

Figure 7 Mayo Clinic experience of carcinoma of the anorectal region: survival by stage (41).

as squamous carcinomas at other sites and dose is limited by the sensitivity of normal perianal tissues. Studies have tested both external beam and implantation therapy, though many have reported high complication rates (38, 44). Papillon (45) has, however, using protracted fractionation, claimed improved results with high 5-year survival rates (68%) and a low incidence (4%) of radionecrosis requiring radical surgery. Green et al. (46) have also claimed improved results using external beam therapy alone. A number of reports of favourable results of preoperative irradiation and chemotherapy (5-FU and mitomycin C) have also appeared, though none of these studies has an appropriate control owing to the rarity of the tumour (47).

Chemotherapy

Anecdotal reports of various single agents and combinations, have often appeared though there is no definitive therapy for advanced disease (5-FU and mitomycin C (47, 48), vincristine and bleomycin (49, 50), doxorubicin, cisplatin, methyl-CCNU (51)).

There is no current consensus regarding management at presentation, some authors having recommended radical surgery in the past (52) whilst more recently conservative procedures with radiation and/or chemotherapy have been advanced.

Cloacogenic Carcinoma at the Anorectal Junction (Junctional, Basosquamous or Basiloid Carcinoma)

Grinvalsky and Helwig (53) drew attention to the unusual histology and embryology of the epithelium of the pectinate line in 1956, though Hermann and Desforses (54) described the transitional nature of these tissues as early as 1880

The mucosa in between that of the anus and rectum has histological characteristics similar to that of the cloacal entoderm. It is similar to that of the urinary tract and can give rise to cancers with similar histological appearances.

Such tumours represent about 2.5% of all anal and rectal tumours (55, 56) though some authors regard them as part of a continuum with squamous carcinomas of this region (57).

There is a predominance in women, the female/male sex ratio being at least 2:1 (58). Most cases are seen between the sixth and eighth decades, though one patient was, at presentation, as young as 29 years (55).

Presentation and Histology

Clinically, they are indistinguishable from other carcinomas of the same region. Most are exophytic, though they can occasionally present as areas of submucosal thickening or more rarely as anal fissures (55, 56).

Histologically some are indistinguishable from transitional carcinomas of the urinary tract. These tumours, accounting for two-thirds of the cases, are composed of circumscribed clusters of fairly uniform cells with ovoid or spherical nuclei and infrequent mitoses (56). The remainder present a different pattern with nests of small cells exhibiting greater polymorphism and hyperchromatic nuclei. Clusters of cells are separated by thin bands of stroma and peripheral cell layers show 'palisading'. The general appearance is similar to basal cell carcinoma and the term 'basaloid carcinoma' has been used for this type of tumour. Other variations have been reported in tumours of this region (55). Some may resemble squamous cell, mucoepidermoid, adenocystic or anaplastic small cell (oat cell) carcinoma (See WHO classification of tumours of the anal canal above).

The commonest mode of presentation is rectal bleeding with or without rectal pain (55, 56). Constipation or change in bowel habit also occur. Most tumours (nearly 40%) involve the anterior rectal wall and they may extend into the rectovaginal septum, so that vaginal involvement is present in about 20% of women with this tumour. Prostatic involvement is less common at presentation (5%), though advanced disease may go on to involve the bladder, urethra and sacrum. Involvement of draining lymph nodes occurs in about a third of cases (55–58). Distant metastases are less common though up to 20% of patients have had such involvement in some series (55–

58). The common sites of involvement have been liver, lungs, bones and peritoneum.

Treatment

Many series have combined data on this tumour with that from squamous carcinomas of this region (41) so that many of the comments in that section may apply to clonogenic tumours (19). Surgery was said to be the treatment of choice, the type and extent of the operation being dictated by the stage of the tumour. The commonest operation reported has been an abdominoperineal resection (about 50% of patients). One of the most frequent sites of relapse has been the posterior vaginal wall in women (56, 59, 60) with tumours of the anterior rectal wall and because of this some surgeons have extended their operation to include posterior vaginectomy and node dissection as this is the next commonest relapse site (56).

Postoperative radiotherapy has been used in some series but its contribution is difficult to assess because of the anecdotal experience. In one study, 9 of 11 patients with basaloid tumours treated by abdominoperineal resection and radiotherapy survived 5 years (61).

⌐rapy with or without chemotherapy ⌐as also been used—see preceding section on squamous carcinomas.

Survival may be related to the histological sub-type (Figure 8) though Bowman et al. (41) did not confirm this: basaloid tumours in women being reported to have a median survival of 5 years compared with 2.5 years for adenocystic and mucoepidermal tumours in man (61). Tumours of 'oat' cell type are reported to be invariably fatal (62). In one report the overall median survival for all cloacogenic tumours was 96 months with survival rates of 56% at 5 years, 49% at 10 years, 47% at 15 years and 46% at 20 years (63). Survival at 15 years by stage was : A-77%; B-59%; C-37%; D₁ (invasion of adjacent organs)—9%; D₂ (distant metastases)— 0%. Chemotherapy has no established role in this tumour though there is one report of a

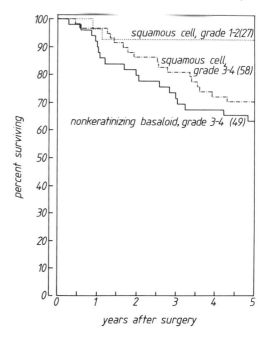

Figure 8 Mayo Clinic experience of carcinoma of the anorectal region: survival by histology (41).

prolonged response to BCNU (64) and there is anecdotal experience in conjunction with radiotherapy (47, 51).

Basaloid carcinomas should be differentiated from basal cell carcinoma of the anus. When treated with wide excision with or without radiation alone these tumours have a good outlook with a 5-year survival rate of 72%—most deaths not being due to basal cell carcinoma (65).

Malignant Melanoma

This rare tumour of the anorectal region only accounts for 1% of all anal tumours or 1.6% of all malignant melanomas (66). It was originally described by Laënnec and Virchow, and to date over 200 cases have been recorded in the literature.

Mason and Helwig (67) in a review of the Armed Forces Institute of Pathology experience concluded that malignant melanoma was always derived from pigmented cells; since such cells are absent above the pectinate line they considered all rectal malignant melanomas as metastatic.

Clinical Features

The lesion is usually small and polypoid (2–4 cm) and projects into the lumen of the anal canal. The commonest presenting symptoms are bleeding and pain with an awareness of a lump. In one series from St Mark's Hospital (68) the mean duration of symptoms was 3–4 months. Nine of 21 tumours were located below the dentate line, 11 were above but within the anal canal and one was in the rectum. In a small proportion of cases the presenting feature is an inguinal lymph node mass.

The diagnosis is suggested by the dark coloured lesion seen at the anal verge or on proctoscopy, though gross appearance can be deceptive and many are initially diagnosed as thrombosed haemorrhoids. Early lesions are usually flat and superficial, nodularity suggesting advanced disease. Most are solitary but up to 15% are multiple (67, 71, 72). Biopsy is necessary to confirm the diagnosis and not infrequently the true nature is revealed only after histological examination of an unusual haemorrhoidectomy specimen. In one series the diameter of the tumours varied from 2 to 10 cm and were all nodular. Tumours of this size are all within Clark's Level V and such classification does not help in treatment planning. Tumour extensions may be along the submucosal plane, laterally into the perineal tissues and via the lymphatics to inguinal nodes (4).

Histology

The histology is very similar to melanoma elsewhere in the body. The cells vary from spindle to polyhedral shaped—the cytoplasm is generally abundant (Figure 9). The nuclear pattern is variable and multinucleated cells are found. Mitotic rates vary from case to case, but they are often frequent. Pigmentation is very variable though up to half of cases have strong

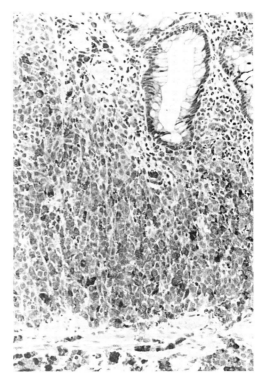

Figure 9 Histological appearance of malignant melanoma of the anal canal (original magnification: ×160). Sheets of pleomorphic cells are present in the lamina propria and are beginning to surround the crypts (top right). Elsewhere the tumour has destroyed crypts and ulcerated through the mucosal surface.

pigmentation (67). Many are anaplastic, and in one series more than half the cases were initially diagnosed as other anaplastic tumours (67, 68).

Treatment

The best prospect of a cure has always been considered to be wide surgical ablation carried out as a radical abdomino-perineal excision with high ligation of the mesenteric vessels. However, the results of such treatment are generally unsatisfactory. In a recent report of the experience of St Mark's Hospital, an alternative, less radical strategy was described (68). In a review of 21 patients treated over a 44-year period, two groups of patients were assessed, those that were treated by radical excision with or without lymph node dissection and a group treated conservatively by wide local excision. The results suggest that radical surgical treatment by rectal excision offers no more in terms of curative potential than local excision. Survival is related to pathological stage at diagnosis rather than the extent of surgery. Birnstad et al. (71) reviewed 86 cases: 34 with limited surgical excision and 27 abdominoperineal resections. As in the St Marks series, there was no improvement in the results with increasingly radical surgery. The role of radiotherapy is doubtful though implantation therapy has been used for local recurrence. Chemotherapy has no useful role in this disease.

Outlook

Median survival is about one year, survival being closely correlated with tumour extent at presentation. Although in the study of Husa and Hockerstedt (66) 5-year survival was 100% in patients with localized disease compared with 15% for those with nodal extension, the survival curve after this time paralleled that of the more advanced patients.

ACKNOWLEDGEMENTS

I would like to thank Dr H. Millward-Sadler for providing the photomicrographs for this chapter.

REFERENCES

1 Buckle AER, Evans L. Leiomyosarcoma of the rectum. Dis Colon Rectum 1974; 17: 109–11.
2 Warkel RL, Stewart JB, Temple AJ. Leiomyosarcoma of the colon: report of a case and analysis of the relationship of history to prognosis. Dis Colon Rectum 1975; 18: 501–3.
3 Anderson PA, Dockerty MB, Byie LA. Myomatous tumours of the rectum. Surgery 1950; 28: 642–6.
4 Quan SHO. Uncommon malignant anal and rectal tumours. In: Stearns MW ed Neoplasms of the Colon, Rectum and Anus. New York: John Wiley & Sons, 1983: 114–41.
5 Goligher J. Rarer tumours of the colon, rectum and anus. In: Surgery of the Anus, Rectum and Colon. Springfield & Thomas. 1980: 79.
6 Morson BC. In: Dukes CE ed Cancer of the Rectum. Edinburgh: Livingstone, 1960: 92.
7 Omura GA, Blessing JA, Major F et al. A randomised clinical trial of adjuvant adriamycin in extensive sarcoma: A Gynaecological Oncology Group Study. J Clin Oncol 1985; 3: 1240–5.
8 Peskin GW, Orloff MJ. A clinical study of 25 patients with carcinoid tumours of the rectum. Surg Gynecol Obstet 1959; 109: 673–6.
9 Zakarias YM, Quan SH, Hajdu SI. Carcinoid tumours of the gastrointestinal tract. Cancer 1975; 35: 588–91.
10 Quan SHO. Uncommon malignant anal and rectal tumours. In: Stearns MW ed Neoplasms of the Colon, Rectum and Anus. New York: John Wiley & Sons, 1983; 115–41.
11 Hadju SI, Winawer SJ, Laird Myers WP. Carcinoid tumours: a study of 204 cases. Am J Clin Pathol 1975; 61: 521–8.
12 Morton WA, Johnstone FRC. Rectal carcinoids. Br J Surg 1965; 52: 391–5.
13 Sanders RJ, Axtell HK. Carcinoids of the gastrointestinal tract. Surg Gynecol Obstet 1964; 119: 369–80.
14 Lipsett MB. Endocrine neoplasms. In: Calabresi P, Schein PS, Rosenberg SA eds Medical Oncology: Basic Principles and Clinical Management of Cancer. New York: McMillan 1985: 476–95.
15 Oberg K, Norheim I, Lind E et al. Treatment of malignant carcinoid tumours with human leukocyte interferon: Long term results. Cancer Treat Rep 1986; 70: 1297–1304.
16 Goodwin JD II. Carcinoid tumours: An analysis of 2837 cases. Cancer 1975; 36: 560–9.
17 Young JL, Percy CL, Asive AJ. Surveillance, epidemiology and end results: Incidence and mortality data 1973–1977. Nat Cancer Inst Monograph 1981: 57.
18 Morson BC. The pathology and results of treatment of squamous cell carcinoma of the anal canal and margin. Proc R Med 1960; 53: 416–20.
19 Stearns MW, Quan SHO. Epidermoid carcinoma of the ano-rectum. Surg Gynecol Obstet 1970; 113: 953–7.
20 Wolfe MRI, Bussey HJR. Squamous carcinoma of the anus. Br J Surg 1968; 55: 295–301.
21 Stearns MW, Urmacher C, Steinberg SS, Woodruff J, Attiyeh F. Cancers of the anal canal. Curr Problm Cancer 1980; 4: 4–44.
22 Singh R, Nime F, Mittleman A. Malignant

epithelial tumours of the anal canal. Cancer 1981; 48: 411–15.

23 Lee SH, McGregor DH, Kuziez MN. Malignant transformation of perianal condyloma accuminatum: A case report with review of the literature. 1981; Dis Colon Rectum 24: 462–7.

24 Brennan JT, Stewart CF. Epidermoid carcinoma of the anus. Ann Surg 1972; 176: 787–90.

25 Bretlau P. Carcinoma arising in anal fistula. Acta Chir Scand 1967; 133: 496–500.

26 McAnally AK, Dockerty MB. Carcinoma developing on chronic draining cutaneous sinuses and fistulas. Surg Gynecol Obstet 1949; 88: 87–96.

27 Getz SB, Ough YD, Patterson RB, Kovaleik PJ. Mucinous adenocarcinoma developing in chronic anal fistula: report of two cases and review of the literature. Dis Colon Rectum. 1981; 24: 562–566.

28 Daling JR, Weiss NS, Klopfenstein LL, Cochran LE, Chow WH, Daifuk R. Correlates of homosexual behaviour and the incidence of anal carcinoma. JAMA 1982; 247: 1988–90.

29 Cabera A, Tsukada Y, Pickren JW, Moore R, Bross DJ. Development of lower genital carcinomas in patients with anal carcinoma. Cancer 1966; 19: 470–80.

30 Comer TP, Beahrs OH, Dockerty MB. Primary squamous carcinoma and adeno acanthoma of the colon. Cancer 1971; 28: 1111–17.

31 Goligher J. Rarer tumours of the colon, rectum and anus. In: Surgery of the Anus, Rectum and Colon. Springfield & Thomas, 1980; 79.

32 Morson BC. The pathology and result of treatment of squamous carcinoma of the anal canal and margin. Proc R Soc Med 1960; 53: 414–20.

33 Kuehn PG, Eisenberg H, Reed JF. Epidermoid carcinoma of the perianal skin and anal canal. Cancer 1968; 22: 932–8.

34 Woolfe HRI, Bussey HJR. Squamous cell carcinoma of the anus. Br J Surg 1968; 55: 245–301.

35 Welch JP, Malt RA. Appraisal of the treatment of carcinoma of the anus and anal canal. Surg Gynecol Obstet 1977; 145: 837–41.

36 Sugarbaker PH, Gunderson LL, Macdonald JS. Cancer of the anal canal. In: De Vita VT, Hellman S, Rosenberg SA. eds Cancer: Principles and Practice of Oncology. Philadelphia: Lippincott 1982: 724–31.

37 MacLean MD, Murray FH, Bacon HE. Hepatic metastases of squamous carcinoma of the anal canal: Review of literature and case report. Dis Colon Rectum 1961; 4: 51–5.

38 Montague ED. Squamous cell carcinoma of the anus. In: Fletcher GH ed Textbook of Radiotherapy, 3rd edition. Philadelphia: Lea & Febiger, 1980.

39 Richards JC, Beahrs OH, Woomer LB. Squa-

mous cell carcinoma of the anus, anal canal and rectum in 109 patients. Wurg Gynecol Obstet 1962; 114: 475–82.

40 Paradis P, Douglas HO, Holyoke ED. The clinical implications of a staging system for carcinoma of the anus. Surg Gynecol Obstet 1975; 41: 411–16.

41 Boman BM, Moertel CG, O'Connell MJ, Scott M, Weiland GH, Beart RW, Gunderson LL, Spencer RJ. Carcinoma of the anal canal: A clinical and pathological study of 188 cases. Cancer 1974; 54: 114–25.

42 Morson BC, Sobin LH. Histological typing of intestinal tumours. International Histological Classification of Tumours, No. 15, Geneva: WHO, 1976.

43 Sawyers JL. Squamous cell carcinoma of the perianus and anus. Surg Clin N Am 1972; 52: 475–82.

44 Moertel CG. The anus. In: Holland JF, Frie E eds Cancer Medicine, 2nd edition. Philadelphia: Lea & Febiger, 1982.

45 Papillon J. Radiation therapy in the management of epidermoid carcinoma of the anal region. Dis Colon Rectum 1974; 7: 181–7.

46 Green JP, Schaupp WC, Cantril ST, Schall G. Anal carcinoma: current therapeutic concepts. Am J Surg 1980; 140: 151–5.

47 Cummings BJ, Rider WD, Harwood AR, Kenne TJ, Thomas GM, Erlichmann C, Fine S. Combined radical radiation therapy and chemotherapy for primary squamous cell carcinoma of the anal canal. Cancer Treat Rep 1982; 66: 484–92.

48 Nigro ND, Vaikevicius VK, Buroker T, Bradley GT, Considine B. Combined therapy for cancer of the anal canal. Dis Colon Rectum 1981; 24: 73–5.

49 Quan SHO, Magill GB, Leaming RH, Hajdu SI. Multidisciplinary preoperative approach to the management of epidermoid carcinoma of the anus and anorectum. Dis Colon Rectum 1978; 20: 89–90.

50 Livingstone RB, Bodley GP, Gottlieb JA, Frei J. Kinetic scheduling of vincristine and bleomycin in patients with lung cancer and other malignant tumours. Cancer Chemo Rep 1973; 57: 219–24.

51 Fisher WB, Herbst KD, Simms JE, Critchfield CF. Metastatic cloacogenic carcinoma of the anus: Sequential responses to adriamycin and cis-dichlorodamnineplatinum. Cancer Treat Rep 1978; 62: 91–7.

52 Grinnell RS. Squamous cell carcinoma of the anus. In: Turrell ed Diseases of Colon and Rectum. Philadelphia: Saunders, 1959: 1019–28.

53 Grinvalsky HT, Helwig EB. Carcinoma of the

anorectal junction. I. Histological considerations. Cancer 1956; 9: 480–5.

54 Hermann G., Desforses L. Sur la muqueuse de la
    région cloacle du rectum: Acad Sci (D) (Paris)
    1880; 90: 1301–2.

55 Klotz RJ Jr, Pamukoglu T, Souilliard DH.
    Transitional clonogenic carcinoma of the anal
    canal. Clinicopathologic study of 373 cases.
    Cancer 1967; 20: 1727–32.

56 Kheir S, Hickey RC, Martin RG, MacKay B,
    Gallager HS. Cloacogenic carcinoma of the anal
    canal. Arch Surg 1972; 104: 407–15.

57 Coffey RJ, Gunderson LL. Neoplasms of the
    anus. In: Calabresi P et al eds Medical Onco-
    logy: Basic Principles and Clinical Management
    of Cancer. New York: Macmillan 1985.

58 Khan MH, Barron J. Cloacogenic carcinoma: A
    study of six cases and review of the literature.
    Am J Gastroenterol 1982; 77: 137–40.

59 Singh R, Nime F, Mittelman A. Malignant
    epithelial tumours of the anal canal. Cancer
    1981; 48: 411–15.

60 Svenson EW, Montague ED. Results of treat-
    ment in transitional cloacogenic carcinoma.
    Cancer 1980; 46: 828–30.

61 Serota AJ, Weil M, Williams RA, Wolfman JJ,
    Wilson SE. Anal cloacogenic carcinoma: Classi-
    fication and clinical behaviour. Arch Surg 1981;
    116: 456–9.

62 Grodsky L. Current concepts on clonogenic

63 Pihl E, Hughes EJ, McDermott F, Milne BJ,
    Kovner JM, Price ABI. Carcinoma of the
    rectum and rectosigmoid: Cancer specific long-
    term survival. Cancer 1980; 45: 2902–7.

64 Zimm S, Wampler GL. Response of metastatic
    cloacogenic carcinoma to treatment with semus-
    tine. Cancer 1981; 48: 2575–6.

65 Nielsen OV, Jensen SL. Basal cell carcinoma of
    the anus—a clinical study of 34 cases. Br J Surg
    1981; 68: 856–7.

66 Husa A, Hockerstedt K. Anorectal malignant
    melanoma. A report of fourteen cases, Acta Chir
    Scand 1974; 140: 68–72.

67 Mason JK, Helwig EB. Ano-rectal melanoma.
    Cancer 1966; 19: 39–50.

68 Morson BC, Volkstadt H. Malignant melanoma
    of the anal canal. J Clin Pathol 1963; 16: 126–32.

69 Pack GT, Martins FG. Treatment of anorectal
    malignant melanomas. Dis Colon Rectum 1960;
    3: 15–21.

70 Pack GT, Oropeza R. A comparative study of
    melanoma and epidermoid cancer of the anal
    canal. Dis Colon Rectum. 1967; 10: 161–76.

71 Birnstad FW, Dockerty MB, Dixon CF.
    Melano-epithelioma of the anus and rectum.
    Surgery 1949; 25: 82–8.

72 Singh W, Madaan TR. Malignant melanoma of
    the anal canal. Am J Proc 1976; 27: 49–53.

transitional cell anorectal tumours. JAMA
1969; 207: 2057–61.

Section V

Tumours of the Nervous System

Textbook of Uncommon Cancer
Edited by C.J. Williams, J.G. Krikorian, M.R. Green and D. Ragavan
© 1988 John Wiley & Sons Ltd

Chapter **29**

Uncommon Tumors of the Nervous System

Alan Hirschfeld* and
Paul Kornblith†
*Assistant Professor, Department of Neurosurgery, Albert
Einstein College of Medicine, Bronx, New York, USA and
†Professor and Chairman, Department of Neurosurgery,
Albert Einstein College of Medicine, Bronx, New York,
USA

TUMORS OF THE BRAIN AND SPINAL CORD

INTRODUCTION

The most frequently encountered primary tumors affecting the central nervous system (CNS) are: glioblastomas and astrocytomas, which are derived from glial cells, meningiomas, which arise from rests of arachnoidal cells and are therefore mesenchymal in origin, pituitary adenomas, and the neurilemoma–schwannoma group of tumors, which arise from the Schwann cells of cranial and spinal nerves. Together these tumors comprise about 60% of all intracranial and intraspinal tumors found in persons greater than 15 years old (1). In the pediatric age group, medulloblastomas, arising from primitive, multipotential, neuro-epithelial cells, and the glial cell-derived tumors, are about equally prevalent.

A wide variety of less frequently encountered tumors also exist. These will be the subject of this chapter. They will be discussed in terms of their incidence, origin, pathology, diagnosis and treatment. When available, data from reports on the basic biology of the tumors will also be presented. These reports come mainly from immunocytochemical, tissue culture and molecular biological studies. Unfortunately these tumors have been the subject of relatively few studies of this nature, compared to the more common tumors, of which biological specimens are more readily available, and for some of which animal models have been developed and played a major research role.

Any attempt to classify CNS tumors is fraught with nosological pitfalls. This is partly due to the number of synonymous appellations which have been given to specific histological entities through the years, partly to the not infrequent coexistence of more than one cell type within a single tumor (2), and partly to the difficulty in assigning a cell of origin to many tumors (3). With the development of immunohistochemical and electron microscopic technology, this latter hurdle has been lowered somewhat.

The ideal classification should not only be based upon a tumor's predominant cell type or cell of origin, as has been the general practice, but should also provide a system for determining a patient's prognosis and selecting his or her therapy (4, 5). At present there are not enough clinical and biological data available on the uncommon tumors to attain these goals. The tumors discussed in this chapter will be categorized in approximate conformity with the World Health Organization Classification (WHO) (6). General categories will be neuroepithelial, vascular and mesenchymal tumors, primary lymphomatous tumors, malformative tumors and intracranial extension of regional tumors (Table 1). As in the WHO classification, some nosological entities have been included which are not tumors in the strict sense of a mass caused by uncontrolled cellular proliferation.

TUMORS OF NEUROEPITHELIAL ORIGIN

Ependymoma

Incidence and Location

Of the uncommon tumors reviewed in this chapter ependymomas are perhaps the most common. They comprise about 2–9% of all intracranial tumors (7, 8), but also accounted for 12.8% of 1322 tumors of the spinal cord seen at the Mayo Clinic (9). Two-thirds of intracranial ependymomas occur infratentorially (10), accounting for approximately 25% of tumors in the region of the fourth ventricle (11). The majority of spinal ependymomas are found at the level of the cauda equina. Those which are wholly intramedullary are situated with roughly equal frequency in the cervicothoracic, thoracic, and thoracolumbar areas. Occasionally they may involve the entire length of the cord (9).

The average age of patients with intracranial ependymomas is approximately 20 years (12), with a reported range between one week and 72 years (13). There is a slight male preponderance (14), and there appears to be a higher incidence among populations of the Far East (15). Spinal ependymomas tend to

TABLE 1 UNCOMMON CNS TUMORS

Tumors of neuroepithelial origin
  Ependymoma
  Pineal cell tumors
  Choroid plexus tumors
  Astrocytic tumors
    Astroblastoma
    Gemistocytic astrocytoma
    Subependymal giant cell astrocytoma
  Poorly differentiated and embryonal tumors
    Primitive polar spongioblastoma
    Medulloepithelioma
    Gliomatosis cerebri
  Neuronal tumors
    Neuroblastoma
    Ganglioglioma
    Gangliocytoma
    Ganglioneuroblastoma, anaplastic gangliocytoma
    and anaplastic ganglioglioma

Tumors and malformations of vascular origin
  Hemangioblastoma
  Vascular malformations
    Venous angioma
    Capillary telangiectasia
    Sturge–Weber disease
    Cavernous angioma

Tumors of mesenchymal origin
  Hemangiopericytoma
  Sarcomas
    Fibrosarcoma and its variants
    Other primary de novo sarcomas
    Gliosarcoma
    Malignant meningioma

Primary melanotic tumors

Tumors of lymphoreticular origin
  Primary lymphomas
  Miscellaneous lymphoreticular disorders
    Histiocytosis X
    Lymphosarcoma
    Plasmacytoma

Tumors of maldevelopmental origin
  Craniopharyngioma
  Dermoid and epidermoid cysts
  Colloid cyst of the third ventricle
  Rathke cleft cyst
  Neurenteric cyst
  Choristoma
  Intracranial lipoma

Intracranial extension of regional tumors
  Primary bone tumors
  Chordoma

become symptomatic at a later age, the average patient being in his mid-thirties (7, 10, 16). Roughly three-fifths are male. As with other tumors of glial origin, ependymomas may occur in neurofibromatosis (17); their occurrence in patients with tuberous sclerosis is, on the other hand, a matter of debate (18). The association of ependymoma and syringomyelia has been reported (19).

Origin and Pathology

By Rubinstein's definition, ependymomas are 'neoplasms composed of, and usually derived from, differentiated ependymal cells' (17). They tend to be well demarcated at surgery and, on gross examination, appear to be soft, pale and, occasionally, nodular. About 40% of supratentorial ependymomas are cystic, but such is not the case in the posterior fossa tumors (14). Many of the latter extend into the subarachnoid space, to present as a mass in the cerebellopontine angle (20), and may even encase the medulla or upper cervical spinal cord.

The classification of ependymomas has been controversial. Previously designated histological varieties include the cellular, papillary, myxopapillary, epithelioid, subependymoma, and mixed types (10), as well as the more aggressive looking 'ependymoblastoma' (21). Kernohan, as with astrocytomas, advocated a four-grade classification, based upon the degree of histologically anaplastic appearance (22). These classification schemes are felt to be not only cumbersome, but impractical in terms of relating histological type to outcome. Most tumors containing ependymal elements will behave either as very slowly-growing, hamartomatous lesions (subependymomas), as well-differentiated tumors (papillary ependymomas), or as more aggressive, anaplastic neoplasms, still frequently referred to as 'ependymoblastomas' (23).

Subependymomas, which consist of mature, fibrillary astrocytes and ependymal cells, arise from the ventricular walls, mimicking the normal architecture of the embryonic sube-

pendymal glia (24). As the majority are encountered incidentally, at autopsy, in middle-aged or elderly people (25), they are of less clinical importance than papillary or anaplastic ependymomas.

Non-anaplastic ependymomas are fairly cellular neoplasms, though their features are regular, with little evidence of pleomorphism, multinucleation, hyperchromatism, mitotic figures, necrosis or vascular endothelial proliferation (17). Characteristic features include ependymal rosettes, which may contain cilia and blepharoplasts, and perivascular pseudo-rosettes. Approximately one-third contain calcification. Immunohistochemical staining with monoclonal antibodies usually reveals the presence of glial fibrillary acidic protein (GFAP) in some cells (26). This may be due to an admixture of astrocyte-derived cells within the tumor. Evidence for this has been found in tissue culture studies, as well (27).

Malignant or anaplastic ependymomas may have invasive properties, have a greater propensity to metastasize within the subarachnoid pathways (21), and, histologically, contain mitotic figures, multinucleated giant cells, and areas of necrosis (17).

Clinical and Radiological Findings

The presenting features of intracranial ependymomas are typical of expanding intraventricular masses. The average duration is 16 months (23). The most common symptom is headache (80%), and the most common sign, papilledema (90%) (28). Supratentorial tumors, half of which are not intraventricular, may also present with focal findings, such as paresis, and one-third will have seizures. Infratentorial tumors, on the other hand, tend to present with vomiting, ataxia, vertigo and dysmetria. Cranial nerve palsies are also common (7).

Spinal cord and nerve root findings may arise because of either disseminated subarachnoid disease, from an intracranial source, or from a primary intramedullary or filum terminale tumor. Approximately half of the tumors which metastasize are of the anaplastic variety (21), and most originate in the fourth ventricle (14). The incidence of metastases varies from series to series, but may be as high as 30% (12, 14, 28).

Spinal cord ependymomas typically will present with vertebral or radicular pain and limb weakness (7). Lesions involving the cauda equina may also frequently cause loss of sphincter control (9). They characteristically have an exophytic component, and may produce a markedly elevated cerebrospinal fluid (CSF) protein content (7), which has been associated with papilledema. Uncommon findings are seeding of the nervous system from a primary spinal cord lesion (29), and the sudden onset of acute sciatica from a spinal subarachnoid hemorrhage (30).

Radiological evidence of chronically increased intracranial pressure and intratumoral calcium may be found in the skull x-rays of patients with intracranial ependymomas (28, 31). In the last 10 years, computed tomography (CT) scanning has become the radiographic procedure of choice for the detection and localization of these tumors. Calcification and cystic components are features of many of the supratentorial lesions, and both infratentorial and supratentorial lesions show diffuse enhancement of their solid portion. Both cystic and calcific components may be detected by this method. Magnetic resonance imaging (MRI) may provide further diagnostic capability and anatomical information, particularly in delineating the relationship of the tumor to the ventricular system.

For spinal ependymomas, myelography has been the procedure of choice. It is likely, though, that MRI will prove a valuable, and certainly less invasive, procedure. Intramedullary lesions, on myelography, appears as diffuse cord swelling over several or many segments, and cauda equina tumors are seen to have exophytic, often multiloculated, components. Often, plain x-rays may provide the preliminary evidence of a cord tumor, as 15–36% show an increased interpedicular distance of scalloping of vertebral bodies (9, 32).

Treatment and Outcome

The treatment of intracranial ependymomas differs from that of the spinal variety, mainly because the latter are more readily excised, but also because malignant characteristics occur less frequently in spinal lesions.

Surgical resection is recommended as the initial treatment of both intracranial and spinal ependymomas (16). Ventricular shunting or drainage may also be necessary in patients with hydrocephalus. Operative mortality in craniotomies for intracranial tumors, defined as death occurring prior to discharge from hospital, was 31.9% in the 47 patients reported by Barone and Elvidge in 1970 (7). Curiously, the mortality in the benign group was 36.1% while it was only 18.1% in the group of malignant tumors. More recently, combined operative mortalities of 17% have been reported (33). Unfortunately, the complete removal of fourth ventricular and supratentorial ependymomas is usually not possible; the former often adhere to the floor of the ventricle, and the latter tend to be large and invasive (12). Therefore some form of postoperative irradiation is usually employed. Next to medulloblastomas, ependymomas are the most radiosensitive of all intracranial tumors (34). Because of the propensity of these tumors to metastasize throughout the neuraxis, spinal radiation is often included. In Barone and Elvidge's group (7), there were no examples of spinal spread of tumors, in contrast to the 34% reported by Kim and Fayos (35). Pierre-Kahn et al. (33) have shown that, in pediatric patients, the risk of seeding depends upon the histological type and the location of the original tumors. They therefore recommend craniospinal irradiation (55 Gy) for all children with infratentorial tumors, whether benign or malignant, whole brain irradiation for malignant, supratentorial tumors, and irradiation of only the tumor bed in benign, supratentorial ependymomas. The dose given to infants (less than 2 years old) was between 40 and 50 Gy, to avoid adverse neuropsychological sequelae. Infants with infratentorial tumors did not receive supratentorial irradiation for the same reason. The routine use of CSF cytology or myelography for staging purposes has not achieved wide acceptance in deciding when to use whole neuraxis radiation. The use of CSF filtration (36) and cell culturing techniques may give more accurate results.

With the aggressive use of postoperative radiation therapy, a 69% 10-year survival rate was reported by Salazar et al. in 51 patients (37). This is considerably better than most other series. Benign histological features and a supratentorial location impart only a slightly better chance of survival.

Using microsurgical techniques, even the largest, non-anaplastic, spinal intramedullary tumors can be totally removed, leading to improved neurological function and prolonged survival (16). Anaplastic tumors are not, in general, amenable to total removal, because of their infiltrating nature. In a recent report (16) of 16 cases treated with microsurgical technique, there were no operative mortalities, but both patients with malignant tumors died within 3 years, of brain stem disease. The other patients survived without recurrence, despite the fact that no radiation therapy was given. The two with anaplastic lesions had had spinal cord irradiation up to, but not including, the brain stem. It would therefore seem that radiation therapy is not necessary in totally resected, benign ependymomas of the spine, but that entire neuraxis radiation should be employed in patients with malignant, infiltrating lesions. The efficacy of chemotherapy has not been adequately investigated to support its use. Intrathecal methotrexate and *intravenous* vincristine and cyclophosphamide have been tried (16). Incompletely removed 'benign' ependymomas tend to progress, and reoperation is difficult and may lead to increased neurological deficits because of the disappearance of tissue planes.

Pineal Cell Tumors

This section presents data on pineal tumors of parencymal and glial origin. Chapter 34 discusses these tumors in more detail as well as germ cell tumors and non-neoplastic cysts and vascular lesions.

Incidence

Approximately 0.4 to 1.0% of all intracranial tumors arise from the pineal gland (38). These comprise a family of tumors with different cells of origin, histological appearance, and clinical behaviour. The most common of these, the germinomas, were, in the past, referred to as pinealomas. It is now felt that germinomas do not arise from pineal parenchymal cells but from primitive germ cells (39). Pineal parenchymal cells give rise to two types of tumor, the pineocytoma, and the more malignant pineoblastoma. Intermediate forms have been described. Roughly 20% of pineal region tumors are of pineal parenchymal origin (38, 40). In the 40 cases compiled by Herrick and Rubinstein (40), from their personal experience and from the literature, 43% were pineoblastomas. These tumors usually appear before the age of 20, have been found in newborn infants, and have an overall incidence in the pediatric population of 0.1/million. Males are more frequently affected than females. Tumors seen in older age groups are more likely to be pineocytomas (40).

Lesnick et al. (41) reported two familial pineoblastomas, the first in a 12 year old girl, and the second, discovered only 20 months later, in the girl's 43 year old mother. Knudsen's (42) 'two-hit theory' was evoked to explain this clustering of an extremely rare tumor. Some pineoblastomas may, therefore, arise due to a combined effect of genetic and environmental factors. Another curious entity, which has become known as the 'trilateral retinoblastoma' has been described in a number of children (43–45). This consists of retinoblastomas of both eyes, and a third, retinoblastoma-like tumor of the pineal parenchyma. Seven of the 11 cases reported by Bader et al. (46) had a familial incidence of retinoblastoma. The pineal location of the third tumor is of interest because of the phylogenetic role of the pineal gland as a photoreceptor organ. The relationship of pineoblastoma to retinoblastoma will be discussed further in the following section. The coexistence of a pineoblastoma and a malignant rhabdoid tumor of the kidney has been reported in a single patient (47).

Origin and Pathology

The organ, or gland, from which pineocytomas and pineoblastomas arise, contains not only pineal cells, but also glial and other supportive cells. It is not surprising, therefore, that several varieties of glioma, as well as meningiomas and benign cysts have been described in this region (48). The most common class of tumors, the germ cell tumors, develop from abnormal rests of germ cells, which are not normally found in the pineal gland. The effector cells of the pineal gland are the pineocytes, which are a specialized type of neuroepithelial cell, closely related to neurons. In mammals, they act, not as transmitters of electrochemical signals, but as secretors of melatonin, which is synthesized from tryptophan in a metabolic pathway which involves serotonin and the enzyme hydroxyindole-o-methyltransferase (HIOMT). The role of melatonin is not as well known in humans as in other animals, but changes in serum melatonin concentration have been related to sexual development, sleep induction and mood alteration (49).

Grossly, pineal parenchymal tumors are often indistinguishable from other pineal tumors. The benign ones, pineocytomas, tend to be well-circumscribed masses, while the malignant ones, pineocytomas, are locally invasive and frequently metastasize along the neuraxis (40). Some pineocytomas may behave in this malignant fashion, but their metastases usually have a pineoblastic appearance (40). One instance of metastasis of a pineoblastoma outside the neuraxis has been reported.

In the adult, the normal pineal parenchyma consists of lobules of pineocytes separated by thin connective tissue septa containing blood vessels. Pineocytomas often retain this general architectural appearance. A silver carbonate impregnation technique can be used to help identify tumor cells as having originated from pineal parenchyma (17). The development of a radioimmunoassay for melatonin may also be of diagnostic usefulness in the future. Immunohistochemical staining for placental alkaline phosphatase has been utilized to distinguish between certain germ cell tumors and pineal cell tumors, which do not stain for this enzyme (50).

Pineoblastomas are highly cellular tumors which resemble medulloblastomas, and contain rosettes similar to those found in neuroblastomas (Homer–Wright rosettes), and areas of focal necrosis, hemorrhage and cyst formation. In some cases, retinoblastomatous features may be found, such as Flexner-Wintersteiner rosettes, and fleurettes. It is felt that these may represent abortive attempts towards photoreceptor development within the tumor (40). Further evidence for the relationship between the human pineal gland and retina, and between the malignant tumor arising in these tissues is the finding of immunoreaction of both normal human pineal cells and some pineocytoma cells to a polyclonal antibody against bovine retinal S-antigen (51).

Areas of pineocytic differentiation may also be seen in some pineoblastomas. These tumors will nonetheless behave malignantly. Two cases with both ganglionic and glial differentiation have been reported as well (52). Pineocytomas may contain areas of astrocytic differentiation, neuronal differentiation or both ('ganglioglioma of the pineal'), as ascertained by light and electron microscopy, and by staining for the cell markers neuron-specific enolase, S-100 protein and GFAP (53). Those with astrocytic differentiation may behave malignantly, whereas the other two varieties are generally benign. These histological variants have been well described by Herrick and Rubinstein (40). A malignant variety of pineocytoma, with papillary features, has been described in a single patient (54) (Table 2).

TABLE 2 PINEAL CELL TUMORS

Tumor type	Features of differentiation	Degree of malignancy
Pineoblastoma	None	High
	Pineocytic	High
	Retinoblastomatous	High
	Neuronal and glial	High
Pineocytoma	None	High
	Astrocytic	High or low
	Neuronal	Low
	Mixed glial/neuronal	Low
	Papillary	High

Modified from reference 65.

Clinical and Radiological Findings

The presentation of patients with pineal parenchymal tumors is generally the same as that of patients with other pineal tumors. Expanding masses in this area will compress the midbrain tectum and the sylvian aqueduct. Tectal compression will produce varying degrees of paralysis of upward gaze (Parinaud's syndrome), but may also produce pupillary abnormalities, convergence spasm and retraction nystagmus (55). Aqueductal compression produces signs and symptoms of obstructive hydrocephalus. As tumors continue to grow posteriorly and inferiorly, the cerebellum and superior cerebellar peduncles may be affected, leading to dysmetria, hypotonia and intention tremor (56). Anterior third ventricular spread of malignant tumors, leading to diabetes insipidus, hypopituitarism, precocious puberty and visual field disturbances, has remained only a theoretical possibility for pineablastomas, though it is known to occur in germinomas (38, 55, 56).

Roentgenological studies may be useful in detecting and localizing these tumors, but are often not of great diagnostic specificity (56–58). Plain skull x-rays may show changes of increased intracranial pressure, such as widened cranial sutures, increased digital markings and sellar demineralization. Calcification of greater than 1 cm diameter in the pineal region is suggestive of a pineal tumor as is any calcification in a child less than 6 years old (59). Computed tomography of both pineocytomas and pineoblastomas shows an isodense tumor, with frequent parenchymal calcification and variable areas of contrast enhancement, which may also be seen in germinomas (38, 60). Coronal sections, sagittal reconstruction and metrizamide cisternography may help to identify tentorial meningiomas in this area. Magnetic resonance imaging is as sensitive in detecting pineal region masses as is CT scanning, and is better at delineating anatomical detail, but it is somewhat limited by its inability to detect calcium, and its anticipated tissue specificity has not yet been realized (61). The CT scan remains the preferred modality at present. Angiography in most pineal region tumors will show only vascular displacement, such as posterior shift of the medial posterior choroidal arteries, elevation and stretching of the internal cerebral veins, and posterior shift of the precentral cerebellar vein, due to the mass itself, and stretching of the lateral posterior choroidal arteries from obstructive hydrocephalus (58). The detection of these changes requires both carotid and vertebral angiography.

CSF cytology may be useful in the management of pineal region tumors, in general (38, 62). The sensitivity of this test is increased by culturing Millipore-filtered specimens (63). Differentiation between malignant pineal lesions may be possible, but positive results have not been reported in more than 60% of serially examined cases, more commonly in germinomas than pineoblastomas (38). The measurement of plasma levels of alpha-fetoprotein (AFP) and the beta chain of human chorionic gonadotrophin (beta-hCG) may also, when they are elevated, help to differentiate between germ cell tumors, which produce AFP and beta-hCG, to varying degrees, and pineal parenchymal tumors, which do not (38, 64). Infrequent attempts have been made to measure serum levels of HIOMT and melatonin, as specific markers for pineal cell tumors.

These have met with inconclusive results (64–66). As with the measurement of AFP and beta-hCG in germ cell tumors, these markers may find more usefulness in the detection and management of tumor recurrence or progression, than as an initial diagnostic modality.

Echography has been useful in detecting pineal tumors, which later proved to be pineoblastoma, in two infants reported by Lilue et al. (67).

Treatment and Outcome

The major controversy in the management of pineal tumors in general has been the role of radical surgery, radiation therapy and CSF diversion, in their management (56, 57, 64, 68, 69). As recently as 1973, operative mortality in the resection of pineal tumors was as high as 60%, and 33% for open biopsy alone (70). Since up to 70% of all pineal region tumors are radiosensitive, many surgeons, at that time, favored some form of shunting procedure, to alleviate hydrocephalus, followed by radiation therapy (70–72). However, with the use of the operating microscope, corticosteroids and CSF drainage, operative mortality now approaches 4%, less than the chance of radiating a non-sensitive tumor (38, 68, 73, 74). Several operative approaches to the pineal region have been advocated in the past, but the two most commonly employed today are the infratentorial, supracerebellar approach and the occipital, transtentorial approach, depending on the exact anatomical location and extension of the tumor. A parietal, transcallosal approach is also occasionally utilized. Through these procedures a definitive diagnosis can be made, and as many as 60% of the tumors may undergo gross total excision. Surgical procedures have not been shown to increase the incidence of spinal seeding in malignant pineal tumors (57, 74).

In the absence of sensitive bioassays and specific imaging methods, the diagnosis of pineoblastoma or pineocytoma usually requires histological verification. This may be accomplished in several ways: through open

operations for total resection of tumor, tumor debulking, or biopsy, and by CT-guided stereotactic biopsy. The gross total excision of malignant pineablastomas or pineocytomas does not obviate the use of postoperative craniospinal irradiation. Recently some have recommended stereotactic biopsy, rather than an open procedure, to establish a diagnosis, followed by definitive surgery or radiation (69). However, because of the known intratumoral histological variability (40), and the small amount of tissue obtained via a stereotactic approach, the chance of sampling error is theoretically considerable, and the usefulness of this procedure has yet to be proven. It may not be necessary to obtain a histological diagnosis if there is evidence of CNS or extraneural metastasis, if CSF cytology is positive for malignant cells, or if there is elevated beta-hCG. In these cases a malignant and, therefore, radiosensitive tumour may safely be presumed.

Although there is not enough data concerning the usefulness of radiation therapy in benign pineocytomas, there is considerable support for its use in malignant pineal tumors, which would include pineoblastomas and some pineocytomas, as discussed above (38, 64, 68, 71, 72, 75). Sung et al. (75) have recommended entire neuraxis irradiation for all locally invasive tumors, and have achieved an overall 79% 5-year survival rate in all pineal tumors using a tumor dose of 50 Gy. Others have recommended cranial irradiation alone unless postoperative CSF cytology is positive (76). The caveat is that CSF cytology may be positive in only 25% of patients who have meningeal seeding (75), and the majority of pineoblastomas develop spinal metastases (69). Doses of less than 50 Gy are associated with a higher recurrence rate. Wood et al. (57) have found that the response of pineal cell tumors to radiation therapy was good, but not as dramatic as that of germinomas.

The usefulness of chemotherapy in the treatment of pineal parenchymal tumors has not been established. Regimens of varying combinations of vincristine, methotrexate, cyclophosphamide and CCNU have been attempted, but have not been successful in producing long-term cures (64).

Cerebrospinal fluid diversion, in the form of a shunt or a ventricular drain, has been recommended by many in the management of patients with pineal tumors (68). A potential complication of this is extraneural seeding along shunt pathways. This has not yet been reported in pineal parenchymal tumors. Jooma and Kendall (38) have reported the onset of paraplegia in a 4 year old boy, 3 days after placement of a V-P shunt, from multiple spinal pineoblastoma metastases. A causal relationship between these two events is only speculative. An approach taken by some is to place a ventricular drain preoperatively, for the acute control of intracranial pressure (ICP), which can be either removed or converted into a shunt, if the need for CSF diversion continues postoperatively (68).

Choroid Plexus Papilloma

Incidence and Location

Although choroid plexus papillomas (CPP) comprise less than 1% of tumors arising in people of all ages (17), their distinct tendency to arise in very young patients makes them the second most frequent tumor in infants less than one year of age (12.5 to 17.5%) (77, 78). There may be a slight male preference (79), and genetic factors appear not to play a role (81). Their incidence is said to be increased in neurofibromatosis, in which familial CPPs have been noted (81). Scattered case reports have also been published on the coincidence of CPP with Arnold–Chiari malformation (82), Aicardi's syndrome (agenesis of the corpus callosum, chorioretinal lacunae, seizure disorder, vertebral anomalies and mental retardation) (83, 84), and mumps encephalitis (85). Interestingly, animal models of CPP have been developed in transgenic mice by injecting fertilized eggs with DNA molecules containing both SV40 enhancers and large T-antigen genes (86).

The most frequent location of CPPs is the ventricular system. Lateral ventricular tumors are most common (87, 88) (left greater than right in the older series (89)) followed by fourth ventricular tumors (mostly in adults (90)), and the relatively rare third ventricular tumor (90, 91). Growing from tufts of choroid plexus extending through the foramen of Luschka, papillomas may also present as cerebellopontine (CP) angle tumors (92). These have been reported to invade the adjacent petrous pyramid. Bilateral lateral ventricular tumors are distinctly unusual, occurring in only 7% of the 83 CPPs in Matson and Crofton's review (93).

Origin and Pathology

Choroid plexus papilloma cells have ultra-structural features similar to normal cuboidal and columnar choroidal epithelial cells (94). Aggressive varieties do occur (82, 94–96), some of which have microscopic similarities to embryonal choroid plexus cells and to the Matushima type III cells in adult choroid plexus. These flat cells, lining the papillary crypts, may be underdeveloped type I cells which have not developed the latter's cuboidal or columnar appearance, and secretory differentiation.

The gross appearance of a benign CPP is that of a soft, vascular, purplish or gray, papillary mass which may fill the ventricular cavity it arises in, expand it and protrude from its foramina, but does not invade the surrounding brain (17). Enlarged ventricles may also occur from overproduction of CSF by the tumor, beyond the ability of the normal CSF absorptive pathways to compensate (97), or from repeated bleeding from the tumour causing basal subarachnoid scarring and obstruction of CSF pathways (96, 98), or by blockage of the ventricular foramina by the tumor itself (80, 99).

Microscopically, benign choroid plexus tumors maintain the overall structure of normal choroid plexus, with its delicate papillary formations of single layers of epithelial cells on a stroma of slender, vascular connective tissue.

Small intratumoral hemorrhages and foci of calcification may also be seen (17). A variant with mucus-secreting cells has also been reported (100), as have 3 cases of CPPs containing bone (101). This later occurrence may be the end stage of mucoid degeneration of the tumor stroma (101). Two cases of an oncocytic variant, whose cells were identical to oncocytes of the thyroid, bronchus, kidney and salivary gland, have also been described (102). Some tumors also have cells with cilia and blepharoplasts on electron microscopy.

Exact criteria for the histological diagnosis of malignant, or aggressive, choroid plexus tumors, also known as choroid plexus carcinoma, have been difficult to agree upon, because their morphology frequently fails to predict their biological behavior (82). Commonly accepted criteria include the local invasion of brain, an ill-defined growth pattern, loss of papillary architecture at the site of invasion, a transition from normal to abnormal choroidal epithelium, mitoses, and areas of cellular pleomorphism (82, 96, 103). The same tumor may, therefore, possess both benign and malignant-looking regions. However, tumors which are otherwise histologically benign may invade brain, while malignant ones may behave benignly (93, 104), and either may seed throughout the CSF pathways. Two CPPs have been reported to seed to extraneural locations, in the lungs (105) and bone (106). The lateral ventricular tumors of children tend to be more malignant, and metastasize more frequently, than the fourth ventricular tumors of adults.

The histological differential diagnosis of choroid plexus papillomas includes papillary ependymoma, xanthogranuloma of the choroid plexus and adenocarcinoma metastatic to the choroid plexus (17).

Clinical and Radiological Findings

Childhood choroid plexus papillomas usually present with hydrocephalus, leading to increased ICP, papilledema, macrocephaly, irritability, and vomiting. Tumors in the lateral ventricles may produce hemiparesis (80). Those expanding in the fourth ventricle may cause cerebellar dysfunction, and if extending into the CP angle, cranial nerve dysfunction (92). Third ventricular tumors may present with diencephalic autonomic seizures, Parinaud's syndrome, obesity, precocious puberty and diabetes insipidus (91). Seizures and psychomotor retardation have been the presenting symptoms in some infants. In adult patients, the progression of hydrocephalus and increased ICP may be gradual, leading to headaches and problems with mentation (80). The presentation may also be acute, with intraventricular hemorrhage (107).

Elevated CSF protein levels are found in over two-thirds of patients (108). Low CSF protein has also been reported, however. Xanthochromia of the CSF is often found, and an elevated CSF pressure is almost universal (108). The overproduction of CSF has been causally related to the development of rhinorrhea in one patient (109). CSF cytology has not been successfully used to predict CSF metastases, which occur in 20% of all tumors, and in 44% of the malignant ones (82). The metastases from benign tumors tend to be benign clinically as well as histologically and often are detected only as incidental findings on postmortem examinations.

The radiological procedure of choice is the CT scan (79), which has almost entirely replaced the poorly tolerated pneumoencephalogram (110). Choroid plexus tumors enhance strikingly with contrast. The enhancement is usually homogeneous. Benign and aggressive CPP can be differentiated with CT, the former being of more uniform density on pre-contrast examination, and better delineated from brain parenchyma (110, 111). The degree of hydrocephalus is usually less in malignant than benign tumors. Plan skull x-rays often reveal non-specific changes of increased ICP, and 21% of pediatric cases may show tumor calcification (80).

Angiography usually shows a tumor blush and feeding through the choroidal arteries (110). Because of its usefulness in planning the operative approach, it should be performed in all suspected cases. Early draining veins, a sign of arteriovenous shunting, may be indicative of a malignant tumor (112).

With the combination of real-time and pulsed Doppler sonography, the detection of a CPP in an infant, and its differentiation from an intraventricular hematoma, has been possible. The tumor was uniformly echogenic on real-time ultrasound, and the pulsed Doppler technique revealed the tumor neovascularity (111).

The value of MRI in the evaluation of these tumors is still unknown.

Treatment and Outcome

As with all intraventricular tumors, the primary therapeutic modality is surgery. Microsurgical technique and the early interruption of the tumor's blood supply are important for a successful outcome. The complete removal of fourth ventricular tumors may be expected in most cases (80). This may be difficult in those growing through the foramen of Luschka into the CP angle. Tumors of the lateral ventricles may also be difficult to remove totally, as they can invade adjacent brain. Operative mortalities as low as 9% have been reported (88). This is less with fourth ventricular than with lateral ventricular tumors. Morbidity is also dependent on tumor location, upon the amount of operative damage to adjacent structures, and the degree and duration of hydrocephalus (113). Hydrocephalus is alleviated in many patients following surgery, but in roughly 50% it will persist, requiring the placement of a permanent shunt (88, 114). Shunting, in lieu of tumor resection, is not only ineffective, but was associated with the accelerated growth of a third ventricular tumor reported by Safdari et al. (115).

The role of radiation therapy in the treatment of CPP is somewhat controversial. Because of the high incidence of spinal metastases in histologically malignant tumors, craniospinal irradiation has been recommended for all such lesions (82). If a benign tumour can be totally removed, there appears to be little to gain by radiation therapy, as the spinal metastases originating from benign tumors usually remain asymptomatic, and the risk of radiation-induced damage to the nervous system is significant, particularly in younger patients (108). In patients with histologically benign tumors which cannot be totally removed, or are found, at operation, to be invasive, a good argument can be made for close observation and radiation if tumor growth or recurrence is detected. Radiation therapy as a primary modality does not reduce tumor bulk but may decrease its vascularity (116).

The outcome in infants with CPP tends to be poor, with only one of the 14 infants reported by Pascual-Castroviejo et al. (79) leading a normal life. Nine had died within 3 years. Persistent hydrocephalus, mental retardation and tumor recurrence were the major reasons for poor outcome. Postoperative seizures may also occur in patients following the removal of supratentorial tumors. Adults and older children have a better chance of obtaining a satisfactory result. Recurrences have been reported after disease-free intervals of as long as 19 years (117). Therefore, any study of the effectiveness of any treatment modality must utilize a long follow-up period.

Astrocytic Tumors

Astroblastoma

An unusual tumor felt to arise from mature astrocytes, the astroblastoma comprises 0.45 to 5% of all gliomas (118). The first description of the tumor, by Bailey and Cushing, was in 1926 (119). Bailey and Bucy's series (120) consisted of 25 case reports some of which may not have been pure astroblastomas (17). It is important to differentiate between the pure tumor and anaplastic astrocytomas or glioblastomas with astroblastomatous regions, because the former has a more benign clinical course (121). The exact origin of the astroblast is still uncertain. The original view was that it arose at an intermediate stage between spongioblast and astrocyte (120), but the possibility of its dedifferentiation from mature astroglial cells cannot be, at present, ruled out (96).

Astroblastomas are usually found in the cerebral hemispheres of young adults (120, 121), but they have been reported in all age groups from infancy to middle age (122). Unusual locations for astroblastomas are the corpus callosum (123), cerebellum (120, 124), optic nerve (118), brain stem (118) and cauda equina (125). Tsuchida et al. have reported an astroblastoma as one of four brain tumors found in patients with tuberous sclerosis (18).

Grossly the tumors are well circumscribed, pink or gray, and soft. Large cysts may be present (17). Microscopically, a characteristic feature are uniform cells, arranged in perivascular pseudorosettes, which may be confused with those seen in ependymomas. Unlike ependymomas, however, silver impregnation stains show foot processes extending to the vessel walls, true rosettes are never found, and there is no ultrastructural evidence of a ciliary apparatus. The tumors are highly cellular and vascular. Mitoses are infrequent but large areas of necrosis may be present accompanied by mesenchymal proliferation. Unlike gemistocytic astrocytomas, which may also have perivascular pseudorosettes, the cells in astroblastomas are poorly fibrillated (17). However, abundant glial intermediate filaments have been described on GFAP staining (121, 122), and ultrastructurally (121, 126), in some cases.

The biological behavior of pure astroblastomas is hard to define because of the scarcity and elusiveness of this tumor. A variety of different outcomes have been reported and recommendations made (18, 124, 127). A fairly consistent theme has been the ease of their gross total resection because of their circumscribed nature. Postoperative radiation therapy to the tumor site is generally recommended, as well as surgery, but recurrence after only 16 months has been reported despite radiation therapy (121). On the other hand, at least one tumor has failed to recur after 5 years, without radiation (124).

Gemistocytic Astrocytomas

As with the astroblastoma, a controversy exists about the occurrence of this tumor in a pure form. They share certain histological and biological features, in that the gemistocytic astrocytoma is found primarily in the cerebral hemispheres of adults, is well circumscribed and soft, and may contain perivascular pseudorosettes. However, these are not as prominent as in astroblastomas (17). The cells are not as uniform in appearance, have more prominent and eccentric nuclei, are more angular in shape, frequently have the characteristic swollen appearance of gemistocytes, and contain more neuroglial fibers. Experimental evidence suggests that gemistocytes arise in areas of relatively intense cellular proliferation with an attendant, rapid utilization of nutrients, which become insufficient for normal growth (128). They are therefore associated with biologically aggressive tumors. Rubinstein has found that many gemistocytic astrocytomas do undergo malignant transformation (17), and surgical resection followed by irradiation has been recommended for them. He has also reported an example associated with long-standing multiple sclerosis (17).

Subependymal Giant Cell Astyrocytomas

These unusual tumors are typically encountered in patients with tuberous sclerosis. They originate from the 'candle gutterings' found lining the lateral ventricular walls (17, 129). Giant, irregular cells are seen microscopically, often forming a streaming pattern, or even perivascular pseudorosettes. Some tumors contain cells which resemble ganglion cells, but neurofibrils cannot be demonstrated, and neoplastic nerve cells are rarely, if ever, present. The giant cells have been identified as monstrous astrocytes in tissue culture studies (130). Many features bespeak a benign biological behavior, such as infrequent mitoses, lack of vascular endothelial proliferation, and focal deposits of calcium (17).

Subependymal giant cell astrocytomas

generally remain asymptomatic but may present with obstructive hydrocephalus due to blockage of the foramen of Monro. Plain x-rays show calcification in two-thirds of the tumor. They are easily discerned on contrast enhanced CT. Surgical resection of the symptomatic tumors has been recommended (129). This may not even be necessary, if a ventricular shunt is placed. There is no role for radiation or chemotherapy in the treatment of these tumors. The stigmata of tuberous sclerosis will, of course, remain, even if the tumor is totally resected.

Poorly Differentiated and Embryonal Tumors

Primitive Polar Spongioblastoma (PPS)

Very few examples of pure primitive polar spongioblastoma have been reported in the world literature. It is a tumor of childhood, almost always arising before the age of 20. Most examples have been located near the third or fourth ventricles, and they may be attached to the ventricular wall (17, 124, 131).

Grossly the tumors usually appear well demarcated, though they tend to be focally invasive, making their total removal impossible. Like other primitive CNS tumors, they also have a tendency to metastasize, via CSF pathways, throughout the neuraxis (132). Histologically, they have a highly recognizable appearance, in which the cells are lined up in characteristic, parallel arrays, which form bands separated by a vascular connective tissue stroma (17). Tumors in which similar palisading may be found, and from which PPS must be differentiated, are medulloblastomas and oligodendrogliomas. The cells are morphologically similar to the migrating spongioblasts seen in the human embryo cerebrum at 10 to 18 weeks of gestation (17). The tumors may have areas of differentiation, where the picture is akin to the benign cerebellar astrocytoma of childhood, and individual, small, stellate fibrillary astrocytes may also be found (17). Vascular endothelial proliferation and

other signs of malignancy are usually not found, but this belies their aggressive biological behavior.

Their rapid growth, invasive nature, central location, and tendency to metastasize make the primitive polar spongioblastoma a very difficult lesion to treat. Therefore, their prognosis is thought to be poor. However, the tumor described by Steinberg et al. (124) was stable 15 years following subtotal resection and radiation therapy. Since significant tumor resection is usually not achievable, craniospinal irradiation alone may offer the best hope for palliation or cure (17). Rubinstein feels that the presence of extensive areas of differentiation in some tumors may be prognostic of a more favorable outcome (17). There is not enough data on either radiation therapy or chemotherapy to indicate their efficacy in treating this type of tumor.

Medulloepithelioma

An entity about which there has been considerable taxonomic controversy is the medulloepithelioma. This tumor was originally a mere hypothesis of Bailey and Cushing (119), representing the most primitive possible neoplasm of the CNS. Since the first case report in 1957 (133), there have been over twenty acceptable examples in the literature (134). As implied by Bailey and Cushing's definition, this tumor is characterized by the ability to exhibit areas of differentiation to any stage of cytogenesis of any central nervous system cell type, neuronal, glial, ependymal or choroidal (135–137). Metaplasia within the connective tissue stroma of some tumors has been reported, leading to bone, cartilage and muscle formation (139). True myogenic differentiation may also be possible (139), as in the exceedingly rare cerebellar medullomyoblastoma (140). Areas of differentiation may be delineated with monoclonal antibodies to GFAP, neurofilament and desmin, the major intermediate filament proteins of astrocytes, neurons and muscle cells, respectively. The putative anlage from which this tumor develops is the neural tube and primitive medullary plate (17, 138, 140).

Medulloepitheliomas usually arise in early childhood and in the cerebral hemispheres. Congenital examples have been noted (133), as have locations within the cerebellum, brainstem and spine (136, 142). They are usually well demarcated, pink and friable, and have focal areas of hemorrhage and necrosis (17). They may invade the leptomeninges and dura, and distant metastases to lymph nodes have been reported (143). The microscopic picture is reminiscent of the primitive medullary epithelium, with medium or tall columnar cells arranged in papillary and tubular arrays (17). Mitotic figures are numerous and are located more frequently in the nuclei of cells near the luminal side of the tubules. The cellular ultrastructure is also similar to that of the fetal neural tube (138).

Again, the behavior of medulloepitheliomas is typical of embryonal tumors. Both neuraxis and extraneural spread of tumors have been reported. The prognosis is generally poor, and the ability of radiation therapy to improve outcome is unknown.

Gliomatosis Cerebri

This very rare tumor consists of a widespread malignant transformation of glial cells, most commonly found in association with anaplastic astrocytomas (144). It has been found associated with neurofibromatosis and tuberous sclerosis (17). Because of its diffuse nature, it may not cause a focal mass effect. The cells are elongated, and spread beneath the ependyma and along the molecular layer. Its treatment consists of biopsy, radiation and chemotherapy. The prognosis is similar to that of other anaplastic astrocytomas (145).

Neuronal Tumors

Neuronal tumors comprise about 0.5 to 2% of all brain tumors (146, 147). They are far more common as tumors of the paraganglionic and autonomic nervous systems. The WHO has divided neuronal brain tumors into five categories: neuroblastoma, gangliocytoma, ganglioglioma, ganglioneuroblastoma, and anaplastic gangliocytoma and ganglioglioma. The designation of a given tumor depends upon its specific association of immature neuroblasts, abnormal ganglion cells, and normal, neoplastic or anaplastic glial cells. This often proves to be difficult to determine because of the presence of transitional forms, a wide variety of contributions from different cell types, heterogeneity within the same tumor, and the ability of some tumors to undergo spontaneous differentiation or dedifferentiation over time (2, 148). Table 3 shows the predominant cell types involved in the different tumors. A major problem in the histological diagnosis of many of these tumors is the differentiation between neoplastic ganglion cells and normal neurons. Silver impregnation, stains for Nissl substance (17), and immunohistological staining with monoclonal antibodies for intermediate filaments and cell surface antigens (149, 150), are

TABLE 3 TUMORS OF NEURONAL ORIGIN

Tumor type	Neuroblasts	Ganglion cells	Non-neoplastic glial cells	Neoplastic glial cells	Anaplastic glial cells
Neuroblastoma	+	−	−	−	−
Gangliocytoma (ganglioneuroma)	−	+	+	−	−
Ganglioglioma	−	+	−	+	−
Ganglioneuroblastoma	+	+	−	−	−
Anaplastic gangliocytoma (hypothetical)	−	+	+	+	+
Anaplastic ganglioglioma	−	+	−	+	+

useful in delineating the neuronal and glial components of the tumors.

Neuroblastoma

Incidence and location. There are two types of neuroblastoma, peripheral and central. The peripheral tumors are one of the three most common tumors found in children, and will not be discussed in detail. The primary neuroblastoma of the brain, however, is quite rare, and is clinically distinct from its more common relative (151). Bennett and Rubinstein's series of 70 patients (152), compiled through an extensive referral network, is the largest series reported on.

Their tumors arose from any location within the cerebral hemispheres; none were found in the cerebellum, brainstem or spinal cord. Leptomeningeal or ventricular spread was found in 38. A rare case of extraneural metastasis has also been reported (153). Over 80% of the cases were diagnosed in the first decade of life; 26% were younger than 2 years old. There was no sex difference.

Origin and pathology. The cell of origin is the immature neuroblast (17, 151). There are two main histological pictures. In the 'classical' variety, sheets of small cells, with round or oval, darkly staining nuclei, are separated by sparse stroma. They frequently contained Homer–Wright rosettes, and mitotic figures were abundant. In the 'desmoplastic' variant, dense connective tissue stroma divides the tumor into lobules which are often distinguishable grossly. This variety is found more frequently in younger patients, and the fibrous tissue is particularly abundant when the leptomeninges have been invaded (154). It is not of particular prognostic or therapeutic significance (152). Transitional types between the two have been described. Both varieties may contain areas in which the cells have become differentiated into ganglion cells. Ganglionic differentiation is not correlated with increased survival. In the less differentiated areas, cells

tend to be unstainable by the standard silver impregnation techniques for neuroblast processes and neurofibrils. Differentiation from other primitive neuroepithelial tumors may be accomplished using electron microscopic (EM) techniques (155, 156). Characterization may also be done with monoclonal antibody panels, as reported by Coakham and Brownell (150). The tumors, though not encapsulated, do have a distinct border with the surrounding brain (151). A cardinal feature is that of dense reactive gliosis around the lesions (17).

Clinical and radiological findings. Clinically, approximately half of the patients present with signs of increased intracranial pressure. A significant number, about 35% in Bennett and Rubinstein's series (152), presented with focal or generalized seizures, and about 20% had focal neurological deficits. These tumors do not grow as rapidly as the other primitive tumors, so the interval between onset of symptoms and diagnosis may be as long as 9 years. However, most are between a couple of weeks and a couple of months.

Radiographic studies of the tumors are non-specific. CT scans without contrast usually show a hypodense, hemispheric lesion, which may contain cysts or flecks of calcium (152, 157, 158). Enhancement is moderate to marked, and peritumoral edema is highly variable. Erosion of the inner table of the skull may be seen (158) on plain x-rays as well as CT, and tumor calcification on plain x-ray has been reported (159). Angiography usually shows an avascular mass, but may show faint neovascularity (157, 158). Very little data has been published on the MRI appearance of cerebral neuroblastoma.

Of some interest is the fact that, unlike peripheral neuroblastomas, urine and plasma catecholamine and catecholamine metabolite levels have rarely been found to be elevated (152, 157, 159, 160). Only one such case has been reported, to our knowledge (155). Results of CSF measurements have not apparently been reported. CSF cytology may be positive, though the incidence of this finding, and its sensitivity in detecting neuraxis metastases, are unknown.

Treatment and outcome. As this tumor is morphologically similar to other primitive neuroepithelial tumors at operation, gross total resection is the initial treatment of choice, but it may be difficult to achieve. This should be followed by radiation therapy to the tumor bed plus a wide margin (157), although some have recommended entire neuraxis radiation (152). The efficacy of radiation therapy has not been conclusively demonstrated, nor has that of chemotherapy, which, when used, has consisted of a variety of different regimens (152, 157). They have been used primarily when a solid tumor could not be totally resected.

Survival of patients with primary cerebral neuroblastoma depends on the age at diagnosis. As in the medulloblastomas, these tumors, in young children, seem to follow Collins' law (161) for the period of risk of tumor recurrence (152). The 3-year survival rate is approximately 60%, and the 5-year rate may exceed 30% (152). In the series of Berger et al. (157) the 6 patients with cystic tumors had no recurrence and, of the 5 with solid tumors, all recurred, except the one who had received adjuvant chemotherapy; none of these had undergone gross total resection, however.

Ganglioglioma

Incidence and location. Gangliogliomas of the brain are also rarer than their counterparts in the peripheral nervous system. The term was first introduced by Courville in 1930 (162) to describe a group of tumors consisting of a mixture of astrocytic and neuronal cells in varying stages of differentiation. These tumors must be distinguished from those astrocytomas where, at the periphery, normal neurons may be interspersed among infiltrating, neoplastic glial cells. This distinction is important to make because the biological behavior of the two tumors is quite different (17, 163).

Gangliogliomas arise most commonly in

children and young adults. The mean age, 17 years old in one recent series (163), and 27.5 in another (164), is somewhat greater than that of neuroblastomas. They comprised 0.6% of 998 tumors reviewed by Demierre et al. (164) and have been reported in as many as 1.7 to 7.6% of pediatric CNS tumors (163, 165). They are found most frequently in the temporal lobe, but may also be found in the cerebellum, parieto-occipital lobe, frontal lobe, thalamus, pineal region, spinal cord (164, 166, 167), and optic nerve (168). Gangliogliomas have been reported in association with tuberous sclerosis (169).

Pathology and origin. They are usually easy to dissect from brain, though their solid portion may be infiltrative. Cystic areas, and calcification, are frequently found (17). On microscopic examination the appearance may vary considerably, even within a single tumor, depending on the relative proportion of gliomatous and gangliomatous elements. The glial cells are usually GFAP positive, may contain Rosenthal fibers, and are identifiable on PTAH staining (163, 164). Occasionally, oligodendroglial cells may be seen (17). The ganglion cells, in contradistinction to normal neurons, have randomly oriented, often tortuous cell processes, vary in size and shape, and occasionally are binucleated (17). They are recognizable by the presence of Nissl substance, and stain immunohistochemically for neurofilament protein. Paired helical filaments, characteristic of the neurofibrillary tangles seen in neuronal degenerative diseases, have also been described in a single tumor, but not in cell lines derived from it (170). Their significance is unknown. The more primitive, bipolar or unipolar neuroblastic cell may occasionally be found. However, when anaplastic features are encountered, it is usually confined to the glial elements. Recently Van den Berg et al. have described a distinct subgroup of ganglioglioma, characterized by intense desmoplasia, occurrence in infancy, large size, and divergent differentiation potential (171).

Ganglion cells probably represent a stage of arrested neuronal cytogenesis early on in the development of the CNS. There is some controversy about whether ganglioglioma, as well as gangliocytomas, are essentially hamartomatous in nature. This may be the case in patients whose symptoms, usually epilepsy, have been of long standing, since childhood (172), but most of them behave clinically as expanding neoplastic lesions. They may represent hamartomas which have undergone neoplastic transformation (164, 173). An extension of this process would lead to transitional forms of the tumor towards neuroblastomas. Such lesions have been described, but these rare tumors may also be thought of as differentiating neuroblastomas, so the controversy remains (17).

Clinical and radiological findings. Seizure disorders are the most frequent presentation of gangliogliomas (164), though progressive focal neurological deficit, emotional disturbances, diabetes insipidus, obesity, headache and papilledema are not uncommon findings (17, 163, 164).

Radiologically, calcifications may be seen on skull x-ray as well as in CT scans (164). On CT, the lesions may be quite large, but do not necessarily produce mass effect, which is consistent with their slow growth rate (174, 175). More than two-thirds have low density areas on non-contrast scans, and less than half enhance with contrast (176). This may make it difficult to define the tumor border on CT. In a recent series of gangliogliomas, MRI was felt to be superior to CT in discriminating neoplastic from normal tissue, and, therefore, in preoperative planning and postoperative monitoring for tumor recurrence (164). Angiography does not offer much useful information, as most of these tumors are avascular masses, but some of them may demonstrate neovascularity (164, 177).

Treatment and outcome. Total surgical resection, when feasible, is the treatment of choice (163, 164, 174). Operative mortality and morbidity is generally quite low. Electrophysiological recording techniques, such as stereotactic electroencephalography (EEG), may be a useful adjunctive means of resecting epileptogenic regions adjacent to some of the tumors, thereby alleviating their most common symptom, seizures (164). The value of radiotherapy is still not known. Most authors recommend careful follow-up with CT, and local radiation if recurrence is detected (165, 174). These tumors grow slowly and are therefore compatible with long-term survival in most patients. Of interest was the finding by Johannsson, et al. (163), that, even if the tumor shows anaplastic features in the glial cells, it behaves more benignly than a histologically similar astrocytoma would. In four of their cases, they were able to compare specimens of tumors removed at different times, from 1 to 14 years apart. None of the tumors had altered the density or degree of maturation of its ganglion cells, and in only one tumor had the glial cells become more malignant morphologically. In this specimen, vascular proliferation had also occurred. Gangliogliomas may undergo malignant anaplasia after many years (96).

Gangliocytoma

This tumor, also referred to as ganglioneuroma, more closely fits the criteria for a hamartoma. It consists of masses of ganglion cells interspersed with relatively little or no glial component. These glia are non-neoplastic. Rubinstein believes that this tumor merely represents one end of the spectrum of ganglioglioma, but that it is distinct from them in its lack of malignant potential (2, 17). Gangliocytomas comprise about 0.1 to 0.5% of all brain tumors (96, 166, 178). There is no sex preference, and patient's ages may range from 4 to 69 years old, with a tendency towards the younger age groups. Their most frequent site of origin is the floor of the third ventricle, but they may be found elsewhere in the cerebrum, cerebellum and spinal cord (17). Four cases of pineal gangliocytoma have been described (178). Intrasellar gangliocytomas have been found, and the term 'choristoma' has been applied to them (179).

The most frequent clinical symptom, as with gangliogliomas, are seizures. Focal deficits are less common than in the latter tumor. They are frequently found by chance, either at autopsy or on CT scan. An interesting report has been published of six hypothalamic gangliocytomas which were found to produce growth hormone-releasing factors in patients with acromegaly (180).

The CT appearance is as variable as that of gangliogliomas, with inconsistent patterns of cystic and calcified regions, and contrast enhancement. The usefulness of MRI is not yet known. Isotope brain scanning may be helpful in certain cases (178).

The location of these lesions may make any operative procedure, other than a biopsy, too risky to undertake. In this case, the patient should be followed with serial CT scans. Radiation therapy is not thought to be of value with these benign lesions.

An interesting variant of gangliocytoma, the 'dysplastic gangliocytoma of the cerebellum' has been described. It is also known as 'Purkinjioma' and 'Lhermitte–Duclos disease' (181, 182). In this disease, large areas of hyperplastic cerebellar folia are found. Their cytoarchitecture is abnormal. Associated findings are mental retardation and megalencephaly. A diffuse form, affecting most of a cerebral hemisphere, has also been reported (183).

Ganglioneuroblastomas, Anaplastic Gangliocytomas and Anaplastic Gangliogliomas

These extremely uncommon tumors represent forms of the previously mentioned tumors in which one or more element has become either more differentiated or anaplastic. In ganglioneuroblastomas, ganglion cells and neuroblasts coexist. This could represent either a gangliocytoma in which the ganglion cells in some areas have dedifferentiated, or a neuroblastoma with areas of maturation (17). Similar derivations may be postulated for the anaplastic gangliocytoma and the anaplastic ganglioglioma (2, 17). The former tumor, so far, remains hypothetical, as no examples which would fit its criteria have, to our knowledge, been reported.

On Primitive Neuroectodermal Tumors

Throughout this chapter, there has been a recurrent theme. Several tumors have been discussed which have similar histological and clinical characteristics: ependymoblastoma, pineoblastoma, primitive polar spongioblastoma, medulloepithelioma, and cerebral neuroblastoma. These are highly cellular, poorly differentiated tumors which occasionally show signs of ganglionic or glial differentiation, or divergent differentiation, and may contain pseudorosette formation. They arise in infants, young children, or adolescents. They progress rapidly, and frequently metastasize along the neuraxis and, occasionally, extraneurally. They tend to be radiosensitive, but are usually associated with a poor outcome. These tumors are members of a group which also includes the more common medulloblastoma and retinoblastoma. Collectively, they have been called embryonal tumors, or primitive neuroectodermal tumors (PNETs).

We have avoided using this term thus far because of the considerable differences of opinion among neuropathologists about its precise nosological significance. By its most restrictive definition, Hart and Earle, who coined the term in 1973 (1984), indicated a group of supratentorial tumors, in which over 90% of the cells were undifferentiated, but which showed the ability to differentiate along neuronal or glial lines or both. Others have used the term interchangeably with 'cerebral neuroblastoma' (158, 185, 186). Becker and Hinton (187) and Rorke (188) have recommended that until the cytogenetic origin of all embryonal tumors is better understood, the term PNET should be applied to all such tumors, with qualifying descriptors of location and differentiation being used in specific instances.

TABLE 4 PRIMITIVE NEUROEPITHELIAL TUMORS

Cell of origin	Tumor type	Potential differentiation
Primitive ventricular matrix	Medulloepithelioma	Glial, neuronal ependymal
Undifferentiated bipotential or multipotential neuroepithelial cells	Medulloblastoma	Glial, neuronal, muscle, melanin
	PNET of the cerebrum	Glial, neuronal
Ependymoblast	Ependymoblastoma	Ependymal, glial
Pineoblast	Pineoblastoma	Pineocytic, glial, neuronal, photosensory
Glioblast (?radial glia)	Primitive polar spongioblastoma	Astrocytic, oligodendroglial
Neuroblast	Neuroblastoma	Neuronal
Retinoblast	Retinoblastoma	Neuroblastic, photosensory
Primitive olfactory epithelium	Esthesioneuroblastoma	Olfactory, neuronal, APUD

APUD = amine precursor uptake and decarboxylation.
Modified from reference 134.

They cite limitations in sampling by surgical biopsy, and lack of adequate immunological tumor markers as a rationale for this 'lumping'. On the other hand, Rubinstein (134, 189) has favored treating the distinct histological patterns as separate entities because of their different cystogenetic potentials (Table 4).

Thus, among the tumors which would formerly have been called cerebral medulloblastomas, the neuroblastoma is distinguished by its ability to differentiate only into ganglionic forms. Like the medulloblastomas, they occur in a 'desmoplastic' variety. The 'cerebral PNET' of Hart and Earle is similar, but may undergo both glial and ganglionic differentiation, being a supratentorial analog of the cerebellar medulloblastoma (184). Recently electron microscopy has been utilized to define an uncommon variety of neuroblastoma of the cerebellum (190–192). This may represent what would be the equivalent of a medulloblastoma arising from the external granular layer of the cerebellar cortex (where the cells have only neurogenic potential), as opposed to those arising from the more primitive germinal cells of the posterior medullary vellum, considered to be the source of most medulloblastomas (134).

Rubinstein (134) prefers to refer to the group of embryonal tumors as primitive neuroepithelial tumors, with cytogenetic potentials which depend on the developmental stage, or 'window', in which each arose. For some, even mesenchymal differentiation has been found, such as the rare medullomyoblastoma (140). Isolated instances of pigmented pineoblastomas and medulloblastomas have also been documented (193, 194). It seems that both the nosological 'splitters' and 'lumpers' will have to rely upon improved immunohistochemical, electron microscopic, and other diagnostic techniques, before their differences can be resolved.

TUMORS AND MALFORMATIONS OF VASCULAR ORIGIN

Hemangioblastoma

Incidence and Location

In various series, hemangioblastomas constitute 1.0 to 2.5% of all primary CNS tumors (195). As most of them arise in the posterior fossa in adults, they make up 7 to 12% of adult posterior fossa tumors. Although they may occur in any age group, from 3 years to the ninth decade, the average age at diagnosis is in the thirties. There is a definite male preponderance in some series (196–198). From 2 to 8% of hemangioblastomas are found in the supratentorial compartment (195, 199), and a spinal, intramedullary location is also uncommon (200, 201). A single suprasellar tumor which presented with amenorrhea–galactorrhea has been reported (202). Of the posterior fossa tumors, about 70% are located in the cerebellar hemispheres, usually in a paramedian position, 15% are in the vermis, 5% in the floor of the fourth centricle, 5% elsewhere in the brainstem, and about 3% in the CP angle. Frequently the tumors are multiple (198, 203), and there is about a 12% incidence of other members of the patient's family having vascular tumors of the CNS or other organs (198). This latter finding is usually a hallmark of von Hippel–Lindau disease (VHL) (195).

Lindau's tumor is an eponym for a hemangioblastoma of the cerebellum occurring in VHL disease (195). It is associated with different combinations of retinal angiomatosis, renal carcinoma, cysts of the kidney and pancreas, and abnormalities of the epididymis (204). VHL disease is an autosomal dominantly inherited syndrome with incomplete penetrance. Members within the same family may present with either one or a combination of the above-mentioned stigmata. Retinal tumors have been found in about 15% of all patients with cerebellar hemangioblastomas, and cerebellar lesions are found in about 20% of patients with retinal hemangioblastomas. The most widely accepted, minimal criteria for the diagnosis of VHL disease, in patients with cerebellar hemangioblastoma, is the presence of multiple CNS hemangioblastomas, the coexistence of a single CNS tumor with one or more of the other characteristic manifestations, or a familial history of the disease (205–207). About two-thirds of patients with VHL disease will have cerebellar hemangioblastomas (206). A number of less common lesions are seen in VHL disease. These include bilateral pheochromocytoma, cysts of the liver, lung, ovary, spleen, or omentum, syringomyelia in patients with spinal hemangioblastomas, and a variety of angiomas or carcinomas in other visceral locations (208).

Hemangioblastomas are the only primary CNS neoplasms which are associated with polycythemia. This occurs more frequently in the solid variety of hemangioblastoma (196,

209). It is felt that, like renal cell carcinoma, hepatic carcinoma and uterine fibroma, they produce an erythropoietic substance (210).

Origin

Hemangioblastomas have been known by many other names, including hemangioma, hemangioendothelioma, capillary hemangioblastoma, capillary hemangioendothelioma, hemangioperithelioma, and angioreticuloma (17, 208). This is but a small indication of the confusion which has existed over the origin and classification of this tumor. It was felt by Cushing and Bailey (211) to originate from endothelial cells, and was given the name hemangioblastoma to differentiate it from 'hemangiomas' of the CNS, which were felt to be more hamartomatous than neoplastic. The principal issues in the classification of hemangioblastomas have been if, and where, they fit into the subgroup of meningeal tumors called angioblastic meningioma, and how they are related to hemangiopericytomas (17). They have been equated with hemangiopericytoma by some authors (212), but their relatively benign behavior and distinct macroscopic and ultrastructural (213, 214) appearance, and the lack of hemangiopericytomas in cases of VHL disease would imply that they should be considered as a separate entity (195). Some feel that they should be considered the benign variety of angioblastic meningioma, while hemangiopericytomas are the malignant variety (96, 214). In the WHO classification scheme, they are not considered to be of meningeal, but of vascular, origin.

In his original work on hemangioblastomas, Lindau hypothesized that their cells of origin were primordial mesenchymal cells, destined to become the choroid plexus of the fourth ventricle, which somehow became engulfed in the substance of the developing cerebellum (215). In support of this are the facts that the embryonal choroid plexus serves an erythopoietic function, and the vast preponderance of the tumors in the posterior fossa (208). It does not, however, explain their occurrence in other locations. Another hypothesis is that the tumors originate from pial cells which undergo conversion to endothelial cells (216). There is certainly a marked proliferation of endothelial cells in these tumors, and most of the tumors are said to be continuous with a pial surface at some point. However, the actual interconversion of these two cell types has not been documented with currently available techniques, including tissue culture (214), and this theory fails to explain the predominance of tumors in the posterior fossa. There is, in effect, no satisfactory explanation of the origin of these tumors.

Pathology

Four morphological forms of the tumor have been described: (198) the simple cyst (6%), with clear cyst fluid and no evidence of a mural nodule, the macrocystic form, with a mural nodule (65%), the microcystic form, with cysts only a few millimeters in diameter (4%), and the solid form, which is found in a greater percentage of the supratentorial tumors (217), and has less well-defined borders (25%). Rarely do these tumors give rise to neuraxis metastases, and then only after a surgical procedure (218). Solid posterior fossa tumors are more likely to involve the cerebellar peduncles and the brainstem (219). In cystic lesions, the cyst fluid may contain over 5 g/ml protein (220), and erythropoietin (221).

Histologically the tumors have a benign appearance which contradicts their name. Mitoses are not seen but some cells may be binucleated. With light microscopy, the cells can be differentiated into endothelial cells, lining the closely packed blood vessels, and intervening stromal cells, which are large, oval, and frequently filled with a foamy, fat-laden cytoplasm (208). The vascular architecture is outlined by a rich reticular network on connective tissue stains, and fat strains reveal the foamy cells to be filled with lipid droplets (17). By electron microscopy, a third cellular element, the pericytes, can be distinguished (222, 223). The degree to which each of the

three cell types participates in the neoplastic process is uncertain. So is the exact origin of the stromal cells, though several hypotheses have been put forth (208). About 10% of hemangioblastomas contain areas which have the histological appearance of meningiomas (214), indicating some degree of plasticity. Eight tumors associated with polycythemia stained positively with antisera against pure human erythropoietin and renin substrate (angiotensinogen) (210).

Clinical and Radiological Findings

The most frequent presenting symptom of cerebellar hemangioblastoma is headache (80–95%). This is followed by vomiting, vertigo, gait disturbance, diplopia and motor weakness (195, 198). Neck stiffness and pain, hiccups, dementia and paresthesias are also reported. Most of these are caused either by obstructive hydrocephalus or by nervous system dysfunction due to direct mass effect. The most frequent signs are papilledema, ataxia and other cerebellar signs, nystagmus, cranial nerve weakness and hemiparesis (198). The average duration of symptoms was 11 months in the 36 series reviewed by Constans et al. (198), though it has probably been less since the advent of the CT scan. The presenting picture in patients with multiple lesions in different compartments of the CNS can be very confusing (195, 224). Conversely, if the clinical picture indicates multiple sites of pathology, radiological evaluation of the supratentorial, infratentorial and spinal compartments should be performed (224). Only rarely do these tumors present with acute subarachnoid or intraparenchymal hemorrhage (225–227), which is interesting for such vascular neoplasms.

Careful evaluation of the retina and other locations of peripheral stigmata of VHL disease should be performed in all patients with suspected hemangioblastoma of the cerebellum. A full blood count may show an elevated hemoglobin level in 9 to 20% of patients with intracranial neoplasms, more frequently in solid tumors (195, 198, 208), but is generally normal in spinal cord tumors. Screening of the patient's urine for catecholamines and their metabolites may help in the diagnosis of a coexistent pheochromocytoma (208). An abdominal CT should also be performed as part of the general workup of VHL disease.

The CT scan and angiogram complement each other in the workup of CNS hemangioblastoma (198, 203, 228, 229). Contrast enhanced CT scan may show a cystic cavity with a mural nodule, or a uniformly enhancing mass. It was felt to be diagnostic in only 31% of the cases reported by Beltramella et al. (228). Because of possible involvement of the cervicomedullary area, CT scan should include the high cervical spine. Angiography, though it may not delineate the cystic component, is virtually pathognomonic when the vascular mural nodule is seen. Vertebral angiography was diagnostic in 80% of the cases of Beltramella et al. (228). Besides a small mural nodule, a ring of abnormal vessels, a large, solid, vascular mass, or multiple, small, widely spaced, vascular nodules may be seen. Occasionally the tumor has no abnormal vascularity. If syringomyelia or a spinal tumor is suspected, myelography should be performed. Spinal arteriography is highly sensitive and specific for spinal hemangioblastoma (224).

Treatment and Outcome

Surgical excision is the treatment of choice for most hemangioblastomas (17, 198, 203). As they are extremely vascular tumors, this was hard to accomplish, without significant morbidity and mortality, prior to the routine use of microsurgical techniques. In patients with cystic lesions and a mural nodule, removal of the nodule alone is probably sufficient, but the entire wall should be removed in cystic lesions where a nodule cannot be located (198). Solid lesions should be completely removed, when possible, but this is often a problem because of their involvement of deeper structures, such as the cerebellar peduncles and brainstem, and their relatively indistinct margins (219). It has

been reported that preoperative irradiation can facilitate removal of solid tumors by shrinking them and creating better planes of dissection between tumor and surrounding brain (230, 231).

The surgical results in infratentorial tumors depends upon their morphological type and their location. Morbidity and mortality are considerably higher for the solid and microcystic types: 25% (50% in one series) (219), compared to 7% for the cystic varieties (198). For selected, non-irradiated, solid tumors involving the cord or brainstem, an internal decompression may be the wiser course of action (219), though there is a risk of postoperative hemorrhage from the remaining portion. Some surgeons have advocated the use of hypothermia and circulatory arrest in the treatment of vascular, solid lesions of the brainstem (230). With microsurgical techniques, tumors of the brainstem and fourth ventricle can be completely removed (230, 231), and operative mortalities of as low as 8% are achievable (203). Upon the removal of solid hemangioblastomas, any preoperative polycythemia usually resolves (210). This may also be suppressed with radiation therapy (208).

Because of the incidence of multiple lesions, and the high mortality of brainstem lesions (40%), the overall mortality in the series reviewed by Constans et al. (198) ranged from 26 to 35%, with an average of 29%. The recurrence rate was 16%, with tumors appearing either at the site of a previous resection or in a distant location, indicating a multicentric lesion. These recurrences were reported to happen as long as 24 years postoperatively but usually arose within 5 to 7 years (232). The possible benefit of radiation therapy is, therefore, an important issue. No prospective controlled studies of its use are available, but there is evidence that, at doses above 45 Gy, tumor size may be diminished, regrowth retarded and symptom-free interval increased (230, 233). It may therefore be a viable alternative treatment of brainstem tumors with or without biopsy.

Of patients who survive an initial operation for hemangioblastoma, the 10-year survival rate is approximately 80% if these tumors are totally removed, but 50% die of tumor regrowth if their initial removal is subtotal (195). Recurrent tumors may be operated on repeatedly. The likelihood of recurrence, and rate of growth of residual tumors cannot be predicted by their histological appearance.

Vascular Malformations

The WHO classification of brain tumors considers 'vascular malformations' as a distinct group of vascular lesions, separate from hemangioblastoma and from tumors of mesenchymal origin. Although they may behave clinically like tumors, they are not true neoplasms. Vascular malformations, as their name implies, are hamartomatous collections of blood vessels, which show no evidence of cellular proliferation. Cushing and Bailey (211), in 1928, attempted to differentiate between 'vascular tumors' and 'vascular malformations' on the basis of the absence or presence, respectively, of brain parenchyma between the vascular elements. By this criterion, the entity known as 'cavernous angioma' would be classified as a tumor. However, Bergstrand (234) pointed out that, though these lesions do not contain a neural component, and may expand to cause compression and dysfunction of the surrounding brain, they are totally devoid of proliferating elements. Most investigators, therefore, consider them among the vascular malformations. Five distinct lesions are now included in this category: venous angiomas, arteriovenous malformations (AVMs), capillary telangiectases, cavernous angiomas and Sturge–Weber disease (6, 235). Cavernous angiomas will be described in some detail at the end of this section, and AVMs, being relatively common clinically, will not be discussed.

Venous Angioma

In a prospective autopsy series, referred to by Sarwar and McCormick (236), venous angiomas were by far the most common of the vascular malformations, roughly five times as common as AVMs. Other autopsy series, however, have shown them to be less common (237, 238). The vast majority never attain clinical significance (236, 239, 240). Those that do usually present with intracerebral hematoma, cerebellar ataxia, subarachnoid hemorrhage or a seizure disorder (239, 241). Although they may grossly resemble AVMs, microscopically they are found not to contain any arterial elements. Instead, they consist of collections of irregularly shaped vessels, lacking an internal elastic lamina, in which calcification, hyalinization and thrombosis are frequent (17, 235, 239). Between the vessels normal or gliotic neural tissue is found. Common sites of occurrence are the cerebral hemispheres, the spinal cord (17, 242) and the cerebellum (241).

Since the advent of CT scanning, the antemortem diagnosis of venous angioma has been made with greater frequency (241), as they are often found serendipitously on contrast studies. They appear as single, or multiple, short, curvilinear streaks of enhancement, representing the most prominent vascular channels (239, 241). Angiographically, they have a characteristic appearance, which has been referred to as a spider, sunburst, umbrella, or caput medusae: in the deep white matter a myriad of veins are arranged in a radial array around a larger, central vein which drains into either a cortical vein, a subependymal vein, or the galenic system (239, 241). They generally are not visualized in the arterial or capillary phases. A single cavernous hemangioma with this appearance has also been described (243). Seven percent of angiographically occult angiomas were venous angiomas, in a recent survey (244).

The management of these lesions is usually conservative, as they generally are asymptomatic, have a low blood-flow rate, and cannot be surgically excised without causing unacceptable damage to surrounding brain (239, 245). The incidence of bleeding from a venous angioma is unknown, but probably low enough to warrant conservative therapy even when they have already bled. The most significant indication for operative intervention is probably to treat a causally related, intractable seizure disorder. Recently Berenstein and Choi have reported the successful treatment of venous angiomas by direct, percutaneous puncture and injection with 95% ethanol (246).

Capillary Telangiectasia

These vascular malformations are also more frequent than their clinical incidence would indicate (17, 235). As their name implies, they are composed of pathologically dilated capillary vessels (239). These are separated from each other by apparently normal neural parenchyma. Although telangiectases may be found anywhere in the brain, their most common site, for unknown reasons, is in the pons, near the midline (17, 239). The blood flow through these vessels is so low that they usually are not detectable on angiography. However, punctate calcification may occur within the lesion, which can be seen on CT or plain x-rays (247). There may be other, associated malformations, such as cavernous angiomas (17, 235), and there has been some debate as to whether the latter may develop from telangiectases (248). Capillary telangiectases may be multiple (17, 249, 250) and, when multiple lesions arise in the cerebellum, may be associated with conjuctival and facial telangiectases, loss of cerebellar Purkinje cells, and a defect in the humoral immune system (Louis-Bar syndrome, or ataxia telangiectasia) (235).

If a capillary telangiectasia causes clinical symptoms, it is usually because of intraparenchymal bleeding which, in the pons, may produce devastating deficits or death (251). Extensive lesions have been known to present with gradually progressive neurological deterioration, probably due to numerous, small bleeds (252). Little can be done to treat these lesions when they become symptomatic, other than evacuating the hematoma. At the time of operation, suspicious areas on the wall of the hematoma should be carefully biopsied, or the diagnosis of capillary telangiectasia may be missed (239).

Sturge–Weber Disease

Also known as 'encephalotrigeminal angiomatosis' (17, 235), this syndrome, in its complete form, consists of a port-wine nevus in the distribution of one or more branches of the trigeminal nerve, buphthalmus, mental retardation, epilepsy and cerebral cortical calcified angioma (253). Most of these findings are present at birth, though the buphthalmus may develop post-natally (1). Incomplete forms of the disease have been reported (254). Rare vascular anomaly syndromes involving the extremities and the spinal cord (Klippel–Trenauney–Weber syndrome), the retina, face and midbrain (Wyburn-Maston syndrome), or the skin, mucous membranes and nervous system (Osler–Rendu–Weber syndrome) also exist (1, 255, 256). All of these syndromes appear to involve somatic mutations which lead to defects in the primitive vasculature, prior to its separation into skin, meningeal, and CNS components (253). Occasionally, an inherited basis may be inferred in these cases.

The leptomeningeal angioma of Sturge–Weber disease is usually associated with gliosis and atrophy of the underlying cerebral cortex (17). The angioma itself is usually located in the pia, in the parieto-occipital region. Extensive calcium deposits in the underlying gliotic cortex are often seen as characteristic 'double contours', or 'tramtracks', on plain skull x-rays (235, 254). The subcortical white matter frequently shows demyelination.

Aggressive treatment of this syndrome is usually reserved for those infants with intractable seizures. Total or subtotal hemispherectomy has, in some cases, been of benefit (257).

Cavernous Angioma

This vascular malformation, also known as cavernous hemangioma or cavernoma (17), is more deserving of discussion in a text on CNS tumors than the previously mentioned lesions. Cavernous angiomas are more likely to present as mass lesions (239, 258) and they contain no neural parenchyma between the vascular elements.

Incidence and location. Though previously considered rare, a recent series of 138 cases, culled from the literature since 1960, has been published by Simard et al. (258). These authors had themselves treated 12 patients with cavernous angioma since 1976. In another, large, prospective autopsy study (259), they comprised 7% of all vascular malformations.

Cavernous angiomas occur most frequently in the cerebral hemispheres, typically in the peri-rolandic region, but they may be located anywhere in the nervous system, including the pituitary fossa, pineal region, cranial nerves, spinal epidural space, spinal roots, dura matter, skull, vertebral body, scalp and peripheral nerves (239, 258, 260). The age at diagnosis ranges from newborn to the eighth decade, but is most frequently in the third and fourth decades (258). The sex distribution is roughly equal. Cavernous angiomas usually are solitary lesions, but may be multiple; as many as 42 have been reported in a single patient (96). Multiple cavernous angiomas may be associated with similar lesions in the liver, kidneys or skin. As mentioned before, they may also be associated with capillary telangiectases (17, 235), and transitional forms between the two types of malformation have been reported. It has been hypothesized that, in such cases, as the neural stroma within a capillary telangiectasia atrophies, the vascular channels increase in size, giving rise to a cavernous angioma. There is insufficient histological or clinical evidence to support this theory, however. A familial incidence of capillary angiomas has rarely been reported (250, 261, 262), as have associations with other CNS (263, 264) and non-CNS neoplasms (17). Lesions resembling cavernous angiomas can be produced in rats by exposure to polyoma virus (265). A single case in a patient with Turner's syndrome has been reported (266).

Pathology. Cavernous angiomas are usually well-circumscribed, dark red, multilobulated lesions (17, 235, 238). They range in size from a few millimeters to several centimeters in diameter. There is often a surrounding area of gliotic brain, which may facilitate removal at the time of operation (238). There are no discernible abnormal vessels feeding or draining the lesions (96). They often contain areas of hemorrhage and thrombosis. Hemosiderin deposition in the surrounding brain is usually, but not universally found. Some of the middle fossa lesions have a dural base, and may even arise from within the cavernous sinus, making their removal difficult (258), though not impossible (266). Some of the extradural angiomas may be hard to differentiate grossly from aneurysmal bone cysts (258).

Microscopically, cavernous angiomas consist of honeycomb-like arrays of irregular, sinusoidal vessels, up to 1 mm or more in diameter, lined by a single layer of endothelial cells (239). These are non-neoplastic in appearance, and may help to differentiate the lesion from certain tumors (258). The vascular channels may be contiguous, sharing the same wall, or may be separated by a thin collagenous stroma. Except at their extreme periphery, they contain no neural tissue, which is a main differentiating feature from telangiectases and venous angiomas (239). The channels may have a lamellated appearance, felt to be caused by repeated thrombosis and recanalization (258, 267). Hyalinized tissue, calcium deposits and even areas of ossification may be found within the lesions. Elastic fibers are occasionally present, in a scattered and disorganized fashion, at the periphery of the lesions and should not, as some authors have argued (268, 269), preclude the diagnosis of cavernous angioma. They were present in 28% of the cases reviewed by Simard et al. (258), and in 58% of their own 12 cases.

Clinical and radiological findings. Cavernous angiomas usually do not manifest themselves clinically until early adulthood. They present, with either seizures, hemorrhage, or as a mass lesion, with roughly equal frequency (258). Many are diagnosed incidentally on enhanced CT, performed in the workup of chronic headaches. A causal relationship with these headaches has not always been demonstrable (239).

When cavernous angiomas present with a seizure disorder, the seizures may have been of long duration, often more than 3 or 4 years (258). The nature of the seizure disorder depends on the location of the lesion. The pathogenesis of these seizures is uncertain, but is felt to differ from those caused by AVMs. In the latter, it is felt that the high-flow state of the lesion may steal blood away from the surrounding brain, thus rendering the neurons hypoxic and, therefore, prone to uncontrolled synchronous depolarization (239). However, such a high-flow situation does not occur in cavernous angiomas; instead it has been hypothesized that the stasis of blood within the lesion leads to the intraluminal breakdown of red cells and the subsequent diffusion of iron-containing pigments into the surrounding parenchyma. This may also occur as the result of multiple microscopic hemorrhages within the lesion. These compounds, as hemosiderin deposits, then cause gliosis of the adjacent brain. There is experimental evidence which suggests that such iron-containing compounds are potent inducers of epileptogenic foci (270, 271).

Patients presenting with hemorrhage may have devastating neurological deficits, even though the hematomas are usually not very large, if the angioma is situated in the basal ganglia or fourth-ventricular region. If a preoperative contrast CT scan is not performed, and if the hematoma wall is not biopsied at the time of evacuation, the diagnosis may be missed. In Simard's series (258), 11 of the 40 patients presenting with hemorrhage were not diagnosed until autopsy. Nine of these patients were never operated upon, but, in the other 2, the diagnosis was missed at operation.

The presentation of cavernous angiomas as mass lesions occurs in approximately 36% of cases (155). The mechanism for this probably differs from case to case. As some symptoms are of insidious onset, it is unlikely that hemorrhage into the lesion caused a rapidly expanding mass in these cases. However, cystic cavities of liquified blood, probably the result of multiple, small hemorrhages, have been frequently found in patients operated on for slowly growing mass lesions. In the more indolent cases, gradual expansion of the vascular channels has also been hypothesized, because of documented cases in which there has been radiological evidence of growth of the lesion over time (262, 272). Midline lesions may present with hydrocephalus, resulting from the obstruction of CSF pathways. Other presenting findings are specific to the anatomical location of the angiomas. These include cranial nerve deficits and proptosis in lesions invading the cavernous sinus (273), deafness and facial weakness in CP angle lesions (274), Parinaud's syndrome in those in the pineal region (275), and endocrinopathies in diencephalic lesions (276). Brainstem lesions have been misdiagnosed as multiple sclerosis, glioma, or encephalitis, leading to inappropriate treatment, and an unfavorable outcome (258). Twelve of the 13 reported cases of middle fossa lesions were female, and many came from Japan (258, 273, 277, 278). They were frequently misdiagnosed preoperatively as medial sphenoid wing meningiomas, because of their characteristic, homogeneous enhancement with contrast on CT and their prolonged clinical course.

Patients with large canvernous angioma may be found to have a bleeding diathesis (239, 279). The etiology of this is unknown, but it may be due to a consumptive coagulopathy secondary to excessive spontaneous thrombosis within the lesion (279), or to a currently uncharacterized, qualitative defect in platelet function, the so-called 'storage pool disease of platelets' (280). This occurs infrequently in the angiomas encountered in the brain, but may be seen in the more extensive lesions involving the middle fossa, base of the skull and face, making their surgical treatment especially hazardous.

Computerized tomography is the most sensitive radiological study for the detection of cavernous angiomas (258, 281). Only 3% show no abnormality, and 70% demonstrate contrast enchancement, although, except for middle fossa lesions, that enchancement is usually not homogeneous. Of the remaining 27%, cystic or hypodense areas, fresh blood, and calcification were the most frequent abnormalities (258, 281, 282). The lesions often did not produce a mass effect. Cavernous angiomas may, therefore, be difficult to differentiate, on CT criteria, from low-grade astrocytomas and thrombosed AVMs.

Skull x-rays are positive in 46%, mottled calcification being the most frequent finding in those patients presenting with seizures, and calcification and sellar erosion being the most common abnormalities in patients presenting with mass lesions (251).

Angiographic abnormalities were reported in 61% of the review series of Simard et al. (258), but these were, in general, quite non-specific. Most of the abnormal angiograms just showed an avascular mass, but, in some cases, widened veins, a vascular blush, puddling of contrast, and neovascularity were seen. A tumor stain was found frequently in middle cranial fossa lesions. Rarely, a highly vascular, malignant-looking lesion is seen (283). Angiography is also, therefore, non-specific in the diagnosis of cavernous angiomas. From the study of Simard et al. (258), there is insufficient evidence for the inclusion of all cavernous angiomas in the category of angiographically occult angiomas (AOAs), though many of them (39%) could, indeed, be so classified. In the series of AOAs reported by Wakai et al. (244), only one of their 13 cases had a cavernous angioma, although their literature review produced an overall incidence of 38% among 159 AOAs.

Treatment and outcome. The natural history of cavernous angiomas remains obscure (258). The current indications for operating on these lesions are for the control of seizures, the evacuation of hematomas, the resection of a mass lesion, and the establishment of a tissue diagnosis. It is unknown whether the prevention of further, potential hemorrhages is sufficient indication to operate on them. Most of the hemispheric lesions can be removed without significant morbidity, because of their relatively well-defined boundaries and low blood-flow rate. Those lesions along the midline, and those involving the cavernous sinus, base of skull, skull and scalp present specific surgical challenges, but they may be successfully extirpated (239), sometimes with the help of preoperative emobolization for blood-flow reduction.

The outcome in patients with seizures is generally favorable. At one year after surgery, 52% were said, by Simard et al. (258), to be seizure free, and 39% were noted to have a 'satisfactory' course. In patients who presented with hemorrhage, only 73% ever underwent surgery; the rest died and were diagnosed at autopsy. Those who made it to surgery generally did well, however. The outcome in patients presenting with a mass, varied according to the location of the lesion. In the subgroup of 13 lesions involving the cavernous sinus, complete resection was accomplished in only 5, and there were 3 operative mortalities (258). Presumably this was due to the lesions' vascularity and intimate involvement with the carotid artery and cranial nerves. Diffuse intravascular coagulopathy is one of the hazards of removing these tumors. Most of the patients with hemispheric, cerebellar or intraventricular tumors did well following surgery, but the prognosis in patients with brainstem lesions was dismal.

Other forms of therapy, such as ionizing radiation and chemotherapy, have not been sufficiently evaluated.

TUMORS OF MESENCHYMAL ORIGIN

Hemangiopericytoma

Incidence and Location

The hemangiopericytoma has been the subject of considerable nosological controversy. It is now felt by most pathologists to represent a variant of the angioblastic meningoma first described by Bailey, Cushing and Einsenhardt in 1928 (284). It is a rare tumor, occurring in 1.6% of the meningiomas reviewed by Jellinger and Slowik (285), and 2.0% of those seen in a 30-year period by Jaaskelainen et al. (286). It appears to arise in males more frequently, and can occur at any age, but with a mean age which tends to be lower than that of the more common types of meningioma (286–288).

Hemangiopericytomas are found primarily in the supratentorial compartment, most frequently in the parasagittal region (286). They are also found along the tentorium and the petrous and sphenoidal ridges, where they are intimately associated with dural sinuses. Other locations include the CP angle 214, 286), choroid plexus (289), foramen magnum and spine (214). In contrast to conventional meningiomas, the parieto-occipital region seems to be the preferred location (286). Almost all are attached to the dura at operation, but there have been occasional reports of tumors with no obvious dural connection (214).

Origin and Pathology

The term 'hemangiopericytoma' was first coined by Stout and Murray, in 1942 (290), to describe an extra-axial tumor composed of masses of capillaries with apparently normal endothelial cells, surrounded by neoplastic cells which were felt to be derived from pericytes. It was Begg and Garrett, in 1954 (291), who first suggested that this entity, and the 'angioblastic meningioma' of Bailey, Cushing and Eisenhardt were one and the same. Since then, the concept of this tumor's being classifiable in the meningioma family has had varying support from light microscopic (214), ultrastructural (287, 292–294), and tissue culture evidence (214, 295). The question has still not been definitively answered. Rubinstein postulated (296) that all angioblastic meningiomas originate from polyblastic mesenchymal cells in the leptomeninges. Tumors dis-

playing areas of both classical meningiomatous and either hemangioblastic or hemangiopericytic histology have been described (214), and cell cultures of purely hemangiopericytic angioblastic meningiomas have developed clearcut whorls and intercellular imbrications, providing further evidence for the related cytogenesis of hemangiopericytomas and meningiomas (295). Progestin receptors, which are commonly found in classical meningiomas (297), have not yet been described in hemangiopericytomas (298).

Despite the histological similarity of intracranial hemangiopericytomas with hemangiopericytomas of the soft tissue, the pericyte may not be the direct cell of origin in the former, because they lack a well-defined pericytoplasmic basal lamina (296). However, the focal condensation of cytoplasmic filaments, termed dense bodies, which are evidence of attempted smooth muscle differentiation frequently found in pericytes, supports their derivation from these cells (293).

In sum, the evidence available to date favors the retention of the term angioblastic meningioma as a family of tumors with two principal varieties, the hemangioblastic and the hemangiopericytic (287, 296). This division carries important clinical implications, as will be seen below. Other, rare varieties include those transitional forms between hemangiopericytoma, hemangioblastoma and the classical meningioma; the clinically aggressive tumor known as 'papillary meningioma' may also be a subvariety of the hemangiopericytic variant of the angioblastic meningioma (300).

Hemangiopericytomas usually present as highly vascular tumors attached to the dura. Like meningiomas, they tend to compress, rather than invade the underlying brain (287). They typically receive their blood supply both from the dura and from cortical vessels. The tumors are spongy in consistency.

Microscopically they consist of masses of closely packed cells containing innumerable, thin-walled vascular channels, giving the tumor a spongy appearance, as well. Mitotic figures are frequent (17, 286, 287, 292). Pleo-morphic, binucleated and multinucleated cells are also seen, as are areas of necrosis. Reticulin stains show an extensive fibrous tissue network surrounding groups of cells or single cells (286). Electron microscopy fails to show the intercellular digitations and prominent desmosomes which are characteristic of more benign forms of meningioma (295), and whorls are not seen on light microscopy (286). The cells contain abundant, 9–10 nm diameter filaments and an electron-dense extracellular matrix is frequently seen.

Clinical and Radiological Findings

Hemangiopericytomas present most commonly with headache (287). The next most frequent symptom is focal weakness, followed by seizures. In general, the presentation is that of meningiomas arising in the same location, but tends to be shorter in duration, due to the relatively rapid growth of hemangiopericytomas.

The radiological workup of these tumors should include a contrast enhanced CT scan and angiography (286, 301). On CT they have the appearance of meningiomas, slightly hyperdense without contrast, with a broad-based dural attachment, and well-defined margins, which are usually smooth. However, the enhancement is usually inhomogeneous, or ring-like, and calcification and peri-tumoral edema are usually not seen (286, 302, 303). The CT sign of 'mushrooming', dural nodules spreading from the main mass, is felt to be a sign of malignancy in recurrent tumors (286, 304). On angiography the tumor is usually found to receive blood supply from cortical vessels, as well as from the meninges, and a dense long-lasting tumor stain is almost always seen. Early draining veins are uncommon. The tumor vessels have a typical corkscrew-like appearance (305).

Plain skull x-rays may show bony destruction, due to direct pressure from the tumor rather than invasion (286). The hyperostosis frequently seen with common meningiomas is absent.

Treatment and Outcome

Surgery, hopefully for a complete removal, is the treatment of choice for hemangiopericytomas (195, 286, 306). This is often a hazardous undertaking because of the tumor's extreme vascularity, which, because of the extensive cortical contribution, cannot always be decreased by interruption of the dural feeders. In the series of Jaaskelainen's et al. (286), intra-operative bleeding caused the death of 3 out of 21 patients at primary resection and of 2 additional patients at reoperation. It also made total resection impossible in 6 of the 21 patients. Sixty percent of the incompletely removed tumors recurred, but took as long as 7 years to do so. Almost 50% of those tumors presumed to have been totally removed also recurred, after a mean interval of 78 months. Other series have shown up to an 87% recurrence rate (287). Metastases, to liver or bone, occurred in 3 patients. The lung has also been found to be a common organ of metastasis (287, 288).

The role of radiation therapy in the prevention of recurrences is not known, though it may have been of use in some tumors (307, 308). Yamakawa et al. (309) and Fukui et al. (308) recommend preoperative radiation therapy to reduce tumor vascularity.

Because of the long mean interval to recurrence, and the scarcity of these tumors, it is evident that an extended follow-up period, and a study period of several decades, would be necessary to determine, in a prospective study, the efficacy of such adjunctive measures as radiation therapy and chemotherapy. The mean survival of the patients in the Mayo Clinic series was 7.3 years (287), but recurrence-free survivals of 14 to 20 years have been reported (286).

Sarcomas

Intracranial sarcomas are uncommon tumors,

comprising between 1 and 2% of all primary, intracranial neoplasms (310). There are several distinct varieties of sarcoma, making it difficult to determine their behavior and optimal treatment. Sarcomas of the brain bear a histological resemblance to those found elsewhere in the body, and are presumed to be derived from anaplastic cells of mesenchymal origin, as are their extraneural counterparts (310, 311). Some intracranial sarcomas also may contain non-mesenchymal elements. Immunohistochemical techniques, in particular staining for GFAP, have helped resolve several issues about certain tumors previously felt to be sarcomas. For example, the entity known as 'monstrocellular sarcoma' is now widely recognized to be a giant cell variant of glioblastoma multiforme, because of the GFAP content of its component cells (310). The GFAP content of the 'meningeal fibrous xanthosarcoma' has brought about its reclassification as a xanthoastrocytoma. Similarly the 'circumscribed sarcoma of the cerebellum', so-called because of its extensive reticulin formation, is now felt to be a subgroup of medulloblastoma which has stimulated leptomeningeal desmoplasia (312).

The most common primary sarcoma arising de novo in the brain is the fibrosarcoma. This tumor accounts for 0.1 to 0.6% of all intracranial neoplasms (313, 314). The other most common sarcomatous lesions are those which arise in association with a malignant glioma (gliosarcoma, or Feigin's tumor) or with an anaplastic meningioma (meningeal sarcoma). The former is probably more common than fibrosarcoma, and may be seen in up to 8% of malignant gliomas (315). Less common primary de novo sarcomas include the rare fibromyxosarcoma, chondrosarcoma, mesenchymal chondrosarcoma, liposarcoma, osteogenic sarcoma, osteochondrosarcoma and rhabdomyosarcoma (316). A couple of cases of sarcoma arising within a metastatic carcinoma have been reported (317, 318). Primary lymphomas of the brain and microgliomas, formerly referred to as reticulum cell sarcomas, share few characteristics with non-lymphoma-

tous sarcomas, and will be discussed in a separate section. Limitations of space and data make it impossible to discuss each of these entities at length, so they will be grouped as follows: fibrosarcoma and its variants, other primary de novo sarcomas, gliosarcoma, and malignant meningioma.

Fibrosarcoma and Its Variants

Sarcomas of the brain may arise from any intracranial structure containing mesenchymal elements, which includes the dura mater, subarachnoid blood vessels, tela choroidea and the pia-arachnoid, including those sleeves accompanying blood vessels into the brain parenchyma. It is probably from the latter anlage that those examples of entirely intra-axial tumors arise (310, 314). Most commonly, they are located intracerebrally, but with a dural attachment (316). There have been rare reports of intraventricular sarcomas (319–321). The well-recognized ability of therapeutic ionizing radiation to induce sarcomas of the soft tissues has also been reported in the brain (322–324). Except for these rare cases, there are no known etiological agents. A viral etiology is conceivable, as has been found and exploited scientifically in other animals (325). There is no evidence that head trauma can lead to the induction of sarcomas.

Fibrosarcomas vary widely in their degree of anaplasia. Christensen and Lara (320) have applied to them a subclassification scheme which has been generally accepted because of its clinical utility. The least anaplastic subclass is the 'fibrous' variant, which consists of bipolar fibroblast-like cells in a network of reticulin and collagen. There is little pleomorphism, and few mitotic figures are found. Of intermediate malignancy are the 'spindle cell' sarcomas, which are more cellular, with less collagen, and have areas of pseudopalisading and necrosis. The least differentiated variety are the 'polymorphic cell' sarcomas in which large, pleomorphic cells with little reticulin stroma are interspersed within extensive areas of necrosis. In Christensen and Lara's series

(320), patients with fibrosarcoma survived an average of 74 months, while those with spindle cell sarcoma lived for an average of 27 months, and those with pleomorphic cell sarcoma for only 12 months. There was also a correllation between the age of the patient, the histological type of the tumor, and its gross appearance and degree of invasiveness of the underlying brain. Younger children and infants tended to have pleomorphic cell sarcomas, which were reddish-gray in color, fairly friable, soft, and poorly demarcated from the brain. Adults more frequently had the fibrous variety, which were firmer, whitish, and easier to dissect from brain, thus making their gross total excision easier. Invasion of the brain, when it occurs, is principally as tongues of tumor penetrating into adjacent parenchyma, often surrounding islands of neuroglia, and as perivascular cuffs of sarcoma cells (310). This may be associated with marked gliosis at the tumor border, and the possibility of this inducing an astrocytoma, making a 'sarcoglioma', has been hypothesized, and rarely reported (96, 326, 327).

An unusual presentation of fibrosarcoma, seen almost exclusively in infants, is as a sheet of anaplastic tumor cells extending over much of the intracranial and spinal dura. This is termed 'meningeal sarcomatosis' and leads inexorably to the death of the patient within a few months (310, 328). Fibrosarcomas may also arise following cranial irradiation for other neoplasms (322–324). They may be located in the same area as the original tumor, or in a completely separate region. As many as 20 years may pass before the sarcoma manifests itself, and the mean latency is around 10 years (17).

Clinical findings are non-specific. Evidence of increased intracranial pressure, especially in the more malignant tumors, is the most common finding. This may include headache and papilledema. Seizures occur in about one-fourth of patients (320), and spontaneous hemorrhage has been reported (329). Neuraxis metastases may occur in 10% (320), and there have been isolated instances of systemic spread following surgical resection (330, 331).

As with other forms of sarcoma, there are no recognized pathognomonic findings on radiographic studies, although arterial encasement may be seen on angiography (316, 332). The diagnosis is, therefore, usually made at the time of surgery. The goals of surgery should include total resection of the tumor, but, especially for the pleomorphic cell sarcoma this is rarely, if ever, attainable (320). There is little evidence for the usefulness of either radiotherapy or chemotherapy in the treatment of sarcomas (310). Meningeal sarcomatosis is not at all amenable to surgical therapy, but for this tumor, there is at least a good rationale, if no corroborative data, for the intrathecal administration of chemotherapeutic agents via an Ommaya reservoir.

Other Primary De Novo Sarcomas

Presumably due to the multipotential nature of the primitive mesenchymal cells from which sarcomas arise, some of these tumors may contain areas of apparent differentiation, into mature mesodermal tissue (96, 316, 326, 333–335). On occasion more than one different tissue type may be present in a given tumor. The tumors are then designated according to this histological appearance (326). Ultrastructural studies and immunohistochemical techniques may sometimes help to identify differentiating regions within a tumor (334, 336–341). For example, rhabdomyosarcomas will be seen to possess mixed thin and thick filaments or transverse densities reminiscent of 'Z-band' material (316, 334). Other tumors in which such rhabdomyoblastic differentiation may occur are teratomas and medullomyoblastomas (316, 342). Leiomyosarcomas are felt to be derived from the smooth muscle cells of blood vessels (336). Chondrosarcomas, osteogenic sarcomas, osteochondrosarcomas and mesenchymal chondrosarcomas, containing varying combinations of neoplastic cartilage, bone, and undifferentiated mesenchymal cells, have become firmly established as distinct nosological entities (316, 333, 335, 338, 339, 343). Three other sarcomas which have only rarely been reported intracranially are the liposar-coma (344, 345), fibrous histiocytoma (337), and myxosarcoma (326, 346), considered to be the most primitive type of sarcoma. The existence of angiosarcomas, though reported in a single case by Mena and Garcia (340), has not achieved universal acceptance (347).

The overall survival in this group of tumors is not good, as few patients survive for more than 5 years. Autopsy and CSF cytology confirm the high incidence of neuraxis seeding in the younger patients, and there have been several reports of extraneural metastases (320, 335, 339, 348). Again, the treatment of choice, when feasible, is total surgical removal (316, 320).

Gliosarcoma

These tumors are felt to arise as the result of the influence of a pre-existing glioblastoma (315, 349). The nature of this influence is not known, but there is an active effort to isolate a soluble, diffusible factor by which vascular endothelial and adventitial cells may be transformed. This may merely represent the end-effect of a 'tumor angiogenesis factor', believed to be secreted locally by glioblastoma cells to pro-duce vascular proliferation and endothelial hyperplasia (350–352). Once the neoplastic process begins among the mesenchymal ele-ments within the glioblastoma, they continue to proliferate until separate areas of pure sarcoma can be distinguished (310, 315). These areas are characterized by an abun-dance of reticulin and collagen, and by the absence of GFAP. Cellular pleomorphism and frequent mitoses are also seen. If the growth of the sarcomatous element is rapid enough, the pre-existing glioblastoma may be obscured. Myogenic, chondroid and osteoid differentia-tion may occur within the sarcomatous ele-ments (310, 315). Both the gliomatous and the sarcomatous elements have been known to metastasize.

Clinically, a gliosarcoma resembles the par-ent glioblastoma, though, at operation, they tend to be firmer because of their collagenous

and reticulin stroma, and are often found attached to the dura, making it occasionally difficult to differentiate grossly from men-ingioma. The survival time is also similar to that of glioblastomas and their clinical mana-gement has been generally the same as that more common, malignant tumor (315).

Malignant Meningioma (Anaplastic Meningioma)

Rarely, anaplastic changes may occur within an otherwise benign meningioma, which imparts to the tumor a new, malignant, clinical behavior (17, 347). These are not to be confused with angioblastic meningiomas, the hemangiopericytic variant of which also behaves in an aggressive fashion. The WHO classification does not include these tumors among the sarcomas, however. In the malig-nant meningioma, frankly sarcomatous fea-tures are found, and there is infiltration of the underlying brain, numerous mitoses, and a typical papillary epithelioid pattern (310). Occasionally the changes are so widespread that the more benign portions can no longer be identified. The distinction between malignant meningioma and fibrosarcoma is sometimes unclear (195, 347, 353). Many of these neo-plasms are diagnosed at the time of a second resection of a tumor initially felt to be totally benign, leading to the possibility that there may have been an evolution in the tumor's behavior during the follow-up period (320, 354). These tumors produce a much more marked astroglial reaction, or hyperplasia, in the adjacent brain, than do benign meningio-mas (310). Again, the treatment of choice is radical surgical resection, when feasible, and little is known about the possible benefit of radiotherapy or chemotherapy. Cerebrospinal fluid-borne metastases (355) and, more fre-quently, extraneural metastases have been reported (96). Rubinstein distinguishes this tumor from the other primary meningeal sarcomas, and classifies it among the meningio-mas (17).

PRIMARY MELANOTIC TUMORS

Virchow first described a case of 'diffuse mela-nosarcomatosis of the central nervous system' in 1859 (356). Since then, over 220 well-documented cases of primary melanotic tumors of the CNS have been reported (357). The metastasis of a peripheral melanoma to the brain is a much more common occurrence, so the existence of peripheral lesions must be assiduously ruled out to establish the CNS as the tumor's primary location. Of the published cases, the majority (63%) were either diffuse or multifocal melanoblastomas. Thirty-seven percent were solitary primary leptomeningeal melanomas. Twenty-six percent of the 220 patients collected by Bamborschke et al. (357) had melanoblastosis or melanoses associated with giant hairy nevi of the skin, the so-called 'neurocutaneous melanosis syndrome'. The 'nevus of Ota', which occurs in the iris, choroid, uveal tract and skin, has been reported in association with diffuse melanosis of the skull, dura, and pia-arachnoid (358). This patient also had an intracranial, extra-axial melanoma.

Leptomeningeal melanoblastosis, or mela-nomatosis, affects males more commonly than females, and has a peak age incidence in the fourth and fifth decades (357, 359). Pathologi-cally it consists of a diffuse infiltration of the leptomeninges by blastoma cells containing melanin. These cells fill the basal cisterns, where they may form large masses, and spread down the Virchow–Robin spaces, often com-pressing small subcortical vessels and growing as nodular deposits (357). Infiltration of the cranial nerves may take place.

Symptomatology is appropriate to the loca-tion and pattern of tumor involvement, and may include seizures, headaches, drowsiness, psychotic syndromes, cranial nerve palsies and meningismus. Signs of increased intracranial pressure from edema or hydrocephalus, and focal deficits due to compression of small cortical, spinal or radicular arteries are com-mon (357). Contrast enhanced CT may reveal diffusely increased density in the subarachnoid spaces, enhancing cortical gyri as the tumor invades further and, eventually, tumor nodules, but the best non-operative method of establishing a diagnosis is examination of the CSF (360, 361). The color alone may be non-specific. It may be clear, but is often xanthoch-romic due to either a high protein content, repeated small tumor hemorrhages (362), or a high melanin content. Cytology, however, will show cells which, by special staining tech-niques, such as the Masson silver stain, can be shown to contain melanin. However, ultra-structural studies may be needed to distinguish between melanoma cells and melanophages (361, 363). Myelography sometimes demon-strates non-specific abnormalities similar to those seen in arachnoiditis (364).

As with other, widespread leptomeningeal neoplastic processes, surgery serves no purpose, except for CSF diversion and intrathecal drug administration, and for establishing a diagno-sis. This tumor is notoriously unresponsive to any form of therapy (357, 365). The mean survival time is 4–5 months (366).

The diagnosis of primary melanoblastosis, as opposed to metastatic, requires a complete autopsy to examine all potential primary sources, such as the retinae and any melanotic skin nevi. Diagnosis may be complicated by the fact that malignant melanoblasts may them-selves metastasize to extraneural locations (367). In metastatic disease there is usually a mass lesion seen on CT, though primary melanoblastosis cells may also pile up over time to create a large tumor mass, as in the case reported by Aichner and Schuler (361). Con-versely, solitary primary melanotic lesions can subsequently spread throughout the neuraxis. Recovery of melanoma cells from the CSF in a patient with a normal CT scan is, therefore, suggestive of, though not diagnostic for, pri-mary leptomeningeal melanoblastosis (361).

Solitary, primary melanomas of the brain are occasionally encountered without wide-spread CSF invasion. Their propensity to spread, and difficulty of total excision is so great, however, that surgery is rarely more than palliative (357, 368). They are histologically malignant, with frequent mitoses. Local invasion of the skull has been reported (369). Melanomas may occasionally be more benign and circumscribed. Melanotic tumors can arise from any location in the CSF which normally contains melanin-producing cells, which are derived from the neural crest. These cells are most common in the pia-arachnoid, particularly the basal pia, ventral to the medulla (17), but may also be found in the pars nervosa of the pituitary gland. Primary melanomas of the pituitary gland have been reported (370, 371), as has a chromophobe adenoma containing pigmented cells (371). Common tumors which may rarely contain melanin-producing cells include schwannomas and meningiomas (372). Primary melanomas arising within the parenchyma of the spinal cord have also been reported (373, 374). They may have a relatively indolent course (374).

Eleven cases of 'meningeal melanocytoma' (375) have recently been reviewed by Winston et al. (376). On the basis of ultrastructural and immunohistological studies, they were felt to be of Schwann cell or melanocytic rather than meningeal origin. They are benign-appearing tumors found in the subarachnoid space associated with a cranial or spinal nerve. Unlike most meningiomas, they stain positively for S-100 protein and are negative for epithelial membrane antigen (377). Ultrastructurally they also differ from schwannomas, in that there is no external lamina around the cells, and micropinocytic activity is not detected. In sum, the evidence indicated a leptomingeal melanocytic, rather than a meningothelial fibroblastic or Schwann cell origin. The biological behavior of these tumors is variable, and survival of 28 years has been reported (378).

The pigmented papillary medulloblastoma (379) and the melanotic neuroectodermal tumor of infancy (380) are entities of debated cytogenesis. The latter tumor, also known as 'retinal anlage tumor', 'melanotic progonoma' and 'melanotic adamantinoma', is felt by Rubinstein to be a tumor of maldevelopmental origin (17). It usually arises in the maxilla of

infants, is locally invasive, but usually benign, and amenable to surgical treatment, unlike primary intracranial melanomas. It has been suggested that the pigmented papillary medulloblastoma is a variant of this tumor (17, 380), because of their similar histologies, but its biological behavior is far more malignant.

Neurocutaneous melanosis is a syndrome in which giant nevi are associated with a broad spectrum of leptomeningeal melanocytic abnormalities (381, 382). These range from a non-neoplastic, diffuse pigmentation of the leptomeninges (the familial condition known as 'neurocutaneous pigmentation' (383)) to a highly malignant proliferation of melanin-containing cells. It is found most commonly in infants and young children, unlike primary malignant melanomas, and may lead to hydrocephalus because of involvement of the leptomeninges at the base of the brain. It has been reported in association with multiple peripheral neurofibromas (17). Again, in the more malignant varieties, the prognosis is always poor.

TUMORS OF LYMPHORETICULAR ORIGIN

Although derived from mesenchymal cells, the behaviour and histology of these tumors differs so much from other sarcomas that they are generally given separate consideration. The tumors discussed in this section will be (1) primary lymphomas of the CNS and (2) miscellaneous lymphoreticular disorders.

Primary Lymphomas

There has been so much semantic confusion about these tumors that it is appropriate to begin our discussion of them with a brief review of their history and nomenclature. The mesenchymal origin of these tumors was appreciated by Bailey who, in 1929 (384), described them as perivascular and perithelial sarcomas, because of their distinct tendency to spread along perivascular spaces. The term 'reticulum cell sarcoma' was first used by Yuile, in 1938

(385), because of their resemblance to tumors of the same name occurring outside the CNS. This connoted an origin from the primitive reticulum cell of the reticuloendothelial system. The term 'microglioma' was used by Russell et al. (386) because of the affinity of the tumor cells for the silver carbonate stain, which was felt to be more characteristic of microglia than of reticulum cells. Both sides agreed that the tumors originated from histiocytes of the lymphoreticular system, located within the brain, so the terms 'reticuloendothelial cell sarcoma' and 'reticulum cell sarcoma–microglioma' were devised as compromises (17, 387). With the development of immunohistochemical and electron microscopic techniques, the derivation of these tumors from the reticular portion of the lymphoreticular system has come into serious question and been abandoned by most (388–393). It is now felt that nearly all of these tumors develop from lymphocytes (394). The detection of intracytoplasmic immunoglobulin, by immunoperoxidase staining, has frequently indicated a B-cell origin (395, 396). Thus far, no tumors of T-cell origin have been positively identified using lymphocytic markers (390). Ultrastructural features of immature immunoblasts have also been detected by electron microscopy (388). Nonetheless, the terms 'microglioma' and 'reticulum cell sarcoma' are still encountered in the recent literature (397–400).

A subset of these tumors bears so much resemblance to histiocyte-derived tumors outside the CNS, that the term 'histiocytic lymphoma' is still used to describe them (388, 391, 401, 402). Most of the recent series have attempted to subdivide primary CNS lymphomas by analogy to their peripheral counterparts (391, 402–409). The classification schemes that have been utilized most frequently are the Kiel (410) classification of non-Hodgkin's lymphomas, the Working Formulation of the National Cancer Institute (411), the Rappaport (412), and the Lukes–Collins classifications (413). According to these, what was previously called a reticulum cell sarcoma would now be classified as histiocytic lymphoma, or immunoblastic sarcoma, but B-cell markers have been detected on these tumors as well. Few practical results, in terms of the treatment of prognosis of these tumors, have been obtained by these efforts at categorization (402, 405, 409, 414). Malignant lymphomas of the CNS have proven stubbornly resistant to treatment, no matter what their type or degree of histological malignancy. This is in contradistinction to their behaviour as extraneural tumors. The ensuing discussion will, therefore, refer to these tumors simply as primary CNS lymphomas.

Incidence and Location

In various sizes, the incidence of primary CNS lymphoma has ranged between 0.5 and 2.3% of all primary brain tumors (326, 403, 414–416). As reported by Spaun et al. (403), in the population of three Danish counties there were 1.83 primary CNS lymphomas per million people per year. Among large groups of lymphoma patients, between 0.2 and 0.7% have disease which is confined to the CNS (407, 417). Levitt et al. (418) reported involvement of the CNS in 9% of their 592 patients with non-Hodgkin's lymphoma. In these patients, involvement of the meninges and epidural space was far more common than of the brain parenchyma, which is not the case with primary tumors. It is not, therefore, justifiable to assert that primary lymphomas of the brain merely represent examples of systemic disease in which the extraneural component has been completely controlled by the patient's 'immune surveillance' system.

In most (389, 391, 394, 402, 404, 419), but not all (403), of the series, there is a distinct male predominance. The most extensive collection of reports from the literature, published by Murray et al. (394), found a male:female ratio of 1.5:1 in 693 cases. The age incidence ranged from 2 months to 90 years, with a mean age of 52 years. A second, minor peak has been reported in the first decade as well (402, 419). No detailed information is available on racial or geographical incidence.

In the last decade, there has been an apparent increase in the interest taken in this tumor, which may be, in part, due to the now universally recognized association between primary CNS lymphoma and disorders of the immune system (394–396, 402, 404, 419). The most common situation is that in which a patient has been chronically immunosuppressed following renal (420) or cardiac (402) transplant, but it has also been reported in patients undergoing immunosuppressive therapy for autoimmune diseases such as systemic lupus erythematosus (421), Sjögren's syndrome (422), rheumatoid arthritis (423), and necrotizing vasculitis (424). Their occurrence in these patients may be due to the failure of B-cell regulation by T-lymphocytes (425), to chronic antigenic stimulation or to stimulation through a B-cell growth factor (426). Most recently, there have been reports of the occurrence of primary CNS lymphoma in patients with acquired immune deficiency syndrome (AIDS) (396, 427–429). The exact incidence in AIDS is unknown at present but it will probably become an increasingly important problem in the future. Finally, primary CNS lymphoma has been reported in patients with such congenital immunological disorders as Mikulicz's syndrome (1), Wiskott–Aldrich syndrome (430, 431), Waldenström's macroglobulinemia (432), immunoglobulin A deficiency (433) and hyperimmunoglobulinemia-E (434). It is unknown if the development of primary CNS lymphoma in these various disorders involves a common pathway, or different mechanisms. One possible culprit, at least in the immunosuppressed patients, is felt to be the Epstein–Barr virus (EBV), which is trophic for B-lymphocytes (435, 436). In most patients infected by the EBV, the infection is controlled, at least in part, by the T-cell-mediated immune system. The virus becomes latent, with viral genomes remaining in the patient's B-cells. The suppression of a patient's T-cells could lead either to reactivation of a latent EBV infection or to the deficient control of new infections, in turn leading to a variety of lymphoproliferative disorders, including pri-

mary CNS lymphoma (437, 438). Hochberg et al. (438) have reported finding EBV genomes in the DNA preparation of an apparently spontaneously occurring CNS lymphoma, but not from the adjacent normal brain tissue, suggesting the induction of the tumor by EBV. Further evidence is the report of intracranial tumors showing the coexistence of 'Burkitt-type lymphoma' areas and areas of 'reticulum cell sarcoma' (439). The reason that some of these immunopathy or EBV-related tumors arise in the CNS is unclear, but may involve the status of the CNS as an immunologically 'privileged' or isolated organ, in which the cell-mediated immune response is normally weak (440, 441).

Most primary CNS lymphomas are found in the cerebral hemispheres, usually in the frontal lobe (394, 404), but often involving multiple lobes or deep structures, and the corpus callosum (389, 442). They have a definite tendency to spread through this structure into both hemispheres, and it has been estimated that 9% of all bi-hemispheric, or 'butterfly' tumors are lymphomas. They usually arise as single masses, but approximately one-third have multiple lesions, either of the same hemisphere (57%) or in different compartments (43%) (394). About 22% of the single lesions occur infratentorially. These tumors arise in the spine only rarely (394, 443) (one out of 30 tumors reported by Helle et al. (402)). Extra-neural spread of the tumor is uncommon, usually occurring in axillary lymph nodes, kidney, testicle and lungs (402).

Origin and Pathology

One of the major questions yet to be answered concerning primary CNS lymphomas is how isolated lesions can occur in an organ which normally has no lymphatic system. This has become more pointed, now that it has been accepted that the endogenous phagocytic cells of the CNS, the microglia, are not the cells of origin of these tumors. To answer this question, the concept of the CNS as an immunologically 'privileged' organ has been evoked (440, 441).

The tumors may have arisen elsewhere in the body, but their growth in the CNS could be selected for to such an extent that they become undetectable anywhere else. The lack of agreement between the reported locations of primary CNS lymphomas and the anticipated locations of metastatic tumors from regional blood flow studies, is against this hypothesis (402, 444).

It has been noted by many pathologists that the tumors arising in the CNS tend to recapitulate, in appearance, if not in overall prognosis, the spectrum of disease found outside the CNS. There are a couple of notable exceptions to this rule. The first is that 'follicular' tumors are rarely reported in the CNS, though some sections of tumors may have a follicular center cell appearance (391, 404, 414). More significant is the lack of well-proven occurrences of primary CNS Hodgkin's lymphomas. The largest series, reported by Henry et al. (407) of 83 cases from the Armed Forces Institute of Pathology (AFIP) files of lymphoma patients, does include 23 tumors designated as Hodgkin's lymphomas, based on the finding of Reed–Sternberg cells. However, subsequent immunohistochemical studies by Taylor et al. (391), of many of the same tumors, have shown them to be immunoblastic sarcomas (Lukes–Collins classification) or diffuse histiocytic lymphomas (Rappaport). The Reed–Sternberg-like cells were interpreted, in these cases, as representing bizarre neoplastic immunoblasts. These authors also found a greater intratumoral morphological diversity among CNS lesions than among their systemic counterparts, as well as a more variable pattern of functional capacity (i.e. ability to produce immunoglobulin components). Thirdly, the percentage of B-cell-derived tumors, particularly among those associated with immune deficient states, 53% in the group of Kawakami et al. (395), 54% in that of Taylor et al. (391), and 5/5 in the report by So et al. (396) of homosexual men, is higher than in the systemic tumors (391, 455–447).

The most common gross appearance of the tumor nodule, is that of a pink or gray mass which is relatively firm and well delineated from the surrounding brain, in which there is often appreciable edema (387, 438). Less commonly, an ill-defined area of less pathological-looking tissue may be seen (415).

Microscopically, the central portions of the tumors are highly cellular, and there are areas of necrosis. At their border, the tumors have a characteristic appearance of perivascular infiltration, with distension of the Virchow–Robin spaces, infiltration of the vessel wall itself, and increased reticulin formation (17, 407, 448). These invasive borders are often found beyond the macroscopically discernible limits of the tumor. Other modes of spread are leptomeningeal, subpial and diffuse parenchymal (17, 407, 448). Areas of plasmacytoid differentiation may be found in otherwise malignant-looking tumors. Reactive gliosis may be prominent at the periphery. It is often difficult to differentiate primary CNS lymphoma from other dense, small cell tumors, such as glioblastoma and undifferentiated adenocarcinoma, but examination of the tumor periphery, and the use of special staining techniques for reticulin, GFAP, immunoglobulin, and lymphocyte cell surface markers, makes the diagnosis more certain (388, 395, 396).

Clinical and Radiological Findings

Due to the different ways the tumor may involve the brain, the presenting symptom complexes may vary considerably (449). Those with circumscribed lymphoma and surrounding edema present with focal or non-focal signs and symptoms of a rapidly growing mass lesion (450). Those with more diffuse disease, or slowly progressive disease, may be misdiagnosed as having viral encephalitis (385, 450), with fever and malaise; demyelinating disease, with a long, remitting and relapsing course of focal deficits (447, 450), or cerebrovascular disease, as vascular patency is compromised by perivascular tumor infiltrates. Patients with primarily meningeal involvement will often present with a picture similar to other diseases with diffuse meningeal involvement, i.e. headache, nausea, nuchal rigidity, and cranial nerve palsies (447). The first type of presentation is most common (about 60%) (449). Disturbances of behavior and intellect, progressive hemiparesis, headaches and papilledema, and seizures are the most common findings of supratentorial lesions (409). There is a generally short average duration of symptoms before diagnosis is made, only 1–3 months in several large series (394, 403, 407–409, 414).

The sign of Leser–Trélat, accepted as an indicator of underlying malignancy, has now been reported in a single case of primary CNS lymphoma (451). This sign is defined as the sudden appearance of numerous seborrheic keratoses in association, usually, with adenocarcinomas of the gastrointestinal or genitourinary tracts, but also with some leukemias (451, 452).

The radiological findings in these tumors are as non-specific as the clinical findings. CT scanning is currently the procedure of choice (401, 404, 453, 454), with the contrast-enhanced scan often showing single or multiple areas of uniform enhancement. These areas may or may not be well defined. They may easily be confused with metastases, meningiomas or hemangiopericytomas. Studies done early in the course of the disease may either be normal or show only areas of decreased attenuation which do not enhance, resembling cerebral infarction.

Angiography is frequently normal, or shows only an avascular mass. Less common, though more specific, vascular findings are vessel narrowing or occlusion, presumably due to arterial encasement, and hypervascularity, with 'shaggy' arteries and veins (397, 449). Skull x-rays, if abnormal, will show evidence of elevated intracranial pressure. Radionuclide scintigraphy shows homogeneous, increased activity (397). MRI findings are uncertain at present.

The preoperative or antemortem diagnosis of lymphoma is often impossible (401). Some authors have recommended examining the CSF in patients in whom a lumbar puncture is not contra-indicated by the presence of a tumor mass (401, 402, 406, 408, 414, 456). The most common CSF abnormality, seen in 81% of the patients collected by Hobson et al. (409), is increased protein. An increased cell count was found in 42%. When CNS lymphoma is suspected, cytological examination is essential. It has a reported sensitivity as high as 70% (449), and immunohistochemical staining of the cells for immunoglobulin may be positive in as many as 25% of patients. A higher level of beta-2-microglobulin in the CSF than in the serum is highly suggestive of CNS lymphoma (457).

The existence of lymphoma elsewhere in the body should be ruled out preoperatively. This preoperative workup may consist of a full blood count, liver-spleen scan, chest and abdominal CT scan, and where indicated a bone marrow aspirate/trephine or a biopsy of abnormal lymph nodes (449).

Treatment and Outcome

Progress in treating lymphomas of the CNS, whether primary or secondary, has been more disappointing than the treatment of systemic lymphoma. Most authors still feel that aggressive treatment, with surgery, radiation, and chemotherapy, offers at least palliative relief to many patients (394, 401–403, 409, 419).

The various surgical interventions include open or stereotactic biopsies, subtotal or gross resection, and placement of an Ommaya reservoir for the administration of chemotherapy. Often some form of operation is necessary to establish a diagnosis, and more radical procedures may be performed in well-localized tumors in accessible locations. However, because of their infiltrative nature, even these tumors cannot be totally removed, and they will recur rapidly, usually at the original site. Without specific treatment, post-diagnosis survival averages between 2 and 3 months (402, 414); surgery can increase survival by about 1–2 months (407), but there is no evidence that the results with radical surgery are better than biopsy alone, especially once radiation therapy is added to the treatment algorithm. The operative mortality for appropriate procedures in properly selected patients should be no more than 5%.

Radiation therapy has been shown to prolong the average life expectancy of patients with primary CNS lymphoma, although few long-term survivals have been reported (387, 399, 407, 447). Several reports have confirmed a dose–response relationship for radiotherapy (394, 458, 459) and minimum doses of 45 to 55 Gy are now usually given (394, 399, 458–460). From their review, Murray et al. (394) recommended more than 50 Gy to the primary tumor. With radiotherapy, mean survivals of up to 45 months have been reported (387). The role of craniospinal radiation is not yet known, as there have been few reports of its use, or of postoperative CNS staging of the extent of tumor. The reported recurrences are usually at the site of the primary lesion, and very few patients have evidence of spinal seeding at initial presentation, despite the presence of malignant cells in the CSF in about 25% of patients, so Leavens et al. (449) feel that craniospinal radiotherapy is unjustified, and recommend intrathecal chemotherapy to sterilize a positive CSF. However, as many as 25% have CSF seeding as the first sign of disease progression, so there may be a role for craniospinal irradiation in selected patients (461). Tumor size may be important for the effectiveness of local radiation, as reported by Mendenhall et al. (462), whose 2 patients with tumors less than 3.5 cm in diameter were free of disease at 38 and 48 months post-radiation.

Chemotherapy has often been reserved for patients with disease progression or recurrence, and not given at the time of initial treatment. The most favorable documented response to a chemotherapeutic agent is to corticosteroids, which seem to have a direct tumoricidal effect, in addition to the usual anti-edema response (394, 463, 464). Recurrence of clinical and radiological abnormalities following the discontinuation of steroids is the rule, however. High-dose, intravenous methotrexate (MTX) has been used, with good results (460, 465), but, especially when used in conjunction with radiation, it can cause devastating encephalomalacia (406, 466). Another regimen which has been reported is alternating doses of MTX and cytosine arabinoside (ara-C), intrathecally or intravenously (406, 449, 467). The major side effects are seizures, dementia and paraplegia (449). Kawakami et al. (395) have recommended a regimen of Cytoxan, Adriamycin, vincristine and prednisone (CHOP) as an adjunctive treatment with subtotal resection and irradiation. Neuwelt et al. (468) have successfully used blood–brain barrier (BBB) modification, with intra-carotid mannitol, followed by intra-carotid MTX, and systemic cyclophosphamide and procarbazine. The pre-treatment discontinuation of steroids was felt by them to enhance BBB opening and, therefore, drug delivery. Dexamethasone, and leucovorin rescue, were instituted the day after MTX was given.

Despite the temporary effectiveness of radiation, and the recent advances in chemotherapy, the prognosis for most patients with primary CNS lymphoma remains poor. In the review of Murray et al. (394) of 693 cases, only 8% survived for more than 3 years and of these 56 patients, only 21 survived for 5 years, 10 of these relapsing between 5 and 12.5 years. The longest survival was for 16.5 years, in an infant. These figures may be somewhat improved with the use of high-dose radiation and innovative forms of chemotherapy, but this tumor, when arising in the CNS, remains a difficult one to treat.

It has not been possible to determine, in advance, which patients are most likely to benefit from aggressive treatment. Woodman et al. (401) and Helle et al. (402) have observed heterogeneous behavior of CNS lymphomas. In the latter series, those patients with either a diffuse, mixed lymphoma or an infratentorial tumor had poorer prognoses, but these two factors alone could not account for the above-mentioned disparity. Survival time also did not appear to correlate well with the extent of surgical resection of the tumor.

Miscellaneous Conditions

Other lesions which may affect the CNS primarily are histiocytosis X, lymphosarcoma and plasmacytoma.

Histiocytosis X

Cerebral histiocytosis X refers to a condition in which a granulomatous mass is found within the infundibulum (17, 469, 470). It has also been called hypothalamic granuloma, Ayala's disease and Gagel's granuloma. Patients generally present with diabetes insipidus or, less frequently, a history of hypogonadism or obesity. The histology consists primarily of large, pale cells which, because of their 'foamy' appearance, are reminiscent of the histiocytes of Hand–Schüller–Christian disease. There is a gliotic border containing reactive astrocytes, so its differentiation from an inflammatory response within an astrocytoma is occasionally difficult. Its differentiation from localized lymphoma is also, on occasion, not easy.

Several cases of primary intracerebral eosinophilic granuloma have been reported. In addition to the hypothalamus, they have been found in the cerebellum and the frontal lobe (470, 471). Moscinski and Kleinschmidt-deMasters (471) have found staining for S-100 protein to be useful in confirming the lesion's histiocytic nature, and in differentiating it from reactive or infectious granulomas.

Lymphosarcoma (see section on lymphoma, above)

Unusual cases have been reported in which lymphosarcoma, a condition which usually has a generalized distribution, has remained isolated to the CNS for many years, either in the spinal epidural space (472), or in the cranial epidural, subdural or subarachnoid space (473). This lesion appears to respond more favorably than most sarcomas to radiation therapy. Rubinstein has reported a patient who presented with a 30-year history of recurrent polyneuropathy, and was found at autopsy to have diffuse leptomeningeal, perivascular and radicular (both cranial and spinal) infiltration by a lymphosarcoma (17, 474).

Plasmacytoma

Primary involvement of the CNS by plasmacytoma can also be distinguished from secondary involvement by multiple myeloma. These isolated lesions are found either in the hypothalamic region, or attached to the frontal dura and falx (475, 476). Total removal of the dural lesions is achievable, and, in the case reported by Moossy and Wilson (476), there was no evidence of recurrence or dissemination after 5 years of follow-up. Treatment of the hypothalamic lesions with radiation therapy may be beneficial, but little data concerning this entity exists.

TUMORS OF MALDEVELOPMENTAL ORIGIN

Craniopharyngioma

Perhaps no other tumor discussed in this chapter has been the subject of as much controversy as the craniopharyngioma. Many questions have been raised concerning its origin, natural history, resectability, and optimal treatment. In this section we will not be able to give as thorough a treatment of this fascinating subject as it deserves, but hope to point out some of its most salient features, in particular, some of the differences in the disease as it presents in children and adults.

Incidence and Location

Craniopharyngiomas comprise less than 4% of all intracranial tumors (17, 477, 478). Roughly 40% occur before the age of 15, but there is a second, lesser peak incidence in the fifth and sixth decades (479). Because of their relatively high incidence in children, they are the most common non-glial tumor of childhood (105). The sex distribution appears to be equal in all age groups (478, 480), though some series report a male preponderance in children (481–483). Most craniopharyngiomas arise in the subarachnoid space between the optic chiasm and the diaphragma sellae. As they grow, they may displace the chiasm posteriorly or superiorly, the floor of the third ventricle superiorly, and the pituitary stalk posteriorly (484). Some may be partially, or even totally, within the sella (485). Another, more unusual location is within the third ventricle (486). Exceptionally, tumors have been found in the sphenoid bone, sphenoid sinus and nasopharynx, along the developmental pathway of Rathke's pouch, for the remnants of which these tumors are felt to arise (487, 488). Steno (489) studied the anatomical relationship of craniopharyngiomas to the surrounding structures and felt that this relationship dictates the direction of growth of the tumor. The radiological delineation of this relationship preoperatively can aid in the choice of an operative approach. When small carniopharyngiomas are found at autopsy, they usually are attached to the tuber cinereum (96). This is also the site of firmest attachment, and occasional invasion, of symptomatic tumors (480, 484). They tend not to attach themselves to the optic apparatus (484). Although most tumors remain in the suprasellar region, some extend under the frontal or temporal lobes or even into the posterior fossa (490).

Origin

Since the end of the 19th century, the epithelial nature of certain intra- and suprasellar tumors has been appreciated. In 1899, Matt and Barrett hypothesized that these lesions arise from remnants of Rathke's pouch (491). This structure develops from an upward diverticulum of the primitive buccal cavity, and normally matures into the anterior lobe and the pars intermedia of the pituitary gland (492). This theory of the origin of carniopharyngiomas has gained widespread acceptance. In support of it is the histological resemblance of craniopharyngiomas to the adamantinoma (a

tumor of the primitive buccal cavity) (492, 493), the discovery of examples along the developmental route taken by Rathke's pouch, and the finding of rudimentary teeth in at least one such tumor (494). The dissimilarity of craniopharyngioma epithelium from that of the rare, Rathke's cleft cyst has been cited as evidence against the theory, but several explanations have been proposed to reconcile these findings. One is that Rathke's cleft cysts may not really be derived from Rathke's pouch (495). Another is that craniopharyngioma and Rathke's cleft cysts merely represent neoplastic and non-neoplastic variants respectively, of the same developmental abnormality (490). Thirdly it has been suggested that the absence of adjacent notochordal remnants and posterior pituitary permits the squamous metaplasia of epithelial cells in the suprasellar area to become, eventually, craniopharyngiomas (490). Very rare tumors, containing elements of both Rathke cleft cyst and craniopharyngioma, support the last two hypotheses (96, 496, 497).

Nearly half of the adult tumors are comprised of squamous epithelium, without the papillary and palisading features seen in childhood tumors (498). This subtype of craniopharyngioma may be related to the rests of squamous epithelial cells which have been found, in increasing frequency with age, in the adenohypophysis at autopsy (499, 500). Such cells may be derived from the metaplasia of pituitary cells and give rise to some of the adult tumors which, therefore, need not be considered of embryological origin (491). Kahn et al. (498) consider these tumors to have a better prognosis than the pediatric variety.

Another theory is that craniopharyngiomas are variants of 'inclusion' cysts, such as epidermoids and dermoids (see below) (96). A tumor sharing the characteristics of both has been reported, but its precise classification has been debated (502).

Pathology

Craniopharyngiomas characteristically contain both solid and cystic components, in varying proportions. The exact mechanism of cyst formation is unknown, but, in many instances, is probably related to degenerative changes (490). Smaller cysts may coalesce to form large ones. They are filled with a turbid fluid, white or brownish in color, which contains birefringent cholesterol crystals. The cyst walls vary in thickness and firmness (96): some are so diaphanous that they may rupture spontaneously, causing a severe chemical meningitis (492). This is a rare occurrence, though, compared to the iatrogenic meningitis caused by the spillage of cholesterol crystals into the subarachnoid space at operation. The tumors vary in size from a few millimeters to over 10 cm in diameter (477, 503). Small intrasellar craniopharyngiomas have been mistaken for prolactin-secreting pituitary adenomas (477). As mentioned above there is usually an area of attachment to the tuber cinereum, and further adhesion may also be found to neighboring arteries, from which the tumor derives its blood supply. This is the most frequent cause of incomplete removal of these otherwise benign tumors (479, 480).

Microscopically, stratified squamous epithelium is seen in the cystic areas, and the solid regions have calcium deposits and cholesterol clefts. In areas of cystic degeneration, foreign body giant cells and lymphocytic infiltration may be found. There is an external layer of high columnar epithelium. Epithelial bands within the tumor are supported by a mesodermal stroma, and palisading and papillary structure are often seen (477). In adults, the above-mentioned squamous variety lacks these characteristics, mimicking instead the epithelium of the buccal cavity (498). They usually do not exhibit areas of calcification. Approximately half of adult tumors, and nearly all pediatric tumors, will show some calcification (478, 484). At the site of attachment to the brain, a gliotic reaction, with Rosenthal fibers, may occur (492, 504). Finger-like projections of tumor, up to 6 mm long, may be found in the brain (484, 505). Nonetheless, these tumors are not felt to be invasive (498, 504), and clearcut

signs of anaplasia have not been reported (17). In tissue culture some aggressive, or 'atypical', tumors may produce rapidly growing cell populations, with microvilli and the ability to synthesize cholesterol crystals (506, 507).

Clinical and Radiographic Findings

The presenting signs and symptoms of craniopharyngioma are different in children than in adults (479, 490, 507–512). In the former, headache, nausea and vomiting are more frequent than visual disturbance, whereas, in the adult, the reverse is true. This may be, in part, due to the degree to which children will tolerate visual loss without complaining (477). Symptoms may be present for as short as one month or as long as 30 years before a diagnosis is made. Endocrine dysfunction, usually on a hypothalamic basis (483, 513, 514), is present in as many as 90% of children and 70% of adults. In the latter, the amenorrhea/galactorrhea syndrome, combined with a small intrasellar tumor may lead to the diagnosis of prolactinoma (477). However, growth hormone deficiency was the most common finding in the series published by Barreca et al. (515). As the tumors may become quite large before being detected, papilledema is a common finding, especially in children. With expansion of the tumors upwards, the foramina of Monro may become obstructed, leading to hydrocephalus. Concomitant frontal lobe dysfunction is frequently manifested as disturbed mentation or a psychiatric disorder, such as apathy, depression, Korsakoff's syndrome, somnolence and incontinence (498). It is prognostic of a poor outcome (505). Signs of meningeal irritation are produced when cyst contents are spontaneously released into the subarachnoid space (516). With recurrent episodes of aseptic meningitis, the diagnosis of craniopharyngioma should be suspected (517).

Calcification on plain skull x-rays is considered a hallmark of craniopharyngioma, although it is found in only 40% of adult patients (478, 484, 509, 517, 518). Another common plain film finding is erosion of the anterior clinoid or dorsum sellae, or expansion of the sella turcica (498, 508, 519). About two-thirds of adult patients, and nearly all children, manifest some abnormality on plain x-ray (498, 509, 519). CT is useful in delineating cystic components of the tumors, though the density of the cyst fluid may vary considerably (520, 21). Solid portions of the tumor tend to enhance with contrast. Of major importance in detecting extension of the tumor into the sella, and delineating its relationships to the third ventricle, circle of Willis and cranial fossae, has been the coronal CT scan (477). The operative approach is often modified based on these findings (489). Angiography may be helpful in determining the regional vascular anatomy (522), but usually does not show the tumor's vascular supply well enough to assist the surgeon (477, 484). In patients who do not have raised intracranial pressure, the use of positive contrast cisternography/CT may provide additional anatomical information, especially in tumors with isodense cysts or non-enhancing areas (477). Prior to the development of this technique, pneumoencephalography was used because of its high degree of sensitivity for suprasellar masses (489, 498, 504).

Preoperative endocrinological assessment is important to determine those patients at risk for hypothyroidism or hypoadrenalism (479, 515). If already present, these should be corrected, time permitting, before attempting to remove the tumor. At times, ventricular drainage or shunting is employed to permit enough time for the workup to be completed and replacement therapy to be instituted (477).

Treatment and Outcome

The greatest controversy concerning cranio-pharyngiomas has been focused on their optimal treatment (479). This has been one of the more long-lasting debates in all of neurosurgery. Cushing stated, in 1932, that craniopharyngiomas 'offer the most baffling problem which confronts the neurosurgeon' (523). Despite the subsequent development of microsurgical techniques, reliable CSF shunt systems, focused radiation therapy, and steroid replacement therapy, they remain a surgical challenge. The controversy centers around three main issues: (1) how safely, and to what extent, can craniopharyngiomas be totally excised; (2) can radiation therapy kill craniopharyngioma tissue at doses which are tolerated by the surrounding neural structures; (3) does postoperative irradiation, following subtotal resection, help prevent symptomatic recurrences (480, 524)?

Some feel that, despite their histologically benign appearance, craniopharyngiomas should be regarded as malignant tumors, especially in children, because of the difficult and hazardous nature of their excision (525, 526). This is supported by the accumulating data concerning the radiosensitivity of cranio-pharyngioma cells relative to other benign neoplasms, such as meningiomas, whose sensitivity has been harder to demonstrate (478, 479, 508, 527, 528). It has been well recognized, since the report by Kahn et al. (498), that tumors arising in children have biological characteristics which make them more difficult to manage than adult tumors. Within the last decade, the authors of several major series have advocated a variety of approaches, from radical excision of all tumors, so that the side-effects of radiation (greatest in children) can be avoided (480, 522), to subtotal resection of selected tumors followed by radiotherapy, in order to avoid operative injury to the hypothalamus and optic apparatus (482, 524, 527), to partial resection or biopsy of all tumors followed by radiotherapy (525, 526, 529–531). Other therapeutic strategies which have been attempted, in isolated series, with qualified success, have been cyst aspiration followed by radiotherapy (498, 518), stereotactic, intracystic injection of a colloidal suspension of radioactive gold or yttrium (532–534), and the intratumoral injection of bleomycin (535). Radiation therapy may decrease the production of fluid by the tumor cyst (480). One of the weaknesses of most of the recent series is their relatively short mean follow-up period, 3–4 years. Tumor recurrences have been reported as late as 20 and 30 years postoperatively (479, 498, 535, 536), but most will recur within 10 years (479). Later recurrences may represent de novo growths of new tumor cell populations (524).

In Hoffman's recent report (522) of 29 pediatric patients, treated between 1976 and 1985, total removal was felt to be achieved, at operation, in 25. There was no clinical evidence of recurrence in 21 despite areas of residual calcification in 14. Three out of the 7 patients whose CTs showed areas of enhancement had recurrences. These patients were treated with reoperation followed by an unspecified dose of radiation. In this series, as in others (478, 479), the main deterrent to total excision was adherence to surrounding vessels, rather than to the hypothalamus or tuber cinereum. Of the 4 patients with a known subtotal resection at the time of operation, all had symptomatic recurrences within a year. All of these responded to radiotherapy, but 2 of the 4 later became mentally retarded.

It is evident, from a review of the recent literature, that the therapeutic approach must be individualized for each patient. Surgeons who have considerable familiarity with the numerous microsurgical approaches to this area should be able to perform a total excision in the majority of cases (504, 523, 537, 538). With enough experience, he or she can tell when further surgical manipulation is likely to produce postoperative deficits, and at that time the operation should be stopped. Residual tumors, whether present at operation, or detected as enhancing masses on CT, should be irradiated with roughly 50–60 Gy in fractions of less than 200 cGy (524). On the other hand, Fischer et al. (529) infer, from their data, that fewer complications are encountered in biopsied and irradiated patients than in patients undergoing gross total excision. Second surgical procedures for recurrences are associated with a greater rate of complications (537, 539, 540), and may therefore be of limited useful-

ness except as the second part of a two-staged procedure, or for residual tumor detected on CT. There appears to be no need to irradiate tumors which have been totally removed or which do not demonstrate residual enhancing areas on CT (522, 524). The routine use of CT should decrease the incidence of 'false cures' reported in some series (477, 524).

A large percentage of patients undergoing microsurgical excision of craniopharyngiomas will experience postoperative hypothalamic or pituitary dysfunction. Diabetes insipidus has been a particularly frequent sequela (480, 504, 518). Delayed coma, associated with a chronic, hyperosmolar state, is one of the more serious complications (529, 539). Growth hormone deficiency was detected in 22 of 28 patients studied by Stahnke et al. (483), following radical surgery. Most endocrinological complications are treatable with replacement therapy. Visual and neuropsychological deficits may occur following both irradiation and radical removal. According to Fischer et al. (529), they are more common in the latter.

Operative procedures for suprasellar masses include subfrontal approaches between the optic nerves, between the optic nerve and carotid artery or through the lamina terminalis. A transcallosal approach is used for intra-third ventricular tumors, and the trans-sphenoidal route is best for primarily intrasellar tumors (477). Other procedures which play a role in the management of craniopharyngiomas are stereotactic biopsies, cyst drainage, placement of Ommaya reservoirs for repeated aspiration of cyst contents or instillation of radioactive or chemotherapeutic substances, and ventricular shunts for hydrocephalus.

In their review of recent series, Stahnke et al. (483) report a recurrence rate of 22% in 'totally' resected tumors, 72% in non-irradiated, partially resected tumors, and 26% in patients with subtotal resection plus radiation therapy. By now, therefore, the efficacy of radiotherapy in treating craniopharyngiomas has been widely accepted. It is more effective when given within a short time of operation, for residual tumor, than for recurrences, but

25% of patients with subtotal resection have long-term control even without radiation (524). The percentage of tumors amenable to total resection has varied between 24 and 83% of patients in various series (480, 482, 498, 512, 537–539). This figure depends upon the criteria used to define total resection, as well as on the skill and experience of the surgeon, and the patient population (tumors in adults being generally easier to remove). Operative mortality in radical procedures, in recent series, has been between 0 and 12% (482, 508, 522). There is ongoing debate about whether the morbidity from radical procedures (i.e. visual loss, endocrinopathies, delayed coma, neuropsychological deficits and seizures) is less than that from radiation therapy (optic neuritis, diminished IQ in younger children, radiation necrosis of brain, memory disturbances, occlusive intracranial arteriopathy and the development of secondary brain tumors (e.g. sarcomas, gliomas and meningiomas)) (484, 524, 526, 529, 541–543). With management which is tailored to the individual patient, many long-term 'useful' survivals are achievable (482, 524, 539, 540, 544), but this tumor still remains a challenge to the clinician.

Dermoid and Epidermoid Cysts

Because of the similarities in their origin, appearance, treatment and outcome, dermoids and epidermoids will be considered together. Whenever appropriate, their differences will be discussed. They both belong to a family of tumors of maldevelopmental origin, which are often referred to as 'inclusion tumors' because of their supposed origin in skin elements 'included' within the neuraxis during embryogenesis (17, 490, 545), or as the result of trauma. Some teratomas which contain well-developed dermal elements may also be included in this category, but, as they also contain regions derived from other embryonal layers, they will not be considered here.

Incidence and Location

Together, dermoids and epidermoids comprise approximately 1% of all intracranial tumors (546). Intracranially, epidermoids are roughly five times as common as dermoids (490), though in the spine they occur with a more equal frequency (547). Both epidermoids and dermoids probably occur with equal frequency in males and females (490, 548–551). The peak incidence of epidermoids is in the third and fourth decades (552, 553), though they may be encountered at any age. Dermoids tend to occur in the first two decades of life (549, 550). The reason for this discrepancy in age incidence is probably the relatively slow rate of growth of epidermoids, which enlarge mainly through the intracystic accumulation of desquamated cellular debris (546, 554). The enlargement of dermoid cysts, on the other hand, is augmented by the glandular secretions of the sebaceous glands found within their walls. Unlike solid tumors, epidermoid cysts tend to have a linear growth rate (555).

The location of epidermoids shows a greater variety than that of dermoids. The former have more of a tendency to be found away from the midline. Epidermoids are most frequently found in the cerebellopontine angle and in the parasellar region of the middle fossa (549, 551, 552, 556), where they may involve the mesial temporal lobe and hypothalamus. In these locations, they may be associated with primary, intracranial, squamous cell carcinoma (557–559). Another common location is the cranial diploic space, usually in the parietal or frontal regions. These epidermoid lesions occur about half as frequently as intradural tumors (548–550). When they occur in the paratrigeminal region of the apex of the temporal bone, their resection may be particularly complicated and has been associated with intracerebral abscess (560). Less common locations are the spinal canal (561), the third (546), fourth (562) and lateral ventricles (96), the cerebral hemispheres (563, 564), optic chiasm, brainstem (565) and pineal region (566). Dermoids are found most frequently in the cerebellar vermis and fourth ventricle (549, 550) and in the spinal canal but may be found at other locations along the midline, and in the scalp, orbit and paranasal region (546). Both dermoids and epidermoids, when located in the spinal canal, are more frequently in the lumbosacral region than elsewhere (547). This may be explained embryologically, through the existence of a spinal–cutaneous attachment at this level during fetal life (547). Dermoids in the spinal cord are often associated with cutaneous abnormalities such as tufts of hair, dermal sinuses, areas of skin pigmentation, and with spina bifida (546, 550) and, more rarely, syringomyelia (17). Cerebellar dermoids have also been associated with dermal sinuses in the occipital region (567). These sinuses may predispose the patient to pyogenic meningitis (568). A case has been reported of an association between Goldenhar's syndrome (oculoauriculovertebral dysplasia) and intracranial dermoid cyst (569).

Epidermoids have been found in patients undergoing repeated spinal taps for intrathecal antibiotic administration (570), or even after a single spinal tap (571). These were felt to arise from small fragments of skin carried through the dura by spinal needles, when used without stylets. This pathogenetic mechanism has been supported by experimental data (572, 573). An unusual case has been reported of multiple intraspinal epidermoids and lipomas following a shotgun injury to the spine (574). In the past, an inflammatory etiology has been hypothesized for some epidermoid-like masses occurring in the middle ear and temporal bone (575). These tumors, known as 'cholesteatomas', were found in patients with chronic otitis media and mastoiditis. This etiology has been questioned because there has been no concomitant decline in the incidence of cholesteatomas with the decreased incidence of chronic otitis media since the introduction of antibiotics (554). Also, cholesteatomas rarely occur in conjunction with other chronic, closed-space infections.

Origin and Pathology

Both dermoids and epidermoids are felt to originate from ectopic epithelium. As mentioned above, this may be due to traumatic or inflammatory mechanisms, but is usually on the basis of dysembryogenesis, either during the closure of the midline neural groove, the subsequent upward migration of the spinal cord from its area of attachment to the skin, or in the formation of the 'secondary vesicles' (i.e. optic and otic) (545, 547, 554, 567, 576). The developmental stage of the ectopic epithelium will then dictate whether an epidermoid, with only epidermal cells, or a dermoid, with its additional components of dermal adnexal structures, will form. The inclusion of epithelium might also occur, after closure of the neural tube, during the formation of the flexures of the brain (577). A theory of metaplastic genesis for middle ear epidermoids has recently been proposed by Sade (578). Whatever the origin of these tumors, it is different from that of craniopharyngiomas, which also probably arise as the result of disturbed embryogenesis, but at a different stage and location (i.e. Rathke's pouch) (555, 579). Still, both craniopharyngiomas and teratomas may contain squamous epithelium, on microscopic examination, and are often included in the differential diagnosis of dermoids and epidermoids (96, 546, 580).

Grossly, both dermoids and epidermoids are usually well-demarcated, smooth, lobulated masses (17, 546). They may have a pinkish or whitish sheen, because of which both have been referred to as 'pearly tumors' (581). As they grow relatively slowly, they often attain a large size before being diagnosed. Focal calcification may be present in both, and, within the cyst, a thick, soft, waxy or flakey material is usually found. This is fluid and yellowish in dermoids, due to the secretions of sebaceous glands in the cyst walls, and white in epidermoids (17, 96, 546). Cholesterol crystals are often found, a product of desquamated keratin. Hair may be encountered in dermoids (546).

The pathognomonic microscopic finding, in both types of tumor, is stratified squamous epithelium, containing not only the basal, but also the granular and cornified layers (not found in craniopharyngioma) (546). The basal layer is anchored to a basement membrane in a fibrous, connective tissue capsule. This capsule tends to be thinner in epidermoid tumors. In dermoids, well-formed sweat and sebaceous glands, hair follicles and adipose tissue are also seen (17). Malignant changes are not found in most of the cysts, but, rarely, squamous cell carcinomas may arise, with invasion of the adjacent brain parenchyma (557–559), and a single example of hidradenoma has been reported (582). Exceptionally, leptomeningeal carcinomatosis has been reported (583, 584). Epidermoids may appear to invade the brain, but usually there is only insinuation into the cortical sulci, or burrowing into the parenchyma (552, 553, 563, 567), with a thickening of the overlying pia-arachnoid, and an adjacent fibrillary gliotic reaction (583). If the contents of a cyst spill into the adjacent subarachnoid space, there may be a violent, granulomatous, meningitic reaction, with the formation of foreign body giant cells (17, 553).

Clinical and Radiological Findings

The clinical findings in both dermoid and epidermoid tumors are rarely specific. They are usually the same as any slowly growing mass in the specific locations they arise in. These tumors also produce symptoms through the obstruction of CSF pathways, and through the spillage of their cyst contents into the subarachnoid space (553, 585). The duration of symptoms is typically lengthy, with 8–10 years being not uncommon (550, 552, 553). The average is less for dermoids than epidermoids (549, 585).

Both types of tumor, when arising in the diploic space or scalp, may present as a slowly growing, rubbery, painless, palpable mass. These patients usually seek medical attention because of the cosmetic appearance of the mass (586, 587). Orbital tumors may also produce a cosmetic abnormality, before other symptoms, by the downward and medial displacement of the globe (567, 586). Cysts in the petrous bone may present with a slowly progressive facial nerve paresis.

Intracranial lesions also produce symptoms through slow expansion. In the basal cisterns, these tumors, because of their soft contents and pliable capsules, may extend a considerable distance through the subarachnoid space before causing enough deformation of, or pressure upon, neural structures to become symptomatic (586). Suprasellar tumors usually produce compression of the optic apparatus (588), but have been reported to present with hypothalamic or pituitary dysfunction (579, 586, 589). In the parasellar region of the middle fossa, they can produce either grand mal or temporal lobe seizure disorders and, when growing into the sylvian fissure, compress the internal capsule and thalamus, producing a hemiparesis (564). Seizures are less common in dermoids because of their more frequent midline location (549, 550). In the CP angle, cranial nerve dysfunction, particularly trigeminal neuralgia, occurs (549, 550, 552, 586). Hemifacial spasm, along with other deficits of the fifth, seventh and eighth cranial nerves, are associated with cerebellar findings and pyramidal tract deficits (552). Because of the relative frequency of trigeminal neuralgia and hemifacial spasm, it has been recommended that any young person presenting with these findings be studied for the presence of an epidermoid cyst (586). Lower cranial nerve deficits arise from tumors in more basal locations (565).

Tumors in the ventricles and midline cerebellum produce a variety of symptoms related to their location, or to the obstruction of CSF pathways (562, 586, 590). This latter finding is less common in tumors of the basal cisterns (552), than with those in the pineal region. Obstruction occurs slowly, and the resultant waxing and waning symptomatology has occasionally been ascribed to multiple sclerosis. Eventually, as the tumors attain a large size, headache and dementia may become prominent features of the presentation, with papilledema found on fundoscopic examination.

As the majority of spinal dermoids and epidermoids are in the lumbosacral region, symptoms are those of intramedullary, conus medullaris or cauda equina compression, with slowly progressive paraparesis, sensory disturbance and loss of sphincter control, and/or back and leg pain and numbness (547, 561, 586, 591). Dermoids may present with the clinical and radiographic picture of a tethered spinal cord.

Dermoid cysts, as they are often associated with dermal sinus tracts which are open to the environment, may present with repeated episodes of bacterial meningitis (549, 586, 593). As mentioned above, both dermoids and epidermoids may also cause aseptic meningitis if their contents leak out of their capsules into the subarachnoid space. This reaction may be severe enough to kill the patient (17). Therefore any physician treating a patient with repeated episodes of bacterial or aseptic meningitis should maintain a high index of suspicion for these tumors. CSF findings are similar to those found in Mollaret's meningitis (594).

The radiographic appearance of dermoids and epidermoids, though somewhat characteristic, is not entirely diagnostic. Skull x-rays of patients with intradiploic tumors will typically show erosion and expansion of the calvarial tables on tangential views, and a lucency with sclerotic borders on orthogonal views (587, 595, 596). Soft tissue skull films will verify the presence of a scalp mass in dermoids of the scalp, and may help rule out a more malignant process. Erosion of the temporal bone may be seen in cholesteotomas. In intradural tumors, skull films are usually normal, and the diagnosis rests upon the findings on CT (596). There is usually a cystic mass in the posterior fossa or parasellar region, whose contents are of CSF density (556, 562, 597) though higher attenuation and fat fluid levels have been reported (598–600). There is usually no enhancing rim seen after contrast administration (556), so arachnoid cysts are often considered in the preoperative diagnosis. If contrast enhancement is found, a malignant component may be present (601). Parasitic cysts usually have some enhancing component, as do craniopharyngiomas. Intraventricular and intraparen-

chymal lesions may usually be distinguished from ependymomas, meningiomas and choroid plexus papillomas, and from cystic gliomas, by their lower attenuation values and lack of contrast enhancement. Other parenchymal lesions such as porencephalic cysts may pose difficulties, for which CSF contrast studies can be helpful. Dermoid tumors can sometimes be distinguished from epidermoids by their location and also by the more frequent observation of calcium in the former (596, 598, 601). Coronal sections and post-cisternography CT can be especially helpful in delineating the regional anatomy (602).

Intraspinal lesions are best studied by water-soluble contrast myelography followed by CT (561). This may reveal not only the tumor, usually in an intradural, extramedullary location, but also an associated developmental abnormality such as spina bifida, tethered cord or syringomyelia. Plain x-rays will often show widening of the interpedicular distance because of the chronic nature of the expanding spinal mass (596). Intramedullary tumors may also be found (591, 604). In this location, dermoids cannot be distinguished from epidermoids. The differential diagnosis includes neurofibroma, meningioma, astrocytoma, ependymoma and lipoma. Again, these tumors, except for lipomas, usually have slightly higher attenuation values than dermoids and epidermoids.

Treatment and Outcome

Surgery is the only known effective treatment for these tumors (586). Benign as they are, surgery is still associated with a significant mortality rate (549, 605). Because of the size they attain before detection, and their ability to insinuate themselves between and around neural and vascular structures, their complete removal can be a difficult undertaking (551). Approximately 50 to 80% of intracranial and intraspinal tumors, and nearly all calvarial and scalp tumors, can be removed completely (586). Very few, however, can be removed intact. Extreme care should be taken to prevent the intraoperative escape of cyst contents into the basal cisterns or ventricle (549, 567). The development of microsurgical, and neuro-anesthetic techniques, along with earlier detection and better delineation of the tumors by improved radiological techniques, are the main factors which have brought the operative mortality down from over 70% before 1936 (606), to less than 10% in the 1970s (549). The microsurgical removal of thickened arachnoid bands from nerve roots in the CP angle and spinal subarchnoid space may also help to restore function in some cases (607).

Clinical recurrences of dermoids and epidermoids have become infrequent since the routine use of the surgical microscope. This is probably because of the ability to detect unremoved portions of the cyst wall, permitting the excision of all portions except those most tenaciously adherent to important neural and vascular structures (586). Despite all precautions, aseptic meningitis will occur in about 40% of patients, more frequently when the cyst removal has been incomplete (549, 586). This can lead to basal arachnoiditis, with hydrocephalus and cranial nerve involvement, or to spinal arachnoiditis in tumors in the conus region. No entirely satisfactory means of reducing this reaction is available, though the anti-inflammatory effects of corticosteroids may be of use in some cases. In spinal, intramedullary lesions, the most common, long-lasting complication is sphincter dysfunction (550).

Arachnoid and Ependymal Cysts

Although these lesions are not tumors, in the sense of a neoplastic process, they are frequently considered in the differential diagnosis of some tumors, such as epidermoids. We feel, therefore, that it is not inappropriate to include at least a brief discussion of them in a chapter about unusual CNS tumors.

Incidence and Location

Arachnoid cysts are generally thought of as a

disease of childhood, but may be seen later in adult life (608). Over 60% of patients in most series are in the pediatric age group (609–611). Some are symptomatic, but many are discovered incidentally (608, 610). According to Robinson (612) they constitute approximately 1% of all intracranial space-occupying lesions, but with the advent of CT scans, they have been reported to represent 4.8% of all non-traumatic mass lesions. In the series of Galassi et al. (610) and Robinson (612), there was a four-to-one male predominance. There is also an apparent predilection for the left side. In Rengachary and Watanabe's review of the 208 intracranial cases reported in the literature from 1831 through 1980 (613), almost half were in the sylvian fissure. The next most frequent locations were the CP angle (11%), supracollicular area (10%), vermian area (9%), and sellar and suprasellar region (9%). They may also be located in the interhemispheric fissure, over the cerebral convexity, and adjacent to the clivus. They must be differentiated from other cystic lesions, such as porencephalic cysts, arachnoid diverticuli, post-traumatic leptomeningeal cysts, Dandy–Walker malformations, the CSF collections occasionally seen following meningitis and basilar arachnoiditis, and ependymal cysts (614). Spinal arachnoid cysts may be divided into intradural, extradural and spinal root cysts (615, 616).

Origin and Pathology

The pathogenesis of arachnoid cysts has been somewhat controversial in the past, but there is now a reasonable consensus about their origin. There is little evidence for either a traumatic or an inflammatory etiology, though, in the past, post-traumatic leptomeningeal cysts (growing skull fractures of children), were considered a variant of arachnoid cyst (608). Evidence in favor of a developmental origin is the finding of bilateral cysts, cysts arising in siblings (617), occurrence of cysts in the neonatal period and childhood (608, 610, 611), association of the cysts with other developmental abnormalities, e.g. agenesis of the corpus callosum (608), and the total absence of inflammatory or neoplastic findings on histological examination (612, 614). The underlying brain shows no evidence of agenesis (618), and the weight of the affected hemisphere is the same as that of the contralateral hemisphere (619), implying that arachnoid cysts do not arise secondarily to developmental abnormalities of the brain. In some sylvian fissure cysts, opercular development is absent, indicating cyst formation at an early stage of development (608). The currently recognized mechanism of formation of arachnoid cysts is that minor abnormalities of CSF flow between the two layers of the embryological 'perimedullary mesh' (which later differentiate into the arachnoid and pial membranes), creates a diverticulum in the outer layer which, in time, expands and may or may not remain in communication with the subarachnoid space (610, 611). A ball-valve-like mechanism, along with the pulsatile fluctuation of CSF pressure and flow, or secretion of fluid from cells in the cyst wall, or the action of an increased colloid osmotic pressure, could each facilitate this enlargement (608, 621–626). Maldevelopment of the underlying brain is the result, not the cause of the cyst's enlargement. Also seen is a bulging of the bone overlying the cysts (612, 614, 624, 627). From the juxtaposition of most arachnoid cysts with the basal cisterns, they appear to be, specifically, developmental abnormalities of these structures (613). The cysts usually contain clear, colorless fluid.

The principal pathological finding is splitting of the arachnoid membrane (613, 620, 628). The pia is not directly involved in the cyst wall. The wall contains a collagenous layer; hyperplastic (but not anaplastic) arachnoid cells, mesenchymal in origin, are found in clusters; and there are no bridging trabecular processes between the inner and outer walls, in contradistinction to the normal subarachnoid space (613). Small bridging veins within the cysts, or over its surface, may rupture spontaneously or as the result of minor trauma (629, 630). An osmolar gradient could then be created by blood within the cyst and further

facilitate its growth (623). Xanthochromic fluid has, indeed, been reported, though most cysts' fluid is clear (620, 631).

Ependymal cysts, which are about one-tenth as common as arachnoid cysts (613), are usually but not always (632) found within the brain parenchyma (633, 634). Unlike porencephalic cysts, they have no demonstrable connection to the ventricular system. They are lined with cuboidal or columnar epithelium, and cilia and blepharoplasts may be present. The cyst fluid is often more proteinaceous than that of arachnoid cysts. Several different pathogenetic theories for ependymal cysts have been proposed (633, 635–637).

Clinical and Radiological Findings

Clinically, arachnoid cysts present as slowly growing masses in the subarachnoid cisterns. Those in the relatively capacious sylvian fissure tend to attain a large size before causing symptoms, and are often found incidentally (608, 610), while those in the suprasellar and collicular cisterns become clinically evident at a smaller size. In children, craniomegaly, developmental delay, seizures and precocious puberty are not uncommon, though most present with signs and symptoms of intracranial hypertension (614, 624). These findings coexist with localizing signs and symptoms. The 'bobble-head doll' syndrome has been reported with suprasellar cysts (614, 624, 638, 639). Cysts in adults may additionally present with an expanding intrasellar mass causing pan-hypopituitarism (608, 640, 641). This subset of the 'empty sella' syndrome may be mistaken for a pituitary tumor until the proper radiological studies are performed. Lang et al. (642) reported an association between arachnoid cysts of the middle and anterior fossae and neuropsychological disturbances in 10 adult patients. Extension into the suprasellar cistern produced hyperprolactinemia in 2 of their patients. Adjacent subdural hematomas have been reported, probably secondary to tearing of veins stretched over the cyst (610, 630, 643). Rapid increase in the mass of the cyst may also occur as a result of subdural hygroma formation if the outer membrane ruptures (610).

The most common finding on plain x-ray is upward displacement, hypertrophy and pneumatization of the lesser sphenoid wing (608, 624, 626). Localized expansion of the temporal bone, calvarial enlargement and thinning, and splitting of the coronal sutures may also be found, the latter primarily in younger patients. CT is the diagnostic procedure of choice (608, 609, 611, 624), but some authors also advocate contrast cisternography, or isotope cisternography, to try to identify a communication between the cyst and subarachnoid space (610, 626, 644–646). The utility of this finding in treating patients with arachnoid cysts is yet to be defined. After intravenous contrast, there is no enhancement, and the cyst fluid has the same attenuation value as ventricular fluid. Cysts of medium size may have a triangular or quadrilateral shape, which helps to distinguish them from epidermoid tumors (610).

Treatment and Outcome

There are currently two main schools of thought concerning the optimal treatment of arachnoid cysts. The oldest advocates removal of the cyst's outer membrane and/or marsupialization with the subarachnoid space (608, 609, 611, 612). The more recent, exemplified by Harsh et al. (624), has found that, in children, at least, cyst-peritoneal shunting is the primary procedure of choice (647, 648). In their series, this was also successfully employed in all 4 cases where fenestration as the primary procedure had failed. With shunting of the cyst, the morbidity and recurrence rates were low, and neurological recovery good. Some authors use a combination of the two approaches (626). Whichever method is used, the placement of a ventriculo-peritoneal shunt may also be necessary (610, 624, 647, 649). Ventriculomegaly develops because of CSF malabsorption secondary to occlusion of the subarachnoid space by the cyst (613), or due to

ventricular outflow obstruction (650). Because of the long-standing nature of the compression of the brain underlying a cyst, the brain often is slow to expand once the cyst is treated, so a residual cavity on postoperative CT scans does not necessarily indicate inadequate treatment (608). The treatment of ependymal cysts has usually consisted of drainage of the cyst contents into the ventricle or, when feasible, removal of the cyst wall (608, 637).

Colloid Cysts of the Third Ventricle

Incidence and Location

Colloid cysts, sometimes referred to as 'paraphyseal' or 'neuroepithelial' cysts, are benign tumors of neuroepithelial origin which are of particular clinical interest because they have been an unrecognized cause of sudden death in young and middle-aged adults (651, 652). They are also of historical interest to neurosurgeons, because Harvey Cushing was found, at autopsy, to have an asymptomatic colloid cyst. They comprised only 0.5% of the 1295 intracranial tumors in Poppen's series (653). Since the advent of CT scanning, the diagnosis of colloid cyst is being made with greater frequency, as many are now found incidentally with this technique (654, 655). Symptomatic colloid cysts are usually diagnosed in patients between 20 and 50 years old, but may be found at any age (655–657). Some series show no sex predominance, but three recent reports, totaling 86 patients, showed 64% to be male (654, 655, 658). The usual location is in the anterior half of the third ventricle, where they are attached to its roof (usually to the tela choroidea, but occasionally to the choroid plexus) by a pedicle (659). In this location they eventually come into juxtaposition with the foramina of Monro. Uncommonly colloid cysts may be located in the posterior third ventricle, where they may obstruct the aqueduct of Sylvius (660), superiorly, between the leaves of the septum pellucidum (661) or in the fourth ventricle (662).

Origin and Pathology

The pathogenesis of colloid cysts is still a matter of some controversy. There is general agreement that they are developmental tumors of neuroepithelial origin, but the exact structure from which they derived has been unclear. The three possibilities most frequently cited are the choroidal epithelia (663), the paraphysis (664), or an abnormal infolding of the ependyma of the diencephalic roof (665, 666). Hirano and Ghatak (667), however, feel that the presence of cilia, atypical microvilli, an electron-dense surface coat, and a prominent basal lamina, makes these sites of origin unlikely. They favor an endodermal derivation for colloid cysts. On the other hand, the existence of mixed colloid cyst–xanthogranulomas has been cited as evidence for a neuroepithelial origin (668), because of the known phagocytic potential of neuroepithelial cells and the assumption that the foamy (xanthoma) cells seen in these tumors are lipid-laden macrophages resulting from the degeneration of phagocytes which have phagocytosed desquamated cells (668–670). As these cells disintegrate and release their lipid content, a response of multinucleated giant cells and macrophages is provoked, and a xanthogranuloma is created. Pure xanthogranulomas of the choroid plexus may have a similar pathogenesis (669, 670).

Macroscopically the tumors are round, unilocular masses, usually measuring 1–3 cm in diameter (17, 659). The capsule is smooth, and grayish or greenish in color. Upon entering the capsule a highly viscous fluid is usually found, but a fibrous component and, rarely, blood (671) may be present. The capsule is often fairly vascular. On histological examination, an inflammatory reaction and evidence of previous hemorrhage is often found. The cavity is lined by either a simple or a pseudostratified layer of cuboidal or columnar epithelium, which is frequently ciliated (659).

Clinical and Radiological Findings

Three different, typical clinical presentations of colloid cysts have been described (658, 672). Most commonly, patients will present with a variably long history of headaches, and with papilledema. The headaches often begin suddenly, mimicking a subarachnoid hemorrhage. There are no localizing signs. The next most frequent presentation, in Nitta and Symon's series (658), was the 'classical' presentation, with paroxysmal obtundation, or loss of consciousness, with headache, or a loss of lower extremity tone (drop attacks). In a minority of patients, these may be precipitated by specific changes in head position (654, 658). The third presentation is that of a progressive, or fluctuating, organic mental syndrome (OMS), with or without signs of increased ICP. This is often confused with normal pressure hydrocephalus. Lobosky et al. (673) have shown that these behavioral changes can occur, even in the absence of dilated ventricles, due to direct compression or vascular compromise of diencephalic or limbic structures. Rarely, patients can present with recurrent aseptic meningitis (due to leakage of cyst contents) (654, 655), CSF rhinorrhea (probably secondary to hydrocephalus) (658), seizures (655, 656) or extrapyramidal symptoms (658). Some remain asymptomatic. The duration of symptoms varies from instantaneous, with sudden coma or death, to 20 years of headaches, drop attacks or OMS (659).

Prior to the use of air ventriculography, these lesions were rarely diagnosed antemortem. The first surgical approach to a colloid cyst was not undertaken until Walter Dandy had introduced this technique (674). Currently, CT is the diagnostic procedure of choice (654, 655, 675). Colloid cysts are usually hyperdense, and enhance slightly with contrast. Isodense cysts have been described and may easily be overlooked (676). Mixed colloid cyst–xanthogranulomas are heterogeneous in appearance (668). There is often an associated widening of the septum pellucidum. Coronal cuts may also be helpful in defining the anatomical relationship of the mass to the ventricular system and the floor of the frontal fossa. Angiography typically shows a focal elevation and downward concavity of the anterior portion of the internal cerebral veins, with downward displacement of their posterior portion if there is associated hydrocephalus (654, 658, 677). Magnetic resonance imaging shows characteristic findings: high signal on both T1 and T2-weighted images (678).

Treatment and Outcome

The treatment of choice is total cyst removal, through the foramen of Monro, which is usually performed by the transcortical (654, 658, 660) or transcallosal routes (674, 679, 680). Complications include amnesia, if even one of the fornices is damaged, hypothalamic dysfunction, and ventricular collapse with subdural hygroma formation (659). If the attachment to the roof of the third ventricle cannot be visualized, and if the cyst wall is highly vascular, a small portion of it may have to be left in situ. An attractive alternative to craniotomy is the stereotactic drainage or endoscopic removal of colloid cysts (655, 681–683). There is no evidence that postoperative radiotherapy or chemotherapy are of any benefit in these cases, and they are generally not employed. Tumor recurrence after excision has rarely been reported (658). Ninety-four percent of the patients in Nitta and Symon's series had a good or excellent operative result (658). Five percent of patients undergoing a transcortical procedure will have postoperative epilepsy (660, 684). The transcallosal route is preferable when the ventricles are small (654), but many result in venous infarction of the retracted hemisphere (680). For colloid cysts found incidentally on CT, if there is no ventriculomegaly, and the patient is asymptomatic, it may be appropriate to observe the patient clinically, and with serial CT scans, though some recommend removal of all such tumors (651, 685). Preoperative or postoperative CSF drainage or shunting may also be necessary (654, 655, 680).

Rathke Cleft Cyst

Rathke cleft cysts have been mentioned before,

in our discussion of craniopharyngiomas, because of their presumably related histogenesis and the transitional forms between the two which have been found. They are benign, intrasellar cysts found at autopsy in 13 to 22% of randomly examined pituitary glands (686, 687). However, only about seventy have been reported in the clinical literature, so they rarely attain sufficient size to cause symptoms (688). They have been called by various other names, including 'pituitary cysts', 'intrasellar epithelial cysts', 'dysontogenic pituitary cysts', and 'mucoid epithelial cysts'. Most of the reported cases have been in adults, and there may be a slight female predominance (689). They appear to arise within the sella turcica but may extend into the suprasellar cistern. The embryological distinction between Rathke cleft cysts and craniopharyngiomas is unclear (690). Both are believed to arise from remnants of Rathke's pouch, but, in their pure form, have quite different histologies. However, lesions with mixed characteristics have been encountered (691–695). Russell and Rubinstein have reported a dumb-bell shaped tumor, with its waist at the level of the diaphragma sellae, above which the cyst was lined by the typical stratified squamous epithelium of a craniopharyngioma, and below which the single layer of columnar and cuboidal epithelium, characteristic of Rathke's cleft and Rathke cleft cysts, was found (96). According to Shuangshoti et al. (696), suprasellar epidermoid cysts and colloid cysts of the third ventricle may also be developmentally related tumors, arising, not necessarily from Rathke's pouch, but from the neuroepithelial precursor of the posterior lobe of the pituitary gland.

In Rathke cleft cysts, the columnar or cuboidal epithelium sits on a basement membrane (689). Goblet cells and cilia are frequently present, as in the normal cleft. Rathke cleft cyst fluid usually contains mucoid, opalescent material but it may also be clear, yellow, green or dark brown and contain cholesterol crystals, like craniopharyngiomas (689, 694, 697). A single case containing pus has also been reported (698). Unlike craniopharyngiomas, they almost never contain areas of calcification (699).

The clinical presentation of Rathke cleft cysts is usually that of any intrasellar mass which compresses the pituitary gland (689). It may, therefore, be confused with cystic pituitary adenoma, the empty sella syndrome, arachnoid cyst, aneurysm, cysticercosis, craniopharyngioma and pituitary abscess, even after CT scanning. Hypopituitarism results, with failure of gonadotrophin, growth hormone, thyroid-stimulating hormone and adrenocorticotrophic hormone secretion, and, occasionally, diabetes insipidus and hyperprolactinemia. About one-third of cases have clinically evident suprasellar extension, with visual field abnormalities, and obstructive hydrocephalus. Occasionally they are entirely suprasellar (694, 700). Aseptic meningitis has also been reported in several cases (688, 695, 701).

On plain skull films, abnormal sellar findings are reported in more than half of the cases (688, 689). Angiography may be able to detect a significant suprasellar extension (688). CT scanning, especially when augmented by coronal cuts or contrast cisternography, is, so far, the best means of defining the anatomical boundaries and relationships of the lesions, and of ruling out an empty sella (688, 695, 697, 702, 703). MRI should also prove highly accurate in their delineation, and may also be more specific in the differential diagnosis of these masses than is the CT scan. Since contrast enhancement has been reported in Rathke cleft cysts (700, 704), it is often impossible to differentiate them preoperatively from craniopharyngiomas and cystic pituitary adenomas (695).

The diagnosis of Rathke cleft cyst is usually not made until a surgical specimen is obtained (689). Both the trans-sphenoidal and the subfrontal approach have been used, depending on the degree of suprasellar extension (688, 697). Following the former type of procedure, two cysts have been reported to recur (705), possibly due to the inability to marsupialize the

cysts to the subarachnoid space by this approach. Five of the seven cysts which have been reported to recur have had some features of craniopharyngioma (689). Therefore cysts which represent transitional forms between Rathke cleft cysts and craniopharyngiomas, appear to behave biologically more like the latter. The usefulness of radiation therapy in recurrent lesions has not been adequately assessed (695, 706).

Neurenteric Cyst

There have been only about 50 reported cases of enteric cysts involving the nervous system (707). Of these, only about 20 have been reported in enough detail to be analysed (708). They are embryologically related to, and sometimes associated with, malformations of the foregut, such as posterior mediastinal enteric cysts (709), and ileal enteric duplication (710, 711). Several theories of the origin of neurenteric cysts have been proposed (707, 708, 712–718). Though they differ in their specifics, a common theme is that, at an early stage in embryogenesis, an abnormal fusion occurs between the endodermal and neuroectodermal layers, which causes a split in the mesodermal layer and developing notochord (712, 716, 717). If this persists, completely or in part, various prevertebral, vertebral and postvertebral abnormalities may develop, such as intraspinal cysts, bands or other connections with the alimentary or respiratory tracts, vertebral body anomalies, posterior vertebral defects, and dermal sinus tracts (712). Pathologically, neurenteric cysts appear to comprise a spectrum of lesions which, themselves, fit into the spectrum of maldevelopmental lesions from the simple dermoid cysts to the more complex teratomatous cysts (719). Because they derive from endodermal tissue displaced posteriorly into the spine, they are sometimes referred to as foregut, enteric or enterogenous cysts (709, 711). A purely teratomatous origin has also been hypothesized, but this fails to account for the frequent associated soft tissue and bony anomalies (720).

They are usually located in the cervical or thoracic spinal cord, and may be either intramedullary or extramedullary–intradural (707, 708, 721). Occasionally they are located in the lumbar spinal canal (722, 723). Rare cases of enterogenous cysts of the fourth ventricle have been reported (724), and Hirano and Ghatak feel (667) that colloid cysts of the third ventricle are also of endodermal origin, and, therefore, embryologically related. The cyst fluid varies from black and mucoid, to clear and colorless (708). The histology also varies from the simpler lesions, with a single layer of simple or pseudostratified columnar epithelial cells, some of which contain mucin, to the more complex, containing other elements of the respiratory or gastrointestinal tracts, such as smooth muscle and gastric, esophageal or intestinal epithelium (709, 719, 725). In about one-third, there is a communication with a posterior mediastinal cyst, and in almost all of these there is an anterior vertebral defect. Vertebral body defects were found, altogether, in 69% of patients. Other abnormalities that have been found include Klippel–Feil anomalies (726), myelomeningocele (723), dermal sinus (505), diastematomyelia (722), and lipoma (707, 721, 722).

Most patients present before the age of five, and about four-fifths are male (708). The more anatomically complex lesions tend to present at an early age. The most common presentation is that of gradual spinal cord compression, which may produce intermittent symptomatology. Some patients present with meningitis (710, 727), or with respiratory symptoms secondary to an associated posterior mediastinal mass (728). As few of the cases reported so far have involved levels below T7, symptoms referable to cauda equina or conus medullaris compromise are uncommon. The case reported by Mann et al. (722) presented with an acute history suggestive of a herniated lumbar disc.

The diagnosis of neurenteric cyst may be suspected on the basis of plain x-rays of the chest and spine, if widened interpedicular distance, anterior spina bifida, or a mediastinal mass are found in a patient with a history and signs of gradual spinal cord compression (708, 729). Neurogenic tumors and schwannomas are among the differential diagnosis. The best anatomical definition of the lesion is obtained with water-soluble contrast myelography followed by a CT scan. The value of MRI is, as yet, unknown.

The treatment of choice is surgical, but the exact approach is dictated by the specific anatomical considerations of each individual case. In cases without a prevertebral abnormality, a laminectomy with intradural exploration may be sufficient, but a thoracotomy, or two-staged procedure involving both a thoracotomy and a laminectomy may be required for the more complex lesions. It is generally considered advisable to ligate or occlude any anterior defect (708, 722, 730). The cyst need not be completely removed to achieve a good result (708). This will depend primarily on the patient's preoperative neurological status.

Choristoma

This is a rare tumor of the neurohypophysis. The cell of origin is unknown but may arise from pituicytes, which are neuroglial in origin (731). However, the 'granular cell myoblastoma', another name which has been applied to the choristoma, is felt to derive from Schwann cells which have a disturbed lipid metabolism (732). It is so named because of its similar appearance to peripheral tumors of the same name (see Chapter 32) (733). Special staining techniques have not led to a greater understanding of this cytogenesis as yet. Recent immunohistochemical staining of a suprasellar lesion was negative for GFAP, S-100 protein, and intermediate filament, suggesting a 'multicellular origin' (734). They are usually found incidentally at autopsy. Only 30 clinically symptomatic examples have been reported (735). The initial symptoms include visual loss, dementia, pituitary insufficiency and diabetes insipidus (736, 737). One such tumor has been associated with the multiple endocrine neoplasia, type 2 (738). On radiological investigation CT demonstrates a hyperdense, enhancing, smoothly demarcated lesion extending upward from the sella into the suprasellar cistern (735). Angiography often reveals a vascular blush. These findings distinguish the lesion from most optic gliomas and pituitary adenomas, but may suggest a meningioma. The sella may not be expanded on plain x-ray.

The course of symptomatic tumors is uncertain, but long-term survival, following either subfrontal or trans-sphenoidal resection, has been reported (735). Their highly vascular nature and adhesion to the optic apparatus and hypothalamus sometimes makes complete removal risky. Some may require several re-operations for local recurrence (735). The effectiveness of radiotherapy on these tumors is unknown.

Rare instances of intracerebral granular cell tumors have been studied (739, 740). Staining for GFAP has yielded equivocal evidence for a glial cell origin. As S-100 protein is absent, a Schwann cell origin is unlikely.

Intracranial Lipoma

Another tumor which, before the CT era, was usually discovered incidentally at autopsy, is the intracranial lipoma (741, 742). As the name implies, they consist of mature fat. They grow so slowly that some consider them hamartomas rather than tumors (741, 743). They are generally felt to arise as a result of abnormal CNS embryogenesis. The malformative nature of these lesions is supported by the presence of neuroglia and ganglion cells in some of them (17, 96), and by their association with other congenital abnormalities, such as cerebellar microgyria, cranium bifidum, hypertelorism, agenesis of the cerebellar vermis, and, most frequently, agenesis of the corpus callosum (744–748). They may also contain microcalcifications, cartilage, bone, smooth or striated muscle, and hematopoietic plaques (17, 96, 743, 747, 748). They have also been reported as part of the Goldenhar–Gorlin syndrome (oculoauriculo-vertebral dysplasia)

(749), and encephalocraniocutaneous lipomatosis (750).

The exact cell of origin of these tumors has been controversial (744). Since all lipomas have been found to have some attachment to the leptomeninges, and since adipose cells are felt to exist in the pia mater, most theories involve these cells in some way (490, 744). An opposing view is that intracranial lipomas derive from dermal elements enclosed within the CNS during embryogenesis. This is more likely to be true of lipomas of the spinal cord found in dysraphic conditions such as myelomeningocele. The process through which intracranial lipomas arise has never led to anaplastic, malignant or metastatic forms (741, 744, 746).

Most intracranial lipomas are located in the midline, primarily in the corpus callosum (741, 751), but also in the tuber cinereum, quadrigeminal plate, brainstem, suprasellar and retrosellar areas, hypothalamus and third ventricle (741, 742). Paramedian lipomas, in the middle fossa, sylvian region and CP angle have also been described (741, 744, 752–754).

Histologically, most are comprised of mature fat cells with varying amounts of a collagenous and vascular stroma (17). Other cell types, as noted above, may also be present. There may be attachment to the brain as well as to the leptomeninges (490).

About 50% of patients with lipomas remain asymptomatic (742, 746, 755). Sixty-five percent of symptomatic patients with corpus callosum lipomas present with seizures (755, 756). Other symptoms are mental retardation, headache, and hemiparesis (742, 746, 755, 757). Occasionally the midline tumors cause CSF pathway obstruction (96, 742, 746, 747), and CP angle lipomas may present with trigeminal neuralgia and other cranial nerve deficits (744, 754, 759). Intracranial lipomas are found slightly more frequently in females (490, 742, 753, 756).

A characteristic sign is seen on the plain skull x-rays of patients with corpus callosum lipomas. A thin rim of calcification at the borders of the tumor forms a shell which, to some, has the appearance on anteroposterior films of a 'wine-glass' (756, 757, 760). The CT findings are an area of very low density surrounded by a rim of calcification (742, 746, 753). Lipomas of the corpus callosum in infants have been detected and diagnosed by ultrasound (761). Magnetic resonance imaging, because of the characteristic appearance of fat on various pulse sequences, is an ideal method for the diagnosis of lipomas (762).

Because of their vascularity and adherence to surrounding structures, it has been recommended that lipomas outside the CP angle not be approached surgically unless severely symptomatic (742, 754, 759). Frequently the anterior cerebral arteries are embedded within the mass (746, 756, 757). Patel, in 1965, reported a 64% mortality rate with such operations (763). Many of the most commonly associated symptoms, such as seizures and mental retardation, are probably due to associated cerebral and callosal abnormalities, and improvement would not be anticipated with resection of the tumor (742); lipomas of the CP angle, however, have not been reported in association with other intracranial abnormalities, and produce symptoms mainly by direct compression (744, 754, 759, 764). Therefore, when CP angle tumors cause symptoms, surgical decompression should be considered, but, since their growth is so slow, radical excision, if it endangers functional neural elements, should be avoided. Cerebrospinal fluid shunting procedures, in themselves, may be appropriate in treating the hydrocephalus associated with lipomas, but are not uniformly successful (742, 743, 746, 755).

INTRACRANIAL EXTENSION OF REGIONAL TUMORS

There are several uncommon tumors which arise in structures at the base of the skull, in the soft tissues of the head, or from the calvarium, which can, because of their locally invasive nature, extend within the cranial cavity. Of these, adenoid cystic carcinoma and esthesioneuroblastoma (olfactory neuroblastoma), are discussed elsewhere in this book.

Primary Bone Tumors (Chapter 54)

Some of the malignant tumors of mesenchymal origin which can affect the CNS by local extension have been mentioned earlier as primary intracranial tumors. These originate in the bony skull and spinal column. Chondrosarcomas of the base of the skull, though they frequently invade the dura, rarely extend intradurally (17). They comprise only about 0.15% of all intracranial tumors (765). Osteosarcomas, the most common primary malignant tumor of the skull (766), also tend not to involve the brain through local extension (17), but, because of local recurrence and a tendency to metastasize, they have a poor prognosis (767). Fibrosarcoma of the skull, and other primary malignant bone tumors, are rare, usually occurring in children and young adults (17). Exceptionally, they may arise in older patients as a complication of advanced Paget's disease (768). Osteochondromas may arise from the dura of the falx, as well as the cerebral convexity, and tend to be well-encapsulated masses which do not invade the underlying brain (769). Occasionally osteochondrosarcomas arise from the falx as well, but they tend to be more invasive into the adjacent brain (770). Rhabdomyosarcomas originating in the ear may extend through the internal auditory canal and grow as a CP angle mass (96, 771). Osteosarcomas and chondrosarcomas may also arise in the spine, extend into the canal, and cause spinal cord or nerve root compression.

Benign tumors of the skull which may produce neurological signs include osteoma, ossifying fibroma, osteoblastoma, chondroma, chondroblastoma, hemangioma and the more aggressive giant cell tumors (772). Osteomas are the most frequent primary tumor of the cranium (758). They occur in the paranasal and mastoid sinuses, and can extend into the anterior and posterior fossae (17, 773). Osteomas of the skull arise sporadically or as a part of

Gardner's syndrome: intestinal polyps, soft tissue fibromas, sebaceous cysts and multiple osteomas. Ossifying fibromas usually arise in the frontal bone or paranasal sinuses and extend into the anterior fossa (774, 775). Osteoblastomas are vascular tumors with a potential for spontaneous or radiation-induced malignant transformation (772). They usually occur in the spinal canal, but may arise in the skull (776, 777). Postoperative recurrences may be reduced by radiation therapy. Chondromas may occur in the paranasal sinuses, parasellar area of petro-occipital synchondrosis. From the latter location they extend into the CP angle (778, 779). They may also arise from the dura of the cerebral convexity and falx, from the choroid plexus, arachnoid, and brain. The occurrence of intracranial extension of chondromas in patients with Ollier's disease (multiple enchondromatosis) and Maffucci's syndrome (Ollier's disease plus multiple hemangiomas) has been reported (780). The risk of malignant transformation in these syndromes is felt to be significant (776). Chondroblastomas rarely arise in the skull, may produce neurological signs, and may also undergo radiation-induced malignant transformation (776, 781). They also have a significant recurrence rate (772, 776). Hemangiomas are more frequently located in the spinal column than in the skull (782). They tend to be highly vascular, and the value of preoperative angiography, ebolization and even carotid ligation has been noted (783). Giant cell tumors also involve the spine more frequently than the skull, where the most common sites are the sphenoid and temporal bones (784, 785). They often arise in the setting of Paget's disease. Their biological behavior is difficult to predict on histological grounds. They tend to be locally invasive and to recur after removal by curettage (772, 776). The role of radiotherapy in these tumors is uncertain, as they may undergo malignant transformation.

The treatment for all of these tumors is surgical extirpation. This is especially difficult when the site of origin is at the base of the skull, and treatment failures, especially in this location, will be due to local recurrence at the margin of resection (772, 786). The role of radiation therapy in the treatment of primary malignant tumors of the skull base is still controversial (765, 772, 786–788). Proton beam therapy has been employed to achieve a finer spatial distribution of high doses of radiation, thereby sparing the adjacent brain (788). Preoperative chemotherapy has been recommended to decrease tumor size and facilitate resection in paraspinal sarcomas (789). Its effectiveness in cranial tumors is not proven.

Chordomas

Origin and Pathology

Chordomas are malignant tumors which arise in the axial skeleton, anywhere from the sellar and parasellar region to the sacrum (790–792). The clivus and the sacrum are the two favored sites. The earliest known description of a clivus chordoma was made by Virchow, in 1856, at autopsy (793). Subsequent descriptions came in the 1850s, and, at the end of that decade, Muller noted their histological resemblance to the notochord (794). This structure, whose blastodermal layer of origin is uncertain (795), forms, in early embryogenesis, the long cylindrical nidus around which the mesodermal tissue which will eventually become the skull base and vertebral column condenses. By the seventh week of gestation, the notochord regresses, leaving behind, as its only known remnant, the centrum of the nucleus pulposus of the intervertebral discs (790, 796). Ribbert in 1894 (797) and Congdon in 1952 (798) were able to induce tumors with similar features to chordomas by puncturing the intervertebral discs of rabbits. Since early this century, the theory of the derivation of chordomas from remnants of the embryonal notochord has had general acceptance (799). Recent ultrastructural comparisons (800, 801), between normal nucleus pulposus and chordomas have provided further support for it. It has been remarked, however, that, for a tumor of embryonal tissue, chordomas tend to appear relatively late in life. The mean age in most series is in the fifth or sixth decade (790–792, 802–804), and only about 5% of the cranial chordomas in the Mayo Clinic's experience occurred in patients less than 20 years old (805). In the rare tumors found in infants, the biological behavior is particularly aggressive (806). Another point which appears inconsistent with the generally accepted theory is that chordomas rarely arise where notochord remnants are found most frequently, in the intervertebral discs, but rather in the clivus or the sacrum. However, microscopic remnants of notochord and hyaline cartilage have been found by Ulich and Mirra within a vertebral body (807). Willis noted that rests of notochordal tissue were identified within the clivus and sacrum in 0.5 to 2.0% of autopsies (808). About 2–5% of chordomas are found incidentally at autopsy (792). These have been classified separately as a benign variant of chordoma. Histologically, however, they are similar to more aggressive tumors.

At surgery, chordomas are multilobulated masses of variable size (790). Sacral lesions may attain a diameter of over 15 cm before coming to medical attention. The portions which expand into soft tissue usually are demarcated by a pseudocapsule, unless the tumor has been operated upon previously. The osseous portion, on the other hand, has no distinct limits. Its invasion into the surrounding bone is often well beyond its grossly discernible boundary, which is why even en bloc, radical resections may have local recurrences, especially in the skull base (809). The mechanism of tumor extension into bone and soft tissue is unknown, but strong proteolytic enzymes have been found in several human chordoma studies in our laboratory (C. Cummins and P. L. Kornblith, unpublished data). The consistency of the tumor varies from soft and gelatinous to firm and gritty (795). Areas of necrosis and hemorrhage may be prominent (776, 790).

The microscopic appearance is typically that of homogeneous tumor cells arranged in cords, sheets or lobules (790). On light microscopy, the characteristic cell has been called 'physaliphorous', meaning 'bubble-bearing', because of its vacuolated cytoplasm. Using appropriate staining techniques, the vacuoles may be found to contain either glycogen or mucin (795). The ability to produce mucin is a known property of notochordal cells during development (810). However, this ability is shared by some adenocarcinomas, with which a chordoma may be confused. Other tumors which may have similar histological appearances to chordomas include myxosarcomas, chondrosarcomas and spindle cell sarcomas (795). Spindle cell anaplasia may be found in chordomas which have been treated with radiation therapy following resection (804, 809). Reticulin staining may be useful in differentiating chordomas from mucinous adenocarcinomas and other tumors (792). The phosphotungstic acid–hematoxylin and silver impregnation stains may be helpful in differentiating chondrosarcoma, which stains positively, from most chordomas (811). The validity of these methods has been questioned (812). Immunohistochemical staining with monoclonal antibodies to intermediate filaments has also proved useful (795, 813). In a significant number of chordomas, cartilagenous elements are found, leading to the division of chordomas into physaliphorous and chondroid subtypes (809). Absence of this feature is the only known histological indicator of aggressiveness (792, 809). The series of Heffelfinger et al. (809), from the Mayo Clinic, indicated a 15.8-year average survival for patients with chondroid chordoma, while those without chondroid elements lived an average of only 4.1 years. 'Cording' (805), cellularity, and mitoses are not of prognostic significance.

The 'signet cell' often described in chordomas is a descriptive term for a physaliphorous cell in which the vacuoles have forced the cell nucleus over to the cell membrane. Dense fibrous septa, occasionally infiltrated with lymphocytes, divide the tumors into lobules. Mitoses are rarely seen in chordomas, but giant cells may be found (790, 814, 815). Recently, ultrastructural studies (800, 814, 815) have found a second cell type in these tumors, called a stellate cell, from which the physaliphorous cell is thought to develop. Intracytoplasmic, virus-like particles have also been noted (814). One striking feature of these cells are regularly observed, alternating arrays of mitochondria and single rough endoplasmic reticulum cisternae (800). These arrays have not to our knowledge been described in other tumors, and may, therefore, be used as markers for chordoma.

Incidence and Location

Chordomas represent about 1–4% of all primary osseous tumors (790), and should be strongly considered when a mass lesion of the sacrum or clivus is encountered in a person of 35–55 years old. In a retrospective study (816), 40% of all primary tumors of the sacrum were chordomas. In the other vertebral bodies, however, the higher incidence of metastatic bone lesions in this age group makes the diagnosis of chordoma less likely. The male:female ratio in most series is about 2:1 (785, 809, 817), but, in the pediatric age group, there is no sex preference (805).

About 50% of chordomas arise in the sacrococcygeal region, 15% in the other vertebrae, and 35% in the spheno-occipital portion of the base of the skull (792, 802, 809, 818). Although the lesions are similar in pathology and origin, there are significant clinical differences which make their consideration as two separate entities, cranial and spinal, appropriate. Sacrococcygeal and other vertebral lesions are similar to each other in presentation, radiographic features, treatment and outcome, and will be discussed together. There are more young patients with cranial tumors, and these appear to behave more aggressively (805). All 12 patients below 20 years of age in Wold and Laws' series had tumors of the base of the skull (805).

Cranial Chordomas

Notochordal remnants may be found in the dorsum sellae, body of the clivus, and basion of the occipital bone (which forms the inferior clivus) (810). Therefore chordomas, as expected, will occur in the sella, parasellar region, and upper and lower clivus. They can arise off the midline in the parasellar and lateral clivus or petrous areas (803, 805). This is due to the sinuous course which the notochord takes in the base of the skull (810). When arising in the ventral aspect of the clivus, the tumors may present as nasopharyngeal masses prior to eroding upward and posteriorly into the cranial cavity (803). Rare examples of chordomas arising in the facial bones and paranasal sinuses have also been reported (817, 819, 820).

Cranial chordomas represent about 0.2% of all primary brain tumors. The average age at diagnosis is somewhat younger (around 40 years) than that of sacrococcygeal tumors (803), probably because of the higher number of patients in the pediatric age group (805), alluded to above. The size that these tumors may grow to, before detection, is also less than that of sacrococcygeal tumors, because of the relatively small space for expansion available to them (820). All three of these findings, as well as the lower incidence of metastases from cranial lesions (817, 821–823), are probably interdependent. There is a higher incidence of chondroid chordomas in the cranium (802, 805, 809), which should lead to an increased disease-free survival. This has not been observed, in part due to the greater difficulty in effecting a radical resection of these tumors than of sacrococcygeal lesions.

Because of the slow growth of most chordomas, the progression of symptoms may be quite gradual. The duration of symptoms in the series of Raffel et al. varied between one month and 15 years (803), averaging about 20 months. The most frequent presenting symptom is diplopia, caused by stretching of the abducens nerve as it courses within the dura

(810). Next in frequency is headache (803). Other symptoms and signs depend on the location and direction of growth of the tumor. Most commonly, midclival lesions will cause deficits of the third, fifth and seventh cranial nerves, ataxia, vertigo, and pyramidal signs from brainstem compression, and obstructive hydrocephalus. Rarely pathological laughter may be seen with a retroclival tumor (803). Inferior clival tumors present with lower cranial nerve findings and a foramen magnum syndrome. Sellar and parasellar tumors may have visual disturbance, a cavernous sinus syndrome, or an endocrinopathy.

The diagnosis of chordoma is often strongly suspected on the basis of the plain skull x-ray alone (810, 824). Destruction of bone, and expansion of the eroded region are prominent features. A 'ground glass' appearance may be present and is due to residual calcium in sequestered fragments of bone. A soft tissue mass in the nasopharynx may also be seen. Angiography, and CT scanning with contrast-cisternography and sagittal reconstruction, have both been useful in the further anatomical delineation and operative planning for these lesions (810, 825, 826). MRI may be even more helpful in the future, and has already been used to advantage by Raffel et al. (803).

The two treatment modalities of choice are surgery and radiation therapy. Surgery should be undertaken with the goal of total tumor removal, since local tumor recurrence is the principal cause of death in these patients (809). The operative approach varies according to the location of the tumor and the experience of the surgeon. The preferred approaches for sellar lesions and lesions of the ventral midclivus are the trans-septal, trans-sphenoidal route; for parasellar lesions, the pterional route; for rostral, dorsal clivus lesions, the subtemporal route; and for caudal, dorsal clivus lesions, a suboccipital craniectomy (809). With the use of microsurgical technique, and a combined team approach with ENT and neurosurgery, wider exposures of the base of the skull have been possible, making radical tumor excision more feasible (803, 810, 827–

831). Repeated surgical resection may, in many cases, be necessary for control of local recurrences, and a number of patients undergo three, or even four, operations (800). The time interval for successive recurrences decreases, however, so even this approach has its limitations.

The role of radiation therapy for the treatment of chordomas is still controversial (817, 819, 832–834). Being slowly growing tumors, they are generally considered to be radioresistant, but there have been enough reports of long-term survival of patients treated with biopsy followed by radiation, that most authors recommend it, some in almost every case (805, 810, 834), and others only in those patients in whom radical excision is not possible (792). Radiotherapy is usually delivered as high-dose, megavoltage, photon radiation (50–70 Gy over 5–7 weeks) (791, 817). Hyperfractionation (833), proton beam radiation (788), and combinations of photon and heavy ion radiation (803, 835) have also been used with encouraging results, but follow-up periods have been short. Because of the relatively localized nature of these tumors, interstitial brachytherapy is an attractive possibility, but, due to difficulty in gaining access to the tumor bed, and determining the exact extent of tumors, the few efforts to date have not been promising (803, 827, 836). There have been no reports of the successful use of chemotherapeutic agents in treating these tumors (790).

The mean time to recurrence (defined as symptomatic tumor regrowth requiring reoperation) was 38 months in 14 of the 26 patients reported by Raffel et al. (803). This occurred as late as 17 years after the initial operation. None of the 6 patients with the chondroid variant had a recurrence, and all were alive after an average of more than 6 years. Only 6 of the 20 patients with the physaliphorous tumor had no recurrence. Tewfik et al., in 1977 (791), reported that only 10% of all cranial chordoma patients will experience a prolonged disease-free survival. Currently the 5-year survival rate may be as high as 50% (809, 834), and the 10-year survival, 40%, but short follow-up periods and small numbers of patients make statistical evaluation difficult.

Spinal and Sacrococcygeal Chordomas

Chordomas represent the most common primary neoplasm of the sacrum, accounting for 40% in the series of Cody et al. (816), but they are frequently misdiagnosed as metastatic carcinoma. There are no definite, predisposing factors or genetic predispositions, but, interestingly, there is a history of trauma to the sacral region in about 40% of patients (790). The presenting signs and symptoms are non-specific and related to the area of involvement. Pain in the low back or sacrum is by far the most frequent complaint (804), with an average duration of about one year (792, 795, 837). There may be incontinence, dysuria, perineal hyperesthesia and constipation. Vertebral lesions present most commonly with pain (100%) and with lower extremity weakness (25%) but may also have bladder dysfunction and, in cervical spine tumors, a palpable cervical mass, hoarseness, dysphagia and pharyngeal bleeding (792). Presenting signs are those of a soft tissue mass and spinal nerve or cord compression. The most frequent misdiagnoses are degenerative disc disease, hemorrhoids and coccygodynia. For sacral lesions, the single most important aspect of the examination is the rectal examination, since all of the cases reported by Sundaresan et al. (804) had palpable presacral masses. In general, sacral tumors take longer to diagnose than vertebral lesions, because, in the latter, spinal cord compression occurs relatively early, usually preceded by radicular pain and sensory findings (790). Vertebral lesions also occur at a younger age, have a predilection for the cervical region (823), and tend to behave more aggressively (790, 804, 818).

Radiological findings on plain x-ray are those of bony destruction by an expanding mass (804, 823, 824). Especially in those tumors involving the vertebral bodies, there may be a sclerotic margin to the defect (790). Unlike other neoplastic processes, involvement of the disc space is typical of chordomas (824). The most significant finding is that of a paravertebral, soft tissue mass. This may be more difficult to appreciate in sacral lesions than in those of the cervical spine. The radiographic procedure of choice is CT, which usually delineates the extent of the prevertebral mass and destruction of bone (838), though some doubt its ability to delineate infiltration of the gluteal muscles (839). Calcification is frequently seen and may be used to identify epidural tumor extension. It tends to be located peripherally, and is more frequent in sacral lesions (838). Adjunctive procedures which may be useful include myelography, to document the extent of epidural tumor, angiography to detect encasement of arteries, and barium enemas and esophagrams, to look for involvement of the rectum or esophagus (790). Contrast enhanced CT scans were not felt to be useful by Krol, because the soft tissue extensions do not enhance, and are clearly distinguishable in unenhanced studies because of the distorted but preserved fat and fascial planes (838). Magnetic resonance may be a useful imaging modality in the future (840).

As with cranial chordomas, the major treatment modalities for sacral and spinal lesions are radical surgery and radiation therapy (792, 795, 804, 841). For small sacrococcygeal lesions, transperineal or transcoccygeal approaches may suffice (790), but more radical procedures are necessary for more extensive lesions. One approach which has been used for tumors involving S2, with a large intra-abdominal mass, is the abdominosacral procedure of Localio et al. (842). It has a 5% operative mortality, and most tumors recur locally because of their large size and invasive nature. Resection of the sacrum above the S2 level has several risks. If both S2 nerve roots are damaged at surgery, the patient will lose control of both bowel and bladder continence (790, 823). The stability of the vertebral column may also be jeopardized, and sinking of the lumbar spine into the pelvis has been reported. The radical sacrectomy reported by Stener and Gunterberg (844) was used successfully to treat five chordomas. They reported good postoperative stability, and sphincteric function was preserved if the S2 nerve root was sacrificed on only one side.

Surgical treatment of vertebral body chordomas has been relatively unsatisfactory, because it usually consists of posterior or postero-lateral approaches to debulk tumor. Radical excision is almost never achieved (795). Sundaresan has pointed out that anterior approaches afford better exposure of the pathological areas and increase the likelihood of a radical resection (790, 804). In the upper cervical region, the median labiomandibular glossotomy has been devised for this purpose (845). It requires splitting the lower lip, mandible and tongue in the midline, as well as the uvula and posterior pharynx. Thoracotomy and retroperitoneal approaches are used in thoracic and lumbar vertebral lesions, respectively (846). As with cranial chordomas, reoperation may afford palliation and relief of pain in many recurrent lesions (792).

Recurrent lesions, and those in which radical removal has not been possible, are usually treated with radiation therapy (790, 791, 817, 832). Methods used to deliver radiation to the tumor more precisely include the wedge filter and rotational beam techniques (790). Conventional photon, proton beam and interstitial radiation have all been used. Their effectiveness is still undergoing evaluation. Cryosurgery (816) and chemotherapy (795, 804) have also been employed.

The median survival rate, following both surgery and radiation, was 5 years in the Memorial Sloan-Kettering patients (804). At 10 years 40% were still alive, but only 10% were free of disease. No statistically significant difference could be detected in those patients treated with surgery alone. This was not a randomized trial, so facts of tumor size and inaccessibility might have counterbalanced any beneficial effect of radiation that would have been seen in such a study. Although vertebral lesions appeared to be associated with a poorer prognosis, no statistically valid statement to that effect could be made. The problems of tumor rarity and long time to recurrence would make randomized, prospective studies difficult, except possibly on a multi-institutional, cooperative basis.

Metastatic Potential

Both cranial and sacrococcygeal chordomas may metastasize. Initially, the reported incidence was low (813), but recent series have found that 30–40% of sacral and spinal lesions, taken as a group, metastasize at some point in their course (804, 822). The incidence for cranial lesions is somewhat less (810, 820, 822), possibly due to their smaller size and shorter duration of illness. The principal sites of metastasis are lung, bone, muscle, lymph nodes and liver (809, 817, 822, 843, 847, 848). Chambers and Schwinn also found three patients with dermal metastases (822). These superficial lesions may be observed by the patient and biopsied before the primary site is symptomatic, permitting an early diagnosis. Interestingly, the presence of metastases, even if widespread, does not appear to significantly affect life expectancy (790). Spread of tumor within the CNS is distinctively rare. Less than 10 cases have been reported (803, 822, 849–852). In one recent instance, the diagnosis was made by the finding of vacuolated cells on cytological examination of the CSF (852).

UNCOMMON PERIPHERAL NERVE TUMORS

INTRODUCTION

The most common tumors of the peripheral nervous system are those which arise from Schwann cells (neurofibroma and schwannoma), or from the nerve cells themselves (neuroblastoma, and ganglioneuroblastoma). A number of uncommon tumors also occur

(Table 5). Some are variants of the more common tumors. Our discussion will include, under the heading of 'Miscellaneous Tumors', two uncommon neurocutaneous phakomatoses, multiple mucosal neuroma syndrome and neurocutaneous melanosis. For an excellent discussion of the pathology of these tumors and syndromes, the reader is referred to the monograph of Harkin and Reed (853).

PRIMARY MALIGNANT NERVE SHEATH TUMORS

Malignant Schwannomas

A fuller description of malignant schwannomas is given in Chapter 31. Though this section has been included in order to place other primary nerve sheath tumors in the context of unusual nervous system tumors. On histological and ultrastructural grounds, these tumors derive from Schwann cells, and are generally benign (96, 853–855). This histogenesis has been supported by tissue culture studies (856), and by finding S-100 protein on immunocytochemical staining (857). S-100 protein is a marker for cells of neuroectodermal origin (858), so it is unlikely that fibroblasts, as was once believed, are the cell of origin of neurofibromas. Some schwannomas and most neurofibromas are seen in the setting of von Reckl-

inghausen's disease, but they also arise de novo. Even solitary lesions may be precursors, or 'formes frustes', of the complete syndrome (859, 860). As will be discussed below, some malignant nerve sheath tumors may arise from fibroblasts. For now though malignant schwannomas will be considered.

The cell of origin of these tumors has been quite controversial, which has led to a number of synonymous appellations, such as 'perineurial fibrosarcoma', 'neurogenic sarcoma', 'neurofibrosarcoma', 'fibromyxosarcoma of nerve', 'neurilemosarcoma', 'malignant peripheral glioma' and the less committal 'malignant peripheral nerve sheath tumor', or 'MPNST' (853, 861). The reason for this uncertainty is that these tumors have lost many of the ultrastructural (862) and immunocytochemical features (such as positive staining for S-100 protein (858)) which associate the benign forms with Schwann cells. Therefore, most of the evidence for the Schwann cell as the cell of origin is circumstantial: they arise within the perineurium of peripheral nerves, they may be contiguous with a plexiform neurofibroma in the setting of von Recklinghausen's disease, or they may show at least some features of Schwann cell differentiation (853). Ultrastructural evidence which has been cited includes elongated, interdigitating cytoplasmic processes, pericellular basal lamina, cytoplasmic granular material and extracellular long-spacing collagen (862).

These tumors can occur in any peripheral nerve. Rarely, they arise in an area which has been previously irradiated (863, 864). Most patients with malignant Schwannomas are over 30 years old, but as many as 17% may be in the pediatric age group (861, 865). The age of onset of benign schwannomas is usually before 20 years old (866). The incidence of malignant schwannomas in patients with von Recklinghausen's disease has been estimated at 29%, if a long enough follow-up period is used (866). These patients are more likely to develop further malignant schwannomas than patients who have not yet had one (861, 863). The neurofibromas in patients with von Recklinghausen's disease have an increased tendency toward malignant transformation than solitary lesions (860, 866). However, the chance of malignant transformation per neurofibroma is so slim in these patients, that only those tumors which show a rapid change in growth pattern or symptomatology need be investigated or excised. Renal cell carcinomas, and thyroid carcinoma, amyloid type, have been rarely reported in associated with malignant schwannomas.

The gross description of these tumors, at operation, is very important to the pathologist. It may help to differentiate a malignant schwannoma from the rare primary soft tissue fibrosarcoma which secondarily involves a peripheral nerve (861). They are fusiform swellings or lobulated masses which appear to be limited to the nerve itself. There is an apparent capsule separating the tumor from surrounding, non-neural tissue, but extensive invasion of these tissues is usually present microscopically. These cells extend along fascial planes and around nerve sheaths (867, 868). Macroscopically it is often difficult to differentiate malignant from benign schwannomas. Because of their increased cellularity, the former may appear a little grayer, and areas of hemorrhage or necrosis may be present on sectioning the tumor (853, 867). Differentiation depends more upon microscopic examination of the tumor and of the adjacent nerve. Because of the radical treatment advocated for malignant tumors, as opposed to benign ones, intraoperative frozen sections are, therefore, essential.

The characteristic picture is that of invasion along the involved nerve, sometimes up to a considerable distance, which is often appreciated only microscopically (868, 869). This invasion, if it occurs in a tumor of the brachial or lumbosacral plexuses, may extend through intervertebral foramina to involve the CNS (867, 870, 871). Tumors of the cranial nerves may, likewise, spread intracranially. Harkin and Reed (853) have divided these tumors into three histological subtypes: malignant schwannomas, proper; malignant epithelioid schwan-

nomas; and malignant melanocytic schwannoma. Malignant schwannomas contain plump sindle-shaped cells which are occasionally arranged in fascicles resembling Schwann cell cords, or in whorls. Areas of plexiform neurofibroma are often found. Microscopically they may be indistinguishable from soft tissue fibrosarcoma. Malignant cells may be found both within and outside the perineurium. Divergent differentiation of these cells has been well described to give areas of chondroid and osteoid appearance (872). Glandular, squamous epithelial, angiomatous (with positive staining for factor VIII) (872), and even rhabdomyablastic differentiation have been reported (865, 867, 870, 872–878). The latter, rare cases have been given the name 'Triton tumor' (see Chapter 31), referring to Locatelli's work on experimentally induced supernumerary limbs in the Triton salamander (879). They may be associated with poorer prognosis than other malignant schwannomas, but their number is too small to state this positively (872).

Malignant epithelioid schwannomas are very rare tumors which resemble malignant melanoma histologically, except for an absence of melanin pigmentation (853). The cells are round or polygonal, wih scanty cytoplasm, and are arranged in nests or ribbons. The diagnosis is difficult to make and is impossible if the tumor is not confined to a nerve grossly. Rarely they will arise in a pre-existing neurofibroma.

Malignant melanocytic schwannomas are also quite rare and are comprised of cells which resemble melanocytes (853). Spindle-shaped cells arranged in interlacing fascicles are present, and, unlike malignant epithelioid schwannomas, mitoses are common. Despite this malignant appearance, there is evidence of a benign clinical course in some patients (853).

The clinical presentation of malignant schwannomas depends on the location in which they arise (861, 866, 867, 880). Usually there is a superficial, rapidly growing mass associated with tenderness and pain along the course of the involved nerve. They may be asymptomatic, though, or only produce paresthesias. Most occur in the proximal portion of an extremity, 40% in Das Gupta's series arising in the leg (866). Here, and in the retroperitoneum, the symptoms may be suggestive of a herniated lumbar disc (880, 881). Twelve percent arise in the head and neck region, and the rest on the trunk. Here they are almost always associated with von Recklinghausen's disease (866). They may occur in any location within the thorax and abdomen. In the mediastinum they present with chest discomfort and a pericardial effusion and have an extremely poor prognosis (882). They may arise from the sympathetic chain and vagus nerves, as well as from non-autonomic peripheral nerves (866, 882, 883).

Palpation of peripheral nerves is important in detecting tumors of the extremities. Where the brachial or lumbosacral plexuses or cranial nerves are involved, plain x-rays may detect a widening of bony foramina, but, among radiological studies, the CT scan is most useful. Gallium scanning has been helpful in detecting malignant schwannomas in patients with von Recklinghausen's disease (884). MRI of the plexuses may prove to be more sensitive than CT scan, in the future. If the possibility of CNS extension exists, it may be confirmed by the finding of malignant cells on CSF cytology or tissue culture, or by myelography (880).

The treatment of choice for malignant schwannomas is radical excision (866, 867, 869, 885). Subtotal resection, often necessitated because of direct invasion of vital structures, as in the posterior mediastinal tumors, is associated with a greater than 40% recurrence rate (868). Because of the ability of the tumors to spread great distances along the involved nerve, complete removal cannot be assured without good microscopic analysis of the proximal and distal limits of the resected portion of the nerve (880). Because of the adjacent soft tissues are also invaded amputation of the extremity must often be considered. With repeated proximal recurrences, patients often undergo, as a final procedure, complete forequarter amputation of the upper extremity, or hemipelvectomy. There is a higher cure rate in

patients with distally located tumors than with proximal lesions (886). Before a radical procedure, such as amputation, is performed, an extensive search for distant metastases should be performed. Metastasis is a frequent cause of death in patients with malignant schwannoma, and the chance for metastasis increases if radical excision is not accomplished at the primary procedure (866, 880, 886). The most common site of metastases are the lungs (861, 880), but the lymph nodes and skeleton may also become involved. Metastases are universally associated with a poor prognosis, so any operative procedure performed on the primary site, in the presence of known metastases, should only be palliative.

Radiation therapy alone is probably ineffective, but some have recommended its use adjunctively with radical resection (887). Few reports of the efficacy of chemotherapy have been published (863, 888). The mean survival in one large series was only 2.5 years (872), but with radical excision patients with greater than 20 years survival have been reported.

Fibrosarcomas and Malignant Mesenchymoma

Fibrosarcomas of the nerve sheath are the most common malignant tumor to arise in patients with von Recklinghausen's disease (853). They are felt to be of fibroblastic, rather than Schwann cell, origin. Their matrix is often mucinous rather than collagenous, as with the malignant schwannomas. They may undergo varying amounts of mesenchymal differentiation and are then termed 'malignant mesenchymoma'. They have many other features in common with malignant schwannomas, both histologically and clinically, with a tendency to local recurrence, spread along nerve trunks, infrequent metastases, and an overall poor outcome unless radical excision is performed. Their separation as a distinct nosological entity seems somewhat of a fine point, with little clinical relevance (880), and a number of workers have felt that malignant schwannomas and nerve sheath fibrosarcomas should both be known by the common term 'malignant peripheral nerve sheath tumor' (MPNST) (861).

SOLITARY BENIGN NERVE SHEATH TUMORS

Nerve Sheath Myxoma

This rare tumor arises in the endoneurium of peripheral nerves (853). The cell of origin is uncertain, but may either be mucin-producing mesodermal cells or modifed Schwann cells. In either case, the tumors characteristically contain an abundant mucoid matrix. Schwann cells have been demonstrated to be capable of synthesizing collagen, and the overgrowth of endoneurium seen in neurofibromas often has myxomatous areas, so myxomas may be considered a variant of that tumor. Harkin and Reed (853) have separated them provisionally. They usually arise in the skin, are lobulated, and occupy most of the thickness of the dermis, sparing the epidermis. They may be confused with focal cutaneous mucinosis and mucin-filled ganglion cysts which are rarely found within the perineurium of peripheral nerves (889, 890). The tumor cells are plump and stellate, multinucleated giant cells may be seen, and there may be areas of hypercelluarity and scantier mucoid matrix. No mitoses are seen and the tumors behave completely benignly. Once excised, these tumors do not recur.

TUMORS OF PERIPHERAL NERVE CELL ORIGIN

Ganglioneuroma

As with most peripheral nerve cell tumors, ganglioneuromas arise mainly from neurons of the sympathetic nervous system. They are, essentially, well-differentiated forms of the neuroblastoma (891), but occur with one-sixth the frequency (880). Because of their prominent Schwann cell component, these tumors have also been called gangliogliomas. Indeed

Schwann cells form the principal cell type, with ganglion cells distributed irregularly among the Schwann cell fascicles (853). This picture may mimic that of a neurofibroma which has involved a neighboring sympathetic ganglion. Points of differentiation are the absence of satellite cells, and the presence of binucleated or multinucleated cells, in ganglioneuromas. These tumors frequently are hormonally active, secreting catecholamines (892), unlike their intracranial counterparts (see above). Elevated catecholamine metabolite levels may be found in the urine (893).

Their growth is slow and the appearance of symptoms insidious. Unlike the more aggressive neuroblastomas, they tend to occur more frequently in adults than in children. In the thorax they tend to occur in the posterior mediastinum, where they may first be noticed as an incidental mass on chest x-ray. Scoliosis may be a presenting symptom, as is spinal cord compression when the tumor extends, in a dumb-bell fashion, through the intervertebral foramen. Rarely they cause respiratory symptoms due to bronchial compression. Intra-abdominal tumors may arise from the lumbar paravertebral plexus, adrenal glands and even from Meissner's and Auerbach's plexuses in the intestines. The most frequent symptoms are abdominal discomfort and changes in bowel habit. As they may achieve a very large size before causing symptoms, they may also be found incidentally as a mass, either on physical examination or on x-ray.

These tumors are usually well encapsulated, and amenable to total resection (894). However, they may become adherent to major vessels, permitting only subtotal resection. The dumb-bell tumors within the canal may also be difficult to excise, requiring a two-staged or combined anterior and posterior procedure. The prognosis is, in general, quite good, most recurrences being from partially removed intraspinal portions. Ganglioneuromas have shown no sensitivity at all to radiation therapy or chemotherapy. Tumors with the histological appearance and biological behavior of MPNST have been known to arise within pre-

existing ganglioneuromas, following radiotherapy (895).

TUMORS OF PARAGANGLIONIC CELL ORIGIN

The paraganglionic system, which is derived
from the neural crest, consists of the adrenal
glands, the brachiomeric and intravagal paraganglia, aorticosympathetic ganglia, and vis-
ceral-autonomic paraganglia (853, 896). As
their name implies, they develop as a separate,
but interconnected system with the sympathetic and parasympathetic nervous systems.
Most paraganglia have the ability to synthesize and store catecholamines. Some act as
chemoreceptors on major blood vessels (880).
The relatively common pheochomocytoma,
originating usually in the adrenal medulla,
and the glomus jugulare and tympanic tumors,
which are discussed fully in Chapter 36, are
examples.

Chemodectomas

Although some authors classify glomus jugulare tumors as chemodectomas (897), here
chemodectomas will signify the rare tumors of
the carotid body. They arise from endocrinologically inactive paraganglion cells, like glomus
jugulare tumors, and have been referred to,
therefore, as 'nonchromaffin paragangliomas'.
Other sites where they may occur are the
glomus aorticum, glomus typanicum, and glomus intravagale (897, 898).

Women are affected more frequently than
men. They may occur at any age between 7
and 70, but the average age is 45 years (896).
Interestingly, it has been said that their incidence is greater in people living at high
altitudes, or who are chronically hypoxic,
because of the chemoreceptor role of their cells
of origin (897). About 6% will develop second
paragangliomas, frequently of the contralateral carotid body, and an autosomal domi-
nent pattern of familial transmission has been
reported (899, 900).

Carotid body tumors, because of their location at the carotid bifurcation, cause a separa-
ration of the internal and external carotid
arteries. Grossly the tumors are vascular, well-
demarcated masses. They obtain their vascular
supply from the external carotid artery (901).
Shamblin et al. (902) have subdivided them
into three categories, according to the degree
to which they are adherent to and surround
adjacent vessels. This grade can often be
determined on preoperative angiography. On
microscopic examination, carotid body tumors
are similar to glomus jugulare tumors (897).
They consist of polygonal, epithelioid 'chief'
cells with finely granular cytoplasm. A rich
vascular network is seen.

In general, carotid body tumors are benign
and slow-growing, but about half may have
aggressive histological characteristics, and distant metastasis to lymph nodes, lung and bone
occur in 2% (902–905). Farr has estimated
that most carotid body tumors grow at a rate of
about 2 cm every 5 years (905). They usually
present as painless masses on the side of the
neck, and must be differentiated from other
masses occurring in this region. They are easy
to move from side to side but not in a vertical
direction. Other symptoms are hoarseness,
from vocal cord paralysis, and Horner's syndrome, dysphagia, local pain and transient
ischemic attacks (904). Although they are
considered inactive endocrinologically, some
may secrete catecholamines, and present with
hypertension and the typical picture of
pheochromocytomas (896). Because of their
slow growth, symptoms are often present for up
to 2 years before a diagnosis is made.

Radiologically the diagnosis is best made
with angiography, which can also be used to
grade the tumor and, thereby, plan the operative approach (901, 902). The angiographic
picture is of separated, and occasionally compressed, carotid bifurcation branches, and a
tumor blush which is often very intense. CT
scanning and radionuclide studies can also
detect the tumors (901, 906), but do not reveal
their relationship to vascular structures as well
as angiography, which may also demonstrate a

second, or even a third, unsuspected chemo-dectoma.

As radiation therapy and chemotherapy are of no known benefit in the treatment of these tumors, their primary therapy consists of surgical resection (903–905, 907). This should be undertaken with some circumspection, however, because of the benign nature of the tumors and the relatively great risk of operating on them. Mortality has been as high as 13%, stroke may occur in up to 20%, and damage to the vagus or hypoglossal nerves has been reported in 32 to 44%. Since one of the surgical options may require sacrifice of the internal carotid artery in order to obtain a total removal of tumor, a contralateral injection with ipsilateral cross-compression should be performed routinely at preoperative angiography, to check the patency of the circle of Willis (897). Carotid artery replacement or bypass grafts are also options in removing large, Grade III tumors. In older patients it may be most prudent to withhold surgery, unless rapid growth or other aggressive behavior of the tumor is noted or suspected. Radiation therapy should be reserved for poor risk patients and for inoperable tumors. With the increased use of microsurgical techniques, the more experienced centers are reporting decreasing operative morbidity and mortality (897).

MISCELLANEOUS TUMORS

Melanotic Neurofibroma

We have already seen that some forms of malignant schwannomas contain varying proportions of melanin-producing cells. Both Schwann cells and melanocytes are of neural crest origin. It is not surprising to encounter dermal tumors, with a close anatomical relationship to nerves, which slow melanocytic differentiation (96). Harkin and Reed (853) have therefore included such tumors, called melanotic neurofibroma, blue nevus, neuronevus, cellular blue nevus, or pacinian neurofi-

broma in their monograph. Their exact pathogenesis, though, is still too uncertain to state definitely that they originate from nerves. The term melanocytic neurofibroma was first employed by Willis (908) to describe three tumors that had features of both blue nevi and plexiform neurofibroma. They are characterized by numerous multinucleated giant cells in clusters and scattered through a hyaline matrix.

Granular Cell Tumor (Myoblastoma)
(see Chapter 32 for a full description)

This tumor is the peripheral variant of the choristoma discussed earlier (909). It is a tumor of unknown origin. Its derivation from primitive muscle cells is not generally accepted (853). The cells are compactly arrayed, and contain numerous acidophilic granules in their cytoplasm. Ultrastructural studies have shown a basement membrane, as is found around Schwann cells. There are also many interdigitating cytoplasmic extensions (910). Five cases studied immunohistochemically by Armin et al. stained for S-100 protein (911). This finding has been verified by others (912–914). Therefore, some of these tumors may be of Schwann cell origin. It is still unclear whether they represent a truly neoplastic process, or arise through a disturbance in lipid metabolism in Schwann cells (909, 915). Markesbery et al. (915) have suggested that more than one cell type may be involved in the CNS tumors. Reticulin stains are positive. There is often a fascicular arrangement of the cells. They are benign tumors, usually found in the dermis, tongue, submucosa of the gastrointestinal tract, breast, bronchi and peritoneum (853, 914). Anatomical relationship between the tumors and peripheal nerves is always present.

Dermatofibrosarcoma Protuberans

This is the name given to an uncommon, nodular, locally invasive skin tumor (853, 916). Spindle-shaped cells in intertwined fascicles are found infiltrating the dermis and subcuticular fat. Frequently the tumors have a myxomatous matrix, and small nodules of lamellated, hyalinized fibrous tissue are seen interspersed in a field which is similar in its appearance to a plexiform neurofibroma. Often small peripheral nerves with a thickened perineurium, infiltrated by tumor cells, are found at the tumor's margins. An unusual variant of this tumor, which often contains melanocytes, is called a 'storiform neurofibroma' (917). The term 'storiform' refers to the star-like pattern made by the interlacing fascicles of tumor cells as they meet and bend at acute angles. The origin of these tumors is unknown, but Schwann cells and nerve sheath fibrocytes have both been implicated (853).

Multiple Mucosal Neuroma Syndrome

This syndrome is similar to von Recklinghausen's syndrome, but the lesions are neuromas rather than neurofibromas (853). Cutaneous lesions do not occur in this syndrome, but there is an association with intestinal ganglioneuromatosis, carcinoma of the thyroid, and pheochromocytoma. A familial incidence of this syndrome has been described.

Neurocutaneous Melanosis Syndrome

This syndrome, alluded to in the discussion of melanotic tumors of the CNS, is a disorder of melanocytes in which giant pigmented nevi of the skin are associated with focal or generalized melanosis in the leptomeninges. Malignant tumors may arise in either location, and may be multiple. The melanosis of the CNS is generally greatest around the medulla, but may involve the cerebellum and other areas (17, 918, 919). The CNS tumors associated with this syndrome include melanoma, primitive neuroepithelial tumors with pigmented cells, and rarely, sarcoma (381, 853). Other neurological complications encountered in this disease include hydrocephalus, spinal cord compression from thickened leptomeninges, seizures and cranial nerve palsies (918, 919). Syringomyelia has also been reported (920). Attempts to shunt hydrocephalic patients often leads to dissemination of melanoma cells in the peritoneal cavity (919, 921). The dermal lesions include cellular nevus, blue nevus, neurofibroma, melanocytic neurofibroma, and malignant melanoma. Portions may be histologically similar to malignant schwannoma or malignant epithelioid schwannoma (853, 918).

CONCLUSIONS AND FUTURE DIRECTIONS

An attempt has been made, in this chapter, to show the variety of tumors which may arise in the central nervous system. Many of the complex issues concerning their origins, biological behavior, diagnosis and therapy have been discussed. The importance of refining existing classification schemes, based on new information acquired through such technological advances as monoclonal antibodies, tissue culturing, and molecular biology, has been stressed (3, 5).

A major impediment to the elucidation of the nature of these tumors is their scarcity. Most studies of their behavior and treatment have been through the retrospective collection of data from the literature or from the case records of the reporting institution. Greater progress would be possible through prospective studies, which, of necessity, would involve multi-institutional, randomized trials. For tumors characterized by long, symptom-free intervals before recurrence, these trials would require lengthy follow-up periods.

The application of developing technologies to basic scientific, taxonomic, and clinical questions concerning these tumors has been somewhat scanty, when compared to the more common tumors, such as glioblastoma and peripheral neuroblastoma. This may be due to the relative lack of tissue to study. To this end, a national, centralized system of tissue banking and distribution to investigators could maximize the scientific utilization of material which would ordinarily be discarded. The ability of some tumor cells to grow in tissue culture has been utilized by both basic and clinical researchers in the study of glioblastoma (922–927). This has been demonstrated to have direct clinical application through the in vitro testing of potential chemotherapeutic agents on these tumors (928, 929). The full potential of this technique in studying the tumors discussed in this chapter has yet to be explored.

The use of polyclonal and monoclonal antibodies directed at specific antigenic determinants on tumor cells may also have both basic research and clinical applications in uncommon tumors (150, 858, 930–935). Some of the markers currently being employed for taxonomic purposes are listed in Table 6. With enough specificity, such antibodies could complement present diagnostic imaging modalities, as well as guide toxins to target cells (933, 936, 937). There have been no series reported of the immunological therapy of any of the uncommon tumors discussed in this chapter. In

TABLE 6 TAXONOMIC MARKERS IN TUMORS OF THE NERVOUS SYSTEM

	Cell or tumour type
Intermediate filament proteins:	
Glial fibrillary acidic protein	Astroglial
Neurofilament	Neuronal
Vimentin	Fibroblast, neuronal, Glial, meningioma
Desmin	Smooth, skeletal and cardiac muscle
Cytokeratins	Simple epithelium, carcinoma, chordoma
Myelin related antigens:	
Myelin basic protein	Central myelin
PO and P2 protein	Peripheral myelin
Myelin associated glycoprotein	Central and peripheral myelin
Carbonic anhydrase	Oligodendroglia
Other biochemically defined antigens:	
S-100 protein	Neuroectodermal
Neuron-specific enolase	Neuronal
Glutamine synthetase	Astroglial
Alpha-2 glycoprotein	Astrocytoma, mixed astro/oligo tumors
Gangliosides	Neuroepithelial, ESP glioma, melanoma
Factor VIII-related antigen	Endothelial
Placental alkaline phosphatase	Germinoma
Pan neurectodermal antigen	Neuroectodermal
B 1 antigen, immunoglublin components	B-lymphocytes
Neuroblastic cell membrane antigen	Fetal brain, neuroblastoma, medulloblastoma
Human chorionic gonadotrophin	Choriocarcinoma, germinoma, Embryonal cell carcinoma
Alpha-fetoprotein	Malignant teratoma, endodermal sinus tumor, embryonal cell carcinoma
Epithelial membrane antigen	Meningioma

From references 26, 50, 149, 150, 377, 858, 913, 931, 934, 935.

the future, immunotherapy with, for example, interleukin-2-induced LAK (lymphokine-activated killer) cells, may establish a position for itself in the clinician's armamentarium (938).

Electron microscopic techniques have provided ultrastructural information which has aided in the classification of uncommon tumors of uncertain cytogenesis. Molecular genetic and molecular biological studies (939–943) may also help answer questions concerning the pathogenesis of certain tumors, as well as suggest innovative ways of treating them, for example, with 'differentiating' agents to make malignant tumors behave less aggressively (944–947). Elucidation of the role of growth factors in the proliferation of normal and anaplastic neuroepithelial cells, and of angiogenic and related factors in the development of solid tumors, may also suggest ways to control tumor growth (350, 352, 948–950).

Data is accumulating on the magnetic resonance characteristics of many of the uncommon tumors. This imaging modality may aid in their non-operative diagnosis, and provide anatomical definition which will complement information obtained by CT.

Although these tumors comprise the minority of all CNS tumors, the insight to be gained into neoplastic processes from their study certainly makes the scientific effort spent on them worthwhile.

ACKNOWLEDGEMENTS

The authors wish to acknowledge, with gratitude, the unstinting efforts of Ms Esther Turull in the preparation of this chapter.

REFERENCES

1 Adams RD, Victor M. Principles of Neurology, 3rd edition. New York: McGraw Hill, 1985.
2 Rubinstein LJ. Morphological problems of brain tumors with mixed cell population. Acta Neurochir 1964; Suppl 10: 141–65.
3 Becker LE. An appraisal of the World Health Organization classification of tumors of the central nervous system. Cancer 1985; 56: 1858–64.
4 McComb RD, Burger PC. Pathologic analysis

of primary brain tumors. Neurologic Clin 1985; 3: 711–28.
5 Burger PC. The 'ideal' classification of pediatric central nervous system neoplasms. Cancer 1985; 56: 1865–8.
6 Zulch KJ. Histologic Typing of Tumors of the Central Nervous System. Geneva: World Health Organization, 1979.
7 Barone BM, Elvidge AR. Ependymomas: a clinical survey. J. Neurosurg 1970; 33: 428–38.
8 Dohrman GJ. Ependymomas. In: Wilkins RH, Rengachary SS eds Neurosurgery. New York: McGraw-Hill, 1985: 767–71.
9 Sloof JL, Keruchera JW, MacCarty CS. Primary Intramedullary Tumors of the Spinal Cord and Filum Terminale. Philadelphia: WB Saunders, 1964.
10 Fokes EC, Earle KM, Ependymomas: clinical and pathological aspects. J Neursourg 1969; 30: 585–94.
11 Craig WM, Kernohan JW. Tumors of the fourth ventricle. JAMA 1938; 111: 2370–7.
12 Kricheff IL, Becker M, Schneck SA, Taveras JM. Intracranial ependymomas: a study of survival in 65 cases treated by surgery and irradiation. AJR 1964; 91: 167–75.
13 Sagerman RH, Bagshaw MA, Hanbery J. Considerations in the treatment of ependymoma. Radiology 165; 84: 401–8.
14 Svien HJ, Mabon RF, Kernohan JW, Craig WM. Ependymoma of the brain: pathologic aspects. Neurology (Minneapolis) 1953; 3: 1–15.
15 Shuangshoti S, Panyathanya R. Ependymomas: a study of forty-five cases. Dis Nerv Syst 1973; 34: 307–14.
16 Fischer G, Mansuy L. Total removal of intramedullary ependymomas: follow-up study of 16 cases. Surg Neurol 1980; 14: 243–9.
17 Rubinstein LJ. Tumors of the Central Nervous System. Bethesda, Md: AFIP, 1972.
18 Tsuchida T, Kamata K, Kawamata M, Okada K, Tanaka R, Oyake Y. Brain tumors in tuberous sclerosis: report of 4 cases. Child's Brain 1981; 8: 271–83.
19 Poser CM. The Relationship Between Syringomyelia and Neoplasm. Springfield, Illinois: Charles C. Thomas, 1956.
20 Woltman HW, Kernohan JW, Adson AW. Gliomas of the cerebellopontine angle. Mayo Clin Proc 1949; 24: 77–82.
21 Shuman RM, Alvord EC, Leech RW. The biology of childhood ependymomas. Arch Neurol (Chicago) 1975; 32: 731–9.
22 Kernohan JW. Ependymomas. In: Minckler J ed Pathology of the Nervous System. New York: McGraw-Hill, 1971: 1976–1993.

23 Mabon RF, Svien HJ, Kernohan JW, Craig WM. Ependymomas. Mayo Clin Proc 1949; 25: 65–70.

24 Globus JH, Kuhlenbeck H. The subependymal cell plate (matrix) and its relationship to brain tumors of the ependymal type. J Neuropathol Exp Neurol 1944; 3: 1–35.

25 Godwin JT. Subependymal glomerate astrocytoma: report of two cases. J Neurosurg 1959; 16: 385–9.

26 Garson JA. The production and characterization of monoclonal antibodies for use in neuropathology. MD Thesis; University of Birmingham 1983.

27 Kersting G. Tissue culture of human gliomas. Progr Neurol Surg 1968; 2: 165–202.

28 Philips TL, Sheline GE, Boldrey E. Therapeutic considerations in tumors affecting the central nervous system: ependymomas. Radiology 1964; 83: 98–105.

29 Rubinstein LJ. The definition of the ependymoma. Arch Pathol 1970; 90: 35–45.

30 Fincher EF. Spontaneous subarachnoid hemorrhage in intrathecal tumors of the lumbar sac: a clinical syndrome. J Neurosurg 1951; 8: 576–84.

31 Martin F, Lemmen LJ. Calcification in intracranial neoplasms. Am J Pathol 1952; 28: 1107–32.

32 Guidetti B, Fortuna A. Surgical treatment of intramedullary hemangioblastoma of the spinal cord. J. Neurosurg 1967; 27: 530–40.

33 Pierre-Kahn A, Hirsch JF, Roux FX, Renier D, Sainte-Rose C. Intracranial ependymomas in childhood: survival and functional results of 47 cases. Child's Brain 1983; 10: 145–56.

34 Schulz MD, Wang C-C, Zinninger GF, Tefft GF. Radiotherapy of intracranial neoplasms: with a special section on the radiotherapeutic management of central nervous system tumors in children. Progr Neurol Surg 1968; 2: 318–79.

35 Kim YH, Fayos JV. Intracranial ependymomas. Radiology 1977; 124: 805–8.

36 Rich JR. A survey of cerebrospinal fluid cytology. Bull LA Neurol Soc 1969; 34: 115–31.

37 Salazar OM, Castro Vita H, Van Houtte P, Rubin P, Aygun C. Improved survival in cases of intracranial ependymoma after radiation therapy: late report and recommendations. J Neurosurg 1983; 59: 652–9.

38 Jooma R, Kendall BE. Diagnosis and management of pineal tumors. J Neurosurg 1983; 58: 654–65.

39 Gonzales-Crussi F. Extragonadal Teratomas. Bethesda, Md: AFIP, 1982.

40 Herrick MK, Rubinstein LJ. The cytological differentiating potential of pineal parenchymal

neoplasms (true pinealomas): a clinicopathological study of 28 tumors. Brain 1979; 102: 289–320.

41 Lesnick JE, Chayt KJ, Bruce DA, Rorke LB, Trajanowsky J, Savino PJ, Schatz NJ. Familial pineoblastoma: report of two cases. J Neurosurg 1985; 62: 930–2.

42 Knudsen AG, Jr. Mutation and cancer: statistical study of retinoblastoma. Proc Natl Acad Sci 1971; 68: 820–3.

43 Bader JL, Miller RW, Meadows AT, Zimmerman LE, Champion LAA, Voute PA. Trilateral retinoblastoma. Lancet (letter) 1980; ii: 582–3.

44 Tarkkanen A, Haltia M, Karjalainen K. Trilateral retinoblastoma. Pineoblastoma (ectopic intracranial retinoblastoma) associated with bilateral retinoblastoma. Ophthal Pediatr Genet 1984; 4: 1–6.

45 Jakobiec FA, Tso MOM, Zimmerman LE, Dannis P. Retinoblastomas and intracranial malignancy. Cancer 1977; 39: 2048–58.

46 Bader JL, Meadows AT, Zimmerman LE, Rorke LB, Voute PA, Champion LA, Miller RW. Bilateral retinoblastoma with ectopic intracranial retinoblastoma: trilateral retinoblastoma. Cancer Genet Cytogenet 1982; 5: 203–13.

47 Bonnin JM, Rubinstein LJ, Palmer NF, Beckwith JB. The association of embryonal tumors originating in the kidney and in the brain: a report of seven cases. Cancer 1984; 54: 2137–46.

48 DeGirolami U. Pathology of tumors in the pineal region. In: Schmidek HH ed Pineal Tumors. New York: Masson Publishing, 1977: 1–19.

49 Mullen PE, Smith I. The endocrinology of the human pineal. Br J Hosp Med 1981; 25: 248, 253–6.

50 Shinoda J, Miwa Y, Sakai N, Yamada H, Shima H, Kato K, Takahashi M, Shimokawa K. Immunohistochemical study of placental alkaline phosphatase in primary intracranial germ-cell tumors. J Neurosurg 1985; 63: 733–9.

51 Korf HW, Klein DC, Zigler JS, Gery I, Schachenmayr W. S-antigen-like immunoreactivity in a human pineocytoma. Acta Neuropathol 1986; 69: 165–7.

52 Sobel RA, Trice JE, Nielsen SL, Ellis WG. Pineoblastoma with ganglionic and glial differentiation: report of two cases. Acta Neuropathol 1981; 55: 243–6.

53 Okeda R, Song SJ, Nakajima T, Matsutani M. Pineocytoma. Observation of an autopsy case by electron microscopy and cell markers. Acta Pathol Japan 1984; 34: 911–18.

54 Trojanowsky JQ, Tascos NA, Rorke LB. Malignant pineocytoma with prominent papillary features. Cancer 1982; 50: 1789–93.

55 Wray SH. The neuro-ophthalmic and neurologic manifestations of pinealomas. In Schmidek HH ed Pineal Tumors. New York: Masson Publishing, 1977: 21–59.

56 Stein BM. Tumors of pineal region. In: Youmans JR, ed Neurological Surgery (2nd edition). Philadelphia: WB Saunders Company 1982: 2863–2871.

57 Wood JH, Zimmerman RA, Bruce DA, Bilaniuk LT, Norris DG, Schut L. Assessment and management of pineal-region and related tumors. Surg Neurol 1981; 16: 192–210.

58 Zimmerman RA. Pineal region masses: radiology. In: Wilkins RH, Rengachary SS eds Neurosurgery. New York: McGraw-Hill, 1985: 680–7.

59 Zimmerman RA, Bilaniuk LT. Age-related incidence of pineal calcification detected by computed tomography. Radiology 1982; 142: 659–62.

60 Zimmerman RA, Bilaniuk LT, Wood JH, Bruce DA, Schut L. Computed tomography of pineal, para-pineal and histologically related tumors. Radiology 1980; 137: 669–77.

61 Kilgore DP, Strother CM, Starshak RJ, Haughton VM. Pineal germinoma: MR imaging. Radiology 1986; 158: 435–8.

62 Sano K. Pinealoma in children. Child's Brain 1976; 2: 67–72.

63 Black PM, Callahan LV, Kornblith PL. Tissue cultures from cerebrospinal fluid specimens in the study of human brain tumors. J Neurosurg 1978; 49: 697–704.

64 Neuwelt EA. An update on the surgical treatment of malignant pineal region tumors. Clinical Neurosurgery 1985; 32: 297–428.

65 Herrick MK. Pineal tumors: classification and pathology. In: Wilkins RH, Rengachary SS eds Neurosurgery. New York: McGraw-Hill, 1985: 674–80.

66 Barber SG, Smith JA, Hughes RC. Melatonin as a tumor marker in a patient with pineal tumor. Br Med J 1978; ii: 328.

67 Lilue RE, Jequier S, O'Gorman AM. Congenital pineoblastoma in the newborn: ultrasound evaluation. Radiology 1985; 154: 363–5.

68 Schmidek HH, Waters A. Pineal masses: clinical features and management. In: Wilkins RH, Rengachary SS eds Neurosurgery. New York: McGraw-Hill 1985: 688–93.

69 Chapman PH, Lingood RM. The management of pineal area tumors: a recent reappraisal. Cancer 1980; 46: 1253–7.

70 Di Girolami U, Schmidek HH. Clinicopatho-

logical study of 53 tumors of the pineal region. J Neurosurg 1973; 39: 455–62.

71 Suzuki J, Hori S. Evaluation of radiotherapy of tumors in the pineal region by ventriculographic studies with iodized oil. J Neurosurg 1969; 30: 595–603.

72 Cummins FM, Taveras JM, Schlesinger EB. Treatment of gliomas of the third ventricle and pinealomas: with special reference to the value of radiotherapy. Neurology (Minneapolis) 1960; 10: 1031–6.

73 Ventureyra ECG. Pineal region: surgical management of tumors and vascular malformations. Surg Neurol 1981; 16: 77–84.

74 Neuwelt EA, Glasberg M, Frenkel E, Clark WK. Malignant pineal region tumors: a clinicopathological study. J Neurosurg 1979; 51: 597–607.

75 Sung DI, Harisiadis L, Chang CH. Midline pineal tumors and suprasellar germinomas: highly curable by irradiation. Radiology 1978; 128: 745–51.

76 Wara WM, Fellows CF, Sheline GE, Wilson CB, Townsend JJ. Radiation therapy for pineal tumors and suprasella germinomas. Radiology 1977; 144: 221–3.

77 Jooma R, Hayward RD, Grant DN. Intracranial neoplasm during the first year of life: analysis of one hundred consecutive cases. Neurosurgery 1984; 14: 31–41.

78 Tomita T, McLone DG. Brain tumors during the first twenty-four months of life. Neurosurgery 1985; 17: 913–15.

79 Pascual-Castroviejo I, Villarejo F, Perez-Higueras A, Morales C, Pascual-Pascual SI. Childhood choroid plexus neoplasms: a study of 14 cases less than 2 years old. Eur J Pediatr 1983; 140: 51–6.

80 James HE. Choroid plexus papillomas. In: Wilkins RH, Rengachary SS eds Neurosurgery. New York: McGraw-Hill, 1985: 783–5.

81 Komminoth R, Woringer E, Baumgartner J, Braun JP, LeMaistre D. Papillome intraventriculaire familial. Neurochirurgie 1965; 11: 267–72.

82 Ausman JO, Shroutz C, Chason J, Knighton RS, Pak H, Patel S. Aggressive choroid plexus papilloma. Surg Neurol 1984; 22: 472–6.

83 Robinow M, Johnson GF, Minella PA. Aicardi syndrome, papilloma of the choroid plexus. cleft lip, and cleft of the posterior palate. J Pediatr 1984; 104: 404–5.

84 Tachibana H, Matsui A, Tamai T. Aicardi's syndrome with multiple papilloma of the chorid plexus. Arch Neurol 1982 (Chicago); 39: 194.

85 Katznelson D, Gross S, Hiss Y. Mumps en-

cephalitis and bilateral papillomas of the choroid plexus. Isr J Med Sci 1982; 18: 649–51.

86 Palmiter RD, Chen HY, Messing A, Brinster RL. SV40 enhancer and large-T antigen are instrumental in development of choroid plexus tumors in transgenic mice. Nature 1985; 316: 457–60.

87 Rovit RL, Schechter MM, Chondraff P. Choroid plexus papillomas. Observations on radiographic diagnosis AJR 1970; 110: 608–17.

88 Raimondi AJ, Gutierrez FA. Diagnosis and treatment of choroid plexus papillomas. Child's Brain 1975; 1: 81–115.

89 von Wagenen WP. Papillomas of the choroid plexus: report of two cases, one with removal of tumor at operation, and one with 'seeding' of the tumor in the ventricular system. Arch Surg (Chicago) 1930; 20: 199–231.

90 Gradin WC, Taylon C, Fruin AH. Chorid plexus papilloma of the third ventricle: case report and review of the literature. Neurosurgery 1983; 12: 217–20.

91 Jooma R, Grant DN. Third ventricular choroid plexus papillomas. Child's Brain 1983; 10: 242–50.

92 Chan RC, Thompson GB, Durity FA. Primary choroid plexus papilloma of the cerebellopontine angle. Neurosurgery 1983; 12: 334–6.

93 Matson DD, Crofton FDL. Papilloma of the choroid plexus in childhood. J Neurosurg 1960; 17: 1002–27.

94 Matsushima T. Choroid plexus papillomas and human choroid plexus: a light and electron microscopic study. J Neurosurg 1983; 59: 1054–62.

95 McComb RD, Burger PC. Choroid plexus carcinoma: report of a case with immunohistochemical and ultrastructural observation. Cancer 1983; 51: 470–5.

96 Russel D, Rubinstein LJ. Pathology of Tumors of the Nervous System, 4th edition. Baltimore: Williams and Wilkins, 1977.

97 Milhorat TH, Hammock MK, Davis DA, Fenstermacher JL. Choroid plexus papilloma. I. Proof of cerebrospinal fluid overproduction. Child's Brain 1976; 2: 273–89.

98 McDonald JV. Persistent hydrocephalus following removal of papillomas of the choroid plexus of the lateral ventricles: report of two cases. J Neurosurg 1969; 30: 736–40.

99 Sahar A, Feinsod M, Beller AJ. Choroid plexus papilloma: hydrocephalus and cerebrospinal fluid dynamics. Surg Neurol 1980; 13: 476–8.

100 Davis Rl, Fox GE. Acinar choroid plexus adenoma: report of a case. J Neurosurg 1970; 33: 587–90.

101 Cardozo J, Cepeda F, Quintero M, Mora E. Choroid plexus papilloma containing bone. Acta Neuropathol 1985; 68: 83–5.

102 Stefanko S, Vuzevski VD. Oncocytic variant of choroid plexus papilloma. Acta Neuropathol 1985; 66: 160–2.

103 Dohrman GJ, Colias J. Choroid plexus carcinoma. J Neurosurg 1975; 43: 225–32.

104 Lana-Peixoto MA, Lagos J, Silbert SW. Primary pigmented carcinoma of the choroid plexus. J Neurosurg 1977; 47: 442–50.

105 Vraa-Jensen G. Papilloma of the choroid plexus with pulmonary metastases. Acta Psych Neurol 1950; 25: 299–306.

106 Valladares JB, Perry RH, Kalbag RM. Malignant choroid plexus papilloma with extraneural metastasis. J Neurosurg 1980; 52: 251–5.

107 Matsushima M, Yamamoto T, Motomochi M, Ando K. Papilloma and venous angioma of the choroid plexus causing primary intraventricular hemorrhage: report of two cases. J Neurosurg 1973; 39: 666–70.

108 Matson D. Neurosurgery of Infancy and Childhood, 2nd edition. Springfield, Ill: Charles C. Thomas, 1969.

109 Lamberts AE. Choroid plexus papilloma with cerebrospinal fluid rhinorrhea. Surg Neurol 1984; 22: 576–8.

110 Spallone A, Guidetti G, Mercuri S, Russo A, Ierardi A, Silipo P. Choroid plexus papillomas: neuroradiological diagnosis. Neurochirurgia (Stuttgart) 1982; 25: 165–9.

111 Chow PP, Horgan JG, Burns PN, Weltin G, Taylor KJW. Choroid plexus papilloma: detection by real-time and Doppler sonography. AJNR 1986; 7: 168–70.

112 Harwood-Nash DC, Fitz CR. Neuroradiology in Infants and Children. St Louis: Mosby, 1976.

113 Koos WT, Miller MH. Intracranial Tumors of Infants and Children. Stuttgart: Georg Thieme Verlag, 1971.

114 Husag L, Costabile G, Probst C. Persistent hydrocephalus following removal of a choroid plexus papilloma of the lateral ventricle. Neurochirurgia (Stuttgart) 1984; 27: 82–5.

115 Safdari H, Bourbotte G, Frerebeau P, Castan P. Possible influence of cerebrospinal fluid pressure on the growth of a third ventricular choroid plexus papilloma. Surg Neurol 1984; 22: 243–8.

116 Carrea R, Palak M. Preoperative radiotherapy in the management of posterior fossa choroid plexus papillomas. Child's Brain 1977; 3: 12–24.

117 Arseni C, Constantinescu A, Danaila L, Istrate C. The choroid plexus papillomas. Neurochirurgia (Stuttgart) 1974; 17: 121–9.

118 Scharenberg K, Liu L. Neuroectodermal Tumors of the Central and Peripheral Nervous System. Baltimore: Williams and Wilkins, 1969.

119 Bailey P, Cushing H. Tumors of the Giloma Group. Philadelphia: JB Lippincott, 1926.

120 Bailey P, Bucy P. Astroblastomas of the brain. Acta Psychiatr Neurol 1930; 5: 339–61.

121 Husain AN, Leestma JE. Cerebral astroblastoma: immunohistochemical and ultrastructural features: case report. J Neurosurg 1986; 64: 657–61.

122 Yamashita J, Handa H, Yamagami T, Haebara H. Astroblastoma of pure type. Surg Neurol 1985; 24: 218–22.

123 De Rueck J, Van de Velde E, Vander Eeken H. The angioarchitecture of the astroblastoma. Clin Neurol Neurosurg 1975; 78: 89–98.

124 Steinberg GK, Shuer LM, Conley FK, Hanbery JW. Evolution and outcome in malignant astroglial neoplasms of the cerebellum. J Neurosurg 1985; 62: 9–17.

125 Elridge AR, Penfield W, Cone W. Gliomas of the central nervous system: study of 210 verified cases. Assoc Res Nerv Ment Dis Proc 1937; 16: 107–81.

126 Kubota T, Hirano A, Sato K, Yamamoto S. The fine structure of astroblastoma. Cancer 1985; 5: 745–50.

127 Jellinger K. Pathology of brain tumors with relation to prognosis. Zentralbl Neurochir 1978; 39: 285–300.

128 Hoshino T, Wilson CB, Ellis WG. Gemistocytic astrocytes in gliomas: an autoradiographic study. J Neuropathol Exp Neurol 1975; 34: 263–81.

129 Kapp JP, Paulson GW, Odom GL. Brain tumors with tuberous sclerosis. J Neurosurg 1967; 26: 191–202.

130 Kersting G. Tissue culture of human gliomas. Progr Neurol Surg 1968; 2: 165–202.

131 Rubinstein LJ. Discussion on polar spongioblastomas. Acta Neurochir 1964; 10: 126–40.

132 Russel DS, Cairns H. Polar spongioblastomas. Arch Histol Norm Pathol 1947; 3: 423–41.

133 Treip CS. A congenital medulloepithelioma of the midbrain. J Pathol Bacteriol 1957; 74: 357–63.

134 Rubinstein LJ. Embryonal central neuroepithelial tumors and their differentiating potential. A cytogenetic view of a complex neuro-oncological problem. J Neurosurg 1985; 62: 795–805.

135 Deck JHN. Cerebral medulloepithelioma with maturation into ependymal cells and ganglion cells. J Neuropathol Exp Neurol 1969; 28: 442–54.

136 Soto T, Shimoda A, Takahashi T, Daita G,

Goto S, Takamura H, Hirama M. Congenital cerebellar neuroepithelial tumor with multiple divergent differentiations. Acta Neuropathol 1980; 50: 143–6.

137 Scheithauer BW, Rubinstein LJ. Cerebral medulloepithelioma: report of a case with multiple, divergent neuroepithelial differentiation. Child's Brain 1979; 5: 62–71.

138 Pollak A, Fried RL. Fine structure of medulloepithelioma. J Neuropathol Exp Neurol 1977; 36: 712–25.

139 Auer RN, Becker LE. Cerebral medulloepithelioma with bone, cartilage and striated muscle: light microscopic and immunohistochemical study. J Neuropathol Exp Neurol 1983; 42: 256–67.

140 Boffin PJ, Ebels E. A case of medullomyoblastoma. Acta Neuropathol 1963; 2: 309–11.

141 Tennyson VM. The fine structure of the developing nervous system. In: Himwich W ed Developmental Neurobiology. Springfield, Illinois: Charles C. Thomas, 1970.

142 Karch SB, Urich H. Medulloepithelioma: definition of an entity. J Neuropathol Exp Neurol 1972; 31: 27–53.

143 Van Epps RR, Samuelson DR, McCormick WF. Cerebral medulloepithelioma: case report. J Neurosurg 1967; 27: 568–73.

144 Dunn J Jr, Kernohan JW. Gliomatosis cerebri. Arch Pathol (Chicago) 1957; 64: 82–91.

145 Grant N. Diffuse glioblastosis. In: Vinken PJ, Bruyn GW, eds Handbook of Clinical Neurology, Vol 18: Amsterdam: North Holland, 1975: 73–80.

146 Bailey P. Cellular types in primary tumors of the brain. In: Penfield W ed Cytology and Cellular Pathology of the Nervous System. Reprinted 1932. New York. Hafner, 1965: 903–51.

147 Christensen E. Nerve Cell tumors: central and peripheral. In: Minckler J ed Pathology of the Nervous System. New York: McGraw-Hill, 1971; 2081–93.

148 Kernohan JW, Learmouth JR, Doyle JB. Neuroblastoma and gangliocytoma of the central nervous system. Brain 1932; 55: 287–310.

149 Trojanowski JQ, Lee VMY, Schlaepfer WW. An immunohistochemical study of human central and peripheral nervous system tumors, using monoclonal antibodies against neurofilaments and glial filaments. Hum Pathol 1984; 15: 248–57.

150 Coakham HB, Brownell B. Monoclonal antibodies in the diagnosis of cerebral tumors and cerebrospinal fluid neoplasia. In: Cavanagh J ed Recent Advances in Neuropathology, Vol 3.

Edinburgh: Churchill Livingstone, 1986: 25–53.

151 Horten BC, Rubinstein LJ. Primary cerebral neuroblastoma: a clinicopathological study of 35 cases. Brain 1976; 99: 735–56.

152 Bennett JP Jr, Rubinstein LJ. The biological behavior of primary cerebral neuroblastoma: a reappraisal of the clinical course in a series of 70 cases. Ann Neurol 1984; 16: 21–7.

153 Henriquez AS, Robertson DM, Marshall WJS. Primary neuroblastoma of the central nervous system with spontaneous extracranial metastases. J Neurosurg 1973; 38: 226–31.

154 Miller AA, Ramsden F. A cerebral neuroblastoma with unusual fibrous tissue reaction. J Neuropathol Exp Neurol 1966; 25: 328–40.

155 Azzarelli B, Richards DE, Anton AH, Roessmann U. Cerebral neuroblastoma. Electron microscopic observations and catecholamine determinations. J Neuropathol Exp Neurol 1977; 36: 384–97.

156 Rhodes RH, Davis RL, Kassell SH, Klague BH. Primary cerebral neuroblastoma: a light and electron microscopic study. Acta Neuropathol 1978; 41: 119–24.

157 Berger MS, Edwards MSB, Wara WM, Levin VA, Wilson CB. Primary cerebral neuroblastoma: long-term follow-up review and therapeutic guidelines. J Neurosurg 1983f; 59: 418–23.

158 Kingsley DPE, Harwood-Nash CDF. Radiological features of the neuroectodermal tumors of childhood. Neuroradiology 1984; 26: 463–7.

159 Grisoi F, Vincentelli F, Boudouresques G, Delpuech F, Hassoun J, Raybaud C. Primary cerebral neuroblastoma in adult man. Surg Neurol 1981; 16: 266–70.

160 Ahdevaara P, Kalimo H, Torma T, Haltia M. Differentiating intracerebral neuroblastoma: report of a case and review of the literature. Cancer 1977; 40: 784–8.

161 Collins VP. Wilms' tumor: its behavior and prognosis. J Louisianna Med Soc 1955; 107: 474–80.

162 Courville CB. Ganglioglioma, tumor of the nervous system: review of the literature and report of two cases. Arch Neurol Psychiatry 1930; 24: 439–91.

163 Johannsson JH, Rekate HL, Roessmann U. Gangliogliomas: pathological and clinical correlation. J Neurosurg 1981; 54: 58–63.

164 Demierre B, Stichnoth FA, Hori A, Spoerri O. Intracerebral ganglioglioma. J Neurosurg 1986; 65: 177–82.

165 Garrido E, Becker LF, Hoffman HJ, Hendrick EB, Humphreys R. Gangliogliomas in children: a clinicopathological study. Child's Brain 1978; 4: 339–46.

166 Henry JM, Heffner RR, Earle KM. Ganglioglioma of CNS: a clinicopathological study of 50 cases. J Neuropathol Exp Neurol 1978; 37: 626 (abstract).

167 Albright L, Byrd RP. Ganglioglioma of the entire spinal cord. Child's Brain 1980; 6: 274–80.

168 Gritzman MCD, Snyckers FD, Proctor NSF. Ganglioglioma of the optic nerve: a case report. S Afr Med J 1983; 63: 863–5.

169 Davis RL, Nelson E. Unilateral ganglioglioma in a tuberosclerotic brain. J Neuropathol Exp Neurol 1961; 20: 571–81.

170 Oberc-Greenwood MA, McKeever PE, Kornblith PL, Smith BH. Human ganglioglioma containing paired helical filaments. Hum Pathol 1984; 15: 834–8.

171 Vanden Berg SR, May EE, Rubinstein LJ, Herman MM, Perentes E, Vinores SA, Collins VP, Park TS. Desmoplastic supratentorial neuroepithelial tumors of infancy with divergent differentiation potential ('desmoplastic infantile gangliomas'). J Neurosurg 1987; 66: 58–71.

172 Steegman AT, Winer B. Temporal lobe epilepsy resulting from ganglioglioma. Neurology 1961; 11: 406–12.

173 Cavanagh JB. On certain small tumors encountered in the temporal lobe. Brain 1958; 81: 389–405.

174 Rossi E, Vacquero J, Martinez R, Garcia-Sola R, Bravo G. Intracranial gangliogliomas. Acta Neurochir 1984; 71: 255–61.

175 Nars R, Whelan MA. Gangliogliomas. Neuroradiology 1981; 22: 67–71.

176 Dorne HL, O'Gorman AM, Melanson O. Computed tomography of intracranial gangliogliomas. AJNR 1986; 7: 281–5.

177 Katz MC, Kier EL, Schechter MM. The radiology of gangliogliomas and ganglioneuromas of the central nervous system. Neuroradiology 1972; 4: 69–73.

178 Ebina K, Suzuki S, Takahashi T, Iwabuchi T, Takei Y. Gangliocytoma of the pineal body: a case report and review of the literature. Acta Neurochir 1985; 74: 134–40.

179 Rhodes RH, Dusseau JJ, Boyd AS, Knigge KM. Intrasellar neural-adenohypophyseal choristoma: a morphological and immunocytochemical study. J Neuropathol Exp Neurol 1982; 41: 267–80.

180 Ara SL, Scheithauer BW, Bilbao JM, Horvath E, Ryan N, Kovacs K, Randall R, Laws ER Jr, Singer W, Linfoot JA, Thorner MO, Vale W. A case for hypothalamic acromegaly: a clinico-

pathological study of six patients with hypothalamic gangliocytomas producing growth hormone-releasing factor. J Clin Endocrinol Metab 1984; 58: 796–803.

181 Ambler M, Pogacar S, Sidman R. Lhermitte-Duclos disease (granule cell hypertrophy of the cerebellum). Pathological analysis of the first familial case. J Neuropathol Exp Neurol 1969; 28: 622–47.

182 Oppenheimer DR. A benign 'tumor' of the cerebellum: report on two cases of diffuse hypertrophy of the cerebellar cortex with a review of nine previously reported cases. J Neurol Neurosurg Psychiatry 1955; 18: 199–213.

183 Dom R, Brucher J-M. Hamartoblastome (gangliocytome diffus) unilaterale de l'ecore cérébrale associé à une dégénérescence soudanophile de la substance blanche du côte oppose. Rev Neurol 1969; 120: 307–18.

184 Hart MN, Earle KM. Primitive neuroectodermal tumors of the brain in children. Cancer 1973; 32: 890–7.

185 Kosnik EJ, Boesel CP, Bay J, Sayers MP. Primitive neuroectoderal tumors of the central nervous system in children. J Neurosurg 1978; 48: 741–6.

186 Duffner PK, Cohen ME, Heffner RR, Freeman AI. Primitive neuroectodermal tumors of childhood. An approach to therapy. J Neurosurg 1981; 55: 376–81.

187 Becker LE, Hinton P. Primitive neuroectodermal tumors of the central nervous system. Hum Pathol 1983; 14: 538–50.

188 Rorke LB. The cerebellar medulloblastoma and its relationship to primitive neuroectodermal tumors. J Neuropathol Exp Neurol 1983; 42: 1–15.

189 Rubinstein LJ. Cytogenesis and differentiation of primitive central neuroepithelial tumors. J Neuropathol Exp Neurol 1972; 31: 7–26.

190 Pearl GS, Takei Y. Cerebellar 'neuroblastoma'. Nosology as it relates to medulloblastoma. Cancer 1981; 47: 772–9.

191 Shin WY, Laufer H, Lee YL, Aftalion V, Hirano A, Zimmerman HM. Fine structure of a cerebellar neuroblastoma. Acta Neuropathol 1978; 42: 11–13.

192 Yagishita S, Itoh Y, Chiba Y, Kuwana N. Morphological investigation on cerebellar 'neuroblastoma' group. Acta Neuropathol 1982; 56: 22–8.

193 Fowler M, Simpson DA. A malignant melanin-forming tumor of the cerebellum. J Pathol Bacteriol 1962; 84: 307–11.

194 Borello ED, Gorlin RJ. Melanotic neuroectodermal tumor of infancy—a neoplasm of neural crest origin. Report of a case associated with high urinary excretion of vanilmandelic acid. Cancer 1966; 19: 196–206.

195 Cobb CA, Youmans JR. Sarcomas and neoplasms of blood vessels. In Youmans JR ed Neurological Surgery, 2nd edition. Philadelphia: WB Saunders, 1982: 2845–62, 1982.

196 Jeffreys R. Clinical and surgical aspects of posterior fossa hemangioblastomata. J Neurol Neurosurg Psychiatry 1975; 38: 105–11.

197 Obrador S, Martin-Rodriguez JG. Biological factors involved in the clinical features and surgical management of cerebellar hemangioblastomas. Surg Neurol 1977; 7: 79–85.

198 Constans J-P, Meder F, Maiuri F, Donzelli R, Spazante R, de Devitiis E. Posterior fossa hemangioblastomas. Surg Neurol 1986; 25: 269–75.

199 Tomasello F, Albanese V, Iannotti F, Di Iorio G. Supratentorial hemangioblastoma in a child. J Neurosurg 1980; 52: 578–83.

200 Browne TR, Adams RD, Robertson GH. Hemangioblastoma of the spinal cord. Arch Neurol 1976; 33: 435–41.

201 Richardson RG, Griffin TW, Parker RG. Intramedullary hemangioblastoma of the spinal cord: definitive management with irradiation. Cancer 1980; 45: 49–50.

202 Grisoli F, Gambarelli D, Raybaud C, Giubout M, Leclerq T. Suprasellar hemangioblastoma. Surg Neurol 1984; 22: 257–62.

203 Ferrante L, Celli P, Fraioli B, Santoro A. Hemangioblastomas of the posterior cranial fossa. Acta Neurochir 1984; 71: 283–94.

204 Lindau A. Capillary angiomatosis of the central nervous system. Acta Genet (Basel) 1957; 7: 338–40.

205 Hardwig P, Robertson DM. von Hippel-Lindau disease: a familial, often lethal, multisystem phakomatosis. Ophthalmology 1984; 91: 263–70.

206 Horton WA, Wong V, Eldridge R. von Hippel-Lindau disease: clinical and pathological manifestations in nine families with 50 affected members. Arch Intern Med 1976; 136: 769–77.

207 Melmon KL, Rosen SW. Lindau's disease: review of the literature and study of a large kindred. Am J Med 1964; 36: 595–617.

208 Rengachary SS. Hemangioblastomas. In: Wilkins RH, Rengachary SS, eds Neurosurgery. New York: McGraw-Hill, 1985: 772–82.

209 Singounos EG. Haemangioblastomas of the central nervous system. Acta Neurochir 1978; 44: 107–13.

210 Rosenlof K, Fyhrquist F, Gronhagen-Riska C, Bohling T, Haltia M. Erythropoietin and renin

substrate in cerebellar hemangioblastoma. Acta Med Scand 1985; 218: 481–5.

211 Cushing H, Bailey P. Tumors Arising From the Blood Vessels of the Brain. Springfield, Illinois: Charles C Thomas, 1928.

212 Bailey OT, Ford R. Sclerosing hemangiomas of the central nervous system. Progressive tissue changes in hemangioblastomas of the brain and in so-called angioblastic meningiomas. Am J Pathol 1942; 18: 1–27.

213 Ramsey HJ. Fine structure of hemangiopericytoma and hemangio-endothelioma. Cancer 1966; 19: 2005–18.

214 Horten BC, Urich H, Rubinstein LJ, Montague SR. The angioblastic meningioma: a reappraisal of a nosological problem: light-, electron microscopic, tissue and organ culture observations. J Neurol Sci 1977; 31: 387–410.

215 Lindau A. Discussion on vascular tumors of the brain and spinal cord. Proc R Soc Med 1931; 24: 363–388.

216 Bailey P, Cushing H, Eisenhardt L. Angioblastic meningiomas. Arch Pathol Lab Med 1928; 6: 953–90.

217 McDonnell DE, Pollock P. Cerebral cystic hemangioblastoma, Surg Neurol 1978; 10: 195–9.

218 Mohan J, Brownell B, Oppenheimer DR. Malignant spread of hemangioblastoma: report on two cases. J Neurol Neurosurg Psychiatry 1976; 36: 515–525.

219 Okawara S-H. Solid Cerebellar hemangioblastoma. J Neurosurg 1973; 39: 514–18.

220 Silver ML, Hennigar G, Cerebellar hemangioma (hemangioblastoma): a clinicopathological review of 40 cases. J Neurosurg 1952; 9: 484–92.

221 Waldman TA. Polycythemia and cancer. In: Fifth National Cancer Congress Proceedings— Philadelphia 1964. Philadelphia: JB Lippincott, 1965: 437–43.

222 Ho KL. Ultrastructure of cerebral capillary hemangioblastoma. IV. Pericytes and their relationship to endothelial cells. Acta Neuropathol 1985; 67: 254–64.

223 Cancilla PA, Zimmerman HM. The fine structure of a cerebellar hemagioblastoma. J Neuropathol Exp Neurol 1965; 24: 621–8.

224 Rawe SE, Van Gilder JC, Rothman SLG. Radiographic diagnostic evaluation and surgical treatment of multiple cerebellar, brain stem, and spinal cord hemangioblastomas. Surg Neurol 1978; 9: 337–41.

225 Mondkar VP, McKissock W, Russell DS. Cerebellar haemangioblastomas. Br J Surg 1967; 54: 45–9.

226 Adegbite AB, Rozdilski B, Varughese G. Supratentorial capillary hemangioblastoma presenting with fatal spontaneous intracerebral hemorrhage. Neurosurgery 1983; 12: 327–30.

227 Matsumura A, Maki Y, Munekata K, Kobayashi E. Intracerebellar hemorrhage due to cerebellar hemangioblastoma. Surg Neurol 1985; 24: 227–30.

228 Beltramella A, Tognetti F, Gaist G, Rosta L. Posterior fossa hemangioblastomas: angiography versus computed tomography. Acta Neurochir 1985; 76: 23–7.

229 Seeger JF, Burke DP, Krake JE, Gabrielson TO. Computed tomographic and angiographic evaluation of hemangioblastomas. Radiology 1981; 136: 65–73.

230 Helle TL, Conley FK, Britt RH. Effect of radiation therapy on hemangioblastoma: a case report and review of the literature. Neurosurgery 1980; 6: 82–6.

231 Nishimoto A, Kawakami Y. Surgical removal of hemangioblastomas in the fourth ventricle. Surg Neurol 1980; 13: 423–7.

232 Pennybacker J. Recurrence of cerebellar hemangiomas. Zentralbl Neurochir 1954; 14: 63–73.

233 Sung DI, Chang CH, Harisiadis L. Cerebellar hemangioblastomas. Cancer 1982; 49: 553–5.

234 Bergstrand H. On the classification of the hemangiomatous tumors and malformations of the central nervous system. Acta Pathol Microbiol Scand 1936; 26 (Suppl): 89–95.

235 Bebin J, Smith EE. Vascular malformations of the brain. In: Smith RR, Haerer AF, Russel WF eds Vascular Malformations and Fistulas of the Brain. New York: Raven Press, 1982: 13–29.

236 Sarwar M, McCormick WF. Intracerebral venous angioma: case report and review. Arch Neurol 1978; 35: 323–5.

237 Courville CB. Pathology of the Central Nervous System, 2nd edition. Mountain View, Calif: Pacific Press Pub Assoc, 1945.

238 Jellinger K. The morphology of centrally situated angiomas. In: Pia HW, Gleave JRW, Grote E, Zierski J eds Cerebral Angiomas. Berlin: Springer-Verlag, 1975.

239 Rengachary SS, Kalyan-Raman UP. Other cranial intradural angiomas. In: Wilkins RH, Rengachary SS eds Neurosurgery. New York: McGraw-Hill, 1985: 1465–73.

240 Saito Y, Kobayashi N. Cerebral venous angioma: clinical evaluation and possible etiology. Radiology 1981; 139: 87–94.

241 Numaguchi Y, Kitamura K, Fukui M, Ikeda J, Hasuo K, Kishikawa T, Okudera T, Uemura

K, Matsuura K. Intracranial venous angiomas. Surg Neurol 1982; 18: 193–202.

242 Wyburn-Mason R. The Vascular Abnormalities and Tumors of the Spinal Cord and Its Membranes. London: Kimpton, 1943.

243 Bogren H, Svalander C, Wickbom I. Angiography in intracranial hemangiomas. Acta Radiol (Diagn) (Stockholm) 1970; 10: 81–9.

244 Wakai S, Ueda Y, Inoh S, Masakatsu N. Angiographically occult angiomas: a report of thirteen cases with analysis of the cases documented in the literature. Neurosurgery 1985; 17: 549–56.

245 Biller J, Toffol GJ, Shea JF, Fine M, Azar-Kia B. Cerebellar venous angiomas: a continuing controversy. Arch Neurol 1985; 42: 367–70.

246 Berenstein A, Choi IS. Treatment of venous angiomas by direct alcohol injection. AJNR 1983; 4: 1144 (abstract).

247 Vaquero J, Manrique M, Oya S, Cabezudo JM, Bravo G. Calcified telangiectatic hamartomas of the brain. Surg Neurol 1980; 13: 453–7.

248 Russel DS. Discussion on vascular tumors of the brain and spinal cord. Proc R Soc Med 1931; 24: 383–5.

249 Burke EC, Winkelman RK, Strickland MK. Disseminated hemangiomatosis. Am J Dis Child 1964; 108: 418–24.

250 Michael JC, Levin PM. Multiple telangiectases of the brain (discussion of the hereditary factors in their development). Arch Neurol 1936; 36: 514–29.

251 Tielmann K. Hemangiomas of the pons. Arch Neurol 1953; 69: 208–23.

252 Farrell DF, Forno LS. Symptomatic capillary telangiectasis of the brainstem without hemorrhage: report of an unusual case. Neurology 1970; 20: 341–6.

253 Alexander GL, Norman RM. The Sturge-Weber Syndrome. Bristol: Wright, 1960.

254 Wohlwill FJ, Yakovlev PI. Histopathology of meningofacial angiomatosis (Sturge-Weber's disease). Report of four cases. J Neuropathol Exp Neurol 1957; 16: 341–64.

255 Heffner RR Jr, Solitaire GB. Hereditary hemorrhagic telangiectasia: neuropathological observations. J Neurol Neurosurg Psychiatry 1969; 31: 604–8.

256 Wyburn-Mason R. Arteriovenous aneurysm of the midbrain and retina, facial nevi and mental changes. Brain 1943; 66: 163–203.

257 Hoffman HJ, Hendrick EB, Dennis M, Armstrong D. Hemispherectomy for Sturge Weber syndrome. Child's Brain 1979, 5: 233–48.

258 Simard JM, Garcia-Bengochea F, Ballinger WE Jr, Mickle JP, Quisling RG. Cavernous

angioma: a review of 126 collected and 12 new clinical cases. Neurosurgery 1986; 18: 162–72.

259 McCormick WF, Hardman JM, Boulter TR. Vascular malformations ('angiomas') of the brain, with special reference to those occurring in the posterior fossa. J Neurosurg 1968; 28: 241–51.

260 Voigt K, Yarargil MG. Cerebral cavernous hemangiomas or cavernomas. Neurochirurgia (Stuttgart) 1976; 19: 59–68.

261 Bicknell JM, Tarlow TJ, Kornfeld M, Stovring J, Turner P. Familial cavernous angiomas. Arch Neurol 1978; 35: 746–9.

262 Hayman LA, Evans RA, Ferrell RE, Fahr LM, Ostrow P, Riccardi VM. Familial cavernous angiomas: natural history and genetic study over a 5 year period. Am J Med Genet 1982; 11: 147–60.

263 Chee CP, Johnston R, Doyle D, Macpherson P. Oligodendroglioma and cerebral cavernous angioma: case report. J Neurosurg 1985; 62: 145–7.

264 Fischer EG, Sotrel A, Welch K. Cerebral hemangioma with glial neoplasia (angioglioma?). J Neurosurg 1982; 56: 430–4.

265 Flocks JS, Weis TP, Kleinman DC, Kristen WH. Dose-response studies to polyoma virus in rats. J Nat Cancer Inst 1965; 35: 259–84.

266 Rosenblum B, Rothman AS, Lanzieri C, Song S. A cavernous sinus cavernous hemangioma. J Neurosurg 1986; 65: 716–18.

267 Bhaskaran S, Rao DR. Cavernous angiomatous malformation of the brain. Indian J Pathol Bacteriol 1968; 11: 202–6.

268 Loeb L, Meyer JS. Pontine syndromes. In: Vinken PJ, Bruyn GW eds Handbook of Clinical Neurology, Vol 2. Amsterdam: North Holland, 1969: 238–71.

269 McCormick WF. The pathology of vascular ('arteriovenous') malformations. J Neurosurg 1966; 24: 807–16.

270 Chusid JG, Kopeloff LM. Epileptogenic effect of pure metals implanted in motor cortex of monkey. J Appl Physiol 1962; 17: 697–700.

271 Sypert GW, Willmore LJ. A new model of post-traumatic epilepsy: iron cations. Presented at the 28th Annual Meeting of the Congress of Neurological Surgeons, Washington, D.C., Dec 28, 1978.

272 Ishikawa M, Handa H, Moritake K, Mori K, Nakano Y, Alii H. Computed tomography of cerebral cavernous hemangiomas. J Comput Assist Tomogr 1980; 4: 587–91.

273 Namba S. Extracerebral cavernous hemangioma of the middle cranial fossa. Surg Neurol 1983; 19: 379–88.

274 Sundaresan N, Eller T, Ciric I. Hemangiomas

of the internal auditory canal. Surg Neurol 1976; 6: 119–21.

275 Fukui M, Matsuoka S, Hasuo K, Numaguchi Y, Kitamura K. Cavernous hemangioma in the pineal region. Surg Neurol 1983; 20: 209–15.

276 Mizutani T, Goldberg HI, Kerson LA, Murtagh F. Cavernous hemangioma in the diencephalon. Arch Neurol 1981; 38: 379–82.

277 Kawai K, Fukui M, Tanaka A, Kuramoto S, Kitamura K. Extracerebral cavernous hemangioma of the middle fossa. Surg Neurol 1978; 9: 19–25.

278 Mori K, Handa H, Gi H, Mori K. Cavernomas in the middle fossa. Surg Neurol 1980; 14: 21–31.

279 Wacksman SJ, Flessa HC, Glueck HI, Will JJ. Coagulation defects and giant cavernous hemangioma. Am J Dis Child 1966; 111: 71–4.

280 Khurana MS, Lian ECY, Harkness DR. 'Storage pool disease' of platelets. JAMA 1980; 244: 169–71.

281 Servo A, Porras M, Rainink R. Diagnosis of cavernous hemangiomas by computed tomography and angiography. Acta Neurochir 1984; 71: 273–82.

282 Savoiardo M, Strada L, Passerini A. Intracranial cavernous hemangiomas: neuroradiological review of 36 operated cases. AJNR 1983; 4: 945–950.

283 Rao VRK, Pillai SM, Shenog KT, Radharkrishnan VV, Matthews G. Hypervascular cavernous angioma at angiography. Neuroradiology 1979; 18: 211–14.

284 Bailey P, Cushing H, Einsenhardt L. Angioblastic meningiomas. Arch Pathol Lab Med 1928; 6: 953–90.

285 Jellinger K, Slowik F. Histological subtypes and prognostic problems in meningiomas. J Neurol 1975; 208: 279–98.

286 Jaaskelainen J, Servo A, Haltia M, Wahlstrom T, Valtonen S. Intracranial hemangiopericytoma: radiology, surgery, radiotherapy, and outcome in 21 patients. Surg Neurol 1985; 23: 227–36.

287 Goellner JR, Laws ER Jr, Soule EH, Okazaki H. Hemangiopericytoma of the meninges: Mayo Clinic experience. Am J Clin Pathol 1978; 70: 375–80.

288 Pitkethly DT, Hardman JM, Kempe LG, Earle KM. Angioblastic meningiomas. Clinicopathological study of 81 cases. J Neurosurg 1970; 32: 539–44.

289 McDonald JV, Terry R. Hemangiopericytoma of the brain. Neurology (Minneapolis) 1961; 11: 497–502.

290 Stout AP, Murray MR. Hemangiopericytoma: a vascular tumor featuring Zimmerman's pericytes. Ann Surg 1942; 116: 26–33.

291 Begg CF, Garrett A. Hemangiopericytoma occurring in the meninges. Case report. Cancer 1954; 7: 602–6.

292 Nunnery EW, Kahn LB, Reddick RL, Lipper S. Hemangiopericytoma: a light microscopic and ultrastructural study. Cancer 1981; 47: 906–14.

293 Popoff NA, Malinin TI, Rosomoff HL. Fine structure of intracranial hemangiopericytoma and angiomatous meningioma. Cancer 1974; 34: 1187–97.

294 Kruse F Jr. Hemangiopericytoma of the meninges (angioblastic meningioma of Cushing and Eisenhardt): clinicopathological aspects and follow-up study in 8 cases. Neurology (Minneapolis) 1961; 11: 771–7.

295 Muller J, Mealey J Jr. The use of tissue culture in differentiation between angioblastic meningioma and hemangiopericytoma. J Neurosurg 1971; 34: 341–8.

296 Rubinstein LJ. Tumors of the Central Nervous System. Supplement. Bethesda. MD: AFIP, 1982.

297 Markwalder TM, Zava DT. Goldhirsch A, Markwalder RV. Estrogen and progesterone receptors in meningiomas in relation to clinical and pathological features. Surg Neurol 1983, 20: 42–7.

298 Hayward E, Whitewell H, Paul KS, Barnes DM. Steroid receptors in human meningioma (Congress abstract). J Steroid Biochem 1983; 19 (Suppl): 164.

299 Pena CE. Intracranial hemangiopericytoma. Ultrastructural evidence of its leiomyoblastic differentiation. Acta Neuropathol 1971; 33: 279–84.

300 Ludwin SK, Rubinstein LJ, Russell DS. Papillary meningioma: a malignant variety of meningioma. Cancer 1975; 36: 1363–73.

301 Yagishita A, Hassoun J, Vincentelli F, Jiddane M, Salamon G. Neuroradiological study of hemangiopericytomas. Neuroradiology 1985; 27: 420–5.

302 Osborne DR, Dubois P, Drayer B, Sage M, Borger P, Heinz ER. Primary intracranial meningeal and spinal hemangiopericytoma: radiological manifestations. AJNR 1981; 2: 69–74.

303 Nadjini M, Piepgras U, Vogelsang H. Kranielle Computertomographie. Ein Synoptischer Atlas. Stuttgart: Georg Thieme Verlag, 1981.

304 New PFJ, Hesselink JR, O'Carroll CPO, Kleinman GM. Malignant meningiomas: CT

and histological criteria, including a new CT sign. AJNR 1982; 3: 267–76.

305 Marc JA, Takei Y, Schechter MM. Intracranial hemangiopericytomas (angiography, pathology and differential diagnosis). Radiology 1975; 125: 823–32.

306 Backwinkel KD, Diddams JA. Hemangiopericytoma: report of a case and comprehensive review of the literature. Cancer 1970; 25: 896–901.

307 Mira JG, Chu FCH, Forther JG. The role of radiotherapy in the management of malignant hemangiopericytomas. Cancer 1977; 39: 1254–9.

308 Fukui M, Kitamura K, Nakagaki H, Yamakawa Y, Kinoshita K, Hayabuchi N, Jingu K, Numaguchi Y, Matsuura K, Watanabe K. Irradiated meningiomas. A clinical evaluation. Acta Neurochir 1980; 54: 33–43.

309 Yamakawa Y, Kinoshita K, Fukui M, Mihara K, Koga K, Kitamura K. Radiosensitive meningioma. Surg Neurol 1980; 13: 471–5.

310 Fleming JFR, Deck JHN, Bernstein M. Intracranial sarcomas. In: Wilkins RH, Rengachary SS eds Neurosurgery. New York: McGraw-Hill, 1985: 1030–6.

311 Hiu YK. Primary intracranial sarcomas. Arch Neurol Psychiatry 1940; 43: 901–924.

312 Rubinstein LJ, Northfield DWC. The medulloblastoma and the so-called 'arachnoidal cerebellar sarcoma': a critical re-examination of a nosological problem. Brain 1964; 87: 379–412.

313 Bingas B. On the primary sarcomas of the brain. Acta Neurochir 1963; Suppl 10: 186–9.

314 Nichols P, Wagner JA. Primary intracranial sarcoma: report of nine cases with suggested classification. J Neuropathol Exp Neurol 1952; 11: 215–34.

315 Morantz RA, Feigin I, Ransohoff J. Clinical and pathological study of 24 cases of gliosarcoma. J. Neurosurg 1976; 45: 398–408.

316 Tomita T, Gonzalez-Crussi F. Intracranial nonlymphomatous sarcomas in children: experience with eight cases and review of the literature. Neurosurgery 1984; 14: 529–40.

317 Feigin I, Budzilovich GN. Sarcoma arising in metastatic carcinoma of the brain. A second instance. Lancet 1984; ii: 2047–50.

318 Schwartz I. Feigin I. Sarcoma arising in metastatic carcinoma of the brain. Acta Neuropathol 1963; 3: 74–8.

319 Abbott KH, Kernohan JW. Primary sarcomas of the brain: review of the literature and report of twelve cases. Acta Neurol Psychiatr 1943; 50: 43–66.

320 Christensen E, Lara DE. Intracranial sarcomas. J Neuropathol Exp Neurol 1953; 12: 41–56.

321 Rueda-Franco F, Lopez-Corella E. Sarcomas in the central nervous system of children. Concepts Pediatr Neurosurg 1982; 2: 188–204.

322 Schrantz JL, Araoz CA. Radiation-induced meningeal fibrosarcoma. Arch Pathol (Chicago) 1972; 93: 26–31.

323 Waltz TA, Brownell V. Sarcoma: a possible late result of effective radiation therapy for pituitary adenoma. Report of two cases. J Neurosurg 1966; 24: 901–7.

324 Noetzli M, Malamud N. Postirradiation fibroid sarcoma of the brain. Cancer 1962; 15: 617–22.

325 Walker JS, Bigner DD. Virus induced brain tumors. In: Wilkins RH, Rengachary SS eds Neurosurgery. New York: McGraw-Hill, 1985: 522–5.

326 Kernohan JW, Uihlein A. Sarcomas of the brain. Springfield, Ill.: Charles C Thomas, 1962.

327 Lalitha VS, Rubinstein LD. Reactive glioma in intracranial sarcoma: a form of mixed sarcoma and glioma ('sarcoglioma'). Report of eight cases. Cancer 1979; 43: 246–57.

328 Onofrio BM, Kernohan JW, Uihlein A. Primary meningeal sarcomatosis: a review of the literature and report of 12 cases. Cancer 1962; 15: 1197–1208.

329 Rottino A, Poppiti R. Diffuse meningeal sarcoma. J Neuropathol Exp Neurol 1943; 2: 190–6.

330 Abbott KH, Love JG. Metastasizing intracranial tumors. Ann Surg 1943; 118: 343–52.

331 Caner GC. Case 24312. New Engl J Med 1938; 219: 169–73.

332 Kishikawa T, Numaguchi Y, Fukui M, Komaki S, Ikeda J, Kitamura K, Matsuura K. Primary intracranial sarcomas: radiological diagnosis with emphasis on angiography. Neuroradiology 1981; 21: 25–31.

333 Hassounah M, Al-Mefty O, Akhtar M, Jinkins JR, Fox JL. Primary cranial and intracranial chondrosarcomas. Acta Neurochir 1985; 78: 123–32.

334 Olson JJ, Menezes AH, Godersky JC, Labosky JM, Hart M. Primary intracranial rhabdomyosarcoma. Neurosurgery 1985; 17: 25–34.

335 Kubota T, Hayashi M, Yamamoto S. Primary intracranial mesenchymal chondrosarcoma: case report with review of the literature. Neurosurgery 1982; 10: 105–10.

336 Anderson WR, Cameron JD, Tsai SH. Primary intracranial leiomyosarcoma. J Neurosurg 1980; 53: 401–5.

337 Kalyanaraman UP, Taraska JJ, Fierer JA, Elwood PW. Malignant fibrous histiocytoma of the meninges: histological, ultrastructural and immunocytochemical studies. J Neurosurg 1981; 55: 957–62.

338 Lam RM, Malik GM, Chason JL. Osteosarcoma of meninges: clinical, light and ultrastructural observations of a case. Am J Surg Pathol 1981; 5: 203–8.

339 Rollo JL, Green WR, Khan LB. Primary meningeal mesenchymal chondrosarcoma. Arch Pathol Lab Med 1979; 103: 239–43.

340 Mena H, Garcia JH. Primary brain sarcomas: light and electron microscopic features. Cancer 1978; 42: 1298–307.

341 Yagishita S, Itoh Y, Chiba Y, Fujino H. Primary rhabdomyosarcoma of the cerebrum: an ultrastructural study. Acta Neuropathol 1979; 45: 111–15.

342 Leedham PW. Primary cerebral rhabdomyosarcoma and the problem of medullomyoblastoma. J Neurol Neurosurg Psychiatry 1972; 35: 551–9.

343 Heros RC, Martinez AJ, Ahn HS. Intracranial mesenchymal chondrosarcoma. Surg Neurol 1980; 14: 311–17.

344 Kothandaram P. Dural liposarcoma associated with subdural hematoma. J Neurosurg 1970; 33: 85–7.

345 Sima A, Kindblom L-G, Pellettieri L. Liposarcoma of the meninges. A case report. Acta Pathol Microbiol Scand (A) 1976; 84: 306–10.

346 Hockley AD, Hoffman HJ, Hendrick EB. Occipital mesenchymal tumor of infancy: report of three cases. J Neurosurg 1977; 46: 239–44.

347 Rubinstein LJ. Sarcomas of the nervous system. In: Minckler J ed Pathology of the Nervous System. New York: McGraw-Hill, 1971: 2144–64.

348 El-Gindi S, Abd-El-Hafeez M, Salama M. Extracranial skeletal metastases from an intracranial meningeal chondrosarcoma: case report. J Neurosurg 1974; 40: 651–3.

349 Feigin I, Allen LB, Lipkin L, Gross SW. The endothelial hyperplasia of blood vessels with brain tumors, and its sarcomatous transformation. Cancer 1958; 11: 264–77.

350 Kelly PJ, Suddith RL, Hutchison HT, Werrback K, Haber B. Endothelial growth factor present in tissue cultures of CNS tumors. J Neurosurg 1976; 44: 342–6.

351 Folkman J. Tumor angiogenesis factor. Cancer Res 1974; 34: 2109–13.

352 Folkman J, Klagsbrun M. Angiogenic factors. Science 1987; 235: 442–7.

353 Black VK, Kernohan JW. Primary diffuse tumors of the meninges (so-called meningeal meningiomatosis). Cancer 1950; 3: 805–19.

354 Rubinstein LJ. The development of contiguous sarcomatous and gliomatous tissue in intracranial tumors. J Pathol Bacteriol 1956; 71: 441–59.

355 Hoffman GT, Earle KM. Meningioma with malignant transformation and implantation in the subarachnoid space. J Neurosurg 1960; 17: 486–92.

356 Virchow R. Pigment und diffuse Melanose der Arachnoides. Arch Pathol Anat 1859; 19: 180–2.

357 Bamborschke S, Ebhardt G, Szelies-Stock B, Dreesbach HA, Heiss WD. Review and case report: primary melanoblastosis of the leptomeninges. Clin Neuropathol 1985; 4: 47–55.

358 Sagar HJ, Ilgren EB, Adams CBT. Nevus of Ota associated with meningeal melanosis and intracranial melanoma. J Neurosurg 1983; 58: 280–3.

359 Budka H, Pantucek F. Primare diffuse Melanoblastosen der Meningen und neurokutane Melanosen. Neurochirurgia (Stuttgart) 1973; 16: 90–8.

360 Enzman DR, Krikorian J, Yorke C, Hayward R. Computed tomography in leptomeningeal spread of tumor. J Comput Assist Tomogr 1978; 2: 448–55.

361 Aichner F, Schuler G. Primary leptomeningeal melanoma: diagnosis by ultrastructural cytology of cerebrospinal fluid and cranial computed tomography. Cancer 1982; 50: 1751–6.

362 Dommasch D, Gruninger W, Schultze B. Autoradiographic demonstration of proliferating cells in cerebrospinal fluid. J Neurol 1977; 214: 97–112.

363 Dommasch D, Gaab M, Advanced cytological techniques in the examination of human cerebrospinal fluid. Adv Neurosurg 1977; 4: 261–5.

364 Jacobson HH, Lester J. A myelographic manifestation of diffuse spinal leptomeningeal melanomatosis. Neuroradiology 1970; 1: 30–1.

365 Kaplan AM, Itabishi HH, Hanelin LG, Lu AT. Neurocutaneous melanosis with malignant leptomeningeal melanoma. Arch Neurol (Chicago) 1975; 33: 669–71.

366 Kiel EW, Starr LB, Hansen JL. Primary melanoma of the spinal cord. J Neurosurg 1961; 18: 616–29.

367 Salm R. Primary malignant melanoma of the cerebellum. J Pathol Bacteriol 1967; 94: 196–200.

368 Pappenheim E, Bhattacharji SK. Primary melanoma of the central nervous system. Arch Neurol (Chicago) 1962; 7: 101–13.

369 Tamura M, Kawafuchi J, Nagaya T, Kanoh T, Fukuda T. Primary leptomeningeal melanoma with epipharyngeal invasion. Acta Neurochir 1981; 58: 59–66.

370 Scholtz CL, Siu K. Melanoma of the pituitary gland: case report. J Neurosurg 1976; 45: 101–3.

371 Neilson JM, Moffat AD. Hypopituitarism caused by a melanoma of the pituitary gland. J Clin Pathol 1963; 16: 144–9.

372 Copeland DD, Sink JD, Seigler HF. Primary intracranial melanoma presenting as a suprasellar tumor. Neurosurgery 1980; 6: 542–5.

373 Hirano A, Carton CA. Primary malignant melanoma of the spinal cord. J Neurosurg 1960; 17: 935–44.

374 Larson TC, III, Houser OW, Onofrio BM, Piepgras DG. Primary spinal melanoma. J Neurosurg 1987; 66: 47–9.

375 Limas C, Tio FO. Meningeal melanocytoma ('melanotic meningioma'). Its melanocytic origin as revealed by electron microscopy. Cancer 1972; 30: 1286–94.

376 Winston KR, Sotrel A, Schnitt SJ. Meningeal melanocytoma: case report and review of the clinical and histological features. J Neurosurg 1987; 66: 50–7.

377 Vogel H, Schnitt SJ. Meningiomas: diagnostic value of immunoperoxidase staining for epithelial membrane antigen. Lab Invest 1986; 54: 67A (abstract).

378 Scott M, Ferrara VL, Peale AR. Multiple melanotic meningiomas of the cervical cord: case report. J Neurosurg 1971; 34: 555–9.

379 Fowler M, Simpson DA. A malignant melanin-forming tumor of the cerebellum. J Pathol Bacteriol 1962; 84: 307–11.

380 Borello ED, Gorlin RJ. Melanotic neuroectodermal tumor of infancy—a neoplasm of neural crest origin. Report of a case with high urinary excretion of vanilmandelic acid. Cancer 1966; 19: 196–206.

381 Fox H. Neurocutaneous melanosis. In: Vinken PJ, Bruyn GW eds Handbook of Clinical Neurology, Vol 14. Amsterdam: North-Holland, 1972: 414–28.

382 Slaughter JL, Hardman JM, Kempe LG, Earle KM. Neurocutaneous melanosis and leptomeningeal melanomatosis in children. Arch Pathol 1969; 88: 298–304.

383 Touraine A. Les mélanoses neuro-cutanées. Ann Derm Syph 1949; 9: 489–524.

384 Bailey P. Intracranial sarcomatous tumors of the leptomeningeal origin. Arch Surg 1929; 18: 1359–402.

385 Yuile Cl. Case of primary reticulum cell sarcoma of the brain. Relationship of microglia cells to histiocytes. Arch Pathol 1938; 26: 1036–44.

386 Russell DS, Marshall AHE, Smith FB. Microgliomatosis: a form of reticulosis affecting the brain. Brain 1948; 71: 1–15.

387 Burstein SD, Kernohan JW, Uihlein A. Neoplasms of the reticuloendothelial system of the brain. Cancer 1963; 16: 289–305.

388 Varadachari C, Palutke M, Climie ARW, Weise RW, Chason JL. Immunoblastic sarcoma (histiocytic lymphoma) of the brain with B-cell markers: case report. J Neurosurg 1978; 49: 887–92.

389 Houthoff HJ, Poppema S, Ebels EJ, Elema JD. Intracranial malignant lymphomas: a morphologic and immunocytologic study of twenty cases: Acta Neuropathol 1978; 44: 203–10.

390 Miyoshi I, Kubonishi I, Yoshimoto S, Hikita T, Dabasaki H, Tanaka T, Kimura I, Tabuchi K, Nishimoto A. Characteristics of a brain lymphoma cell line derived from primary intracranial lymphoma. Cancer 1982; 49: 456–9.

391 Taylor CR, Russell R, Lukes RJ, Davis RL. An immunohistological study of immunoglobulin content of primary central nervous system lymphomas. Cancer 1978; 41: 2197–205.

392 Horvat B, Pena C, Fisher ER. Primary reticulum cell sarcoma (microglioma) of brain. An electron microscopic study. Arch Pathol 1969; 87: 609–16.

393 Ishida Y. Fine structure of primary reticulum cell sarcoma of the brain. Acta Neuropathol 1975; Suppl 6: 147–53.

394 Murray K, Kun L, Cox J. Primary malignant lymphoma of the central nervous system. Result of treatment of 11 cases and review of the literature. J Neurosurg 1986; 65: 600–7.

395 Kawakami Y, Tabuchi K, Ohnishi R, Asari S, Nishimoto A. Primary central nervous system lymphoma. J Neurosurg 1985; 62: 522–7.

396 So YT, Beckstead JH, Davis RL. Primary central nervous system lymphoma in acquired immune deficiency syndrome: a clinical and pathological study. Ann Neurol 1986; 20: 566–72.

397 Kishikawa T, Numaguchi Y, Fukui M, Komaki S, Ikeda J, Kitamura K, Matsuura K. Primary intracranial sarcomas: radiological diagnosis with emphasis on arteriography. Neuroradiology 1981; 21: 25–31.

398 Purvin V, Van Dyk HJ. Primary reticulum cell sarcoma of the brain presenting as steroid-sensitive optic neuropathy. J Clin Neuro-ophthalmol 1984; 4: 15–23.

399 Sagerman RH, Collier CH, King GA. Radia-

tion therapy of microgliomas. Radiology 1983; 149: 567–70.

400 Routh A, Kapp J, Smith EE, Hickman BT. Microglioma. J Miss State Med Assoc 1982; 23: 99–101.

401 Woodman R, Shin K, Pineo G. Primary non-Hodgkin's lymphoma of the brain. Medicine 1985; 64: 425–30.

402 Helle TL, Britt RH, Colby TV. Primary lymphoma of the central nervous system. Clinicopathological study of experience at Stanford. J Neurosurg 1984; 60: 94–103.

403 Spaun E, Midholm S, Pedersen NT, Ringsted J. Primary malignant lymphoma of the central nervous system. Surg Neurol 1985; 24: 646–50.

404 Letendre L, Banks PM, Reese DF, Miller RH, Scanlon PW, Kiely JM. Primary lymphoma of the central nervous system. Cancer 1982; 49: 939–43.

405 Jardon-Jeghers C, Reznik M. Etude immunohistochimique de 16 lymphomes primitifs du système nerveux central. J Neurol Sci 1982; 53: 331–46.

406 Mackintosh FR, Colby TV, Podolsky WJ, Burke JS, Hoppe RT, Rosenfelt FP, Rosenberg SA, Kaplan HS. Central nervous system involvement, in non-Hodgkin's lymphoma: an analysis of 105 cases. Cancer 1982; 49: 586–95.

407 Henry JM, Heffner RR, Dillard SH, Earle KM, Davis RL. Primary malignant lymphoma of the central nervous system. Cancer 1974; 34: 1293–302.

408 Frank G, Ferracini R, Spagnolli F, Frank F, Gaist G, Lorenzini P, Ricci R. Primary intracranial lymphomas. Surg Neurol 1985; 23: 3–8.

409 Hobson DE, Anderson BA, Carr I, West M. Primary lymphoma of the central nervous system: Manitoba experience and literature review. Can J Neurol Sci 1986; 13: 55–61.

410 Lennert K. Histopathology of the non-Hodgkin's lymphomas. (Based on the Kiel Classification). Berlin: Springer-Verlag, 1981.

411 The non-Hodgkin's lymphoma pathologic classification project: National Cancer Institute—sponsored study of classification of non-Hodgkin's lymphomas. Summary and description of a working formulation for clinical usage. Cancer 1982; 49: 2112–35.

412 Rappaport H. Tumors of the hematopoietic system. In: Atlas of Tumor Pathology, Section 3, Fascicle 8. Washington, DC: AFIP 1966.

413 Lukes RJ, Collins RD. New approaches to the classification of the lymphomata. Br J Cancer 1975 (Suppl II); 31: 1–28.

414 Jellinger K, Radaskiewicz T, Slowik F. Primary malignant lymphoma of the central

415 nervous system in man. Acta Neuropathol 1975; Suppl 6: 95–102.

415 Zimmerman HM. Malignant lymphomas of the nervous system. Acta Neuropathol 1975; Suppl 6: 69–74.

416 Kepes JJ, Chen WYK, Pang I-C, Kepes M. Tumors of the central nervous system in Taiwan, Republic of China. Surg Neurol 1984; 22: 149–56.

417 Freeman C, Berg JW, Cutler SJ. Occurrence and prognosis of extranodal lymphomas. Cancer 1972; 29: 252–60.

418 Levitt LJ, Dawson DM, Rosenthal DS, Moloney WC. CNS involvement in the non-Hodgkin's lymphomas. Cancer 1980; 45: 545–52.

419 Jiddane M, Nicoli F, Diaz P, Bergvall U, Vincentelli F, Hassoun J, Salamon G. Intracranial malignant lymphoma. Report of 30 cases and review of the literature. J Neurosurg 1986; 65: 592–9.

420 Kersting G, Neumann J. 'Malignant lymphoma' of the brain following renal transplant. Acta Neuropathol 1975; Suppl 6: 1–16.

421 Lipsmeyer EA. Development of malignant cerebral lymphoma in a patient with systemic lupus erythematosus treated with immunosuppression. Arthritis Rheum 1972; 15: 183–6.

422 Klassen SS, Hoover R, Kimberly R, Budman OR, Decker JL, Chused TM. Increased incidence of malignancy in Sjøgren's syndrome (SS). Arthritis Rheum 1977; 20: 123 (abstract).

423 Good AE, Russo RH, Schnitzer B, Weatherbee L. Intracranial histiocytic lymphoma with rheumatoid arthritis. J Rheumatol 1978; 5: 75–8.

424 Jellinger K, Kothbauer P, Weiss R, Sunder-Plassman E. Primary malignant lymphoma of the CNS and polyneuropathy in a patient with necrotizing vasculitis treated with immunosuppression. J Neurol 1979; 220: 259–68.

425 Louie S, Schwartz RS, Immunodeficiency and the pathogenesis of lymphoma and leukemia. Semin Hematology 1978; 15: 117–38.

426 Kay HEM. Immunosuppression and the risk of brain lymphoma. N Engl J Med 1983; 308: 1099–100.

427 Snider WD, Simpson DM, Aronyk KE, Nielsen SL. Primary lymphoma of the nervous system associated with acquired immune-deficiency syndrome. N Engl J Med 1983; 308: 45.

428 Pitlik SD, Fainstein V, Bolivar R, Guarda L, Rios P, Mansell PA, Gyorkey F. Spectrum of central nervous system complications in homosexual men with acquired immune deficiency syndrome. J Infect Dis 1983; 148: 771–2.

429 Gill PS, Levine AM, Meyer PR, Boswell WD,

Burkes RL, Parker JW, Hofman FM, Dworsky RL, Lukes RJ. Primary central nervous system lymphoma in homosexual men. Clinical, immunologic and pathologic features. Am J Med 1985; 78: 742–7.

430 Model LM. Primary reticulum cell sarcoma of the brain in Wiskott-Aldrich syndrome: report of a case. Arch Neurol (Chicago) 1977; 34: 633–5.

431 Heidelberger KP, Le Golvan DP. Wiskott-Aldrich syndrome and cerebral neoplasia: report of a case with local reticulum cell sarcoma. Cancer 1974; 33: 280–4.

432 Gunderson CH, Henry J, Malamud N. Plasma globulin determinations in patients with microglioma. Report of five cases. J Neurosurg 1971; 35: 406–15.

433 Gregory MC, Hughes JT. Intracranial reticulum cell sarcoma associated with immunoglobulin A deficiency. J Neurol Neurosurg Psychiatry 1973; 36: 769–76.

434 Bale JF Jr, Wilson JF, Hill HR. Fatal histiocytic lymphoma of the brain associated with hyperimmunoglobulinemia-E and recurrent infections. Cancer 1977; 39: 2386–90.

435 Pattengale PK, Taylor CR, Panke T, Tatter D, McCormick RA, Rawlinson DG, Davis RL. Selective immunodeficiency and malignant lymphoma of the central nervous system. Acta Neuropathol 1979; 48: 165–9.

436 Purtilo DT. Epstein-Barr virus-induced oncogenesis in immune deficient individuals. Lancet 1980; i: 300–3.

437 Hanto DW, Frizzera G, Purtilo DT, Sakamoto K, Sullivan JL, Saemundsen AK, Klein G, Simmons RL, Najarian JS. Clinical spectrum of lymphoproliferative disorders in renal transplant recipients and evidence for the role of Epstein-Barr virus. Cancer Res 1981; 41: 4253–61.

438 Hochberg FH, Miller G, Schooley RT, Hirsch MS, Feorino P, Henle W. Central nervous system lymphoma related to Epstein-Barr virus. N Engl J Med 1983; 309: 745–8.

439 Hegedus K. Burkitt-type lymphoma and reticulum-cell sarcoma. An unusual mixed form of two intracranial primary malignant lymphomas. Surg Neurol 1984; 21: 23–9.

440 Giovanella B, Nilsson K, Zech L, Yim O, Klein G, Stehlin JS. Growth of diploid, Epstein-Barr virus-carrying human lymphoblastoid cell lines heterotransplanted into nude mice under immunologically privileged conditions. Int J Cancer 1979; 24: 103–13.

441 Epstein AL, Herman MM, Kim H, Dorfman RF, Kaplan HS. Biology of the human malignant lymphomas: III. Intracranial heterotransplantation in the nude, athymic mouse. Cancer 1976; 37: 2158–76.

442 Ebels EJ. Reticulosarcomas of the brain presenting as butterfly tumors. Possible implication for treatment. Eur Neurol 1972; 8: 333–8.

443 Mitsumoto H, Breuer AC, Lederman RJ. Malignant lymphoma of the central nervous system: a case of primary spinal intramedullary involvement. Cancer 1980; 46: 1258–62.

444 Kindt GW. The pattern of location of cerebral metastatic tumors. J Neurosurg 1964; 21: 54–7.

445 Frizzera G, Rosai J, Dehner LP, Spector BD, Kersey JH. Lymphoreticular disorders in primary immunodeficiencies: new findings based on an up-to-date histologic classification of 35 cases. Cancer 1980; 46: 692–9.

446 Matos AJ, Hertel BF, Rosai J, Simmons RL, Najarian JS. Post-transplant malignant lymphoma. Am J Med 1976; 61: 716–20.

447 Schaumberg H, Plank C, Adams R. The reticulum cell sarcoma-microglioma group of brain tumors. Brain 1972; 95: 199–212.

448 Barnard RO, Scott T. Patterns of proliferation in cerebral lymphoreticular tumors. Acta Neuropathol 1975; Suppl 6: 125–30.

449 Leavens ME, Manning JT, Wallace S, Maor MH, Velasquez WS. Primary lymphoma of the central nervous system. In: Wilkins RH, Rengachary SS eds Neurosurgery. New York: McGraw-Hill, 1985: 1022–9.

450 Samuelsson SM, Werner I, Ponten J, Nathorst Windahal G, Thorell J. Reticuloendothelial (perivascular) sarcoma of the brain. Acta Neurol Scand 1966; 42: 567–80.

451 Kaplan DL, Jegasothy B. The sign of Leser-Trelat associated with primary lymphoma of the brain. Cutis 1984; 34: 164–5.

452 Dantzig PI. Sign of Leser-Trelat. Arch Dermatol 1973; 108: 700–1.

453 Tadmor R, Davis KR, Roberson GH, Kleinman GM. Computed tomography in primary malignant lymphoma of the brain. J Comput Assist Tomogr 1978; 2: 135–40.

454 Cellerier P, Chiras J, Gray F, Metzger J, Bories J. Computed tomography in primary lymphoma of the brain. Neuroradiology 1984; 26: 485–92.

455 Holtos SL, Kido DK, Simon JH. MR imaging of spinal lymphomas. Case report. J Comput Assist Tomogr 1986; 10: 111–15.

456 Matsuda M, McMurria H, Van Hale P, Miller C. CSF findings in primary lymphoma of the CNS. Arch Neurol (Chicago) 1981; 38: 397.

457 Mavligit GM, Stuckey SE, Cabanillas FF, Keating MJ, Tourtellotte WW, Schold SC, Freireich EJ. Diagnosis of leukemia or lymphoma in the central nervous system by beta-2-

microglobulin determination. N Engl J Med 1980; 303: 718–22.

458 Cox JD, Koehl RH, Turner WM, King FM. Irradiation in the local control of malignant lymphoreticular tumors (non-Hodgkin's malignant lymphoma). Radiology 1974; 112: 179–85.

459 Berry MP, Simpson WJ. Radiation therapy in the management of primary malignant lymphoma of the brain. Int J Radiat Oncol Biol Phys 1981; 7: 51–9.

460 Loeffler JS, Ervin TJ, Mauch P, Skarin A, Weinstein HJ, Canellos G, Cassady JR. Primary lymphomas of the central nervous system: patterns of failure and factors that influence survival. J Clin Oncol 1985; 3: 490–4.

461 Rampen FJH, van Andel JG, Sizoo W, van Unnik JAM. Radiation therapy in primary non-Hodgkin's lymphomas of the CNS. Eur J Cancer 1984; 16: 177–84.

462 Mendenhall RP, Thar TL, Agee FD, Harty-Golder B, Ballinger WF, Jr., Million RR. Primary lymphoma of the central nervous system: computerized tomography scan characteristics and treatment results for 12 cases. Cancer 1983; 52: 1993–2000.

463 Vaquero J, Martinez R, Rossi E, Lopez R. Primary cerebral lymphoma: the 'ghost tumor'. Case report. J Neurosurg 1984; 60: 174–6.

464 Weingarten KL, Zimmerman RD, Leeds NE: Spontaneous regression of intracerebral lymphoma. Radiology 1983; 149: 721–4.

465 Ervin T, Canellos GP. Successful treatment of recurrent primary central nervous system lymphoma with high-dose methotrexate. Cancer 1980; 45: 1556–7.

466 Rubinstein LJ, Herman MM, Long TF, Wilbur JR. Leukoencephalopathy following combined therapy of central nervous system leukemia and lymphoma. Acta Neuropathol 1975; Suppl 6: 251–5.

467 Jacobs A, Clifford P, Kay HEM. The Ommaya-reservoir in chemotherapy for malignant disease in the CNS. Clin Oncol 1981; 7: 123–9.

468 Neuwelt EA, Balaban E, Diehl J, Hill S, Frenkel E. Successful treatment of primary central nervous system lymphomas with chemotherapy after osmotic blood-brain barrier opening. Neurosurgery 1983; 12: 662–71.

469 Bernard JD, Aguilar MJ. Localized hypothalamic histiocytosis X. Report of a case. Arch Neurol 1969; 20: 368–72.

470 Kepes JJ, Kepes M. Predominantly cerebral forms of histiocytosis X. A reappraisal of 'Gagel's hypothalamic granuloma', 'granuloma infiltrans of the hypothalamus' and 'Ayala's disease' with a report of four cases. Acta Neuropathol 1969; 14: 77–98.

471 Moscinski LC, Kleinschmidt-deMasters BK. Primary eosinophilic granuloma of the frontal lobe. Diagnostic use of S-100 protein. Cancer 1985; 56: 284–8.

472 Bucy PL, Jerva MJ. Primary epidural spinal lymphosarcoma. J Neurosurg 1962; 19: 142–52.

473 Jernstrom P, Crockett HG, Bachhuber RG. Primary lymphosarcoma of cerebral meninges. J Neurosurg 1966; 24: 679–83.

474 Borit A, Altrocchi P. Recurrent polyneuropathy and neurolymphomatosis. Arch Neurol 1971; 24: 40–9.

475 French JD. Plasmacytoma of the hypothalamus: clinical pathological report of a case. J Neuropathological Exp Neurol 1947; 6: 265–70.

476 Moossy J, Wilson CB. Solitary intracranial plasmacytoma. Arch Neurol 1967; 16: 212–16.

477 Carmel PW. Craniopharyngiomas. In: Wilkins RH, Rengachary SS eds Neurosurgery. New York: McGraw-Hill, 1985: 905–16.

478 Sung DI, Chang CH, Harisiadis L, Carmel PW. Treatment results of craniopharyngiomas. Cancer 1981; 47: 847–52.

479 Carmel PW, Antunes JL, Chang CH. Craniopharyngiomas in children. Neurosurgery 1982; 11: 382–9.

480 Hoffman HJ, Hendrick EB, Humphreys RP, Buncic JR, Armstrong DL, Jenkin RD. Management of craniopharyngiomas in children. J Neurosurg 1977; 47: 218–27.

481 Koos WT, Miller MH. Intracranial Tumors of Infants and Children. Stuttgart: Thieme, 1971.

482 Shapiro K, Till K, Grant DN. Craniopharyngiomas in childhood. A rational approach to treatment. J Neurosurg 1979; 50: 617–23.

483 Stahnke N, Grubel G, Lagenstein I, Willig RP. Long-term follow-up of children with craniopharyngioma. Eur J Pediatr 1984; 142: 179–85.

484 Pertuiset B. Craniopharyngiomas. In: Vinken RJ, Bruyn GW eds Handbook of Clinical Neurology, Vol 18, Tumors of the Brain and Skull. Amsterdam: North Holland, 1975: 531–72.

485 Svein HJ. Surgical experience with craniopharyngiomas. J Neurosurg 1965; 23: 148–55.

486 Cashion EL, Young JM. Intraventricular craniopharyngioma. Report of two cases. J Neurosurg 1971; 34: 84–7.

487 Podoshin L, Rolan L, Altman MM, Peyser E. 'Pharyngeal' craniopharyngioma. J Laryngol Otol 1970; 84: 93–9.

488 Cooper PR, Ransohoff J. Craniopharyngioma

originating in the sphenoid bone. Case report. J Neurosurg 1972; 36: 102–6.

489 Steno J. Microsurgical topography of craniopharyngiomas. Acta Neurochir 1985; Suppl 35: 94–100.

490 Cobb CA, Youmans JR. Brain tumors of disordered embryogenesis in adults. In: Youmans JR ed Neurological Surgery, 2nd edition Philadelphia: WB Saunders, 1982; 2899–935.

491 Matt FW, Barrett JOW. Three cases of tumor of the third ventricle. Arch Neurol (London) 1899; 1: 417–40.

492 Critchley M, Ironside RN. The pituitary adamantinomata. Brain 1926; 49: 437–81.

493 Erdheim J. Ueber Hypophysengangsgeschwulste und Hirncholesteatome. Sitzungsber Akad Wiss (Wien) 1904; 113: 437–726.

494 Seemayer TA, Blundell JS, Wiglesworth FW. Pituitary craniopharyngioma with tooth formation. Cancer 1972; 29: 423–30.

495 Shuangshoti S, Netsky MD, Nashold BS. Epithelial cysts related to sella turcica: Proposed origin from neuroepithelium. Arch Pathol (Chicago) 1970; 90: 444–50.

496 Yoshida J, Kobayashi T, Kageyama N, Kanzaki M. Symptomatic Rathke's cleft cyst: morphological study with light and electron microscopy and tissue culture. J Neurosurg 1977; 47: 451–8.

497 Steinberg GK, Koenig GH, Golden JB. Symptomatic Rathke's cleft cysts: report of two cases. J Neurosurg 1982; 56: 290–5.

498 Kahn EA, Gosch HH, Seeger JF, Hicks SP. Forty-five years experience with the craniopharyngiomas. Surg Neurol 1973; 1: 5–12.

499 Luse SA, Kernohan JW. Squamous cell rests of the pituitary gland. Cancer 1955; 8: 623–8.

500 Goldberg GM, Eshbaugh DE. Squamous cell rests of the pituitary gland as related to the origin of craniopharyngiomas. A study of their presence in the newborn and infants up to age four. Arch Pathol Lab Med 1960; 70: 293–9.

501 Hunter IJ. Squamous metaplasia of cells of the anterior pituitary gland. J Pathol Bacteriol 1955; 69: 141–5.

502 Weber FP, Worster-Drought C, Dickson WEC. Cholesterol tumor (craniopharyngioma) of the pituitary body. J Neurol Psychopath 1934; 15: 39–45.

503 Al-Mefty O, Hassounah M, Weaver P, Sakati N, Jinkins JR, Fox JL. Microsurgery for giant craniopharyngiomas in children. Neurosurgery 1985; 17: 585–95.

504 Matson DD, Crigler JF. Management of craniopharyngioma in childhood. J Neurosurg 1969; 30: 699–704.

505 Bartlett JR. Craniopharyngiomas: an analysis of some aspects of symptomatology, radiology and histology. Brain 1971; 94: 725–32.

506 Cobb JP, Wright JC. Studies on a craniopharyngioma in tissue culture. I. Growth characteristics and alterations produced following exposure to two radiometric agents. J Neuropathol Exp Neurol 1959; 18: 563–8.

507 Liszczak T, Richardson EP, Phillips JP, Jacobson S, Kornblith PL. Morphological, biochemical, ultrastructural, tissue culture, and clinical observations of typical and aggressive craniopharyngiomas. Acta Neuropathol 1978; 43: 191–203.

508 Hoff JT, Patterson RH Jr. Craniopharyngiomas in children and adults. J Neurosurg 1972 36: 299–302.

509 Banna M. Craniopharyngiomas in adults. Surg Neurol 1973; 1: 202–4.

510 Banna M, Hoare RD, Stanley P, Till K. Craniopharyngiomas in children. J Pediatr 1973; 83: 781–5.

511 Arseni C, Maretsin M. Craniopharyngioma. Neurochirurgia (Stuttgart) 1972; 1: 25–32.

512 Svolos DG. Craniopharyngiomas: a study based on 108 verified cases. Acta Chir Scand 1969; 403: 1–44.

513 Korsgaard O, Lindholm J, Rasmussen P. Endocrine function in patients with suprasellar and hypothalamic tumors. Acta Endocrine (Copenhagen) 1976; 83: 1–84.

514 Barbarino A, DeMarinis L, Mancini A, Menini E, D'Amico C, Passeri M, Sambo P, Anile C, Maira G. Prolectin dynamics in patients with non-secreting tumors of the hypothalamic-pituitary region. Acta Endocrinol (Copenhagen) 1985; 110: 10–16.

515 Barreca T, Perria C, Francaviglia N, Rolandi E. Evaluation of anterior pituitary functions in adult patients with craniopharyngiomas. Acta Neurochir 1984; 71: 263–72.

516 Patrick BS, Smith RR, Bailey TO. Aseptic meningitis due to spontaneous rupture of a craniopharyngioma cyst. Case report. J Neurosurg 1974; 41: 387–90.

517 Ross-Russell RW, Pennybacker JB. Craniopharyngioma in the elderly. J Neurol Neurosurg Psychiatry 1961; 24: 1–13.

518 Garcia-Uria J. Surgical experience with craniopharyngioma in adults. Surg Neurol 1978; 9: 11–14.

519 Michelsen WJ, Mount LA, Renaudin J. Craniopharyngioma: a thirty-nine year survey. Acta Neurol Lat Amer 1972; 18: 100–106.

520 Naidich TP, Pinto RS, Kushner MJ, Lin JP, Kricheff II, Leeds NE, Chase NE. Evaluation of sellar and parasellar masses by computed tomography. Radiology 1976; 120: 91–9.

521 Fitz CR, Wortzman G, Harwood-Nash DC, Holgate RC, Barry JF, Boldt DW. Computed tomography in craniopharyngiomas. Radiology 1978; 127: 687–91.

522 Hoffman HJ. Craniopharyngiomas. Can J Neurol Sci 1985; 12: 348–52.

523 Cushing HW. Papers Relating to the Pituitary Body, Hypothalamus, and Parasympathetic Nervous System. Springfield, Illinois: Charles C Thomas, 1932.

524 Amacher AL. Craniopharyngiomas: the controversy regarding radiotherapy. Child's Brain 1980; 6: 57–64.

525 Mori K, Handa H, Murata T, Takeuchi J, Miwa S, Osaka K. Results of treatment of craniopharyngioma. Child's Brain 1980; 6: 303–12.

526 Kramer S. Craniopharyngioma: the best treatment is conservative surgery and post-operative radiation therapy. In: Morley TP ed Current Controversies in Neurosurgery. Philadelphia: WB Saunders, 1976: 336–43.

527 Richmond IL, Wara WM, Wilson CB. Role of radiation therapy in the management of craniopharyngiomas in children. Neurosurgery 1980; 6: 513–17.

528 Onoyama Y, Ono K, Yabumoto E, Takeuchi J. Radiation therapy of craniopharyngioma. Radiology 1977; 125: 799–803.

529 Fischer EG, Welch K, Belli JA, Wallman J, Shillito JJ Jr, Winston KR, Cassady R. Treatment of craniopharyngiomas in children: 1972–1981. J Neurosurg 1985; 62: 496–501.

530 Bloom HJG, Harmer CL. Craniopharyngiomas. Br Med J 1972; ii: 288–9.

531 Lichter AS, Wara WM, Sheline GE, Townsend JJ, Wilson CB. The treatment of craniopharyngiomas. Int J Radiat Oncol Biol Phys 1977; 2: 675–83.

532 Backlund E-O. Studies on craniopharyngiomas. IV. Stereotactic treatment with radiosurgery. Acta Chir Scand 1973; 139: 344–51.

533 Backlund E-O. Studies on craniopharyngiomas. III. Stereotactic treatment with intracystic yttrium 99. Acta Chir Scand 1973; 139: 237–247.

534 Nakayama T, Kodama T, Matsukado Y. Treatment of inoperable craniopharyngioma with radioactive gold. No To Shinkei 1971; 23: 509–13.

535 Takahashi H, Nakazawa S, Shimura T. Evaluation of postoperative intratumoral injection of bleomycin for craniopharyngioma in children. J. Neurosurg 1985; 62: 120–7.

536 Bartlett JR. Craniopharyngiomas—a summary of 85 cases. J Neurol Neurosurg Psychiatry 1971; 34: 37–41.

537 Sweet WH. Radical surgical treatment of craniopharyngiomas in children. Clin Neurosurg 1976; 23: 52–79.

538 Symon L, Sprich W. Radical excision of craniopharyngioma. Results in 20 patients. J Neurosurg 1985; 62: 174–81.

539 Katz EL. Late results of radical excision of craniopharyngiomas in children. J Neurosurg 1975; 42: 86–90.

540 Sweet WH. Recurrent craniopharyngiomas: therapeutic alternatives. Clin Neurosurg 1980; 27: 206–29.

541 Cavazzuti V, Fischer EG, Welch K, Belli JA, Winston KR. Neurological and psychophysiological sequelae following different treatments of craniopharyngioma in children. J Neurosurg 1983; 59: 409–17.

542 Waga S, Handa H. Radiation-induced meningioma: with review of literature. Surg Neurol 1976; 5: 215–19.

543 Danoff BF, Cowchock FS, Kramer S. Childhood craniopharyngioma: survival, local control, endocrine and neurologic function following radiotherapy. Int J Radiat Oncol Biol Phys 1983; 9: 171–5.

544 Manaka S, Teramoto A, Takakura K. The efficacy of radiotherapy for craniopharyngioma. J Neurosurg 1985; 62: 648–656.

545 Bostroem E. Ueber die pialen Epidermoide, Dermoide und Lipome und duralen Dermoide. Zentralbl Allg Path Path Anat 1897; 8: 1–98.

546 Baxter JW, Netsky MG. Epidermoid and dermoid tumors: pathology. In: Wilkins RH, Rengachary SS eds Neurosurgery. New York: McGraw-Hill, 1985: 655–61.

547 List CF. Intraspinal epidermoids, dermoids and dermal sinuses. Surg Gynecol Obstet 1941; 73: 525–38.

548 Grant FC, Austin GM. Epidermoids: clinical evaluation and surgical results. J Neurosurg 1950; 7: 190–8.

549 Guidetti B, Gagliardi FM. Epidermoid and dermoid cysts: clinical evaluation and late surgical results. J Neurosurg 1977; 47: 12–18.

550 McCarty CS, Levens ME, Love JG, Kernohan JW. Dermoid and epidermoid tumors in the central nervous system of adults. Surg Gynecol Obstet 1959; 108: 191–8.

551 Berger MS, Wilson CB. Epidural cysts of the posterior fossa. J Neurosurg 1985; 62: 214–19.

552 Obrador S, Lopez-Zafra JJ. Clinical features of the epidermoids of the basal cisterns of the brain. J Neurol Neurosurg Psychiatry 1969; 32: 450–4.

553 Ulrich J. Intracranial epidermoids. A study on their distribution and spread. J Neurosurg 1964; 21: 1051–8.

554 Taglia JU, Netsky MG, Alexander E Jr. Epithelial (epidermoid) tumors of the cranium. J Neurosurg 1965; 23: 384–93.

555 Alvord EC. Growth rates of epidermoid tumors. Ann Neurol 1977; 2: 367–70.

556 Chambers AA, Lukin RR, Tomsick TA. Cranial epidermoid tumors: diagnosis by computed tomography. Neurosurgery 1977; 1: 276–80.

557 Garcia CA, McGarry PA, Rodriguez F. Primary intracranial squamous cell carcinoma of the right cerebellopontine angle. J Neurosurg 1981; 54: 824–8.

558 Lewis AJ, Cooper PW, Kassel EE, Schwartz ML. Squamous cell carcinoma arising in a suprasellar epidermoid cyst. Case report. J Neurosurg 1983; 59: 538–41.

559 Giangaspero F, Manetto V. Ferracini R, Piazza G. Squamous cell carcinoma of the brain with sarcoma-like stroma. Virchows Arch (Pathol Anat) 1984; 402: 459–64.

560 Kohno K, Sakaki S, Nakano K, Yano M, Matsuoka K. Brain abscess secondary to intracranial epidural epidermoid cyst. Surg Neurol 1984; 22: 541–6.

561 Donoghue V, Chuang SH, Chilton SJ, Fitz CR, Harwood-Nash DCF. Intraspinal epidermoid cysts. J Comput Assist Tomogr 1984; 8: 143–144.

562 Rosario M, Becker DH, Conley FK. Epidermoid tumors involving the fourth ventricle. Neurosurgery 1981; 9: 9–13.

563 Peyton WB, Baker AB. Epidermoid, dermoid and teratomatous tumors of the central nervous system. Arch Neurol Psychiatry 1942; 47: 890–917.

564 Chandler WF, Farhat SM, Pauli FJ. Intrathalamic epidermoid tumor. J Neurosurg 1975; 43: 614–17.

565 Leal O, Miles J. Epidermoid cyst in the brain stem. Case report. J Neurosurg 1978; 48: 811–13.

566 Kirsch WM, Stears JL. Radiographic identification and surgical excision of an epidermoid tumor of the pineal gland. J Neurosurg 1970; 33: 708–13.

567 Tytus JS, Pennybacker J. Pearly tumors in relation to the central nervous system. J Neurol Neurosurg Psychiatry 1956; 19: 241–59.

568 Logue V, Till K. Posterior fossa dermoid cysts with special reference to intracranial infection. J Neurol Neurosurg Psychiatry 1952; 15: 1–12.

569 Murphy MJ, Risk WS, Van Gilder JL. Intracranial dermoid cyst in Goldenhar's syndrome. Case report. J Neurosurg 1980; 53: 408–10.

570 Choremis C, Economos D, Papadatos C, Gargoulas A. Intraspinal epidermoid tumors (cho-

lesteatomas) in patients treated for tuberculous meningitis. Lancet 1956; ii: 437–9.

571 Tabaddor K, Lamorgese JR. Lumbar epideroid cyst following single lumbar puncture. J Bone Joint Surg (Am) 1975; 57: 1168–9.

572 Spencer AT, Smith WT. Behavior of intracerebral autografts of mouse tail skin pretreated with a single application of 20-methylcholanthrene. Nature 1965; 207: 649–50.

573 Van Gilder JL, Schwartz HG. Growth of dermoids from skin implants to the nervous system and surrounding spaces of the newborn rat. J Neurosurg 1967; 26: 14–20.

574 Smith CML, Timperley WR. Multiple intraspinal and intracranial epidermoids and lipomata following gunshot injury. Neuropathol Appl Neurol 1984; 10: 235–9.

575 Juers AL. Cholesteatoma genesis. Arch Otolaryngol 1965; 81: 5–8.

576 Fleming JFR, Botterell EH. Cranial dermoid and epidermoid tumors. Surg Gynecol Obstet 1959; 109: 403–11.

577 Critchley M, Ferguson FR. The cerebrospinal epidermoids (cholesteatomata). Brain 1928; 51: 334–84.

578 Sade J. Pathogenesis of attic cholesteatomas. JR Soc Med 1978; 71: 716–32.

579 Rhodes RH, Davis RL, Beamer YB, Marantz C. A suprasellar epidermoid cyst with symptoms of hypothalamic involvement: case report and a review of pathogenetic mechanisms. Bull L A Neurol Soc 1981; 46: 26–32.

580 Frazier CH, Alpers BJ. Adamantinoma of the craniopharyngeal duct. Arch Neurol Psychiatry 1931; 26: 905–65.

581 Cruveilhier J. Anatomie Pathologique du Corps Humain, Vol 2: Paris, JB Bailliere, 1829: 341.

582 Keogh AJ, Timperley WR. Atypical hidradenoma arising in a dermoid cyst of the spinal canal. J Pathol 1975; 117: 207–9.

583 Yamanaka A, Hinohara S, Hashimoto T. Primary diffuse carcinomatosis of the spinal meninges accompanied with a cancerous epidermal cyst of the base of the brain. Report of a case of autopsy. Gan 1955; 46: 274–6.

584 Wong SW, Ducker TB, Powes JM. Fulminating parapontine epidermoid carcinoma in a four-year-old boy. Cancer 1976; 37: 1525–31.

585 Love JG, Kernohan JW. Dermoid and epidermoid tumors (cholesteatomas) of central nervous system. JAMA 1936; 107: 1876–83.

586 Conley FK. Epidermoid and dermoid tumors: clinical features and surgical management. In: Wilkins RH, Rengachary SS eds Neurosurgery. New York: McGraw-Hill, 1985: 668–73.

587 Bucy PC. Intradiploic epidermoid (cholestea-

toma) of the skull. Arch Surg (Chicago) 1935; 31: 190–9.

588 Olivecrona H. On suprasellar cholesteatomas. Brain 1932; 55: 122–34.

589 Mohanty S, Bhattacharya RN, Tandon SC, Shukla PK. Intracerebral cystic epidermoid: report of two cases. Acta Neurochir 1981; 57: 107–13.

590 Bailey P. Cruveilhier's 'tumeurs perlees'. Surg Gynecol Obstet 1920; 31: 390–401.

591 Manno NJ, Uihlein A, Kernohan JW. Intraspinal epidermoids. J Neurosurg 1962; 19: 754–65.

592 Bailey IC. Dermoid tumors of the spinal cord. J Neurosurg 1970; 33: 678–81.

593 Matson DD, Ingraham FD. Intracranial complications of congenital dermal sinuses. Pediatrics 1951; 8: 463–74.

594 Szabo M, Majtenyi C, Guseo A. Contribution to the background of Mollaret's meningitis. Acta Neuropathol 1983; 59: 115–18.

595 Haig PV. Primary epidermoids of the skull: including a case with malignant change. AJR 1956; 76: 1076–80.

596 Osborne DR. Epidermoids and dermoid tumors: radiology. In: Wilkins RH, Rengachary SS eds Neurosurgery. New York: McGraw-Hill, 1985: 662–7.

597 Dee RH, Pishore PRS, Young HF. Radiological evaluation of cerebello-pontine angle epidermoid tumor. Surg Neurol 1980; 13: 293–6.

598 Braun IF, Naidich TP, Leeds NE, Koslow M, Zimmerman HM, Chase NE. Dense intracranial epidermoid tumors: computed tomographic observations. Radiology 1977; 122: 717–19.

599 Hasegawa H, Bitoh S, Nakata M, Fujiwara M, Yasuda H. Intracranial epidermoid mimicking meningioma. Surg Neurol 1981; 15: 372–4.

600 Cornell SH, Grof CJ, Dolan KD. Fat-fluid level in intracranial epidermoid cyst. AJR 1977; 128: 502–3.

601 Nosaka Y, Nagao S, Tabuchi K, Nishimoto A. Primary intracranial epidermoid carcinoma. J Neurosurg 1979; 50: 830–3.

602 Fawcitt RA, Isherwood I. Radiodiagnosis of intracranial pearly tumors with particular reference to the value of computer tomography. Neuroradiology 1976; 11: 235–42.

603 Fein JM, Lipow K, Taati F, Lansem T. Epidermoid tumor of the cerebellopontine angle: diagnostic value of computed tomographic metrizamide cisternography. Neurosurgery 1981; 9: 179–82.

604 King AB. Intramedullary epidermoid tumor of the spinal cord. J Neurosurg 1957; 14: 353–7.

605 Hamel E, Frowein RA, Karemi-Nejad A.

Intracranial intradural epidermoids and dermoids. Surgical results of 38 cases. Neurosurg Rev 1980; 3: 215–19.

606 Mahoney W. Die Epidermoide des Zentralnervensystems. Z Ges Neurol Psychiat 1936; 155: 416–471.

607 Baumann CHH, Bucy PC. Paratrigeminal epidermoid tumors. J Neurosurg 1956; 13: 455–68.

608 Rengachary SS. Intracranial arachnoid and ependymal cysts. In: Wilkins RH, Reganchary SS eds Neurosurgery. New York: McGraw-Hill, 1985: 2160–72.

609 Anderson FM, Segall HD, Caton WL. Use of computerized tomography scanning in supratentorial arachnoid cysts. A report on 20 children and four adults. J Neurosurg 1979; 50: 333–8.

610 Galassi E, Piazza G, Gaist G, Frank F. Arachnoid cysts of the middle cranial fossa: a clinical and radiological study of 25 cases treated surgically. Surg Neurol 1980; 14: 211–19.

611 Hoffman HJ, Hendrick EB, Humphreys RP, Armstrong EA. Investigation and management of suprasellar arachnoid cysts. J Neurosurg 1982; 57: 597–602.

612 Robinson RG. Congenital cysts of the brain: arachnoid malformations. Prog Neurol Surg 1971; 4: 133–74.

613 Rengachary SS, Watanabe I. Ultrastructure and pathogenesis of intracranial arachnoid cysts. J Neuropathol Exp Neurol 1981; 40: 61–83.

614 Menzes AH, Bell WE, Perret GE. Archnoid cysts in children. Arch Neurol 1980; 37: 168–72.

615 Galzio RJ, Zenobii M, Lucantoni D, Cristuib-Grizzi L. Spinal intradural arachnoid cyst. Surg Neurol 1982; 17: 388–91.

616 DiSclafani A 2nd, Canale DJ. Communicating spinal arachnoid cysts: diagnosis by delayed metrizamide computed tomography. Surg Neurol 1985; 23: 428–30.

617 Handa J, Okamato K, Sato M. Arachnoid cyst of the middle cranial fossa: report of bilateral cysts in siblings. Surg Neurol 1981; 16: 127–30.

618 Go KG, Houthoff H-J, Blaauw EH, Havinga P, Hartsuiker J. Arachnoid cysts of the Sylvian fissure. Evidence of fluid secretion. J Neurosurg 1984; 60: 803–13.

619 Shaw CM. 'Arachnoid cysts' of the Sylvian fissure versus 'temporal lobe agenesis' syndrome. Ann Neurol (Chicago) 1979; 5: 483–5.

620 Starkman SP, Brown TL, Linell EA. Cerebral arachnoid cysts. J Neuropathol Exp Neurol 1958; 17: 484–500.

621 Rengachary SS, Watanabe I, Brackett CE.

Pathogenesis of intracranial arachnoid cysts. Surg Neurol 1978; 9: 139–44.

622 Smith RA, Smith WA. Arachnoid cysts of the middle cranial fossa. Surg Neurol 1976; 5: 246–52.

623 Dyck P, Gruskin P. Supratentorial arachnoid cysts in adults. A discussion of two cases from a pathophysiologic and surgical perspective. Arch Neurol 1977; 34: 276–9.

624 Harsh GR, IV, Edwards MB, Wilson CB. Intracranial arachnoid cysts in children. J Neurosurg 1986; 64: 835–42.

625 Go KG, Houthoff H-J, Hartsuiker J, Blaauw EH, Havinga P. Fluid secretion in arachnoid cysts as a clue to cerebrospinal fluid absorption at the arachnoid granulation. J Neurosurg 1986; 65: 642–5.

626 Sato K, Shimoji T, Yaguchi K, Sumie H, Kuru Y, Ishii S. Middle fossa arachnoid cyst: clinical, neuroradiological and surgical features. Child's Brain 1983; 10: 301–16.

627 Robinson RG. Intracranial collections of fluid with local bulging of the skull. J Neurosurg 1955; 12: 345–53.

628 Bright R. Serous cysts in the arachnoid. In: Diseases of the Brain and Nervous System, Part I. London; Longman, Rees, Orme, Brown and Green, 1831: 437–9. (Cited in reference 608.)

629 Oliver LC. Primary arachnoid cysts. Report of two cases. Br Med J 1958; 1: 1147–9.

630 La Cour F, Trevor R, Carey M. Arachnoid cyst and associated subdural hematoma. Arch Neurol (Chicago) 1978; 35: 84–9.

631 Weinman DF. Arachnoid cysts in Sylvian fissure of brain. J Neurosurg 1965; 22: 185–7.

632 Patrick BS. Ependymal cyst of the sylvian fissure. J Neurosurg 1971; 35: 751–4.

633 Friede RL, Yasargil MG. Supratentorial intracerebral epithelial (ependymal) cysts: review, case reports and fine structure. J Neurol Neurosurg Psychiatry 1977; 40: 127–37.

634 Bouch DC, Mitchell I, Maloney AFJ. Ependymal lined paraventricular cerebral cysts: a report of three cases. J Neurol Neurosurg Psychiatry 1973; 36: 611–17.

635 Jakubiak P, Dunsmore RH, Beckett RS. Supratentorial brain cysts. J Neurosurg 1968; 28: 129–36.

636 Ghatak NR, Hirano A, Kasoff SS, Zimmerman HM. Fine structure of an intracerebral epithelial cyst. J Neurosurg 1974; 41: 75–82.

637 Markwalder T-M, Markwalder RV, Slongo T. Intracranial ciliated neuroepithelial cyst mimicking arachnoid cyst. Surg Neurol 1981; 16: 411–14.

638 Obenchain TG, Becker DP. Head bobbing associated with a cyst of the third ventricle: case report. J Neurosurg 1972; 37: 457–9.

639 Albright L. Treatment of bobble-head doll syndrome by transcallosal cystectomy. Neurosurgery 1981; 8: 593–5.

640 Baskin DS, Wilson CB. Transsphenoidal treatment of non-neoplastic intrasellar cysts. A report of 38 cases. J Neurosurg 1984; 60: 8–13.

641 Spaziante R, de Devitiis E, Stella L, Cappabianca P, Donzelli R. Benign intrasellar cysts. Surg Neurol 1981; 15: 274–82.

642 Lang W, Lang M, Kornhuber A, Gallwitz A, Kriebel J. Neuropsychological and neuroendocrinological disturbances associated with extracerebral cysts of the anterior and middle cranial fossa. Eur Arch Psychiatr Neurol Sci 1985; 235: 38–41.

643 Auer LM, Gallhofer B, Ladurner G, Sager WD, Heppner F, Lechner H. Diagnosis and treatment of middle fossa arachnoid cysts and subdural hematomas. J Neurosurg 1981; 54: 366–9.

644 Murali R, Epstein F. Diagnosis and treatment of suprasellar arachnoid cysts. Report of three cases. J Neurosurg 1979; 50: 515–18.

645 Wolpert SM, Scott RM. The value of metrizimide CT cisternography in the management of cerebral arachnoid cysts. AJNR 1981; 2: 29–35.

646 Handa J, Nakano Y, Aii H. CT cisternography with intracranial arachnoid cysts. Surg Neurol 1977; 8: 451–4.

647 Kaplan BJ, Mickle JP, Parkhurst R. Cystoperitoneal shunting for congenital arachnoid cysts. Child's Brain 1984; 11: 304–11.

648 Stein SC. Intracranial developmental cysts in children: treatment by cystoperitoneal shunting. Neurosurgery 1981; 8: 647–50.

649 Serlo W, van Wendt L, Heikkinen E, Saukkonen A-L, Heikkinen E, Nystrom S. Shunting procedures in the management of intracranial cerebrospinal fluid cysts in infancy and childhood. Acta Neurochir 1985; 76: 111–16.

650 di Rocco C, Caldarelli M, di Tropani G. Infratentorial arachnoid cysts in children. Child's Brain 1981; 8: 119–33.

651 Ryder JW, Kleinschmidt-DeMasters BK, Keller TS. Sudden deterioration and death in patients with benign tumors of the third ventricular area. J Neurosurg 1986; 64: 216–23.

652 Chan RC, Thompson GB. Third ventricular colloid cysts presenting with acute neurological deterioration. Surg Neurol 1983; 19: 358–62.

653 Poppen JL, Reysr V, Horrax G. Colloid cysts of the third ventricle. Report of seven cases. J Neurosurg 1953; 10: 242–63.

654 Antunes JL, Louis KM, Ganti SR. Colloid

cysts of the third ventricle. Neurosurgery 1980; 7: 450–5.

655 Hall WA, Lunsford LD. Changing concepts in the treatment of colloid cysts. An 11-year experience in the CT era. J Neurosurg 1987; 66: 186–91.

656 Yenerman MH, Bowerman CI, Hymaker W. Colloid cyst of the third ventricle: a clinical study of 54 cases in light of previous publications. Acta Neuroreg 1958; 17: 211–77.

657 Buchsbaum HW, Colton RP. Anterior third ventricular cysts in infancy: case report. J Neurosurg 1967; 26: 264–6.

658 Nitta M, Symon L. Colloid cysts of the third ventricle. A review of 36 cases. Acta Neurochir 1985; 76: 99–104.

659 Antunes JL. Masses of the third ventricle. In: Wilkins RH, Rengachary SS eds Neurosurgery. New York: McGraw-Hill, 1985: 935–8.

660 Little JR, McCarty CS. Colloid cysts of the third ventricle. J Neurosurg 1974; 40: 230–5.

661 Ciric I, Ziwin I. Neuroepithelial (colloid) cysts of the septum pellucidum. J Neurosurg 1975; 43: 69–73.

662 Parkinson D, Childe AE. Colloid cyst of the fourth ventricle: report of a case of two colloid cysts of the fourth ventricle. J Neurosurg 1952; 9: 404–9.

663 Shuangshoti S, Netsky MG. Neuroepithelial (colloid) cysts of the nervous system. Further observations on pathogenesis, location, incidence and histochemistry. Neurology 1966; 16: 887–903.

664 Sjovall E. Uber eine Ependymcyste embryalen Charakters (Paraphyse?) im dritten Hirnventrikel mit todlichem Ausgang. Beitr Path Anat 1910; 47: 248–69.

665 Ariens Kappers J. The development of the paraphysis cerebri in man with comment on its relationships to the intercolumnar tubercle and its significance for the origin of cystic tumors in the third ventricle. J Comp Neurol 1955; 102: 425–510.

666 Coxe WS, Luse SA. Colloid cyst of third ventricle. An electron microscopic study. J Neuropathol Exp Neurol 1964; 23: 431–45.

667 Hirano A, Ghatek NR. The fine structure of colloid cysts of the third ventricle. J Neuropathol Exp Neurol 1974; 33: 333–41.

668 Antunes JL, Kvam D, Ganti SR, Louis KM, Goodman J. Mixed colloid cysts-xanthogranulomas of the third ventricle. Surg Neurol 1981; 16: 256–61.

669 Shuangshoti S, Netsky MG. Xanthogranuloma (xanthoma) of choroid plexus: the origin of foamy (xanthoma) cells. Am J Pathol 1966; 48: 503–33.

670 Shuangshoti S, Phongprasert C, Suwanwela N, Netsky MG. Combined neuroepithelial (colloid) cyst and xanthogranuloma (xanthoma) in the third ventricle. Neurology 1975; 25: 547–52.

671 Malik GM, Horoupian DS, Boulos RS. Hemorrhagic (colloid) cyst of the third ventricle and episodic neurological deficits. Surg Neurol 1980; 13: 73–7.

672 Kelly R. Colloid cysts of the third ventricle. Analysis of 29 cases. Brain 1951; 74: 23–65.

673 Lobosky JM, Van Gilder JC, Damasio AR. Behavioral manifestations of third ventricular colloid cysts. J Neurol Neurosurg Psychiatry 1984; 47: 1075–80.

674 Dandy WE. Benign Tumors in the Third Ventricle of the Brain. Springfield, Illinois: Charles C Thomas, 1933.

675 Ganti SR, Antunes JL, Louis KM, Hilal SK. Computed tomography in the diagnosis of colloid cysts of the third ventricle. Radiology 1981; 138: 384–91.

676 Powell MP, Torrens MJ, Thomson JLG, Horgan JG. Isodense colloid cysts of the third ventricle: a diagnostic and therapeutic problem resolved by ventriculoscopy. Neurosurgery 1983; 13: 234–7.

677 Batnitsky S, Sarwar M, Leeds NE, Schechter MM, Behrog A-K. Colloid cysts of the third ventricle. Radiology 1974: 112: 327–41.

678 Kjos BO, Brant-Zawadzki M, Kucharczyk W, Kelly WM, Norman D, Newton TH. Cystic intracranial lesions: magnetic resonance imaging. Radiology 1985; 155: 363–9.

679 Greenwood J. Paraphysial cysts of the third ventricle: with report of eight cases. J Neurosurg 1949; 6: 153–9.

680 Shucart WA, Stein BM. Transcallosal approach to the anterior ventricular system. Neurosurgery 1978; 3: 339–43.

681 Bosch DA, Rahn T, Backlund EO. Treatment of colloid cysts of the third ventricle by stereotactic aspiration. Surg Neurol 1978; 9: 15–18.

682 Apuzzo MLJ, Chandrasoma PT, Zelman V, Gianotta SL, Weiss MH. Computed tomographic guidance stereotaxis in the management of lesions of the third ventricular region. Neurosurgery 1984; 15: 502–8.

683 Rivas JJ, Lobato RD. CT-assisted stereotaxis aspiration of colloid cysts of the third ventricle. J Neurosurg 1985; 62: 238–42.

684 McKissock W. The surgical treatment of colloid cysts of the third ventricle. A report based upon twenty-one personal cases. Brain 1951; 74: 1–9.

685 Lane CD, Lignelli GJ. Colloid cyst of the third ventricle. Penn Med 1985; 88: 40–4.

686 Shanklin WM. On the presence of cysts in the human pituitary. Anat Rec 1949; 104: 397–407.

687 Bayoumi ML. Rathke's cleft and its cysts. Edinb Med J 1948; 55: 745–9.

688 Shimoji T, Shinohara A, Shimizu A, Sato K, Ishii S. Rathke cleft cysts. Surg Neurol 1984; 21: 295–310.

689 Eisenberg HM, Weiner RL. Benign pituitary cysts. In: Wilkins RH, Regachary SS eds Neurosurgery. New York: McGraw-Hill, 1985: 932–4.

690 Shanklin WM. Incidence and distribution of cilia in the human pituitary with a description of micro-follicular cysts derived from Rathke's cleft. Acta Anat 1951; 11: 361–82.

691 Kepes JJ. Transitional cell tumor of the pituitary gland developing from a Rathke's cleft cyst. Cancer 1978; 41: 337–43.

692 Matsushima T, Fukui M, Ohta M, Yamahawa Y, Takaki T, Okano H. Ciliated and goblet cells in craniopharyngioma: light and electron microscopic studies at surgery and autopsy. Acta Neuropathol 1980; 50: 199–205.

693 Verhijk A, Bots GT. An intrasellar cyst with both Rathke's cleft and epidermoid characteristics. Acta Neurochir 1980; 51: 203–7.

694 Yoshida J, Kobayahi T, Kageyama N, Kanzaki M. Symptomatic Rathke's cleft cyst: morphologic study with light and electron microscopy and tissue culture. J Neurosurg 1977; 47: 451–8.

695 Steinberg GK, Koenig GH, Golden JB. Symptomatic Rathke's cleft cysts: report of two cases. J Neurosurg 1982; 56: 290–5.

696 Shuangshoti S, Netsky MG, Nashold BS, Jr. Epithelial cysts related to sella turcica: proposed origin from neuroepithelium. Arch Pathol Lab Med 1970; 90: 444–50.

697 Martinez LJ, Osterholm JL, Berry RG, Lee KF, Schatz NJ. Trans-sphenoidal removal of a Rathke's cleft cyst. Neurosurgery 1979; 4: 63–5.

698 Oberchain TG, Becker DP. Abscess formation in a Rathke's cleft cyst. Case report. J Neurosurg 1972; 36: 359–62.

699 Adelman LS, Post KD. Calcification in Rathke's cleft cysts. J Neurosurg 1977; 47: 641.

700 Kapcala LP, Molitch ME, Post KD, Billen BJ, Prager RJ, Jackson IMD, Richlin S. Galactorrhea, oligoamenorrhea and hyperprolactinemia in patients with craniopharyngiomas. J Clin Endocrinol Metab 1980; 51: 798–800.

701 Menault F, Sabouraud O, Javalet A, Madigand M. Kyste de la fente de Rathke. Rev Otoneuroophthalmol 1979; 51: 383–90.

702 Baldini M, Mosea L, Princi L. The empty sella

syndrome secondary to Rathke's cleft cyst. Acta Neurochir 1980; 53: 69–78.

703 Byrd SE, Winter J, Takahashi M, Joyce P. Symptomatic Rathke's cleft cyst demonstrated on computed tomography. J Comput Assist Tomogr 1980; 4: 411–14.

704 Izeki H, Imanaga H, Himuro H, Ginbo M, Kitamura K, Okino M, Fukuyama S. A case of Rathke's cleft cyst. Nervous System in Children 1980; 5: 235–42.

705 Marcincin RP, Gennarelli TA. Recurrence of symptomatic pituitary cysts following trans-sphenoidal drainage. Surg Neurol 1982; 18: 448–51.

706 Eisenberg HM, Sarwar M, Schlochet S Jr. Symptomatic Rathke's cleft cyst. J Neurosurg 1976; 45: 585–8.

707 Wilkins RH, Odom GH. Spinal intradural cysts. In: Vinken PJ, Bruyn GW eds Handbook of Clinical Neurology, Vol 20, Tumors of the Spine and Spinal Cord, Part II. Amsterdam: North-Holland, 1976: 55–102.

708 French BN. Midline fusion defects and defects of formation. In: Youmans JR ed Neurological Surgery. Philadelphia: WB Saunders, 1982: 1236–1380.

709 Dorsey JF, Tabrisky J. Intraspinal and mediastinal foregut cyst compressing the spinal cord: report of a case. J Neurosurg 1966; 24: 562–7.

710 Millis RR, Holmes AE. Enterogenous cyst of the spinal cord with associated intestinal reduplication, veretebral anomalies and a dorsal dermal sinus. Case report. J Neurosurg 1973; 38: 73–7.

711 Rhaney K, Barclay GPT. Enterogenous cysts and congenital diverticula of the alimentary canal with abnormalities of the vertebral column and spinal cord. J Pathol Bacteriol 1959; 77: 457–71.

712 Bentley JFR. Smith JR. Developmental posterior enteric remnants and spinal malformation: the split notochord syndrome. Arch Dis Child 1960; 35: 76–86.

713 Bell HH. Anterior spina bifida and its relation to a persistence of the neurenteric canal. J Nerv Ment Dis 1923; 57: 445–62.

714 Gardner WJ. The Dysraphic States From Syringomyelia to Anencephaly. Amsterdam, Exerpta Medica, 1973.

715 Prop N, Frensdorf EL, van de Stardt FR. A postvertebral entodermal cyst associated with axial deformities: a case showing the entodermal-ectodermal adhesion syndrome. Pediatrics 1967; 39: 555–62.

716 Burrows FDG, Sutcliffe J. The split notochord syndrome. Br J Radiol 1968; 41: 844–7.

717 Saunders RL de CH. Combined anterior and

posterior spina bifida in a living neonatal human female. Anat Rec 1943; 87: 255–78.

718 Bremer JL. Dorsal intestinal fistula; accessory neurenteric canal; diastematomyelia. Arch Pathol Lab Med 1952; 54: 132–8.

719 Wilkins RH. Intraspinal cysts. In: Wilkins RH, Rengachary SS eds Neurosurgery. New York: McGraw-Hill, 1985: 2061–70.

720 Adams RD, Wagner W. Congenital cyst of the spinal meninges as cause of intermittent compression of the spinal cord. Arch Neurol Psychiatry 1947; 58: 57–69.

721 D'Almeida AC, Stewart DH Jr. Neurenteric cyst: case report and literature review. Neurosurgery 1981; 8: 596–9.

722 Mann KS, Khosla VK, Gulati Dr, Malik AK. Spinal neurenteric cyst. Association with vertebral anomalies, diastematomyelia, dorsal fistula and lipoma. Surg Neurol 1984; 21: 358–62.

723 Odake G, Yamaki T, Naruse S. Neurenteric cyst with meningomyelocele: case report. J Neurosurg 1976; 45: 353–6.

724 Afshar F, Sholtz CL. Enterogenous cyst of the fourth ventricle: case report. J Neurosurg 1981; 54: 836–8.

725 Knight G, Griffiths T, Williams I. Gastrocytoma of the spinal cord. Br J Surg 1955; 42: 635–8.

726 Levin P, Antin SP. Intraspinal neurenteric cyst in the cervical area. Neurology (Minneapolis) 1964; 14: 727–30.

727 Jackson FE. Neurenteric cysts. Report of a neurenteric cyst with associated chronic meningitis and hydrocephalus. J Neurosurg 1961; 18: 678–82.

728 Holcomb GW Jr, Matson DD. Thoracic neurenteric cyst. Surgery 1954; 35: 115–21.

729 Neuhauser EBD, Harris GBC, Berrett A. Roentgenographic features of neurenteric cysts. ARJ 1958; 79: 235–40.

730 Gimeno A, Arachnoid, neurenteric and other cysts. In: Vinken PJ, Bruyn GW eds Handbook of Clinical Neurology, Vol 32. Amsterdam: North-Holland, 1978: 393–448.

731 Liss L, Kahn EA. Pituicytoma: tumor of the sella turcica: a clinicopathological study. J Neurosurg 1958; 15: 481–8.

732 Kobrine AI, Ross E. Granular cell myoblastoma of the pituitary region. Surg Neurol 1973; 1: 275–9.

733 Burston J, John R, Spencer H. 'Myoblastoma' of the neurohypophysis. J Pathol Bacteriol 1962; 83: 455–61.

734 Liwnicz BH, Liwnicz RG, Huff JS, McBride BH, Tew JM Jr. Giant granular cell tumor of the suprasellar area: immunocytochemical and electron microscopic studies. Neurosurgery 1984; 15: 246–51.

735 Becker DH. Parasellar granular cell tumors. In: Wilkins RH, Rengachary SS eds Neurosurgery. New York: McGraw-Hill, 1985: 930–2.

736 Becker DH, Wilson CB. Symptomatic parasellar granular cell tumors. Neurosurgery 1981; 8: 173–80.

737 Schlachter LB, Tindall GT, Pearl GS. Granular cell tumor of the pituitary gland associated with diabetes insipidus. Neurosurgery 1980; 6: 418–21.

738 Cusick JF, Ho K-C, Hagen TL, Kun LE. Granular cell pituicytoma associated with multiple endocrine neoplasia type II. Case report. J Neurosurg 1982; 56: 594–6.

739 Dickson DW, Suzuki KI, Kanner R, Weitz S, Horoupian DS. Cerebral granular cell tumor: immunohistochemical and electron microscopic study. J Neuropathol Exp Neurol 1986; 45: 304–14.

740 Lechevalier B, Mandard JC, Adam Y, Da Silva DC, Bazin C, Courtheoux P. Tumeur à cellules granuleuses d'une hémisphère cérébral: intérêt de la recherche de la proteine acide gliofibrillaire. Rev Neurol 1982; 138: 619–29.

741 Budka H. Intracranial lipomatous hamartomas (intracranial 'lipomas'): a study of 13 cases including combinations with medulloblastoma, colloid and epidermoid cysts, angiomatosis and other malformations. Acta Neuropathol 1974; 28: 205–22.

742 Kazner E, Stochdorph O, Wende S, Grumme T. Intracranial lipoma. Diagnostic and therapeutic considerations. J Neurosurg 1980; 52: 234–45.

743 Ehni GW, Adson AW. Lipoma of the brain. Report of cases. Arch Neurol Psychiatry 1945; 53: 299–304.

744 Stcimle R, Pageaut G, Jacguet G, Bourghli A, Godard J, Bertaud M. Lipoma in the cerebellopontine angle. Surg Neurol 1985; 24: 73–6.

745 Pascual-Castroviejo I, Pascual-Pascual SI, Perez-Higueras A. Frontonasal dysplasia and lipoma of the corpus callosum. Eur J Pediatr 1985; 144: 66–71.

746 Tahmouresie A, Kroll G, Shucart W. Lipoma of the corpus callosum. Surg Neurol 1979; 11: 31–4.

747 Vonderahe AR, Niemer WT. Intracranial lipoma: a report of four cases. J Neuropathol Exp Neurol 1944; 3: 344–54.

748 Schmid AH. A lipoma of the cerebellum. Acta Neuropathol (Berlin) 1973; 26: 75–80.

749 Aleksic S, Budzilovich G, Greco MA, McCarthy J, Reuben R, Margolis S, Epstein F, Feigin I, Pearson J. Intracranial lipomas,

hydrocephalus and other CNS anomalies in occulo-auriculo vertebral dysplasia (Goldenhar-Gorlin Syndrome) Child's Brain 1984; 11: 285–97.

750 Miyao T, Saito T, Yamamoto T, Kamoshita S. Encephalocraniocutaneous lipomatosis: a recently described neurocutaneous syndrome. Child's Brain 1984; 11: 280–4.

751 Manganiello LOJ, Daniel EF, Hair LQ. Lipoma of corpus callosum. Case report. J Neurosurg 1966; 24: 892–4.

752 Hatashita S, Sakakibara T, Ishii S. Lipoma of the insula. J Neurosurg 1983; 58: 300–2.

753 Hayashi T, Shojima K, Moritaka K, Utsunomiya H, Konishi J, Maehara F, Kuratomi A. Intracranial lipomas. Case presentations and CT features. Kurume Med J 1983; 30: 133–41.

754 Leibrock LG, Deans WR, Bloch S, Schuman RM, Skultety FM. Cerebellopontine angle lipoma: a review. Neurosurgery 1983; 12: 697–9.

755 Gastaut H, Regis H, Gastaut JL, Yermenos E, Low MD. Lipomas of the corpus callosum and epilepsy. Neurology (NY) 1980; 30: 132–8.

756 Zettner A, Netsky MG. Lipoma of the corpus callosum. J Neuropathol Exp Neurol 1960; 19: 337–59.

757 Graham DG. Lipoma of the corpus callosum. In: Wilkins RH, Rengachary SS eds Neurosurgery. New York: McGraw-Hill, 1985: 1036–8.

758 Halmagyi GM, Evans WA. Lipoma of the quadrigeminal plate causing progressive obstructive hydrocephalus: case report. J Neurosurg 1978; 49: 453–6.

759 Pensak ML, Glasscock ME, Gulya AJ, Hays JW, Smith HP, Dickens JRE. Cerebellopontine angle lipomas. Arch Otolaryngol Head Neck Surg 1986; 112: 99–101.

760 Sosman MC. Discussion of Echternacht AP, Campbell JA. Midline anomalies of the brain. Their diagnosis by pneumoencephalography. Radiology 1946; 46: 119–31.

761 Boechat MI, Kangarloo H, Diament MJ, Krauthamer R. Lipoma of the corpus callosum: sonographic appearance. J Clin Ultrasound 1983; 11: 447–8.

762 Kean DM, Smith MA, Douglas RHB, Martyn CN, Best JJK. Two examples of CNS lipomas demonstrated by computed tomography and low field (0.08T) MR imaging. J Comput Assist Tomogr 1985; 9: 494–6.

763 Patel AN. Lipoma of the corpus callosum: a non-surgical entity. N C Med J 1965; 26: 328–35.

764 Graves VB, Schemm GW. Clinical characteristics and CT findings in lipoma of the cerebel-

lopontine angle. Case report. J Neurosurg 1982; 57: 839–41.

765 Kveton JF, Brackmann DE, Glasscock ME, III, House WF, Hitselberger WE. Chondrosarcoma of the skull base. Otolaryngol Head Neck Surg 1986; 94: 23–32.

766 Vandenberg HJ, Coley BL. Primary tumors of the cranial bones. Surg Gynecol Obstet 1950; 90: 602–12.

767 Caron AS, Hajdu SI, Strong EW. Osteogenic sarcoma of the facial and cranial bones: a review of 43 cases. Am J Surg 1971; 122: 719–25.

768 Kirshbaum JD. Fibrosarcoma of the skull in Paget's disease. Arch Pathol 1943; 36: 74–9.

769 Forsythe RW, Baker GS, Dockerty MB, Camp JD. Intracranial osteochondroma. Mayo Clin Proc 1947; 22: 350–6.

770 Wolf A, Ecklin F. Osteochondrosarcoma of the falx invading frontal lobes of the cerebrum. Bull Neurol Inst New York 1936; 5: 515–25.

771 Berry MP, Jenkin RDT. Parameningeal rhabdomyosarcoma in the young. Cancer 1981; 48: 281–8.

772 Voorhies RM, Sundaresan N. Tumors of the skull. In: Wilkins RH, Rengachary SS eds Neurosurgery. New York: McGraw-Hill, 1985: 984–1001.

773 Van Dellen JR. A mastoid osteoma causing intracranial complications. A case report. S Afr Med J 1977; 51: 597–8.

774 Schwartz E. Ossifying fibromas of the face and skull. AJR 1964; 91: 1012–16.

775 Tomita T, Huvos AG, Shah J, Sundaresan N. Giant ossifying fibroma of the nasal cavity with intracranial extension. Acta Neurochir 1981; 56: 65–71.

776 Huvos AG. Bone Tumors: Diagnosis, Treatment and Prognosis. Philadelphia: WB Saunders, 1979.

777 Williams RN, Boop WC Jr. Benign osteoblastoma of the skull. Case report. J Neurosurg 1974; 41: 769–72.

778 Minagi H, Newton TH. Cartilagenous tumors of the base of the skull. AJR 1969; 105: 308–13.

779 Kragenbuhl H, Yasargil MG. Chondromas. Prog Neurol Surg 1975; 6: 435–53.

780 Imagawa K, Hayashi M, Toda I, Asai A, Nomura T. Intracranial chondroma. Surg Neurol 1978; 10: 167–70.

781 Cares HL, Terplan KL. Chondroblastoma of the skull. Case report. J Neurosurg 1971; 35: 614–18.

782 Wyke BD. Primary hemangioma of the skull: a rare cranial tumor. AJR 1949; 61: 302–16.

783 Schneider RC, Gabrielsen TO, Hicks SP. Calvarial hemangioma: the value of selective

external carotid angiography in surgical excision of the lesion. Neurology 1973; 23: 352–6.

784 Arseni S, Horvath L, Maretsis M, Carp N. Giant cell tumors of the calvaria. J Neurosurg 1975; 42: 535–40.

785 Epstein N, Whelan M, Reed D, Aleksic S. Giant cell tumor of the skull: a report of two cases. Neurosurgery 1982; 11: 263–7.

786 Mansfield JB. Primary fibrosarcoma of the skull. Case report. J Neurosurg 1977; 47: 785–7.

787 Bahr AL, Gayler BW. Cranial chondrosarcomas: report on four cases and review of the literature. Radiology 1977; 124: 151–6.

788 Suit HD, Goitien M, Munzenrider J, Verhey L, Davis KR, Kochler A, Lingood R, Ojemann RG. Definitive radiation therapy for chordoma and chondrosarcoma of base of skull and cervical spine. J. Neurosurg 1982; 56: 377–85.

789 Sundaresan N, Rosen G, Fortner J, Lane JH, Hilaris B. Preoperative chemotherapy for paraspinal sarcomas. J Neurosurg 1983; 58: 446–50.

790 Sundaresan N, Chordomas, Clin Orthop Rel Res 1986; 204: 135–42.

791 Tewfik HH, McGinnis WL, Nordstrom DG, Latourette HB. Chordoma. Evaluation of clinical behavior and treatment modalities. Int J Radiat Oncol Biol Phys 1977; 2: 959–62.

792 Rich TA, Schiller A, Suit HD, Mankin HJ. Clinical and pathological review of 48 cases of chordoma. Cancer 1985; 56: 182–7.

793 Virchow RLK. Untersuchungen über die Entwickelung des Schadelgrundes in gesunden und Krankhaften Zustande und über den Einfluss derselben auf schadelform. Gesichtsbildung und Gehirnbau. Berlin: G Reimer, 1857: 128.

794 Muller H. Ueber das Vorgommen von Resten der Chordodorsalis bei Menschen nach der Geburt und über ihr Verhaltniss zu den Gallertgesch wulsten am Clivus. Z Rat Med 1858; 2: 202.

795 Risio M, Bagliani C, Leli R, Dio Girolamo P, Del Pero M, Coverliza S. Sacrococcgeal and vertebral chordomas. Report of three cases and review of the literature. J Neurosurg Sci 1985; 29: 211–27.

796 Horwitz T. The Human Notochord. A Study of Its Development and Regression, Variations and Pathological Derivative, Chordoma. Indianapolis, Limited Private Printing, 1977.

797 Ribbert H. Ueber die Echondrosis Physaliphora sphenooccipitalis. Zentralbl Allg Pathol 1894; 5: 457–61.

798 Congdon CF. Proliferative lesions resembling chordoma following puncture of nucleus pulposus in rabbits. J Nat Cancer Inst 1952; 12: 893–907.

799 Alezais H, Peyron A, Sur l'histogenese et l'origine des chordomes. CR Acad Sci (Paris) 1922; 174: 419–21.

800 Erlandson RA, Tandler B, Lieberman PH, Higinbotham N. Ultrastructure of human chordoma. Cancer Res 1968; 28: 2115–25.

801 Pena CE, Horvat BL, Fisher ER. The ultrastructure of chordoma. Am J Clin Pathol 1970; 53: 544–51.

802 Dahlin DC. Bone Tumors: General Aspects and Data on 6221 cases. Springfield, Illinois: Charles C Thomas, 1978: 329–343.

803 Raffel C, Wright DC, Gutin PH, Wilson CB. Cranial chordomas: clinical presentation and results of operative and radiation therapy in twenty-six patients. Neurosurgery 1985; 17: 703–10.

804 Sundaresan N, Galicich JH, Chu FCH, Huvos AG. Spinal chordomas. J Neurosurg 1979; 50: 312–19.

805 Wold LE, Laws ER Jr. Cranial chordomas in children and young adults. J Neurosurg 1983; 59: 1043–7.

806 Occhipinti E, Mastrostefano R, Pompili A, Carapella CM, Caroli F, Riccio A. Spinal chordomas in infancy. Report of a case and analysis of the literature Child's Brain 1981; 8: 198–206.

807 Ulich TR, Mirra JM. Ecchordosis physaliphora vertebralis. Clin Orthop 1982; 163: 282–9.

808 Willis RA. Pathology of Tumors, 4th edition. London: Butterworth, 1967.

809 Heffelfinger MJ, Dahlin DC, MacCarty CS, Beabout JW. Chordomas and cartilaginous tumors at the skull base. Cancer 1973; 32: 410–20.

810 Laws ER Jr. Cranial chordomas. In: Wilkins RH, Rengachary SS eds Neurosurgery. New York: McGraw-Hill, 1985: 927–30.

811 Crawford T. The staining reactions of chordoma. J Clin Pathol 1958; 119: 110–13.

812 Batsakis JG. Tumors of the Head and Neck. Clinical and Pathological Consideration, 2nd edition, Baltimore: Williams and Wilkins, 1975.

813 Miettinen M, Lehto VP, Dahl D, Virtanen I. Differential diagnosis of chordoma, chondroid and ependymal tumors as aided by antiintermediate filament antibodies. Am J Pathol 1983; 112: 160–9.

814 Mured TM, Murthy MSN. Ultrastructure of a chordoma. Cancer 1970; 25: 1204–15.

815 Pena CE, Horvat BL, Fisher ER. The ultras-

tructure of chordoma. Am J Clin Pathol 1970; 53: 544–51.

816 Cody HS, Marcove RC, Quan SH. Malignant retrorectal tumors: 28 years' experience at Memorial Sloan-Kettering Cancer Center. Dis Colon Rectum 1981; 24: 501–6.

817 Higinbotham NL, Philips RF, Farr HW, Husto HO. Chordoma: thirty-five year study at Memorial Hospital. Cancer 1967; 20: 1841–50.

818 Mabray RE. Chordoma: a study of 150 cases. Am J Cancer 1935; 25: 501–17.

819 Kamrin RP, Potanos JN, Pool JL. An evaluation of the diagnosis and treatment of chordoma. J Neurol Neurosurg Psychiatry 1964; 27: 157–65.

820 Wright D. Nasopharyngeal and cervical chordoma—Some aspects of their development and treatment. Laryngol Otol 1967; 81: 1337–55.

821 Ariel IM, Verdu C. Chordoma: An analysis of 20 cases treated over a 20 year span. J Surg Oncol 1975; 7: 27–44.

822 Chambers PW, Schwinn CP. Chordoma: a clinicopathological study of metastasis. Am J Surg Pathol 1979; 72: 765–76.

823 Utne JR, Pugh DJ. The roentgenologic aspects of chordomas. AJR 1955; 74: 593–608.

824 Firooznia H, Pinto RS, Lin JP, Baruch HH, Zausner J. Chordoma: radiological evaluation of 20 cases. AJR 1976; 122: 797–805.

825 Kendall BE, Lee BCP. Cranial chordomas. Br J Radiol 1977; 50: 687–98.

826 Krayenbuhl H, Yasargil MG. Cranial chordomas. Prog Neurol Surg 1975; 6: 380–434.

827 Guiot G, Rougerie J, Bouche J. The rhinoseptal route for the removal of clivus chordomas. Johns Hopkins Med J 1968; 122: 329–35.

828 Derome PJ, Guiot G. Surgical approaches to the sphenoidal and clival area. Adv Tech Stand Neurosurg 1979; 6: 101–36.

829 Decker RE, Malis LI. Surgical approaches to midline lesions at the base of the skull, A review. Mt Sinai J Med 1970; 37: 84–102.

830 Stevenson GC, Stoney RJ, Perkins RK, Adams JE. A transvervical transclival approach to the ventral surface of the brainstem for the removal of clivus chordomas. J Neurosurg 1966; 24: 544–51.

831 Derome PJ. The transbasal approach to tumors invading the base of the skull. In: Schmidek HH, Sweet WH eds Operative Neurosurgical Techniques: Indications, Methods and Results. New York: Grune and Stratton, 1982: 357–80.

832 Pearlman AW, Friedman M. Radical radiation therapy of chordoma. AJR 1970; 108: 333–41.

833 Cummings BJ, Hodson ID, Bush RS. Chordoma: the results of megavoltage radiation therapy. Int J Radiat Oncol Biol Phys 1983; 9: 633–42.

834 Amendola BE, Amendola MA, Oliver E, McClatchey KD. Chordoma: role of radiation therapy. Radiology 1986; 158: 839–43.

835 Saunders WM, Castro JR, Chen GTY, Gutin PH, Collier JM, Zink SR, Phillips TL, Gauger GE. Early results of ion beam radiation therapy or sacral chordoma. J Neurosurg 1986; 64: 243–7.

836 Zoltan L, Fenyes I. Stereotactic diagnosis and radioactive treatment in a case of sphenoccipital chordoma. J Neurosurg 1960; 17: 888–900.

837 Kaiser TE, Pritchard DS, Unni KK. Clinicopathological study of sacrococcygeal chordoma. Cancer 1984; 54: 2574–8.

838 Krol G, Sundaresan N. Computerized tomography in axial chordomas. J Comput Assist Tomogr 1983; 7: 286–9.

839 Hudson TM, Galceran M. Radiology of sacrococcygeal chordoma. Clin Orthop Rel Res 1983; 175: 237–42.

840 Mapstone TP, Kaufman B, Ratcheson BA. Intradural chordoma without bone involvement: nuclear magnetic resonance (NMR) appearance. Case report. J Neurosurg 1983; 59: 535–7.

841 Mindell ER. Chordoma. J Bone Joint Surg 1981; 63: 501–5.

842 Localio SA, Eng K, Ranson JHC. Abdominosacral approach for retro-rectal tumors. Ann Surg 1980; 191: 555–60.

843 Dahlin DC, MacCarty CS. Chordoma: a study of fifty-nine cases. Cancer 1952; 5: 1170–8.

844 Stener B, Gunterberg B. High amputation of the sacrum for extirpation of tumors. Principles and techniques. Spine 1978; 3: 351–66.

845 Arbit E, Patterson RH. Combined transoral and median labiomandibular glossotomy approach to the upper cervical spine. Neurosurgery 1981; 8: 672–4.

846 Gregorius FK, Batzdorf U. Removal of thoracic chordoma by staged laminectomy and thoractomy. Case report. Am Surg 1979; 45: 535–7.

847 Wang CC, James AF Jr. Chordoma: brief review of the literature and report of a case with widespread metastases. Cancer 1968; 22: 162–7.

848 Fox JE, Batsakis JG, Owano LR. Unusual manifestations of chordoma: a report of two cases. J Bone Joint Surg 1968; 50A: 1618–28.

849 Stough DR, Hatzog JT, Fisher RG. Unusual

intradural metastasis of a cranial chordoma. J Neurosurg 1971; 34: 560–2.

850 Holzner H. Ungewohnliche metastasierung eines Chordoms. Zentralbl Pathol Anat 1954; 92: 12–58.

851 Aleksic S, Budzilovich GN, Nirmel K, Ransohoff J, Feigin I. Subarachnoid dissemination of thoracic chordoma. Arch Neurol 1979; 36: 652–4.

852 Marigil MS, Pardo-Mindan FJ, Joly M. Diagnosis of chordoma by cytologic examination of cerebrospinal fluid. Am J Clin Pathol 1983; 80: 402–4.

853 Harkin JC, Reed RJ. Tumors of the peripheral nervous system. In: Atlas of Tumor Pathology. Bethesda, MD: AFIP, 1969.

854 Cravioto H. Studies on the normal ultrastructure of peripheral nerve: axis cylinders, Schwann cells and myelin. Bull L A Neurol Soc 1965; 30: 1698–90.

855 Cravioto H. The ultrastructure of acoustic nerve tumors. Acta Neuropathol 1969; 12: 116–40.

856 Cravioto H, Lockwood R. The behavior of acoustic neuroma in tissue culture. Acta Neuropathol 1969; 12: 141–57.

857 Jacque CM, Kujas M, Poreau A, Raoul M, Collier P, Racadot J, Baumann N. GFA and S-100 protein levels as an index of malignancy in human gliomas and neurinomas J Nat Cancer Inst 1979; 62: 479–83.

858 Steffanson K, Wollmann R, Jerkovic M. S-100 protein in soft-tissue tumors derived from Schwann cells and melanocytes. Am J Pathol 1982; 106: 261–8.

859 Riccardi VM. Von Recklinghausen neurofibromatosis. N Engl J Med 1981; 305: 1617–27.

860 Asbury AK, Johnson PK. Tumors of peripheral nerve. In: Pathology of Peripheral Nerve. Philadelphia: WB Saunders, 1978: 206–29.

861 Ducatman BS, Scheithauer VW, Piepgras DG, Reiman HM. Malignant peripheral nerve sheath tumors in childhood. J Neuro-oncol 1984; 2: 241–8.

862 Taxy JB, Battifiora H. Trujillo Y, Dorfman HO. Electron microscopy in the diagnosis of malignant schwannoma. Cancer 1981; 48: 1381–91.

863 Sordillo PP, Helson L, Hajdu SI, Magill GB, Kosloff C, Golbey RB, Beattie EJ. Malignant schwannoma: clinical characteristics, survival and response to therapy. Cancer 1981; 47: 2503–9.

864 Foley KM, Woodruff JM, Ellis FT, Posner JB. Radiation-induced malignant and atypical peripheral nerve sheath tumors. Ann Neurol 1980; 7: 311–18.

865 Guccion JG, Enziger FM. Malignant schwannoma associated with von Recklinghausen's neurofibromatosis. Virchow's Arch (Pathol Anat) 1979; 383: 43–57.

866 Das Gupta TK. Tumors of the peripheral nerves. Clin Neurosurg 1977; 25: 574–90.

867 D'Agostino AN, Soule EH, Miller RH. Primary malignant neoplasms of nerves (malignant neurilemomas) in patients without manifestations of multiple neurofibromatosis (von Recklinghausen's disease). Cancer 1963; 16: 1003–14.

868 Cantin J, McNeer GP, Chu FL, Booker RJ. The problem of local recurrence after treatment of soft tissue sarcoma. Ann Surg 1968; 168: 47–53.

869 White HR Jr. Survival in malignant schwannoma: an 18-year study. Cancer 1971; 27: 720–9.

870 Vieta JO, Pack GT. Malignant neurilemomas of peripheral nerves. Am J Surg 1951; 82: 416–31.

871 Snyder M, Batzdorf U, Sparks FL. Unusual malignant tumors involving the brachial plexus. A report of two cases. Am Surg 1979; 45: 42–48.

872 Ducatman BS, Scheithauer BW. Malignant peripheral nerve sheath tumors with divergent differentiation. Cancer 1984; 54: 1049–57.

873 Krumerman MS, Stingle W. Synchronous malignant glandular schwannomas in congenital neurofibromatosis. Cancer 1978; 41: 2444–51.

874 Michel SL. Epithelial elements in a malignant neurogenic tumor of the tibial nerve. Am J Surg 1967; 113: 404–8.

875 Woodruff JM. Peripheral nerve tumors showing glandular differentiation (glandular schwannomas). Cancer 1976; 37: 2399–413.

876 MacCaulay RAA. Neurofibrosarcoma of the radial nerve in von Recklinghausen's disease with metastatic angiosarcoma. J Neurol Neurosurg Psychiatry 1978; 41: 474–478.

877 Foraker AG. Gland like elements in a peripheral neurosarcoma. Cancer 1948; 1: 286–293.

878 Woodruff JM, Chernik NL, Smith MC, Millett WB, Foote FW, Jr. Peripheral nerve tumors with rhabdomyosarcomatous differentiation (malignant 'Triton' tumors). Cancer 1973; 32: 426–439.

879 Locatelli P. Formation des Membres Supernumeraires. CR Assoc des Anatomistes, 20e reunion, Turin 1925; 279–282.

880 Youmans JR, Ishida WY. Tumors of peripheral and sympathetic nerves. In: Yourmans JR, ed Neurological Surgery, 2nd ed. Philadelphia: W B Saunders 1982: 3299–3315.

881 Richards JL, Matolo NM. Malignant schwannoma: report of a case mimicking lumbar disk disease. Am Surg 1979; 45: 49–51.

882 Ingels GW, Campbell DC Jr, Giampetro AM, Kozub RE, Bentlage CH. Malignant schwannomas of the mediastinum: report of two cases and review of the literature. Cancer 1971; 27: 1190–1201.

883 Sarin CL, Bennett MH, Jackson JW. Intrathoracic neurofibroma of the vagus nerve. Br J Dis Chest 1974; 68: 46–50.

884 Hammond JA, Driedger AA. Detection of malignant change in neurofibromatosis (von Recklinghausen's disease) by gallium-67 scanning. Can Med Assoc J 1978; 119: 352–353.

885 Ghosh BC, Ghosh L, Huvos AG, Fortner JG. Malignant schwannoma: a clinocopathologic study. Cancer 1973; 31: 184–190.

886 Shiu MH, Castro EB, Hajdu SI, Fortner JG. Surgical treatment of 297 soft tissue sarcomas of the lower extremity. Ann Surg 1975; 182: 597–602.

887 Das Gupta TK, Brasfield RD, Strong EW, Hajdu SI. Benign solitary schwannomas (neurilemomas). Cancer 1969; 24: 355–66.

888 Goldman RL, Jones SE, Heusinkveld RS. Combination chemotherapy of metastatic malignant schwannoma with vincristine, Adriamycin, cyclophosphamide, and imidazole carboxamide: a case report. Cancer 1977; 39: 1955–8.

889 Johnson WC, Helwig EB. Cutaneous focal mucinosis. A clinicopathological and histochemical study. Arch Dermatol 1966; 93: 13–20.

890 Barrett R, Cramer F. Tumors of the peripheral nerves and so-called 'ganglia' of the peroneal nerve. Clin Orthop 1963; 27: 135–146.

891 Feigin I, Cohen M. Maturation and anaplasia in neuronal tumors of the peripheral nervous system; with observations on the glia-like tissues in the ganglioneuroblastoma. J. Neuropathol Exp Neurol 1977; 36: 748–763.

892 Rosenstein BJ, Engleman K. Diarrhea in a child with a catecholamine-secreting ganglioneuroma. J Pediatr 1963; 63: 217–226.

893 Weinblatt ME, Heisel MA, Siegel SE. Hypertension in children with neurogenic tumors. Pediatrics 1983; 71: 947–951.

894 Hamilton JP, Koop CE. Ganglioneuromas in children. Surg Gynecol Obstet 1965; 121: 803–12.

895 Ricci A, Jr, Parham DM, Woodruff JM, Callihan T, Green A, Erlandson RA. Malignant peripheral nerve sheath tumors arising from ganglioneuromas. Am J Surg Pathol 1984; 8: 19–29.

896 Glennen GG, Grimley PM. Tumors of the extra-adrenal paraganglion system. In: Tumors of the Peripheral Nervous System. Washington, DC: AFIP, 1974.

897 Robertson JT. Chemodectomas. In: Wilkins RH, Rengachary SS eds Neurosurgery. New York: McGraw-Hill, 1985: 785–90.

898 Murphy TE, Huvos AG, Frazell EL. Chemodectomas of the glomus intravagale: vagal body tumors, non-chromaffin paragangliomas of the nodose ganglion of the vagus nerve. Ann Surg 1970; 172: 246–55.

899 Grufferman S, Gillman MW, Pasternak LR, Peterson CL, Young WG. Familial carotid body tumors: case report and epidemiological review. Cancer 1980; 46: 2116–22.

900 Veldman JE, Mulder PHM, Ruijs SHG, de Haas G, van Waes PFGM, Hoekstra A. Early detection of asymptomatic hereditary chemodectoma with radionuclide scintiangiography. Arch Otolaryngol 1980; 106: 547–52.

901 O'Callaghan J, Timperley WR, Ward P. The CT scan and subtraction angiography in chemodectomas. Clin Radiol 1979; 30: 575–80.

902 Shamblin WR, ReMine WH, Sheps SG, Harrison EG. Carotid body tumors (chemodectomas): clinicopathologic analysis of ninety cases. Am J Surg 1971; 122: 732–9.

903 Poster DS, Schapiro H, Woronoff R. Chemodectomas: review and report of nine cases. J Med 1979; 10: 207–23.

904 Lees CD, Levine HL, Bevin EG, Tucker HM. Tumors of the carotid body: experience with 41 operative cases. Am J Surg 1981; 142: 362–5.

905 Farr HW. Carotid body tumors: a 40-year study. CA 1980; 30: 260–5.

906 Peters JL, Ward MW, Fisher C. Diagnosis of a carotid body chemodectoma with dynamic radionuclide perfusion scanning. Am J Surg 1979; 137: 661–4.

907 Krupski WC, Effeney DJ, Ehrenfeld WK, Stoney RJ. Cervical chemodectoma: technical considerations and management options. Am J Surg 1982; 144: 215–20.

908 Willis RA. Some uncommon and recently identified tumors. In: Collins DH ed Modern Trends in Pathology. London: Butterworth, 1959: 106–31.

909 Budzilovich GN. Granular cell 'myoblastoma' of vagus nerve. Acta Neuropathol 1968; 10: 162–5.

910 Fisher ER, Wechsler H. Granular cell myoblastoma—a misnomer. Electron microscopic and histochemical evidence concerning its Schwann cell derivation and nature (granular cell schwannoma). Cancer 1962; 15: 936–54.

911 Armin A, Connelly EM, Rowden G. An immunoperoxidase investigation of S-100 pro-

tein in granular cell myoblastomas: evidence for Schwann cell derivation. Am J Clin Pathol 1983; 79: 37–44.

912 Bedetti CD, Martinez AJ, Beckford NS, May M. Granular cell tumor arising in myelinated peripheral nerves. Light and electron microscopy and immunoperoxidase study. Virchows Arch (A) 1983; 402: 175–83.

913 Mukai M. Immunohistochemical localization of S-100 protein and peripheral nerve myelin protein (P2 protein, PO protein) in granular cell tumor. Am J Pathol 1983; 112: 139–46.

914 Seo IS, Azzarelli B, Warner TF, Goheen MP, Senteneve GE. Multiple visceral and cutaneous granular cell tumors. Ultrastructural and immunocytochemical evidence of Schwann cell origin. Cancer 1984; 53: 2014–10.

915 Markesbery WR, Duffy PE, Cowen D. Granular cell tumors of the central nervous system. J Neuropathol Exp Neurol 1973; 32: 92–109.

916 Burkhardt BR, Soule EH, Winkelman RK, Ivins JL. Dermatofibrosarcoma protuberans. Study of 56 cases. Am J Surg 1966; 111: 638–44.

917 Bednar B. Storiform neurofibromas of the skin, pigmented and non-pigmented. Cancer 1957; 10: 368–76.

918 Fox H, Emery JL, Goodbody RA, Yates PO. Neurocutaneous melanosis. Arch Dis Child 1964; 39: 508–16.

919 Faillace WJ, Okawara S-H, McDonald JV. Neurocutaneous melanosis with extensive intracerebral and spinal cord involvement. J Neurosurg 1984; 61: 782–5.

920 Leaney BJ, Rowe PW, Klug GL. Neurocutaneous melanosis with hydrocephalus and syringomyelia. J Neurosurg 1985; 62: 148–52.

921 Hoffman HJ, Freeman A. Primary malignant leptomeningeal melanoma in association with giant hairy nevi. Report of two cases. J Neurosurg 1967; 26: 62–71.

922 Bressler J, Smith BH, Kornblith PL. Tissue culture techniques in the study of human gliomas. In: Wilkins RH, Rengachary SS, eds Neurosurgery. New York: McGraw-Hill, 1985: 542–8.

923 Bigner DD, Bigner SH, Ponten J, Westermark B, Mahaley MS Jr, Ruoslahti E, Herschman H, Eng LF, Wickstrand CJ. Heterogeneity of genotypic and phenotypic characteristics of fifteen permanent cell lines derived from human gliomas. J Neuropathol Exp Neurol 1981; 40: 201–29.

924 Rosenblum ML, Gerosa MA, Wilson CB, Barger GR, Pertuiset BF, de Tribolet N, Dougherty DV. Stem cell studies of human malignant brain tumors. Part 1: Development of the stem cell assay and its potential. J Neurosurg 1983; 58: 170–6.

925 Black P McL, Kornblith PL. Biophysical properties of human astrocytic brain tumor cells in cell culture. J Cell Physiol 1980; 105: 565–70.

926 Kornblith PL. Role of tissue culture in prediction of malignancy. Clin Neurosurg 1978; 25: 346–76.

927 Brdar B. Induction of plasminogen activator by alkylating agents in a repair defective human glioblastoma cell strain. Cancer Res 1986; 46: 2282–4.

928 Kornblith PL, Smith BH, Leonard LA. Response of cultured human brain tumors to nitrosoureas: correlation with clinical data. Cancer 1981; 47: 255–65.

929 Kimmel DW, Shapiro JR. In vitro drug sensitivity testing in human gliomas. Review Article. J Neurosurg 1987; 66: 161–71.

930 Lee Y, Bigner DD. Aspects of immunobiology and immunotherapy and uses of monoclonal antibodies and biological immune modifiers in human gliomas. Neurol Clin 1985; 4: 901–17.

931 Gullotta F, Schindler F, Schmutzler R, Weeks-Seifert A. GFAP in brain tumor diagnosis: possibilities and limitations. Pathol Res Pract 1985; 180: 54–60.

932 Bourdon MA, Wikstrand CJ, Furthmayr H, Matthews TJ, Bigner DD. Human glioma-mesenchymal extracellular matrix antigen defined by monoclonal antibody. Cancer Res 1983; 43: 2796–805.

933 Phillips J, Alderson T, Sikora K, Watson J. Localization of malignant glioma by a radiolabelled human monoclonal antibody. J Neurol Neurosurg Psychiatry 1983; 46: 388–92.

934 Bonnin JM, Rubinstein LJ. Immunohistochemistry of central nervous system tumors. Its contribution to neurosurgical diagnosis. J Neurosurg 1984; 60: 1121–33.

935 McLendon RE, Vick WW, Bigner SH, Bigner DD. The application of monoclonal antibodies to the In Vitro diagnosis of brain neoplasms. In: Kupchik HZ ed In Vitro Diagnosis of Human Tumors Using Monoclonal Antibodies. New York: Marcel Dekker (in press).

936 Frankel AE, Houston LL, Issell BF, Fathman. Prospects for immunotoxin therapy in cancer. Ann Rev Med 1986; 37: 125–42.

937 Weil-Hillman G, Uekun FM, Manske JM, Vallera DA. Combined immunochemotherapy of human solid tumors in nude mice. Cancer Res 1987; 47: 579–85.

938 Jacobs SK, Wilson DJ, Kornblith PL, Grimm EA. Interleukin-2 and autologous lymphokine-

activated killer cells in the treatment of malignant glioma. J Neurosurg 1986; 64: 743–9.

939 Klein G, Klein E. Evolution of tumors and the impact of molecular oncology. Review article. Nature 1985; 315: 190–5.

940 Scott RE, Wille JJ Jr. Mechanism for the initiation and promotion of carcinogenesis: a review and a new concept. Mayo Clin Proc 1984; 59: 107–17.

941 Bishop MJ. The molecular genetics of cancer. Science 1987; 235: 305–11.

942 Buick RN, Pollak MN. Perspective on clonogenic tumor cells, stem cells and oncogenes. Cancer Res 1984; 44: 4909–18.

943 Kingler KW, Bigner SH, Bigner DD, Trent JM, Law ML, O'Brien SJ, Wong AJ, Vogelstein B. Identification of an amplified, highly expressed gene in a human glioma. Science 1987; 236: 70–3.

944 Bullard DE, Bigner SH, Bigner DD. The morphologic response of cell lines derived from human gliomas to dibutyryl adenosine 3′:5′-cyclic monophosphate. J Neuropathol Exp Neurol 1981; 40: 231–46.

945 Kruh J. Effects of sodium butyrate, a new pharmacological agent, on cells in culture. Molec Cell Biochem 1982; 42: 65–82.

946 Schneider FH. Effects of sodium butyrate on mouse neuroblastoma cells in culture. Biochem Pharmacol 1976; 25: 2309–17.

947 Kumar S, Weingarten DP, Callahan JW, Sachar K, de Vellis J. Regulation of RNAs for three enzymes in the glial cell model C6 cell line. J Neurochem 1984; 43: 1455–63.

948 Vinores SA, Perez-Polo JR. Nerve growth factor and neural oncology. J Neurosci Res 1983; 9: 81–100.

949 Pantazis P, Pelicci PG, Dalla-Favera R, Antoniades HN. Synthesis and secretion of proteins resembling platelet-derived growth factor by human glioblastoma and fibrosarcoma cells in culture. Proc Natl Acad Sci 1985; 82: 2404–8.

950 Miyagami M, Smith BH, McKeever PE, Chronwall BM, Greenwood MA, Kornblith PL. Immunocytochemical localization of factor VIII-related antigen in tumors of the human central nervous system. J Neuro-Oncol 1987; 4: 269–85.

Textbook of Uncommon Cancer
Edited by C.J. Williams, J.G. Krikorian, M.R. Green and D. Raghavan
© 1988 John Wiley & Sons Ltd

Chapter **30**

Esthesioneuroblastoma

F. Marc Stewart,*
Henry F. Frierson,†
Paul A. Levine‡ and
Cynthia A. Spaulding§

*Assistant Professor of Medicine, University of Virginia School of Medicine, Charolottesville, Virginia, USA, †Assistant Professor of Pathology, University of Virginia School of Medicine, Charolottesville, Virginia, USA, ‡Vice Chairman, Otolaryngology Head and Neck Surgery Department, Associate Professor of Surgery, University of Virginia School of Medicine, Charlottesville, Virginia, USA and §Assistant Professor of Radiology, Department of Radiotherapy, University of Virginia School of Medicine, Charlottesville, Virginia, USA

HISTORY

Esthesioneuroblastoma is an uncommon neoplasm arising from the nasal-olfactory epithelium high in the nasal cavity and bears histopathologic resemblance to neuroblastomas from other sites. The French physician Berger first described this tumor in 1924 as 'l'esthésioneuroépithéliome olfactif' (1) and later in 1951 Schall and Lineback reported the same tumor in the United States (2). From these early observations, pathologists defined a variety of tumor subtypes based on the presence or absence of rosettes and type of rosettes. As a result, other terms reflecting these features have been used to describe this tumor including esthesioneurocytoma, olfactory neuroblastoma, olfactory neuroneoplasm, olfactory esthesioneuroblastoma, and esthesioneuroepithelioma (1, 3, 4). However, these terms have had little practical usefulness for predicting prognosis or patterns of spread. Esthesio-

neuroblastoma is the most widely accepted term used by otolaryngology head and neck surgeons while olfactory neuroblastoma is used more commonly by surgical pathologists.

Esthesioneuroblastoma has become recognized increasingly by surgical pathologists with over 200 cases now reported. Obert et al., in 1960, summarized the important light microscopic features which form the basis for our current histopathologic diagnostic criteria (4). In 1966 Skolnik et al. reported the first major clinical review of the world literature for cases described from 1924 to 1966 (5). Reviews by Cantrell et al. (6), Shah and Feghali (7) and Elkon et al. (8) have described the natural history of esthesioneuroblastoma and reported more recent treatment results with surgery and radiation therapy. In 1976 Kadish et al. (9) proposed a staging classification for esthesioneuroblastoma based on extent of disease. Homzie and Elkon (10) in 1980 made an extensive analysis of important prognostic factors in patients with esthesioneuroblastomas. Wade et al., in 1984, reviewed the role of chemotherapy in esthesioneuroblastoma (11) and O'Conor et al. reported the first use of high dose chemotherapy and autologous bone marrow transplantation in a patient with refractory tumor who subsequently achieved a 5-year disease-free survival (12).

From the knowledge and experienced gained over the past 30 years a general approach to esthesioneuroblastoma has emerged. In the evaluation of nasal cavity tumors, a careful review of the pathology with consideration of important differential diagnoses is essential prior to confirming the presence of an esthesioneuroblastoma. Treatment is based on the extent of disease present at diagnosis and, although late relapses may occur even after 5 to 10 years, cure may be possible in a large number of patients who present with early stage disease. Most investigators agree that proper use of therapeutic modalities including surgery, radiation therapy and in advanced disease, chemotherapy, is required to achieve long-term control of the disease.

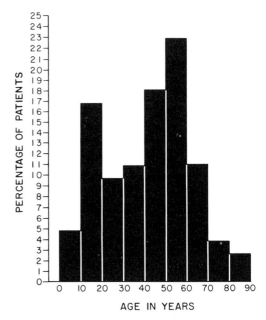

Figure 1 Age distribution of 97 patients with esthesioneuroblastoma. (*Reproduced with permission from Elkon et al (8)* (p.1089, Figure 1).)

EPIDEMIOLOGY AND ETIOLOGY

Epidemiology

Esthesioneuroblastoma is a very rare tumor. Data from the Los Angeles County Cancer Surveillance Program over 10 years identified 13 cases with an average of 1–2 incident cases per year in a population of 7 000 000 people (13). The tumor comprises about 3% of nasal fossa tumors when nasal polyps are excluded. In a major review of thirteen series with a total of 97 patients, Elkon et al. noted a slight male predominance (54% vs 46%) (8). The age incidence showed a bimodal distribution with a peak in the age group of 11–20 years and a second higher peak in the age group 51–60 years (Figure 1). Although the disease has been reported in patients as young as 3 years (14) and as old as 88 years (15), the tumor is

unusual in patients less than age 10 or older than age 70.

Etiology

No specific causative agents have been identified in humans. Data for occupation and industry exposure at diagnosis were available for 10 patients in one series, but no common predisposing etiologic factors were found (13). Esthesioneuroblastoma may be induced in Syrian hamsters by administering nitrosodiethylamine systemically (16). The mechanism of tumor induction in this model is unknown. No hereditary patterns have been described for this tumor.

PATHOLOGY

Esthesioneuroblastoma arises as a polypoid, fleshy mass in the portion of the nasal cavity lined by olfactory mucosa. This sensory mucosa is confined largely to the upper one-third of the nasal septum, the superior turbi-

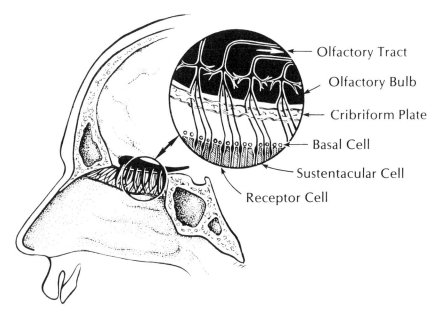

Olfactory Tract

Olfactory Bulb

Cribriform Plate

Basal Cell

Sustentacular Cell

Receptor Cell

Figure 2 Anatomy of the nasal olfactory region.

nate, and the cribriform plate (17). It is composed of sensory receptor cells, sustentacular cells, and basal cells (Figure 2). The olfactory receptor cells lie between the sustentacular cells and their cytoplasmic processes emerge to form the olfactory nerves, which penetrate the cribriform plate, eventually reaching the olfactory bulb. In adults, the olfactory epithelium undergoes degeneration with replacement of respiratory epithelium (17). The zonal distribution of sustentacular, sensory receptor, and basal cells is disrupted with depletion of the receptor and sustentacular cells.

Microscopically, esthesioneuroblastoma is readily recognized when there are intercellular fibrils and Homer Wright rosettes (4, 18). Either the presence of an intercellular fibrillary background or Homer Wright rosettes in a sinonasal neoplasm is diagnostic for esthesioneuroblastoma. Formerly, esthesioneuroblastomas were classified according to the presence or absence of rosettes and the type of rosette (19, 20). Neuroepitheliomas contained Flexner rosettes (a round cluster of cells surrounding a central avascular lumen), neuroblastomas had Homer Wright rosettes (an

annular array of cells around a central zone of eosinophilic fibrils), and neurocytomas lacked rosettes. Such designations were abandoned when subsequent data showed a lack of correlation between morphologic features and prognosis (21–24). Flexner rosettes, uncommonly observed in esthesioneuroblastoma, were not identified in any of the 21 neoplasms studied by Mills and Frierson (18). Well-formed Homer Wright rosettes were only identified in approximately one-third of their cases (18). Perivascular pseudo-rosettes may be found in esthesioneuroblastoma, but they are a completely nonspecific finding and are not helpful for diagnosis.

The most common histologic feature necessary for the diagnosis of esthesioneuroblastoma is the presence of intercellular fibrils. A fibrillary background is usually conspicuous in hematoxylin and eosin-stained sections, but may be enhanced with staining techniques for neuronal cell processes (18). The cells are arranged in discrete nests and are separated by thin or wide bands of fibrovascular tissue or edematous stroma (Figure 3). Occasionally, a diffuse pattern may be present and tumors forming both nests and sheets of cells are not

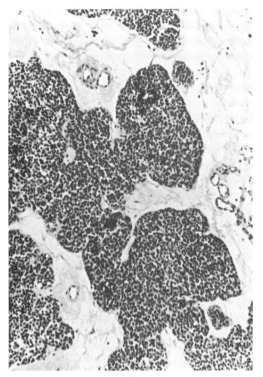

Figure 3 Esthesioneuroblastoma is composed of interconnecting nests of cells separated by bands of fibrovascular tissue (courtesy of D.J. Innes).

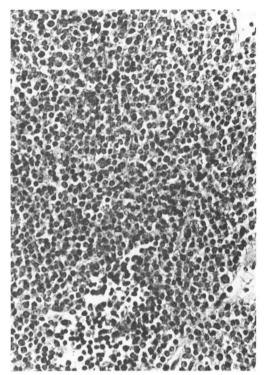

Figure 4 The cells of esthesioneuroblastoma typically have small uniform nuclei and scant cytoplasm. The diagnosis is secure when intercellular fibrils or Homer Wright rosettes are observed (courtesy of D.J. Innes).

uncommon. The cells typically have small to medium-sized, round hyperchromatic nuclei with uniform chromatin and inconspicuous nucleoli (Figure 4). Nuclear pleomorphism may be variable, but is usually minimal. The cytoplasm is generally scant. The mitotic rate, although variable, is often low. Ganglion cells are rarely observed (25), but were noted in 15% of cases in one study (18). Vascular invasion occurs in approximately half of the cases (18) and focal or, occasionally, larger areas of necrosis may be present. Argyrophilic cells may be seen after staining with one of several silver techniques; however, only a few scattered, weakly positive cells are characteristically identified. Rare examples of pigmented esthesioneuroblastoma (26) and esthesioneuroblastomas with glandular or squamous differentiation have been reported (25, 27).

Most authors who have examined various microscopic features of esthesioneuroblastoma agree that such features do not correlate with prognosis (18, 21–24). Hyams (28), however, developed a grading system for esthesioneuroblastoma and found that the prognosis correlated with the assigned grade. Histologic features that were evaluated included architectural pattern, mitotic activity, nuclear pleomorphism, fibrillary matrix, rosettes, and necrosis. None of 7 Grade I neoplasms were fatal, but 3 of 29 patients with Grade II, 6 of 11 with Grade III, and each of 4 patients with Grade IV tumors died of disease. The findings from this study have not been confirmed and there has not been universal acceptance of this grading scheme.

Electron microscopy and immunoperoxidase techniques are often helpful for the diag-

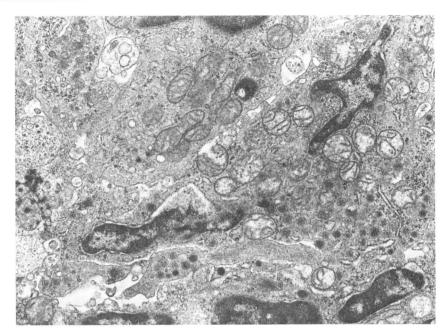

Figure 5 Ultrastructurally, esthesioneuroblastoma contains cell processes, cytoplasmic filaments, and dense-core granules. Uranyl aetate and lead citrate, original
magnification: ×20 000.

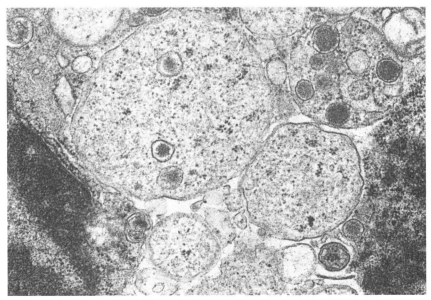

Figure 6 Membrane-bound granules located in transverse sections of cell processes
have central dense cores surrounded by clear spaces or 'halos'. Uranyl acetate and
lead citrate, original magnification: ×38 000.

nosis of a poorly differentiated sinonasal tumor, including poorly differentiated examples of esthesioneuroblastoma. Ultrastructurally, esthesioneuroblastoma contains dense-core neurosecretory granules, dendritic cell processes, filaments, and microtubules (Figures 5 and 6) (29–34). Neurosecretory granules and cell processes are usually abundant and only one grid is often sufficient for their identification (34). Schwann cell differentiation has also been identified ultrastructurally (25, 33–35). Immunocytochemically, esthesioneuroblastoma is marked with antibodies to neuronspecific enolase (34–36) and often with antibodies to S-100 protein (34, 35). S-100 protein, although nonspecific, identifies Schwann cells that are present singly at the periphery of cell nests. Occasionally, esthesioneuroblastoma may be immunoreactive with antikeratin (27, 34, 36) or antineurofilament antibodies (34, 37). Sometimes both cytokeratin and neurofilament will be expressed in the same neoplasm (34).

Formaldehyde-fume-induced fluorescence, a method to identify membrane-bound granules containing biogenic amines, has been noted in esthesioneuroblastoma (25, 38, 39), but this technique is nonspecific and is used rarely for diagnostic confirmation. A few esthesioneuroblastomas have been shown to contain dopamine-beta-hydroxylase, norepinephrine, and vasopressin (38, 40). In contrast to adrenal neuroblastoma, assays of urinary catecholamines are not markedly abnormal in patients with olfactory tumors (33).

Esthesioneuroblastoma, at times, may be difficult to distinguish microscopically from other poorly differentiated sinonasal neoplasms. Such neoplasms include lymphoma, melanoma, rhabdomyosarcoma, and sinonasal undifferentiated carcinoma (41). Sinonasal lymphoma forms sheets of noncohesive lymphoid cells without intervening stroma. Multiple paranasal sinuses are often involved but the cribriform plate is spared (42). Immunohistochemical stains and Southern blot hybridization studies for immunoglobulin and T-cell receptor gene rearrangements may be useful for the diagnosis of sinonasal lymphoreticular neoplasms. The diagnosis of sinonasal melanoma is secure when melanin pigment is observed. In amelanotic tumors, the presence of junctional melanocytic change and cells with eosinophilic cytoplasm and prominent nucleoli suggest the diagnosis. A Fontana stain is helpful to identify small amounts of pigment that may not be detected in hematoxylin and eosin-stained sections. Premelanosomes may be observed ultrastructurally. Also, melanoma typically is strongly immunoreactive for S-100 protein. Rhabdomyosarcoma should be considered in the differential diagnosis of a poorly differentiated sinonasal neoplasm in a child with a malignant nasal tumor. In some instances, electron microscopy and immunocytochemistry may be helpful for diagnosis. Finally, esthesioneuroblastoma must be distinguished from sinonasal undifferentiated carcinoma (41), a more aggressive neoplasm that also arises from the superior portion of the nasal cavity. Unlike undifferentiated carcinoma, esthesioneuroblastoma less often shows orbital encroachment and cranial nerve involvement at initial diagnosis. A high mitotic rate, tumor necrosis, and extensive vascular invasion are characteristic for sinonasal undifferentiated carcinoma. This neoplasm can be distinguished from esthesioneuroblastoma by its lack of Homer–Wright rosettes and the absence of an intercellular fibrillary background.

CLINICAL FEATURES

Patients initially present with nasal symptoms, most frequently unilateral nasal obstruction and epistaxis. Other symptoms such as rhinorrhea and anosmia may be noted. These symptoms may have been present for long periods prior to diagnosis (6). Perforation into the subarachnoid space infrequently may occur leading to cerebrospinal fluid (CSF) rhinorrhea, distinguished from other nasal secretions by its clear watery nature and high glucose content. Headache often correlates with intracranial involvement. Over one-half of patients in one series of 38 cases presented with symptoms referable to the orbit such as tearing, periorbital pain, decreased vision (blurring), and diplopia. Proptosis, eyelid edema, globe injection, and cranial nerve palsies were noted less frequently (43).

Not uncommonly, the initial clinical diagnosis is incorrect with nasal carcinoma, nasal polyps, benign nasal mass, and sinusitis suspected (43). The differential diagnosis of a nasal tumor also includes lymphoma, rhabdomyosarcoma, melanoma, lymphoepithelioma, squamous cell carinom, sinonasal undifferentiated carcinoma and metastatic carcinoma, particularly renal cell carcinoma.

Physical examination reveals a pink, fleshy, polypoid mass in the nasal cavity. Its friability results in a tendency to bleed when touched and adequate vasoconstriction is necessary to allow full examination of the nose and nasopharynx. Biopsy may result in excessive bleeding and one should be prepared to pack the nose, particularly if the biopsy is performed in an outpatient setting. For nasal cavity masses preservation of a portion of tissue in glutaraldehyde allows electron microscopy to be used should difficulty arise in establishing a diagnosis. Cervical lymph node metastases occur in 10% of cases. Distant disease is unusual at presentation, but may occur subsequently at the time of relapse in bone, bone marrow, lung, or skin. A careful evaluation for areas of bony tenderness and subcutaneous nodules should be performed prior to surgery.

INVESTIGATION AND STAGING

The laboratory evaluation should include a complete blood count and differential count. Unexplained cytopenias should prompt a bone marrow aspiration and biopsy. Also, on differential cell count nucleated red blood cells with a shift toward immature white cells (leukoerythroblastic smear) may suggest bone marrow involvement. Abnormalities of screening chemistries including SGOT, SGPT, lactate dehydrogenase, and alkaline phosphatase require a search for metastatic disease.

Radiologic examination includes a routine chest x-ray to exclude the unusual occurrence of lung metastases and plain films of the paranasal sinuses which may show involvement of the ethmoid, maxillary or sphenoid sinuses with bony destruction. The use of computed tomography (CT) with or without magnetic resonance imaging (MRI) to further define the primary lesion is indicated in every patient. CT scanning usually delineates a well circumscribed mass that enhances after contrast medium injection (Figure 7). Intracranial involvement, which may occur eventually in up to 20%, may be detected either as locoregional extension through the cribriform plate or, less commonly, as metastatic disease. Differentiation of tumor extension from secondary obstruction and sinusitis may be difficult. Opacification of the ethmoid sinuses, maxillary antrum, and nasal fossae, are nonspecific, but frequent findings (14). However, bony destruction identified by CT scanning strongly favors tumor extension (44). An additional role for CT or MRI scanning is its use in the therapeutic management of the patient, for example, by radiotherapists to plan treatment portals, or by otolaryngology head and neck surgeons and neurosurgeons to determine operability and plan surgery. Preoperative assessment by CT scan is accurate in determining disease extent; however, two cases of extension along the olfactory nerve requiring neurosurgical intervention have been reported which CT scans failed to identify (45). Finally, CT scanning is useful for all physicians of multimodality specialties to assess response to treatment (Figure 7). MRI (Figure 8) is an alternative or supplement to CT scanning (46). Although MRI scanning provides excellent visualization of soft tissue structures, its advantage for optimal differentiation between tumor invasion into sinuses and fluid retention due to tumor compression of the sinus orifices needs to be established.

For the evaluation of a nasal tumor CT scanning is recommended as an initial study since it provides more accurate information about bony involvement than MRI. If the

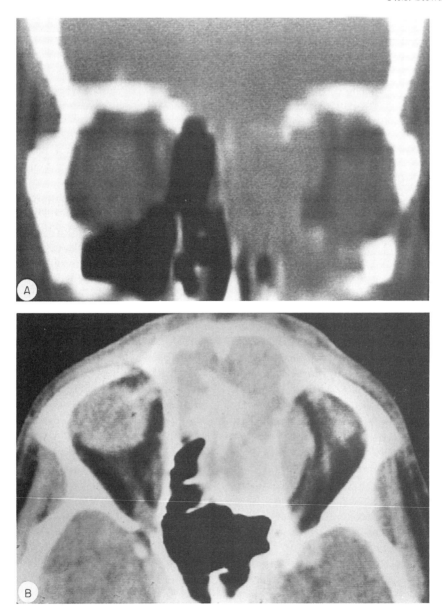

Figure 7A, B CT scan demonstrates esthesioneuroblastoma involving ethmoid sinus with extension to the right orbit.

cribriform plate and other sinus bones are intact, no further studies are indicated. If erosion of the cribriform plate or other bony sites by tumor is observed, MRI scanning may give a more accurate assessment of soft tissue extent into the brain (47) or other vascular structures (Figure 8). Angiography has been used to complement the preoperative CT scan particularly when intracranial involvement is noted and further delineation of the tumor and blood supply is required.

Due to the rarity of this tumor, no single institution has enough experience to make conclusions about factors influencing prog-

TABLE 1 ESTHESIONEUROBLASTOMA: STAGING

A. Tumor confine to the nasal cavity
B. Tumor involving the nasal cavity and paranasal sinuses
C. Tumor spread beyond the nasal cavity and paranasal sinuses including intracranial and/or orbital extension, lymph node and other distant metastases

---

Adapted from Kadish et al. (9)

nosis. Correlations between extent of local involvement, or the presence or absence of metastatic disease, with disease-free survival form the basis for published staging systems. Based on a study of 17 patients, Kadish et al. in 1976 proposed the system (Table 1) most commonly referred to by otolaryngology head and neck surgeons (9). In the series of 97 patients Elkon et al. reported 30% had Stage A disease, 42% had Stage B disease, and 28% had Stage C disease (8). Five-year survival rates for patients receiving treatment were 75% for Stage A, 60% for Stage B, and 41% for Stage C (Table 2). Other prognostic factors have been reviewed. In a multivariate analysis Homzie and Elkon reviewed 113 patients from two series (10). Factors found to predict a poor outcome (disease-free survival less than 3 years) included intracranial tumor extension, lymph node involvement, orbital extension, and ethmoid sinus extension. No patient who remained disease-free for greater than 3 years had more than two sites of local tumor involvement at diagnosis. Extension to the maxillary antrum or sphenoid sinus was not found to be an adverse prognostic factor. The presence of metastatic disease was associated significantly

with an inability to achieve a 3-year disease-free survival. However, the absence of metastatic disease did not correlate with disease-free status at 3 years. Furthermore, the presence of disease after treatment failure did not necessarily portend an immediate poor prognosis. Eight of 62 patients were reported alive with disease for 3, 4, 7, 7, 8, 10, 20, and 20 years and 2 of these patients had metastatic disease remaining alive with disease at 4 and 8 years (10).

Finally, patients over age 60 had a 29% 3-year disease-free survival rate compared with 53% for patients aged 60 or less (10).

MANAGEMENT

Overview

The treatment of esthesioneuroblastoma is a multidisciplinary endeavor which requires the expertise of the otolaryngology head and neck surgeon, neurosurgeon, radiation oncologist, and medical oncologist. Close collaboration with the pathologist and diagnostic radiologist is essential. Treatment with a curative intent is advised in all cases, although achievement of this goal is much less likely in the face of metastatic disease or multiple local recurrences. Nevertheless, as noted above, even patients with metastatic tumor or extensive local tumor occasionally may live years with stable or slowly progressive disease (10).

The optimal treatment for esthesioneuroblastoma remains controversial. Some authors recommend radiotherapy or surgery alone for early stage disease, reserving the alternative

TABLE 2 CRUDE AND DETERMINATE SURVIVAL RATES
(reproduced with permission from Elkon et al. (8)
p. 1093 Table 8)

Stage	Crude 3-year survival			Crude 5-year survival		
A	16/18	88.9%	(94.1%)[a]	9/12	75%	(90.0%)
B	25/30	83.3%	(83.3%)	17/25	60%	(70.8%)
C	9/17	52.9%	(56.3%)	7/17	41.2%	(46.7%)

[a]Determinant survival in parentheses.

modality as salvage therapy for treatment failures (5, 8). Others prefer a combined modality approach with radiotherapy and surgery as initial therapy. In series published to date, comparison of the diverse treatment options for each of the three stages of disease is difficult due to the small numbers of patients in each subgroup. As might be anticipated with an unusual tumor, no prospective controlled studies have been done and absolute conclusions regarding therapy cannot be made.

Skolnik et al. reviewed the 97 cases reported in the literature up to 1966. They found an advantage in 5-year survival rates for patients treated with surgery (64%) as compared with radiotherapy (38%). Patients receiving combined therapy had more advanced disease with a 50% 5-year survival (5). In 1979 Elkon et al. reviewed the patients in the literature subsequent to 1966 (8). He noted that for both Stage A and B disease, single modality therapy with alternative modality salvage treatment at the time of relapse was equivalent to a combined modality approach. For Stage C disease, combined modality therapy with radiation and surgery provided the best results (Table 3).

Thirty patients with esthesioneuroblastoma have been treated at the University of Virginia from 1959 through 1986. Over this time period there has been a gradual evolution of treatment policy and technique, with the introduction of craniofacial resections (1976) and complex field megavoltage radiation in the initiation of treatment with chemotherapy, prior to radiotherapy and surgery (1979).

Twenty-five patients were available for analysis after a 2-year minimum follow-up. The majority were treated with radiotherapy (50 Gy) followed 4 to 6 weeks later by surgery; however, 4 patients were treated with palliative intent without surgery. Chemotherapy, cyclophosphamide and vincristine, was given prior to radiotherapy in the 5 patients with Stage C disease treated since 1978. Overall 2- and 5-year determinate survival rates were

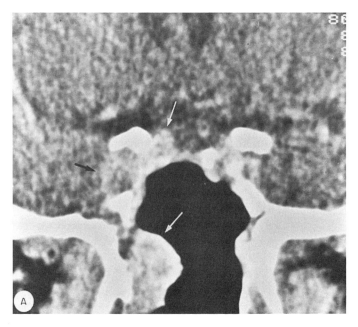

Figure 8A CT scan demonstrates tumor adherent to the lateral nasopharyngeal wall.

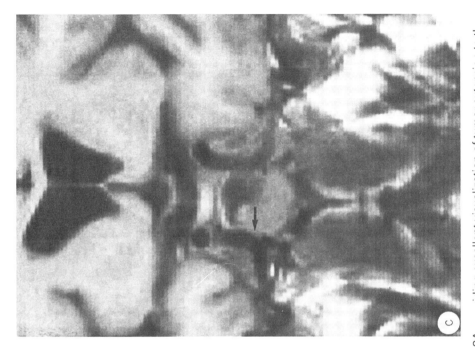

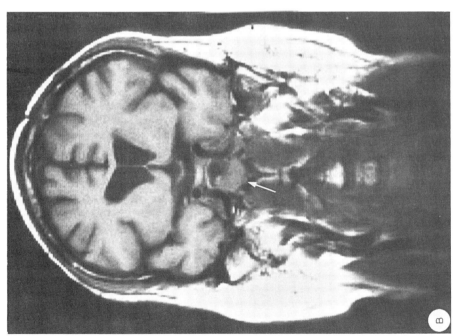

Figure 8B, C MRI scans of same region as that shown in Figure 8A, providing excellent visualization of tumor extension to the left carotid siphon.

TABLE 3 RESULTS OF TREATMENT BY MODALITY AND STAGE: 78 CASES WITH 6 MONTHS TO 32 YEARS
FOLLOW-UP (reproduced with permission from Elkon et al. (8) p. 1092, Table 6)

Modality	Stage A			Stage B			Stage C		
	Initial treatment	For recurrence	Total control rate	Initial treatment	For recurrence	Total control rate	Initial treatment	For recurrence	Total Control rate
Radiotherapy alone	2/5	5/5	70%	4/7	3/4	64%	1/5	1/1	33%
Surgery alone	5/9	4/4	69%	3/6	1/2	50%	1/1	—	—
Radiotherapy and surgery	7/10	—	70%	12/20	0/1	57%	7/15	—	47%

80% (20/25) and 61% (11/18) respectively. Two-year determinate survival rates by stage were 100% (1/1) for Stage A, 83% (10/12) for Stage B, and 75% (9/12) for Stage C disease. For Stage C disease, there was a definite trend towards increased overall survival with aggressive modern therapy 2-year determinate survival rates of 50% (2/4) from 1959 through 1975 versus 88% (7/8) from 1976 through 1985, although relapses were not circumvented. Excluding 1 Stage C patient who died with persistent disease several days after surgery, 58% (14/24) of patients failed initial therapy. Thirty-three per cent (4/12) of Stage B and 91% (10/11) of Stage C patients relapsed. With more aggressive initial therapy, isolated relapses were in primary, nodal, or metastatic sites, as opposed to the pattern of predominantly local failures in earlier years, suggesting an improvement in local control. Most relapses presented within 2 years with the longest interval (93 months) between treatment and initial recurrence occurring in a patient with Stage C disease treated with radiotherapy and craniofacial resection. Multiple relapses with temporary salvage were not uncommon. Salvage therapy has an important role in prolonging survival in this disease. Five recurrences were salvaged for a period of 29 to 96 months, with 2 of these patients still disease-free at 65 and 68 months. An aggressive approach to salvage, which in our experience has included surgery, radiotherapy, or chemo-therapy (with bone marrow transplantation in 1 case) appears worthwhile.

Surgery

A neurosurgical consultation should be obtained in every case since occasionally pre-operative CT scans fail to identify extension along the olfactory nerve and into the cribriform plate and brain (46). Since the tumor often extends into the cribriform plate; orbital apex, or sphenoid sinus, in the past surgical management has been quite difficult.

The most significant advance in surgery for esthesioneuroblastoma has been the development of the craniofacial resection. From past experience, the head and neck surgeon has recognized that the limiting factor for tumor excision using the lateral rhinotomy approach (48), was the inability to remove tumor extending into the cribriform plate and anterior cranial fossa (49, 50). Previously, the lateral rhinotomy with ethmoidectomy and maxillectomy has been associated with a high rate of local recurrence. The supraorbital rim approach provides excellent exposure of the anterior cranial fossa, cribriform plate, superior portion of the orbit and ethmoid roof allowing more complete excision of locally advanced nasal tumors (Figure 9). The other important improvement has been the accuracy of the high resolution CT scan and the additional information that is now potentially available with MRI (47).

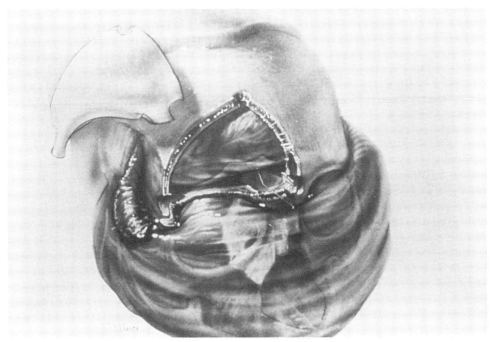

Figure 9 Removal of the bone flap incorporating the supraorbital rim. (*Reproduced with permission from Johns et al.* (*54*) (p. 1138 Figure 4).)

As mentioned earlier, the treatment approach to Kadish Stage A and Stage B disease at the University of Virginia is to treat preoperatively with 50 Gy of radiotherapy, and to Stage C disease, to treat preoperatively with chemotherapy followed by 50 Gy external beam radiation. All three stages have a craniofacial resection performed after a 4 to 6 week respite from their preoperative treatment. The craniofacial resection involves the removal of the cribriform region in conjunction with both ethmoid complexes and all the involved nasal and paranasal sinus structures. On occasion, this may additionally include resection of the dura and small portions of the frontal lobe. We utilize the high resolution CT scan to evaluate the extent of all lesions and the MRI scan to further evaluate those that have erosion of the cribriform plate or intracranial involvement on CT (47).

Due the procedure length, central venous pressure, arterial pressure, esophageal temperature, urine output, and end tidal carbon dioxide are continuously monitored. Additionally, a lumbar subarachnoid drain is paced at the beginning of the procedure and is left in place for 24 to 48 hours to monitor intracranial pressure. This provides easy access for cerebrospinal fluid removal to allow frontal lobe retraction, and to remove cerebrospinal fluid, as needed, in the postoperative period. The patient is then placed supine on the operating room table with the head extended to bring the floor of the anterior cranial fossa in a vertical position. This position is secured in a Mayfield skeletal fixation head holder.

Because the limitation of the craniofacial resection is the extent of intracranial involvement, the neurosurgeon begins the procedure with the exposure and evaluation of the floor of the anterior cranial fossa. A transcoronal incision is used, and skin flaps elevated, preserving the periosteum under the galea. The pericranial flap, based on the supraorbital vessels, is created, to be employed at the end of the case to help seal the separation of cranial cavity and nose (51). The bone flap for the craniotomy stays attached to the temporalis muscle and extends 4 cm in height and 4 cm across the midline.

Two modifications of the standard bone flap have been employed. The first, the supraorbital rim approach described by Jane et al. (52), permits excellent exposure with less frontal lobe retraction (Figure 9). Because of the occasional indentation in the mid-forehead from a burr hole using this technique, a modification of the frontal sinus osteoplastic flap has also been used (53). This permits similar exposure but prevents an anterior midfrontal burr hole depression by creating a bone flap from the front wall of the frontal sinus for bony access.

After the creation of the bone flap, the olfactory nerves are cut, the dura retracted and elevated from the cribriform plate. Because of its many invaginations into the roof of the cribriform plate, clips are applied along these dural extensions before resecting to prevent multiple defects in the dura and a subsequent cerebrospinal fluid leak. If necessary, cerebrospinal fluid is removed via the previously placed lumbar drain to facilitate frontal lobe retraction. If the tumor involves dura or small portions of the frontal lobe, these areas are resected, and the dura is repaired either by primary closure or with a lyophilized dural graft. Chisels or a drill are then used to resect the cribiform plate and ethmoid region from above.

The facial resection then begins after the upper resected area is covered with the appropriate saline soaked dressing. A Weber–Ferguson type incision is used; extension of the incision across the roof of the nose is not mandatory. The osteotomy across the nasal bridge can be made with elevation of the soft tissues but without the incision. The incision can be modified to allow exenteration of the orbital contents, which is rarely performed. The rest of the ethmoidectomy, septectomy, or partial or complete maxillotomy can be performed as necessary through this incision. Once the head and neck surgeon has freed the tumor from all neural, muscular, and bony attachments, the specimen is delivered from below. The specimen usually contains both ethmoid labyrinths with cribriform plate and superior and middle turbinates with upper nasal septum.

The surgical site is then inspected for any suspicious areas. It should be remembered that with this procedure, standard oncologic surgical margins may be difficult to attain. Therefore, what is left in the cavity becomes more important than what is in the surgical specimen.

In our series, the orbital contents have not been sacrificed (53). After the preoperative therapy, the tumor may have to be dissected from the tumor-resistant periorbita, but the eye does not have to be sacrificed unless there is significant neoplastic penetration of this tumor-resistant membrane. Also, neck dissections are not performed for neck disease. Initially, one patient receive a bilateral neck dissection, but since that time, the practice has been to remove the node for diagnosis and irradiate the neck. With the advent of fine needle aspiration cytology, the neck is no longer violated. After fine needle aspiration cytologic confirmation, the neck is then irradiated. Utilizing this technique, we have had no tumor persistence in the neck (53).

After the resection has been completed, the pericranial flap is sutured to cover the midline dura, providing a sling, an additional layer of closure to prevent a cerebrospinal fluid leak, and a satisfactory vascular bed for the skin graft placed intranasally. The epithelial side of the graft is placed on a piece of Gelfoam, the graft and Gelfoam are cut to slightly larger than the size of the defect, and they are held in place with antibiotic ointment impregnated nasal packing for 7 to 10 days. The Gelfoam permits easier handling of the graft intraoperatively and prevents accidental removal when removing the nasal packing. The patient is placed on broad spectrum antibiotic coverage while the packing is in place. The bone flap is then replaced and held in position with stainless steel wire, and the craniotomy and facial wounds are closed in the appropriate layers.

The patient is monitored in an intensive care unit setting for 24 to 48 hours. In most situations, all monitor lines are removed on the second postoperative day, and the packing is removed between the seventh and tenth postoperative days. While the complications may be significant (53), the majority of patients are discharged on the fourteenth postoperative day.

A disadvantage of the supraorbital rim approach is the possible sacrifice of the supraorbital nerve and artery leading to hypalgesia of the forehead. Usually this is transient and often disappears within 6 months (54). In an earlier series of patients with far advanced disease Ketcham et al. reported the complications of craniofacial resection which included meningitis, subdural abscess, cerebrospinal fluid leak, diplopia, and hemorrhage. One-third of patients required intensive care support and prolonged hospitalization with a mortality rate of 4% (50).

The approach defined above has the advantage of obtaining excellent exposure of the tumor both inferiorly and superiorly, less brain retraction than conventional techniques and an excellent cosmetic result.

Radiation Therapy

Esthesioneuroblastomas are both radioresponsive and radiocurable lesions. Evidence for radiosensitivity includes cures with radiotherapy alone in early stage disease, salvage of surgical recurrences by radiotherapy, and the occasional sterilization of surgical specimens following 45 to 50 Gy (55). The recommended dose of radiation in the setting of combined modality therapy is 50 Gy in 25 fractions, although this varies in the literature from 40 to 60 Gy. If the patient has distant metastases at presentation or remains inoperable, the dose of radiation is increased to 60 Gy in 30 fractions. For combined modality therapy, it remains a moot point whether preoperative or postoperative radiotherapy is best. Theoretical advantages of preoperative radiotherapy are the potential of rendering an unresectable lesion resectable, prevention of tumor seeding at surgery, better oxygenation of tissues permitting a lower dose of irradiation, and utilization of a smaller treatment volume, as it is not necessary to encompass the entire surgical field. Potential advantages of postoperative radiotherapy include accurate surgical staging and, although debatable, no interference with wound healing.

In the past, radiation technique was quite rudimentary, consisting of a single anterior beam, usually of conventional x-rays. Today, megavoltage radiotherapy delivered via multiple fields necessitates complex, individualized treatment planning. CT scans before and after chemotherapy are reviewed with the diagnostic radiologist in order to accurately localize the tumor extent. Selected CT cuts, for example, through the orbits, are taken in the treatment position. At the time of simulation and again at dosimetric planning, the target volume is carefully mapped in three dimensions.

The irradiation technique is well described by Million et al. (56). A critical early decision is whether it is possible to spare the eye from the field of irradiation. With extensive orbital involvement, the entire orbit, including the eyeball and lacrimal tissue, is irradiated. When orbital invasion is minimal, it is possible to shield most of the lacrimal gland. In the absence of orbital invasion, the medial one-fourth of the eyeball (1 cm from the medial canthus) is within the high dose volume in order to adequately encompass the ethmoids.

As esthesioneuroblastomas are centrally located tumors, a three-field technique, consisting of an anterior and two lateral wedged fields, usually provides the best dosimetry (Figure 10). This differs from the situation in antral tumors which are more lateralized and can be treated with a wedge pair technique. Due to the anterior location of esthesioneuroblastomas, the anterior field is heavily weighted in a ratio of from 6:1:1 to 8:1:1. The 6 MV linear accelerator is the treatment machine of

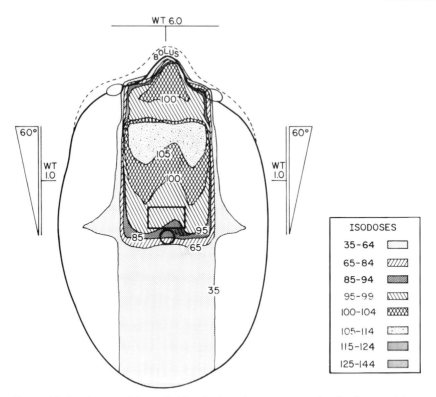

Figure 10 Dosimetry of three-field technique for treatment of esthesioneuroblastoma in the absence of orbital involvement.

choice because of the sharpness of its beam edges. However, bolus is frequently required over the nasal bridge, ethmoids, and orbit (if invaded by tumor), in order to compensate for skin sparing.

In the absence of orbital involvement, the anterior field is rectangular, or, with antral involvement, L-shaped, with a width at eye level of 4 to 5 cm, which covers the ethmoid sinuses adequately without irradiating the lens of either eye. Superiorly the field encompasses the cribriform plate and any intracranial tumor extension, while inferiorly it includes the floor of the nasal cavity. In this situation, the anterior border of the lateral fields is located at the lateral bony canthus and the posterior border will, of course, depend on the tumor extent, but is frequently just anterior to the external auditory canal, ensuring coverage of the sphenoid sinus. Some authors recom-

mend tilting the lateral fields posteriorly by 5 degrees to reduce contralateral eye irradiation, but this may result in dose fall-off anteriorly (56). Thermoluminescent dosimeters are placed over both lenses at the time of the first treatment to directly measure the amount of lens irradiation. If the doses are of concern, lens blocks may be added, providing the tumor dose is not compromised by their addition.

When the orbit is extensively involved with tumor, then no attempt is made to shield the eye. An oblique wedge pair technique is utilized with the addition of a small third field as a boost which compensates for the posterior-medial cold spot from the wedge pair (Figure 11). The anterior field encompasses the ipsilateral orbit as well as the entire ethmoid complex. The anterior border of the lateral field is 1 to 2 cm anterior to the orbit. In the situation where there is only minimal orbital involvement, it may be possible to place a lacrimal gland block without shielding tumor.

Cervical nodal metastases from esthesioneuroblastoma are unusual, but when present, are treated primarily with radiotherapy. Careful attention must be paid to the junction between the primary and neck fields. Tangential neck portals with a midline block is a common technique for this special situation.

Sequelae from radiation for esthesioneuroblastomas consist of skin telangiectases, hair loss, serous otitis media, and nasal synechiae. Cataracts, a serious complication in the past, are now surgically correctable. The major complication is loss of vision after the entire orbit has been irradiated. Parsons has summarized the ophthalmic syndromes after orbital irradiation (57). Irradiation of the entire orbit produces a dry eye with corneal ulceration and opacification, resulting in progressive loss of vision over 6 to 10 months. If the lacrimal gland is spared, blindness may occur secondary to radiation retinopathy after a latent period of 2 to 3 years, but is unusual with doses less than 50 Gy.

In a series of 37 patients with a variety of nasal cavity and ethmoid/sphenoid sinus malignancies treated with radiation therapy, complications reported by Parsons included a transient nervous system syndrome, characterized by headache, lethargy, vertigo, and diminished cerebration lasting 1 to 2 months, noted in 3 patients (56). Lhermitte's syndrome occurred in 2 patients. Other complications included symptomatic sinusitis, nasal synechiae, serous otitis media requiring myringotomy, and bone necrosis. Many of these patients received more than 50 Gy, however.

Radiation therapy in our own experience with esthesioneuroblastoma has resulted in only minor complications, other than the anticipated visual loss in patients in whom the eye could not be shielded. Looking specifically at complications from combined therapy, the review by Newbill et al. of our initial group of cases noted few postoperative sequelae (45). Levine et al. reviewed our more recent experience with aggressive combination therapy and found significant morbidity, including 1 perioperative death, 1 patient with seizures and coma, and 2 patients with infected bone flaps resulting in epidural abscesses (53).

Chemotherapy

The use of chemotherapy for esthesioneuroblastoma evolved naturally from its efficacy in childhood neuroblastomas. In esthesioneuroblastomas chemotherapy has induced significant regression of disease in over 50% of patients treated. In a review of the literature Wade et al. noted objective responses in 8 of 13 patients treated with a variety of different drugs (11). Most responses occurred after a single course but lasted only a short time.

Chemotherapeutic agents which have shown anecdotal single agent activity in esthesioneuroblastoma include cyclophosphamide, vincristine, thiotepa, doxorubicin, dacarbazine (DTIC), and nitrogen mustard (11). Cyclophosphamide and vincristine with or without doxorubicin have been used in combination in several patients.

The experience with childhood neuroblastomas provides a guide for future combination chemotherapy approaches for esthesioneuroblastoma. Information derived from cell kinetic studies have provided the rationale for constructing effective combination chemotherapy regimens in some tumors. The fraction of proliferating cells in disseminated neuroblastoma is approximately 10–15%. Theoretically, a non-phase specific drug such as cyclophosphamide may be used to kill nonproliferating cells and recruit cells into S phase where an S phase specific drug such as doxorubicin may maximize the elimination of cells (58). In 70 Stage IV patients with childhood neuroblastoma treated with cyclophosphamide, 150 mg/m^2, days 1–7, and doxorubicin, 35 mg/m^2, day 8, given every 21 days, a complete response rate of 52% was noted (59). In patients with neuroblastomas resistant to cyclophosphamide and doxorubicin, VM-26, 100 mg/m^2, and cisplatin, 90 mg/m^2, in a 21-day cycle, produced complete responses in 6 of 22 patients (27%) (58).

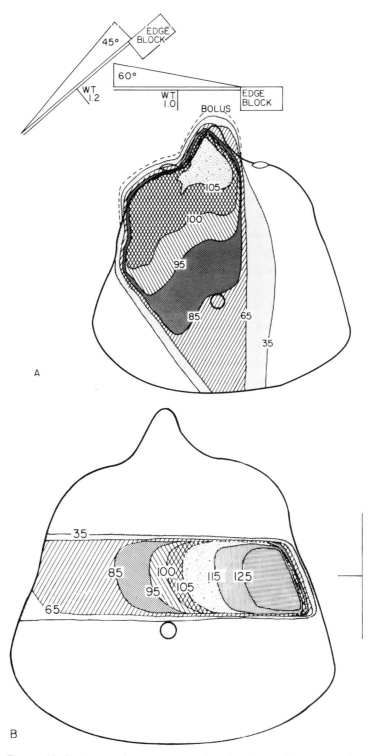

Figure 11 Dosimetry for treatment of esthesioneuroblastoma with extensive orbital involvement. A. Oblique wedge pair (50 Gy to 95% isodose line) with posterior-medial cold spot. B. Single field boost of 4 Gy to compensate for cold spot.

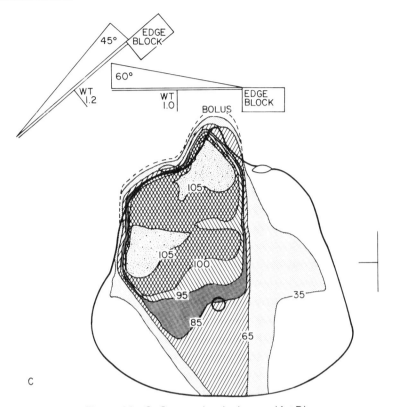

C

Figure 11   C. Composite dosimetry (A+B).

At present we recommend a 28-day cycle of chemotherapy with cyclophosphamide 650 mg/m² intravenously (IV) given on days 1 and 8 and vincristine 1.5 mg/M² IV given on days 1 and 8 for patients with Stage C disease prior to definitive local therapy. Alternatively, we are now exploring a more aggressive regimen given every 21 days which includes on day 1 cyclophosphamide 1000 mg/m² IV, vincristine 1.5 mg/m² IV and doxorubicin 40 mg/m² IV. Serial CT scans are obtained to monitor the response prior to initiation of radiotherapy. Usually after two courses, the CT scan is repeated and if no response or progression is noted, the patient receives radiation therapy. If a significant partial response has been obtained one or two additional courses are administered prior to radiotherapy. Postoperatively, chemotherapy may be given as adjunctive therapy to patients with Stage C disease

who responded to the initial chemotherapy (11).

The toxicity of these regimens is tolerable. Cyclophosphamide and vincristine produce few side-effects in most patients. Mild nausea and vomiting occur 6 to 10 hours after treatment. Transient alopecia and myelosuppression are observed infrequently. Vincristine often causes paresthesias in the extremities and occasionally transient interosseous muscle weakness of the hands, 'foot drop', or ileus. The addition of doxorubicin increases the intensity of nausea and vomiting although this is manageable with aggressive antiemetic therapy. Rare side-effects include a dose dependent risk of cardiac failure, particularly if the total dose exceeds 550 mg/m².

The use of conventional chemotherapy regimens in esthesioneuroblastoma may prove beneficial. However, it is disappointing that chemotherapy has not resulted in more effective prolongation of long-term disease-free survival in children with disseminated neuroblastoma or in children with localized neuroblastoma treated with adjuvant chemotherapy.

Finally, the use of high dose chemotherapy followed by autologous marrow transplantation has been attempted in a number of patients with esthesioneuroblastoma. Four patients who were otherwise refractory to standard chemotherapy and radiation and were considered inoperable, underwent intense therapy with high dose doxorubicin, vinblastine, and cyclophosphamide followed by infusion of previously cryopreserved autologous bone marrow. Two patients achieved a complete remission and one patient with distant intracranial metastases had partial tumor regression. One patient is alive with residual CT scan abnormalities without evidence of progression. Survival times for all 4 patients are $7+$, 9, $11+$, and 60 months. One patient relapsed after 5 years of continuous disease-free survival and underwent a second autologous transplant without tumor regression and died of her disease. The toxicity of this approach is significant with sepsis and moderate to severe mucositis experienced by most patients. In general, intense therapy followed by autologous marrow transplantation is associated with a 10% risk of acute mortality. Accordingly, for treatment of esthesioneuroblastoma, its use at present is limited to patients who fail conventional therapy. The technique is usually limited to patients under the age of 55–60.

Autologous marrow transplantation has been used with some success in childhood neuroblastomas (60). Marrow procured for autologous transplantation usually requires that the marrow show no evidence of tumor involvement after bilateral iliac crest bone marrow aspirations and biopsies. Allogeneic transplantation from an HLA and MLC compatible sibling for esthesioneuroblastoma remains an important alternative for patients with marrow involvement (61). More recently, in vitro techniques to 'clean' neuroblastoma

tumor cells from bone marrow with monoclonal antibodies and complement have been utilized in patients undergoing autologous transplantation. Another technique involves the physical separation of tumor cells from the normal marrow cells. After the addition of anti-neuroblastoma cell monoclonal antibodies such as anti-H-11 and anti-VJ-13A attached to metal colloid particles, the treated marrow is transferred past a magnetic field allowing the retention of malignant cells in the magnetic field and the collection of normal marrow cells which pass through (62, 63). Currently, these techniques may be applied to selected patients with esthesioneuroblastomas who demonstrate minimal bone marrow involvement (63).

SUMMARY

Esthesioneuroblastoma remains a challenging tumor from the standpoint of both diagnosis and treatment. It is deceptively responsive to therapy, yet characterized by late recurrences and deaths. Progress is being made, albeit slowly. While it is difficult to prove from the literature, we recommend radiotherapy combined with surgery for Stage A and B disease, in an effort to provide maximum disease-free survival, as the ultimate salvage rate after recurrence is not high. The addition of chemotherapy to the treatment regimen for Stage C disease appears to delay recurrence and enhance survival, although a longer period of observation would permit a more realistic assessment.

ACKNOWLEDGEMENT

We would like to express appreciation to Lynda James for her excellent secretarial assistance.

REFERENCES

1 Berger L, Luc et Richard. L'esthésioneuroépithéliome olfactif. Bull Assoc Franc Etude Cancer 1924; 13: 410–21.

2 Schall LA, Lineback M. Primary intranasal neuroblastoma. Ann Otol Rhinol Laryngol 1951; 60: 221–9.

3 Berger L, Coutard H. L'esthésioneurocytome olfactif. Bull Assoc Franc Etude Cancer 1926; 15: 404–14.

4 Obert GJ, Devine KD, McDonald JR. Olfactory neuroblastoma. Cancer 1960; 13: 205–15.

5 Skolnik EM, Massari FS, Tenta LT. Olfactory neuroepithelioma: Review of the world literature and presentation of two cases. Arch Otolaryngol 1976; 84: 84–93.

6 Cantrell RW, Ghorayeb BY, Fitz-Hugh GS. Esthesioneuroblastoma: Diagnosis and treatment. Ann Otol Rhinol Laryngol 1977; 86: 760–5.

7 Shah JP, Feghali J. Esthesioneuroblastoma. CA 1983; 33: 155–9.

8 Elkon D, Hightower SI, Lim ML, Cantrell, RW, Constable WC. Esthesioneuroblastoma. Cancer 1979; 44: 1087–94.

9 Kadish S, Goodman M, Wang CC. Olfactory neuroblastoma. Cancer 1976; 37: 1571–6.

10 Homzie MJ, Elkon D. Olfactory esthesioneuroblastoma—Variables predictive of tumor control and recurrence. Cancer 1980; 46: 2509–13.

11 Wade PM, Smith RE, Johns ME. Response of esthesioneuroblastoma to chemotherapy. Cancer 1984; 53: 1036–41.

12 O'Conor GT Jr, Drake CR, Johns MF, Cail WS, Winn HR, Niskanen E. Treatment of advance esthesioneuroblastoma with high dose chemotherapy and autologous bone marrow transplantation. A case report. Cancer 1985; 55(2): 347–9.

13 Preston-Martin S, Henderson BE. Esthesioneuroblastoma. CA 1984; 34(6): 356(letter).

14 Momose KJ, Weber AL, Goodman ML. Radiological and pathological findings of esthesioneuroblastoma. Adv Oto-Rhino-Laryng 1978; 24: 166–9.

15 Tyler TC, Chandler JR, Wetli C, Moffitt BM. Olfactory neuroblastoma. South Med J 1974; 67: 640–3.

16 Herrold KMcD. Induction of olfactory neuroepithelial tumors in Syrian hamsters by diethylnitrosamine. Cancer 1964; 17: 114–21.

17 Nakashima T, Kimmelman CP, Snow JB Jr. Structure of human fetal and adult olfactory neuroepithelium. Arch Otolaryngol Head Neck Surg 1984; 110: 641–6.

18 Mills SE, Frierson HF Jr. Olfactory neuroblastoma. A clinicopathologic study of 21 cases. Am J Surg Pathol 9: 317–27, 1985.

19 Mendeloff J. The olfactory neuroepithelial tumors. A review of the literature and report of six additional cases. Cancer 1957; 10: 944–56.

20 Gerard-Marchant R, Micheau C. Microscopical diagnosis of olfactory esthesioneuromas: General review and report of five cases. J Nat Cancer Inst 1965; 35: 75–82.

21 Hutter RVP, Lewis JS, Foote FW Jr, Tollefsen HR: Esthesioneuroblastomna: A clinical and pathological study. Am J Surg 1963; 106: 748–53.

22 Bailey BJ, Barton S: Olfactory neuroblastomas. Management and prognosis. Arch Otolaryngol Head Neck Surg 1975; 101: 1–5.

23 Oberman HA, Rice DH: Olfactory neuroblastomas. A clinicopathologic study. Cancer 1976; 38: 2494–502.

24 Djalilian M, Zujko RD, Weiland LH, Devine KD. Olfactory neuroblastoma. Surg Clinic North Am 1977; 57: 751–62.

25 Silva EG, Butler JJ, Mackay B, Goepfert H. Neuroblastomas and neuroendocrine carcinomas of the nasal cavity. A proposed new classification. Cancer 1982; 50: 2388–405.

26 Curtis JL, Rubinstein LJ. Pigmented olfactory neuroblastoma: A new example of melanotic neuroepithelial neoplasm. Cancer 1982; 49: 2136–43.

27 Miller DC, Goodman ML, Pilch BZ, Shi SR, Dickersin GR, Halpern H, Norris CM Jr. Mixed olfactory neuroblastoma and adenocarcinoma. A report of two cases. Cancer 1984; 54: 2019–28.

28 Hyams VJ. Olfactory neuroblastoma (case 6). In: Batsakis JG, Hyams VJ, Morales AR eds. Special Tumors of the Head and Neck. Chicago: ASCP Press, 1982; 24–9.

29 Chaudhry AP, Haar, JG, Koul A, Nickerson PA. Olfactory neuroglastoma (esthesioneuroblastoma). A light and ultrastructural study of two cases. Cancer 1979; 44: 564–79.

30 Kahn LB. Esthesioneuroblastoma. A light and electron microscopic study. Hum Pathol 1974; 5: 364–71.

31 Mackay B, Luna MA, Butler JJ. Adult neuroblastoma. Electron microscopic observations in nine cases. Cancer 1976; 37: 1334–51.

32 Osamura RY, Fine G: Ultrastructure of the esthesioneuroblastoma. Cancer 1976; 38: 173–9.

33 Taxy JB, Hidvegi DF. Olfactory neuroblastoma. An ultrastructural study. Cancer 1977; 39: 131–8.

34 Taxy JB, Bharani NK, Mills SE, Frierson HF Jr, Gould VE. The spectrum of olfactory neural tumors. A light-microscopic immunohistochemical and ultrastructural analysis. Am J Surg 1986; 10: 687–95.

35 Choi HSH, Anderson PJ. Immunohistochemical diagnosis of olfactory neuroblastoma. J Neuropathol Exp Neurol 1985; 44: 18–31.

36 Silva EG, Battifora H. Immunoreactivity for

keratin and neuron specific cavity. Lab Invest 1985; 52: 62A–3A.

37 Trojanowski JQ, Lee V, Pillsbury N, Lee S. Neuronal origin of human esthesioneuroblastoma demonstrated with antineurofilament monoclonal antibodies. N Engl J Med 1982; 307: 159–61.

38 Micheau C, Guerinot F, Bohuon C, Brugere J. Dopamine-B-hydroxylase and catecholamines in an olfactory esthesioneuroma. Cancer 1975; 35: 1309–12.

39 Judge DM, McGavron MH, Trapukdi S. Fume-induced fluorescence in diagnosis of nasal neuroblastoma. Arch Otolaryngol Head Neck Surg 1976; 102: 97–8.

40 Singh W, Ramage C, Best P, Angus B. Nasal neuroblastoma secreting vasopressin: A case report. Cancer 1980; 45: 961–6.

41 Frierson HF Jr, Mills SE, Fechner RE, Taxy JB, Levine PA. Sinonasal undifferentiated carcinoma. An aggressive neoplasm derived from Schneiderian epithelium and distinct from olfactory neuroblastoma. Am J Surg Pathol 1986; 10: 771–9.

42 Frierson HF Jr, Mills SE, Innes DJ Jr. Non-Hodgkin's lymphomas of the sinonasal region: Histologic subtypes and their clinicopathologic features. Am J Clin Pathol 1984; 81: 721–7.

43 Rakes SM, Yeatts RP, Campbell RJ. Ophthalmic manifestations of esthesioneuroblastoma. Ophthalmology 1985; 92: 1749–53.

44 Manelfe C, Bonafe A, Fabre P, Pessey JJ. Computed tomography in olfactory neuroblastoma: One case of esthesioneuroepithelioma and four cases of esthesioneuroblastoma. J Comput Assist Tomogr 1978; 2: 412–20.

45 Newbill ET, Johns ME, Cantrell RW. Esthesioneuroblastoma: Diagnosis and management. South Med J 185; 78(3): 275–82.

46 Schroth G, Gawehn J, Marquardt B, Schabet M. MR Imaging of esthesioneuroblastoma. J Comput Assist Tomogr 1986; 10(2): 316–19.

47 Levine PA, Paling MR, Black WC, Cantrell RW. MRI versus high resolution CT scanning: Evaluation of the anterior skull base in Otolaryngol Head Neck Surg. 1987; 96: 260–7.

48 Elner A, Koch A. Combined radiological and surgical therapy of cancer of the ethmoid. Acta Otolaryngol 1974; 78: 270–6.

49 Clifford P. Transcranial approach for cancer of the antroethmoidal area. Clin. Otolaryngol 1977; 2: 115–30.

50 Ketcham AS, Chretien PB, VanBuren JM, Hoye RC, Bezley RM, Herdt JR. The ethmoid sinuses: A re-evaluation of surgical resection.

Am J Surg 1973; 126: 469–76.

51 Johns ME, Winn HR, McLean WC, Cantrell RW. Percranial flap for the closure of defects of craniofacial resections. Laryngoscope 1981; 91: 952–9.

52 Jane JA, Park TS, Pobereskin AH. The supraorbital rim approach. Neurosurgery 1982; 211: 537–42.

53 Levine PA, McLean WC, Cantrell RW. Esthesioneuroblastoma: The University of Virginia experience 1960–1985. Laryngoscope 1986; 96: 742–6.

54 Johns ME, Kaplan MJ, Jane JA et al. Supraorbital rim approach to the anterior skull base. Laryngoscope 1984; 94: 1137–9.

55 Elkon D. Olfactory neuroblastoma. In: Reznik G, Stinson SF eds. Nasal Tumors in Animals and Man. Vol II. CRC Press 1983: 129–47.

56 Million RR, Cassisi NJ, Hamlin DJ. Nasal vestibule, nasal cavity, and paranasal sinuses. In: Million RR, Cassisi NJ eds. Management of Head and Neck Cancer—A Multidisciplinary Approach. JB Lippincott, 1984: 407–44.

57 Parsons JR. The effect of radiation on normal tissues of the head and neck. In: Million RR, Cassisi NJ eds. Management of Head and Neck Cancer—A Multidisciplinary Approach. JB Lippincott, 1984: 173–208.

58 Hayes FA, Green AA, Mauer AM. The correlation of cell kinetics and clinical response to chemotherapy in disseminated neuroblastoma. Cancer Res 1977; 37: 3766–70.

59 Green AA, Hayes FA, Hushu HO. Sequential cyclophosphamide and doxorubicin for induction of complete remission in children with disseminated neuroblastoma. Cancer 1981; 48: 2310–17.

60 Urban C, Slace I, Kaulfersch W, Greinix H, Hocker P. Treatment of stage IV neuroblastoma with high-dose melphalan and preliminary treatment of the bone marrow with the active cyclophosphamide derivative Asta Z-7654. Paediatr Paedol, 1986; 21(3): 275–82.

61 Clark J, Dana Farber Cancer Center. Personal communication.

62 Reynolds CP, Seeger RC, Vo DD, Ugelstad J, Well J. Purging of bone marrow with immunomagnetic beads: studies with neuroblastoma as a model system. In: Dicke KA, Spitser G, Zander AR eds. Autologous Bone Marrow Transplantation. The University of Texas M.D. Anderson Hospital and Tumor Institute at Houston.

63 Gee A. University of Florida, Gainesville, Fla. Personal communication.

Textbook of Uncommon Cancer
Edited by C.J. Williams, J.G. Krikorian, M.R. Green and D. Raghavan
© 1988 John Wiley & Sons Ltd

Chapter **31**

Malignant Schwannomas with Divergent Differentiation Including 'Triton' Tumor

John J. Brooks
Associate Professor of Pathology, Department of Pathology and Laboratory Medicine, University of Pennsylvania, Philadelphia, Pennsyslvania, USA

INTRODUCTION

The vast majority of sarcomas arising from peripheral nervous tissue exhibit only a single cell type histologically. Most such tumors can be found in the literature under the designation 'malignant schwannomas', despite the fact that not all tumors of this category display clear-cut schwannian differentiation. For that reason, a number of authors have proposed the term 'malignant peripheral nerve sheath tumors' (MPNST) for lesions of this category. Regardless, this particular subgroup of soft tissue appears unique in that occasionally other non-neural elements may be found within them. The most common of these is the so-called 'Triton' tumor defined as a malignant schwannoma or MPNST with rhabdomyoblastic differentiation. However, other types of differentiated tissues may be found in these tumors including glandular or squamous epithelium, cartilage, bone, vascular tissue and adipose tissue. Malignant peripheral nerve sheath tumors or malignant 'schwannomas' with such divergent differentiation account for approximately 16% of all MPNSTs according to Ducatman et al. (1). The various theories which might explain this peculiar phenomenon are detailed later in this chapter.

Importantly, although the divergent differentiation may include epithelial elements such as glands or squamous epithelium, '*epithelioid*' malignant schwannomas (2) are *not* included under this designation. Epithelioid MPNSTs are pure tumors whose neural element has taken the form of rounded cells giving them an 'epithelioid' appearance. Similarly, tumors referred to as 'neuroepitheliomas' are also excluded from discussion (2); these are primitive neural tumors which are again uniform, lack true epithelial elements, and are similar to but not identical with neuroblastomas. Lastly, a nerve sheath tumor need not be malignant to contain diverse elements; occasional benign schwannomas and neurofibromas with other mesenchymal tissues have been described (see below).

This chapter will summarize in detail the literature on 95 cases of MPNST with divergent differentiation in an effort to (1) define important clinical information; (2) describe the natural history of these lesions; and (3) assess their clinical significance.

TABLE 1 LITERATURE SUMMARY: MALIGNANT TRITON TUMORS

No	Year	Author and reference	Age	Sex	VRN	Size	Site	Surgery	CRx	LR Time to LR (months)	Mets Time to Mets (months)	Site-Mets	Survival	Comment
1	1932	Masson (3)	23	M	+	?	Neck	?	No	?	?		?	
2	1938	Masson and Martin (5)	18	F	+	?	Thigh	IE	?	Yes 7	No		AND 120 mo	Died of breast cancer
3	1938	Masson and Martin (5)	32	M	+	?	Back	IE	No	No	Yes 3	Lungs	DOD 3 mo	
4	1955	Agustsson et al. (6)	14	M	+	5	Thigh	CE	No	No	Yes 76	Lungs	DOD 15 mo	Also reported by D'Agostino
5	1963	D'Agostino et al. (7)	57	M	+	5	Forearm	CE	No	Yes ?	Yes	Lungs	DOD 20 mo	
6	1963	D'Agostino et al. (7)	29	M	+	?	Chest	Bx	No	Yes 3	?		DOD 3 mo	
7	1969	Harkin and Reed (8)	?	F	+	?	Forehead	?	?	?	?		?	Osteoid element; no other info.
8	1971	White (9)	35	M	+	?	Neck	IE	?	Yes 5	No		DOD 5 mo	
9	1973	Despres et al. (10)	38	F	+	?	Buttock	IE	?	Yes 13	No		DOD 19 mo	Glandular, and rhabdomyoblast elements
10	1973	Woodruff et al. (11)	31	M	+	9	Neck	CE	Yes	Yes 15	Yes 15	Lung, heart	DOD 18 mo	Cartilaginous element; Autopsy
11	1973	Woodruff et al. (11)	53	F	–	2	Back	CE	No	Yes 6	No		DOD 7 mo	Autopsy, died of intracerebral extension
12	1973	Woodruff et al. (11)	41	F	–	2	Back	CE	No	No	No		AND 12 mo	
13	1974	Pertschuk (12)	67	M	?	?	Thigh	?	?	?	?		?	
14	1977	Karcioglu et al. (13)	0.5	F	?	6	Face	IE	Yes	Yes 8	No		AND 15 mo	
15	1978	Averback (14)	45	M	+	10	Sciatic	CE	?	No	No		AND 36 mo	
16	1978	Krumerman and Stingle (15)	8	F	+	7	Neck	–	No	No	No		DOD 0 mo	Glandular element; died at operation
17	1978	Raney (16)	7	M	–	?	Thigh	CE	Yes	No	No		AND 15 mo	
18	1979	Guccion and Enzinger (17)	63	M	+	?	Pelvis	?	?	?	?			No specific info.
19	1979	Guccion and Enzinger (17)	37	M	+	?	Buttock	?	?	?	?			No specific info.
20	1979	Guccion and Enzinger (17)	?	?	+	?		?	?	?	?			1 of 5 other cases, no info.
21	1979	Guccion and Enzinger (17)	?	?	+	?		?	?	?	?			1 of 5 other cases, no info.
22	1979	Guccion and Enzinger (17)	?	?	+	?		?	?	?	?			1 of 5 other cases, no info.
23	1979	Guccion and Enzinger (17)	?	?	+	?		?	?	?	?			1 of 5 other cases, no info.
24	1979	Guccion and Enzinger (17)	?	?	+	?		?	?	?	?			1 of 5 other cases, no info.
25	1979	Shuangshoti and Chongchet (18)	8	M	–	2	Forearm	CE	No	Yes 5	?			
26	1980	Bambirra and Miranda (19)	43	F	?	?	Aorta	No	No	No	No		DOD 0 mo	Patient died on admission due to erosion of aorta and hemorrhage
27	1980	Foley et al. (20)	53	F	–	?	Brachial	?	No	?	Yes mo	Lungs, meninges	DOD 8 mo	+autopsy
28	1980	Inoue et al. (21)	4	M	+	?	Abd. wall	?	?	?	?		?	In Daimaru
29	1981	Mizoguchi et al. (22)	31	F	+	?	Mediast.	?	?	?	?		?	In Daimaru
30	1981	Taxy et al. (23)	10	F	–	Lg	Face	IE	?	?	?		DOD 15 mo	
31	1981	Taxy et al. (23)	?	?	?	?		?	?	?	?		?	2nd case no info.
32	1983	Ducatman and Scheithauer (24)	9	M	+	?	Temple	CE	Yes	Yes 15	No		AND 20 mo	Post-radiation case; osteo- and chondrosarcoma elements
33	1983	Warner et al. (25)	29	M	+	6	Thigh	CE	?	?	?		?	Glangular with endocrine cells
34	1984	Daimaru et al. (26)	0.4	F	+	14	Bladder	CE	No	Yes 3	Yes 3	Brain, lymph nodes	DOD 3 mo	Botryoid-like lesion on bladder

Case	Year	Reference	Age	Sex	VRN	Size	Site	Excision	CRx	LR	Mets	Mets site	Outcome	Comments
35	1984	Daimaru et al. (26)	4	M	+	?	Abd. wall	CE	No	Yes 12	Yes 21	Liver, nodes, abdomen	DOD 21 mo	Autopsy done
36	1984	Daimaru et al. (26)	30	F	+	10	Thigh	?	No	?	Yes ?	Lungs	DOD 24 mo	Primary not excised; autopsy; mediastinal disease
37	1984	Daimaru et al. (26)	22	F	+	10	Back	CE	No	No	No		DOD 0 mo	Operative death
38	1984	Daimaru et al. (26)	29	M	+	25	Buttock	?	No	Yes ?	Yes 7	Lungs	DOD 7 mo	Post-radiation for neurofibroma of buttock at 10; MTT of buttock and continous local disease; also glandular
39	1984	Daimaru et al. (26)	27	F	+	8	Sacral	IE	No	?	Yes 4	Peritoneum, adjacent bones	DOD 4 mo	
40	1984	Daimaru et al. (26)	20	M	−	6	Thigh	CE	No	No	No		AND 36 mo	Case added in note
41	1984	Daimaru et al. (26)	53	F	+	?	Axilla	?	No	?	?		?	Case added in note
42	1984	Daimaru et al. (26)	58	M	−	?	Arm	?	?	?	?		?	
43	1984	Daimaru et al. (26)	18	F	−	10	Buttock	CE	No	Yes >6	Yes ?		?	Local recurrences 3× in 3 yrs; total of 6
44	1984	Daimaru et al. (26)	35	F	−	10	Thigh	CE	Yes	No	Yes 12	Lungs	?	?
45	1984	Ducatman and Scheithauer (27)	33	M	−	?	Sciatic n.	CE	No	Yes 2	?		DOD 23 mo	Chondrosarcoma areas too
46	1984	Ducatman and Scheithauer (27)	48	M	−	?	Leg	?	No	Yes 15	?		DOD 34 mo	Chondrosarcoma areas too
47	1984	Ducatman and Scheithauer (27)	12	F	+	?	Retroper.	CE	No	Yes 2	?		DOD 15 mo	Angiosarcoma areas too
48	1984	Ducatman and Scheithauer (27)	49	F	+	?	Neck	CE	No	No	No		Died 18 mo	Said to have died of renal cancer
49	1984	Ducatman and Scheithauer (27)	31	F	+	?	Mediast.	IE	No	Yes 0	?		DOD 3 mo	Osteosarcoma and chondrosarcoma elements
50	1984	Ducatman and Scheithauer (27)	34	M	+	?	Neck	CE	No	No	?		DOD 19 mo	
51	1984	Ducatman and Scheithauer (27)	24	F	−	?	Forearm	CE	No	?	?		AWD 33 mo	Nodular fibromatosis 7 yrs earlier
52	1984	Ducatman and Scheithauer (27)	13	M	−	?	Facial n.	CE	Yes	No	?		No follow-up	
53	1985	Brooks et al. (28)	12	F	+	5	Neck	CE	Yes	No	No		AND 156 mo	
54	1985	Brooks et al. (28)	63	M	+	12	Buttock	IE	Yes	Yes 0	Yes mo	Lung, bone	DOD 5 mo	
55	1985	Brooks et al. (28)	25	F	+	11	Neck	IE	No	Yes ?	?		DOD 16 mo	
56	1985	Brooks et al. (28)	40	F	−	37	Thigh	CE	No	No	No		AND 18 mo	
57	1985	Brooks et al. (28)	22	M	−	8	Esophagus	IE	No	No	No		AND 23 mo	
58	1985	Brooks et al. (28)	70	F	−	3	Mediast.	IE	No	No	No	Lung	AWD 54 mo	No autopsy
59	1985	Brooks et al. (28)	33	M	+	Lg	Retroper.	IE	?	Yes 36	Yes ?		DOD 36 mo	
60	1985	Brooks et al. (28)	50	F	−	7	Back	CE	No	No	No		AND 4 mo	
61	1985	Buck et al. (29)	0	F	?	9	Retroper.	IE	Yes	Yes 0	Yes wk	Liver, pleura	DOD 4 mo	Autopsy done; case also in Brooks et al.
62	1986	Dewit et al. (30)	32	M	+	13	Calf	IE	No	Yes 15	Yes 15	Brain	DOD 20 mo	+des, myo myosin S-100, no autopsy
63	1986	Dewit et al. (30)	20	F	−	8	Pelvis	IE	Yes	Yes 1	Yes 0	Liver, bowel	DOD 6 mo	+des, −myo −myosin +S-100, +autopsy
64	1986	Dewit et al. (30)	12	M	−	6	Calf	CE	Yes	No	Yes 12	Lung	DOD 24 mo	+des, +myo +myosin +S-100, no autopsy
65	1986	Ducatman et al. (1)	?	?	?	?	?	?	?	?	?		?	2 more MTTs without information, over prior paper
66	1986	Konishi et al. (31)	31	F	+	18	Pelvis	Bx	No	Yes 0	Yes 0	Umbilicus, liver, lungs, gallbladder	DOD 4 mo	+autopsy, +S-100, +myo
67	1987	Brooks (32)	20	M	−	10	Mediast.	IE	Yes	Yes 0	?		DOD 6 mo	

Abbreviations: VRN, von Recklinghausen's neurofibromatosis; CRx, chemotherapy; LR, local recurrence; Mets, metastases; DOD, dead of disease; AWD, alive with disease; AND, alive, no disease; mo, months; IE, incomplete excision; CE, complete excision; Bx, biopsy.

MPNST WITH DIVERGENT DIFFERENTIATION: MALIGNANT 'TRITON' TUMOR

In 1932 Masson (3) originally described a malignant schwannoma containing rhabdomyoblastic differentiation. At that time, he was aware of experiments by Locatelli (4) on the 'Triton' salamander (genus *Triturus*). Locatelli observed the formation of a supernumerary limb containing both neural and muscular elements after transplanting the sciatic nerve onto the dorsal surface of this salamander. In this way she demonstrated an intimate developmental relationship between neural and muscular tissues. Masson thus gave his peculiar tumor the pseudonym 'Triton' since it appeared to recapitulate this normal interrelationship between nerve and muscle tissues. Since then, a number of series and case reports (1, 5–32) of malignant Triton tumor (MTT) have been reported. In 1973 Woodruff and his co-workers (11) brought this entity to the attention of modern pathologists by summarizing 10 cases including 3 of their own. In 1979, Guccion and Enzinger (17) mentioned an additional 7 cases. By 1985, Brooks et al. (28) described 9 additional cases and summarized the literature to that date, noting a total of

36 cases. Since then, other series have been reported (1, 26, 27, 30) including an extensive review of malignant peripheral nerve sheath tumors by Ducatman et al. (1, 27). At the present time, a total of 68 cases have been located in the literature, the details of which are summarized in Table 1. Only 67 are listed there, since the 1986 summary by Ducatman et al. (1) provided no information on 2 cases (see Table 1, number 65). It should be mentioned that a benign counterpart to MTT does exist, the so-called 'neuromuscular hamartoma' (33–35).

Clinical Features

Although all reports were summarized, not all had complete information. Of the 68 total MTT patients, there were 30 males and 30 females for a male/female ratio of 1.0. The mean age at diagnosis was 29.8 years, in the center of the age peak from 20 to 40 years as shown in Figure 1.

The patients may be further divided into two groups: those with von Recklinghausen's neurofibromatosis (VRN cases); and those without neurofibromatosis (sporadic or non-VRN cases). VRN patients accounted for over

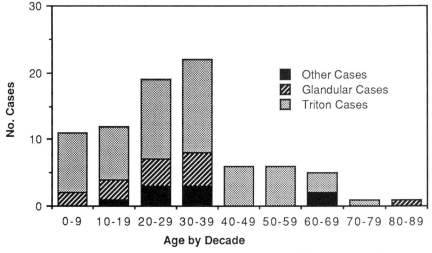

Figure 1 Age distribution of MPNST with divergent differentiation: three tumor categories.

65% of cases and displayed a slight male predominance, with a male/female ratio of 1.2. Unexpectedly and in contrast to our previous study (28), there is now little difference in the average age of VRN and non-VRN patients. The age *range* of the two groups likewise overlaps completely.

Clinically, the majority of patients complained of a mass or swelling as their only symptom. Interestingly, two MTTs, both in VRN patients, occurred after prior radiation (24, 26). Available information on the size and location of tumors in both VRN and non-VRN cases showed a similar distribution and, indeed, similar as well to the combined number of MPNSTs with all types of divergent differentiation. Therefore, these data will be discussed in the summary section.

Pathology of MTT

The histology of MTT is that of a dense tightly packed proliferation of spindle cells with elongated nuclei representing the nerve sheath element. The cells are bipolar and the nuclei often are wavy or comma-shaped (Figure 2). In many cases, clear-cut schwannian morphology is noted: densely hypercellular Antoni A areas alternate with more myxoid loose regions (Antoni B areas). As is true of malignant schwannomas in general, thick-walled blood vessels are noted together with whorled clusters of tumor cells resembling nerves.

The rhabdomyoblastic differentiation within these tumors is often found at the junction between the hypercellular and the more myxoid areas. Here, groups and aggre-

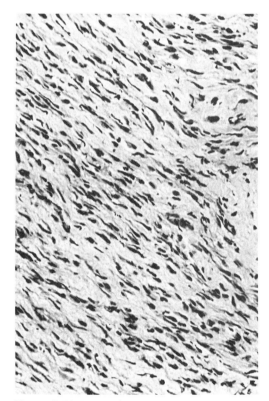

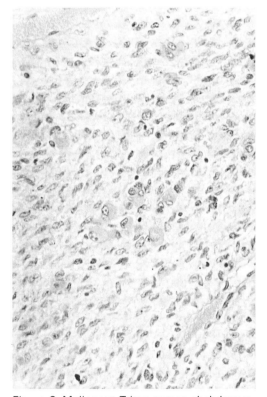

Figure 2 Malignant Triton tumor, nerve sheath element. Note the elongated and wavy nuclei with pointed ends.

Figure 3 Malignant Triton tumor, rhabdomyoblastic element. The plump cells in the center represent the muscle element.

gates of cells with prominent eosinophilic cytoplasm may be identified (Figure 3). On closer inspection, the cytoplasm of these cells may be fibrillar in appearance; indeed cross-striations may be identified in a subpopulation of these cells. Identification of rhabdomyoblasts in a spindle cell sarcoma is essentially only observed in MTT, and is thus helpful in putting such a sarcoma into the nerve sheath category.

Immunohistochemically, the MTT is unique. First of all, the nerve sheath element may be defined by immunoreactive S-100 protein (30, 31). This protein is found in about 50–70% of all malignant schwannomas or peripheral nerve sheath tumors. In particular, it appears to decorate the spindle cell population, particularly in the more differentiated areas with whorls or nerve-like structures.

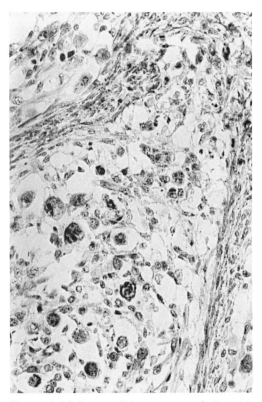

Figure 4 Malignant Triton tumor. Cells with immunoreactive myoglobin appear darkened (center and left).

Hypocellular areas more commonly express this marker than hypercellular areas. Secondly, the rhabdomyoblastic element may be defined by immunoreactive desmin (30) and myoglobin (28, 30, 31). Although myoglobin has been adequate in identifying a number of cases, clearly immunoreactive desmin is superior and more sensitive in this regard. Once again, this immunoreactivity tends to highlight the more differentiated rhabdomyoblasts (Figure 4).

Ultrastructurally, the Schwann cell nature of the spindle component is typified by the presence of numerous overlapping and interdigitating cell processes (23). Spindle cells contain an interrupted basal lamina together with scattered cell junctions. Occasional dense core granules are noted. Within the rhabdomyoblastic element, numerous cytoplasmic filaments are noted together with the occasional formation of z-band material (23).

Like the other MPNSTs described here, the MTT is a high grade (Grade 3) sarcoma for two reasons. First, the nerve sheath element practically always exhibits a high mitotic rate, areas of necrosis, and nuclear pleomorphism. Secondly, any tumor with a rhabdomyoblastic element is generally classified as a high grade sarcoma.

Interestingly, a number of MTTs have also demonstrated other types of divergent differentiation. For example, 4 cases had glandular elements (10, 15, 25, 26), 5 contained cartilaginous areas either benign (11) or malignant (24, 27), 3 showed regions of benign osteoid (8) or frank osteosarcoma (24, 27), and one unusual case had an angiosarcoma component (27). Of these 13 cases, all but 2 occurred in neurofibromatosis patients.

Natural History of MTT

As can be seen from the literature summary (see Table 4), MTT is an extremely aggressive tumor. Seventy-two percent of all patients died of disease, mostly within 2 years of diagnosis. The local recurrence rate was high (60%) despite the claim of adequate excision in many.

TABLE 2 LITERATURE SUMMARY: MALIGNANT GLANDULAR SCHWANNOMAS

	Year	Author	Age	Sex	VRN	Size	Site	Surgery	CRx	LR Time to LR (months)	Mets Time to Mets (months)	Site-Mets	Survival	Comment
1	1892	Garre (36)	31	F	+	15	Knee, sciatic	CE	No	Yes 6	?		DOD 6 mo	Glandular, first case report
2	1927	Lanford and Cohn (39)	35	M	+	6	Arm, med. n.	CE	No	Yes 12	No		AND 48 mo	Glandular, amputation post recurrences
3	1948	Foraker (40)	8	F	+	?	Brach. plex.	CE	No	Yes 120	?		DOD 120 mo	Glandular, mediastinal recurrence
4	1976	Woodruff (37)	8	F	+	11	Neck	CE	No	Yes 12	No		DOD 125 mo	Glandular
5	1976	Woodruff (37)	15	F	+	6	Back	CE	No	No	No		AND 126 mo	Glandular
6	1976	Woodruff (37)	32	F	+	4	Thigh	CE	No	No	Yes 42	Lung	DOD 65 mo	Glandular
7	1976	Woodruff (37)	27	M	−	10	Retroper.	CE	Yes	Yes 4	No		DOD 7 mo	Glandular, post-radiation for lymphoma
8	1979	Hadju (38)	35	M	+	?	Retroper.	?	?	?	?		DOD 12 mo	Glandular
9	1979	Takahara et al. (41)	89	F	+	5	Chest wall	CE	No	Yes 4	Yes 11	Lungs	DOD 15 mo	Glandular element; benign tumor at same site for 76 yrs
10	1984	DeSchryver et al. (42)	26	M	+	4	Neck	CE	?	?	?	?	?	Glandular, said to have ependymal EM
11	1984	Ducatman and Scheithauer (43)	35	F	+	?	Flank	CE	No	Yes 2	Yes 28	Lung, pleura, retroperit.	DOD 28 mo	Glandular and squamous elements
12	1984	Ducatman and Scheithauer (43)	19	M	−	?	Retroper.	CE	No	No	?		No follow-up	Glandular elements
13	1984	Uri et al. (44)	16	M	+	?	Retroper.	IE	Yes	Yes	No		AWD 17 mo	EM of glandular element—not ependymal but intestinal-like
14	1985	Daimaru et al. (45)	28	F	+	8	Buttock	CE	No	?	?		DOD 4 mo	Glandular element
15	1986	Lodding et al. (46)	?	?	?	?	?	?	?	?	?		?	Glandular differentiation, no info.; 1 met. had cartilage
16	1987	Brooks (47)	23	M	+	12	Neck	CE	Yes	Yes 6	No		DOD 14 mo	glandular, with osteoid and cartilaginous metaplasia

Abbreviations as in Table 1.

The average time to local recurrence was 7.5 months and only one patient had a late local recurrence beyond 15 months. While a number of patients died as a result of uncontrolled local growth in critical bodily regions, many died from progressive metastatic disease. Nearly half of all patients (48%) described in the literature had metastases. Metastases were mainly to lungs, liver, and brain where details were provided. Only occasional patients had radiation (mostly to bulky unresected disease) and/or chemotherapy, with little apparent effect.

Whether the presence of neurofibromatosis or divergent differentiation affects the prognosis of MPNST will be addressed in the summary section.

MPNST WITH DIVERGENT DIFFERENTIATION: 'GLANDULAR' SCHWANNOMAS

Epithelial differentiation in nerve sheath tumors was first noted long ago by Garre (36). Once again, it was Woodruff (37) at Memorial Sloan-Kettering Hospital in New York who brought this phenomenon to the attention of modern oncology. While both he (37) and his colleague Dr Hadju (38) each describe a single case of benign schwannoma with glands, the vast majority of these tumors have been malignant. In a recent summary of epithelial PNST, DiCarlo et al (2) mention 20 glandular schwannomas in the literature. Since at least 3 of their cases also had rhabdomyomatous differentiation, these have been listed and analyzed here under MTT in Table 1. Therefore, only pure glandular (non-MTT) cases are summarized in Table 2 in an effort to define the natural history of this tumor and separate it from those cases with potentially more aggressive elements. With that condition in mind, the author has identified 16 pure *malignant* glandular schwannomas (MGS). (Excluded are unconvincing cases by Vieta and Pack (48) and Michel (49).)

Clinical Features

Like MTT, MGS occurred at a young age (28.5 years on the average). However, a wide age distribution is seen as illustrated in Figure 1. In this subtype, females outnumbered males nine to six (M/F = 0.66). Nearly all tumors were large (average 8.1 cm) and the main locations were the retroperitoneum (4 cases), neck (13 cases), and trunk (3 cases). An overwhelming majority of patients (87%) had the stigmata of neurofibromatosis. Few symptoms or signs pointed to a clinical diagnosis of a neural tumor other than the occasional patient with paresthesias.

Pathology of Malignant Glandular Schwannoma

The predominant cell population of these tumors is the spindle cell nerve sheath element identical to that previously described under MTT. Concerning glandular differentiation, it can be an extremely focal finding as it was in the author's case. In fact, Krumerman and Stingle (15) located glands (in one recurrent MTT–glandular case) only after submitting 27 blocks of tissue. This unusual case only serves to emphasize the characteristic rarity of the glands in these tumors.

Histologically, the glands may occur singly or in small groups. For the most part, the glands were round to oval or tubular in shape (Figure 5). Only in a few instances were complex glandular structures resembling carcinoma described. In one case (43) squamous elements were found nearby. While the glandular structures were originally postulated to be similar to ependymal cells, no blepharoplasts are found. Instead, goblet cells and absorptive-type columnar cells with a brush border have been identified. Intraluminal secretions are often present an exhibit PAS and mucicarmine positivity. If other special stains are applied, occasional neuroendocrine cells can also be located, as reported by Warner et al. (25). In fact, specific polypeptides such as somatostatin were located immunohistochemically in these glands by the same authors.

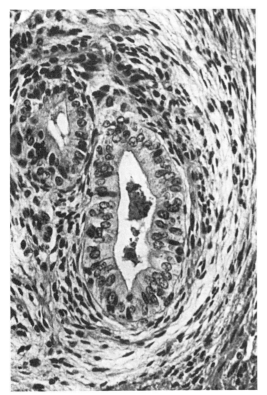

Figure 5 Malignant glandular schwannoma. Tall columnar cells line a glandular structure. The luminal aspect is darker, representing a brush border. The periglandular stroma of tumor cells is looser than in other areas.

Ultrastructure of the glandular element has been performed by two groups—DeSchryver et al. (42) and Uri et al. (44). While the former group argued for similarity to ependymal cells, the argument is weak. They describe a case with less than complete gland formation and histochemical and ultrastructural similarities to ependymal cells. Yet, a number of these are clearly non-specific findings. In contrast Uri et al. (44) noted the lack of cilia and blepharoplasts ordinarily found in ependymal cells. Instead, characteristics of intestinal-type epithelium were observed, including microvilli with core rootlets, a glycocalyx, and R-bodies (probable progenitors of glycocalyceal bodies). This evidence, together with the microscopic appearance with goblet and endocrine cells, strongly supports the intestinal-like nature of the glands.

As mentioned above, some MGSs have displayed other types of differentiation: four with rhabdomyosarcomatous elements (10, 15, 25, 26); two with benign cartilaginous elements (46, 47); and one case with focal osteoid formation (47).

Natural History of MGS

Like MTT, the malignant glandular schwannoma (MGS) is a highly malignant tumor. From the summarized data on the 16 cases in Table 4, one notes that over three-fourths (10/13) of the patients died of this tumor. While the deaths were usually within a 2 year period, there were 2 long-term survivors who finally succumbed 10 years after diagnosis. Local recurrences were noted in 75% of patients and metastatic disease in 33%.

OTHER TYPES OF DIVERGENT DIFFERENTIATION IN MPNST

The phenomenon of mesenchymal differentiation in nerve sheath tumors may take forms other than skeletal muscle tissue (50–56). These other malignant soft tissue elements are detailed in Table 3 and, as can be seen, chondro-osseous differentiation is the most common neoplastic mesenchymal element in this group. Seven cases had a malignant cartilaginous component and osteosarcoma was identified in 4. One patient's tumor (54) contained both chondrosarcoma and osteosarcoma. Interestingly, angiosarcoma was also observed to occur in one case. Unlike chondro-osseous tissue, neoplastic vascular tissue is not ordinarily found accompanying any other tumor, much less nerve sheath lesions. In fact, Chaudhuri et al. (57) reported the only other example of angiosarcoma associated with nerve tissue, actually arising in a neurofibroma. *Benign* mesenchymal elements within neural tissues have included a neurofibroma with angioma, lipoma, cartilage and bone (58), and fibro-fatty tissue in the so-called

TABLE 3 LITERATURE SUMMARY: OTHER CASES OF DIVERGENT DIFFERENTIATION.

	Year	Author	Age	Sex	VRN	Size	Site	Surgery	CRx	LR Time to LR (months)	Mets Time to Mets (months)	Site-Mets	Survival	Comment
1	1963	D'Agostino et al. (50)	33	M	–	8	Thigh	IE	No	Yes 8	No		DOD 13 mo	Chondrosarcoma element; amputation at 8 mo, died of local disease
2	1978	Macaulay (51)	18	M	+	15	Axilla	CE	No	No	Yes 0	Lungs, brain	DOD 2 mo	Angiosarcoma element
3	1979	Guccion and Enzinger (52)	21	M	–	?	Sciatic n.	?	?	?	?		?	No specific info.; malignant cartilaginous element
4	1983	Chitale and Dickersin (53)	64	F	?	5	Pelvis	IE	No	?	?		?	Epithelial element, but poorly differentiated
5	1983	Ducatman and Scheithauer (54)	32	M	–	?	Neck	CE	Yes	Yes 8	?		DOD 10 mo	Osteo- and chondrosarcoma elements
6	1984	Ducatman and Scheithauer (55)	28	F	+	?	Axilla	CE	No	Yes 13	?		?	Osteosarcoma
7	1984	Ducatman and Scheithauer (55)	31	F	+	?	Retroper.	CE	No	No	?		DOD 64 mo	Osteosarcoma element
8	1984	Ducatman and Scheithauer (55)	20	F	+	?	Sciatic n.	CE	No	No	Yes 14	Lung, liver	DOD 34 mo	Osteosarcoma element
9	1984	Ducatman and Scheithauer (55)	62	F	+	?	Buttock	CE	No	Yes 9	?		DOD 14 mo	Chondrosarcoma element
10	1985	Matsunou et al. (56)	?	?	+	?	?	?	?	?	?		?	Cartilaginous element, no other info.
11	1985	Matsunou et al. (56)	?	?	+	?	?	?	?	?	?		?	Cartilaginous element, no other info.
12	1985	Matsunou et al. (56)	?	?	+	?	?	?	?	?	?		?	Cartilaginous element, no other info.

Abbreviations as in Table 1.

'fibrolipomatous hamartoma' of nerve (59). When pigmentation occurs in nerve sheath tumors, it frequently (but not always) signals an aggressive course (60). However, pigmentation per se is not considered divergent differentiation due to the close relationship between the melanocyte and the Schwann cell.

The natural history of MPNSTs with these other types of divergent differentiation resembles that of the 'Triton' tumor and malignant glandular schwannomas. All reports with survival data relate the unfortunate ultimate outcome; that is, 100% of patients died of disease.

SUMMARY—ALL MPNSTs WITH DIVERGENT DIFFERENTIATION

Once this data was collected and compiled, it was readily apparent that all nerve sheath tumors with divergent differentiation were similar clinically and biologically regardless of specific element. For that reason, a number of aspects of this entire group can be discussed together (Table 4).

Most remarkable was the high frequency of association of divergent differentiation with neurofibromatosis (VRN). Overall, 70% of all cases had VRN, definitely an overrepresentation since only 30–40% of all usual MPNSTs are related to that inherited disease. Ordinarily, tumors with a genetic basis occur earlier than sporadic cases, but that was not observed here; the average age for VRN and non-VRN cases was nearly identical. Although both these groups show a peak age incidence in the 20–40 year range (Figure 6), the non-VRN cases appear to have a flatter distribution by age at presentation. The sex of patients was also remarkably similar between the two groups, with only the MTT cases showing a slight male predominance in VRN cases.

As far as tumor size and location, this was influenced little by either tumor type, or the presence of VRN. Whether in VRN patients or not, the majority of tumors were in more centrally located sites; there was only a modest increase of central location in VRN patients

TABLE 4 SUMMARY OF LITERATURE ON MPNST WITH DIVERGENT DIFFERENTIATION

	MTT	MGS	Other	Totals
Number of cases	67	16	12	95
%VRN	66%	87%	73%	70%
Average age	29.8	28.5	34.3	30.0
with VRN				30.1
no VRN				29.9
M/F ratio	1.0	0.66	0.44	0.83
with VRN	1.2			
Average size	9.5	8.1	9.1	9.2
% less than 6 cm				39%
Location				
Head/neck				18
Lower extremity				19
Pelvis/retroperitoneum				13
Buttock/sacral				8
Trunk				11
Axilla				5
Mediastinal				4
Upper extremity				4
Visceral				2
% Central (non-extremity)				73%
with VRN				80%
no VRN				60%
Specific elements				
Rhabdomyosarcoma	67	0	0	67
Glandular	4	16	0	20
Chondroid	5	1	7	13
Osteoid	3	1	4	8
Angiosarcoma	1	0	1	2
Post radiation	2	0	0	2 (2%)
% Local recurrence	60%	75%	57%	63%
(no. with data)	(45)	(12)	(7)	(64)
VRN cases (40)				68%
non-VRN cases (24)				54%
Time to local recurrence (mo)				
Average, all cases				10.7
Average, VRN cases				13.6
Average, non-VRN cases				7.6
% Metastases	48%	33%	67%	41%
(no. with data)	(36)	(9)	(3)	(48)
VRN cases (31)				55%
non-VRN cases (17)				29%
Time to metastases (mo)				
Average, all cases				10.8
Average, VRN cases				12.2
Average, non-VRN cases				6.2
Sites metastases (22 cases)				
Lungs/pleura				19
Liver				5
Brain				4
GI				3
Lymph nodes				2
Bone				2
Survival data				
% Dead of disease (DOD)	72%	77%	100%	75%
(no. with data)	(46)	(13)	(6)	(65)
VRN, DOD				84%
non-VRN, DOD				59%
% Alive with disease	4%	7%	0%	5%
% Alive, no disease	24%	16%	0%	20%
Crude 2-yr survival				27%
Crude 5-yr survival				13%

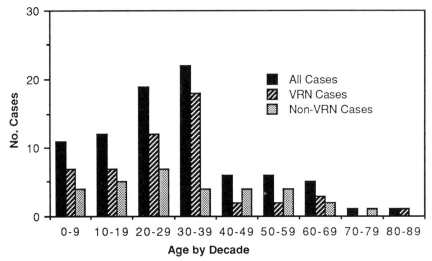

Figure 6 Age distribution of MPNST with divergent differentiation: presence or absence of neurofibromatosis (VRN).

(80% vs 60% in non-VRN cases). Oddly enough, however, these figures almost exactly parallel the death rates in the two groups—a fact which underscores the importance of location and the difficulty presented to surgical management of centrally placed neoplasms.

Local recurrence rates were fairly close in the three tumor categories, and the overall rate of 63% is certainly high by today's standards. This is a likely reflection of poorer surgical technique in the distant past and the lack of modern postoperative adjuvant radiotherapy. No major differences were noted in either the percentage of recurrence or the time to recurrence when VRN patients were compared to others.

The metastatic rate of 41% approximates that found in large studies of malignant 'schwannomas' in general (61–65). Interestingly, neurofibromatosis patients had nearly double the metastatic rate of sporadic cases (55% vs 29%). It appears that, even in this highly aggressive group of tumors, differences between VRN and non-VRN patients are still found. As with most sarcomas, the lungs were the most common site of metastasis, followed by the liver. An unusually high proportion of brain metastases occurred.

In terms of survival in patients harboring MPNST with divergent differentiation, it is uniformly dismal. Seventy-five percent of all patients died of disease and no differences were identified among the three tumor categories. Further, those patients yet alive were followed for only short periods of time, with only 2 long-term survivors (at 10 years). However, as noted in the MTT section above, patients may suffer recurrence and death even at such a late time interval. Overall, so-called sporadic cases fared somewhat better with fewer deaths (59% vs 84%).

COMPARISON WITH MPNST LACKING DIVERGENT DIFFERENTIATION

Survival rates for standard cases of malignant schwannoma vary from study to study but show that around half of patients survive for 5 years (40% (62), 66% (63). Obviously, this is much better than the 13% figure compiled here. There are at least two possible explanations for such a miserable survival rate. First, the cases presented here were in a population of patients with a much higher proportion of von Recklinghausen's neurofibromatosis (70%

overall vs 30–40% in most series on standard malignant schwannomas). It is well known that the 5 year survival rates for malignant schwannoma in VRN patients (15% (17), 19% (7), 23% (64), 25% (9), 30% (63)) are clearly inferior to that in sporadic cases (33% (7), 47% (64), and 75% (63)). Only one recent study has a fair survival for VRN patients although it is still below that for sporadic cases (37% vs 48%) (61). While some authors consider the presence of VRN a poor prognostic sign in itself, it is actually quite difficult to separate this factor from those of tumor size and location, a point made by Bojsen-Moller and Myhre-Jensen (61). VRN patients tend to have large and centrally situated tumors making resection difficult. That was certainly the trend seen here in divergent differentiation cases as well. As mentioned above, the frequencies of poor location and of death from disease were quite similar, making location the most likely critical prognostic factor (as opposed to presence of VRN).

The second explanation involves the neoplastic grade. If sarcomas are divided into three grades, all three grades are adequately and evenly represented in most studies of MPNST. In contrast, essentially all MTTs are considered Grade III neoplasms, and tumors in the other two categories here with divergent differentiation also exhibited Grade III histology. Thus, the poorer survival in divergent differentiation cases may be partially caused by their highly proliferative nature, despite the fact that grade has never been clearly shown to be a strong independent prognostic factor in malignant nerve sheath tumors. This exercise apparently refutes prior claims that the presence of heterologous elements does not alter prognosis (22,27).

All in all, *divergent differentiation cases do fare far worse than sporadic malignant schwannomas* and are therefore similar to VRN-associated malignancy for reasons related to tumor location and grade. Better survival in the future may be achieved by an aggressive clinical approach to the primary tumor, with wide local excision and radiation therapy recommended.

THEORIES RELATING TO DIVERGENT DIFFERENTIATION

Non-nerve sheath sarcomas may occasionally contain heterologous elements such as cartilage or bone. These are seen in a small percentage of rhabdomyosarcomas, liposarcomas, and malignant fibrous histiocytomas. However, only nerve sheath tumors display such heterologous elements with a relatively high frequency (16%) (1), and, aside from synovial sarcoma, they are the only sarcomas to form clear epithelial elements. Obviously, this phenomenon deserves an explanation. Theories relating to induction by endoneural cells (Masson (3)), formation from some sort of teratoid influence (Shuangshoti (18)), or a peculiar 'collision tumor' of the various elements (Naka (66)) have little to support them. Masson also originally proposed the metaplastic theory whereby neoplastic Schwann cells might transform into other tissues. This concept has definite validity and has become incorporated into the now generally accepted ectomesenchymal theory (see below). Transdifferentiation of one tissue into another has been realized in the laboratory (67) and might be the actual mechanism involved here.

The origin of this divergent differentiation within tumors arising from peripheral nerve has been most adequately explained by the concept of 'ectomesenchyme' (11, 13, 27). According to the ectomesenchymal theory, developed by Horstadius, neuroectodermal structures develop from migratory stem cells of the neural crest. These neuroectodermal structures include melanocytes, ganglion cells and Schwann cells as well as the remaining mesenchymal tissues of the head and neck including muscle, bone, and cartilage (68, 69). Schwann cells later become dispersed around the body but retain this innate capacity of the neuroectoderm to form various tissues. Therefore, tumors of neuroectodermal origin including peripheral nerve sheath tumors may recapitulate this normal developmental phenonenon to produce neural tumors containing other soft tissue and epithelial elements. While such tumors might be referred to as 'ectomesenchy-momas' or 'malignant mesenchymomas', it is convention to refer to them as malignant schwannomas or MPNSTs since the neural or schwannian element often predominates.

Support for the multipotentiality of neur-oectodermally derived cells is provided by tissue culture studies (discussed by Ducatman (27)), brain tumors with mesenchymal differentiation (70–73) and the previously mentioned benign nerve sheath–mesenchymal combination tumors (34, 35, 58, 59).

ACKNOWLEDGEMENTS

The author is indebted to Dr Virginia A. LiVolsi for helpful suggestions and comments, to Kathy Snyder for typing the manuscript, and to Bethann Gee for performing immuno-histochemical studies.

REFERENCES

Malignant Triton Tumor

1 Ducatman BS, Scheithauer BW, Piepgras DG, Reiman HM, Ilstrup DM. Malignant peripheral nerve sheath tumors. A clinicopathologic study of 120 cases. Cancer 1986; 57: 2006–21.
2 DiCarlo EF, Woodruff JM, Bansal M, Erlandson RA. The purely epithelioid malignant peripheral nerve sheath tumor. Am J Surg Pathol 1986; 10: 478–90.
3 Masson P. Recklinghausen's Neurofibromatosis, Sensory Neuromas and Motor Neuromas. Libman Anniversary Volumes 2. New York: International Press, 1932; 793–802.
4 Locatelli P. Formation de Membres Surnuméraires. C.R. Assoc. es Anatomistes, 20e Reunion Turin, 1925; 279–282.
5 Masson P, Martin J. Rhabdomyomes des Nerfs. Bull Assoc Fr Cancer 1938; 27: 751–67.
6 Agustsson M, Lipsomb P, Mills S, Soule E. Aeltgeng neurofibromatosis hja barni med rhabdomyosarcoma og neurofibrosarcoma. Laeknabladid 1955; 39: 113–23.
7 D'Agostino A, Soule E, Miller R. Sarcomas of the peripheral nerves and somatic soft tissues associated with multiple neurofibromatosis (Von Recklinghausen's disease). Cancer 1963; 16: 1015–27.
8 Harkin JC, Reed RJ. Tumors of the peripheral

nervous system. In: Atlas of Tumor Pathology, Series 2, Fascicle 3. Washington DC: Armed Forces Institute of Pathology, 1969; 126–45.
9 White H. Survival in malignant schwannoma. Cancer 1971; 27: 720–9.
10 Despres S, Doliveux LM, Nezelof C. Neurofibrosarcome à différenciation glandulaire. A propos d'une observation. Arch Anat Pathol 1973; 21: 59–62.
11 Woodruff J, Chernik N, Smith M, Millett W, Foote F. Peripheral nerve tumors with rhabdomyosarcomatous differentiation (malignant 'Triton' tumors). Cancer 1973; 32: 426–39.
12 Pertschuk L. Immunofluorescence of soft-tissue tumors with anti-smooth muscle and anti-skeletal muscle antibodies. Am J Clin Pathol 1975; 6: 332–42.
13 Karcioglu Z, Someren A, Mathes S. Ectomesenchymoma: A malignant tumor of migratory neural crest (ectomesenchyme) remnants showing ganglionic, schwannian, melanocytic and rhabdomyoblastic differentiation. Cancer 1977; 39: 2486–96.
14 Averback P. Spheroidal filamentous inclusion body cells in Von Recklinghausen's disease. Virchows Arch (A) 1978; 377: 363–8.
15 Krumerman MS, Stingle W. Synchronous malignant glandular schwannomas in congenital neurofibromatosis. Cancer 1978; 41: 2444–51.
16 Raney RB. Malignant schwannoma of 'triton' tumor type. Med Pediatr Oncol 1978; 5: 99.
17 Guccion J, Enzinger F. Malignant schwannoma associated with Von Recklinghausen's neurofibromatosis. Virchows Arch (A) 1979; 383: 43–57.
18 Shuangshoti S, Chongchet V. Malignant mesenchymoma of ulnar nerve: Combined sarcoma of nerve sheath and rhabdomyosarcoma. J Neurosurg Psychiatry 1979; 42: 524–8.
19 Bambirra E, Miranda D. Spontaneous aortic rupture in a malignant schwannoma. South Med J 1980; 73: 1533–5.
20 Foley K, Woodruff J, Ellis F, Posner J. Radiation-induced malignant and atypical peripheral nerve sheath tumors. Ann Nuerol 1980; 7: 311–18
21 Inoue K, Muraoka S, Nozima T, et al. A case report of 'triton' tumor (abstract). In Proceedings of 69th Annual Meeting of the Japanese Pathological Society 1980; 69: 442.
22 Mizoguchi Y, Horibe Y, Miki Y et al. An autopsy report of malignant schwannoma of the mediastinum associated with 'triton' tumor (abstract). In: Proceeding at 70th Annual Meeting of the Japanese Pathological Society 1981; 70: 390.

23 Taxy J, Battifora H, Trujillo Y, Dorfman H. Electron microscopy in the diagnosis of malignant schwannoma. Cancer 1981; 48: 1381–91.

24 Ducatman B, Scheithauer B. Postirradiation neurofibrosarcoma. Cancer 1983; 51: 1018–33.

25 Warner TFCS, Louie R, Hafez GR, Chandler E. Malignant nerve sheath tumor containing endocrine cells. Am J Surg Pathol 1983; 7: 583–90.

26 Daimaru Y, Hashimoto H, Enjoji M. Malignant 'Triton' tumors: A clinicopathologic and immunohistochemical study of nine cases. Hum Pathol 1984; 15: 768–78.

27 Ducatman BS, Scheithauer BW. Malignant peripheral nerve sheath tumor with divergent differentiation. Cancer 1984; 54: 1049–57.

28 Brooks JSJ, Freeman M, Enterline HT. Malignant 'Triton' tumors. Natural history and immunohistochemistry of nine new cases with literature review. Cancer 1985; 55: 2543–9.

29 Buck B, Mahboubi S, Raney R. Congenital neurogenous sarcoma with rhabdomyosarcomatous differentiation. J Pediatr Surg 1977; 12: 581–2.

30 Dewit L, Albus-Lutter CE, DeJong ASH, Voute PA. Malignant schwannoma with a rhabdomyoblastic component, a so-called Triton tumor. A clinicopathologic study. Cancer 1986; 58: 1350–6.

31 Konishi N, Hiasa Y, Shimoyama T, Seki A, Mazima M. Malignant 'Triton' tumor with metastatic hemangiopericytoma in a patient associated with von Recklinghausen's disease. Acta Pathol Jpn 1986; 36: 459–69.

32 Brooks JJ. Malignant 'Triton' tumor, unpublished case.

33 Orlandi E Sopra. Un Caso di Rhabdomioma del Nervo Ischiatico. Arch Sci Med (Torino) 1895; 19: 113–37.

34 Markel S, Enzinger F. Neuromuscular hamartoma: A benign 'Triton tumor' composed of mature neural and striated muscle elements. Cancer 1982; 49: 140–4.

35 Azzopardi JG, Eusebi V, Tison V, Betts CM. Neurofibroma with rhabdomyomatous differentiation: benign 'triton' tumor of the vagina. Histopathology 1983; 7: 561–72.

'Glandular' Schwannoma

36 Garre C. Ueber sekundär maligne Neurome. Beitr Klin. Chir. 1892; 9: 465–95.

37 Woodruff J. Peripheral nerve tumors showing glandular differentiation (glandular schwannomas). Cancer 1976; 37: 2399–413.

38 Hadju S. Pathology of Soft Tissue Tumors. Philadelphia: Lea & Febiger 1979: 450.

39 Lanford JA, Cohn I. Ependymal neoplasm of the median nerve, with case report. South Med J 1927; 20: 273–8.

40 Foraker AG. Glandlike elements in a peripheral neurosarcoma. Cancer 1948; 1: 286–93.

41 Takahara O, Nakayama I, Yokoyama S, Moriuchi A, Muta H, Uchida Y. Malignant neurofibroma with glandular differentiation (glandular schwannoma). Acta Pathol Japan 1979; 29: 597–606.

42 DeSchryver K, Santa Cruz DJ. So-called glandular schwannoma: Ependymal differentiation in a case. Ultrastr Pathol 1984; 6: 167–75.

43 Ducatman BS, Scheithauer BW. Malignant peripheral nerve sheath tumor with divergent differentiation. Cancer 1984; 54: 1049–57.

44 Uri AK, Witzleben CL, Raney RB, Electron microscopy of glandular schwannoma. Cancer 1984; 53: 493–7.

45 Daimaru Y, Hashimoto H, Enjoji M. Malignant peripheral nerve-sheath tumors (malignant schwannomas). An immunohistochemical study of 29 cases. Am J Surg Pathol 1985; 9: 434–44.

46 Lodding P, Kindblom L-G, Angervall L. Epitheliod malignant schwannoma. A study of 14 cases. Virchows Arch (A) 1986; 409: 433–51.

47 Brooks JJ. Malignant glandular schwannoma, unpublished case.

48 Vieta JO, Pack GT. Malignant neurilemomas in peripheral nerves. Am J Surg 1951; 82: 416–31.

49 Michel SL. Epithelial elements in a malignant neurogenic tumor of the tibial nerve. Am J Surg 1967; 113: 404–8.

Other Types of Divergent Differentiation in MPNST

50 D'Agostino A, Soule E, Miller R. Primary malignant neoplasms of nerves (malignant neurilemmoma in patients without manifestations of multiple neurofibromatosis (Von Recklinghausen's disease). Cancer 1963; 16: 1003–14.

51 Macaulay RAA. Neurofibrosarcoma of the radial nerve in von Recklinghausen's disease with metastatic angiosarcoma. J Neurol Neurosurg Psychiatry 1978; 41: 474–8.

52 Guccion J, Enzinger F. Malignant schwannoma associated with Von Recklinghausen's neurofibromatosis. Virchows Arch (A) 1979; 383: 43–57.

53 Chitale AR, Dickersin GR. Electron microscopy in the diagnosis of malignant schwannomas. A report of six cases. Cancer 1983; 51: 1448–61.

54 Ducatman B, Scheithauer B. Postirradiation neurofibrosarcoma. Cancer 1983; 51: 1018–33.

55 Ducatman BS, Scheithauer BW. Malignant

peripheral nerve sheath tumor with divergent differentiation. Cancer 1984; 54: 1049–57.

56 Matsunou H, Shimoda T, Kakimoto S, Yamshita H, Ishikawa E, Mukai M. Histopathologic and immunohistochemical study of malignant tumors of peripheral nerve sheath (malignant Schwannoma). Cancer 1985; 56: 2269–79.

Other Lesions in Neural Tumors

57 Chaudhuri B, Ronan SG, Manaligod JR. Angiosarcoma arising in a plexiform neurofibroma. A case report. Cancer 1980; 46: 605–10.

58 Kasantikul V, Brown J, Netsky MG. Mesenchymal differentiation in trigeminal neurilemmoma. Cancer 1982; 50: 1568–71.

59 Silverman TA, Enzinger FM. Fibrolipomatous hamartoma of nerve. A clinicopathologic analysis of 26 cases. Am J Surg Pathol 1985; 9: 7–14.

60 Lowman RM. LiVolsi VA. Pigmented (melanotic) schwannomas of the spinal cord. Cancer 1980; 46: 391–7.

61 Bojsen-Moller M, Myhre-Jensen O. A consecutive series of 30 malignant schwannomas. Survival in relation to clinico-pathological parameters and treatment. Acta Pathol Microbiol Immunol Scand Sect A 1984; 92: 147–55.

62 Storm F, Eilber R, Mirra J, Morton D. Neurofibrosarcoma. Cancer 1980; 45: 126–9.

63 Ghosh B, Ghosh L, Huvos A, Fortner J. Malignant schwannoma: A clinicopathologic study. Cancer 1973; 31: 184–190.

64 Sordillo P, Helson L, Hadju S. Malignant schwannoma: Clinical characteristics, survival and response to therapy. Cancer 1981; 47: 2503–9.

65 Trojanowski JQ, Kleinman GM, Proppe KH. Malignant tumors of nerve sheath origin. Cancer 1980; 46: 1202–12.

66 Naka A, Matsumoto S, Shirai T, Itoh T. Ganglioneuroblastoma associated with malignant mesenchymoma. Cancer 1975; 36: 1050–6.

67 Nathanson MA. Transdifferentiation of skeletal muscle into cartilage: transformation or differ-

entiation? Current Topics Develop Biol 1986; 20: 39–62.

68 Bronner-Fraser M. The neural crest: What can it tell us about cell migration and determination? Curr Top Dev Biol 1980; 15: 1–25.

69 Le Dourain N. Migration and differentiation of neural crest cells. Curr Top Dev Biol 1980; 16: 31–85.

70 Pasquier B, Coudere P, Pasquier D, Hong P, Pellat J. Primary rhabdomyosarcoma of the central nervous system. Acta Neuropathol (Berl) 1975; 33: 333–42.

71 Yagishita S, Itoh Y, Chiba Y, Fujino H. Primary rhabdomyosarcoma of the cerebrum. Acta Neuropathol (Berl) 1979; 45: 11–115.

72 McKeen E, Bodurtha J, Meadows A, Douglass E, Mulvihill J. Rhabdomyosarcoma complicating multiple neurofibromatosis. J Pediatr 1978; 93: 992–3.

73 Zimmerman J, Font R, Anderson R. Rhabdomyosarcomatous differentiation in malignant intraocular medullo-epitheliomas. Cancer 1972; 30: 817–35.

74 Enzinger F, Weiss S. Soft Tissue Tumors. St Louis: CV Mosby, 1983: 625–54.

75 Cozzutto C, Comelli A, Bandelloni R. Ectomesenchymoma. Virchows Arch 1982; 398: 185–95.

76 Hendrickson M, Ross J. Neoplasma arising in congenital giant nevi. Am J Surg Pathol 1981; 5: 109–35.

SUPPLEMENTARY REFERENCES

1 Cozzutto C, Comelli A, Bandelloni R. Ectomesenchymoma. Virchows Arch A 1982; 398: 185–95.

2 Enzinger F, Weiss S. Soft Tissue Tumors. St Louis: CV Mosby, 1983: 625–54.

3 Hendrickson MR, Ross JC. Neoplasms arising in congenital giant nevi: Morphologic study of seven cases and Review of the Literature. Am J Surg Pathol 1981; 5: 109–35.

Textbook of Uncommon Cancer
Edited by C.J. Williams, J.G. Krikorian, M.R. Green and D. Raghavan
© 1988 John Wiley & Sons Ltd

Chapter **32**

Malignant Granular Cell Tumors (Myoblastomas)

John J. Brooks*
Associate Professor of Pathology, University of Pennsylvania, Philadelphia, Pennsylvania, USA

INTRODUCTION

In 1926, Abrikossoff (1) described five examples of an unusual tumor occurring within muscle tissue in various sites of the body. Although he thought that the origin of these tumors was probably muscular, he failed to find any evidence of cross-striations and considered them to be different from other skeletal muscle tumors. Because he described an appearance resembling 'myoblasts', these tumors had come to be known as 'granular cell myoblastomas'. Interestingly, Abrikossoff would not speculate as to whether these tumors were benign or malignant. He mentioned that, while the lack of mitosis and pleomorphism was against a malignant nature, the tumors nonetheless were unencapsulated and infiltrating. His reluctance to consider these tumors malignant was certainly well founded; the vast majority of these tumors behave in a benign fashion with only occasional local recurrences. More recently, with the advent of immunohistochemical techniques, the cellular composition of the granular cells has been shown to be not myogenic at all, but rather schwannian in nature. For that reason, the name of the tumor has changed to the currently accepted form—

namely benign 'granular cell tumor' (BGCT).

While most BGCTs clearly behave in a benign but occasionally locally aggressive manner, there are clear reports of a malignant variant. In fact, it was only about 20 years after Abrikossoff's original description that Ravich et al. (2) (1945) described the first example of a malignant granular cell tumor (MGCT). It should be noted however that this entity is exceedingly rare, perhaps the rarest of all soft tissue sarcomas. For example, to date the author has been able to identify a total of 36 reports of MGCT in the literature, to which he has added another case. Not all the reports described under this name are acceptable (see below). The full details concerning all acceptable reports of MGCT are summarized here in an effort to understand the natural history of this extremely unusual and rare tumor.

Granular Cell Tumor—General Comments

Some description of the characteristics of the usual benign granular cell tumor are in order. This is a tumor which is fairly common and is usually diagnosed after biopsy. Although it may occur in patients of any age, it is most common in patients in the fourth, fifth and sixth decades of life. Interestingly, it is about

* Dr Brooks is a member of the Eastern Cooperative Oncology Group Committee on Soft Tissue Pathology.

twice as common in women as in men. It is also apparently more frequent in black patients. For the most part, the tumor presents itself as a solitary painless lump usually within the dermis of the skin. One of the more common nondermal locations is the tongue, but the tumor may also be found in the viscera. Examples of the tumor involving the gastrointestinal tract, larynx and trachea, bile duct, and rarely other organs have been reported.

Somewhat more unusual are patients presenting with multiple BGCTs; this is not a rare finding and may occur in anywhere from 7 to 16% of all patients, according to Moscovic and Azar (3). Very rarely, BGCT may also be familial. Although its nature is now known to be of Schwann cell origin (see below), multiple BGCTs are almost never found in von Recklinghausen's neurofibromatosis (4).

The histology of the standard BGCT is quite straightforward (Figure 1). The vast majority

of lesions are small, usually less than 3 cm. The characteristic histologic feature is the presence of abundant eosinophilic and *granular* cytoplasm coupled with a small often pyknotic nucleus. The tumor cells tend to grow in clusters, sheets or trabeculae and for the most part have indistinct cell borders. The presence of nucleoli is quite unusual; mitotic figures and necrosis are essentially never found. The tumor characteristically invades surrounding structures and may often show neurotropism (involvement of local small nerves). The granules, ultrastructurally shown to be autophagosomes (modified lysosomes), are PAS positive and diastase resistant and may vary quite a lot in size.

Therapy for the BGCT includes total surgical excision. When this is not possible, local recurrences will develop. These are unusual, accounting for perhaps 6% of cases.

In summary, the BGCT is a benign occasio-

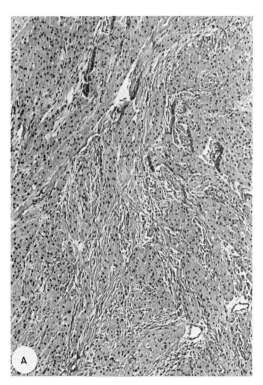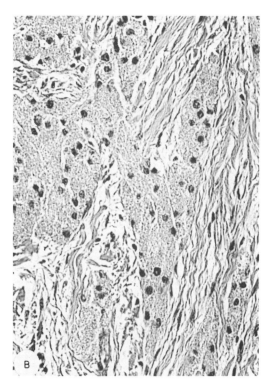

Figure 1 Benign or usual granular cell tumor. At left (A), tumor cells occur in groups and cords. Pyknotic nuclei without nucleoli are present at high power (B); no mitoses are identified.

nally local recurrent tumor with no evidence of malignant features and a characteristic ultrastructural appearance. Recently, immunohistochemical techniques have demonstrated that essentially all BGCTs contain immunoreactive S-100 protein as well as 'neuron-specific' enolase (NSE). All tumors tested have lacked myogenic markers such as myoglobin and desmin. The immunohistochemical profile is that of an altered schwannian cell, a fact in keeping with the occasional observance of granular morphology focally within schwannomas and neurofibromas.

Malignant Granular Cell Tumor— Definition

Unquestionably, a malignant counterpart to the granular cell tumor does exist, although it may be confused with other entities. In general, a case of MGCT is considered to be one in which metastases have occurred from an original lesion nearly identical to the benign granular cell tumor. For a more strict definition, the following criteria ought to be met: (1) an original lesion with histology *exactly* similar to the ordinary granular cell tumor; (2) the presence of a low mitotic rate, prominent nucleoli, and/or necrosis may be present; (3) the occurrence of metastatic disease; and (4) in the absence of metastatic disease, prominent nuclear pleomorphism and anaplasia together with mitoses and necrosis, at least focally. Importantly, a number of histologic mimickers of MGCT can be eliminated if one also requires the absence of: (1) any alveolar histology; (2) any lesion with prominent cell borders; (3) any lesion with extremely bizarre nuclei; (4) any lesion without *variably* sized eosinophilic granules; and (5) any lesion failing to show growth in sheets or long trabeculae. Further corroboration of the appropriate diagnosis would be the ultrastructural presence of the classic autophagosomes found in the cytoplasm of the usual granular cell tumor.

From a clinical point of view, it is extremely important to recognize that the diagnosis of MGCT is essentially always *after the fact*. That is, in the majority of cases, diagnosis of MGCT is made only after metastatic disease has been discovered. There is little evidence for any reliable diagnostic criteria for the prediction of metastatic disease, when viewing a granular cell tumor (see below). Rare lesions may harbor fully malignant histology in the primary lesions; these may then be initially approached as malignancies.

Literature Review

An extensive search of the literature disclosed 36 previous reports of putative MGCT. To these prior reports, a further case is added here, for a total of 37 cases. Only 23 of these 37 cases were deemed acceptable after full review of these reports. There are a variety of reasons for not accepting 14 previous reports of MGCT (Table 1). Three cases had a clear-cut alveolar pattern visible in the photomicrographs and most likely represent examples of another tumor with eosinophilic and granular cytoplasm—namely alveolar soft part sarcoma (ASPS). Another 3 cases failed to demonstrate cohesive sheets characteristic of granular cell tumor; rather these were interpreted as probably examples of rhabdomyosarcoma. In the report by Caby et al. (9) there are no photomicrographs to enable accurate evaluation; however, this may be a possible case of MGCT. In 4 cases (10, 11, 14, 16) the photographs clearly did not show the characteristic pattern of a granular cell tumor. Some of these tumors are either myxoid or extremely spindly with rounded cells. Others had prominent cell borders and argyrophilia unlike a granular cell tumor. Indeed, in the report by Remaggi et al. (14) the authors specifically state that it did *not* have features of a granular cell tumor. Two other cases (those by Salvadori and Talamazzi (13) and Madhavan et al. (17)) lack any biologic aggressiveness in the form of local recurrence or metastatic disease. Further, there was no mention of necrosis or mitoses nor cell atypic within these lesions. Rather, they are merely large granular cell tumors locally invasive. Last, in the 1985 paper by Khansur et

TABLE 1 MGCT: UNACCEPTABLE CASES IN LITERATURE

Year	First author and reference no.	Comments
1946	Ackerman (5)	Probable alveolar soft part sarcoma (ASPS)
1948	Dunnington (6)	Probable rhabdomyosarcoma (RMS), seen by Stout
1951	Schwidde (7)	NA by Robertson; probable ASPS
1958	Meredith (8)	Probable ASPS
1960	Caby (9)	NA by Robertson; no pictures (but a possible case from description)
1960	Hunter (10)	Pictures not MGCT, resemble Ca with prominent cell borders, argyrophilia; no metastases
1962	Kirschner (11)	Pictures not MGCT, spindly and round cells, negative PAS; no pathologist, no clear conclusion
1962	Krieg (12)	NA by Robertson; probable RMS
1967	Salvadori (13)	Non-metastatic, no mention of necrosis, mitoses
1968	Remaggi (14)	Pictures not MGCT, authors say it did not have GCT features, really myogenic
1969	McCabe (15)	NA by Robertson; probable RMS (vs Ca)
1971	Kuchemann (16)	Pictures not MGCT, myxoid tumor with spindly cells, much inflam., no granules
1974	Madhavan (17)	No mitoses, necrosis, cell atypia; no recurrence; large and invasive into mandible
1985	Khansur (18)	?Carcinoma; EM lacked prominent autophagosomes, had cell junctions, microvilli

NA, not accepted

al. (18) the ultrastructural features were certainly not classic MGCT; microvilli and prominent cell junctions raise the possibility of a poorly differentiated carcinoma. In a previous report on MGCT summarizing the literature, Robertson et al. (19) specifically excluded some of the cases referred to above (7, 9, 12, 15). This author agrees with Dr Robertson concerning these cases and also his inclusion of cases by Magoi et al. (20), Haustein et al. (21) and Usui et al. (22). However, Dr Robertson also included reports by Kirschner et al. (11), Salvadori and Talamazzi (13), Remaggi et al. (14) and Madhaven et al. (17); these were deemed unacceptable by this author for the above stated reasons.

A listing of cases of MGCT can be found in Table 2. The only unusual cases in this listing is that by Powell et al. (23) in which a patient developed lesions consistent with granular cell tumor in multiple sites of the body including within numerous visceral organs. However, due to the long survival (as mentioned within the paper by Crawford et al. (26)), one naturally suspects the diagnosis of malignancy in this case. The only other possible explanation would be that it represents the most unusual example of widespread multi-focal benign lesions ever described.

CLINICAL DATA

As can be seen in Figure 2, MGCT may occur in a very wide age range (23–82 years). Like its benign counterpart, the majority of cases occurred within the fourth to sixth decades of life. The average age of all 23 patients was 45.7 years. Information concerning the patient's sex also paralleled that seen in the benign granular cell tumor: the female/male ratio is 2.3, approximating the 2 : 1 ratio seen in the benign counterpart. Concerning symptomatology, this was largely a function of the site of the lesion. Most patients present with an asymptomatic solitary nodule on the external body. Occasional patients experienced pain, particularly when the lesion encroached upon or involved local nerves. The patient with an esophageal tumor experiences severe dysphasia and difficulty breathing was noted by the patient with the laryngeal lesion. Only the single case reported by Finkel and Lane (4) exhibited the stigmata of von Recklinghausen's neurofibromatosis.

The symptoms and signs are otherwise nonspecific. While most lesions were located on the external surfaces, either in the superficial skin or deep soft tissues, 4 cases were located in the viscera (including the case by Powell et al.

TABLE 2 MGCT: CHARACTERISTICS OF ACCEPTED CASES

Year	First author	Age	Sex	Size	Site	Surgery	CRx	LR Time to LR (months)	Mets Time to Mets (months)	Sites-Mets	Survival	Comment
1945	Ravich (2)	31	M	12	Bladder	1		10	1	14 · Lung, liver, spleen, prostate	DOD 17	First case
1946	Powell (23)	26	F	4	Multiple	0		1	0 · Retroperit, ovaries, neck	AWD 264	Long survival (over 22 years as per Crawford) leads one to suspect malignancy
1949	Ceelen (24)	45	F	10	Arm, multiple	1	3	1	28 · Breast lung	DOD 36	Mitoses numerous; necrosis also present
1952	Ross no. 1 (25)	60	M	2	Sacro-iliac	1	36	1	12 · Lymph nodes, lungs later	AWD 36	Mitoses numerous; necrosis not mentioned
1952	Ross no. 2 (25)	58	F	2	Ankle	1	8	1	30 · Lymph nodes, skin, CNS	DOD 78	Mitoses and necrosis not mentioned; melanoma also present and metastatic
1952	Ross no. 3 (25)	33	F	2	Thigh	1	5	0		AND 63	Mitoses and necrosis not mentioned; atypism cause for malignant designation
1953	Crawford (26)	50	F	4	Breast	0		1	0 · Lung, liver	DOD 9	Mitoses—several; necrosis not mentioned
1955	Gamboa (27)	30	F	15	Thigh	0		1	37 · Lymph nodes, lung	AWD 61	Mitoses occasional, necrosis not mentioned; outlines cases benign and malignant histology
1958	Busanny-Caspari (28)	40	M	3	Larynx	1	5	1	24 · Lymph nodes	DOD 24	No mitoses or necrosis in original biopsy; occasional mitoses in recurrence
1958	Svejda (29)	48	F	2	Groin	1	36	1	36 · Generalized, liver, nodes, lung, heart	DOD 42	Pictures=MGCT; mitoses not seen either in biopsy or at autopsy; necrosis not noted
1961	Obiditsche-Mayer (30)	23	F	10	Eosphagus	1	0	1	6 · Lymph nodes	DOD 6	No mitoses, necrosis not mentioned; autopsy: well-documented case
1966	Nitze (31)	66	M	3	Cheek	0		1	0 · Lymph node, retrobulbar later	DOD 18	No mitoses, necrosis not mentioned
1967	Mackenzie (32)	82	F	6	Lumbar	1	24	1	24 · Lymph node, lungs, breast	DOD 39	No features of malignancy in biopsy; no mitoses at post
1971	Al-Sarraf (33)	35	M	15	Perio-rectal	1	18	1	18 · Lymph nodes	AWD 96	Mitoses infrequent, necrosis not mentioned; good histochemistry and EM
1973	Magori (20)	49	F	3	Vulva	1	16	1	20 · Lymph nodes	AWD 33	Mitoses and necrosis not mentioned; good EM
1974	Haustein (21)	73	F	2	Multiple	1	0	1	0 · Lymph node, pharynx, breast, spleen	DOD 0	Mitoses present; necrosis not mentioned; EM=muscle only; questionable case by photos
1974	Cadotte (34)	60	F	10	Thigh	1	0	1	0 · Lymph nodes, lung	DOD 9	Mitoses and necrosis not mentioned; case seen by Stewart and Stout
1977	Usui (22)	34	M	17	Radial nerve	1	3	1	3 · Lymph nodes, lungs	DOD 20	Mitoses virtually absent; necrosis not mentioned; good EM
1981	Robertson (19)	33	F	3	Vulva	0		1	61 · Lymph nodes	AND 68	Mitoses and necrosis not seen initially; occasional mitosis in recuts; good EM
1982	Finkel (4)	39	M		Thigh	0		1	12 · Lymph node	AND 29	Mitoses scattered; necrosis not mentioned; good EM; VRN associated
1982	Steffelaar (35)	58	F	4	Chest	0		1	21 · Lymph node, lungs, skin, heart	DOD 35	Mitoses occasional; necrosis not mentioned; good EM; CEA− after absorbed; Alk phos+
1984	Shimamura (36)	43	F	9	Sciatic nerve	1	5	1	5 · Lung	DOD 13	Mitoses virtually absent; necrosis not mentioned; good EM; autopsied; S-100 positive
1986	Brooks (37)	36	F	2	Pre-auricular	1	12	1	24 · Lungs	DOD 42	Mitoses present at 1/10 HPF; necrosis seen; EM and IHC

Abbreviations: LR, local recurrence; Mets, metastases; DOD, died of disease; AWD, alive with disease; AND, alive no disease; IHC, immunohistochemistry.

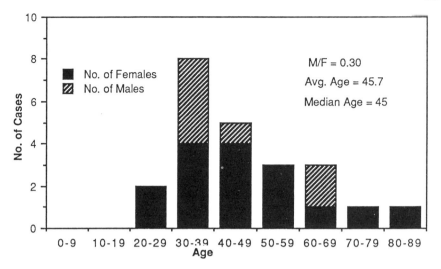

Figure 2 MGCT: age and sex distribution.

(23)). Once again, a parallel was noted here regarding location in comparison to the benign variant.

PATHOLOGY

Gross Features

On section, MGCTs are characteristically yellow-tan to pale grey-tan in appearance. Necrosis has never been noted grossly and only rarely have lesions contained apparent hemorrhage. Like the benign counterpart, a large proportion of cases are fairly small. In 22 of the 23 cases with data, 13 (or 59%) were less than or equal to 4 cm in size. On the other hand, 8 cases were quite large (greater than 9 cm). One case was intermediate in size at 6 cm. In fact, this turned out to be quite close to the average tumor size, being 6.4 cm. With this size distribution, there is considerable overlap with the benign variant and no conclusions may be drawn about this tumor based solely on size.

Histology

All the accepted cases were extremely similar microscopically. Each contained the charac-teristic features seen in the benign granular cell tumor including the presence of a sheet-like growth pattern with occasional nests and trabeculae; the presence of small nuclei with occasional nucleoli, the presence of prominent eosinophilic granular cytoplasm; the presence of variable granules within the cytoplasm; and the lack of any prominent cell borders for the most part (Figure 3). Importantly, the gra-nules are of different sizes (2–10 μm), grainy as opposed to glassy, appearing as spherical inclusions surrounded by a clear halo. In occasional cases, areas may be seen where the tumor cells round up almost resembling large histiocytes or macrophages. If just these areas are viewed, the possibility of a carcinoma might be suspected. In about 25% of the cases, involvement of local nerves or neurotropism was described. In two or three cases, vascular invasion was noted upon review of the original sections, after metastatic disease became evi-dent. However, such features are not promi-nent. Indeed, practically all of the acceptable cases exhibited the so-called 'benign' histology described by Gamboa (27) in the original biopsy specimens. In only one case (Ross et al. (25) no. 3) was there sufficient nuclear atypia so as to suggest a malignant neoplasm. As this

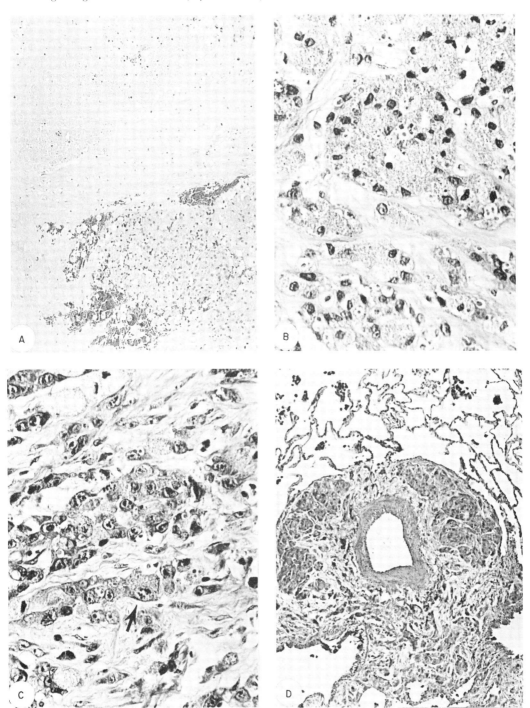

Figure 3 MGCT. At low power (A), this recurrent skin lesion had large areas of necrosis (top); some areas had typical histology with only rare cells with nucleoli (B); much of the tumor had nucleolated cells and rare mitotic figures (arrow, C); an interstitial and perivascular pattern was observed in the lung metastases (D). Note the variably sized granules in B and C.

case lacked metastatic disease, pleomorphism was the feature which made it acceptable as an MGCT. Nonetheless, in contrast to previous summaries, this review emphasizes the benign appearance of practically all cases of MGCT. Although Gamboa (27) had a second category of so-called 'malignant' appearing cases, these were (with the one exception above) not noted in this review. The reason for this is the likely exclusion of other cases in the literature failing to show characteristic histology.

Are there any clues to a malignant diagnosis in a granular cell tumor? This question is difficult to answer. The presence of any significant mitotic rate and/or necrosis should lead one to suspect malignancy in a granular cell tumor. However, as can be seen from the summary in Table 2, mitotic counts are not given in any of the published reports. Indeed, in 10 cases, no mitoses were mentioned at all. Curiously, in one example, occasional mitoses were seen only in recuts, after the appearance of metastatic disease. For the most part, mitoses are noted to be either 'virtually absent' or 'occasional' or 'present'. Similarly, no necrosis was noted in any of the reported cases. In the author's case, the mitotic rate was noted to be approximately one per ten high power fields in the initial biopsy and necrosis was seen only in the local recurrences. Since it is well recognized that the benign granular cell tumor lacks necrosis, if this feature is seen it should be extremely worrisome to the pathologist. Likewise, the presence of any mitotic figures at all shoul also raise suspicion of malignancy. Only an extremely rare mitotic figure (perhaps at the rate of one per section) may be identified in a benign granular cell tumor. Therefore, it is stressed that any mitotic rate at all in such a lesion should be cause for alarm on the part of the pathologist; further, this ought to be communicated to the clinician. It is also stressed, however, that there are no criteria concerning the mitotic rate to be put forward for a diagnosis of clear-cut malignancy. Naturally, any lesion suspected of being an MGCT ought to contain PAS positive diastase resistant granules within the cytoplasm.

Immunohistochemistry

Only a few cases of MGCT have been subjected to immunohistochemistry techniques. Immunoreactive S-100 antigen was noted in the case described by Shimamura et al (36). However, in a large study examining the usefulness of S-100 antibodies, Weiss et al. (38) disclosed a single case of MGCT which was S-100 negative. The author's case here was S-100 positive, although there was considerable negativity reflecting tumor heterogeneity (37). Carcinoembryonic antigen (CEA), occasionally reactive in the benign granular cell tumor (39, 40), had originally been noted in MGCT by Steffelaar et al. (35). However, this reaction disappeared after the antisera was absorbed with cross-reacting antigen. Further, they noted positivity with antisera to alkaline phosphotase. Additional studies were performed by the author on the single case reported here. The tumor was clearly negative for a host of antigens including monoclonal cytokeratin, the putative fibrohistiocytic marker alpha-l-antichymotrypsin, the muscle proteins myoglobin and desmin, and endothelial markers factor VIII and Ulex lectin. Tumor cells gave a weak positive reaction with vimentin antibody and numerous positive cells were seen with antisera to NSE. Although immunoreactive myelin basic protein (41) has been reported in the benign variant (42), the author's case was negative. Interestingly, a monoclonal antibody raised to melanoma (MEL 491) gave an extremely strong reaction in essentially all tumor cells. Although initially confusing, this antibody has also decorated subsequently tested benign granular cell tumors, as well as a host of other neoplasms (43, 44). Suffice to say that the immunohistochemical nature of this lesion is sufficiently similar to the benign granular cell tumor. Thus, it is also considered to be a malignancy of an altered Schwann cell.

Differential Diagnosis

Depending upon the site, there are a number of other tumors which may mimic malignant granular cell tumor. Among lesions which may present in the skin or soft tissue, rhabdomyosarcoma (RMS) and alveolar soft part sarcoma (ASPS) must be considered (concerning RMS, only those tumors with abundant cytoplasm which may appear similar to MGCT). However, in addition to an eosinophilic and granular cytoplasm, RMS quite frequently contains a filamentous texture within its cytoplasm, representing abortive cross-striations. Occasionally, actual cross-striations can also be seen. Importantly, however, RMS will not have the cohesive sheets and trabeculae of MGCT. Rather, in most examples of RMS with a sheet-like pattern, the cells are actually somewhat rounded to polygnal and have well-defined cell borders. Again, this is true for those more differentiated tumors which may cause confusion with MGCT. Further, the muscle antigens myoglobin and desmin characterize RMS.

Granular eosinophilic cytoplasm is also seen in ASPS. However, the hallmark of this tumor is its alveolar pattern, something which is never seen in a MGCT. The alveolar pattern of ASPS consists of a group of cells outlined by an endothelial cell layer, giving it an organoid appearance. Furthermore, although PAS positivity is also seen, it is usually in the form of elongated crystalline structures. Occasional examples of paraganglioma may also have an eosinophilic and granular cytoplasm; however, once again the cells form a distinctive pattern consisting of nests or 'Zellballen'. Rarely, peripheral nerve sheath tumors may contain granular cell morphology, but this is usually present only focally and the main lesion is usually evident. In the skin, a variant of angiosarcoma may be quite granular (45). In this lesion, the cytoplasm of the vascular tumor is eosinophilic and granular. However, evidence of vascular formation is evident, either in the heart of the lesion or at its peripheral edge. In other words, vascular channels will be formed in some portion of the tumor. Also, immunohistochemical stains for factor VIII related antigen will be positive in angiosarcoma. Occasionally, histiocytes may mimic

those areas of MGCT which have circular cells outside of sheets and trabeculae. Histiocytes may also contain PAS positive diastase resistant material. However, in such reactive histiocytic processes, no sheets or trabeculae of such cells are evident; rather they are often accompanied by other inflammatory cells and fibrosis.

In the skin as well as in sites of metastatic disease, melanoma may mimic MGCT. Although most melanomas have an eosinophilic cytoplasm, it is commonly glassy or nongranular in appearance. However, occasional cases of melanoma may be seen with granular cytoplasm. One helpful feature distinguishing melanoma from MGCT is the presence in melanoma of intranuclear cytoplasmic inclusions. Furthermore, the intracytoplasmic granules seen in melanoma are often quite small and uniform if present. It should be noted that both melanoma and MGCT may be S-100 positive and indeed MGCT may also express melanoma associated antigens, as described here. Ultrastructurally, however, these two tumors are vastly different; melanomas do not contain autophagosomes but rather premelanosomes or melanosomes.

When one encounters a granular cell lesion in the lung, there are a number of possibilities. These include metastatic hepatoma, thyroid carcinoma, renal cell carcinoma, acinar cell carcinoma of the pancreas, the bronchial oncocytoma, and the oncocytic type of carcinoid tumor. For the most part, all of these lesions will have prominent cell borders although some may display a trabecular-like pattern growth. Within the cytoplasm, the granules present in these neoplasms are due mainly to the presence of mitochondria and are small and quite uniform. Those in acinar cell carcinoma of the pancreas, for example, are somewhat coarse and smaller than the largest ones seen in MGCT. In hepatoma, eosinophilic hyaline globules may be noted, but these are quite uniform glassy structures as opposed to the granular-like globules seen in MGCT. Lastly, a variety of special stains may aid in the differential diagnosis of these epithelial lesions from MGCT; as epithelial lesions, all should express immunoreactivity with monoclonal cytokeratin and/or epithelial membrane antigen. One further differential diagnostic point is the pattern of disease within the lung. If multiple, the bronchial oncocytoma and oncocytic carcinoid are essentially automatically excluded from consideration.

NATURAL HISTORY OF MGCT

Although the biologic aggressiveness of MGCT was stressed in the past, this summary emphasizes the extremely variable natural history of this tumor. Occasional patients present with widespread disease and die within months. Others only develop metastatic disease after a significant period of time. Still other patients continue with active disease for variable periods of time. It is true, however, that it is only the rare patient who escapes the ultimate outcome in this disease. In this summary, there are 3 such patients who remained alive with no evidence of disease at 29, 63 and 68 months. Two of these cases had metastatic disease to local lymph nodes only; apparently lymphadenectomy was curative although one may not know for sure until longer follow-ups in the unusual disease are available. The other case (Ross et al. (25) no. 3) had no evidence of

metastatic disease. This tumor, the only one considered malignant in the absence of metastatic disease, did have a high degree of nuclear atypism consistent with malignancy.

Concerning specific tumor attributes, 16 of 23 patients (70%) had evidence of local recurrence (Figure 4). All but 3 of these occurred within 2 years after diagnosis. The average time to local recurrence was 11.3 months, and the median time to local recurrence was 5 months.

Concerning metastatic disease, all but one of the 23 patients had metastatic disease, since this is nearly a requirement for the diagnosis. All but 5 patients developed metastatic disease within 24 months. The latest time to the development of metastasis was 61 months, and this case was the only one to do so after 37 months. The average time to the development of metastasis was 17.1 months and the median time was 14 months. The most frequent site of metastasis was the regional lymph nodes, followed by the lungs; other common sites included the liver and skin. Interestingly, 2 patients developed cardiac metastasis, 3 patients developed breast metastasis, and 2 had metastatic disease to the spleen. Therefore, it is incumbent upon clinicians caring for a patient with a potential MGCT to repeatedly examine the originally resected site and the

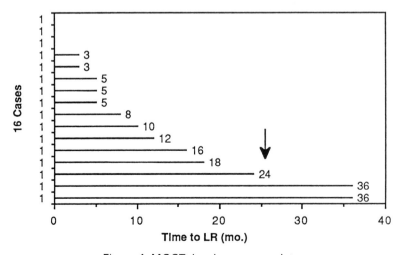

Figure 4 MGCT: local recurrence data.

regional lymph nodes, and obtain periodic chest x-ray to search for lung metastases.

Survival data was available on all 23 patients (Figure 5). In this regard, the only case which stands out as being odd is that reported by Powell et al (23). As mentioned above, this patient has survived over 22 years in the presence of widespread disease. There appears to be no particular explanation for this and the alternative of interpreting this patient's numerous tumors as benign seems untenable.

Fifteen of 23 patients (65%) ultimately died of their disease. In this group, the average survival time was 25.9 months. A further 5 patients (22%) are alive with disease at an average time interval of 98 months (56 months excluding Powell cases). Only 3 patients (13%) remain alive with no evidence of disease, for an average of 53.3 months. The overall average survival was 45.1 months and the median survival 35 months. When examining the data on these 23 patients, it seemed that the status at the 2-year point was critical: those surviving over 24 months (14 cases) had an average survival of 65.9 months compared with those 8 cases dying before 2 years with an average survival of 11.5 months. Although some patients developed metastatic disease after local recurrence, it was more common for

metastatic tumor to develop either simultaneously with or occasionally before the presence of local recurrence.

RECOMMENDATIONS FOR THERAPY

Due to the small number of cases over an extended period of time, the therapeutic manipulations varied widely. Thus, no conclusions can be drawn as to the efficacy of any particular therapeutic manipulation. Nonetheless, it is recommended that this rare sarcoma be approached in the same manner as one would the more common sarcomas. Namely, wide local excision should be attempted wherever possible, followed by postoperative radiation therapy. Once again, this therapeutic approach can only be attempted in those lesions where the initial histology is worrisome enough for a potentially malignant granular cell tumor. As mentioned above, the vast majority of lesions reported in the literature were benign appearing at the initial excision. It is further recommended that, when metastases do develop, consideration be given to an aggressive approach involving resection, due to the occasional indolent growth rate of MGCT. Certainly if only lymph node metastases are present, these should be completely

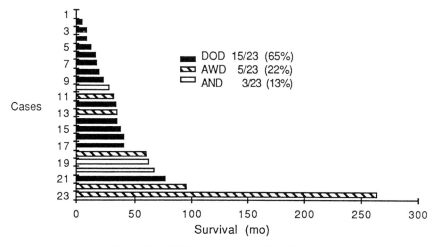

Figure 5 MGCT: survival data for 23 cases.

excised. If only a single or small number of pulmonary metastases are present, again consideration ought to be given to resection, depending upon the status of the patient and an assessment of the growth rate of the tumor. There is no current evidence that chemotherapy has any effect on this unusual sarcoma variant.

SUMMARY

In conclusion, malignant granular cell tumor is perhaps the rarest of all sarcoma types and can only be diagnosed with certainty after the development of metastatic disease. A number of lesions may mimic it histologically, compounding the problem of definitive diagnosis. Its natural history is variable but progressive and emphasis is placed upon an aggressive surgical approach to metastatic disease where possible.

ACKNOWLEDGEMENTS

A debt of gratitude is owed to Dr Guisseppe G. Pietra, Director of Anatomic Pathology at HUP, for translating a large number of previous reports. The author would like to thank Dr Roger Schinella of New York University Medical Center for supplying material, and Dr Virginia A. LiVolsi, Director of the Division of Surgical Pathology at HUP, for her comments and suggestions. Also, the author is indebted to Dr Masanori Shiraki, Chairman of the Eastern Cooperative Oncology Group Soft Tissue Committee, and other committee members with whom he has investigated this unusual tumor. A word of thanks is also due to Kathy Snyder for typing the manuscript and to Bethann Gee for performing immunohistochemical studies.

REFERENCES

1 Abrikossoff A. Über Myome, ausgehend von der quergestreiften wilülkrlichen Muskulatur. Virchows Arch Pathol Anat Physiol 1926; 260: 215–33.

2 Ravich A, Stout AP, Ravich RA. Malignant granular cell myoblastoma involving the urinary bladder. Ann Surg 1945; 121: 361–72.

3 Moscovic EA, Azar HA. Multiple granular cell Tumors ('Myoblastomas'): Case report with electron microscopic observations and Review of the Literature. Cancer 1967; 20: 2032–47.

4 Finkel G, Lane B. Granular cell variant of neurofibromatosis: Ultrastructure of benign and malignant tumors. Hum Pathol 1982; 13: 959–63.

5 Ackerman LV, Phelps CR. Malignant granular cell myoblastoma of the gluteal region. Surgery 1946; 29: 511–19.

6 Dunnington JH. Granular cell myoblastoma of the orbit. Arch Ophthalmol 1948; 40: 14–22.

7 Schwidde JT, Meyers R, Sweeney DB. Intracerebral metastatic granular cell myoblastoma. J Neuropathol Exp Neurol 1951; 10: 30–9.

8 Meredith JM, Kay S, Bosher LH. Case of granular cell myoblastoma (organoid type) involving arm, lung, and brain, with twenty years' survival. J Thorac Surg 1958; 35: 80–90.

9 Caby F, Duperrat B, Ecochard JC. Un cas de tumeur d'Abrikossof a évolution maligne. Memoires de l'Academie de Chirurgie 1960; 86: 585–9.

10 Hunter DT, Dewar JP. Malignant granula-cell myoblastoma: report of a case and review of literature. Am Surg 1960; 26: 554–9.

11 Kirschner H. Uber einen fall von maligne entartetem Myoblastenmyom der Mamma Bruns' Beitr Klini Chir 1962; 204: 87–94.

12 Krieg AF. Malignant granular cell myoblastoma. A case report. Arch Pathol 1962; 74: 251–6.

13 Salvadori B, Talamazzi F. Sul mioblastomioma granulocellulare maligno. Tumori 1967; 53: 645–9.

14 Remaggi PL, Galetti G, Balli R. Considerazioni istomorfologiche sui mioblastomiomi maligni in occasione di uni caso interessante il massiccio maxillo-facciale. Minerva Otorinolaringologica 1968; 18: 275–86.

15 McCabe MM, Harman JW. Malignant myoblastoma. A case report. J Irish Med Assoc 1969; 62: 284–6.

16 Kuchemann von K. Malignes Granuläres Neurom (Granularzell-myoblastom). Fallbericht und Literaturübersicht. Zentralbl Pathol Pathol Anat 1971; 114: 426–34.

17 Madhavan M, Aurora AL, Sen SB. Malignant granular cell myoblastoma—report of a case. Indian J Cancer 1974; 11: 360–3.

18 Khansur T, Balducci L, Tavassoli M. Identification of desmosomes in the granular cell tumor. Am J Surg Pathol 1985; 9: 898–904.

19 Robertson AJ, McIntosh W, Lamont P, Guthrie

W. Malignant granular cell tumor (myoblastoma) of the vulva: report of a case and review of the literature. Histopathology 1981; 5: 69–79.

20 Magoi von A, Szegvari M. Rezidivierender und metastasierender Abrikossoff Tumor der Vulva. Zentralb Pathol Pathol Anat 1973; 117: 265–73.

21 Haustein von UF. malignes metastasierendes Granularzellmyblastom Abrilosow mit symptomatischer Dermatomyositis. Dermatologische Monatsschrift 1974; 160: 318–28.

22 Usui M, Ishii S, Yamawaki S, Sasaki T, Minami A, Hizawa K. Malignant granular cell tumor of the radial nerve. Cancer 1977; 39: 1547–55.

23 Powell EB. Granular cell myoblastoma. Arch Pathol 1946; 42: 517–24.

24 Ceelen von W. Über die Natur der sogenannten Myoblastenmyome (zugleich ein Bericht über eine malignane Myoblastengeschwulst). Zentralbl Pathol Pathol Anat 1949; 85: 289–300.

25 Ross RC, Miller TR, Foote FW. Malignant granular cell myoblastoma. Cancer 1952; 5: 112–21.

26 Crawford ES, DeBakey ME. Granular cell myoblastoma: Two unusual cases. Cancer 1953; 6: 786–9.

27 Gamboa LG. Malignant granular cell myoblastoma. Arch Pathol 1955; 60: 663–8.

28 Busanny-Caspari von W., Hammar CH. Zur Malignitat der sogenannten Myoblastenmyome. Zentralbl Pathol Pathol Anat 1958; 98: 401–6.

29 Svejda J, Horn V. A disseminated granular cell pseudotumor; so-called metastasizing granular cell myoblastoma. J Pathol Bateriol 1958; 76: 343–8.

30 Obiditsche-Mayer I, Salzer-Kuntschik M. Malignes, 'getörntzelliges Neurom' sogenanntes, 'Myoblastenmyom', des Oesophagus. Beitr Pathol Anat 1961; 125: 357–73.

31 Nitze von H. Das sogenannte Myoblastenmyom und seine Maligne Verlaufsform. Z Laryngol Rhinol Otol Greggebiete 1966; 45: 740–7.

32 Mackenzie DH. Malignant granular cell myoblastoma. J Clin Pathol 1967; 20: 739–42.

33 Al-Sarraf M, Loud AV, Vaitkevicius VK. Malignant granular cell tumor. Arch Pathol 1971; 91: 550–8.

34 Cadotte M. Malignant granular cell myoblastoma. Cancer 1974; 33: 1417–22.

35 Steffelaar JW, Nap M, v. Haelst UJGM. Malignant granular cell tumor. Report of a case with special reference to carcinoembryonic antigen. Am J Surg Pathol 1982; 6: 665–72.

36 Shimamura K, Osamura RY, Ueyama Y et al. Malignant granular cell tumor of the right sciatic nerve. Report of an autopsy case with electron microscopic, immunohistochemical,

and enzyme histochemical studies. Cancer 1984; 53: 524–9.

37 Brooks JJ, Shiraki M, Cooper NS, Hirschl S, Leipa E, Rao UN, Roth JA, Schinella R, Greco MA, Fazzini EP. Malignant granular cell tumor: Detailed immunohistochemical study and review. Arch Pathol Lab Med (submitted).

38 Weiss SW, Langloss JM, Enzinger FM. Value of S-100 protein in the diagnosis of soft tissue tumors with particular reference to benign and malignant Schwann cell tumors. Lab Invest 1983; 49: 299–308.

39 Shousha S, Lyssiotis T. Granular cell myoblastoma: positive staining for carcinoembryonic antigen. J Clin Pathol 1979; 32: 219–24.

40 Matthews J, Mason G. Granular cell myoblastoma: An immunoperoxidase study using a variety of antisera to human carcinoembryonic antigen. Histopathology 1983; 7: 77–82.

41 Hickey WF, Lee V, Trojanowski JQ et al. Immunohistochemical application of monoclonal antibodies against myelin basic protein and neurofilament triple protein subunits: Advantages over antisera and technical limitations. J Histochem Cytochem 1983; 31: 1126–35.

42 Penneys N, Adachi K, Ziegels-Weissman J, Nadji M. Granular cell tumors of the skin contain myelin basic protein. Arch Pathol Lab Med 1983; 107: 302–3.

43 Atkinson B, Ernst CS, Ghrist BFD et al. Identification of melanoma-associate antigens using fixed tissue screening of antibodies. Cancer Res 1984; 44: 2577–81.

44 Atkinson B, Ernst CS, Ghrist BFD et al. Monoclonal antibody to a highly glycosylated protein reacts in fixed tissue with melanoma and other tumors. Hybridoma 1985; 4: 243–55.

45 McWilliams LJ, Harris M. Granular cell angiosarcoma of the skin: histology, electron microscopy and immunohistochemistry of a newly recognized tumor. Histopathology 1985; 9: 1205–16.

SUPPLEMENTARY REFERENCES

Armin A, Connelly EM, Rowden G. An immunoperoxidase investigation of S100 protein in granular cell myoblastomas: Evidence for Schwann cell derivation. Am J Clin Pathol. 1983; 79: 37–44.

Dhillon AP, Rode J. Immunohistochemical studies of S100 protein and other neural characteristics expressed by granular cell tumor. Diagnostic Histopathol 1983; 6: 23–8.

Enzinger F, Weiss S. Soft Tissue Tumors. St Louis: CV Mosby, 1983.

Gilliet F, MacGee W, Stoian M, Delacretaz J. Zur histogenese granuliertzelliger Tumoren. Der Hautarzt 1973; 24: 52–7.

Hsu S-M, Raine L, Fanger H. Use of avidin-biotin-peroxidase complex (ABC) in immunoperoxidase techniques: A comparison between ABC and unlabeled antibody (PAP) procedures. J Histochem Cytochem 1981; 29: 577–80.

Manivel JC, Dehner LP, Wick MR. Non-vascular sarcomas of the skin. In: Wick MR ed Pathology of Unusual Malignant Cutaneous Tumors. New York: Marcel Dekker, 1985.

Mogollon R, Penneys N, Albores-Saavedra J, Nadji M. Malignant schwannoma presenting as a skin mass. Confirmation by the demonstration of myelin basic protein within tumor cells. Cancer 1984; 53: 1190–3.

Mukai M. Immunohistochemical localization of S-100 protein and peripheral nere proteins (P2 protein, PO protein) in granular cell tumors. Am J Pathol 1983; 112: 139–46.

Nakajima T, Kameya T, Watanabe S, Hirota T, Sato Y, Shiosato Y. An immunoperoxidase study of S100 protein distribution in normal and neoplastic tissues. Am J Surg Pathol 1982; 6: 715–27.

Nakazato Y, Ishizeki J, Takahashi K, Yamaguchi H. Immunohistochemical localization of S100 protein in granular cell myoblastoma. Cancer 1982; 49: 1624–8.

Rode J, Dhillon AP, Papadaki L. Immunohistochemical staining of granular cell tumor for neurone specific enolase: Evidence in support of a neural origin. Diagnostic Histopathol 1984; 5: 205–11.

Stefansson K, Wollman RL. S100 protein in granular cell tumors (granular cell myoblastomas). Cancer 1982; 49: 1834–8.

Textbook of Uncommon Cancer
Edited by C.J. Williams, J.G. Krikorian, M.R. Green and D. Raghavan
© 1988 John Wiley & Sons Ltd

Chapter **33**

Peripheral Neuroepithelioma

Mark A. Israel

Head, Molecular Genetics Section, Pediatric Branch,
National Cancer Institute, National Institutes of Health,
Bethesda, Maryland, USA

HISTORY

Peripheral neuroepithelioma (PN), first described by Stout in 1918 (1), remains an evolving nosologic entity. The term can now be applied to various neuroectodermal tumors that arise outside the central nervous system and show evidence of neuronal differentiation. On the basis of recent genetic and biochemical data, such tumors as neuroepithelioma (2–8), peripheral neuroectodermal tumor (9), adult neuroblastoma (10), primitive neuroectodermal tumor (occurring outside the central nervous system) (11, 12), malignant neuroepithelioma (13), primitive neuroectodermal tumor of bone (14–16), and the malignant small round-cell tumor the thoracopulmonary region (Askin's tumor) (17–19) are now recognized as probable members of a group of tumors best regarded as a single biologic entity. These are ontologically related to but clearly distinguishable from childhood neuroblastoma.

EPIDEMIOLOGY AND ETIOLOGY

The incidence of PN is unknown. Because this tumor has been perhaps most commonly regarded as a subgroup of childhood neuroblastoma, it may represent as much as 10% of these cases, or approximately 50 cases in the United States per year. On the other hand, numerous biologic and genetic features of this tumor now suggest that it is closely related to Ewing's sarcoma (see below). Ongoing reviews at a number of clinical centers suggest that perhaps as much as 50% of tumors previously diagnosed as Ewing's sarcoma, both those occurring in bone (20) and those occurring in soft tissue (21), may have recognizable neural features. In view of these observations, the actual incidence may be as high as 200 to 300 cases per year in the United States.

The etiology of PN is also unknown. Nonetheless, this tumor is recognized in virtually all cases to be associated with either a t(11;22) (q24;q12) chromosomal rearrangement or a related, complex cytogenetic change (Figure 1) (8, 22). These translocations are indistinguishable from the chromosomal rearrangements reported in Ewing's sarcoma (23, 24), and initial molecular analysis of this translocation breakpoint confirms their similarity (25). Interestingly, a rearrangement which is cytogenetically indistinguishable but molecularly distinct from the translocation found in PN has been identified as a constitutional abnormality in a large number of families (26); however, an evaluation of those families does not indicate any evidence for an increased incidence of cancer in general or PN in particular.

683

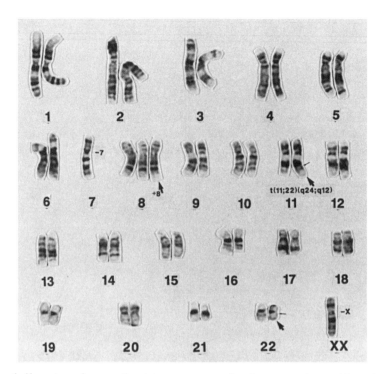

Figure 1 Karyotype from a direct tumor preparation from a patient with peripheral neuroepithelioma, showing the t(11;22) (q24;q12) cytogenetic rearrangement. Arrows indicate breakpoints in the patient's chromosomes to emphasize the chromosomal regions in the reciprocal translocation of genetic material. (Cytogenetic studies courtesy of J. Whang-Peng.)

Site-specific chromosomal rearrangements in human tumors can sometimes be associated with structural or regulatory changes in proto-oncogenes (Figure 2). In PN, the t(11;22) rearrangement results in the translocation of the c-*sis* proto-oncogene from chromosome 22 to chromosome 11 (27), although it has not been possible to demonstrate expression of this proto-oncogene in PN tumor cell lines. Since c-*sis* is located quite distant from the rearrangement, the inability to identify a structural rearrangement in this gene is not unexpected. On the other hand, the proto-oncogene c-*ets*-1 maps to chromosome 11 at precisely the breakpoint observed in PN and Ewing's sarcoma. To date, however, a rearrangement of this proto-oncogene has not been identified. Neuroblastoma tumors and cell lines generally express c-*ets*, although it is usually not expressed in PN

tumor cell lines (28); perhaps the lack of c-*ets* expression in PN is of pathologic significance. Another cytogenetic alteration in PN is the high frequency of trisomy 8, which is of interest in view of the observation that the c-*myc* proto-oncogene is located on chromosome 8 and is expressed at high levels in these tumors (Figure 3) (28).

PATHOLOGY AND BIOLOGY

PN shares not only histopathologic features with the other small round-cell tumors of childhood but also an aggressive, invasive, highly malignant behavior. This tumor can arise throughout the body, most commonly in the chest wall, and metastasizes widely. Biologically, an important feature of tumor cell lines derived from PN is the presence of choline

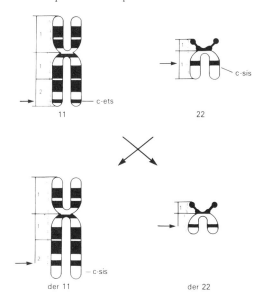

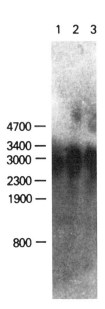

Figure 2 Proto-oncogenes rearranged in association with the reciprocal t(11;22) (q24;q11) translocation of peripheral neuroepithelioma. The genetic rearrangement of material between the long arms of chromosomes 11 and 22 occurs at sites indicated by the arrows in the vicinity of the chromosomal regions known to include c-*ets* and c-*sis* proto-oncogenes. Hybridization in situ confirmed the translocation of c-*sis* proto-oncogenes to the derivative chromosomes, although a complete evaluation of c-*ets* has not been completed.

Figure 3 c-*myc* expression in peripheral neuroepithelioma. Northern blot hybridization analysis of RNA from three peripheral neuroepitheliomas examined for the expression of c-*myc* is shown demonstrated in lanes 1, 2, and 3, where intense hybridization to a 2.7 kb RNA species demonstrates the high level of c-*myc* expression in these tumors.

acetyltransferase, an enzyme important for the synthesis of acetylcholine (27, 28). Cell lines from childhood neuroblastoma typically do not express choline acetyltransferase but do have high levels of enzymes necessary for the synthesis of catecholamines, which are neurotransmitters in the sympathetic nervous system (29). Outside the central nervous system, acetylcholine is largely limited to postganglionic parasympathetic neurons, which can be found throughout the body. These findings suggest that PN may be a tumor of this particular peripheral neuron and complement the observation that most patients with PN do not excrete high levels of urinary catecholamines (although this is a frequent biochemical alteration detectable in childhood neuroblastoma).

Pathologically, PN shows only subtle evidence of neuronal differentiation on light microscopy or immunocytochemical analysis (Figure 4). These neuronal features distinguish PN from other small round-cell tumors such as rhabdomyosarcoma, Ewing's sarcoma, small cell osteogenic sarcoma, and occasionally lymphoma. Ultrastructural features of PN which are important in this regard include dense core granules, neurites, neurotubules, and neurofilaments. Occasionally, ultrastructural studies are also non-diagnostic, and in these cases immunocytochemical evaluation for the expression of neuron-specific enolase can be of importance in establishing the neural origin of this tumor (30). Other special stains are not generally useful; and silver staining for neural secretory granules is virtually always negative. To date, no distinctive pathologic features of PN distinguish this tumor from primitive neur-

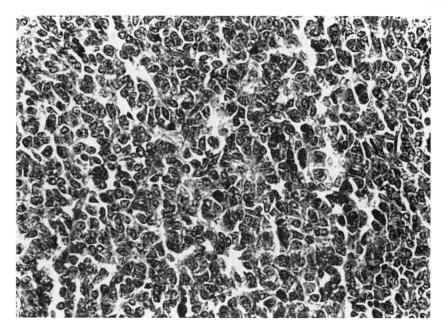

Figure 4 Peripheral neuroepithelioma on light microscopy. Sheets of morphologically undifferentiated cohesive cells separated by coarse trabeculae are seen
throughout the tumor. No firm evidence of neural differentiation is seen, although a
few rosette light clusters are present. H&E, original magnification: ×900. (Photomicrograph courtesy of T. Triche.)

oectodermal tumors of bone (16) or from
Askin's tumor of the chest wall (17–19).

CLINICAL FEATURES

PN typically occurs in adolescents and young
adults, although it has been reported in very
young children (under one year of age) and in
elderly adults. While PN may occur throughout the body, the most common site of presentation is the chest wall. Initial signs an symptoms are typically related to growth of the
primary tumor and metastases. When arising
in bone, pain is a prominent feature of the
clinical presentation. In soft tissue, the mass
may be asymptomatic, and there are rarely
functional neurologic abnormalities at diagnosis.

When PN presents as a chest wall lesion,
pleural effusion may be the most common
complication. If the effusion is contaminated
with malignant cells, there is often evidence of
pleural-based spread. Indeed, metastases are
detectable at presentation in about 25% of
patients. In the largest clinical series reported,
13 of 47 patients presented with metastatic
disease (31); the most common sites of metastatic disease were bone and bone marrow followed by lung, the most common site of
recurrence (31, 32).

INVESTIGATION AND STAGING

Evaluation of patients with PN should focus on
determining the extent of local metastatic
disease. Local evaluation should include radiography as well as computerized tomography
(CT) to define both the extent of invasion into
surrounding tissues and the extent of soft tissue
mass associated with tumors that present in
bone. In this regard, magnetic resonance
imaging (MRI) may become a more effective

technique than CT. Since regional lymph nodes can be involved at presentation, a CT or MRI scan of known sites of disease at presentation should include regional draining lymph nodes. Although the usefulness of lymphangiogram has not been defined, the evaluation of suspicious nodes must be considered, since local therapy plays an important role in the control of known sites of disease.

Metastatic disease at presentation should be investigated by isotopic bone image, bone marrow biopsy and aspiration, chest x-ray, and CT of the chest. These examinations are usually adequate to define all sites of disease, although autopsy studies have revealed diffuse abdominal and spinal metastases. When such metastases are suspected at the time of presentation, further diagnostic studies are obviously required.

There is no tested or agreed upon clinical staging for PN. Small tumor size and the absence of metastases may be important clinical variables and prognostic indicators that can contribute to clinical staging. In the only prospective study reported to date, these were the major features of the clinical staging used (Table 1) (31); however, the impact of such staging remains unknown.

MANAGEMENT AND PROGNOSIS

Recent clinical studies indicate the importance of multimodality treatment, although the optimal therapy remains to be determined (31, 32). PN is responsive to both radiation and chemotherapeutic agents. The particularly good response of patients in these trials who had completely resectable tumors suggests strongly that surgery can make an important contribution to the management of this tumor (31, 32). Complete removal of a small tumor may provide adequate local control, making radiation therapy to the primary tumor unnecessary. This can be particularly important in small children and rapidly growing adolescents for whom the potential toxicity of radiation therapy is enhanced. No current data support the usefulness of surgery to reduce

TABLE 1 CLINICAL STAGING OF PERIPHERAL NEUROEPITHELIOMA USED AT THE NATIONAL CANCER INSTITUTE (31)

Stage 1: Small tumor size (<5 cm in diameter); complete resection performed; no metastases present.

Stage 2: Small tumor size (<5 cm in diameter); gross tumor resection accomplished but microscopic disease remains; no metastases present.

Stage 3: Large tumor size (>5 cm in diameter); gross tumor resection not usually possible; no metastases present.

Stage 4: Primary tumor may be of any size; metastases present.

tumor size when complete resection cannot be achieved or metastatic disease precludes it.

Radiation therapy, in combination with chemotherapy, can provide efficient local treatment of the primary tumor at presentation. In a study reported from the National Cancer Institute (NCI), 5000 to 5500 cGy were administered to patients in 180-cGy fractions five times per week to all known sites of disease after several cycles of chemotherapy (31). In this study, with more than 2 years' follow-up, there have been no local failures. However, such intense radiation delivered over large fields, especially to the chest wall in children, can cause significant long-term toxicity.

On the basis of the natural history of this disease and its propensity to metastasize, the need for adjuvant chemotherapy seems clear, although this has not been definitively established in studies reported to date. Chemotherapy also plays a central role in patients with PN who present with metastatic disease. Only very limited data reporting single-agent chemotherapeutic response are available, but a number of drug combinations are clearly active in the treatment of PN. To date, the most extensively studied is the combination of vincristine, doxorubicin, and cyclophosphamide (31). Other drug combinations for which significant activity has been reported include ifosfamide and etoposide (33), cis-platinum and teniposide (34), and vincristine, cyclophosphamide, and dactinomycin (32). With the exception of the first regimen, experience with these combinations is limited, and only ifosfamide and etoposide provide evidence of activity that may be comparable to that of the combination of vincristine, doxorubicin, and cyclophosphamide.

In a recent NCI study, vincristine, doxorubicin, and cyclophosphamide were reported to be effective in producing an objective tumor response of greater than 50% reduction in tumor volume in more than 90% of patients treated (32). This drug combination, together with radiation therapy and surgery, resulted in complete remission in all patients studied. In a phase 2 evaluation of the efficacy of ifosfamide and etoposide in the treatment of recurrent PN, 50% of patients achieved a partial response, suggesting not only the usefulness of these agents in the relapsed patient but also their potential for use in the treatment of newly diagnosed patients (33).

Clearly, there is a role for multimodality therapy in the management of patients with PN. Initial recommendations for the management of patients include surgery when it is possible to remove the entire tumor and radiation therapy for local control when surgery is not possible. The necessity for radiation when pathologically uninvolved surgical margins can be achieved is unclear. In the recent NCI trial, chemotherapy was administered before radiation therapy to reduce the size of the tumor mass and enhance the opportunity for local control while avoiding the toxicity of large radiation fields. Such an approach also provides for immediate intervention focused on the treatment of micrometastatic disease, which is the most common source of treatment failure. Current chemotherapeutic recommendations must include a multidrug regimen at an intensity and for a duration compatible with the extent of presenting disease. In the prospective NCI series discussed above, Stage 1 and 2 patients were treated with adjuvant chemotherapy of a somewhat more modest intensity and duration than patients with advanced-stage lesions, who received intensive chemotherapy (31).

CURRENT RESEARCH IN NEUROEPITHELIOMA

Ongoing biologic studies should provide insight into the relationship of PN and other, more extensively studied, related tumors. In particular, the relationship of this tumor to Ewing's sarcoma remains enigmatic. PN can easily be confused with Ewing's sarcoma on the basis of their similar clinical presentation and appearance on light microscopy, but electron microscopic and immunocytochemical features defining neural differentiation in PN distinguishes this tumor from Ewing's sarcoma. Recent data demonstrating the expression of selected neuronal antigens (35) and the induction of neural differentiation in cell lines derived from Ewing's sarcoma (36) suggest that both these tumors belong to a common family. Ewing's sarcoma may be somewhat more dedifferentiated than PN or may arise in a slightly less differentiated cell of the same lineage.

Similarly, the relationship of PN to thoracic neuroblastoma is unclear. Thoracic neuroblastoma is a well-described tumor of childhood that is clinically and biologically distinct from childhood neuroblastoma presenting in the abdomen. It is usually asymptomatic when detected and highly curable. In contrast to PN, thoracic neuroblastoma typically involves the sympathetic spinal ganglia, a known site of sympathetic nervous tissue. Further research is required to determine the ontologic and pathologic relationships of these tumors.

Recent recognition of the activity of ifosfamide and etoposide in relapsed patients with PN suggests that new clinical protocos utilizing these agents will enhance the high response rates of current approaches, diminishing the need for extensive radiation therapy and surgery. In this regard, other data suggesting the possible efficacy of teniposide, cis-platinum, and dactinomycin in these tumors may also be of importance. Since most patients with PN who present with bulky or metastatic disease generally relapse at sites distant from where the tumor originally presented, chemotherapy should remain a focal point for attempts to improve treatment outcome.

REFERENCES

1 Stout AP. A tumor of the ulnar nerve. Proc NY Pathol Soc 1918; 18: 2.

2 Stout AP, Murray MR. Neuroepithelioma of the radial nerve with a study of its behavior in vitro. Rev Can Biol 1942; 1: 651.

3 Penfield W. Tumors of the sheaths of the nervous system. In: Cytology and Cellular Pathology of the Nervous System. New York: Hoebe, 1932: 980.

4 Lagerkvist B, Ivemark B, Sylven B. Malignant neuroepithelioma in childhood. A report of three cases. Acta Chir Scand 1969; 135: 641.

5 Ishikawa S, Ohsima Y, Suzuki T, Oboshi S. Primitive neuroectodermal tumor (neuroepithelioma) of spinal nerve root. Report of an adult case and establishment of a cell line. Acta Pathol Jpn 1979; 29: 289.

6 Bolen JW, Thorning D. Peripheral neuroepithelioma: A light and electron microscopic study. Cancer 1980; 46: 2456.

7 Harper PG, Pringle J, Souhami RI. Neuroepithelioma—A rare malignant peripheral nerve tumor of primitive origin. Report of two new cases and a review of the literature. Cancer 1981; 48: 2282.

8 Whang-Peng J, Triche TJ, Knutsen T, Miser J, Douglass EC, Israel MA. Chromosome translocation in peripheral neuroepithelioma. N Engl J Med 1984; 311: 584.

9 Seemayer TA, Thelmo WL, Bolande RP, Wiglesworth FW. Peripheral neuroectodermal tumors. In: Rosenberg HS, Boland RP eds Perspectives in Pediatric Pathology. Chicago: Year Book Medical, 1979: 151.

10 Mackay B, Luna MA, Butler JJ. Adult neuroblastoma. Electron microscopic observations in nine cases. Cancer 1976; 37(3): 1334.

11 Nesbitt KA, Vidone RA. Primitive neuroectodermal tumor (neuroblastoma) arising in the sciatic nerve of a child. Cancer 1976; 37: 1562.

12 Samuel AW. Primitive neuroectodermal tumor arising in the ulnar nerve. A case report. Clin Orthop 1982; 167: 236.

13 Hashimoto H, Enjoji M, Nakajima T, Kryu H, Daimaru Y. Malignant neuroepithelioma (peripheral neuroblastoma): A clinico-pathologic study of 15 cases. Am J Surg Pathol 1983; 7: 309.

14 Willis RA. Metastatic neuroblastoma in bone presenting as Ewing syndrome, with a discussion of 'Ewing's sarcoma.' Am J Pathol 1940; 16: 317.

15 Jaffe R, Santamaria M, Yunis EJ, Tannery NH, RM Agostini Jr, Medina J, Goodman M. The neuroectodermal tumor of bone. Am J Surg Pathol 1984; 8(12): 885.

16 Jaffe N (ed). Bone Tumors in Children. Littleton: PSG Publishing, 1979.

17 Askin FB, Rosai J, Sibley RK, Dehner LP, McAlister WH. Malignant small cell tumor of the thoracopulmonary region in childhood. A distinctive clinicopathologic entity of uncertain histogenesis. Cancer 1979; 43(6): 2438.

18 Scotta MS, DeGiacoma C, Maggiore G, Corbella F, Coci A, Castello A. Malignant small cell tumor of the thoracopulmonary region in childhood: A case report. Am J Pediatr Hematol Oncol 1984; 6(4): 459.

19 Linnoila RI, Tsokos M, Triche TJ, Chandra R. Evidence for neural origin and periodic acid-Schiff-positive variants of the malignant small cell tumors of thoracopulmonary region ('Askin tumor'). Lab Invest 1983; 48: 51A (abstract).

20 Perez-Atayde AR, Grier H, Weinstein H, Belarey M, Neslie N, Vawter G. Neuroectodermal differentiation in bone tumors presenting as Ewing's sarcoma. Proceedings of SIOP Meeting XIX, p. 61, 1985.

21 Shimada H, Newton WA, Soul LA, Qualman SJ, Aoyama C, Mauer HM. Pathologic features of extraosseous Ewing's sarcoma: A report from the Intergroup Rhabdomyosarcoma Study (submitted).

22 Whang-Peng J, Triche TJ, Knutsen T, Miser J, Kao-Shan S, Tsai S, Israel MA. Cytogenetic characterization of selected small round-cell tumors of childhood. Cancer Genet Cytogenet 1986; 21: 185.

23 Turc-Carel C, Philip I, Berger MP, Philip T, Lenoir GM. Chromosomal translocations in Ewing's sarcoma. N Engl J Med 1983; 390: 496.

24 Aurias A, Rimbaut C, Buffe D, Duboussett J, Mazabraud A. Chromosomal translocations in Ewing's sarcoma. N Engl J Med 1983; 309: 496.

25 Griffin CA, McKeon C, Israel MA, Gegonne A, Chysdael J, Stehelin D, Douglass EC, Green AE, Emanuel BS. Comparison of constitutional and tumor-associated 11;22 translocations: Nonidentical breakpoints on chromosomes 11 and 22. Proc Natl Acad Sci USA 1986; 83: 6122.

26 Zachai GH, Emanuel BS. Site-specific reciprocal translocation, t(11;22) (q23;q11), in several unrelated families with a 3:1 meiotic disjunction. Am J Med Genet 1980; 7: 507.

27 Thiele CJ, McKeon C, Triche TJ, Ross RA, Reynolds CP, Israel MA. Differential protooncogene expression characterizes histopatholo-

gically indistinguishable tumors of the peripheral nervous system. Cancer Gen Cytogen 1987;
24: 119.

28 McKeon C, Thiele CJ, Ross RA, Kwan M,
    Triche TJ, Miser JS, Israel MA. Indistinguish-
    able and predictable patterns of proto-oncogene
    expression in two histopathologically distinct
    tumors: Ewing's sarcoma and neuroepithelioma
    (in press).

29 Ross RA, Biedler JL, Spengler BA, Reis DJ.
    Neurotransmitter-synthesizing enzymes in 14
    human neuroblastoma cell lines. Cell Molec
    Neurobiol 1981; 1: 301.

30 Tsokos M et al. Neuron-specific enolase in the
    diagnosis of neuroblastoma and other small,
    round-cell tumors in children. Human Pathol
    1984; 15: 575.

31 Miser JS, Kinsella TJ, Triche TJ, Steis R,
    Tsokos M, Wesley R, Horvath K, Belasco J,
    Longo DL, Glatstein E, Israel MA. Treatment
    of peripheral neuroepithelioma in children and
    young adults. J Clin Oncol 1987; 5: 1752–8.

32 Gobel V, Jurgens H, Beck J, Brandeis W,

Etspuler G, Gadner H, Harms D, Schmidt D,
    Sternschulte W, Treuner J, Gobel U. Malignant
    peripheral neuroectodermal tumors of child-
    hood and adolescence: Retrospective analysis of
    treatment results in 30 patients. Proc ASCO
    1986; 5: 810.

33 Miser JS, Kinsella TJ, Triche TJ, Wesley R,
    Forquer R, Magrath IT. Treatment of recur-
    rent solid tumors of childhood and young adults
    with etoposide, ifosfamide and mensa uroprotec-
    tion. Clin Oncol (in press).

34 Fink I, Kinsella TJ, Cazennave L, Miser JS.
    Radiographic evaluation of peripheral neuroe-
    pithelioma. Am J Radiol (in press).

35 Lipinski M, Braham K, Philip I, Wiels J, Philip
    T, Goridis C, Lenoir GM, Tursz T. Neuroecto-
    derm-associated antigens on Ewing's sarcoma
    cell lines. Cancer Res 1987; 47: 183.

36 Cavazzana AO, Miser JS, Jefferson J, Triche
    TJ. Experimental evidence for a neural origin of
    Ewing's sarcoma of bone. Am J Pathol 1987;
    127: 507–18.

Section VI

Endocrine Tumours

Textbook of Uncommon Cancer
Edited by C.J. Williams, J.G. Krikorian, M.R. Green and D. Raghavan
© 1988 John Wiley & Sons Ltd

Chapter **34**

Tumors in the Pineal Region

Jay S. Loeffler* and
Peter Mauch†
*Instructor, Joint Center for Radiation Therapy, Depart-
ment of Radiation Therapy, Harvard Medical School,
Boston, Massachusetts, USA and †Chief, Brigham and
Women's Hospital Division, Joint Center for Radiation
Therapy; Associate Professor, Department of Radiation
Therapy, Harvard Medical School, Boston, Massachusetts,
USA

INTRODUCTION

Neoplasms arising in the region of the pineal
gland, aound the region of the third ventricle
and in the suprasellar region represent less
than 1% of all intracranial tumors of adults
and between 5% and 11% in children (1–3).
Clinical symptoms at presentation are extremely helpful in reaching a likely diagnosis,
even in the absence of a histologic confirmation
(4). The presence of diabetes insipidus in a
teenage patient with delayed or absent development of secondary sexual characteristics
or other pituitary dysfunction nearly always
indicates a pineal region tumor. Other less
common findings related to the compression of
the dorsal tectum or its projection include
nystagmus, hearing loss and ataxia (5).

ANATOMY AND EMBRYOLOGY

Certain aspects of the anatomy and embryology of the pineal region will be briefly
reviewed to aid in understanding the complicated classification and nature of tumors in this
region.

The pineal body is part of the epithalamus.

The epithalamus also consists of two habenulas
with the habenular commissure and part of the
posterior commissure with nerve cell groups in
and around it. A portion of the ependyma and
subependyma at the third ventricle also belong
in the epithalamus. The leptomeninges en-
velop the pineal gland and also support part of
the ependyma of the third ventricle in the area.

The pineal gland itself is located in the
superior cistern of the subarachnoid space and
is bathed in cerebrospinal fluid (CSF). It is
attached to the rest of the epithalamus by a
glial stalk between the habenular and posterior
commissures and is densely populated by
pinealocytes. Small numbers of astrocytes and
cells containing melanin are also found in this
densely cellular region. The area is well vascularized by blood vessels that course into its
substance from the leptomeningeal capsule of
the body. Innervation of the pineal is by cells of
the autonomic nervous system.

Embryologically, the pineal parenchymal
cells originate from the ventricular cells of the
roof of the diencephalon which continue to
proliferate after leaving the ventricular layer.
Histologically on hematoxylin and eosin
stained sections, the primitive proliferating

cells in the gland resemble small lymphocytes. Subsequently, the cells and their nuclei enlarge and become identifiable pinealocytes and astrocytes. During this phase of cell differentiation, there is a two-cell pattern of primitive, small lymphocyte-like cells with the larger, differentiating cells of various sizes.

PATHOLOGY

Tumors of the pineal region may be classified into four different histogenic groups: (1) tumors of germ cell origin (germinoma, teratoma, embryonal carcinoma, choriocarcinoma, and endodermal sinus tumor); (2) tumors of pineal parenchymal cell origin (pineocytoma and pineoblastoma); (3) tumors originating from glial or other surrounding tissues (glioblastoma, ganglioneuroma, ganglioglioma, meningioma, hemangiopericytoma, chemodectoma, astroblastoma); (4) nonneoplastic cysts and vascular lesions (6). The general pathology classification is outlined in Table 1. The most common tumors of the pineal region are described in detail below.

Germ Cell Tumors

Over 50% of pineal region tumors are germ cell tumors (7). Among the germ cell tumors

.TABLE 1 CLASSIFICATION OF PINEAL TUMORS

Tumors of germ cell origin
  Germinoma (atypical teratoma) and closely related tumors
   Teratoma—typical and teratoid

Tumors of pineal parenchymal cells
  Pineoblastoma:
    with pineocytic differentiation
    with retinoblastomatous differentiation
  Pineocytomas
    with astrocytic differentiation
    with neuronal differentiation

Tumors of glial and other cell origin

Non-neoplastic cysts and masses

---

listed above, only the germinoma and teratomas develop in appreciable numbers. All these tumors both biologically and histopathologically, resemble the germ cell tumors of the gonads and other specific extragonadal sites. The germ cell tumors originate within the pineal gland or in the surrounding leptomeningeal tissues or in the suprasella area.

At the time of surgery, germinomas are often poorly circumscribed, light grey and granular, solid tumors usually 4 cm or less in diameter at the time of diagnosis. The pineal gland can be totally replaced with tumor particularly the posterior third ventricular germinomas. Early seeding of the ventricular system and subarachnoid space, together with focal invasion of the walls of the third ventricle and rostral mesencephalon, are very common. The incidence of clinically apparent cerebrospinal seeding is significant and will be discussed in detail later in this chapter. The increased incidence of seeding seen in operated germ cell tumors is related to tumor spillage at the time of surgery. Ventricular enlargement secondary to obstruction of the aqueduct or third ventricle is common. Germinomas seldom have areas of frank necrosis, hemorrhage or cystic degeneration as is seen commonly in other intracranial tumors.

A less common germ cell tumor of the pineal gland is the well-differentiated teratoma. It is usually partially encapsulated, non-invasive, lobulated, multicystic and solid. The pineal gland itself if often totally replaced and the quadrigeminal plate may be destroyed. As with germinomas, the obstruction of CSF outflow with symmetrical hydrocephalus is an invariable finding. Calcifications are more common in teratomas than germinomas, but are not found in the majority of cases. Rarely, areas of dedifferentiation are found within the teratoma (teratocarcinoma).

Pineal Parenchymal Tumors

Pineocytomas are benign tumors of adults and account for approximately a third of the parenchymal cell tumors of the pineal. They appear to be more frequent among women. The majority of pineocytomas are well-circumscribe tumors that are confined to the posterior third ventricle. The more undifferentiated pineocytomas are more invasive into the ventricular system and tissue surrounding the posterior third ventricle.

The microscopic picture of pineocytomas is very distinctive. In its mature differentiated form the neoplasm is almost indistinguishable from the adult pineal gland (10). The tumor is often moderately cellular and composed of rounded and fusiform cells. The appearance of the tumor cells is not uniform with a great deal of histologic heterogeneity. The glial cells seen in the normal pineal are usually absent from the neoplasm. Mitotic figures, hemorrhage, necrosis, and calcifications are not usually found.

Pineoblastomas are primitive malignant neoplasms which account for approximately two-thirds of the pineal parenchymal cell tumors (11). These tumors usually originate in childhood and are somewhat more common in males. They are usually frankly invasive, gray-white gelatinous tumors that extend into the third ventricle and subarachnoid space and destroy tissues surrounding the posterior third ventricle. Extension of tumor into the posterior fossa, with involvement of the superior surface of the cerebellum and anterior vermis, can be found. Pineoblastomas found in this region have been clinically confused with medulloblastoma because of their location (12). Necrosis, hemorrhage, and calcifications are not ordinarily observed while cystic degeneration is observed occasionally. Microscopically the tumor is densely cellular and composed of cells with round or oval nuclei, rich in chromatin, and with scanty irregular cytoplasm. The presence of rosettes with central argyrophilic fibers is seen in some examples. In these instances the tumor is histologically indistinguishable from medulloblastoma and primitive neuroectodermal tumors. Pineoblastomas and bilateral retinoblastoma (so-called trilateral retinoblastoma) have been described in some patients (13).

Pineal Astrocytoma

Occasional astrocytomas confined to the pineal body have been reported (14). Pineal astrocytomas may occur throughout life, but are more common in young women. The cells are the same as in extrapineal astrocytomas and are similar to the non-neoplastic astrocytes. The majority of these tumors are of the pilocytic and pleomorphic variety. Glioblastoma multiforme is also seen, though rarely, in the pineal region (15). Central nervous system spread may occur with malignant pineal astrocytomas by way of the CSF to which these tumors have direct access because of their location in the superior cistern of the subarachnoid space.

CLINICAL MANIFESTATIONS

Tumors of the pineal region, as described earlier in this chapter, are extremely rare. Although the incidence is low, these tumors have intrigued neurologists, endocrinologists, neurosurgeons, and ophthalmologists for decades because of the characteristic clinical symptoms and signs produced. Regardless of their histologic type, tumors of the pineal region often produce a similar clinical picture characterized by increased intracranial pressure secondary to encroachment upon the posterior aspect of the third ventricle and aqueduct of Sylvius. Eye finding are related to the direct compression of the quadrigeminal plate. This compression interrupts fibers coursing from the cerebral cortex to the superior colliculi and subsequently the oculomotor nuclei. This leads to bilateral paralysis of upward gaze, pupillary areflexia, and the lack of convergence (Parinaud's syndrome).

The most common neuro-ophthalmic manifestation of a tumor in the pineal region is paralysis of upward gaze (16). The presence of vertical eye movement with neck flexion and Bell's phenomenon and simultaneous bilateral caloric stimulation with hot and cold water are evidence that the paralysis in upward gaze is supranuclear in origin. The innervational disturbances responsible for absences of upward gaze have been shown to be related to the impaired facilitation of the agonist elevator muscles and failure of the antagonist depressor muscle to inhibit (17). Recovery from upward gaze paralysis does occur. Full-gaze movements may be restored simply by relieving pressure on the pretectum following a shunt operation for hydrocephalus or rapid tumor reduction by radiation therapy (18).

With rare exceptions, pupillary reflexes are abnormal when paralysis of upward gaze is present (19). The pupils are often moderately dilated and fixed, or poorly reactive to direct light stimulation while pupillary constriction with the near reflex is retained. This type of pupil abnormality seen with pineal region tumors is different from Argyll Robertson pupils by virtue of lack of miosis and the normal responses to atropine.

Paralysis of convergence is the third sign completing the triad of Parinaud's syndrome (20). Convergence palsy is characterized by a failure of convergence with crossed diplopia when the eyes view a near target but with absence of paresis of the medial recti muscles on lateral gaze. To recognize a convergence defect the patient is asked to fix on an object brought rapidly towards the nose. Pupillary constriction indicates that new effort is being made. If complete paralysis of convergence is present, the eyes remain immovable as the object is brought towards the patient's nose. Other less common ocular signs presenting in patients with pineal region tumors include: accommodative control disorder, downward gaze paralysis, Collier's sign, cranial nerve paralysis, reduced visual acuity, and abnormal visual fields (3, 4, 16).

The location of pineal tumors above the aqueduct of Sylvius often leads to obstruction and resultant hydrocephalus even with slow growing tumors. Papilledema is present in over 50% of patients that present with these tumors (16). In addition to papilledema, optic disc swelling may occur and when present, it is usually similar in appearance in both eyes and often is severe.

In addition to the neuro-ophthalmic mani-festations of pineal tumors, other neurologic symptomatology can be present. The most frequent symptom is headache which has been described in up to 80% of patients at presentation (21). Nausea, vomiting and papill-edema are present in the majority of patients with headache. Seizures, not usually associated with pineal region tumors, occur in a few patients with severe hydrocephalus. If the pineal tumor invades the cerebellum, dysmetria, hypotonia and intention tremor can be present. Direct invasion of the brain stem (most common in pineoblastoma) can result in long tract and cranial nerve findings (22).

Endocrine dysfunction is such a frequent concomitant of tumors of the pineal region that the endocrine status of all patients with these tumors must be assessed thoroughly. Although precocious puberty in males is the most widely known endocrine abnormality, it is merely one of several endocrine disturbances that beset patients with such neoplasms. These tumors are not infrequently associated with isolated hypogonadism, diabetes insipidus, and anterior pituitary insufficiency. These findings may be less obvious than precocious puberty, but are more threatening to the survival of the patient.

The reported incidence of sexual precocity among patients with pineal region tumors varies markedly in the literature. In one series of 606 patients with these tumors, 46 cases of precocious puberty were found (23), whereas no cases of precocious puberty were found in 65 patients with confirmed pineal region tumors from Stockholm (24). Pineal region tumors in contrast only make up a small proportion of the children with precocious puberty (15–20%) (25, 26). Precocious puberty associated with tumors of the pineal region was reported in one study to occur mainly in boys (23).

There are presently three theories to explain the occurrence of precocious puberty in boys with tumors of the pineal region (27). The first theory postulates the presence of an antigonadotropic substance released by the pineal gland. Sexual prococity occurs when secretion of this substance is decreased as a result of the destruction of pineal parenchymal cells by a tumor of nonparenchymal origin. The second theory suggests that the expanding tumor produces loss of the inhibiting effects of the diencephalon on the median eminence resulting in augmental secretions of the gonadotropins and precocity. The third hypothesis is that the pineal tumor itself produces an ectopic gonadotropin. Despite these three theories, all of which are supported by indirect evidence, the mechanism of sexual precocity in boys with tumors of the pineal region is not yet established.

Diabetes insipidus is an important clinical manifestation of these tumors. Its presence may herald the diagnosis and it is the most common endocrine abnormality associated with these tumors. The exact incidence is not known because of the different criteria used by previous investigators to make this diagnosis. In most reports the diagnosis is asserted on clinical grounds; however, a few recent studies have used plasma and urine osmolalities and even provocative tests to detect mild cases (28). The exact cause of diabetes insipidus is unknown. It is thought to be probably due to extension of the tumor from the pineal area to the hypothalamus and pituitary (29, 30). Whatever the cause, it is an extremely important clinical finding in these patients. It may precede the potential devastating neurologic and ophthalmologic manifestations of the tumor by months and even years (31, 32). Diabetes insipidus can be reversed if rapid tumor regression occurs secondary to surgery or radiation.

DIAGNOSTIC EVALUATION

Radiography

Radiographic evaluation of the central nervous system is an essential part of the initial work-up of all patients suspected on clinical grounds to be harboring a pineal region tumor. Skull radiographs are abnormal in approximately 25–50% of patients at presentation (33). The abnormalities seen are often the result of changes secondary to chronic intracranial hypertension such as the erosion of the dorsum sellae or widening of the sutures of the cranial vault. There may be changes in the amount and configuration of calcification in the pineal region which may suggest the presence of a space-occupying lesion. While pineal calcifications can be seen in 50% of the normal adult population, their presence in the pediatric population is rare (34). The presence of calcification in the region of the pineal gland in a child should be considered a pineal tumor until proven otherwise (35). Presently, computed tomography (CT) of the cranial contents with intravenous contrast represents the most widely used and perhaps the most useful study for tumors of this region. CT of the head with enhancement can delineate the size and position of the lesion, the presence and degree of calcification, cystic or hemorrhagic component, the degree of hydrocephalus, and whether there is evidence of subependymal extension. Suprasellar extension from a posterior third ventricular mass may be quite subtle and require serial tomographic pictures for its detection.

In addition to defining the size and location of pineal region tumors, CT can also aid in the differential diagnosis. Germinomas have a soft tissue density greater than normal brain tissue. Uniform enhancement is generally the rule (Figure 1). Calcification is not generally found in the tumor matrix of germinomas as seen on CT. Germinomas tend to be better defined and do not appear to invade the surrounding normal brain or subarachnoid spaces. Embryonal cell carcinomas have similar soft tissue density as germinomas, but more commonly contain calcification and cystic areas (37). The benign teratomatous tumors show evidence of tissue derived from all three germinal layers of development, such as fat, ossification, calcification and soft tissue density.

The CT is also helpful in diagnosing pineocytomas and pineoblastomas. These tumors show isodense tumor matrix and a tendency towards parenchymal calcification within the tumor. Contrast enhancement, while generally

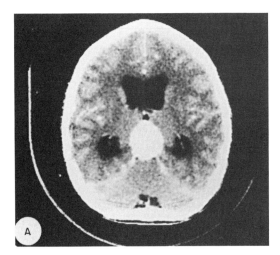 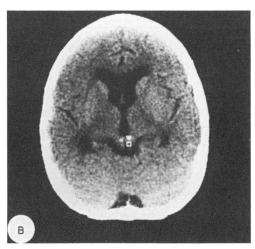

Figure 1 A, Post-enhancement CT image of a 12 year old boy who presented with headaches, diplopia, and a stiff neck. B, After 2000 cGy, the enhancing 3 cm pineal region mass has dramatically responded. The patient went on to receive cranial–spinal irradiation for a presumed germinoma. The patient is currently alive and free of disease 2 years after the completion of therapy.

not as dramatic as seen in germinomas, also tends to be the rule. Astrocytomas can either expand, invade or displace the pineal gland depending on whether the tumor is arising from within the gland or adjacent to it. Astrocytomas often are of decreased density relative to the surrounding brain parenchyma. Inhomogeneous contrast enhancement is generally seen as in astrocytomas outside the pineal region (Figure 2). Direct coronal and reconstructed sagittal sections may help differentiate the pineal from the hypothalamic and mesencephalon astrocytomas.

While it has not been our policy to use cerebral angiography (particularly in children), this can be a useful radiographic study to complement the CT. In tumors of the pineal region, a number of adjacent arterial and venous structures may be displaced or deformed or may provide an abnormal source of blood supply or venous drainage. Abnormalities in angiography appear to depend upon the quality of the examination with particular reference to the use of magnification angiography with subtraction after the deliverance of an adequate volume of contrast material. In a series of 12 patients with pineal

region tumors, 4 patients (33%) had tumor vascularity or stain with the displacement of adjacent arteries and veins (38).

The role of myelography in the examination of the spinal axis in patients with pineal tumors is not clear. It has generally been our policy not to perform this procedure in children with clinical and radiographic evidence of pineal region tumors. If on clinical grounds (i.e. response to radiation therapy) the patient has a germinoma or pineoblastoma, we begin cranial–spinal irradiation to prophylactically treat the axis in these seeding tumors. Thus, the presence of spinal axis metastases would not change our therapy and we do not for purely investigational reasons feel it is worth the expense and morbidity. An advantage of myelography is the collection of CSF. Cytologic examination of the fluid by use of Millipore-filtered and CSF tissue culture techniques may establish the nature and extent of the lesion.

It is difficult to conclude a section on radiographic studies of any brain tumor without a brief discussion of magnetic resonance imaging (MRI). The role of MRI in the diagnosis of pineal region tumors is yet uncertain. CT images are limited to the transverse

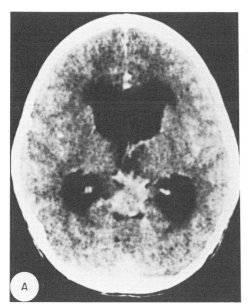
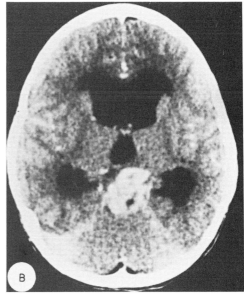

Figure 2 A, Post-enhancement CT image of a 5 year old boy who presented with a left sixth nerve palsy and severe headaches. CT shows an enhancing mass obstructing the aqueduct with secondary acute hydrocephalus. B, After 2000 cGy, little change in the size and enhancement has occurred. A CT guided stereotactic biopsy was obtained which revealed a low grade astrocytoma. The patient received 5400 cGy to a local field and is alive and well 20 months after the completion of therapy.

axial plane (with gantry angulation). MRI can be produced in any of the three orthogonal planes: axial, sagittal, or coronal. This would be particularly helpful in the imaging of tumors in this region and preliminary evidence suggests that MRI may be an effective tool in identifying abnormalities in this region (39, 40). Its ability to differentiate specific histology is at the present unknown although a recent report indicates that the different germ cell tumors of the pineal lesions demonstrate different and distinct MR signals (65). Unfortunately, MR does not image calcification and patients with only calcification are better served with CT. Another advantage of MRI is the ability to scan the spinal axis with good sensitivity for metastases.

Tumor Markers

The use of serum and CSF fluid to measure tumor markers is very helpful in the diagnosis,

quantitative measurement of tumor burden, management, and prognosis in patients with pineal region tumors. As reflection of tumor burden, they may allow evaluation of response to therapy and detection of early tumor recurrence.

Alpha-fetoprotein (AFP) is an oncofetal glycoprotein that has been useful in the evaluation of certain diseases (41). Primary germ cell tumors of the pineal region, specifically endodermal sinus tumors, yolk sac tumors, have been reported to elevate CSF AFP with normal serum levels or have abnormal CSF–serum gradients (42).

Human chorionic gonadotropin (hCG), a placental glycoprotein, is secreted by the placental trophoblastic epithelium. The immunologically specific beta subunit (β-hCG) is found normally only in fetal blood and in the serum of pregnant women. Elevated β-hCG levels have been found to be present in patients with pineal region choriocarcinomas, embryonal cell tumors and teratocarcinomas (41). Forty to fifty percent of germinomas and embryonal carcinomas of the pineal region are β-hCG producing. Cases have been reported in which pineal tumors produce both AFP and β-hCG, although no tumors have been reported, as far as these authors know, that produced AFP alone. In 7 teratomas seen at our institution, in a 10-year period from 1972 to 1982, 5 patients produced elevation of CSF β-hCG, one produced elevation of serum β-hCG and one patient was found to have elevated CSF β-hCG and AFP (44). It has been our experience that plasma levels of these tumor markers correlate well with tumor growth kinetics and regression and have served as a useful tool in assessing response to radiation therapy. Another tumor marker that has been utilized in pineal region tumors is plasma melatonin. However, since there often might be significant extrapineal sources of melatonin, the value of this test has been questioned even when a pineal tumor is present and raised melatonin levels exist (45).

TREATMENT AND RESULTS

Surgery

The exact role of surgery in the diagnosis and treatment of pineal region tumors is highly debated. Pineal region tumors are perhaps the most dangerous of all intracranial masses to excise. It is not clear that surgery is in the patient's best interest. The attempt to explore these lesions has historically been associated with high morbidity and mortality (46). This high rate of morbidity and mortality has been greatly reduced in recent years, however. Schmidek and Waters in a literature review of 128 posterior third ventricle tumors subjected to direct exploration found only 2 operative deaths (47). All these explorations were performed in the last 10 years with the use of modern microsurgical techniques. The 2 deaths in this combined series review were in patients with large, infiltrating glioblastomas that hemorrhaged postoperatively.

While it appears feasible for a neurosurgeon, highly experienced in the exploration of the third ventricle, to operate on these lesions with acceptable risk, we believe not all patients require surgical intervention. Diagnosis may be obtained on the cytologic examination of the CSF, extraneural metastases, or the presence of an elevated tumor marker (AFP, β-hCG) in patients harboring a germinoma or other malignant germ cell tumor. In contrast to the above tumors, there is a strong indication for surgical intervention if the diagnostic studies suggest that a symptomatic benign tumor may be present (teratoma). Another indication for surgery includes patients who have been shunted and irradiated who present with progressive neurologic deterioration despite a well-functioning shunt. A somewhat more controversial role for surgery is in those patients in whom all non-surgical investigations have failed to reveal characterization of the tumor (48). As will be discussed later, the use of response to radiation therapy as judged by serial CT scanning may provide important information concerning the potential histology of the tumor present.

The development of CT guided stereotactic biopsy technology has provided a safe and efficient method in obtaining histologic diagnosis of pineal region tumors. In two separate reports of 50 patients undergoing stereotactic biopsy, 46 (92%) of these biopsies provided diagnostic tissue specimens (48, 49). There were no deaths and no significant morbidity among these 50 patients. The use of a flexible ventriculoscope, has provided a new method to biopsy pineal region masses. The scope is introduced into a lateral ventricle through a burr hole and under direct visualization a biopsy is obtained. Using these new techniques, approximately 50% of patients are able to have a diagnosis established (50).

The description of the variety of operations devised to allow direct surgical exploration of the pineal region is beyond the scope and purpose of this chapter. The authors would like to mention briefly, however, the posterior fossa–supracerebellar approach to the pineal region. This operation, reintroduced to the neurosurgical community by Stein in 1971, has the specific advantage of avoiding the deep venous structures usually situated dorsal and lateral to these tumors (51). In addition, the amount of retraction of important structures is less than required with the supratentorial approach. This procedure is performed in the sitting position (except in children) and allows for adequate decompression. In the encapsulated lesions (teratoma), total excision by dissection can be performed.

Radiation Therapy

The high morbidity and mortality rates of surgery in the past for these tumors, led investigators to explore the use of radiation therapy in these tumors. Rubin and Kramer reviewed the available literature in 1965 and could find no long term survivors in patients with germinomas treated with surgery alone (31). In contrast, the authors reported 50% of their patients alive without disease 5 years after radiation therapy. This early report focused attention on the radiocurability of pineal germinomas. It also encouraged the use of radiation without biopsy for tumors in the pineal and suprasellar locations. This approach was particularly attractive because of the relatively high cure rate with little morbidity.

The interpretation of treatment results in the literature with radiation therapy is difficult. Most series suffer from small numbers of patients treated and the absence of histologic diagnosis. Survival rates at 5 years post-radiation therapy range from 44 to 78% in the literature (52, 53). The incidence of intracranial recurrence range from 6 to 40% depending on the dose, technique, and histology (38, 54).

The Children's Cancer Study Group (CCSG) reported on 118 patients treated with radiation from twelve institutions (7). With follow-up ranging from 2 to 15 years, 65% of patients are alive. The importance of this study is the high rate of histologic confirmation of the diagnosis of the treated patients (see Table 2). A diagnosis was obtained in 57/65 (88%) of patients before the initiation of radiation. Seventy-two percent (26/36) of patients with germinoma survived compared to only 22% (3/14) of patients with a pineal parenchymal tumor or malignant teratoma. The survival of patients with biopsy proven germinoma was comparable to that of patients treated without a biopsy.

It is noteworthy that non-germinomatous tumors appear also to have an excellent prognosis in more recent studies that have used more aggressive therapy. In a report from the Children's Hospital of Philadelphia, 15/22 (69%) of patients with pineoblastoma (5), pineocytoma (3), embryonal cell carcinoma (5), glioma (8), and ganglioneuroblastoma (1) are alive from 6 months to 13 years after radiation (3). Our experience with non-germinomatous tumors is similar with 13 patients (7 malignant teratomas, 6 solitary tumors); 9/13 (69%) are alive 7–127 months (31 months median) following radiation. This compares with 10/11 (91%) in germinomas and multiple midline tumor patients.

Germinomas may infiltrate locally, spread along the ventricular walls or seed throughout the leptomeninges. The exact incidence of seeding at presentation is difficult to determine from the present literature, but it is believed to be less than 15% (55). In the CCSG experience, 9 of 109 (8%) patients with pineal or suprasellar tumors who did not receive spinal

TABLE 2 HISTOLOGIC DIAGNOSIS
OF PINEAL REGION
TUMORS

Germinoma	63%
Germinoma with embryonal	2%
Embryonal	4%
Choriocarcinoma	2%
Teratoma	12%
Parenchymal tumors	12%
Astrocytoma	2%
Glioblastoma multiforme	2%
'Benign'	2%

From Children's Cancer Study Group (7)

irradiation developed metastases in the spine. In the absence of a biopsy or surgical exploration, the incidence of spinal seeding appears low and some authors believe that routine spinal irradiation is not warranted (8, 55). However, the data on spinal recurrence after cranial irradiation alone must be viewed with caution. In the CCSG data, the risk of spinal failure of 8% is a crude value of many patients followed for a relatively short period of time. It would be helpful to know an actuarial value for the risk of spinal failure at a longer follow-up period. If the spinal axis is not going to be treated, the use of myelography is mandatory. CSF cytology with Millipore-filtered preparation and tissue culture techniques should also be performed before the initiation of cranial irradiation. Unfortunately, the correlation between CSF cytology and metastasis to the spinal axis is uncertain (22). We have had 2 patients with negative cytology in the presence of clinical and myelographic evidence of cord involvement. Despite the apparently low risk of spinal axis seeding, it has been our policy to irradiate the spinal axis in all germ cell tumors of the pineal region. With the more widespread use of stereotactic pre-radiation biopsy, there has been an increase in the incidence of seeding of the subarachnoid space. In 8/14 (57%) patients with pre-radiation biopsies, metastases to the subarachnoid space have occurred (53). In a retrospective review of 10 patients with biopsy proven germinoma, Jenkin et al. found 0/5 patients treated with cranial–spinal irradiation developing seeding as compared with 2/5 in whom the spine was not treated (56).

Regardless if spinal axis irradiation is used or not, large brain fields should be used initially in patients with germinomas (8, 31, 44, 55, 57). We recommend the use of opposed lateral cranial fields that encompass the whole brain and the meninges or at least the entire ventricular system. Intracranial recurrences have been reported at the margin of the irradiated volume when less than whole brain fields have been used even with the use of pre-treatment CT scanning (8, 56, 58). In a literature review,

Salazar found that patients treated with whole brain irradiation had a higher survival rate than those treated to the ventricular system or to smaller volumes. The survival rate without evidence of recurrence for patients treated to the whole brain was 76% compared with 61% an 51% for patients treated to the ventricular system or smaller volumes respectively.

The exact dose of radiation needed to control pineal region tumors is dependent on tumor histology. Pure germinomas appear to be similar in their radio-responsiveness as testicular seminomas, while some 'germinomas' contain embryonal cell elements that appear to require a higher dose (56, 59). The intracranial relapse rate in patients receiving 5000 cGy per lesion is substantially less than those patients receiving a lower dose. In a retrospective review, Sung et al. found an intracranial relapse rate of 47% (15/32) for patients receiving less than 5000 cGy compared with 10% (4/40) for those receiving 5000 cGy or more (53). In the experience at the University of Rochester, a survival of 90% was achieved when patients were treated with prophylactic whole brain irradiation and a boost to the primary for a total dose of at least 5000 cGy. This compares to a 33% survival for patients treated to the same dose with smaller fields and 33% of patients who received less than 5000 cGy to the primary site, regardless of field size. Recommended doses for prophylactic whole brain irradiation are 2500–4000 cGy, 2500–3500 cGy for the spinal axis, and 5000–5500 cGy for the primary.

If the histologic diagnosis is unknown, CSF cytology and myelogram are negative, and serum and CSF markers are absent, it is our practice to utilize the radiation response of the tumor by CT as an aid in the diagnosis and a guide to management. CT in verified germinoma has documented rapid tumor response with low dose of radiation (2000 cGy) (60, 61). A rapid response to irradiation has been interpreted as diagnostic of germinoma, thereby obviating the need for histologic confirmation for certain selected cases (Figure 1). The slowly responding or non-responding tumors

include choriocarcinoma, embryonal cell carcinoma, endodermal sinus tumor, malignant
teratoma, pineocytoma, astrocytic tumor and
benign tumors (teratoma). It has been our
policy to deliver 2000 cGy to the tumor and
repeat the CT. If substantial tumor regression
has occurred (presumed germinoma or
pineoblastoma), we then initiate cranial–spinal irradiation. If little or no response is noted
by CT, the smaller field is continued to a dose
of 5500 cGy at 180 cGy per fraction (Figure 2).
If tumor persists after full dose irradiation,
surgical exploration and tumor excision may
salvage some patients (3).

Chemotherapy

There is very little information about the role
of systemic chemotherapy in the treatment of
pineal region tumors. However, there are
special features in this region to suggest that
they might be treated successfully with chemotherapy. The absence of a blood–brain barrier
in the pineal gland suggests that lesions located
there may have an increased vulnerability to
systemic chemotherapy. Non-germinomatous
germ cell tumors that occur in this region are
also known to respond in other extra-gonadal
sites and there is no reason to believe that the
same response would not occur in the pineal
region (62). The use of a vinblastine–bleomycin–cis-platinum regimen has achieved complete responses in patients with systemic metastases and local recurrence of non-
germinomatous germ cell tumors of the pineal
gland (3, 4, 63, 66). A 50% response rate was
found recently using a multi-agent chemotherapy (vinblastine, bleomycin, Adriamycin)
in 8 children with either recurrent local disease
or metastatic disease. The authors conclude
that good palliation with acceptable morbidity
can be achieved and suggest that chemotherapy be used in the histologically confirmed
pineal germ cell tumors as the primary treatment. Recently, Bamberg et al. have proposed
a formal protocol for systemic chemotherapy as
the primary treatment of endodermal sinus
tumors of the pineal region (64). Chemo-

therapy for the pineal parenchymal tumors
can not be recommended at this time except in
very young patients for whom pre-radiation
chemotherapy may enable the delay of radiation to the developing nervous system.

SUMMARY

Tumors of the pineal region are rare and
represent a heterogeneous group of mass
lesions originating in or located adjacent to the
pineal gland. Characteristic eye signs, diabetes
insipidus, and precocious puberty are some of
the distinct clinical findings associated with
these tumors. While the presumptive diagnosis
can often be made on the basis of clinical
findings, the use of CT imagings allows for
more precise diagnosis as well as for differentiating between cysts and malignant tumors. It
also provides an opportunity to evaluate the
responsiveness of the tumor to treatment.
Although treatment varies from one medical
center to another, radiation therapy remains
an integral part of management. While surgical excision has historically been associated
with a high rate of morbidity, the reintroduc-
tion of the posterior fossa–supracerebellar
approach has led to greatly reduced operative
risks. Also, the development of CT guided
stereotactic biopsy has helped in the management of these patients. The exact role of
chemotherapy has not been determined, but,
early results with cis-platinum based regimens
for pineal region germ cell tumors have been
encouraging.

REFERENCES

1 Zulch KJ. Brain Tumors: Their Biology and
   Pathology. New York: Springer Verlag, 1957:
   189–92.
2 Hoffman HJ, Yoshida M, Becker LE et al.
   Experience with pineal region tumours in childhood. Neurol Res 1984; 6: 107–12.
3 Packer RJ, Sulton LN, Rosenstock JG et al.
   Pineal region tumors in childhood. Pediatrics
   1984; 74: 97–102.
4 Swischuk LE, Bryan RN. Double midline intracranial atypical teratomas. Am J Roentgenol
   Radium Ther Nucl Med 1974; 122: 517–24.

5 Milhorat TH. Pediatric Neurosurgery. Contemporary Neurology Series. Philadelphia: FA Davis, 1978; 211–83.

6 Rubinstein LJ. Tumors of the central nervous system. In: Atlas of Tumor Pathology, Series 2, Fascicle 6. Washington DC: Armed Forces Institute of Pathology 1972; 154–284.

7 Wara W, Jenkin DT, Evan A et al. Tumors of the pineal and suprasellar region: Children's Cancer Study Group treatment results 1960–1975. Cancer 1979; 43: 698–701.

8 Salazar OM, Castro-Vita H, Bakos RS et al. Radiation therapy for tumors of the pineal region. Int J Rad Onc Biol Phys 1979; 5: 491–9.

9 Dayan AA, Marshall AHE, Miller AA et al. Atypical teratomas of the pineal and hypothalamus. J Pathol Bacteriol 1966; 92: 1–28.

10 Degirolami U, Schmidek H. Clinicopathological study of 53 tumors of the pineal region. J Neurosurg 1973; 39: 455–62.

11 Borit A, Blackwood W, Mair WGP. The separation of pinecytoma from pineoblastoma. Cancer 1980; 45: 1408–18.

12 Rubinstein LJ. Cytogenesis and differentiation of primitive central neuroepithelial tumors. J Neuropathol Exp Med 1972; 31: 7–26.

13 Bader JL, Miller RW, Meadows AT et al. Trilateral retinoblastoma. Lancet 1980; ii: 582–3.

14 Papasozomenos S, Shapiro S. Pineal astrocytoma: report of a case confined to the epiphysis with immunocytochemical and electron microscope studies. Cancer 1981; 47: 99–103.

15 Zeitlin H. Tumors in the region of the pineal body. A clinicopathologic report of three cases. Arch Neurol Psychiatry 1935; 34: 567–86.

16 Posner M, Horrax G. Eye signs in pineal tumors. J Neurosurg 1964; 3: 15–24.

17 Collins CC, O'Meara D, Scott AB. Muscle tension during unrestrained human eye movement. J Physiol 1975; 245: 351–69.

18 Shallat RF, Pawl RB, Jerua MS. Significance of upward gaze palsy (Parinaud's Syndrome) in hydrocephalus due to shunt malfunction. J Neurosurg 1973; 38: 717–21.

19 Tod PA, Porter AJ, Jamieson KG. Pineal tumors. Am J Roentgenol Ther Nucl Med 1974; 120: 19–26.

20 Parinaud H. Paralysis of the movement of convergence of the eyes. Brain 1986; 9: 330–41.

21 Wray SH. The neuro-ophthalmic and neurologic manifestations of pinealomas. In: Schmidek HH ed, Pineal Tumors. New York: Masson, 1977: 21–59.

22 Jooma R, Kendall BE. Diagnosis and management of pineal tumors. J Neurosurg 1983; 58: 654–65.

23 Kitay JI, Altschule MD. The Pineal Gland. Cambridge, MA: Harvard University Press, 1954.

24 Ringertz N, Nordenstam H, Flyger G. Tumors of the pineal region. J Neuropathol Exp Neurol 1954; 13: 540–61.

25 Bing SF, Globus SH, Simon H. Pubertas praecox: a survey of the reported cases and verified anatomical findings: with reference to tumors of the pineal body. J Mt Sinai Hosp 1938; 4: 935–65.

26 Wilkins L. Diagnosis and Treatmetn of Endocrine Disorders in Childhood and Adolescence, 3rd edition. Springfield, Illinois: CC Thomas 1965; 223.

27 Bourier-Lapierre M, David M, Jeunce M. Manifestations endocriniennes des lésions de la région pinéale chez l'enfant. Oto-Neuro-Ophthalmol 1973; 45: 7–16.

28 Puschett JB, Goldberg M. Endocrinopathy associated with pineal tumors. Ann Intern Med 1968; 69: 203–19.

29 Horrax G. The role of pinealomas in the causation of diabetes insipidus. Ann Surg 1947; 126: 725–39.

30 Stringer SW. Diabetes insipidus associated with pinealoma transplant in the tuber cinereum. Yale J Biol Med 1934; 6: 375–83.

31 Rubin P and Kramer S. Ectopic pinealoma: a radiocurable neuroendocrinologic entity. Radiology 1965; 85: 512–23.

32 Lewis I, Baxter DW, Stratford JG. Atypical teratomas of the pineal. Can Med Assoc J 1963; 89: 103–10.

33 Grossman CB, Gonzalez CF. Neuroradiology of the pineal region. In: HH Schmidek ed Pineal Tumors. New York: Masson 1977: 79–98.

34 Zimmerman RA, Bilanisk LT. Age-relate incidence of pineal calcification detected by computed tomography. Radiology 1982; 142: 659–62.

35 Willich E, Sellier W, Weigel W. Die intraKraniellen Verkalkungen des Kindes alters. Furtschr Geb Roentgenstr Nuklearmed Erganzungsband 1972; 116: 735–50.

36 Weisberg LA. Clinical and computed tomographic correlations of pineal neoplasms. Comput Radiol 1984; 8: 285–92.

37 Zimmerman RA, Bilaniuk LT, Wood JH et al. Computed tomography of pineal, parapineal, and histologically related tumors. Radiology 1980; 131: 669–77.

38 Abay EO, Laws Jr ER, Grado GL et al. Pineal tumors in children and adolescents; treatment by shunting and radiotherapy. J Neurosurg 1981; 55: 889–95.

39 Zimmerman RA. Pineal region masses: radio-

logy. In: Wilkins RH, Rengachary SS eds Neurosurgery, New York: McGraw-Hill, Vol 1 1985: 680–7.

40 Brant-Zawadski M, Norman D, Newton TH et al. Magnetic resonance of the brain: the optimal screening technique. Radiology 1984; 152: 71–7.

41 Schein PS. Tumor markers. In: Wyngaarden JB, Smith LH Jr eds Textbook of Medicine, Philadelphia: WB Saunders, 1982: 1020–2.

42 Seldenfield J, Marton LJ. Biochemical markers of central nervous system tumors measured in cerebrospinal fluid and their potential use in diagnosis and patient management: a review. J Nat Cancer Inst 1979; 63: 919–31.

43 Haase J, Nielsen K. Value of tumor markers in the treatment of endodermal sinus tumors and choriocarcinoma in the pineal region. Neurosurgery 1979; 5: 485–8.

44 Rich TR, Cassady JR, Strand RD, Winston KR. Radiation therapy for pineal and suprasellar germ cell tumors. Cancer 1985; 55: 932–40.

45 Barber SG, Smith JA, Hughes RC. Melatonin as a tumor marker in a patient with pineal tumour. Br Med J 1978; ii: 328.

46 Torkildsen A. Should extirpation be attempted in cases of neoplasms in or near the third ventricle of the brain. J Neurosurg 1948; 5: 269–75.

47 Schmidek HH, Waters A. Pineal masses: clinical management and features. In: Wilkens RH, Rengachary SS eds Neurosurgery. Vol 1. New York: McGraw-Hill, 1985: 688–92.

48 Conway LW. Stereotaxic diagnosis and treatment of intracranial tumors including an initial experience with cryosurgery for pinealomas. J Neurosurg 1973; 28: 483–60.

49 Moser RP, Backlund EO. Stereotactic radiosurgery in pineal region tumors. Presented at the 51st Annual Meeting of the American Assoc of Neurosurg, Honolulu, Hawaii, April 25, 1982.

50 Fukushima T. Endoscopic biopsy of intraventricular tumors with the use of a ventriculofiberscope. Neurosurgery 1978; 2: 110–113.

51 Stein BM. The infratentorial supracerebellar approach to pineal lesions. J Neurosurg 1971; 35: 197–202.

52 Bradfield JJ, Perez CA. Pineal tumors and ectopic pinealomas. Analysis of treatment and failures. Radiology 1972; 108: 399–406.

53 Sung DI, Harisiadis L, Chang CH. Midline pineal tumors and suprasellar germinomas: highly radiocurable by irradiation. Radiology 1978; 128: 745–51.

54 Mincer F, Meltzer J, Botstein C. Pinealoma: a report of twelve cases irradiated. Cancer 1978; 37: 2713–18.

55 Bloom HJG. Intracranial tumors: response and resistance to therapeutic endeavers, 1970–1980. Int J Radiat Onc Biol Phys 1982; 8: 1083–113.

56 Jenkin RDT, Simpson WJK, Keen CW. Pineal and suprasellar germinomas. Results of radiation treatment. J Neurosurg 1978; 48: 99–107.

57 Chapman PH, Linggood RM. The management of pineal area tumors: A recent reappraisal. Cancer 1980; 46: 1253–7.

58 Amendola BE, McClatchey K, Amendola MA. Pineal region tumors: Analysis of treatment results. Int J Radiat Oncol Biol Phys 1984; 10: 991–7.

59 Wara WM, Fellows CF, Sheline GE et al. Radiation therapy for pineal tumors and suprasellar germinomas. Radiology 1977; 124: 221–3.

60 Inove Y, Takeuchi T, Tamaki M et al. Sequential CT observations or irradiated intracranial germinomas. AJR 1979; 132: 361–5.

61 Spiegel AM, DiChiro G, Gorden P et al. Diagnosis of radiosensitive hypothalamic tumors without craniotomy. Ann Intern Med 1976; 85: 290 3.

62 Einhorn LH. Extragonadal germ cell tumors. In: Einhorn (ed) Testicular Tumors: Management and Treatment. New York: Masson 1980: 185–204.

63 Gay JG, Janco RL, Lukens JN. Systemic matastases in primary intracranial germinoma. Cancer 1985; 55: 2688–90.

64 Bamberg M, Metz K, Alberti W et al. Endodermal sinus tumors of the pineal region. Cancer 1984; 54: 903–6.

65 Kilgore DP, Strother CM, Starshak RJ, Haughton UM. Pineal germinoma: MR imaging. Radiology 1986; 59: 435–8.

66 Stein BM, Fetall MR. Therapeutic modalities for pineal region tumors. Clin Neurosurg 1985; 32: 445–55.

67 Allen JC, Bosl G, Walker R. Chemotherapy trials in recurrent primary intracranial germ cell tumors. J Neurol 1985; 3: 147–52.

Textbook of Uncommon Cancer
Edited by C.J. Williams, J.G. Krikorian, M.R. Green and D. Raghavan
© 1988 John Wiley & Sons Ltd

Chapter **35**

Uncommon Tumours of the Thyroid Gland

Christopher J. O'Brien
Attending Surgeon, Department of General Surgery, Royal Prince Alfred Hospital, Sydney, Australia

INTRODUCTION

Malignant thyroid neoplasms account for 1% of new cancers and 0.2% of cancer deaths each year in the United States. Therefore all forms of thyroid cancer are uncommon. Although the overall incidence of this disease has changed little in recent years, there has been some alteration in the pattern of disease and the incidence, or perhaps recognition, of different tumour types (1, 2). Differentiated cancers of thyroid follicle cell origin are the commonest malignant thyroid neoplasms and in most series account for 60–80% of cancers (3–5). Within this group the apparent incidence of papillary carcinoma, which is unrelated to the incidence of goitre, has increased. This may be due to increasing recognition of radiation induced cancers and also to further refinement of diagnostic criteria, with cytological and nuclear characteristics now being the major determinants of the diagnosis of papillary carcinoma, irrespective of architectural growth pattern (1). In contrast, follicular carcinoma is less common probably due to a diminished incidence of endemic goitre (6).

The medical literature is replete with retrospective analyses of the clinical course and prognostic factors associated with differentiated thyroid cancers, to a degree which is disproportionate with the relatively low incidence and indolent course of these tumours. Debate continues to focus on the extent of surgery necessary to adequately treat differentiated carcinomas and the need for adjuvant radioactive iodine therapy.

Medullary (parafollicular cell) carcinoma represents only 5–10% of thyroid cancers, but this tumour has also received widespread attention because of its association with other endocrine neoplasms (multiple endocrine neoplasia, type 2), and the existence of a tumour marker, calcitonin, which facilitates both screening and follow-up.

The present chapter will not deal with these tumours but rather will focus on less common follicle cell neoplasms—Hürthle cell, anaplastic and squamous carcinomas—along with thyroid lymphoma, teratoma and other tumours of doubtful histogenesis.

HÜRTHLE CELL TUMOURS

Among 1161 patients who received their primary treatment for malignant thyroid disease at the Mayo Clinic between 1946 and 1971, 44 Hürthle cell variants of follicular carcinoma were identified and only 29 of these were accepted after re-examination—an incidence of less than 3% of thyroid cancers (7). Clearly,

Hürthle cell malignancies are uncommon. Nonetheless these tumours represent an important subgroup of thyroid neoplasms which continue to attract controversy. A variety of synonyms has been used to describe the predominant cell type: 'eosinophil and granular cell', 'oxyphil cell', 'Askanazy cell', 'oncocyte' but most authors now refer to these neoplasms as Hürthle cell tumours, using the terminology introduced by Ewing in 1928, which gives credit to the nineteenth century German pathologist who described these large eosinophilic cells in the dog thyroid in 1894. In fact, Baber initially described the same cells in several laboratory animals as early as 1877. Askanazy is credited with the first description of these cells in the human thyroid in 1898. Miller et al. reviewed this historical background in 1983 (8).

Hürthle cells are large and acidophilic with hyperchromatic nucleoli. The cytoplasm stains intensely blue with phosphotungstic acid–haematoxylin stain and, ultrastructurally, is seen to be packed with mitochondria. These cells do not concentrate ^{131}I reproducibly and, although Hürthle cell neoplasms were initially believed to represent variants of follicular neoplasms, it is now clear that Hürthle cells are associated with several other tumours and pathological processes in the thyroid gland. Hürthle cell neoplasms are also found in parathyroid and salivary glands.

Two principal areas of controversy are associated with Hürthle cell tumours of the thyroid gland. The first question is whether they represent a distinct pathological entity or whether oncocytic change is an inconsequential degenerative process which can affect thyroid follicle cells and the cells of pre-existing thyroid neoplasms. The second question is that, if neoplasms of Hürthle cell origin are a distinct pathological entity, what is their malignant potential?

That Hürthle cell neoplasms can be found in association with other forms of thyroid pathology is beyond question. Bondeson et al. found Hürthle cell tumours in association with multinodular goitre, chronic thyroiditis, toxic diffuse goitre and follicular adenoma (9). Caplan et al. reported Hürthle cell tumours with coexisting Hashimoto's thyroiditis, follicular carcinoma and nodular hyperplasia (10). Multiple synchronous Hürthle cell tumours have also been described by Bondeson et al. (9) and Miller et al. (8). Microscopically, Hürthle cell neoplasms usually have their cells arranged in a follicular pattern; however, papillary-type Hürthle cell neoplasms have been described by Caplan et al. (10) and Gonzalez-Campora et al. (11). Non-neoplastic Hürthle cell aggregations are also common (12) but the aetiology of Hürthle cell change remains obscure.

Clinically, patients with Hürthle cell tumours may range in age from the second to ninth decades; however a median age from mid 40s to late 50s is most frequently reported. There is some evidence that the incidence of malignancy in these tumours increases with age (13, 14). The reported sex incidence also varies, although the usual female to male ratio is of the order of 5 or 6 to 1. The distribution of malignant Hürthle cell neoplasms between the sexes is approximately equal (1, 14).

There have been several retrospectiive studies of the behaviour of Hürthle cell neoplasms; however, a number of factors limit the interpretation of the available data. Case numbers are relatively small, some series include Hürthle cell aggregations which do not necessarily represent autonomous new growth and definitions of malignancy have not been totally agreed upon.

Clarification of the malignant potential of Hürthle cell tumours has been complicated principally by reports from the University of Michigan, Ann Arbor. In 1974 these workers reported 25 cases of Hürthle cell tumours treated between 1949 and 1972 (12). Thirteen of these were malignant by histological criteria, while 8 were indeterminate and 4 were benign. The most disturbing fact was that 3 patients with pathologically benign neoplasms died of their disease. It was concluded that all Hürthle cell tumours were potentially malignant and that pathological criteria were inadequate to predict clinical behaviour. Bondeson et al. (9) criticized this report because of the inclusion of a large number of previously treated patients, referred from other centres and an apparent failure to verify the source of metastases in patients who were said to have died from their thyroid tumours. Bondeson et al. also reviewed 42 cases of Hürthle cell neoplasms treated at the University of Lund, Sweden. Only 2 of 8 histologically malignant tumours behaved in a clinically malignant fashion while 34 histologically benign tumours behaved in a benign fashion. Median follow-up, however, was only 4 years (range 2–25 years) in that study.

In 1984 the University of Michigan group reviewed a further 33 cases of Hürthle cell tumour treated between 1973 and 1982 (15). Of these, 15 were histologically malignant. A lower recurrence rate and improved survival in this group, when compared to the 29 cases reported 10 years earlier, was attributed to an increased use of total thyroidectomy as surgical treatment. However, mean follow-up was only 3 years and a direct comparison of the patient groups was clearly not valid. Nonetheless these authors concluded that total thyroidectomy is the treatment of choice for all Hürthle cell neoplasms larger than 2 cm in diameter and for those neoplasms with histological evidence of malignancy.

Gosain and Clarke (13) reviewed 84 patients with Hürthle cell neoplasms of which only 4 had microscopic angioinvasion, capsular invasion, lymph node involvement or distant metastases. There were no recurrences or deaths from disease from the histologically benign group at a mean of almost 15 years. These authors support the view of Gonzalez-Campora et al. (11) and Bondeson et al. (9) that histology reliably predicts the clinical behaviour of Hürthle cell tumours and that routine total thyroidectomy is unnecessary. Heppe et al. (16) and the Mayo Clinic group (7) similarly have concluded that the appropriate initial treatment for histologically benign Hürthle cell neoplasms is lobectomy and isthmusectomy, while total thyroidectomy should be reserved for tumours demonstrating microscopic evidence of malignancy.

In contrast Rosen et al. (17) and Miller et al. (8) have supported the University of Michigan view and proposed a surgically aggressive approach for all Hürthle cell tumours despite the fact that such an approach is inconsistent with their reported clinical experience. The view of these two groups that total thyroidectomy should be performed was based, in part, on the fact that Hürthle cell tumours are frequently multifocal, i.e. Hürthle cell foci are often present in the opposite lobe. However, the significance of this finding is unclear since these foci may represent innocent aggregations rather than intrathyroidal dissemination.

Malignant Hürthle cell tumours have a tendency to metastasize to lymph nodes as well as disseminate via the blood stream. In contrast to papillary carcinomas, evidence suggests that the presence of nodal metastases worsens prognosis. There is, however, no evidence that elective neck dissection, i.e. dissection in the absence of clinically enlarged nodes, is of any benefit and therefore this is not recommended. The common sites for distant metastases include bone and lung, as with follicular thyroid cancer.

The relative aggressiveness of malignant Hürthle cell tumours compared to other differentiated thyroid cancers is not entirely clear. Furthermore their inability to reliably concentrate ^{131}I means that this form of therapy cannot be used in an adjuvant or palliative role; consequently death from disease may occur soon after metastases appear.

In summary, the weight of evidence suggests that the vast majority of Hürthle cell neoplasms are benign and that their biological behavior can be predicted from the histological appearance. At this stage, acceptable criteria for malignancy appear to be: the presence of metastatic spread, capsular invasion and vascular invasion. While Hürthle cell neoplasms may be diagnosed by means of fine needle aspiration cytology, a definitive diagnosis to exclude or confirm malignancy would usually require examination of the entire lesion, as with follicular neoplasms. In concert with the surgical management of all thyroid neoplasms, lobectomy and isthmusectomy represent the minimal adequate resection for diagnosis. If a diagnosis of malignancy is made either by frozen section or paraffin section, a 'completion' near-total or total thyroidectomy should be carried out since radioactive iodine (^{131}I) is unlikely to be of benefit in management.

ANAPLASTIC CARCINOMA

Anaplastic carcinomas account for 5–8% of thyroid malignancies (18–20) and these tumours remain among the most lethal of human cancers. In fact, patient survival beyond a year is so uncommon that it should raise the question of an incorrect diagnosis. There is some evidence that the incidence of anaplastic carcinoma is decreasing (21) and this may represent both a genuine decrease in occurrence as well as improved diagnosis with the exclusion of non-anaplastic tumours. It is now clear, for example, that virtually all small cell tumours of the thyroid gland are lymphoma (22, 23) and so this group should be eliminated from the category of anaplastic thyroid cancer. Other neoplasms previously called anaplastic have also been shown by argyrophilia and calcitonin immunoreactivity to be of C-cell origin (24). However, this latter finding and the resultant conclusion that many anaplastic carcinomas are variants of medullary carcinoma has not been widely substantiated (23) and is highly controversial. Nonetheless, an anaplastic variant of medullary carcinoma probably exists (24).

In general, it is now recognized that anaplastic carcinomas are composed of spindle cells or giant cells or a combination of the two, and that they represent de-differentiation or transformation of well differentiated neoplasms (19, 21, 24–26). In a report of 84 cases of giant and spindle cell carcinoma of the thyroid treated at the M.D. Anderson Hospital, Houston, tissue was available for review in 74 cases. In 66 of these (89.2%) differentiated thyroid carcinoma was demonstrated (19). Similarly, differentiated cancers were asso-

ciated with 42 of 53 anaplastic carcinomas reported by Nishayama et al. of the University of Michigan. These included follicular, papillary and Hürthle cell types (27).

Despite anecdotal reports of individual patients surviving for 5 years, anaplastic carcinoma is usually associated with a rapidly fatal outcome. In a review of 10 series totalling 420 cases, Casterline et al. found only 14 patients surviving 2 or more years (28). Aldinger et al. (19) reported a mean survival of 6.2 months from the time of tissue diagnosis and 11.8 months from initial symptoms for patients treated at the M.D. Anderson Hospital. Similarly, Carcangiu et al. (20) reported a mean survival of 4 months among 57 patients from a combined series from the Universities of Florence, Italy and Minnesota, USA, and Jereob et al. (29) described 2.5 months mean survival among 79 patients treated at the Karolinska Institute, Stockholm. The Staging System of the American Joint Committee on Cancer places these tumours in Stage IV regardless of extent.

Factors associated with the development of anaplastic thyroid carcinoma are pre-existing differentiated carcinoma and benign goitre, but the transformation rates are statistically so low that treatment decisions related to these conditions should not be based on the fear of anaplastic change. Of 99 patients who died of differentiated thyroid cancer following treatment at the Lahey Clinic between 1931 and 1970, only 2 had verified anaplastic transformation (21). The administration of radioactive iodine and external radiation have also been implicated as initiating causes of anaplastic transformation (26, 27), but again the association is anecdotal only.

Clinically, females are usually more frequently affected than males by a rate of 1.5 : 1 to 4 : 1; however, of 82 patients treated at the Mayo Clinic between 1966 and 1971, 59% were males. The mean age of diagnosis is usually about 65 years and only 5–10% of patients in most series are younger than 50 years of age. While all patients initially present with thyroid enlargement this is commonly of long standing and initial presentation is often precipitated by rapid recent growth of the thyroid or development of symptoms of compression or invasion of neck structures. The incidence of cervical metastases at presentation varies from 15 to 40% while 15–30% of patients will have distant metastases. Commonest sites for distant metastases are lung and liver; however, kidney, adrenal, pancreas, brain and heart may be affected (27).

Commonly, local disease is so advanced at initial presentation that surgery cannot be carried out. Often, therefore, the diagnosis is made only by a biopsy or at autopsy. Surgical resection with curative intent could be performed in only 34 of the 82 patients in the Mayo Clinic series (18), in 28 of 70 patients reported by Carcangiu et al. (20) and fewer than 20% of the University of Michigan series reported by Nishayama et al. (27).

All forms of therapy have been used in the management of anaplastic thyroid cancer. Retrospective comparison of treatment regimens is inappropriate and usually valueless since patient groups are unmatched and those treated surgically usually have localized or resectable disease while those receiving radiotherapy alone tend to have unresectable disease. It is clear, however, that any possibility of survival is dependent upon complete eradication of local disease (19, 21).

Although treatment is rarely successful in patients with anaplastic thyroid cancer, it is important to appreciate which factors, if any, are associated with survival. The amount of anaplastic disease appears to be one such factor. Tollefsen et al. studied 70 patients who died of papillary carcinoma of the thyroid (26). Among these, 18 had histological evidence of anaplastic giant or spindle cell transformation. The average time from detection of the anaplastic component to death was directly proportional to the size of the anaplastic foci. Eight patients with 'minute' foci survived an average of 5 years; 4 patients with 'small' foci survived an average of 2 years while 6 patients with 'large' foci survived a mean of only 6 months.

Aldinger et al. similarly reported that, among 11 of 84 patients in the M.D. Anderson series who survived more than one year, 8 had only small foci of giant and spindle cell carcinoma (19). Offsetting this apparently hopeful observation, however, were a further 8 patients with small anaplastic foci whose disease was rapidly fatal. In 1985 a 25-year experience at the Mayo Clinic was reported by Nel et al. (18). Although this series of 82 patients included 19 small cell tumours and must therefore be interpreted with caution, the authors reported that, by multifactorial analysis, survival decreased significantly as the extent of disease on presentation increased; when the thyroid could not be resected; when the tumour was larger than 6 cm in diameter; and when both spindle and giant cell components were present.

It remains unclear whether choice of treatment can influence prognosis. Not surprisingly, prospective randomized studies have not been carried out and much of the available data is anecdotal. A 13-year survivor reported by Nishayama et al. was treated by total thyroidectomy and radiotherapy but this patient had only a small focus of spindle cell cancer (27). Spiro and Daniella described a patient who was alive and well 5 years after lobectomy and radiotherapy for anaplastic carcinoma (30). Casterline et al. proposed 'an aggressive multidisciplinary therapeutic approach' based on the 4-year survival of a 54 year old woman treated by total thyroidectomy with central compartment and left neck dissection, followed by 6000 rads radiotherapy and then 10 doses of actinomycin D given twice weekly (28). Simpson, in reporting a series of 94 patients treated at the Princess Margaret Hospital, Toronto, stated that external irradiation should be administered to all patients and that hyperfractionation, a large number of small doses, was the prefered method (31). Aldinger et al. reported improved results using surgical removal of all tumour where possible, irradiation to the neck, both supra-clavicular fossae and mediastinum to 6000 rads combined with actinomycin D chemotherapy. Three of

14 patients so treated were alive and disease free 5 to 7 years after therapy. Again, however, only small foci of disease were present in these patients (19). It is unlikely that radical surgery alone will control disease, although Goldman et al. reported 3-year survival in a 50 year old woman following total laryngectomy with thyroidectomy, partial pharyngectomy and radical neck dissection (32).

The addition of chemotherapy to the management of anaplastic thyroid cancer has not been studied in any systematic way. Several cytotoxic agents have been used and of these, Adriamycin appears to have the most activity. In a review of the role of chemotherapy in thyroid cancer, Poster et al. reported objective responses in 69 of 199 evaluable patients from various series following treatment with Adriamycin (33). However, not all these patients had anaplastic carcinoma. The use of Adriamycin is limited by cardio-toxicity which develops when a cumulative dose of 550 mg/m^2 is exceeded. Hill has stated that anaplastic carcinoma is often so virulent that it is only possible to administer three courses of chemotherapy before spread or death occurs (34). Using a schedule of between 60 and 105 mg/m^2 of Adriamycin every 3 weeks up to a dose of 450 to 550 mg/m^2, Hill described a response rate of only 11%.

Bleomycin is another active single agent with responses recorded in 14 of 32 patients treated by different groups and having various types of thyroid pathology (33).

There remains a need for further phase 2 studies to identify active single agents and combinations of cytotoxic drugs. Chemotherapy may have an adjuvant role and Poster et al. quote several uncontrolled studies in which long term survival in a few patients has been achieved following treatment with surgery, radiotherapy and chemotherapy (33) Overall, however, prognosis remains very poor for patients with giant and spindle cell carcinomas of the thyroid gland with the only hope being that radical treatment can be carried out when disease is minimal.

PRIMARY SQUAMOUS CARCINOMA

Pure squamous cell carcinomas affecting the thyroid gland account for perhaps 0.2% of all thyroid malignancies (35). In 1984, Segel et al. described 4 cases of pure squamous cell carcinoma of the thyroid and 2 cases of adenosquamous carcinomas (36). Two of these patients were alive and disease free over one year after treatment, 3 had died of their disease within a few months of surgery and the sixth patient died of a myocardial infarction within one month of operation. Half of the patients had obstructive symptoms consistent with an invasive tumour while the other half presented with an otherwise asymptomatic nodular goitre. The histological diagnosis was made only following surgery in each case. In the 2 patients who survived, and the one who died of infarction, complete removal of the tumour was achieved at surgery and in one of these postoperative radiotherapy was given. In the other cases complete excision could not be achieved and the addition of 5000 rads of radiotherapy did not stop rapid local recurrence, dissemination and death.

This study exemplifies the possible clinical situations with which this unusual and potentially highly malignant tumour can be associated.

Squamous epithelium has been identified in the normal thyroid and in association with other thyroid neoplasms (37–39). Squamous cells may originate from the ultimobranchial body, thyroglossal duct, or by metaplasia of follicular epithelium. An origin from follicle cell metaplasia seems most likely and may explain the adenosquamous tumours described by Segel et al. (36) and other authors (40, 41).

While primary squamous carcinomas of the thyroid do occur, local extension from adjacent mucosal or metastatic cancer should be excluded. Clinically, the presentation of disease and patient population are similar to those associated with anaplastic thyroid cancer and there is some argument as to whether squamous carcinoma is a variant of giant and spindle cell carcinomas. This debate, however, would appear to be largely academic since the diseases have in common a follicle cell origin and, in the vast majority of cases a rapidly lethal outcome.

The cause of squamous carcinoma of the thyroid gland is of course uncertain although Bakri et al. (40) reported a case of adenosquamous carcinoma occurring in a 61 year old man, 48 years after having radiotherapy for Hodgkin's disease. These authors cited 3 other cases of squamous or adenosquamous thyroid cancer occurring following radiotherapy—the latent period ranged from 3 to 48 years. It also remains unclear whether squamous carcinoma of the thyroid gland evolves from cells demonstrating squamous metaplasia or whether this disease represents direct transition from a pre-existing differentiated adenocarcinoma. Harada et al. from Tokyo, Japan believe that the latter process is more likely and reported 8 autopsy cases in which adenocarcinoma and squamous cell carcinoma coexisted (41). They could not demonstrate associated squamous metaplasia or malignant transformation of squamous metaplasia.

As with anaplastic giant and spindle cell tumours, squamous carcinoma and adenosquamous carcinoma of the thyroid affects principally an elderly population and survival is only likely if all disease can be radically resected.

Rarely, it may be necessary to differentiate squamous carcinoma of the thyroid gland from intrathyroidal epithelial thymoma. Miyauchi et al. from Osaka, Japan recently reported 3 cases of intrathyroidal epithelial thymoma and pointed out that, while this unusual tumour may be readily mistaken for squamous carcinoma of the thyroid, it is a very different entity both histologically and clinically (42). It is believed that the thymic tissue resides within the thyroid due to aberrant descent. The neoplasm of this tissue looks like squamous carcinoma surrounded by many lymphocytes. However, there is no associated differentiated follicle cell carcinoma nor foci of anaplastic cancer, features often seen with squamous carcinoma. Importantly, intrathyroidal thymoma has an excellent prognosis, with 2 patients surviving 17 years and 1 alive and well at 3 years after treatment, in the series reported (42).

THYROID LYMPHOMA

Malignant lymphoma originating in the thyroid gland accounts for fewer than 5% of thyroid malignancies. These neoplasms are predominantly non-Hodgkin's lymphomas and, as such, represent approximately 1.5% of all non-Hodgkin's lymphomas and about 6.5% of primary extranodal lymphoma (43). About one-quarter of non-Hodgkin's lymphomas arise in extranodal sites with the head and neck and gastrointestinal tract being the commonest.

Clarification of the histogenesis and morphology of thyroid lymphomas has occurred over recent years, but the pathological diagnosis may still be difficult in individual cases and several questions remain unanswered.

The important distinction between thyroid lymphoma and anaplastic carcinoma has already been mentioned in this chapter. The weight of pathological evidence appears to convincingly indicate that virtually all small cell thyroid malignancies are lymphoma, and that studies of anaplastic thyroid cancer which include a small cell subgroup should be interpreted with caution.

Of more interest and greater controversy is the question of the association of thyroid lymphoma with, and possible origin from, chronic lymphocytic thyroiditis (Hashimoto's disease). Burke et al. emphasized this association and the difficulty sometimes experienced by pathologists in differentiating the two conditions (44). These authors drew comparison with the reported increased incidence of lymphoma with Sjögren's disease (45) and supported the view of Lukes and Collins (46, 47) that lymphomas originate in these settings from transformed lymphocytes or immunoblasts. Burke et al. demonstrated a definite association between malignant lymphoma of the thyroid and Hashimoto's thyroiditis in 27 of 35 cases (44). The extent of thyroiditis varied from multifocal infiltrates to the presence of reactive germinal centres demonstrating Hürthle cell change. None of the patients reported by Burke et al. had immunological evidence of Hashimoto's disease but thyroid antibodies were only measured in 5 cases. However, Hamburger et al. found anti-thyroglobulin antibodies in 7 and antimicrosomal antibodies in 17 of 29 patients with thyroid lymphoma who were tested (48).

Compangno and Oertel recognized varying degrees of lymphocytic thyroiditis in 95% of 245 cases reviewed at the Armed Forces Institute of Pathology (49) while Anscombe and Wright claimed the association of malignant lymphoma and lymphocytic thyroiditis was 'of the order of 100%' (50). By contrast, the incidence of associated lymphocytic thyroiditis was only 36% among 103 patients with primary lymphoma treated at the Mayo Clinic (51) and although the authors in this latter series admitted that this probably underestimated the true frequency of association of the two diseases, they raised the question of why so few people with Hashimoto's disease go on to develop thyroid lymphoma.

The histological differentiation between chronic lymphocytic thyroiditis and thyroid lymphoma may be difficult. The presence of blood vessel invasion and extrathyroid extension or both can be used to reliably identify the malignant condition. Compagno and Oertel required the following criteria for a diagnosis of lymphoma: architectural effacement and parenchymal replacement by a homogeneous lymphoid infiltrate composed of immature and often pleomorphic cells. Occasionally the thyroid follicles are not completely effaced but packed with lymphoid cells, a feature not seen in lymphocytic thyroiditis (49).

As previously mentioned, the vast majority of thyroid lymphomas are non-Hodgkin's lymphomas and, among these, the commonest histological type is diffuse histiocytic lymphoma (43, 44, 51, 52), according to the

Rappaport classification (53).

The histological picture among lymphoproliferative disorders of the thyroid gland may be quite variable. Compagno and Oertel described 10 histological subgroups of these neoplasms. These were (1) atypical lymphocytic thyroiditis, in which the features suggested lymphoma but where a firm diagnosis could not be made, (2) plasmacytoma, (3) lymphocytic lymphoma (not otherwise specified) with diffusely distributed moderately to poorly differentiated lymphocytes, (4) histiocytic lymphoma, (5) nodular lymphoma, (6) lymphocytic lymphoma with plasmacytoid features, (7) Hodgkin's lymphoma, (8) undifferentiated (Burkitt) lymphoma, (9) lymphocytic lymphoma, well differentiated, (10) unclassifiable group. Categories 1 to 6 accounted for 92% of their series (49).

Diffuse histiocytic lymphoma accounted for 34 of 35 cases reported by Burke et al. (44), and 16 of 21 cases reported by Kapadia et al. (52). Chak et al. similarly found a preponderance of diffuse histiocytic lymphomas among 11 patients treated at Stanford between 1969 and 1978 (43).

The predominance of the diffuse histiocytic subgroup makes histology a poor prognostic discriminant when the Rappaport classification is adhered to. Aozasa et al. from Kobe, Japan recognized this limitation and applied the Kiel classification to a group of 71 patients with extranodal lymphomas of the head and neck, of which 26 originated in the thyroid (54). The Kiel classification divides non-Hodgkin's lymphomas into low grade malignancy, comprising lymphocytic, lymphoplasmacytoid, centrocytic and centroblastic/centrocytic types, and high grade malignancy, comprising centroblastic, lymphoblastic and immunoblastic types. In that study there was a statistically significant difference in survival between patients with high grade and low grade malignancies in non-thyroid sites, and although the survival difference between patients with high and low grade thyroid lymphoma did not reach significance the low grade group was strongly favoured.

Clinically, women are most frequently affected by thyroid lymphoma in contrast to the male predominance among patients with lymphoma in lymphoid sites. The female to male ratio is generally of the order of 3 : 1 (44, 49, 51); however, Anscombe and Wright found an eight-fold female predominance in their series of 76 cases (50). Age at onset may vary from 20 to 90 years with a median of approximately 60–65 years most widely reported (44, 49–51).

Most patients present with recent onset of an enlarging thyroid mass and symptoms are usually present for several weeks before medical attention is sought. Pre-existing goitre is uncommon (43, 51). Features of compression and extrathyroid invasion may be present in 10 to 65% of patients (43, 44, 48, 51, 52) and symptoms include hoarseness, stridor, dysphagia and local pain and tenderness.

Difficulty is usually encountered with the clinical diagnosis of thyroid lymphoma and it is uncommon for this diagnosis to be considered prior to treatment. All patients have a palpable thyroid mass and the goitre is more often nodular than diffuse (48). Concomitant cervical lymphadenopathy may be present in 20 to 35% of cases (44, 49, 52). Needle biopsy, however, has been shown to be useful in preoperative evaluation. Hamburger et al. reported that a diagnosis of lymphoma was suggested in 17 of 28 patients evaluated by fine needle aspiration biopsy and 21 of 23 patients by large needle biopsy (48). These authors addressed the problem of differentiating between lymphoma and lymphocytic thyroiditis by means of fine needle aspiration. They claim that the rate of false negatives, that is either missing a lymphoma or calling it lymphocytic thyroiditis, can be reduced with experience. Hashimoto's thyroiditis can usually be diagnosed on the basis of the clinical picture, reduced thyroid function and elevated antibody titres. These patients usually do not require needle biopsy to screen for lymphoma unless the gland is nodular and does not regress with thyroid hormone treatment.

Clinical stage is both a prognostic factor and a determinant of treatment. Patients staged I or II after a full work-up can usually be treated locally with a high expectation of disease control, while those with Stage III and IV disease require systemic treatment and still are likely to relapse. Patients with neck or systemic dissemination from their thyroid lymphoma tend to fare badly (49); therefore, accurate clinical staging is important. This involves full blood count, biochemical screen, chest x-ray, computed tomography (CT) scanning and bone marrow biopsy. Lymphangiography and gallium scans are also used according to regional and institutional preference. The Ann Arbor staging system which is used for Hodgkin's disease has little applicability in non-Hodgkin's lymphomas since approximately 80% of patients with non-Hodgkin's lymphomas arising from nodal or peripheral lymphatic sites have Stage III or IV disease at presentation and, when thyroid involvement occurs under these circumstances, it is of academic interest whether the disease originated in the thyroid gland or not. Anscombe and Wright (50) pointed out, however, the tendency for thyroid lymphomas and other lymphomas arising from mucosa-associated lymphoid tissue to remain localized for a long time and for patients to present with early stage disease.

The best treatment for thyroid lymphoma has not been clearly defined. Retrospective series which compare treatment modalities used alone or in combination reflect a great degree of bias in patient selection and usually no attempt is made to correct for clinical or pathological prognostic factors. The role of surgery is certainly unclear. In many cases initial diagnosis is only made following a thyroidectomy carried out for what is clinically a neoplastic thyroid nodule. The 'diagnostic biopsy' among the 11 patients in the Stanford University series was a sub-total or total thyroidectomy in 7 cases (43). In the Mayo Clinic series almost all the 29 patients with intrathyroidal lymphoma underwent surgical resection before irradiation (51) and among the 74 patients with extrathyroidal disease, approximately equal numbers were treated with combined surgical resection and radiotherapy or radiotherapy alone. In this latter group, one form of therapy was as effective as the other. Whatever thyroid resection is carried out this should be regarded as a biopsy. Once the diagnosis is confirmed it is appropriate to fully investigate and stage the patient. Thereafter, definitive treatment should be given.

Thyroid lymphomas have a strong propensity for invasion of local neck structures and extrathyroid spread is clearly a poor prognostic factor. Extrathyroid invasion was found in 60% of cases examined by Compagno and Oertel (49) and 72% of cases reported by Anscombe and Wright (50). In reviewing the Mayo Clinic experience, Devine et al. reported that the 5-year survival for 74 patients in whom lymphoma had spread beyond the thyroid capsule was 38% in contrast to 86% for those in whom the disease was intrathyroidal (51). The high frequency of macroscopic or microscopic extrathyroid extension strongly suggests that surgery alone is unlikely to be effective in the treatment of thyroid lymphoma. Local control can certainly be achieved by radiotherapy to a dose of 50–60 Gy, given by standard techniques or an equivalent dose in larger fractions delivered more rapidly (43, 52). There is no clear evidence that patients with thyroid lymphoma should be treated routinely with chemotherapy if, after adequate staging, disease is found to be localized. Chak et al. reported 75% relapse free survival at 2 years and 83% survival at 3 years in a small group of patients treated at Stanford with initial surgery and definitive mantle irradiation (43). However, that institution strongly favours the use of radiotherapy and a valid alternative view would be that, irrespective of the disease being apparently localized, there is a high likelihood that the lymphoma is generalized and that multiagent chemotherapy which includes an anthracycline is appropriate.

Patients dying of their disease invariably have dissemination although some will have resistant local disease which causes asphyxia or pneumonia (52). Dissemination may be to lymph nodes, extranodal lymphoid tissue and non-lymphoid organs and tissues. The overall 5-year survival rate for the Mayo Clinic series was 50% (51), similar to the 54% survival rate at the M.D. Anderson Hospital (44).

Other Lymphoproliferative Tumours

Both Hodgkin's disease and plasmacytoma may have a primary origin in the thyroid gland but these are considerably less common than thyroid lymphoma. Among 103 primary lymphomas treated at the Mayo Clinic to 1968 material was reviewed in 86 cases and only 3 of these were plasmacytomas (51). Compagno and Oertel described 21 plasmacytomas and 7 cases of Hodgkin's lymphoma among 245 cases of lymphoproliferative tumours of the thyroid gland reported in 1980 (49). Of the cases of Hodgkin's disease, 2 were nodular sclerosing and 5 of the lymphocytic depleted type. Both patients with nodular sclerosing tumours were young females with concomitant mediastinal disease and both patients died of their tumour.

Hodgkin's disease usually presents as superficial lymphadenopathy, with cervical nodes being affected in 60–80% of cases. An extranodal presentation of Hodgkin's disease is far less common than with non-Hodgkin's lymphoma and certainly the thyroid gland is an uncommon site (55). The diagnosis of Hodgkin's disease is almost invariably made after resection and examination of the thyroid nodule. Thereafter, treatment should be based on adequate staging and this should include full blood count, serum biochemistry, chest x-ray, bone marrow biopsy, and whole body CT scanning. Gallium scanning and lymphangiography are also used but not in all institutions.

The diagnosis of Hodgkin's disease of the thyroid is so uncommon that clear guidelines for treatment cannot be given. In general, however, where primary extranodal Hodgkin's disease is found to be localized definitive widefield radiotherapy is the treatment of choice. However, for patients with systemic symptoms like weight loss, fever or night sweats and for those with Stage III or IV disease multiagent chemotherapy would offer a greater chance of achieving remission and possible cure.

Plasmacytoma of the thyroid was first reported by Voegt in 1938 (56). Systemic myeloma rarely involves the thyroid gland and Wiltshaw reported an incidence of only 2.6% among 272 patients with multiple myeloma (57). Macpherson et al. had not a single instance of thyroid involvement in 62 consecutively autopsied subjects with myeloma (58).

Fortunately, plasmacytoma limited to the thyroid gland carries a reasonable prognosis. With a mean follow-up of 6.9 years, Compagno and Oertel reported a significantly better outcome for patients with this disease compared with patients with other thyroid lymphomas (49). Similarly, malignant lymphoma with plasmacytoid features carried a better prognosis than histiocytic or lymphocytic lymphoma. Interestingly, the same association with lymphocytic thyroiditis was demonstrated for plasmacytoma as for thyroid lymphoma (44).

Demonstration of paraproteins has not been widely described in thyroid plasmacytoma. Macpherson et al. demonstrated a homogeneous IgG component of the kappa type in the serum of one patient by electrophoresis and in thyroid tissue by immunoperoxidase staining (58). These authors also reviewed 9 previously reported cases and, following treatment by surgery with or without radiotherapy, all patients were alive at follow-up times of 15 months to 10 years. In 1983 Lopez et al. also published a literature review of primary extramedullary plasmacytoma of the thyroid gland (59). They stated that only 12 previous cases of primary extramedullary plasmacytoma of the thyroid had been described. However, like Macpherson et al (58) these authors did not include the 25 cases included in the larger series of lymphomas from the Mayo Clinic (45) and Armed Forces Institute of Pathology (44).

Clinically the sex incidence of patients with thyroid plasmacytoma is equal and ages tend to range from the fifth to seventh decades. In concert with virtually all thyroid neoplasms, plasmacytoma presents as a painless mass in the thyroid gland. Symptoms suggesting invasion are less common than with other lymphomas. Again, the paucity of reported cases precludes firm conclusions about optimal treatment. While thyroidectomy alone has been associated with survival in some cases the addition of definitive radiotherapy has also been shown to be of benefit and is strongly suggested. Selection of patients for chemotherapy should depend on the presence of systemic disease.

THYROID TERATOMA

Thyroid teratomas develop from totipotential cells presumably residing in or around the thyroid gland. These tumours are rare and the vast majority of report cases have involved infants. By 1980 the accumulated literature consisted of approximately 132 cases involving neonates and infants and a further 12 cases involving patients 10 years of age or older (60). In 1982, Fisher et al. added a further 2 infant cases and reviewed the literature in this age group (61). The 2 teratomas reported in that study presented as distinct anterior neck masses causing respiratory distress. In both instances a well encapsulated, histologically benign tumour was resected without difficulty and the children recovered.

Teratomas of infancy are usually located in the median preaxial or paramedian sites (61). The sacrococcygeal region is most commonly affected but these tumours also occur in the ovary and mediastinum. The neck is an uncommon site for teratoma and cervical teratomas account for only 2% of all childhood teratomas (62, 63). While the origin of cervical teratoma is not always clear it has been proposed that they probably originate in the embryonic thyroid anlage.

Macroscopically both solid and cystic areas may be present and histologically these tumours demonstrate derivatives of the three germ cell layers. In infants they are invariably benign and over 90% of cases occur in early infancy with an equal sex incidence (64). Adjacent thyroid tissue is not always recognizable and may be largely effaced by teratoma.

A common clinical presentation is that described in the 2 cases reported by Fisher et al. (61). Thyroid teratomas are often congenital and may be large enough to complicate delivery and necessitate caesarean section. In other cases growth following delivery causes progressive airway obstruction. Unfortunately, stillbirth and neonatal death may occur in up to one-third of affected infants. Large teratomas may have associated polyhydramnios.

While this is an uncommon tumour the diagnosis should be an early consideration in any child under 1 year of age with an anterior neck swelling. The differential diagnosis in this setting includes cystic hygroma, branchial cleft cyst and congenital goitre. Preoperative investigations should include ultrasound and CT scanning. Thyroid scanning is also recommended to define functioning thyroid tissue. Surgical resection should be carried out without delay and may be necessitated by a rapidly deteriorating clinical situation.

Thyroid teratomas occurring in adults present a different clinical picture. They almost invariably affect females and are malignant. Wolvos et al. (60) reviewed 12 previously reported cases and described a further patient, a 72 year old female, with a benign thyroid tumour containing two germ cell elements. These authors felt, however, that the latter case could not be classified as a teratoma or hamartoma. Among previously reported 'adult' thyroid teratomas, a 10 year old boy described by Kingsley et al. (65) was included. The median age among the remaining patients was 28 with a range of 19 to 68 years. Kimmler and Math (66) reported a malignant thyroid teratoma occurring in a pregnant female and speculated that the hormonal changes associated with pregnancy may have stimulated growth of the tumour.

Several forms of therapy have been used in the treatment of this rare malignancy. Median time to death in the 9 fatal cases described was approximately 9 months with a range of 1 to 22 months. Pulmonary metastates were present in most cases and recurrent disease was resistant to chemotherapy and radiotherapy.

HAEMANGIOENDOTHELIOMA

Haemangioendothelioma appears to be an exclusively European disease since the majority of cases have been reported by Swiss authors. In 1983 Egloff of Winterthur, Switzerland, described 65 cases and, in reviewing the clinicopathological characteristics of this tumour, argued strongly for wider acceptance of the existence of haemangioendothelioma. American pathologists have largely disregarded this histological label, preferring to include tumours with features of haemangioendothelioma among anaplastic carcinomas.

Among the cases described by Egloff (67) the male to female ratio was almost 2:1 while the mean age of all patients was 67.3 years. These tumours are said to often lie within an adenomatous goitre but with irregular boundaries and frequent areas of haemorrhage and necrosis. Microscopically tumour development begins with multiplication and widening of capillaries and associated endothelial proliferation. As the neoplastic endothelial cells proliferate and fill the vascular lumina the tumour has the appearance of a carcinoma. Spindle cells may also be present. Individual cells are extremely pleomorphic and may occur in cords, rows or solid clusters. Recognizable thyroid follicles are usually seen nearby.

Egloff found metastases in 22 or 30 patients who died of haemangioendothelioma and underwent autopsy. The lungs and pleura were the most frequently affected sites. The angiomatous pattern is said to be more prominent in the metastases, which are frequently haemorrhagic.

Both Egloff and Ruchti et al. from Bern, Switzerland (68) drew attention to Factor VIII related antigen, a marker for endothelial cells. Egloff found evidence of Factor VIII related antigen in 2 cases while Ruchti et al. using immunohistochemical techniques, demonstrated this antigen in neoplastic cells in 13 of 20 cases of haemangioendothelioma. In both studies the presence of this antigen was proposed by the respective authors to strongly support the endothelial origin of the tumour.

The clinical course of haemangioendothelioma is an aggressive one. Local invasion of trachea and oesophagus readily occur and Egloff quoted a median survival time of 3.2 months from treatment to death. This behaviour is entirely consistent with that of anaplastic carcinoma.

MUCOEPIDERMOID CARCINOMA

Mucoepidermoid carcinoma is the commonest malignancy of salivary gland origin (69, 70). It occurs principally in the parotid glands but is also found in minor salivary gland scattered throughout the upper aerodigestive tract. This tumour was first described in the thyroid gland by Rhatigan et al. in 1977 (71) and since then other authors have reported similar findings (72–74).

The common histological findings from each series have been the presence of squamous cells, which ultrastructurally demonstrate tonofilaments and desmosomes and mucinous material which stains positive with mucicarmine stain and PAS (periodic acid–Schiff). In 2 cases reported by Franssila et al. (73) there were associated psammoma bodies but tumour cells were negative for thyroglobulin. The third case reported by this group demonstrated areas of anaplastic carcinoma associated with the mucoepidermoid features.

The origin of mucoepidermoid carcinoma of the thyroid is unclear. However, Harach (74) described the presence of solid cell nests in the thyroid which may correspond to vestiges of the ultimobranchial body. He pointed out that mucoepidermoid carcinoma of the thyroid presented all the histological and histochemical features shown by solid cell nests and believed there was strong evidence that mucoepidermoid carcinoma originated in these nests. With so few cases reported there appears

to have been no attempt to grade the malignancy of thyroid mucoepidermoid carcinomas. In salivary gland cancers, tumour grade is such an important prognostic determinant that high and low grade mucoepidermoid carcinomas essentially behave as different diseases, representing the far ends of the spectrum of behaviour of salivary malignancies (69).

A prominent clinical feature in all the cases described has been the association of cervical lymph node metastases. These were present either at the time of diagnosis of the thyroid primary or subsequently. In mucoepidermoid carcinomas of salivary gland origin, lymph node metastases are uncommon except in the case of high grade tumours. These high grade tumours are the most lethal salivary malignancies; however, not all the thyroid mucoepidermoid cancers described have behaved in an aggressive fashion. Of the patients report by Franssila et al. 1 was alive and disease free at 17 months, 1 was alive and disease free at 10 years, while the third patient whose tumour demonstrated anaplastic features died 13 months after initial diagnosis. The patient reported by Mizukami et al. (72) was alive and disease free 20 months after treatment. Franssila et al. drew the conclusion that mucoepidermoid carcinoma appears to resemble papillary carcinoma in its natural history on the basis of a high incidence of lymph node metastases and an apparently reasonable prognosis despite this finding. Clearly, however, longer follow-up is needed before firm conclusions can be drawn about the behaviour of this tumour.

METASTASES TO THE THYROID GLAND

Although the thyroid gland is very vascular, haematogenous metastases do not commonly develop in this organ. In the 20-year period to 1980 only 12 patients treated at the Mayo Clinic had thyroidectomy for tumours metastatic to that gland (75). In a later report from that institution, Ivy (76) found 30 cases with thyroid metastates treated between 1946 and 1982. The primary sites, identified in 23 patients, were as follows: kidney 12 cases, breast 6, lung 5, while bladder, pancreas, oesophagus, lungs, nasopharynx and a pelvic teratoma represented 1 case each. Two patients had malignant melanoma although the primary site was not identified.

The sexes were equally represented among these patients and 26 of the 30 were 50 years of age or older. In 19 patients the thyroid metastases became evident before the primary was discovered and in one of these, a lung cancer, the primary was diagnosed 3 years after treatment of the thyroid secondary. Also, in 14 cases the thyroid gland was not the only metastatic site.

Mortensen et al. (77) claimed that metastases to the thyroid were not so uncommon. Among 567 autopsies on patients dying of malignancy 3.9% were found to have metastases in the thyroid. However, these were rarely solitary and mostly occult metastases. Shimaoka et al. (78) reported an incidence of thyroid metastases of nearly 9% among 1999 patients autopsied following death from malignancy. The autopsy incidence of this finding, however, will vary with the thoroughness of pathological examination and multiple sections must be examined if the true incidence of metastatic disease in the thyroid gland is to be determined.

Since the presence of thyroid metastases represents dissemination of a malignant tumour, usually adenocarcinoma, death from disease is virtually inevitable (79). However, the rapidity of this event depends both on the nature of the primary and the presence of other metastatic disease. In the Mayo Clinic series, 9 patients survived 3 years or more after treatment of the thyroid metastases. Three of these had renal cell carcinoma, 3 had breast cancer, 2 had lung cancer and 1 had carcinoma of the oesophagus.

When a diagnosis of metastatic adenocarcinoma is made following needle biopsy or thyroidectomy, subsequent management becomes problematical. Although treatment should be planned on an individual basis, current evidence indicates that investigations

carried out in the absence of specific symptoms are unlikely to uncover a diagnosis and are not cost effective (80). The fact that disease is likely to be disseminated and that prognosis is poor should temper a headlong and expensive search for the primary. However, investigation of specific symptoms is appropriate as this may allow useful palliative treatment to be given and, in the rare instance of the thyroid lesion being the solitary metastatic site, may offer a chance for effective disease control.

REFERENCES

1 Rosai J, Carcangiu ML. Pathology of thyroid tumours: Some recent and old questions. Hum Pathol 1984; 15: 1008.
2 Cady B. Surgery of thyroid cancer. World J Surg 1981; 5: 3.
3 Woolner LB. Thyroid carcinoma: Pathological classification with data on prognosis. Semin Nuc Med 1971; 1: 481.
4 Staunton MD, Greening WP. Treatment of thyroid cancer in 293 patients. Br J Surg 1976; 63: 253.
5 McConahey WM, Hay ID, Wooner LB, Van Heerden JA, Taylor WF. Papillary thyroid cancer treated at the Mayo Clinic, 1946 through 1970: Initial manifestations, pathologic findings, therapy and outcome. Mayo Clin Proc 1986; 61: 978.
6 Harness JK, Thompson NW, McLeod MK, Eckhauser FE, Lloyd RV. Follicular carcinoma of the thyroid gland: Trends and treatment Surgery. 1984; 96: 972.
7 Watson RG, Brennan MD, Van Heerden JA, McConahey WM, Taylor WF. Invasive Hürthle cell carcinoma of the thyroid: natural history and management. Mayo Clin Proc 1984; 59: 851.
8 Miller RH, Estrada R, Sneed WF, Mace ML. Hürthle cell tumours of the thyroid gland. Laryngoscope 1983; 93: 884.
9 Bondeson L, Bondeson AG, Ljungberg O, Tibblin S. Oxyphil tumours of the thyroid. Follow-up of 42 surgical cases. Ann Surg 1981; 194: 677.
10 Caplan RH, Abellera RM, Kisken WA. Hürthle Cell tumours of the thyroid gland. A clinicopathologic review and long term follow-up. JAMA 1984; 251: 3114.
11 Gonzalez-Campora R, Herrero-Zapatero A, Lerma E, Sanchez F, Galera H. Hürthle cell and mitrochondrial rich cell tumours. A clinicopathologic study. Cancer 1986; 57: 1154.

12 Thompson NW, Dunn EL, Batsakis JG, Nishayama RH. Hürthle cell lesions of the thyroid gland. Surg Gynecol Obstet 1974; 139: 555.

13 Gosain AK, Clark OH. Hürthle cell neoplasms. Malignant potential. Arch Surg 1984; 119: 515.

14 Johnson TL, Lloyd RV, Burney RE, Thompson NW. Hürthle cell thyroid tumour. An immunohistochemical study. Cancer 1987; 59: 107.

15 Grundry SR, Burney RE, Thompson NW, Lloyd R. Total thyroidectomy for Hürthle cell neoplasm of the thyroid. Arch Surg 1983; 118: 529.

16 Heppe H, Armin A, Calandra DB, Lawrence AM, Paloyan E. Hürthle cell tumours of the thyroid gland. Surgery 1985; 98: 1162.

17 Rosen IB, Luk S, Katz I. Hürthle cell tumour behaviour: Dilemma and resolution. Surgery 1985; 98: 777.

18 Nel CJC, Van Heerden JA, Goellner JR, McConahey WM, Taylor WF, Grant CS. Anaplastic carcinoma of the thyroid: a clinicopathologic study of 82 cases. Mayo Clin Proc 1985; 60: 51.

19 Aldinger KA, Samaan NA, Ibanez M, Hill CS. Anaplastic carcinoma of the thyroid. A review of 84 cases of spindle and giant cell carcinoma of the thyroid. Cancer 1978; 41: 2267.

20 Carcangiu ML, Steeper T, Zampi G, Rosai J. Anaplastic thyroid carcinoma. A study of 70 cases. Am J Clin Pathol 1985; 83: 135.

21 Rossi R, Cady B, Meissner WA, Sedgwick CE, Werber J. Prognosis of undifferentiated carcinoma and lymphoma of the thyroid. Am J Surg 1978; 135: 589.

22 Rayfield EJ, Nishayama RH, Sisson JC. Small cell tumours of the thyroid. A clinicopathologic study. Cancer 1971; 28: 1023.

23 Rosai J, Saxen EA, Wooner L. Undifferentiated and poorly differentiated carcinoma. Semin Diag Pathol 1985; 2: 123.

24 Kruseman ACN, Bosman FT, Van Bergen Henegouw JC, Cramer Knijnenberg G, de la Riviere GB. Medullary differentiation of anaplastic thyroid carcinoma. Am J Clin Pathol 1982; 77: 541.

25 Mooradian AD, Allam CK, Khalil MF, Salti I, Salem PA. Anaplastic transformation of thyroid cancer: report of two cases and review of the literature. J Surg Oncol 1983; 23: 95.

26 Tollefsen HR, De Cosse JJ, Hutter RVP. Papillary carcinoma of the thyroid: A clinical and pathological study of 70 fatal cases. Cancer 1964; 17: 1035.

27 Nishayama RH, Dunn EL, Thompson NW. Anaplastic spindle-cell and giant-cell tumours of the thyroid gland. Cancer 1972; 30: 113.

28 Casterline PF, Jaques DA, Blom H, Wartofsky L. Anaplastic giant and spindle-cell carcinoma of the thyroid gland. A different therapeutic approach. Cancer 1980; 45: 1689.

29 Jereb B, Stjernsward J, Lowhagen T. Anaplastic giant-cell carcinoma of the thyroid. Cancer 1975; 35: 1293.

30 Spiro RH, Daniella NS. Spindle and giant cell carcinoma of the thyroid: report of a five-year survival after lobectomy and post-operative irradiation. J Surg Oncol 1979; 12: 385.

31 Simpson WJ. Anaplastic thyroid carcinoma: a new approach. Can J Surg 1980; 23: 25.

32 Goldman JM, Goren EN, Cohen MH, Webber BL, Brennan MF, Robbins J. Anaplastic thyroid carcinoma: longer term survival after radical surgery. J Surg Oncol 1980; 14: 389.

33 Poster DS, Bruno S, Penta J, Pina K, Catane R. Current status of chemotherapy in the treatment of advanced carcinoma of the thyroid gland. Cancer Clin Trials 1981; 3: 301.

34 Hill CS. Chemotherapy for thyroid cancer. In: Kaplan EL ed Surgery of the Thyroid and Parathyroid Gland, Chapter 8. Edinburgh: Churchill Livingstone, 120–6.

35 Shimaoka K, Tsukada Y. Squamous cell carcinomas and adenosquamous carcinomas originating from the thyroid gland. Cancer 1986; 46: 1833–42.

36 Segel K, Sidi J, Abraham A, Konichezky M, Ben-Bassat M. Pure squamous cell carcinoma and mixed adenosquamous cell carcinoma of the thyroid gland. Head Neck Surg 1984; 6: 1035–42.

37 Li Volsi VA, Merino MJ. Squamous cells in the human thyroid gland. Am J Surg Pathol 1978; 2: 133–40.

38 Bullock WK, Hummer GJ, Kahler KE. Squamous metaplasia of the thyroid gland. Cancer 1952; 5: 966–74.

39 Meissner WA, Warren S. Tumours of the thyroid gland. Fascicle 4, Second Series, Washington, DC: Armed Forces Institute of Pathology, 1969.

40 Bakri K, Shimaoka K, Rao U, Tsukada Y. Adenosquamous carcinoma of the thyroid after radiotherapy for Hodgkin's disease. A case report and review. Cancer 1983; 52: 465–70.

41 Harada T, Shimaoka K, Yakamuru K, Ito K. Squamous cell carcinoma of the thyroid gland— transition from adenocarcinoma. J Surg Oncol 1982; 19: 36–43.

42 Miyauchi A, Kuma K, Matsuzuha F, Matsubayashi S, Kobayashi A, Tamai H, Katayama S. Intrathyroidal epithelial thymoma: An entity distinct from squamous cell carcinoma of the thyroid. World J Surg 1985; 9: 1228–35.

43 Chak LY, Hoppe RT, Burke JS, Kaplan HS. Non-Hodgkin's lymphoma presenting as thy-

roid enlargement. Cancer 1981; 48: 2712–16.

44 Burke JS, Butler JJ, Fuller LM. Management of lymphomas of the thyroid. A clinical pathologic study of 35 patients including ultrastructural observations. Cancer 1977; 39: 1587–602.

45 Talal N, Bunim JJ. The development of malignant lymphoma in the course of Sjogren's syndrome. Am J Med 1964; 36: 529–40.

46 Lukes RJ, Collins RD. Immunologic characterisation of human malignant lymphomas. Cancer 1974; 34: 1488–503.

47 Lukes RJ, Collins RD. New approaches to the classification of lymphomata. Br J Cancer 1975; 31 (Suppl): 1–28.

48 Hamburger JI, Miller M, Kini SR. Lymphoma of the thyroid. Ann Intern Med. 1983; 99: 685–93.

49 Compagno J, Oertel JE. Malignant lymphoma and other lymphoproliferative disorders of the thyroid gland. Am J Clin Pathol 1980; 74: 1–11.

50 Anscombe AM, Wright DH. Primary malignant lymphoma of the thyroid—a tumour of mucosa-associated lymphoid tissue: review of seventy-six cases. Histopathology 1985; 9: 81–97.

51 Devine RM, Edis AJ, Banks PM. Primary lymphoma of the thyroid: A review of the Mayo Clinic experience through 1978. World J Surg 1981; 5: 33–8.

52 Kapadia SB, Dekker A, Cheng VS, Desai U, Watson CG. Malignant lymphoma of the thyroid gland: a clinicopathologic study. Head Neck Surg 1982; 4: 270–80.

53 Rappaport H. Tumours of the hematopoietic system. In: Atlas of Tumour Pathology, Section 3, Fascicle 8. Washington, DC: Armed Forces Institute of Pathology, 1966: 91–156.

54 Aozasa K, Nara H, Ikeda H, Masaki N, Miyata Y, Matsuzuka F, Shigematsu U. The influence of histologic type on survival in early extranodal non-Hodgkin's lymphoma in head and neck. Oncology 1984; 41: 164–9.

55 Kugler JW, Armitage JO, Dick FR. Hodgkin's disease presenting as a thyroid mass. Postgrad Med 1982; 72: 243–5.

56 Voegt H. Extramedullare Plasmacytome. Virchows Arch (Pathol Anat) 1938; 302: 497–508.

57 Wiltshaw E. The natural history of extramedullary plasmacytoma and its relation to solitary myeloma of bone and myelomatosis. Medicine 1976; 55: 217–38.

58 Macpherson TA, Dekker A, Kapadia SB. Thyroid-gland plasma cell neoplasm (plasmacytoma). Arch Pathol Lab Med 1981; 105: 570.

59 Lopez M, Di Louro L, Marolla P, Medonna V. Plasmacytoma of the thyroid gland. Clin Oncol 1983; 9: 61.

60 Wolvos TA, Chong FK, Razui SA, Tully GL III. An unusual thyroid tumour: a comparison to a literature review of thyroid teratomas. Surgery 1985; 97: 613–17.

61 Fisher KE, Cooney DR, Voorhess ML, Jewett TC. Teratoma of thyroid gland in infancy: review of the literature and two case reports. J Surg Oncol. 1982; 21: 135–40.

62 Mahour GH, Landing BH, Wooley MM. Teratomas in children: clinicopathologic studies in 133 patients. Z Kinderchir Grenzgeb 1978; 23: 365.

63 Grosfeld JL, Ballantine TVN, Lowe D, Baehner RL. Benign and malignant teratomas in children: analysis of 85 patients. Surgery 1976; 80: 297.

64 Stone HH, Henderson WD, Guido FA. Teratomas of the neck. Am J Dis Child 1967; 113: 222–4.

65 Kingsley DPE, Elton A, Bennett MH. Malignant teratoma of the thyroid: A case report and a review of the literature. Br J Cancer 1968; 22: 7–11.

66 Kimler SC, Math WF. Primary malignant teratoma of the thyroid. Cancer 1978; 42: 311–17.

67 Egloff B. The hemangioendothelioma of the thyroid. Virchows Arch (Pathol Anat) 1983; 400: 119–42.

68 Ruchti C, Gerber HA, Schaffner T. Factor VIII-related antigen in malignant hemangioendothelioma of the thyroid. Additional evidence of the endothelial origin of this tumour. Am J Clin Pathol. 1984; 82: 474–80.

69 O'Brien CJ, Soong S-J, Herrera GA, Urist MM, Maddox WA. Malignant salivary tumors—analysis of prognostic factors and survival. Head Neck Surg 1986; 9: 82.

70 Spiro RH. Salivary neoplasms: an overview of a 35 year experience with 2,807 patients. Head Neck Surg 1986; 8: 177.

71 Rhatigan RM, Roque JL, Bucher RL. Mucoepidermoid carcinoma of the thyroid gland. Cancer 1977; 39: 210.

72 Mizukami Y, Matsubara F, Hashimoto T, Haratake J, Terahata S, Noguchi M, Hirose K. Primary mucoepidermoid carcinoma of the thyroid gland. A case report including an ultrastructural and biochemical study. Cancer 1984; 53: 1741.

73 Franssila KO, Harach HR, Wasenius V-M. Mucoepidermoid carcinoma of the thyroid. Histopathology 1984; 8: 847.

74 Harach HR. A study of the relationship between solid cell nests and mucoepidermoid carcinoma of the thyroid. Histopathology 1985; 9: 195.

75 Czech JM, Lichtor TR, Carney A, van Heerden JA. Neoplasms metastatic to the thyroid gland. Surg Gynecol Obstet 1982; 155: 503.

76 Ivy HK. Cancer metastatic to the thyroid: a

diagnostic problem. Mayo Clin Proc 1984; 59: 856.

77 Mortensen JD, Woolner LB, Bennett WA. Secondary malignant tumors of the thyroid gland. Cancer 1956; 9: 306.

78 Shimaoka K, Sokal JE, Pickren JW. Metastatic neoplasms in the thyroid gland: pathological and clinical findings. Cancer 1962; 15: 557.

79 Altman E, Cadman E. An analysis of 1539 patients with cancer of unknown primary site. Cancer 1986; 57: 120.

80 Osteen RT, Kopf G, Wilson RE. In pursuit of the unknown primary. Am J Surg 1978; 135: 494.

Textbook of Uncommon Cancer
Edited by C.J. Williams, J.G. Krikorian, M.R. Green and D. Raghavan
© 1988 John Wiley & Sons Ltd

Chapter **36**

Paraganglioma of the Head and Neck

C.C. Wang

Head, Division of Clinical Services, Department of Radiation Medicine, Massachusetts General Hospital; Professor of Radiation Therapy, Harvard Medical School, Boston, Massachusetts, USA

Glomus tumors or chemodectomas arising from the jugular bulb, nerve of Jacobson and nerve of Arnold are unusual tumors. These vascular lesions are now commonly termed, according to site of origin, as glomus jugulare, glomus tympanicum and glomus vagale respectively and pathologically are best described under the common category of paraganglioma. The great majority of glomus tumors are benign in character, slow growing, and spread by local extension (1). Owing to lack of significant symptoms, the tumors tend to be diagnosed rather late in the course of the disease. Metastases to the regional nodes and distant sites are extremely rare. The frequent otologic symptoms and signs of these tumors originating or extending into the middle ear are pressure sensation in the ear, the presence of an aural polyp, progressive loss of hearing, a sensation of fullness or pulsating tinnitus. The patients with extensive disease extending to the middle cranial fossa may experience vertigo, temporoparietal headache, retro-orbital pain, proptosis and paresis of the fifth and sixth cranial nerves. Other neurologic symptoms and signs include dysphagia, occipital headache, ataxia, hoarseness of voice and paralysis of the cranial nerves IX and XII which may occur if the tumor reaches the posterior cranial fossa and cranial nerves V through VII;

invasion of the jugular foramen causes paralysis.

Glomus tumor may secrete norepinephrine and epinephrine, producing symptoms similar to pheochromocytoma. The catecholamines are rapidly inactivated and their urinary metabolites such as vanillylmandelic acid (VMA) and MHPH can be measured and used as a guide to the success of therapies.

Evaluation of the extent of these lesions is based on careful analysis of the symptoms and neurologic signs, detailed radiologic findings, including polytomes of appropriate projections, and computed tomography (CT) of the brain and temporal bone; selective angiography is the most useful radiographic technique for evaluation of intracranial extension of the disease, and assessment of collateral cerebral blood flow in case ligation of major vessels is necessary and/or embolization, or possible second or third tumors. The role of magnetic resonance imaging (MRI) remains to be evaluated. Biopsy is rarely required if the angiogram is positive and in fact it is quite risky.

SELECTION OF THERAPY

For small tumors limited to the middle ear, the treatment of choice is surgical excision. This is in the form of hypotympanectomy or radical mastoidectomy and temporal bone resection. Because of the intricate anatomy of the temporal bone, the surgical removal of extensive glomus tumors arising from the jugular bulb is often incomplete and followed by local recurrence or persistence of the tumor (2). Large tumors with intracranial extension are rarely amenable to treatment by surgical removal. Since these tumors are generally extremely vascular, radical surgery is often difficult and dangerous, and advocates of surgery frequently recommend postoperative radiation therapy (3). It is therefore difficult to determine whether the treatment results from such surgical extirpation of the large lesions are due to surgery alone or radiation therapy or a combination of these two methods. In our experience, such heroic radical surgery for extensive glomus tumor is rarely advisable.

Intra-arterial embolization of glomus tumors may be carried out either as a preoperative procedure or for palliation. Since most of these tumors are extremely vascular, embolization is seldom complete, and therefore may be carried out prior to radiation therapy during angiographic study. Radiation therapy is effective as a growth restraint procedure (1, 4–9) and may be used for patients with residual or recurrent disease after radical mastoidectomy and/or temporal resection or for inoperable lesions.

RADIOTHERAPEUTIC MANAGEMENT

Since most of the glomus tumors are eccentrically situated in the temporal bone and base of skull, ipsilateral wedged pair techniques employing low megavoltage x-rays, i.e. 4–6 MeV x-rays, or cobalt-60 radiations are used (Figure 1). If the lesions extend to the midline structures, opposed lateral portals would be necessary at least for approximately two-thirds of the total dose and the remaining by lateral

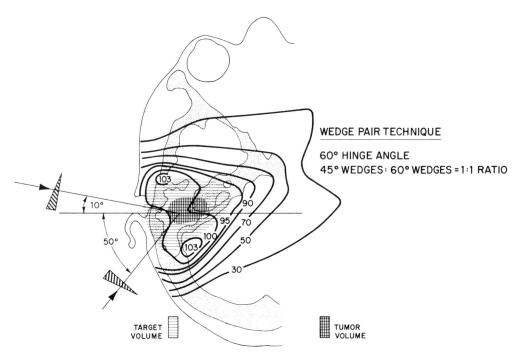

Figure 1 Diagram showing isodose distribution using ipsilateral wedge pair portal technique with cobalt-60 irradiation for glomus tumor within the temperal bone. (*From Wang CC, Radiation Therapy for Head and Neck Neoplasms. John Wright-PSG, Inc. 1983.*)

wedged pair. At times, ipsilateral electron beam radiation therapy is used to supplement external photon radiation therapy.

The radiation therapy dose given postoperatively is 45 Gy in 4.5 to 5 weeks with a daily fraction of 1.8 Gy (5, 10, 11). For the inoperable lesions, a dose of 50 Gy in 5.5 weeks is recommended. Therefore, like ultra-radical surgery high dose radiation therapy is rarely justified for a benign chemodectoma. Under no circumstances should a dose of 60 Gy in 6 weeks be exceeded if temporal bone necrosis is to be avoided (12, 13).

RADIOTHERAPEUTIC RESULTS

Because of the indolent nature of most glomus tumors, it is difficult to assess and/or compare the results of various forms of therapy. The reported series have shown that results after combined surgery and radiation therapy for the lesion in the temporal bone were superior to surgery alone. Local recurrence can be reduced with the use of adjuvant postoperative radiation therapy (2, 8, 11).

MASSACHUSETTS GENERAL HOSPITAL (MGH) EXPERIENCE

From 1958 through 1986, a total of 45 patients with glomus jugulare, tympanicum and vagale were treated by radiation therapy. Of these, 23 received postoperative radiation therapy for residual disease following radical mastoidectomy and/or temporal bone resection and 13 received radiation therapy alone for inoperable or unresectable tumors. Nine patients with gross recurrence after previous surgery had radiation therapy as a salvage procedure. The survival status of this group is summarized in Figure 2. The duration of follow-up ranged from 1 year to 26 years. Table 1 shows the tumor response of this group of patients after radiation therapy.

Of 23 patients receiving postoperative radiation therapy after surgical resection, 21 or 91% were alive and well without progressive

tumor, for periods ranging from 1 to 25 years; 1 died of the disease with osteoradionecrosis at $5\frac{1}{2}$ years. One patient suffered recurrences after 30 Gy, at 11 years, which were subsequently treated by cryotherapy with marginal benefit and 1 patient had osteoradionecrosis but was living and well without tumor at 6 years. Of 9 patients with gross recurrences after surgical resection, 6 were salvaged with no visible growth, one with persistent but smaller growth and 2 died of the disease with persistent tumor. Of 13 patients receiving radiation therapy alone for unresectable tumors, 9 were living without progressive tumors, two with persistent but smaller tumors of glomus vagale.

SUMMARY

Paragangliomas of the head and neck are uncommon tumors. Most of these lesions occur in the temporal bone and are treated by temporal bone resection if the lesions are operable; some occurring in the parapharyngeal space are technically inoperable. For the resectable lesions, postoperative radiation therapy has been found to be effective in reducing the incidence of local recurrence. Therefore, radiation therapy should be considered as an integrated treatment program with a dose of 45 to 50 Gy in 5 to 6 weeks. For the lesion extending into the cranial cavity or arising from the parapharyngeal space, surgical resection has become technically impossible. For such inoperable lesions, radiation therapy alone is the preferred treatment modality with satisfactory local control. The benignity of paragangliomas of the head and neck is well demonstrated by our experience with 45 patients. Very few patients succumbed to the disease and many patients can survive with the disease living reasonably well and symbiotically with their tumors. Therefore, treatment of this disease, either surgical or radiotherapeutic, must be tempered with conservatism. Aggressive radiation therapy with high dose to the tumors, particularly to the temporal bone, is a disservice to patients with this disease.

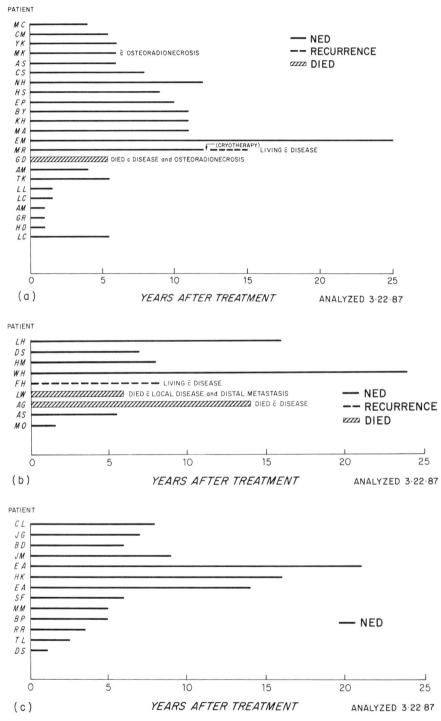

Figure 2 Survival status with glomus tumor after radiation therapy for various conditions: (a) for residual disease; (b) for gross recurrence after surgery; (c) for inoperable tumor. NED, no evidence of disease.

TABLE 1 RESPONSE OF GLOMUS TUMORS AFTER VARIOUS TREATMENT MODALITIES: MGH EXPERIENCE

	Follow-up	Surgery and postop. RT	RT for recurrence after surgery	RT for inoperable tumors
No evidence	<3 yrs	5	1	2
of progressive	4–5 yrs	2	0	3
disease	>5–10 yrs	9	3	5
	>10–15 yrs	4		1
	>15–25 yrs	1	2	2
Total		21	6	13
Local recurrence		1	1	0
Died from tumor		1	2	0
Total		23[a]	9	13

Analyzed 3/26/87.
RT, radiotherapy.
[a]Two were associated with osteoradionecrosis of the temporal bone after radiation therapy.

REFERENCES

1 Fuller AM, Brown HA, Harrison EG et al. Chemodectomas of the glomus jugulare tumors. Laryngoscope 1967; 77: 218–38.

2 Hatfield PM, James AE, Schulz MD. Chemodectomas of the glomus jugulare. Cancer 1972; 30: 1164–8.

3 Jackson CG, Glasscock ME III, Harris PF. Glomus tumors—diagnosis, classification and management of large lesions. Arch Otol 1982; 108: 401–6.

4 Bradshaw JD. Radiotherapy in glomus jugulare tumors. Clin Radiol 1961; 12: 227–34.

5 Hudgins PT. Radiotherapy for extensive glomus jugulare tumors. 1972; Radiology 103: 427–9.

6 Maruyama Y. Radiation therapy of tympanojugular chemodectoma. Radiology 1972; 105: 659.

7 Simko TG, Griffin TW, Gerdes AJ et al. The role of radiation therapy in the treatment of glomus jugulare tumors. Cancer 1978; 42: 104–6.

8 Spector GJ, Compagno J, Perez CA et al. Glomus jugulare tumors: Effects of radiotherapy. Cancer 1975; 35: 1316–21.

9 Grubb WB, Lampe I. The role of radiation therapy in the treatment of chemodectomas of the glomus jugulare. Laryngoscope 1965; 75: 1861–71.

10 Wang CC. What is the optimum dose of radiation therapy for glomus jugulare? (Editorial) Int J Radiat Oncol Biol Phys 1980; 6: 945–6.

11 Tidwell TJ, Montague ED. Chemodectoma involving the temporal bone. Radiology 1975; 116: 147.

12 Schuknecht HF, Karmody CS. Radionecrosis of the temporal bone. Laryngoscope 1966; 76: 1416–28.

13 Wang CC, Doppke K. Osteoradionecrosis of the temporal bone—Consideration of nominal standard dose. Int J Radiat Oncol Biol Phys 1976; 1: 881–3.

Textbook of Uncommon Cancer
Edited by C.J. Williams, J.G. Krikorian, M.R. Green and D. Raghavan
© 1988 John Wiley & Sons Ltd

Chapter **37**

The Diagnosis and Treatment of Neoplastic Disorders of the Adrenal Glands

K. Oberg, A. Goldhirsch and
A. Munro Neville
*Ludwig Institute for Cancer Research, Uppsala, Sweden,
and Bern and Zürich, Switzerland*

INTRODUCTION

Disorders of the adrenal glands have traditionally presented either with endocrine disturbances caused by the increased secretion of steroid hormones or catecholamines or with symptoms relating to an abdominal mass. However, the recent introduction of computed tomography (CT) and ultrasonography has markedly increased the clinician's dilemma as a wide variety of additional asymptomatic adrenal lesions are now being recognized, many when quite small (1). Such lesions include the so-called 'non-functioning' adrenal nodule, the 'non-hormonal' (non-functioning) carcinoma, myelolipoma, metastatic carcinoma, foci of calcification, cysts and pseudocysts. Careful clinical and biochemical analyses are required prior to biopsy or open surgery to establish the correct diagnosis (see below).

Hyperfunction of the adrenal cortex (hypercorticalism) mainly manifests itself in three ways—Cushing's, Conn's and the adrenogenital syndromes. Bilateral adrenocortical hyperplasia, not neoplasia, is usually the cause of Cushing's and the adrenogenital syndrome, while hyperaldosteronism with low plasma

renin (Conn's syndrome) is due generally to an adrenocortical adenoma (2).

While bilateral adrenal medullary hyperplasia may also occur to account for increased catecholamine production, this is more commonly due to a pheochromocytoma, which accounts for 0.05–0.1% of all patients with hypertension (3). The vast majority of pheochromocytomas are benign (4).

Malignant adrenocortical and medullary tumors are, therefore, extremely rare, afflicting approximately two and one per million of the population per year respectively (5–7). Their detection before metastases become overt is difficult. Current therapy for metastases is far from satisfactory. Their early detection while limited to the adrenal gland must be a future goal; surgical removal is the only known effective curative treatment.

ADRENOCORTICAL TUMORS

Symptoms related to tumors of the adrenal cortex depend upon whether the tumors are functional or non-functional (biologically inactive hormone producing) (2). Functional tumors mainly produce cortisol, aldosterone

731

and/or sex steroids. The unregulated hyper-
production of these hormones results in well
defined clinical syndromes. In adult patients
with functioning tumors, the commonest clinical presentation is Cushing's syndrome, whereas in children, the adrenogenital syndrome or
precocious puberty predominates. Feminization is rare and is predominantly diagnosed in
adult men with gynecomastia. An excess of
mineralocorticoids is seldom due to an adrenocortical carcinoma.

'Non-functional' tumors release biologically
inactive hormone precursors and cause symptoms related to the mass, its local extension or
to metastases (8).

Cushing's Syndrome

Cushing's syndrome is due to a chronic incre-
ment in the level of circulating glucocorticoid
hormones, in particular cortisol. Adrenocortical tumors account for about one-quarter of all
adult cases of Cushing's syndrome, occurring
most frequently in females particularly
between the ages of 30 and 60 years. In
children, tumors are more frequent than bilateral hyperplasia as a cause of the syndrome
(Table 1).

Clinical Presentation

Cushing's syndrome manifests itself as truncal
obesity with the characteristic buffalo hump
and florid rounded facies. Increased body
weight, cutaneous striae, ecchymoses, increasing degrees of tiredness and weakness, hyper-

tension, personality changes (depression or
psychotic signs) are also often noted. In
women, hirsutism, amenorrhea and clitorimegaly may occur. Mild glucose intolerance with
polyuria and polydipsia, alterations in
immune function, thinning of the skin, osteoporosis and renal calculi may be evident. These
symptoms and signs, caused by glucocorticoid
excess, are due to increased gluconeogenesis,
inhibition of amino acid uptake and protein
synthesis and accelerated protein breakdown.

Clearly, none of these symptoms or signs is
unique to Cushing's syndrome and classical
cushingoid features can occur with each type of
etiology. Adenomas in adults are generally
associated with a 'pure' form of the syndrome
while, in children, virilism may be an added
feature. Carcinomas, on the other hand, in
addition to the classical stigmata, are frequently associated with virilism and hypertension.

While this chapter is devoted to neoplastic-
induced Cushing's syndrome, it is worth
remembering that the syndrome is more frequently due to bilateral adrenocortical hyperplasia (Table 1), or is an iatrogenic disorder
due to the therapeutic administration of excessive amounts of glucocorticoids or ACTH.
Similar symptoms may also be met in chronic
alcoholism due to defective elimination of
steroid hormones and their metabolites (9).

Pathology

Adenomas. These are generally single and
unilateral. If bilateral and/or multiple, the
possibility of bilateral nodular hyperplasia
should be excluded (10). The appearances of
the attached gland are the clue to the diagnosis. It is atrophic with an adenoma and
hyperplastic with a nodule. Adenomas are
small rounded lesions with a yellow cut surface
in which brown foci are present (2). Rarely will
a black adenoma be found. Necrosis and
hemorrhage are rare. They usually weigh less
than 50 g and often less than 30 g. However,
adenomas weighing up to 250 g have been
recorded.

TABLE 1   INCIDENCE OF ADRENAL
LESIONS IN CUSHING'S
SYNDROME AS A
FUNCTION OF AGE (2)

Adrenal lesions	Incidence (%)	
	Adults	Children
Hyperplasia	78	42
Adenoma	13	12
Carcinoma	9	46

Microscopically, a tenuous capsule surrounds the lesion. The yellow areas correspond to lipid-laden clear cells, morphologically similar to the cells of the zona fasciculata of the normal adrenal cortex (Figure 1). The brown areas consist of compact cells with eosinophilic lipid-poor granular cytoplasm, similar to the cells of the normal zona reticularis. Usually clear cells predominate, but compact cells are the sole component of 'black adenomas'. The tumor cells are arranged in small cords or alveoli. Nuclear or cellular pleomorphism is uncommon. The ipsilateral and contralateral adrenal cortex associated with adenomas is always atrophic (2).

Adrenocortical carcinomas causing Cushing's syndrome. These tend to be large lesions, most weighing in excess of 100 g and measuring

over 6 cm in diameter. This may be related, on a cellular basis, to their relatively ineffective production of cortisol. However, not all carcinomas are large, and weight alone cannot be used rigidly to assist in the differentiation of benign and malignant lesions.

Carcinomas tend to affect the right more often than the left gland and are usually encapsulated, soft in consistency, often with a pink lobulated cut surface (2). Areas of necrosis, hemorrhage, cystic change and calcification are not uncommon and occur more frequently as the lesions increase in size and weight. In larger tumors, there may be obvious microscopic evidence of capsular penetration with infiltration of the related neighboring tissues including the ipsilateral adrenal, kidney, liver, diaphragm and venous system. Satellite tumor nodules may also be present.

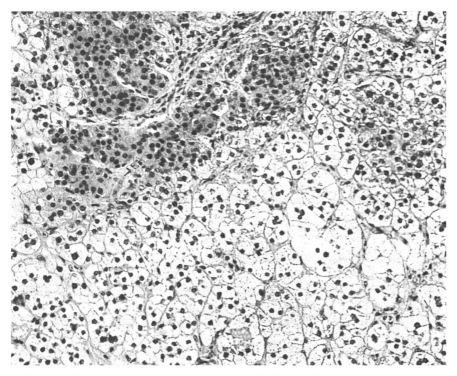

Figure 1   Cushing's syndrome—adrenocortical adenoma (5 g). A typical adenoma is illustrated composed predominantly of clear lipid-laden zona fasciculata type cells arranged in small nests. Such tumors also contain frequently small foci of eosinophilic lipid-sparse compact cells (upper left), similar to those of the normal zona reticularis (H&E, original magnification: ×240).

Microscopically, the typical large carcinoma consists solely of compact-type cells with eosinophilic, granular, lipid-poor cytoplasm, grouped in large alveoli, sheets or trabeculae separated by a fine fibrovascular stroma; in some cases, viable tumor cells form cords or tubules which only surround vessels (Figures 2 and 3). Extensive areas of necrosis may be present. Characteristically, there is cellular and nuclear pleomorphism with marked nuclear vesicularity and one or more prominent nucleoli. Bizarre and giant cellular forms may be present in some lesions while others exhibit little nuclear abnormality. Mitotic figures may or may not be seen. They are not necessarily the best indicators of malignancy. Vascular invasion through the walls of blood vessels is uncommon, although tumor cells may be observed within vessels or thrombi containing cells may be present in the tumor sinusoids or main adrenal vein.

Metastases, when they evolve, are generally detected in the regional and mediastinal lymph nodes, bones, contralateral adrenal gland and, particularly, the lungs and liver.

Prognosis

Adenomas are cured by surgery (12, 13). A few examples of spontaneous remissions in association with adenomas have been recorded. (2, 14). Survival in patients with Cushing's syndrome due to an adrenocortical carcinoma is seldom prolonged beyond 3 years. Long term survivorship (> 5 years) has been described in approximately one-fourth of patients (15). However, the introduction of adjuvant drug therapy may help to improve the prognosis (see below).

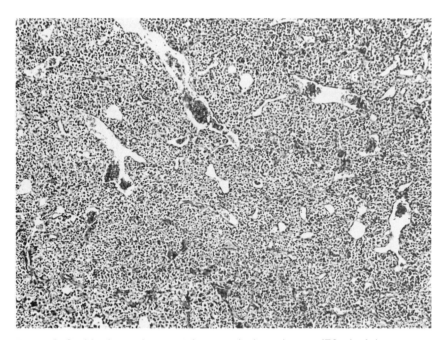

Figure 2 Cushing's syndrome—adrenocortical carcinoma (70 g). A low power view of a typical carcinoma is shown in which there are large sheets of compact eosinophilic cells of the zona reticularis type forming large trabeculae punctuated by vascular sinusoids. This kind of appearance is typical of the large carcinomas of Cushing's syndrome, the adrenogenital syndrome as well as 'non-functioning' carcinomas (H&E, original magnification: ×50).

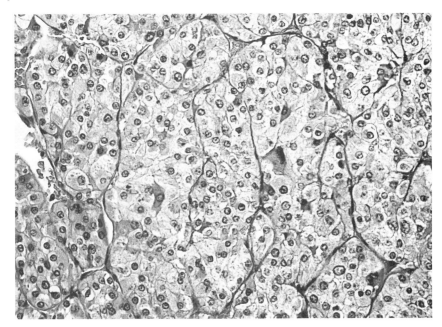

Figure 3 Cushing's syndrome—adrenocortical carcinoma (386 g). The cellular pattern of a typical carcinoma is shown at higher power, where the compact cells form trabeculae punctuated by vascular sinusoids. The cells are compact in type with lipid-sparse eosinophilic cytoplasm. The nuclei show pleomorphism with increased vesicularity and one or more prominent nucleoli (H&E, original magnification: ×240).

Adrenogenital Syndrome

The adrenogenital syndrome is associated with abnormal levels of circulating sex steroid hormones and refers to all cases of sexual precocity and heterosexual abnormalities due to adrenocortical dysfunction. Neoplasms, both benign and malignant, can give rise to the syndrome and are most often detected in children between the ages of 2 and 7 years rather than in adults. Females are more affected than males (F:M = 3:1), and the left gland is involved more frequently (2).

Clinical Presentation

In female children, *virilization* presents with clitorimegaly, hirsutism and enhanced growth. In adult females, oligomenorrhea followed by amenorrhea, 'masculine' baldness, hirsutism, deepening voice, breast atrophy, decreased libido and increased musculature occur. In male children, virilizing tumors are associated with precocious puberty, reduced gonadotrophin levels and often spermatogenic arrest; lesions with corresponding functional properties in adult men usually cause no overt endocrine symptoms (16). In some cases, signs of Cushing's syndrome may be present; hypertension is also a frequent finding in virilizing tumors. Problems in differential diagnosis include late-onset congenital adrenal hyperplasia, gonadal tumors, polycystic ovarian syndromes and central nervous system tumors causing precocious puberty as well as idiopathic sexual precocity, idiopathic hirsutism and ectopic human chronic gonadotrophin (hCG) production.

Feminization is rare; approximately only 80 adrenal carcinomas causing feminization have been recorded (2) (Table 2). Most are diagnosed in men, aged 20 to 50 years, but have

TABLE 2 AGE INCIDENCE OF 80
ADRENOCORTICAL
TUMORS CAUSING
FEMINIZATION (2)

Age (years)	Adenomas	Carcinomas
0–10	7	4
11–20	—	3
21–30	2	14
31–50	2	29
51–60	2	14
>60	—	3
Total	13 (16%)	67 (84%)

been reported in female children and postmenopausal women. The syndrome in adult males presents as bilateral gynecomastia with testicular atrophy. In prepubertal females, the tumors cause isosexual precocity.

Pathology

Unlike tumors associated with Cushing's syndrome, there is a considerable overlap in the size and weight of *virilizing adenomas and carcinomas* (2). Although large tumors are again more likely to be malignant, adenomas have been known to weigh as much as 1.5 kg. All tumors are encapsulated, have a reddish-brown cut surface and, with increasing size, areas of necrosis, hemorrhage, cystic change, and foci of calcification can often be observed.

These tumors contain one or more enzyme deficiencies which tend to channel steroidogenesis towards the production of sex hormones and/or their precursors. Although testosterone synthesis has been recorded in some cases, most tumors produce greater amounts of other C_{19}-steroids and their precursors, such as dehydroisoandrosterone (DHA) and/or its sulfate and androstenedione.

Compact cells generally are the sole cell type in these growths (17). In adenomas the cells, which are arranged in short cords or acini, have single, uniform, vesicular nuclei and may be of normal size (Figure 4). Individual cell

necrosis may be present. Apoptotic features are frequently noted (16). As tumors increase in weight, the component cells and their nuclei enlarge and exhibit increasing degrees of nuclear and cellular pleomorphism (Figure 5). The histological classification of such tumors as benign or malignant is extremely difficult. The relatively clear-cut distinction noted in Cushing's syndrome is not apparent in virilizing lesions.

In proven carcinomas, the compact cells may have a syncytial arrangement or they form large alveoli with prominent vascular sinusoids (Figure 6). In addition, there may be large areas of necrosis, and vesicular, pleomorphic and/or enlarged nuclei with prominent nucleoli are usually found. Bizarre and giant forms may occur; mitoses, however, are seldom prominent. The appearances are, thus, similar to carcinomas causing Cushing's syndrome.

Tumors associated with *feminization* vary in weight from 10 g to more than 2 kg. Their gross and histological features are indistinguishable from large virilizing or cortisol-secreting tumors. Long periods of reappraisal are necessary, as the development of metastases can be delayed for up to 8 years. Consequently, all feminizing tumors, with the possible exception of small prepubertal tumors, should be regarded as carcinomas, irrespective of histology, and managed accordingly.

In functional terms, the differences between tumors causing virilism and feminization are minimal. As with virilizing tumors, the steroid secretion patterns of feminizing tumors reflect various enzyme defects, which channel steroidogenesis towards sex steroid formation. Estrogen excretion rates rise to adult female levels or higher. C_{19}-steroids are also elevated in most patients, with DHA accounting for up to 50% of the total urinary 17-ketosteroids. Occasional tumors of this type also produce cortisol and may be associated with Cushing's syndrome as well as feminization (18). In one case, an adrenal carcinoma, which caused virilism in a child as its primary presenting feature, recurred with feminization after treatment (19).

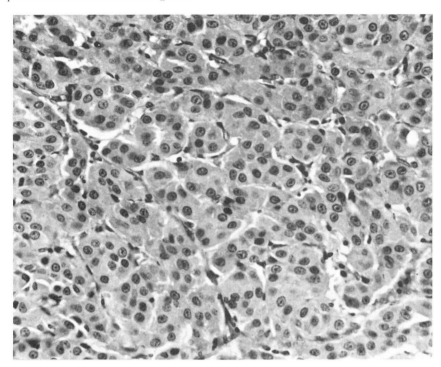

Figure 4 Virilization—adrenocortical adenoma (25 g). A characteristic benign cortical adenoma associated with virilism is shown. It contains compact cells similar to those of the normal zona reticularis arranged in short strands and nests. Nuclear pleomorphism is minimal; most of the nuclei are regular, uniform and hyperchromatic (H&E, original magnification: ×350).

Prognosis

The signs of virilization abate over several months following the curative surgical removal of an adenoma. Recurrences in malignant cases are fatal, but as a group such virilizing carcinomas tend to pursue a slower course than their counterpart causing Cushing's syndrome (16). Metastases from feminizing lesions may also be slow to emerge but with the exception of the small prepubertal lesion, most of which seem to be benign, all other feminizing tumors should be regarded as carcinomas.

The Distinction of Benign from Malignant Adrenocortical Tumors Associated with Cushing's and the Adrenogenital Syndromes

As the above descriptions indicate, there are few, if any, absolute prognostic criteria, apart from the overt presence of metastases. A combination of light morphological and functional criteria represent the best possible present approach (2, 20).

The greatest difficulty is encountered with compact cell tumors between 100 g and 500 g in weight and between 5 cm and 10 cm in diameter. Prominent nuclear pleomorphism, a high nuclear/cytoplasmic ratio, and enlarged vesicular nuclei with one or more prominent nucleoli are valuable criteria, together with distinct areas of necrosis in contrast to single cell apoptosis. The presence of true vascular wall invasion, in contrast to tumor cells in blood vessels, is also helpful but rarely observed (17). Electron microscopic criteria have proved disappointing because they do not assist with ascertaining the functional status or malignant potential (2). Recently in one study (21), the intermediate filament protein,

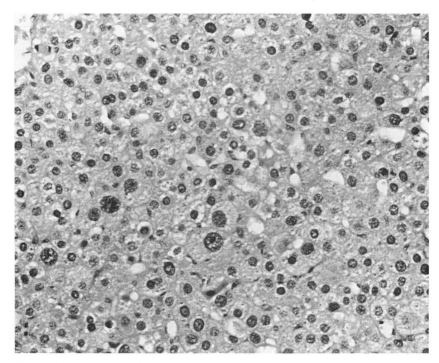

Figure 5 Virilization—adrenocortical adenoma (225 g). This is a compact cell lesion with cells containing eosinophilic lipid-sparse cytoplasm forming large trabeculae. The cells show some pleomorphism, but the nuclei are not vesicular, nor do they have prominent nucleoli. This particular lesion forms one of those which is difficult to diagnose as either benign or malignant. The young man from whom this tumor was removed is alive and well some 20 years after surgery (H&E, original magnification: ×240).

vimentin, has been demonstrated in the cytoplasm of some adrenocortical carcinoma cells but not in those of adenoma cells and may prove helpful. Flow cytometry of DNA profiles may also be valuable, but needs further study (22). Tissue culture and short term in vitro studies reveal functional abnormalities, and although none is individually pathognomonic, they aid collectively in the distinction of benign from malignant lesions (22).

Hyperaldosteronism with Low Plasma Renin (Conn's Syndrome)

The syndrome of hyperaldosteronism with low plasma renin (so-called 'primary' aldosteronism) was recognized as a specific clinicopathological entity by Conn in 1955 (23). It is typified by hypokalemic alkalosis, hypertension and muscle weakness, and is usually referred to as Conn's syndrome, particularly when associated with a solitary aldosterone-secreting adrenal adenoma. Similar symptoms also occur when steroids with mineralocorticoid activity other than aldosterone (e.g. deoxycorticosterone, corticosterone) are secreted in excess, as sometimes occurs in association with adrenocortical tumors.

The hypokalemic state, which often waxes and wanes during the course of the disease, is responsible for most of the symptoms and signs. These include muscular weakness, nocturia, persistent frontal headaches, polydipsia, paraesthesia, visual disturbances, temporary paralysis, cramps and tetany. The volume-dependent hypertension may be quite severe.

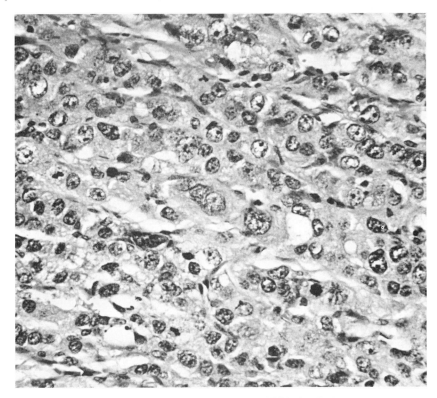

Figure 6 Virilization—adrenocortical carcinoma (1 250 g): a lesion associated with virilism is shown. The cells are of the compact zona reticularis type. The nuclei show considerable pleomorphism, are vesicular and have one or more prominent nucleoli, features associated with malignant adrenocortical lesions (H&E, original magnification: ×350).

However, it is usually not malignant in intensity and does not cause retinopathy. It, nevertheless, causes the major threat to life with ensuing nephrosclerosis, cardiac enlargement and increased risk of cardiovascular or cerebral accidents. The physical signs and symptoms of primary hyperaldosteronism are not, however, always distinguished from 'essential' hypertension without laboratory studies (24). The current consensus is that 1–2% of unselected hypertensive patients have demonstrable primary aldosteronism (25).

Pathology

This syndrome is associated with three types of adrenal change: tumor, nodules and hyperplasia of the zona glomerulosa, which may occur singly or in combination (2, 26). Approximately 65% of patients with this disorder have adrenal tumors (Table 3). Nontumorous hyperaldosteronism accounts for the

TABLE 3 PRIMARY ALDOSTERONISM: ANALYSIS OF 240 PATIENTS WITH BENIGN TUMORS OF THE ADRENAL CORTEX (2)

	Male	Female
Sex incidence	30%	70%
Modal age incidence (years)	30–50	30–50
Site of tumors (left:right)		
Single	1:1	7:4
Multiple	1:4	4:1
Weight of tumors (g)		
<2	34%	
<4	58%	

remainder, tends to affect an older age group and has been discussed elsewhere in detail (2).

Almost all adrenal tumors causing hyperaldosteronism are benign. Ninety-two percent are unilateral and single. When multiple (8%), they are still usually unilateral. Many weigh less than 2 g (Table 3). Nevertheless, a few adenomas can weigh as much as 75 g when they overlap with the weights of carcinomas associated with hyperaldosteronism (26).

The typical small adenoma associated with this syndrome is a circumscribed, encapsulated lesion with a distinctive golden-yellow cut surface. Carcinomas, on the other hand, present gross appearances indistinguishable from those causing other forms of hypercorticalism (2, 26).

As such tumors produce aldosterone, one would anticipate that their component cells would be of the zona glomerulosa type. This is

most often not the case. Adenomas have a characteristic histological appearance typified by their protean cellular morphology. Four cell types occur in such lesions: large and small clear lipid-laden cells, zona glomerulosa type cells and zona reticularis type (compact) cells (Figure 7). Very few adenomas consist of a single cell type; indeed, all four types may be found in one tumor. The commonest pattern consists of large, lipid-laden clear cells similar to those of the normal zona fasciculata in size and nuclear/cytoplasmic ratio; they are arranged in small cords or alveoli separated by fine, fibrovascular connective tissue. The nuclei are vesicular, often with inclusions, and pleomorphism may or may not be seen. Such cells may occur alone but are more commonly found in association with smaller lipid-rich cells which possess a vesicular nucleus and a nuclear/cytoplasmic ratio similar to that of

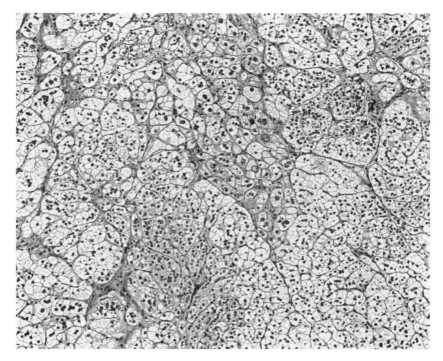

Figure 7 Hyperaldosteronism with low plasma renin—adrenocortical adenoma (1 g). Cells with clear lipid-laden cytoplasm comprise the dominant cell type in this tumor. Large and intermediate clear cell types are both seen together with a small focus of zona glomerulosa type cells in relation to fibrovascular trabeculae at the foot of the photograph (H&E, original magnification: ×200).

zona glomerulosa cells. This cell type, referred to as an intermediate (hybrid) cell, seems to have the cytological characteristics of both zona glomerulosa and zona fasciculata cells.

In many tumors, zona glomerulosa type cells are also present. Rarely, they may be the sole component. Generally, such cells are seen in nests or short cords around the periphery of the lesion dipping in a tongue-like manner into the body of the tumor accompanied by fibrovascular trabeculae (Figure 7). Groups of compact cells are occasionally noted in association with the other cells types. This cellular heterogeneity and occasional foci of nuclear pleomorphism should not mislead one into a diagnosis of malignancy, as these appearances are entirely characteristic of benign lesions causing Conn's syndrome.

Proven carcinomas associated with hyperaldosteronism are rare; only about 30 have been reliably documented (2). Most are large,

weighing more than 500 g although lesions between 30 g and 100 g have subsequently metastasized. Characteristically, the cells are zona glomerulosa in type or are similar to the intermediate (hybrid) cell type found in adenomas and are arranged in large alveoli or trabeculae separated by prominent vascular sinusoids (Figure 8) (26). Necrosis may be marked, and pleomorphism, mitotic activity, and hemorrhage may or may not be present. Some areas may present a remarkably uniform appearance. Other areas may, however, be indistinguishable from carcinomas associated with other forms of hypercorticalism.

Excess deoxycorticosterone and corticosterone production may also cause hypertensive syndromes (2). These steroids are formed by the inner zone cells of the normal cortex. Tumors secreting them are, therefore, probably not of glomerulosa origin but are akin to those associated with Cushing's and the

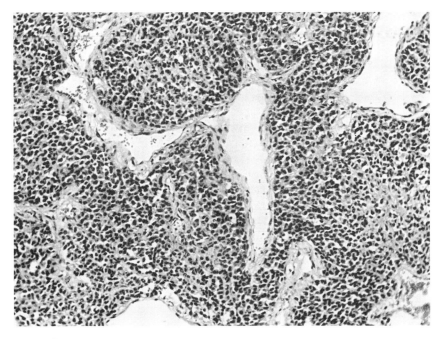

Figure 8 Hyperaldosteronism with low plasm renin—adrenocortical carcinoma (2000 g). The features of a typical adrenocortical carcinoma associated with hyperaldosteronism are shown. The cells are of the hybrid type, and form large trabeculae punctuated by thick-walled fibrovascular trabeculae (H&E, original magnification: ×160).

adrenogenital syndromes, and show typical compact cell carcinoma-like appearances (Figures 2 and 3).

Prognosis

Carcinomas causing this syndrome pursue a most aggressive course. Our personal experience has shown that survival seldom exceeds 1 year. Following 'curative' resection of an adenoma, however, the hypertensive state may persist.

Interpretation of the Structural and Functional Properties of Tumors in Conn's Syndrome

The morphology of Conn's syndrome tumors appears at first glance to be an enigma— composed of zona fasciculata type (cortisol-producing) cells in the main and yet associated with increased aldosterone production. There is no doubt about the tumor being the main source of the raised aldosterone levels, although it also will contain cortisol and corticosterone. Many benign tumors, however, have few recognizable zona glomerulosa type cells and, if present, are usually found in relation to the capsule or those fibrovascular trabeculae which permeate the tumor. Normal zona glomerulosa cells in culture initially produce aldosterone but then rapidly modulate to secrete only glucocorticoids such as cortisol (2). Ultrastructurally, there is also a morphological transition to cells of the zona fasciculata type. Benign aldosterone-producing tumors, irrespective of morphology, behave functionally in a similar manner when introduced into culture, i.e. aldosterone production is not sustained and cortisol becomes the main product (2).

This change from glomerulosa to fasciculata type cells, explains the structural and functional heterogeneity of the benign tumor of Conn's syndrome. This explanation for the cellular heterogeneity of such tumors also raises the intriguing, but probably unprovable, possibility that some non-functioning nodules asso- ciated with hypertension may have been 'Conn's adenomas' to start with, causing established essential hypertension but eventually converting entirely to zona fasciculata type cells.

'Non-hormonal' Adrenocortical Tumors

Adrenocortical tumors are considered 'non-hormonal' if there is no evidence of endocrine signs or symptoms. Such tumors are not steroidogenically inert; rather, they fail to form biologically active hormones, releasing instead inactive precursor steroids and/or their metabolites. Approximately 200 examples have been recorded in the literature, usually being diagnosed during the fifth to seventh decades of life, although children are not exempt. They occur in males twice as often as in females (2, 8).

These tumors have gross features similar to those of functioning adrenocortical carcinomas although they tend to be larger, probably because they fail to produce clinical signs and symptoms of hormonal excess at an early stage. Weights in excess of 1 kg are common. Microscopically, the predominant cell is of the compact type, although occasional tumors contain more clear than compact cells, possibly because of defective cholesterol utilization (Figure 9).

Prognosis

The prognosis is poor. Most patients die within 1 year of diagnosis. About one-third will survive beyond 3 years (8). In the follow-up of patients with carcinomas without overt function, it is essential to characterize the nature of the precursors being released (see below) and to use them as index substances to monitor the clinical course.

Diagnostic Investigative Tests and Staging

Biochemical investigations and imaging techniques form the cornerstone for the differential

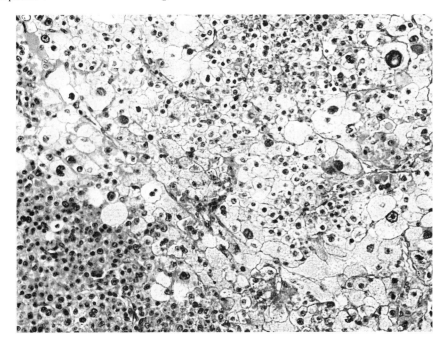

Figure 9 Non-functioning adrenocortical carcinoma (1110 g). An example of a non-functioning adrenocortical carcinoma is shown in which the cells are predominantly of the clear lipid-laden zona fasciculata type. A small group of compact eosinophilic zona reticularis type cells is shown in one corner. Note the significant nuclear ploomorphism, the vesicularity of the nuclei and one or more prominent nucleoli which are present in this lesion (H&E, original magnification: ×240).

diagnosis of all adrenocortical lesions. Detailed discussion of their utility can be found in other texts to which the reader is referred (27–29).

Biochemical Studies

Table 4 illustrates a series of tests of value in *the initial investigation* of any subject suspected of *harboring an adrenal tumor*, while those in use to categorize the basic pathology in a subject with *Cushing's syndrome* are shown in Table 5.

A number of reports have appeared concerning the use of corticotrophin releasing factor (CRF) as a stimulation test in Cushing's syndrome (30, 31). Following intravenous injection of CRF, a definite and exaggerated rise in plasma cortisol and ACTH is noted in patients with pituitary-dependent Cushing's syndrome whereas in adrenocortical tumors,

the responses are blunted or absent (Figure 10).

Biochemical investigation of patients *with virilizing symptoms* and suspected of having an

TABLE 4 SEQUENCE OF INVESTIGATIONS IN PATIENTS SUSPECTED OF HARBORING AN ADRENAL TUMOR DETECTED BY ULTRASOUND OR CT SCAN

Urinary 24-hour cortisol levels
Urinary catecholamine and VMA levels
Serum electrolytes
Plasma aldosterone, testosterone
Serum DHAS
Short overnight dexamethasone test
If tumor >5 cm
Detailed urinary steroid profile
Guided biopsy using ultrasound

TABLE 5 SUGGESTED BIOCHEMICAL INVESTIGATIVE PROCEDURE IN SUSPECTED CASES OF CUSHING'S SYNDROME

Decision	Procedure	Result
Confirmation of suspected diagnosis	Urinary free cortisol	(>300 nmol/24 h)
	Overnight dexamethasone suppression test	
	Plasma cortisol at 08.00	>100 nmol/l
OR	Low dose dexamethasone suppression test (0·5 mg four times a day for 48 h)	
	Plasma cortisol at 48 h	>50 nmol/l
	Urinary cortisol	>100 nmol/24 h
Adrenal hyperplasia or neoplasia?	Basal plasma ACTH	
	100 µg intravenous CRF	
	High dose dexamethasone suppression test (2 mg four times daily for 2 days)	
	Urinary cortisol	>50% suppression in hyperplasia
Suspected adrenal tumor	CRF test	Low basal ACTH with no resulting rise
	High dose dexamethasone suppression test	<50% suppression of urinary cortisol levels
	CT scan	
	Ultrasound	
	Detailed urinary steroid profile	Search for precursor steroids
Suspected ACTH-dependent hyperplasia	Plasma ACTH	Normal or elevated levels
	HPLC analysis	'Big' ACTH (ectopic) ACTH syndrome
	Skull x-ray	
	Magnetic resonance tomography	

HPLC=high-performance liquid chromatography.

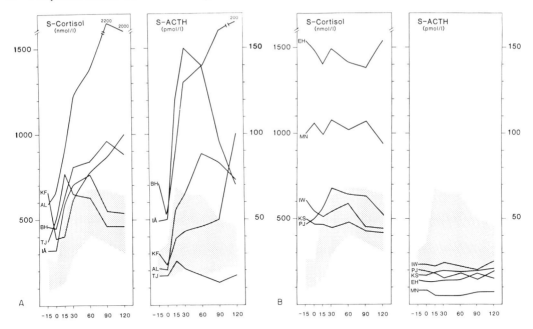

Figure 10 Cushing's syndrome: response to CRF. Four out of 5 patients with pituitary-dependent Cushing's syndrome (A) show exaggerated responses in serum cortisol and ACTH to CRF (1 μg/kg body weight or 100 μg) injected at time 0 (minutes) whereas no significant response is noted in the 5 cases with adrenocortical tumors (B). Three out of 5 patients with adrenocortical adenomas show basal plasma ACTH levels within the reference range (B).

adrenal lesion, should include determination of: serum testosterone; sex hormone binding globulin (SHBG) (to obviate spurious results due to variations in binding capacity, e.g. oral contraceptives, liver disease); dehydroisoandrosterone sulfate (DHAS); and 17α-hydroxyprogesterone an urinary 17-ketosteroids (16, 32, 33).

The steroid secretion patterns of *feminizing tumors* suggest enzyme defects, which channel steroidogenesis towards sex steroid formation (34, 35). Estrogen excretion rates rise to adult female levels, or above. C_{19}-steroids are also elevated in most patients, with DHA accounting for up to 50% of the total urinary 17-ketosteroids.

The following program to confirm *primary aldosteronism* has been suggested (24, 36). Diuretic administration should be discontinued for at least one month, if feasible, prior to biochemical investigations being started. On admission, correct any hypokalemia and keep the patient on a liberal sodium intake (100 mmol/day). When the serum potassium is normal, a 24-hour urine collection is taken to measure aldosterone. Draw supine (08.00 h) and, after 4 hours in an erect position (12.00 h), plasma samples for the determination of aldosterone, renin and 18-hydroxycorticosterone levels.

In patients with primary aldosteronism and adrenocortical adenomas, the aldosterone and 18-hydroxycorticosterone levels are significantly lowered after 4 hours in an erect posture, whereas, in patients with bilateral adrenocortical hyperplasia, the reverse is noted with higher levels in the erect posture compared with the supine position. Plasma renin activity remains suppressed when erect, instead of the increasing levels noted in normal subjects. Recently, the use of the 'captopril test' has been suggested (37). Captopril, an inhibitor of the angiotensin-converting enzyme, decreases renin-mediated aldosterone secretion in patients who do not have primary aldosteronism, whereas in patients with Conn's syndrome, no suppression of plasma aldosterone is noted with this drug.

Urinary Steroid Profiles

Adrenocortical carcinomas often excrete biologically inactive steroid hormone precursor forms (38–40), such as 3β-hydroxy-5-ene steroids, tetrahydro-11-deoxycortisol, etc. These different steroids can be analyzed by gas and high pressure liquid chromatography. The excretion pattern is clearly different in malignant adrenocortical tumors compared to benign tumors or controls (Figure 11).

Determination of such urinary steroid profiles is an important adjunct in the assessment of whether a particular tumor is malignant. Carcinomas as opposed to adenomas often produce percursor steroids as well. Such profiles also indicate the steroids which it would be most useful to measure sequentially in the follow-up phase for monitoring the efficacy of therapy and the earlier detection of recurrences and/or metastases.

Selective Adrenal Venous Sampling

Preoperative localization of hormone-producing adrenocortical tumors, especially valuable in Conn's syndrome, is aided by selective adrenal venous sampling. It employs two catheters, one through each femoral vein to allow concomitant bilateral adrenal blood sampling. There are difficulties in ensuring correct localization of the catheters, especially on the right side. Simultaneous sampling should also be done from both arms. In all cases, cortisol and aldosterone must be determined in each sample and a ratio calculated. In our own series, selective venous sampling correctly localized 80% of tumors and hyperplastic glands. In cases with hyperplasia, it was the single most successful procedure in localizing the site of adrenal hyperfunction (41).

Computerized Tomography (CT)

This is the recommended localizing technique. The normal adrenal gland can usually be visualized by this method (15, 42). Since its introduction, many adrenal masses which hitherto would not have been detected in vivo have been discovered, not least of which is the typical adrenocortical nodule so frequent in elderly obese, diabetic and hypertensive patients. Other lesions found using this technique include adrenal calcification, metastatic neoplasms, myelolipoma and adrenal cysts. Clinical, biochemical and pathological studies are required to distinguish them from primary adrenal tumors. Criteria for distinguishing a carcinoma from other masses involving the adrenal glands include size as well as signs of infiltration. In our own series of 55 consecutive patients operated upon for various adrenal gland disorders between 1976 and 1984, CT correctly localized 94% of all adrenal tumors, while only 42% of hyperplastic glands were recognized (41). Adenomas down to a minimal size of 7 mm can be visualized. Conn's syndrome tumors are often small and undetectable by CT so that bilateral venous sampling is also required. No false positive images were encountered in our series but have been reported in the literature and include intestinal loops, ectopic spleens, the gastric fundus and blood vessels.

Ultrasonography

The preoperative assessment of the nature of an adrenal lesion is best obtained by guided needle biopsy and ultrasonography. The overall sensitivity of this technique in our hands together with guided needle biopsy is about 85% in the series of 55 patients (41). The size of the tumors identified by sonographic examination is usually 1 cm in diameter and above.

Selective Arteriography

In our series, selective arteriography unveiled 75% of all tumors but was unable to demon-

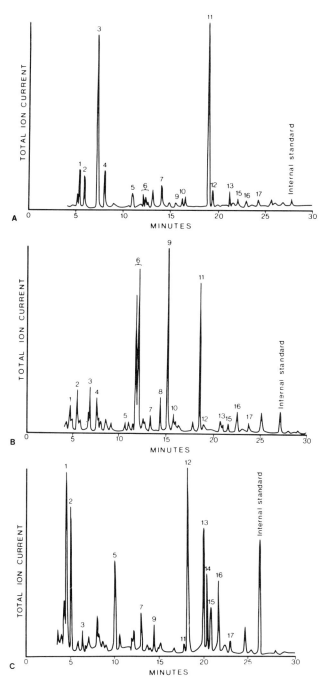

Figure 11 Urinary steroid profile. Panel A illustrates the profile from a patient with an adrenocortical carcinoma and excessive secretion of the cortisol precursors, 3β-hydroxy-5-ene steroids (peak 11) and tetrahydro-11-deoxycortisol (peak 10). In panel B is the urine from the same patient investigated after 7 months' therapy with streptozotocin and o,p'DDD. Note the increase of 16-oxygenated steroids (peak 6 and 9) and the decrease of dehydroisoandrosterone (peak 3) paralleling diminishing tumor size. In panel C a normal profile is demonstrated.

strate adrenal hyperplasia (41). Because of the availability of CT scanning, the use of selective arteriography has become less frequent.

Radionuclide Scanning

The commonest radioisotopes used are ^{131}I-19-iodocholesterol (19-IC) and ^{131}I-6β-iodomethyl-19-norcholesterol (NP-59). Suppression with dexamethasone is required and the thyroid must be blocked with Lugol's solution for 2 weeks. In a comparative study, both ^{131}I-6β-iodomethyl-19-norcholesterol (NP-59) scanning and CT were separately found to be superior as localizing techniques to ^{131}I-19-iodocholesterol (43). Furthermore, CT scanning is faster and less expensive than radionuclide scanning.

Magnetic Resonance Tomography (MRT)

MRT is the newest imaging technique. Early studies indicate its efficacy in outlining the normal adrenal gland as well as its disorders (44). However, it may be marginally less accurate than CT scanning (44); its clinical utility requires further study.

We conclude, therefore, and recommend that CT scanning is used as the primary localizing procedure, but in some cases, mostly adrenocortical hyperplasia, selective venous sampling is also needed.

Staging Procedures

Staging includes, where appropriate, seeking metastases as well as assessing other organ functions. Consequently, it consists of: (a) a search for metastatic lesion with chest x-ray, bone scans and extension of the CT scan or MRT to supradiaphragmatic regions; and (b) an assessment of cardiovascular, renal and hepatic function.

On this basis, four preoperative stages of disease are recognized:

Stage I   Tumor < 5 cm, negative nodes, no local invasion, no metastases;

Stage II   Tumor $\geq$ 5 cm, negative nodes no local invasion, no metastases;

Stage III Tumor of any size, positive nodes and/or local invasion, no metastases; and

Stage IV   Tumor of any size with distant

Treatment of Adrenocortical Tumors

Surgery is the treatment of choice and is curative for all benign tumors. Some signs, however, may persist (e.g. hypertension, hirsutism, etc). For tumors 1–10 cm in size, a unilateral posterior surgical approach is preferred. For larger tumors, an oblique or posterolateral approach should be considered. Bulky tumors may require an anterior or a thoracoabdominal approach. The latter is preferred in the majority of cases of suspected carcinomas since large en bloc resections can be undertaken (45). Perioperative corticosteroid supplementation is needed for all patients undergoing adrenalectomy.

Perioperative Corticosteroid Treatment

The following is recommended:

Day 0 100 mg hydrocortisone (cortisol) intramuscularly or intravenously with the premedication. Then 100 mg hydrocortisone by intravenous infusion over each 8-hour period to give a total of 400 mg on the day of operation.

Day 1 75 mg hydrocortisone intravenously every 8 hours.

Day 2 50 mg hydrocortisone intramuscularly every 8 hours.

Day 3 50 mg cortisone acetate orally, thrice daily.

Day 4 25 mg cortisone acetate orally, thrice daily.

Day 5 25 mg cortisone acetate orally, twice daily.

Cortisone replacement is then gradually decreased to a daily dose of 25 mg in the morning and 12.5 mg in the afternoon following bilateral adrenalectomy or where there is evidence of chronic adrenal suppression. In other patients, cortisone replacement is gradually withdrawn over 3 to 12 months. Individual assessment might indicate the need for a more prolonged withdrawal. In a small number of patients, replacement with a mineralocorticoid such as fludrocortisone acetate (0.05–0.1 mg once daily) may be needed.

Postoperative Follow-up

All patients should be clinically assessed every 3 months for the first year. Patients with malignant or suspected malignant disorders need continued regular surveillance. This not only includes clinical examination but also biochemical and radiographic studies.

Cytotoxic Treatment

o,p'DDD (mitotane, Lysodren). This drug, which exerts a specific cytolytic effect on adrenocortical cells (46), both normal and neoplastic, has been used to treat unresectable as well as metastatic adrenocortical carcinomas. It is currently regarded as the therapy of choice (47–50). Its cytolytic effects may result in hemorrhage and infarction of the tumor.

*o,p'*DDD alters significantly the extra-adrenal metabolism of cortisol (51) and a correct estimate of its effect during treatment of cortisol producing tumors can only be gauged by measurement of plasma or urinary cortisol and *not* from urinary 17-hydroxycorticosteroid levels.

Twenty-five percent to 54% of patients will show objective tumor regressions (47–50). The median duration of response is between 10 and 12 months although remissions lasting over 4 years have been reported. This drug is administered orally in three to four divided daily doses. Our current treatment policy is to start with 2 g daily and gradually increase the daily dose up to 6–8 g. Doses as high as 16 g per day have been administered. Since almost all the patients will develop adrenal insufficiency,

steroid replacement is started simultaneously using dexamethasone (0.5 mg, three times per day). Cortisone is not used because the latter interferes with the cortisol radioimmunoassay. *o,p'*DDD should not be administered with a fat-containing meal because of its lipid solubility and its tendency to concentrate in fats and, thus, not be absorbed. Responses are rarely noted before 6–8 weeks of treatment; 3 months' therapy constitutes an appropriate trial although a minority of patients will not respond until later. Treatment should continue until progression occurs.

Pharmacokinetics of o,p'DDD. Approximately 40% of single oral doses are absorbed, the remainder being excreted unchanged in the feces. A small fraction of the absorbed drug appears in the bile, whereas the remainder is stored primarily in fatty tissue throughout the body, including the nervous system (50).

Most pharmacokinetic studies in man have shown neither a dose–response nor a dose–toxicity relationship. After the single oral administration of 5–15 g, peak blood levels varied from 7 to 90 μg/ml for the unchanged drug, and from 29 to 54 μg/ml for its metabolites. The primary metabolites are oxidation products: the ethene derivative, *o,p'*DDE and the acetate, *o,p'*DDA (50). With typical daily doses, blood levels of the drug steadily increase to a median level around 10 μg/ml, with metabolite levels being 10 times higher.

The prognostic importance of serum levels of *o,p'*DDD measured during therapy has been emphasized by Van Slooten and colleagues (52). In their study, an objective response was achieved in 8 patients, 7 of whom had blood drug levels in excess of 14 μg/ml for at least 6 months. Three patients showed total tumor regression for periods of 23 to 100 months: the blood *o,p'*DDD levels in these cases ranged from 15 to more than 25 μg/ml. No therapeutic response was observed in patients whose blood levels were 10 μg/ml or less. Reversible neuromuscular toxicity was associated with drug concentrations over 20 μg/ml. The authors conclude that monitoring the blood levels of *o,p'*DDD is mandatory for safe and effective treatment.

Hogan et al. (50) have followed blood levels of *o,p'*DDD in several patients noting that measurable drug levels remain in the circulation for up to 8 months after cessation of therapy. Urinary metabolites are still detectable 18 months after discontinuing the drug.

Toxic effects. Eighty percent of patients experience gastrointestinal disturbances such as anorexia, nausea, vomiting and occasional diarrhea. Forty percent of patients exhibit CNS toxicity with lethargy, drowsiness, vertigo or dizziness. Long term use may cause brain damage and repeated neurological behavioral assessments are recommended when treatment is prolonged. Acute adrenal insufficiency can be precipitated by stress. Leukopenia, liver function abnormalities and allergic rashes are frequent. Visual disturbances (blurring, double vision, opacification of the lens, toxic retinopathy), genitourinary (hemorrhagic cystitis, albuminuria, hematuria) and cardiovascular (hypertension, orthostatic hypotension) toxicity have also been observed (50).

Other Agents

Streptozotocin, an alkylating agent, is known to concentrate in the rodent adrenal cortex (53). By combining *o,p'*DDD and streptozotocin, the doses required of each can be reduced and thereby their individual toxicities limited. The toxicity of streptozotocin includes vomiting, renal dysfunction and, less frequently, liver dysfunction. Recommended doses of streptozotocin are 0.5–1.0 g/m^2 body surface intravenously given as a bolus injection every third week, starting with induction therapy of 0.5 mg/m^2 daily intravenously for 5 days. Concomitantly, *o,p'*DDD is started at a dose of 2 g/day, gradually increasing to 4 or 6 g per day.

In a preliminary study we have treated, prior to surgery, 3 patients with adrenocortical carcinomas with a combination of streptozoto-

cin and *o,p'*DDD (54). Two of the 3 patients with Cushing's syndrome showed objective responses with a complete remission in one. At operation after 19 months' therapy, no viable tumor tissue was found. This patient has now been followed for 6 years without evidence of recurrence. CT images before the start of cytotoxic treatment and just before operation and the MRT images for the second patient are illustrated in Figures 12 and 13. The second patient had the remaining tumor tissue surgically removed; 15 months later, there was no evidence of recurrence. The third patient with a non-functioning carcinoma did not respond to this form of cytotoxic treatment.

The number of patients studied so far is small and further investigation of this potentially more promising therapeutic approach is warranted.

The use of conventional cytotoxic chemotherapy has been reported in an anecdotal fashion. The available results are summarized in Table 6.

Adjuvant Therapy

Evidence for the efficacy of post-resection adjuvant therapy for adrenocortical carcinomas has been reported by Schteingardt et al. (58). Twenty-three patients were studied from 1953 to 1981. Six patients had resection of primary disease and/or local irradiation and no adjuvant therapy was administered: the mean survival ($\pm$ SD) in this group was 10.3 ± 8.7 months. Seventeen patients who underwent curative resection received adjuvant *o'p*-DDD, with a mean survival of 46.6 ± 42.7 months. Patients received *o'p*-DDD at maximal doses ranging from 6 g to 12 g daily; the mean duration of therapy was 28 months (range 4 to 96 months). Patients receiving adjuvant therapy exhibited the longest disease-free interval and survival post-resection of recurrent disease (74 ± 33 months). Confirmation of these adjuvant effects of *o'p*-DDD in a randomized prospective trial is required before it can be accepted as a routine procedure.

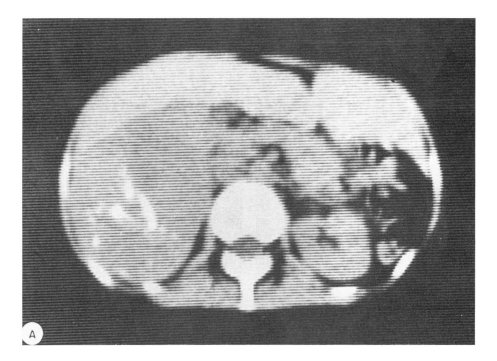

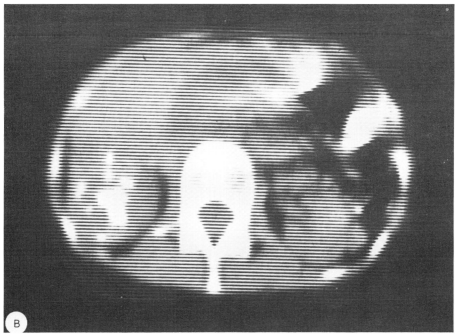

Figure 12 The CT images before (A) and after 18 months' therapy (B). Note the significant decrease in the size of the adrenal tumor.

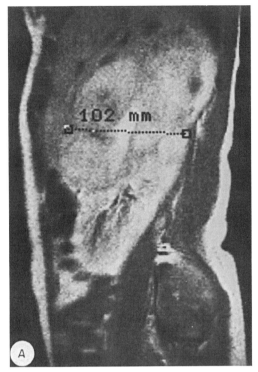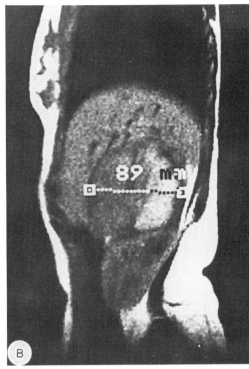

Figure 13 The MRT(NMR) changes in patient no. 2 before (A) and after 5 months' therapy (B). Note the reduction in tumor size.

TABLE 6 RESULTS OF CYTOTOXIC DRUG
THERAPY FOR PATIENTS WITH
ADRENOCORTICAL CARCINOMAS

Authors	Cytotoxic regimen	Reported results
Tattersall et al (55)	DDP[a]	4/4 partial responses; survival for 12 months
Chun et al (56)	DDP	1 minor response/12; survival >12 months in patients with metastases independent of response
Van Slooten et al (57)	CAP[b]	3/11 partial responses; responders survived 12, 18 and 23 months

[a] DDP: cis-platinum
[b] CAP: cyclophosphamide, Adriamycin and cis-platinum.

Radiation Therapy

Radiation therapy has shown little benefit although, in a small number of patients, objective responses have been reported. In general, radiotherapy should be reserved for the palliation of bone pain (8, 59).

Antihormonal Agents

In progressive disease associated with active hormonal excess, drugs blocking steroid synthesis may be used to ameliorate such signs and symptoms.

Metyrapone. An inhibitor of cortisol biosynthesis, acting primarily at the final 11β-hydroxylase step, this drug has been shown to lower plasma cortisol to normal in both short and long term use (60). The oral dose must be adjusted on an individual basis (between 0.75 and 4 g/day). The drug is generally well tolerated, gastric side effects being avoided if taken with food. In females, worsening of hirsutism may occur. The drug may be used preoperatively to reduce the raised steroid levels, thereby diminishing complications from surgery, such as thrombosis and infection.

Aminoglutethimide. This drug, 1 g/day orally in four divided doses with corticosteroid substitution, may also be of value. It primarily inhibits the enzymatic conversion of cholesterol to pregnenolone. The measurement of urinary 17-hydroxycorticosteroid excretion may overestimate its effectiveness because extra-adrenal cortisol metabolism is also altered. Therefore, plasma cortisol concentrations are the best way to assess this medication. Toxicities (61) include skin rashes, somnolence, anorexia, ataxia, thyroid hypofunction and, rarely, thrombocytopenia which can be severe.

ADRENAL MEDULLARY TUMORS

Pheochromocytoma

Pheochromocytomas are tumors of neuroectodermal origin arising from chromaffin tissues which are widespread in their association with sympathetic ganglia during fetal life. Postnatally, most chromaffin tissue degenerates with the predominant exception of the adrenal medulla (4). Pheochromocytomas occur most frequently between the ages of 20 and 50 years although no age is exempt. Congenital lesions have been recorded and, in children, the peak age incidence is between 9 and 14 years of age (62). The incidence in adults shows no sex difference. In children, males are affected more often.

The majority (90%) of pheochromocytomas are adrenal in origin with the right gland being more often involved. The remainder of pheochromocytomas are extra-adrenal and are found in association with the organs of Zuckerkandl and paravertebral sympathetic ganglia although tumors involving the bladder, thorax, neck and brain have also been recorded (4).

Almost all pheochromocytomas are benign; occasionally (up to 20%) multiple benign pheochromocytomas are encountered (e.g. one

in an adrenal gland and another in the organ of Zuckerkandl, etc). Such lesions must not be confused with malignancy. However extra-adrenal pheochromocytomas are more likely to be malignant (63).

Bilateral adrenal pheochromocytomas are the rule in the familial disorder associated with the multiple endocrine neoplasia type 2 (MEN-2) syndromes (64). These familial disorders are inherited as autosomal dominant traits. MEN-2a (Sipple's syndrome) includes medullary thyroid carcinoma, primary hyperparathyroidism and pheochromocytoma, whereas MEN-2b, includes medullary thyroid carcinoma, multiple mucosal neuromas and pheochromocytoma (65). Familial pheochromocytomas also occur with neurofibromatosis (less than 1%) and in the von Hippel–Lindau syndrome affecting up to 25% of some kindreds (66).

Clinical Presentation

The clinical manifestations of pheochromocytomas are due to the effects of the released catecholamines, and seldom due to the tumor mass per se. Common signs and symptoms include headache, palpitation and anxiety, with weakness, visual disturbances, abdominal and chest pain with gastrointestinal upsets such as diarrhea being less frequent. All symptoms are typically paroxysmal, lasting for minutes to hours. In many cases, the hypertension is sustained but exhibits marked fluctuations with peak blood pressures occurring during symptomatic episodes. Rarely, hypotension may be the presenting sign (66, 67).

There should be a high degree of clinical suspicion of pheochromocytoma in patients with accelerated hypertension, unusual blood pressure lability, paroxysmal tachyarrhythmias, hypermetabolism, abnormal carbohydrate metabolism and, finally, abnormal pressure responses to the induction of anesthesia or to antihypertensive drugs (68). Pheochromocytomas have also been reported during pregnancy (4).

However, despite clinical awareness, a significant number of pheochromocytomas are still detected as incidental findings at autopsy or as a result of cardiovascular collapse at the time of an unrelated operation (69).

The majority of pheochromocytomas release noradrenaline and/or adrenaline. The release of the latter in increased amounts is almost always the prerogative of an adrenal gland-sited lesion as oppose to extra-adrenal tumors (4, 66). Pheochromocytomas often contain a variety of peptides, including chromogranin A (69, 70), neuropeptide Y (71), the enkephalins (72), vasoactive intestinal polypeptide (VIP) (73), gastrin-releasing peptide (74), somatostatin (75), growth hormone-releasing factor (76), calcitonin (77), oxytocin (78), vasopression (ADH) (78) and ACTH (79, 80). The clinical relevance of many of these peptides remains to be elucidated. Neuropeptide Y may be involved in the regulation of myocardial perfusion (81). The presence of high circulating levels of neuropeptide Y may, therefore, contribute in part to the cardiovascular features of pheochromocytoma. Raised plasma levels of vasoactive intestinal polypeptide (VIP) are mainly found in extra-adrenal chromaffin tumors and may be responsible for the diarrhea and hypokalemia in these patients (73). Chromogranin A is the major soluble protein stored in the vesicles of the adrenal medulla and sympathetic nerves and secreted along with catecholamines (69). Elevated plasma levels can be found in patients with pheochromocytoma. The release of ACTH may result in Cushing's syndrome.

Pathology

The precise size and weight of a pheochromocytoma is determined by its functional activity. The more hormonally active lesions tend to be found earlier and are, therefore, smaller. While weights of 1.4 g have been noted, most tumors weigh around 100 g. Lesions of 3.5 kg have been recorded. Their size varies from being a small nodule to 14 cm in diameter (4).

Most tumors are encapsulated although small intra-adrenal lesions will result in com-

pression of the surrounding cortex to give a pseudocapsule. Their cut surface is pearly grey or light brown with areas of hemorrhage, necrosis, myxomatous change and cysts in larger lesions.

Microscopically, two dominant morphological patterns, the large or small alveolar types, are found, both frequently occurring in different parts of a single tumor. Both patterns consist of mature pheochromocytes. In the large alveolar type, the tumor cells are arranged in large trabeculae and sheets punctuated by thin-walled vascular sinusoids (Figure 14). In the small alveolar type, the tumor cells form small groups and cords separated by prominent fibrovascular septa (Figure 15). The cellular cytoplasm is granular, basophilic and sometimes vacuolated. While the single nuclei are generally round and vesicular, nuclear and cellular pleomorphism may be marked. Giant and bizarre forms may be seen; these features are *not* equatable with malignancy (4).

It is imperative, in all suspected lesions, to verify the diagnosis of pheochromocytoma by histochemical and/or immunocytochemical techniques. Formerly, the chromaffin reaction was valuable. However, with the demonstration of their specific localization in pheochromocytes, the delineation of neurofilaments (82), neurone-specific enolase (NSE) (83) and/or the peptides discussed previously is a better and more meaningful approach, giving valuable functional data. The presence or absence of these properties, however, does not appear to help with the histological diagnosis of malignancy.

As with other endocrine tumors, a definitive diagnosis of *malignancy* cannot be given by morphological criteria alone. Benign pheochromocytomas can display more pleomorphism and more frequent mitoses than malignant lesions. Minimal capsular invasion and tumor cells in blood vessels are features of benign lesions. A recent review (84) has suggested that malignant lesions tend to be larger, have extensive areas of necrosis and are composed of small cells. However, such features are

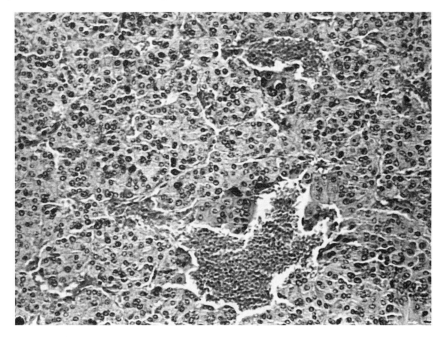

Figure 14 Benign pheochromocytoma. The large alveolar pattern is illustrated with the tumor cells forming solid trabeculae and sheets punctuated by thin-walled vascular sinusoids (H&E, original magnification: ×200).

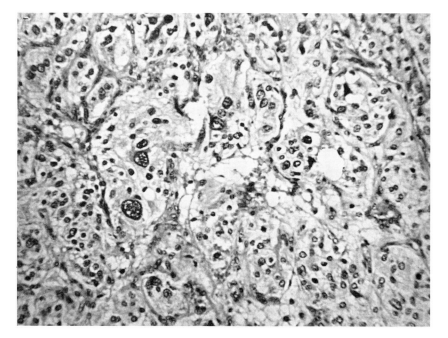

Figure 15 Benign pheochromocytoma. The small alveolar pattern is shown with the tumor cells arranged in small groups separated by prominent fibrovascular trabeculae. Note the marked nuclear and cellular pleomorphism of this benign lesion (H&E, original magnification: ×200).

not absolute criteria for the diagnosis of malignancy.

In view of the lack of accepted criteria of malignancy, it is not surprising that there are such conflicting reports regarding its incidence. Morphological criteria have suggested that 10% of all pheochromocytomas are malignant (85). If the proven ability to metastasize is considered as the sole criterion, only 1% of all pheochromocytomas were found to be malignant (4).

Assistance in reaching a diagnosis of malignancy may be attained from functional studies of the tumor itself or the products in the urine. Most malignant pheochromocytomas produce catecholamines; the metastases may be functionally active or inactive. The tumor content of dopa and/or dopamine and their presence, together with their metabolites, in increased amounts in the urine may be indicative of malignancy (86, 87). Similar phenomena with respect to the production and secretion of precursor steroids were noted for malignant adrenocortical lesions. The commonest sites of metastases are the regional lymph nodes, liver, lung and bones. It is important to distinguish malignancy and metastases from multiple pheochromocytomas. Metastases occur at sites where chromaffin tissue is not normally found (88).

Prognosis

Survival following removal of a malignant pheochromocytoma is variable and depends on the degree of spread noted at operation and the success of any debulking procedure. Generally, recurrences are apparent within 1 year and survival beyond 3 years is exceptional (88).

Diagnostic Investigative Tests and Staging

Biochemical Studies

Measurement of catecholamines, total meta-

nephrines and vanillylmandelic acid (VMA) in 24-hour urine collections are the traditional methods of proven value for the biochemical diagnosis of pheochromocytoma (66, 86, 89). Urinary measurements provide an index of catecholamine production and release integrated over time. Plasma catecholamine determinations have been introduced recently and may be superior because of the lesser overlap in discriminating between pheochromocytoma and essential hypertension (89). However, patients with pheochromocytoma and the intermittent secretion of catecholamines can be missed. It is important to remember that normal plasma and urine catecholamine levels, which may occur when a patient is normotensive and free of symptoms, do not exclude pheochromocytoma.

The current clinical practice of measuring the 24-hour urinary catecholamines and VMA as well as plasma noradrenaline and adrenaline is recommended. Raised adrenaline levels are usually associated with an adrenal gland-sited pheochromocytoma although their being normal does not exclude an adrenal location (66). Physical and mental stress, even venepuncture, increase plasma catecholamine levels. Upright posture doubles plasma catecholamine concentrations. The patient should be at rest in a horizontal position for at least 30 minutes prior to any test, e.g. after insertion of an indwelling intravenous needle. If possible, samples should be obtained when the patient is not receiving antihypertensive therapy (66, 89).

A clonidine suppression test has been suggested to assist in differentiating essential hypertension with elevated basal plasma noradrenaline levels from hypertension due to a pheochromocytoma (90). The utility of this test awaits further experience. False negative tests have been reported (91).

Determination of plasma levels of neuropeptide Y, NSE and chromogranin A may be further adjuncts assisting with the diagnosis of pheochromocytoma. These moieties are relatively stable and may be useful markers for this disease (69–71, 80).

Radiographic Tests

Once biochemical confirmation of the clinical diagnosis is reached, CT or MRT is recommended to localize a pheochromocytoma as these methods detect the vast majority of adrenal pheochromocytomas and have largely superseded angiography (92). External scanning, after injection of [131]-I-m-iodobenzylguanidine (MIBG), which is concentrated in catecholamine-storing tissues, is the procedure of most value in locating extra-adrenal pheochromocytomas (93, 94). Metastases can also be detected by this method.

Staging Procedures

Staging is required to search for metastases as well as to assess the functional integrity of other organ systems. Consequently it consists of:

(a) an assessment of hypertension, cardiovascular and renal function;
(b) localization of the neoplastic lesion(s); and
(c) a search for extra-adrenal sites of involvement.

The following localizing procedures are used:

(a) CT scan or MRT;
(b) ^{131}I-MIBG scan; and
(c) a bone scan, if there is suspicious symptomatology.

Postoperative Follow-up

All patients should be clinically assessed every 3 months during the first postoperative year. Patients with malignant or suspected malignant lesions require continued surveillance including frequent biochemical analytical studies.

Treatment of Pheochromocytomas

Surgery is the treatment of choice and is curative for all benign lesions. It should only be performed after adequate preoperative and intraoperative precautions (88). Treatment of the associated hypertension is mandatory before commencing surgery.

The treatment of associated hypertension in patients with pheochromocytoma should primarily include alpha-adrenergic antagonists. The long-acting, orally effective, antagonist phenoxybenzamine (Dibenzyline) is often used. Starting with 10 mg twice daily, the dose is increased until the blood pressure is controlled. Doses of 60 mg or more might be required. Side effects include postural hypotension and, occasionally, cardiac arrythmias. Another relatively selective alpha-adrenergic antagonist, prazosin, has also been used. An initial dose of 0.5 mg twice daily is recommended.

Beta-adrenergic antagonists, such as propranolol, are generally not administered unless tachycardia or arrhythmias have become a problem. It should be emphasized that beta-blockade should not be given prior to effective alpha-blockade. A starting dose of propranolol might be 20 mg three times a day. In patients with moderate hypertension, labetalol, a combined beta-receptor and weak alpha-receptor blocker might be used, starting with 100 mg twice daily. This drug may not provoke such severe postural hypotension as phenoxybenzamine, but it is not as potent in controlling severe hypertension. Immediately after removal of the tumor mass, the withdrawal of catecholamines will result in a loss of vascular tone which may be associated with hypotension. This will be totally avoided by adequate preoperative preparation.

Although the blood pressure returns to normal following removal of pheochromocytoma, some degree of hypertension can persist during the first postoperative week. This does not preclude cure. Thus, it is better to assess the patient clinically and biochemically one month after surgery. However, 10–30% of patients with sustained hypertension prior to surgery may remain hypertensive. Persistent hypertension can also be the result of a further clinically missed pheochromocytoma, renal ischemia, concomitant renal artery stenosis or essential hypertension (66, 88).

Anti-neoplastic Treatment

Surgery and radiation may be used to palliate metastatic disease and have been recorded as being successful in dealing with isolated, single metastases. Cytotoxic drugs such as thiotepa or cyclophosphamide alone (95, 96) and the combination of cyclophosphamide and Adriamycin (97) have been reported in anecdotal fashion. The results have been poor. Single agent chemotherapy with vincristine (98), Adriamycin (98), methotrexate (99) or streptozotocin (97) is stated to be ineffective.

Radiopharmacological treatment with ^{131}I-MIBG two to four doses of 8–11 Ci/mol at 3 to 10 months intervals has been reported to elicit minor responses (about a 30% reduction in volume) in 5 treated patients (100).

The outcome and prognosis, therefore, at this time is dismal. The assay of dopa, dopamine and their metabolites in the urine together with plasma levels of neuropeptide Y, NSE and chromogranin A can help to monitor therapeutic efficacy.

OTHER ANOMALIES

While this chapter has concentrated upon malignant functioning tumors of the adrenal gland, it is important to realize that other tumors, benign and malignant, but not unique to the adrenal gland, may be detected from time to time, the more so since the introduction of CT scanning.

The commonest lesion will be the so-called 'non-functioning' nodule so common with advancing age and particularly prone to be found in hypertensive populations. The etiology and genesis of such lesions has been discussed in detail previously (2).

Other lesions include myelolipoma, cysts, pseudocysts, tuberculosis, histoplasmosis and amyloid of the adrenal and neonatal hemorrhage (1). Clinical acumen and histological examination serve to identify such conditions.

Neoplasms of the adrenal stroma will occur from time to time arising from connective, vascular or adipose tissues. Their therapy is the same as when they occur at more common sites.

The adrenal is a common site for metastastic carcinoma, particularly of bronchial and mammary origin. Not infrequently, such metastases will be bilateral and involve adrenal nodules. Bilateral adrenal enlargement will also occur in the 'ectopic ACTH' syndrome and MEN-1.

CONCLUSIONS

Adrenocortical and medullary tumors are uncommon lesions. The majority are benign, cured by surgical extirpation.

If overt metastases are not detected, the histological diagnosis of malignancy is difficult. Functional biochemical parameters are more helpful than light or electron microscopy and also provide useful therapy monitoring indices.

Too few malignancies have been seen at any one center to enable useful therapeutic recommendations to be given at this juncture. A multicenter international study group may be one of the best ways to proceed to overcome this problem and derive therapeutic regimens of some value for patients in the future.

REFERENCES

1 Geelhoed GW, Druy EM. Management of the adrenal 'incidentaloma'. Surgery 1982; 92: 866–74.
2 Neville AM, O'Hare MJ. The Human Adrenal Cortex. Berlin: Springer-Verlag, 1982.
3 Kvale WF, Roth GM, Manger WM, Priestley JT. Pheochromocytoma. Circulation 1956; 14: 622–30.
4 Neville AM. The Adrenal Medulla. In: Symington T ed The Functional Pathology of the Human Adrenal Gland. Edinburgh: E&S Livingstone, 1969: 243–71.
5 Ferber B, Hardy VH, Gerhardt PR, Solomon M. Cancer in New York State, exclusive of New York City. Bureau of Cancer Control, New York State, Department of Health. Albany, 1962.

6 Griswold MH, Wilder CS, Cutler SJ, Pollak ES. Cancer in Connecticut 1935–1951. Connecticut State Department of Health. Hartford, 1955.

7 Clemmesen J. Danish Cancer Registry under the National Anti-Cancer League. Copenhagen, 1965.

8 Lewinsky BS, Grigor K, Symington T, Neville AM. The clinical and pathological features of 'non-hormonal' adrenocortical tumors. Cancer 1974; 33: 778–90.

9 Rees LH, Besser GM, Jeffcoate WJ, Goldie DJ, Marks V. Alcohol-induced pseudo-Cushing's syndrome. Lancet 1977; i: 726–8.

10 Neville AM, Symington T. The pathology of the adrenal gland in Cushing's syndrome. J Pathol Bacteriol 1967; 93: 19–35.

11 Hussain S, Belldegrun A, Seltzer SE, Richie JP, Gittes RF, Abrams HL. Differentiation of malignant from benign adrenal masses: predictive indices on computed tomography. Am J Radiol 1985; 144: 61–5.

12 Välimäki M, Pelkonen R, Porkka L, Sivula A, Kahri A. Long term results of adrenal surgery in patients with Cushing's syndrome due to adrenocortical adenoma. Clin Endocrinol 1984; 20: 229–36.

13 Welbourne R. Barber's company symposium on endocrine surgery: current concepts. Some aspects of adrenal surgery. Br J Surg 1980; 67: 723–7.

14 Margulies PL, Imperato-McGinley J, Arthur A, Peterson RE. Remission of Cushing's syndrome during pregnancy. Int J Gynaecol Obstet 1983; 21: 77–83.

15 Scott HW Jr, Naji N, Abumrad MD, Orth DN. Tumors of the adrenal cortex and Cushing's syndrome. Ann Surg 1985; 201: 586–94.

16 McKenna TJ, Cunningham SK, Loughlin T. The adrenal cortex and virilization. Clin Endocrinol Metab 1985; 14: 997–1020.

17 Symington T. Functional Pathology of the Human Adrenal Gland. Edinburgh: E&S Livingstone 1969: 94–8.

18 De Asis DN, Samaan NA. Feminizing adrenocortical carcinoma with Cushing's syndrome and pseudohyperparathyroidism. Arch Intern Med 1978; 138: 301–3.

19 Halmi KA, Lascari AD. Conversion of virilization to feminization in a young girl with adrenal cortical carcinoma. Cancer 1971; 27: 931–5.

20 O'Hare MJ, Monaghan P, Neville AM. The pathology of adrenocortical neoplasia: a correlated structural and functional approach to the diagnosis of malignant disease. Hum Pathol 1979; 10: 137–54.

21 Miettinen M, Lehto VP, Virtanen I. Immunofluorescence microscopic evaluation of the intermediate filament expression of the adrenal cortex and medulla and their tumors. Am J Pathol 1985; 118: 360–6.

22 Klein FA, Kay S, Ratliff JE, White FKH, Newsome HH. Flow cytometric determinations of ploidy and proliferation patterns of adrenal neoplasms: an adjunct to histological classifications. J Urol 1985; 134: 862–6.

23 Conn JW. Presidential address. Part I: Painting the background. Part II: Primary aldosteronism: A new clinical syndrome. J Clin Lab Med 1955; 45: 3–6.

24 Bravo EL, Tarazi RC, Dustan HP et al. The changing clinical spectrum of primary aldosteronism. Am J Med 1983; 74: 641–51.

25 Brown JJ, Frazer R, Lever AF, Robertson JIS. Aldosterone: physiological and pathophysiological variations in man. Clin Endocrinol Metab 1972; 1: 397–449.

26 Neville AM, Symington T. Pathology of primary aldosteronism. Cancer 1966; 12: 1854–68.

27 Howlett TA, Rees LH, Besser GM. Cushing's syndrome. Clin Endocrinol Metab 1985; 14: 911–45.

28 Crapo L. Cushing's syndrome. A review of diagnostic tests. Metabolism 1979; 28: 955–77.

29 Ross EJ, Linch DC. Cushing's syndrome—killing disease. Discriminatory value of signs and symptoms aiding early diagnosis. Lancet 1982; ii: 646–9.

30 Müller OA, Stalla GK, von Werder KV. Corticotropin releasing factor: a new tool for the differential diagnosis of Cushing's syndrome. J Clin Endocrinol Metab 1983; 57: 227–9.

31 Chrousos GP, Nieman L, Nisula B et al. Corticotropin-releasing factor stimulation test. N Engl J Med 1984; 311: 471–3.

32 Vermeulen A. Androgen secretion by the adrenals and gonads. In: Makesh UK, Greenblatt RB eds Hirsutism and Virilism: Pathogenesis, Diagnosis and Management. Bristol: John Wright, 1983: 17–34.

33 Burr IM, Sullivan J, Graham T, Hartman WH, O'Neill J. A testosterone secreting tumour of the adrenal producing virilisation in a female infant. Lancet 1973; ii: 642–4.

34 Gabrilove JL, Sharma DC, Wotiz HH, Dorfman RI. Feminizing adrenocortical tumors in the male. Medicine 1965; 44: 37–79.

35 Boyar RM, Hellman L. Syndrome of benign nodular adrenal hyperplasia associated with feminization and hyperprolactinemia. Arch Intern Med 1974; 80: 389–94.

36 Melby JC. Primary aldosteronism (clinical conference). Kidney International 1984; 26: 769–78.

37 Luderer JR, Demers LM, Harrison TS, Hayes AH Jr. Converting enzyme inhibition with captopril in patients with primary hyperaldosteronism. Clin Pharmacol Ther 1982; 31: 305–11.

38 Drafta D, Franchi F, Luisi M, Stroe E. Urinary, plasma and adrenal tissue steroids in a male patient with Cushing's syndrome due to adrenal carcinoma. Endocrinology 1978; 16: 41–9.

39 Watanobe H, Kamari K, Kimura K, Takebe K. Adrenocortical carcinoma with Cushing's syndrome presenting unusual urinary 17-ketosteroid fractionation. J Endocrinol Invest 1985; 8: 249–52.

40 Minowada S, Kinoshita K, Hara M, Isurugi K, Uchikawa T, Niijima T. Measurement of urinary steroid profile in patients with adrenal tumor as a screening method for carcinoma. Endocrinol Japan 1985; 32: 29–37.

41 Malmaeus J, Lauri A, Oberg K et al. Adrenal gland surgery. Preoperative location of lesions, histologic findings and outcome of surgery. Acta Chir Scand 1986; 152: 577–81.

42 Mitty HA, Cohen BA. Adrenal imaging. Urol Clin North Am 1985; 12: 771–85.

43 Thrall JH, Freitas JE, Beierwaltes WH. Adrenal scintigraphy. Semin Nucl Med 1978; 8: 23–41.

44 Moon KL Jr, Hricak H, Crooks LE et al. Work in progress: nuclear magnetic resonance imaging of the gall bladder. Radiology 1983; 147: 481–4.

45 Brennan MF, McDonald JS. Cancer of the endocrine system. In: DeVita VT, Hellman S, Rosenberg SA, eds. Principles and Practice of Oncology. Philadelphia: Lippincott, 1985; 1179–241.

46 Kaminsky N, Luse S, Hartroft P. Ultrastructure of adrenal cortex of the dog during treatment with DDD. J Nat Cancer Inst 1962; 29: 127–31.

47 Hutter AM, Kayhoe DE. Adrenal cortical carcinoma. Am J Med 1966; 41: 581–92.

48 Lubitz JA, Freeman L, Okun R. Mitotane used in inoperable adrenal cortical carcinoma. JAMA 1973; 223: 1109–12.

49 Van Slooten H, Moolenaar AJ, Van Seters AP, Smeenk D. The treatment of adrenocortical carcinoma with o,p-DDD: prognostic implications of serum level monitoring. Eur J Cancer Clin Oncol 1984; 20: 47–53.

50 Hogan TF, Citrin DL, Johnson BM, Nakamura S, Davis TE, Borden EC. o,p'-DDD

(mitotane) therapy of adrenal cortical carcinoma. Cancer 1978; 42: 2177–81.

51 Koide Y, Inoue S, Murayama H, Kawai K, Yamashita K. Effect of o,p'-DDD on cortisol metabolism in Cushing's syndrome of various etiology. Endocrinol Japan 1985; 32: 615–24.

52 Van Slooten H, Schaberg A, Smeenk D, Moolenaar AJ. Morphologic characteristics of benign and malignant adrenocortical tumors. Cancer 1985; 55: 766–73.

53 Tjälve H, Wilander E, Johansson EB. Distribution of labelled streptozotocin in mice: uptake and retention in pancreatic islets. J Endocrinol 1976; 69: 455–6.

54 Eriksson B, Oberg K, Curstedt T et al. Treatment of hormone-producing adrenocortical cancer with o,p'DDD and streptozocin. Cancer 1987; 59: 1398–1403.

55 Tattersall MHN, Lander H, Bains B. Cisplatinum treatment of metastatic adrenal carcinoma. Med J Aust 1980; 1: 419–21.

56 Chun HG, Yagoda A, Kemeny N, Watson RC. Cisplatin for adrenal cortical carcinoma. Cancer Treat Rep 1983; 67: 513–14.

57 Van Slooten H, van Oosterom AT. CAP (cyclophosphamide, doxorubicin and cisplatin) regimen in adrenal cortical carcinoma. Cancer Treat Rep 1983; 67: 377–9.

58 Schteingardt DB, Motazedi A, Noonan RA, Thompson NW. Treatment of adrenal carcinomas. Arch Surg 1982; 117: 1142–6.

59 Percarpio B, Knowlton AH. Radiation therapy of adrenal cortical carcinoma. Acta Radiol Ther Phys 1976; 15: 288–92.

60 Jeffcoate WJ, Rees LH, Tomlin S, Jones AE, Edwards CRW, Besser GM. Metyrapone in long-term management of Cushing's disease. Br Med J 1977; ii: 215–17.

61 Powles TJ, Ford HT, Nash AG et al. Treatment of disseminated breast cancer with tamoxifen, aminoglutethimide, hydrocortisone, and danazol, used in combination or sequentially. Lancet 1984; ii: 1369–73.

62 Hume DM. Pheochromocytoma in the adult and in the child. Am J Surg 1960; 99: 458–96.

63 Altergott R, Barbato A, Lawrence A, Paloyan E, Freeark RJ, Prinz RA. Spectrum of catecholamine-secreting tumors of the organ of Zuckerkandl. Surgery 1985; 98: 1121–6.

64 Lips KSM, Veer JVDS, Struyvenberg A et al. Bilateral occurrence of pheochromocytoma in patients with the multiple endocrine neoplasia syndrome type 2A (Sipple's syndrome). Am J Med 1981; 70: 1051–60.

65 Carney JA, Go VLW, Sizemore GW, Hayles AB. Alimentary-tract ganglioneuromatosis. A major component of the syndrome of multiple

endocrine neoplasia, type 2B. N Engl J Med 1976; 295: 1287–91.

66 Cryer PE. Phaeochromocytoma. Clin Endocrinol Metab 1985; 14: 203–20.

67 Melicow MM. One hundred cases of pheochromocytoma (107 tumors) at the Columbia-Presbyterian medical center, 1926–1976. A clinicopathological analysis. Cancer 1977; 40: 1987–2004.

68 Manger WM, Gifford RW Jr. Hypertension secondary to pheochromocytoma. Bull New York Acad Med 1982; 58: 139–58.

69 St John Sutton MG, Sheps SG, Lie JT. Prevalence of clinically unsuspected pheochromocytoma. Mayo Clin Proc 1981; 56: 354–60.

70 Wilson BS, Lloyd RV. Detection of chromogranin in neuroendocrine cells with a monoclonal antibody. Am J Pathol 1984; 115: 458–68.

71 Adrian TE, Terenghi G, Brown MJ et al. Neuropeptide Y in phaeochromocytomas and ganglioneuroblastomas. Lancet 1983; ii: 540–2.

72 Yoshimasa T, Nakao K, Li S et al. Plasma methionine-enkephalin and leucine-enkephalin in normal subjects and patients with pheochromocytoma. J Clin Endocrinol Metab 1983; 57: 706–12.

73 Long RG, Bryant MG, Mitchell SJ, Adrian TE, Polak JM, Bloom SR. Clinicopathological study of pancreatic and ganglioneuroblastoma tumours secreting vasoactive intestinal polypeptide (vipomas). Br Med J 1981; 282: 1767–71.

74 Bostwick DG, Bensch KG. Gastrin releasing peptide in human neuroendocrine tumours. J Pathol 1985; 147: 237–44.

75 Berelowitz M, Szabo M, Barowsky HW, Arbel ER, Frohman LA. Somatostatin-like immunoactivity and biological activity is present in a human pheochromocytoma. J Clin Endocrinol Metab 1983; 56: 134–8.

76 Sano T, Saito H, Yamasaki R et al. Production and secretion of immunoreactive growth hormone-releasing factor by pheochromocytoma. Cancer 1986; 57: 1788–93.

77 Weinstein RS, Ide LF. Immunoreactive calcitonin in pheochromocytomas. Proc Soc Exp Biol Med 1980; 165: 215–17.

78 Ang VTY, Jenkins JS. Neurohypophyseal hormones in the adrenal medulla. J Clin Endocrinol Metab 1984; 58: 688–91.

79 Spark RF, Connolly PB, Gluckin DS, White R, Sacks B, Landsberg L. ACTH secretion from a functioning pheochromocytoma. N Engl J Med 1979; 301: 416–18.

80 Hassoun J, Monges G, Henry JF et al. Immu-
nohistochemical study of pheochromocytomas. An investigation of methionine-enkephalin, vasoactive intestinal peptide, somatostatin, corticotropin, beta-endorphin, and calcitonin in 16 tumors. Am J Pathol 1984; 114: 56–63.

81 Allen JM, Bircham PM, Edwards AV, Tatemoto K, Bloom SR. Neuropeptide Y (NPY) reduces myocardial perfusion and inhibits the force of contraction of the isolated perfused rabbit heart. Reg Pept 1983; 6: 247–53.

82 Lehto VP, Virtanen I, Miettinen M, Dahl D, Kahri A. Neurofilaments in adrenal and extra-adrenal pheochromocytoma. Demonstration using immunofluorescence microscopy. Arch Pathol Lab Med 1983; 107: 492–4.

83 Lloyd RV, Shapiro B, Sisson JC, Kalff V, Thompson NW, Beierwaltes WA. An immunohistochemical study of pheochromocytomas. Arch Pathol Lab Med 1984; 108: 541–4.

84 Medeiros LJ, Wolf BC, Balogh K, Federman M. Adrenal pheochromocytoma: a clinicopathologic review of 60 cases. Hum Pathol 1986; 16: 580–9.

85 Remine WH, Chonge GC, Van Heerden JA, Sheps SG, Harrison EG. Current management of pheochromocytoma. Ann Surg 1974; 179: 740–8.

86 Sjoerdsma A, Engelman K, Waldmann TA, Cooperman LH, Hammond WG. Pheochromocytoma. Current concepts of diagnosis and treatment. Ann Intern Med 1966; 65: 1302–26.

87 Anton AH, Greer M, Sayre DF, Williams CM. Dihydroxyphenylalanine secretion in a malignant pheochromocytoma. Am J Med 1976; 42: 469–75.

88 Van Heerden JA, Sheps SG, Hamberger B, Sheedy PF, Poston JG, ReMine WH. Pheochromocytoma: Current status and changing trends. Surgery 1982; 91: 367–73.

89 Bravo EL, Tarazi RC, Gifford RW Jr, Stewart BH. Circulating and urinary catecholamines in pheochromocytoma. Diagnostic and pathophysiologic implications. N Engl J Med 1979; 301: 682–6.

90 Bravo EL, Tarazi RC, Fouad FM, Vidt DG, Gifford RW. Clonidine-suppression test. A useful aid in the diagnosis of pheochromocytoma. N Engl J Med 1981; 305: 623–6.

91 Halter JB, Beard JC, Pfeifer MA, Metz SA. Clonidine-suppression test for diagnosis of pheochromocytoma. N Engl J Med 1982; 306: 49–50.

92 Welch TJ, Sheedy PF, van Heerden JA, Sheps SG, Hattery RR, Stephens DH. Pheochromocytoma: value of computed tomography. Radiology 1983; 148: 501–3.

93 Sisson JC, Frager MS, Valk TW et al. Scinti-

graphic localization of pheochromocytoma. N Engl J Med 1981; 305: 12–17.

94 Francis IR, Glazer GM, Shapiro B, Sisson JC, Gross BH. Complementary roles of CT and ^{131}I-MIBG scintigraphy in diagnosing pheochromocytoma. AJR 1983; 141: 719–25.

95 Moloney GE, Lowdell RH, Lewis CL. Malignant phaeochromocytoma of the bladder. Br J Urol 1966; 38: 461–70.

96 Joseph L. Malignant phaeochromocytoma of the organ of Zuckerkandl with functioning metastases. Br J Urol 1967; 39: 221–5.

97 Hamilton BPM, Cheik ML, Rivera LE.

Attempted treatment of inoperable pheochromocytoma with streptozocin. Arch Intern Med 1977; 137: 762–5.

98 Phillips AF, McMurty RJ, Taubman J. Malignant pheochromocytoma in childhood. Am J Dis Child 1976; 130: 1252–5.

99 Schart Y, Ben Arieh Y, Gellei B. Orbital metastases from extra-adrenal pheochromocytoma. Am J Ophthalmol 1970; 69: 638–40.

100 Sisson JC, Shapiro B, Bierwaltes W et al. Treatment of malignant pheochromocytomas with a new radiopharmaceutical. Clin Res 1983; 31: 547A.

Textbook of Uncommon Cancer
Edited by C.J. Williams, J.G. Krikorian, M.R. Green and D. Raghavan
© 1988 John Wiley & Sons Ltd

Chapter **38**

Parathyroid Carcinoma

Elizabeth Shane and
John P. Bilezikian
Department of Medicine, College of Physicians and Surgeons, Columbia University, New York, USA

HISTORY

Parathyroid carcinoma is a rare cause of primary hyperparathyroidism accounting for less than 3% of patients with hypercalcemia due to parathyroid disease (1–8). Since the original description of parathyroid carcinoma in 1938, several reviews published through 1982 have described its clinical characteristics, natural history and management (2–6). In the 5 years since the most recent account (6), approximately one hundred additional cases have been reported (7–39). This cumulative experience has clearly distinguished malignant parathyroid disease from its much more common benign counterpart. The presence of marked and symptomatic hypercalcemia as well as the presence of both skeletal and renal complications of hyperparathyroidism are particularly important grounds for clinical distinction between malignant and benign disease.

In this chapter we review the natural history, clinical presentation, diagnosis and prognosis of parathyroid carcinoma. Surgical and medical management are also covered. Since a successful outcome of the disease depends in large measure upon early recognition, and appropriate surgical resection, those features of parathyroid cancer that distinguish it from benign parathyroid disease are stressed.

EPIDEMIOLOGY

The incidence of benign primary hyperparathyroidism has increased markedly over the past 15 years, due largely to the routine use of the multichannel autoanalyzer in clinical medicine (40–45). It would appear that the incidence of primary hyperparathyroidism (recognized cases) now more closely reflects its prevalence (total number of cases) in the population (46). No similar population studies of parathyroid carcinoma exist because of its relative rarity. It is thus not possible to know whether, like benign parathyroid disease, its incidence has also changed. The increasing rate at which cases are reported (62 cases: 1968 to 1982, vs 100 cases: 1982 to 1987) does not address this issue because many of these reflect the long term experience from large institutions rather than recently diagnosed patients (7, 8, 11, 16, 22, 36–38). The patients reported by Holmes et al. (3) in the pre-autoanalyzer era (1969) are very similar to those patients described in our review (6) and more recent cases reported since 1982 (Table 1; 7–39). Patients with parathyroid carcinoma tend to be symptomatic and are as likely to seek medical attention now as in the past. Thus, for all these reasons the overall incidence and presentation of the patient with parathyroid carcinoma, has probably not changed appre-

TABLE 1 PARATHYROID CARCINOMA

	Holmes et al. (3)	Shane and Bilezikian (6)	Shane and Bilezikian
Period of review	1933–1968	1968–1981	1982–1987
Number of cases	46	62	104
Female:male ratio	0.8:1	1.2:1	104:1
Average age (years)	44	48	46
Serum calcium (mg/dl)	15.9	15.5	15.0
Renal involvement	15 (32%)	37 (60%)	53 (50%)
Skeletal involvement	34 (73%)	34 (55%)	46 (44%)
No symptoms	—	1 (2%)	—

ciably over the past four decades. Relative to the increased incidence of benign primary hyperparathyrodism, therefore, parathyroid carcinoma is probably an even more uncommon cause of hypercalcemia than it used to be.

ETIOLOGY

The etiology of parathyroid carcinoma is not known. There is no convincing evidence that this tumor develops in previously adenomatous or hyperplastic tissue despite occasional case reports (12, 15, 27, 47, 48). Reports of disease occurring in patients with a history of previous neck irradiation, chronic renal failure (12, 30, 34) or in familial hyperparathyroidism (49–52) exist but no clear pattern of such factors has emerged in the approximately 200 cases described to date. The disease may be somewhat more common in Japan than in Western countries (22).

GROSS PATHOLOGY

In contrast to the typical parathyroid adenoma which is most often soft, round or oval in shape and dark brown or reddish in color, parathyroid carcinoma is frequently a large, very firm, greyish-white mass that is surrounded by a dense, white fibrous capsule. It may be very difficult to separate the tissue from contiguous structures. Gross infiltration of adjacent thyroid tissue, nerve, muscles or esophagus or obvious cervical lymph node

metastases makes the diagnosis apparent at the time of operation. However, any one or all of these features may be absent making the intraoperative diagnosis difficult. Furthermore, examination of frozen sections of tissue is often unreliable. In these cases, careful histological evaluation of the tissue is imperative.

HISTOLOGY

The distinction between benign and malignant parathyroid tumors is difficult to make histologically, a fact true for most endocrine neoplasms. Nevertheless, the guidelines set up by Schantz and Castleman in 1973 are useful (4). The principal histological features of parathyroid carcinoma are (1) a trabecular, lobulated pattern of rather uniform sheets of cells separated by thick fibrous bands that traverse the gland (90% of cases); (2) mitotic figures within parenchymal cells (mitotic activity in parenchymal cells must be distinguished from mitotic activity in endothelial cells which does not have the same significance); (3) capsular or vascular invasion. A histological comparison between normal, hyperplastic, adenomatous and carcinomatous parathyroid tissue is shown in Figure 1. Any parathyroid cell has been reported to become malignant, but the chief cell is most frequently involved. Unfortunately, any or all of these criteria may either be absent or prove to be misleading (53, 54). One thus may still not be certain about the diagnosis even after careful histological examination of the parathyroid tissue.

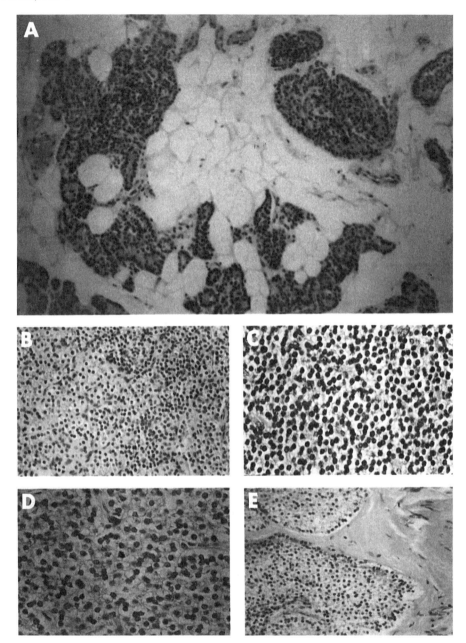

Figure 1 Histology of the parathyroid gland. A, Normal parathyroid tissue characterized by prominent glandular fat surrounding nests of chief cells. B, A parathyroid adenoma characterized by sheets of chief cells and absent glandular fat. C, Parathyroid hyperplasia. All four parathyroid glands are involved in contrast to the histological presentation in B, involving only a single gland. D, Parathyroid carcinoma with a mitotic figure in the center of the field. E, Parathyroid carcinoma demonstrating a trabecular organization with dense acellular fibrous bands traversing the tumor. (Photomicrographs kindly provided by Dr Virginia LiVolsi, Department of Surgical Pathology, University of Pennsylvania School of Medicine.)

ULTRASTRUCTURAL CHARACTERISTICS AND IMMUNOPEROXIDASE STAINING

Electron microscopy of parathyroid cancer has been performed in a limited fashion and does not help further in establishing the diagnosis. Nuclear and mitrochondrial anomalies, increased cellular secretory and metabolic activity, and basement membrane modifications with intramembranous cytoplasmic expansions all have been described (9, 32, 54, 55). In addition to electron microscopy, immunoperoxidase staining of tissue for localization of cellular parathyroid hormone and genetic probes for identification of parathyroid hormone messenger RNA (29) can also be performed but they are primarily research tools at this time and are of dubious value insofar as the diagnosis of parathyroid carcinoma is concerned.

BIOLOGY

Parathyroid carcinoma is a relatively slow growing tumor with generally low malignant potential. Local spread to contiguous structures in the neck may be followed later by distant metastases (cervical lymph nodes, lung, liver, bone and pancreas). Symptoms of parathyroid carcinoma are generally caused by excessive parathyroid hormone production by the functioning tumor rather than by infiltration of vital organs. Thus, signs and symptoms of hypercalcemia are clinical hallmarks of parathyroid cancer and successful attempts to localize and remove tumor deposits may often provide amelioration of symptoms for significant periods of time.

CLINICAL FEATURES

Parathyroid carcinoma presents a diagnostic problem when it is not clinically or histologically distinguishable from the much more common benign disorder. In this setting, the diagnosis may be made only in retrospect when local recurrence or distant metastases are recognized. Several clinical features of parathyroid carcinoma are noteworthy (2–6). The ratio of affected women to men is $1:1$ in comparison to primary hyperparathyroidism $(3:2)$. The average age of the patient with parathyroid carcinoma is in the fifth decade, younger by approximately 10 years than the typical patient with primary hyperparathyroidism. Most patients with primary hyperparathyroidism have mild hypercalcemia (11–12 mg/dl and few if any symptoms of hypercalcemia) (40–45). In contrast, most patients with parathyroid carcinoma have moderate-to-severe hypercalcemia $(>14$ mg/dl) and virtually all are symptomatic. The most frequently cited complaints are fatigue, weakness, anorexia, weight loss, nausea, vomiting, polyuria, polydipsia. Also useful in differentiating benign from malignant disease is the presence of very high parathyroid hormone levels. Extreme elevations of parathyroid hormone are not usually seen in primary hyperparathyroidism, whereas in parathyroid carcinoma parathyroid hormone levels are, on average, greater than three times the upper limit of normal.

A palpable neck mass is reported to be present in up to 76% of patients with parathyroid carcinoma (2–8, 12). This exceptional clinical finding in parathyroid carcinoma contrasts with the virtual absence of a palpable neck mass in patients with benign disease (56). Kidneys and bones, classical target organs for parathyroid hormone, appear to be affected more frequently and more severely than in benign primary hyperparathyroidism. In addition to complaints referable to hypercalcemia (see above) many patients with parathyroid carcinoma present with renal colic, bone pain or pathological fractures. Of those with renal disease (32 to 60%), nephrolithiasis occurs most frequently; nephrocalcinosis and diminished renal function are also commonly observed. Involvement of the skeleton is also more common and more severe in patients with parathyroid carcinoma than in benign disease. In addition to bone pain and pathological fractures, specific radiological evidence of hyperparathyroid bone disease (osteitis fibrosa cystica, subperiosteal bone resorption, 'salt and pepper' skull, diffuse osteopenia, absent lamina dura) is present in 44 to 73% of patients. It is also noteworthy that patients with parathyroid carcinoma often have concomitant renal and skeletal involvement, a clinical presentation very different from that of benign hyperparathyroidism, in which the simultaneous presence of bone and renal involvement is rare. A summary of those features that might lead one to suspect the diagnosis of parathyroid cancer in a patient with hypercalcemia and elevated parathyroid hormone levels is shown in Table 1.

Besides the kidneys and skeleton, other organs are frequently affected by the hyperparathyroid state in parathyroid carcinoma. Recurrent severe pancreatitis, peptic ulcer disease and anemia occur with greater frequency in patients with malignant disease.

INVESTIGATION AND STAGING

Currently there is no reliable preoperative method for making the diagnosis of parathyroid carcinoma. Fine needle aspiration of tumor tissue (13, 32) has no place in the diagnostic approach because seeding can occur. Moreover, the results are unlikely to be diagnostic insofar as the distinction between benign and malignant disease is concerned. Detection of calcification in the parathyroid glands by computed tomography (28) and abnormal accumulation of gallium-67 citrate (31) have been suggested as useful markers of malignancy but the experience with these two techniques is too limited to permit any conclusions to be drawn. Patients with parathyroid carcinoma may have elevated levels of subunits of human chorionic gonadotrophin as compared to patients with primary hyperparathyroidism who do not (57).

Selective venous catherization, computed tomography, ultrasonography and arteriography are all useful in the localization of recurrent tumor deposits or metastases but are rarely necessary prior to the initial operation.

No formal pre- or postoperative staging protocols exist for parathyroid carcinoma.

MANAGEMENT AND PROGNOSIS

Surgery

Surgical resection of parathyroid carcinoma is the only effective therapy. The optimal time for the curative surgery is the initial operation, when extensive local disease or distant metastases are less likely to be present. In this regard, the surgeon should be prepared to perform the definitive operation. At the time of surgery a lobulated, large, grey-white mass, with a dense fibrous capsule, should suggest the presence of parathyroid carcinoma. Local invasion is further proof. These clues are of particular importance in view of the unreliability of frozen sections and the controversy that exists regarding the histopathology of benign versus malignant parathyroid disease (4, 53, 54).

The abnormal gland should be removed en bloc. Great care must be taken to avoid rupture of the capsule and subsequent 'seeding' of the neck with multiple small tumor deposits. If the tumour is adherent to the strap muscles or to the thyroid gland, resection must include these areas. Similarly, the recurrent laryngeal nerve must be sacrificed if it is invaded by tumor. Since there is a 30% incidence of cervical lymph node metastases (3, 5–8), excision of all nodes in the tracheoesophageal groove should be performed. A radical neck dissection is performed only in patients with grossly involved lymph nodes since there is no evidence that prophylactic radical neck dissection alters the course or prognosis of the disease (7, 8).

The natural history of parathyroid carcinoma is one of slow progression. Hypercalcemia may recur months to years following the initial surgery and all too often is the first clue that the patient has recurrent parathyroid carcinoma. The average time from first operation to first recurrence is approximately 3 years (6), but much longer intervals have been reported. Since this tumor has a great propensity for local invasion, the most frequent site of recurrence is the contiguous structures of the neck. The thyroid gland is most commonly involved, followed by the strap muscles of the neck, the recurrent laryngeal nerve, blood vessels, esophagus and trachea.

This tumor metastasizes via both lymphatic and hematogenous routes and invades cervical lymph nodes (30%), lung (40%) and liver (10%). Other distant sites include bone, pleura, pericardium, and pancreas.

In contrast to many other tumors, management of metastatic parathyroid carcinoma is primarily surgical. The generally slow growth of the tumor and the fact that symptoms are generally caused by overproduction of parathyroid hormone rather than by infiltration of vital organs makes surgery to remove metastatic foci often a reasonable approach. Even very small metastases may produce enough parathyroid hormone to cause life-threatening hypercalcemia. Thus, although removal of local or even distant metastases is unlikely to be curative, such action may result in significant periods of remission. In patients with recurrent disease, therefore, vigorous attempts to localize and to remove tumor deposits are often indicated. Arteriography, sampling of selected venous beds for parathyroid hormone, computerized axial tomography are all useful localization aids.

Radiation Therapy

Unfortunately, parathyroid carcinoma is not a radiosensitive tumor. Attempts to control tumor growth or to inhibit parathyroid hormone production by irradiation of the tumor itself have usually been ineffective (3, 6), although occasional successes have been reported.

Chemotherapy

If the carcinoma is widely disseminated and surgery is not feasible, the ultimate prognosis is poor. The 5-year survival of inoperable patients is generally less than 50% (6). Several

chemotherapeutic regimens have been tried without success (nitrogen mustard; vincristine, cyclosphosphamide and actinomycin D; Adriamycin, cyclosphosphamide and 5-fluorouracil; and Adriamycin alone (16, 58, 59). Recently, 2 patients, treated with dacarbazine (DTIC) alone (23, 24, 36) or in combination with other drugs (5-fluorouracil and cyclophosphamide) (17) achieved at least a partial response with amelioration of hypercalcemia and decreases in parathyroid hormone levels. This approach warrants further investigation.

Since chemotherapeutic attempts to control tumour burden in parathyroid carcinoma have proven disappointing, the approach to metastatic parathyroid carcinoma is directed toward management of the hypercalcemia. The marked elevations of parathyroid hormone itself and acceleration of parathyroid hormone mediated bone resorption may make this therapeutic goal difficult to achieve, especially in the long run.

Management of acute hypercalcemia due to parathyroid carcinoma is the same as management of hypercalcemia from any other cause (60, 61). In addition to maneuvers designed to improve hydration and promote urinary calcium excretion, such as saline infusion and the use of loop diuretics, agents that interfere with osteoclast-mediated bone resorption figure most prominently. Mithramycin (62), a specific inhibitor of bone resorption, effectively lowers the serum calcium in parathyroid carcinoma and is the agent most frequently used to control the hypercalcemia of this disease. Mithramycin is administered intravenously as a 4- or 8-hour infusion (15–25 μg/kg) daily until the serum calcium declines to an acceptable range. Unfortunately, the effects of mithramycin are transient and in a disease such as parathyroid cancer that is characterized by relentless bone resorption, hypercalcemia usually recurs within a few days or weeks after a course of therapy. Repeated courses of mithramycin are associated with liver, kidney and bone marrow toxicity. Although one patient whose serum calcium was well controlled with this drug at smaller doses (12.5

mg/kg), received it for several months without any ill effects (38), mithramycin in parathyroid carcinoma should be reserved for special situations of life-threatening hypercalcemia, while sites of surgically accessible metastatic disease are being sought, or when the hypercalcemia of widespread parathyroid cancer cannot be otherwise controlled.

Calcitonin should theoretically be an ideal drug for parathyroid carcinoma because it inhibits osteoclast-mediated bone resorption and increases urinary calcium excretion. However, it lowers serum calcium only transiently, if at all (6, 17, 20, 21, 24, 27, 38). Calcitonin (200–400 MRC units) in combination with glucocorticoids (100–300 mg hydrocortisone) may be more efficacious and deserves further investigation (63). Another group of drugs that inhibit osteoclast-mediated bone resorption are the diphosphonates. Dichloromethylene diphosphonate (Cl_2MDP) lowers serum calcium in patients with parathyroid carcinoma; it is administered intravenously in daily doses until the serum calcium is lowered. Although its effects are temporary and it has not proven to be useful orally yet, the lack of serious toxicities makes it a more likely candidate than mithramycin for the management of chronic hypercalcemia due to parathyroid cancer (21, 64, 65). Another diphosphonate, 3-amino-1-hydroxypropylidene-1-bisphosphonate (APD) has been reported to be effective when administered by both intravenous and oral routes; moreover this drug successfully lowered serum calcium albeit slightly, in a patient in whom Cl_2MDP had proven ineffective (33). Neither Cl_2MDP nor APD is available in the United States. The only diphosphonate available in the United States is etidronate disodium (Didronel). The intravenous form of etidronate, while still experimental, has been shown to lower serum calcium transiently in parathyroid carcinoma (66). If the intravenous form of this drug becomes generally available, it could conceivably be used in conjunction with the oral preparation to treat the chronic hypercalcemia of parathyroid carcinoma.

The use of oral phosphate (2 g/day) may lower serum calcium by 1–2 mg/dl which may be accompanied by symptomatic improvement. However, it has generally proven ineffective for treatment of severe hypercalcemia. A newer hypocalcemic agent, WR-2721 [5-,2-(3- aminopropyl) amino]-ethylphosphorothioic acid, has had limited but promising use in parathyroid cancer (39, 67). This drug, which should be useful in the therapy of parathyroid cancer because of its ability to lower parathyroid hormone levels (67), deserves further investigation.

Because of the relative rarity of parathyroid carcinoma few investigators have an experience with large enough numbers of patients within a workable time frame; thus, large scale organized clinical research trials of therapeutic options for this malignancy do not exist. Perhaps the organization of a tumor registry for patients with parathyroid cancer would lead to the initiation of such clinical investigation by interested researchers.

REFERENCES

1 Aurbach GD, Marx SJ, Spiegel AM. Parathyroid hormone, calcitonin and the calciferols. In: Wilson JD, Foster DW eds Williams Textbook of Endocrinology, 7th edition. Philadelphia: WB Saunders, 1985: 1137.
2 Black BK. Carcinoma of the parathyroid. Ann Surg 1956; 139: 355.
3 Holmes EC, Morton DL, Ketcham AS. Parathyroid carcinoma: A collective review. Ann Surg 1969; 169: 631.
4 Schantz A, Castleman B. Parathyroid carcinoma: A study of 70 cases. Cancer 1973; 31: 600.
5 Van Heerden JA, Werland LH, Remine WH, Walls JT, Purnell DC. Cancer of the parathyroid glands. Arch Surg 1979; 114: 475.
6 Shane E, Bilezikian JP. Parathyroid carcinoma: A review of 62 patients. Endocrine Reviews 1982; 3: 218.
7 Cohn K, Silverman M, Corrado J, Sedgewick C. Parathyroid carcinoma: The Lahey Clinic experience. Surgery 1985; 98: 1095.
8 Wang C, Gaz R. Natural history of parathyroid carcinoma: Diagnosis, treatment, and results. Am J Surg 1985; 149: 522.
9 Holck S, Pedersen NT. Carcinoma of the parathyroid gland. A light and electron microscopic study. Acta Pathol Microbiol Scand 1981.

10 Delikaris P, Poulsen J, Lovgreen NA, Skjold-borg H. Parathyroid carcinoma: A cause of recurrent primary hyperparathyroidism a few years after removal of a parathyroid adenoma. Act Chir Scand 1981; 147: 335.

11 Krudy AG, Doppman JL, Marx SJ, Brennan MF, Spiegel A, Aurbach GD. Radiographic findings in recurrent parathyroid carcinoma. Radiology 1982; 142: 625.

12 Berland Y, Olmer M, Lebreuil G, Grisoli J. Parathyroid carcinoma, adenoma and hyper-plasia in a case of chronic renal insufficiency on dialysis. Clin Nephrol 1982; 18: 154.

13 Guazzi A, Gabriella M, Guadagni G. Cytologic features of a functioning parathyroid carci-noma. Acta Cytol 1982; 26: 709.

14 Love GL, Samuels M. Fatal acute hyperparathyroidism and parathyroid carci-noma. South Med J 1983; 76: 407.

15 Haghighi P, Astarita RW, Wepsic T, Wolf PL. Concurrent primary parathyroid hyperplasia and parathyroid carcinoma. Arch Pathol Lab Med 1983; 107: 349.

16 Anderson BJ, Samaan NA, Vassilopoulou-Sellin R, Ordonez NG, Hickey RC. Parathyroid carci-noma: Features and difficulties in diagnosis and management. Surgery 1983; 94: 906.

17 Bukowski RM, Sheeler L, Cunningham J, Essel-styn C. Successful combination chemotherapy for metastatic parathyroid carcinoma. Arch Intern Med 1984; 144: 399.

18 Young TO, Saltzstein EC, Boman DA. Para-thyroid carcinoma in a child: Unusual presen-tation with seizures. J Pediatr Surg 1984; 19: 194.

19 Menkes AL, Rosenblum J, Modglin FR. Para-thyroid carcinoma with massive parathyroid hormone production and severe mitral incom-petence: Report of a case with review of litera-ture. AOA 1984; 83: 852.

20 Dubost C, Jehanno C, Lavergne A, Charpentier YL. Successful resection of intrathoracic metas-tases from two patients with parathyroid carci-noma. World J Surg 1984; 8: 547.

21 Jungst D. Disodium clodronate effective in management of severe hypercalcaemia caused by parathyroid carcinoma. Lancet 1984; i: 1043.

22 Fujimoto Y, Obara T, Ito Y, Kanazawa K, Aiyoshi Y, Nobori M. Surgical treatment of ten cases of parathyroid carcinoma: importance of an initial en bloc tumor resection. World J Surg 1984; 8: 392.

23 Calandra DB, Chejfec G, Foy BK, Lawrence A, Paloyan E. Parathyroid carcinoma: Biochemi-cal and pathological response to DTIC. Surgery 1984; 96: 1132.

24 Lake MS, Kahn SE, Favus MJ, Bermes EW. Case report: Clinical pathological correlations

in a case of primary parathyroid carcinoma. Ann Clin Lab Sci 1984; 14: 458.

25 McKeown PP, McGarity WC, Sewell CW. Carcinoma of the parathyroid gland: Is it overdiagnosed? A report of three cases. Am J Surg 1984; 147: 292.

26 Shapiro DH, Jurado R. Recurrent parathyroid carcinoma: Value of aggressive surgical approach. J Florida MA 1984; 71: 937.

27 Desch CE, Arsensis G, May AG, Amatruda JM. Parathyroid hyperplasia and carcinoma within one gland. Am J Med 1984; 77: 131.

28 Lineaweaver W, Clore F, Mancuso A, Hill S, Rumley T. Calcified parathyroid glands detected by computed tomography. J Comp Assist Tomogr 1984; 8: 975.

29 Baba H, Kishihara M, Tohmon M, Fukase M, Kisahi T, Okada S, Matsuzuka F, Kobayashi A, Kuma K, Fujita T. Identification of para-thyroid hormone messenger ribonucleic acid in an apparently nonfunctioning parathyroid car-cinoma transformed from a parathyroid carci-noma with hyperparathyroidism. J Clin Endo-crinol Metab 1984; 62: 247.

30 Sherlock DJ, Newman J, Holl-Allen RTJ. Para-thyroid carcinoma presenting as tertiary hyper-parathyroidism. Postgrad Med J 1985; 61: 243.

31 Iwase M, Shimizu Y, Kitahara H, Tobioka N, Takatsuki K. Parathyroid carcinoma visualized by Gallium-67 citrate scintigraphy. J Nucl Med 1986; 27: 63.

32 de la Garza S, de la Garza EF, Batres FH. Functional parathyroid carcinoma: Cytology, histology and ultrastructure of a case. Diag Cytopathol 1985; 1: 232.

33 Mann K. Oral bisphosphonate therapy in metastatic parathyroid carcinoma. Lancet 1985; i: 101.

34 Ireland JP, Fleming SJ, Levison DA, Cattell WR, Baker LRI. Parathyroid carcinoma asso-ciated with chronic renal failure and previous radiotherapy to the neck. J Clin Pathol 1985; 38: 1114.

35 McPheeters GO, Bender CAB. Parathyroid carcinoma: A case report and review. Hawaii Med J 1985; 44: 104.

36 Calandra D, Shah K, Lawrence AM, Paloyan E. Parathyroid carcinoma: A report of five cases. Am Surg 1985; 51: 372.

37 Lillemoe KD, Dudley NE. Parathyroid carci-noma: Pointers to successful management. Ann R Coll Surg Engl 1985; 67: 222.

38 Trigonis C, Cedermark B, Willems J, Ham-berger B, Granberg PO. Parathyroid carci-noma—problems in diagnosis and treatment. Clin Oncol 1984; 10: 11.

39 Hirschel-Scholz S, Jung A, Fischer JA, Trechsel U, Bonjour JP. Suppression of parathyroid

secretion after administration of WR-2721 in a patient with parathyroid carcinoma. Clin Endocrinol 1985; 23: 313.

40 Purnell DC, Scholz DA, Smith LH, Sizemore GW, Black BM, Goldsmith RS, Arnaud CD. Treatment of primary hyperparathyroidism. Am J Med 1974; 56: 800.

41 Purnell DC, Smith LH, Scholz DA, Elveback LR, Arnaud CD. Primary hyperparathyroidism: a prospective clinical study. Am J Med 1971; 50: 670.

42 Mallette LE, Bilezikian JP, Heath DA, Aurbach GD. Primary hyperparathyroidism: clinical and biochemical features. Medicine 1974; 53: 127.

43 Heath III H, Hodgson SF, Kennedy MA. Primary hyperparathyroidism: incidence, morbidity, and potential economic impact in a community. N Engl J Med 302: 189.

44 Mundy GR, Cove DH, Fisken R. Primary hyperparathyroidism: changes in the pattern of clinical presentation. Lancet i: 1317.

45 Rohl PG, Wilkinson M, Clifton-Bigh P, Posen S. Hyperparathyroidism: experiences with treated and untreated patients. Med J Aust 1981; 1: 519.

46 Silverberg SJ, Shane E, De la Cruz L, Jacobs TP, Siris E, Clemens TL, Feldman F, Cafferty M, Dempster DW, Tohme J, Lindsay R, Bilezikian JP. A current view of primary hyperparathyroidism. J Bone Min Res 1987; 2 Suppl I: 107A.

47 Kramer WH Association of parathyroid hyperplasia with neoplasia. Am J Clin Pathol 1970; 53: 275.

48 Murrayama T, Kawabe K, Tagami M. A case of parathyroid carcinoma concurred with hyperplasia: an electron microscopic study. J Urol 1977; 118: 126.

49 Frayha RA, Nassar VH, Dagher F, Salti IS. Familial parathyroid carcinoma. Leban Med 1972; 25: 299.

50 Dinnen JS, Greenwood RH, Jone JH, Walker DA, Williams ED. Parathyroid carcinoma in familial hyperparathyroidism. J Clin Pathol 1977; 30: 966.

51 Mallette LE, Bilezikian JP, Ketcham AS, Aurbach GD. Parathyroid carcinoma in familial hyperparathyroidism. Am J Med 1974; 57: 642.

52 Leborgne J, LeNeel JC, Brizelin F, Malvy P. Cancer familial des parathyroids. J Chir (Paris) 1975; 109: 315.

53 Snover DC, Foucar K. Mitotic activity in benign parathyroid disease. Am J Clin Pathol 1981; 75: 345.

54 Smith JF, Coombs RRH. Histological diagnosis of carcinoma of the parathyroid gland. J Clin Pathol 1984; 37: 1370.

55 Obara T, Fujimoto Y, Yamaguchi K, Takanashi R, Kino I, Sasaki Y. Parathyroid carcinoma of the oxyphil cell type. A report of two cases, light and electron microscopic study. Cancer 1985; 55: 1482.

56 Lejeune E, Deplante JP, Daumont A, Bouvier M. L'hyperparathyroidisme primitiff à propos de 50 cas personnels. Revue Rhum Mal Osteoartic 1975; 42: 747.

57 Stock JL, Weintraub BD, Rosen SW, Aurbach GD, Spiegel AM, Marx SJ, Human chorionic gonadotropin subunit measurement in primary hyperparathyroidism. J Clin Endocrinol Metab 1982; 54: 57.

58 Goepfert H, Smart CR, Rochlin DB. Metastatic parathyroid carcinoma and hormonal chemotherapy: case report and reponse to hexestrol. Ann Surg 1966; 164: 917.

59 Inone H. Ishihara T, Fukai S, Mikata A, Ito K, Mimura T. Parathyroid carcinoma with tracheal invasion and airway obstruction. Surgery 1980, 87: 113.

60 Bilezikian JP. Hypercalcemia. In: Stein JH ed Internal Medicine, 2nd edition. Boston/Toronto: Little, Brown, 1987: 2076.

61 Catherwood BD, Deftos LJ. Hypercalcemia. In: Krieger DT, Bardin CW eds Current Therapy in Endocrinology and Metabolism, 2nd edition. Philadelphia: BC Decker, 1985: 337.

62 Calabresi P, Parks Jr RE. Antiproliferative drugs and drugs used for immunosuppression. In: Gilman AG, Goodman LS, Rall TW, Murad F eds The Pharmacological Basis of Therapeutics, 7th edition New York: Macmillan; 1985; 1287.

63 Au WYW. Calcitonin treatment of hypercalcemia due to parathyroid carcinoma: synergistic effect of prednisone on longterm treatment of hypercalcemia Arch Intern Med 1975; 135: 1594.

64 Jacobs TP, Siris ES, Bilezikian JP, Baquiran DC, Shane E, Canfield RE. Hypercalcemia of malignancy: treatment with intravenous dichloromethylene diphosphonate. Ann Intern Med 1981; 94: 312.

65 Shane E, Jacobs TP, Siris ES, Steinberg SF, Stoddart K, Canfield RE, Bilezikian JP. Therapy of hypercalcemia due to parathyroid carcinoma with intravenous dichloromethylene diphosphonate. Am J Med 1982; 72: 939.

66 Jacobs TP, Gordon AC, Gundberg CM, Silverberg SJ, Shane E, Reich L, Clemens TL. Neoplastic hypercalcemia: physiologic response to intravenous etidronate. Am J Med 1987; 82: 42.

67 Glover D, Riley L, Carmichael K, Spar B, Glick J, Klugerman MM, Agut ZS, Slatopolsky E. Hypercalcemia and inhibition of parathyroid hormone secretion. N Engl J Med 1983; 309: 1137.

Section **VII**

Breast Tumours

Textbook of Uncommon Cancer
Edited by C.J. Williams, J.G. Krikorian, M.R. Green and D. Raghavan
© 1988 John Wiley & Sons Ltd

Chapter **39**

Paget's Disease of the Breast

M.D. Lagios
Department of Pathology, Children's Hospital of San Francisco, California, USA

The popular conception of Paget's disease of the nipple reflects an overwhelming clinical experience with Paget's disease in association with invasive breast carcinoma. This clinical experience, the cytologic resemblance of Paget cells to duct carcinomas, and the historical experience of Paget relating to the subsequent appearance of invasive (scirrhous) cancer in the breast, have been woven into an apocryphal medical theory concerning the origin of these cells. In simple terms this theory states that Paget cells represent breast cancer cells which have migrated into the epidermis either by direct extension or lymphatic invasion, or in the case of underlying in situ carcinomas, have migrated via duct epithelium. Such is the weight of tradition in medicine that much recent evidence which contradicts this theory has been ignored or interpreted in a way which will bolster the orthodox theory of histogenesis.

HISTORY

James Paget (1) described 'about fifteen' cases of a peculiar eczematoid lesion limited to the skin of the nipple–areolar complex which preceded the development of clinical breast cancer by 1–2 years. Although Paget made a number of important histopathologic observations, he did not describe the histology of the lesion bearing his name. Darier (2) first described 'Paget' cells in a case of extramammary

Paget's disease but did not recognize their neoplastic nature. He speculated that Paget cells and their dyskeratotic remnants in the stratum corneum were manifestations of a parasitic infection (psorosperms).

DEFINITION

Paget's disease of the nipple represents an intraepidermal proliferation of neoplastic cells in the skin and adnexa of the nipple and areola. Clinically it commonly masquerades as a chronic eczematoid dermatitis of the nipple, but one with a fixed or expanding topographic distribution. Although some modest clinical improvement may appear to occur with typical emollient creams, the underlying process remains and very slowly progresses. Cases of Paget's disease which have been treated as persistent eczematoid dermatitis without improvement a year or more continue to occur. The vast majority of cases of Paget's disease of the nipple are associated with underlying breast carcinoma, i.e. carcinoma involving the duct system of the breast apart from the skin of the nipple–areolar complex. This amounts to 97% of the series of 214 cases reported by Ashikari et al. (3). Many of these associated carcinomas are noninvasive duct carcinomas which frequently involve the distal lactiferous ducts of the nipple—in direct continuity with the involved nipple epidermis—a feature which supported the Paget cell migration or epidermotrophic theory. Prognosis in Paget's disease is dependent on stage and grade of the underlying carcinoma—if any. The presence of Paget's disease in the nipple does not alter the prognosis of breast carcinomas stratified for similar size, grade and stage.

MICROSCOPY

In less severely involved epidermis Paget cells are typically single large cells, twice the size of normal keratinocytes. A large vesicular nucleus with prominent nucleolus is frequently eccentrically located within the cell. The pale cytoplasm may contain vesicles or lacunae which may contain epithelial mucin as demonstrated by PAS diastase or mucicarmine procedures. However, this feature, although diagnostic when present, occurs in only a minority of cases in the author's personal experience. In more heavily involved epidermis, Paget cells occur in groups, particularly in the suprabasal portion of the epidermis, and in the most severely involved areas such cells may replace the entire population of keratinocytes.

Paget cells are generally rather cohesive within the epidermis. They exhibit both upward migration—through the malpighian layers and stratum corneum, and in addition exhibit a dyskeratotic type of maturation with nuclear condensation and a dense eosinophilic cytoplasm within the stratum corneum. Such cells can be appreciated in simple exfoliative cytologies (scrapings) of the nipple epidermis where they are reminiscent of a keratinizing dysplasia in their cytologic appearance. This appearance, first noted by Darier (2) in extra-mammary Paget's disease, led him to describe the dyskeratotic cells within the stratum corneum as psorosperms, a condition which he thought represented a parasitic infestation. A number of related changes are evident in the epidermis including prominent acanthosis out of proportion to the number of Paget cells identified.

DIFFERENTIAL DIAGNOSIS

The most celebrated differential diagnostic alternative to Paget's disease of the breast is malignant melanoma. This differential is, however, more theoretical than real. Malignant melanoma of the pigmented skin of the nipple–areolar complex of the adult female is exceedingly rare relative to Paget's disease, while the latter was detected in 4% of a consecutive series of 149 mastectomy specimens resected for breast carcinoma and was the clinical presenting sign of that disease in one of those cases (4). Moreover the differential is pertinent only for malignant melanoma in situ (atypical melanocytic hyperplasia) since Paget's disease is virtually confined to the epidermis itself and does not involve the underlying dermis (Table 1). Melanoma and

TABLE 1 DIFFERENTIAL DIAGNOSTIC FEATURES

	Paget's disease	Malignant melanoma
Distribution	Confined to epidermis	Epidermis+dermis
	Intraepidermal groups, predominantly suprabasal	Numerous basal thèques project into papillary dermis
	Dyskeratotic cells in stratum corneum (parakeratosis)	Melanin in stratum corneum
Epidermis	Hyperplastic with hyperkeratosis	Minimally altered
Histochemistry	Variable epithelial mucin present in cells	No mucin
Immunochemistry	S-100− Cytokeratin AEI+	S-100+ Cytokeratin AEI−
Electron microscopy	Intercellular desmosomes, microvilli	No desmosomes or microvilli. Melanosomes and premelanosomes may be identified

Paget's disease exhibit groups of individual neoplastic cells proliferating within a background of non-neoplastic keratinocytes. Bowen's disease (intraepithelial carcinoma) in contrast involves the entire epidermis in a diffuse fashion and represents a neoplasm of keratinocytes which lacks evidence of glandular differentiation and lacks S-100 antigen. All these neoplastic processes, Paget's and Bowen's diseases and malignant melanoma may exhibit melanin in the cytoplasm of neoplastic cells.

CELL REPLICATION

Pierard-Franchimont and Pierard (5) studied 3 cases of Paget's disease (2 mammary) and noted that a tritiated thymidine label was avidly taken up by Paget cells and keratinocytes in the deepest or basal proliferative compartment of the epidermis. Morphologically normal keratinocytes in areas involved with Paget's disease show a four- to five-fold increased rate of tritiated thymidine incorporation. The authors hypothesize a common topographic controlling mechanism for proliferative activity in both populations of cells and parallel processes of maturation. These findings are understandable when Paget's disease is considered as an in situ neoplastic process which arises within the epidermis. The high rate of tritiated thymidine labelling of Paget cells in the basal compartment would reflect their origin there, an origin shared with keratinocytes. The decreasing label noted in Paget cells in the more mature portions of the malpighian layer is consistent with the apparent maturation or keratinization of Paget cells as they enter the stratum granulosum. In corollary fashion these results cannot be explained by a model of Paget's disease which proposes that the neoplasm invades the epidermis. Growth within the epidermis in such a model would be expected to be independent of topography—there would be no greater tritiated thymidine uptake in the basal compartment as compared to other portions of the epidermis.

IMMUNOCYTOCHEMISTRY

The recent development of readily available immunoperoxidase techniques has had a great impact on the field of diagnostic pathology. The successful application of such techniques to specific clinical problems, e.g. the identification of a metastatic 'poorly differentiated' carcinoma as prostatic in origin with prostate specific antigen, has directed a great effort towards resolving the specific origin of poorly differentiated metastases but also has generated an interest in the resolution of histogenetic origin for some tumors. Unfortunately, few applications of the immunoperoxidase technique presently available are so specific as the example cited. While prostate specific antigen is essentially a marker for prostatic origin, the majority of antigenic markers are shared by numerous different epithelial tissues and cannot identify the site of origin of the cell in question. Moreover, it should be recalled that neoplastic processes commonly exhibit antigenic markers completely foreign to their normal tissues of origin, e.g. ACTH and parathormone in lung and pancreatic carcinomas.

Immunoperoxidase techniques have been applied to Paget's disease of the breast and extramammary sites with an interest towards establishing the histogenesis of the Paget cell on the basis of comparative immunocytochemistry. The types of antigens studied can be grouped into several classes.

1 Antigens which are common markers for epithelial differentiation, the cytokeratins, e.g. AE1, etc. (6–10). Such cytokeratins would appear to be common to all epithelial tissues and may occur in a host of different carcinomas. In the context of Paget's disease they have been used to contrast the presence of certain low molecular weight cytokeratin antigens, (e.g. AE1) in Paget cells, with their absence in the specialized keratinocytes of the malpighian layer. Such low molecular weight cytokeratins are also found in normal eccrine, apocrine and other epithelia including ducts of the breast and their neoplastic counterparts.

2 CEA. Carcinoembryonic antigen (CEA) is shared by numerous carcinomas of different histogenetic origin and occurs in actively regenerating epithelia as well, e.g. in the damaged mucosa of chronic inflammatory bowel diseases. It occurs in breast carcinomas and Paget cells as well as in pancreatic and ovarian carcinomas.

3 Relatively specific antigens. Human milk fat globulin antigens (6, 10), alpha lactalbumin (11), casein (12) and gross cystic disease protein (13) are antigens generally considered more specific to mammary epithelium and are shared by Paget cells. However, the majority of these antigens also occur in apocrine epithelium and may occur in the epidermal basal layer in areas involved by Paget's disease, as well as in the clear cells of Toker in patients without Paget's disease (7).

In summary, the available immunocytochemical studies of Paget cells demonstrate the presence of antigenic markers which are shared with many carcinomas including duct carcinoma of the breast. These include low molecular weight cytokeratins, carcinoembryonic antigen and certain lectin binding sites (14). Additionally, Paget cells both of mammary and extramammary origin have been shown to share relatively more specific antigens with breast duct epithelium including human milk fat globulin antigen, alpha lactalbumin, anti-casein, anti-gross cystic disease protein, etc. As noted these antigens are not specific to the mammary duct epithelium and their neoplastic counterparts but also occur in apocrine glands and the basal portion of the epidermis and the epidermal clear cells of Toker. Various authors have proposed on the basis of these studies that Paget cells originate in underlying (parenchymal) breast carcinoma (10, 15) within the epidermis (7), in apocrine epithelium (14) or within eccrine epithelium.

We have previously shown the presence of cytoplasmic bound estrogen in Paget cells which we interpret as consistent with the presence of a specific estrophilin. Of interest, however, was our ability to demonstrate similar bound estrogen in apocrine epithelium and cells intermediate in Paget morphology within the epidermis (16). Similar estrophilins have been identified in many other carcinomas of different histogenetic origin, e.g. melanoma, endometrial and ovarian carcinoma and even certain lung carcinomas.

ULTRASTRUCTURE OF PAGET'S DISEASE OF NIPPLE

Ultrastructural examination of Paget cells demonstrate numerous features which confirm the light microscopic observations of acinar differentiation. These include: deep invaginations of the cell surface, so-called intracytoplasmic acinar structures, which are lined by microvilli and exhibit a prominent glycocalyx; as well as true acini formed by two or more adjacent cells to produce a gland lumen (Figure 1). More significantly, however, ultrastructural examination reveals a series of features which argue for an intraepidermal origin. These are represented by specialized cell attachment structures—desmosomes between Paget cells and keratinocytes, and hemidesmosomes between Paget cells and the epidermal basal lamina; and by a series of cells intermediate in their morphology between Paget cells and keratinocytes. Such intermediate cells are predominantly located in the deeper malpighian layer, lack tonofibrils typical of keratinocytes in similar strata but exhibit a size similar to keratinocytes. These intermediate cells can also be distinguished by the presence of antigens foreign to the normal keratinocyte. Bussolati and Pich (12) demonstrated casein in such intermediate cells and Lagios et al. (16) demonstrated bound estradiol.

Sagami (17) and Sagebiel (18) first identified desmosomes between keratinocytes and Paget cells, and Sagebiel suggested their significance for site of origin. In our own series of 10 mammary and one extramammary Paget's disease examined by electron microscopy, desmosomes were demonstrated in every case between the Paget cell and adjacent keratinocytes. Although occasionally rather simple, a

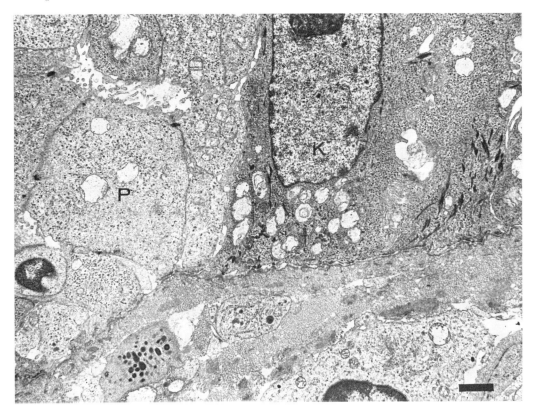

Figure 1 Electron micrograph of basal portion of nipple epidermis. Keratinocyte (K) and Paget cell (P) are both attached to epidermal basal lamina by hemidesmosomes. Numerous desmosomes (maculae adherentes) are seen between adjacent Paget cells which form a common acinus between them. Microvilli project into the acinus. Note the absence of tonofibrils in Paget cells in contrast to keratinocytes of basal layers. Scale: 1 μm.

number of cases exhibited well developed maculae adherentes with mirror-image tonofibrils extending into the attachment from both the keratinocytes and the Paget cells (Figures 2 and 3) of the type typically developed between keratinocytes in the malpighian layer. Although Paget cells are classically described as suprabasal in position, in three instances we demonstrated Paget cells, recognized by their larger size, more open nuclear morphology and absence of tonofibrils, clearly attached to small hemidesmosomal attachments to the epidermal basal lamina (basement membrane) (Figure 4).

SUMMARY: MORPHOLOGIC AND IMMUNOCHEMICAL STUDIES

A comprehensive theory of Paget's disease of the nipple must be able to explain: (1) the morphologic identity of Paget's disease of the nipple with that of other sites; (2) the distribution of Paget's disease in relation to apocrine glands, i.e. breast, anogenital (vulva, perineum, etc.), external auditory canal, palpebra and skin of the axilla; (3) the occurrence of Paget cells without underlying carcinoma—a rare phenomenon in the breast (3%) but the predominant pattern in other sites (75%); (4)

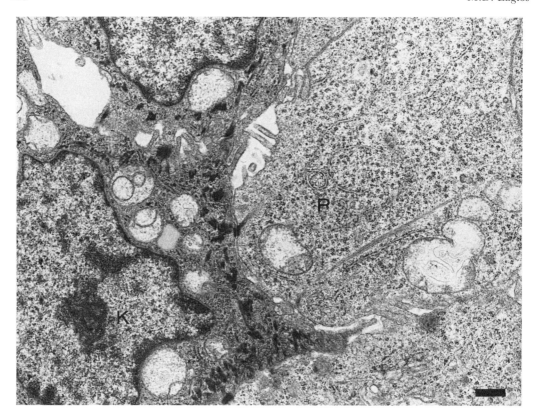

Figure 2 Electron micrograph of small area of microvillous differentiation on the surface of a Paget cell. A well developed macula adherentes locks the Paget cell (P) to the adjacent keratinocyte (K). Scale: 0.5 μm.

the evidence derived from cell kinetic, immunocytochemical, and ultrastructural studies; and (5) the maturation and keratinization of Paget cells within the stratum corneum.

In corollary fashion the popular epidermotrophic theory must explain (1) the ability of duct carcinoma in situ cells distant from the nipple to lose their desmosomal attachments and migrate within the duct system of the breast to the epidermis; (2) the ability of these cells and those of invasive breast cancers to invade intact normal epidermis and establish complex demosomes of the maculae adherentes type with adjacent keratinocytes; (3) the origin of Paget cells in the 75% of extramammary Paget cases without underlying carcinoma and the 3% of mammary Paget's without underlying carcinoma.

These diverse observations of light and electron microscopy, cell kinetic and immunocytochemical studies can be collated and tested against the two available models for Paget cell histogenesis—the prevalent epidermotrophic theory and the autochthonous theory of origin.

The complex desmosomal attachments between Paget cells and keratinocytes, their location in the basal layer attached by hemidesmosomes to the basal lamina, the morphologic evidence of dyskeratotic 'maturation' of Paget cells as they enter the stratum corneum, and the 'intermediate' morphology of the basal–suprabasal population of Paget cells, is most consistent with origin within the epidermis and maturation in a manner reminiscent of keratinocytes. The work of Pierard-Franchimont and Pierard (5) supports this interpretation. An autochthonous origin of Paget cells explains the infrequent cases of mammary

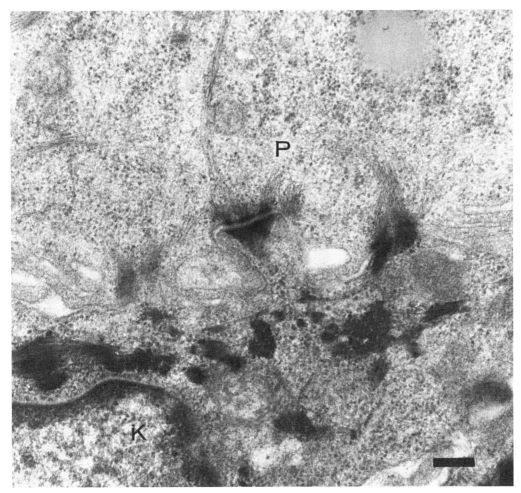

Figure 3 Electron micrograph of adjacent Paget cell (P) and keratinocytes (K) with well-developed maculae adherentes. Note dense tonofilament bundles in cytoplasm of keratinocyte. Scale: 0.5 μm.

Paget's disease and the more numerous cases of extramammary Paget's disease which are unassociated with underlying carcinoma. Furthermore, a substantial number of cases of mammary Paget's disease are associated only with noninvasive duct carcinoma, most frequently involving the larger lactiferous ducts of the nipple.

These ultrastructural observations, the frequent lack of association of extramammary and occasional mammary Paget's disease with underlying carcinoma, the evidence derived from thymidine labelling and the morphology of Paget cells in the stratum corneum cannot be explained by the epidermotrophic theory of origin. One could argue that those cases of mammary Paget's disease in which the mastectomy specimen lacked evidence of parenchymal carcinoma, were in fact cases of overlooked microscopic disease. This argument will not explain the numerous extramammary cases which lack any evidence of any underlying carcinoma.

Given that all cases of Paget's disease of the nipple have occult in situ carcinoma, we have no model which will account for the migration of malignant epithelial cells of a noninvasive duct carcinoma through the desmosomal

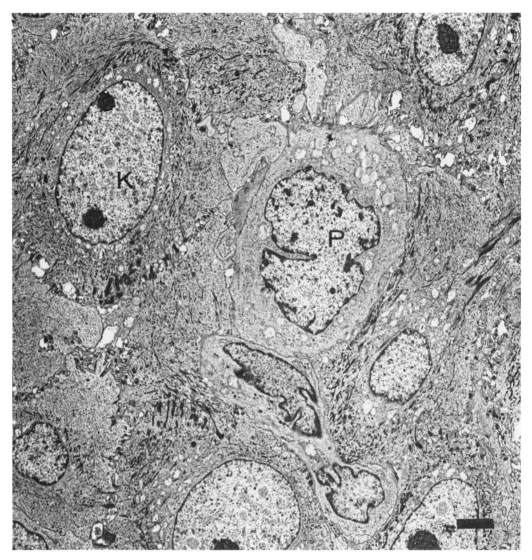

Figure 4 Electron micrograph of suprabasal portion of epidermis with presumptive 'intermediate' Paget cell. Note paucity of tonofibrils in comparison with adjacent keratinocytes. Scale: 2 μm.

attachments of intact duct epithelium and/or through the brambles of maculae adherentes in the malpighian layer to account for the appearance of Paget cells in the skin. Given that there were such a unique mechanism of intraepithelial migration, the apparent 'maturation' of Paget cells and their 'dyskeratosis' in the stratum corneum, would require yet another unique mechanism.

The most recent evidence which has been used to support the epidermotrophic theory of origin derives not from morphology per se, but from comparative immunocytochemistry. A host of specific protein antigens have been shown to be shared between Paget cells and ductal carcinomas. These include casein, lactalbumin, milk fat globulin protein, CEA and low molecular weight cytokeratins. Furthermore, these antigens have been shown to be lacking in the normal keratinocytes of the epidermis. Some investigators have used this shared antigenicity between Paget cells and duct carcinomas and the lack of similar antigens in keratinocytes to argue that Paget cells do not originate within the epidermis but rather from underlying duct carcinoma. This position ignores the presence of these same antigens in epidermal adnexa. Apocrine epithelium normally contains cytokeratins, CEA, and demonstrates bound estradiol similar to duct carcinoma, in a pattern distinctly different from normal keratinocytes.

Furthermore, the normal epidermis may also show similar antigens. Kirkham et al. (10) demonstrated human milk fat globulin antigen in the basal keratinocytes in areas involved by Paget's disease, as well as in Paget cells and mammary duct epithelium. These authors also demonstrated that cytokeratin LE6 was strongly present in morphologically normal basal keratinocytes. Nagle et al. (7) similarly demonstrated reactivity in the clear cells of Toker in the uninvolved epidermis with cytokeratin KA4 in contrast to normal keratinocytes. Lee et al. (11) demonstrated alpha lactalbumin antigen not only in Paget cells and mammary epithelium, but also in a series of epidermal adnexal and salivary gland tumors and some mesotheliomas, and in select cells of normal pancreatic islets. The demonstration of some shared antigens between the basal epidermal cells and various glandular epithelium probably reflects the relative lack of antigenic differentiation in the regenerative layer of the skin. The more mature differentiated keratinocytes may have repressed expression of these antigens.

Finally, the arguments of shared antigenicity to substantiate origin with underlying duct carcinoma ignore the fact that a vast number of different carcinomas express antigens foreign to their tissue of origin. One need only consider bronchogenic carcinoma with its not infrequent production of immunoreactive parathormones, growth hormone, somatomedin and ACTH, to name one specific example, to realize that antigens expressed in a neoplasm cannot be used to derive the histogenesis of the neoplastic cell.

CONSERVATIVE MANAGEMENT OF SELECT CASES OF PAGET'S DISEASE OF THE BREAST

As noted previously (16) the most important implication of the two theories of Paget cell histogenesis relate to the therapeutic options which each permits.

A corollary to the epidermotrophic theory is that all Paget's disease of the nipple is secondary to underlying duct carcinoma, either in situ or invasive. Therapy must address the invariant underlying carcinoma according to the logic of this histogenetic model. At present segmental resection and radiation therapy could be an option for clinically recognizable carcinomas, but when the breast is without palpable masses or mammographically identified lesions then total mastectomy is virtually the only appropriate alternative.

In contrast, the autochthonous theory of Paget cell histogenesis recognizes that some patients presenting with Paget's disease will lack any evidence of underlying carcinoma. Such patients accounted for 6.25% of Paget's disease cases without palpable masses described by Ashikari et al. in 1970 (3). Our own more recent experience would suggest that increased surveillance for breast carcinoma has permitted a larger number of very limited cases of Paget's disease to be detected. Ten such cases have been encountered in the last 7 years, 9 of which were identified in our laboratory. This amounts to a very small fraction of our new breast cancer patients—approximately 0.6%. These patients lack palpable and mammographic abnormalities and reveal a relatively translucent N1/P1 Wolfe parenchymal pattern.

Six of these patients have previously been described (16) and the current information represents an update through August 31, 1986. Their average age is 61 years at diagnosis (range 43–73) and current average follow-up for the 6 patients treated conservatively and who remain at risk is 65 months (range 28–96). Three patients underwent immediate modified radical mastectomy; 2 were studied by serial subgross and correlated radiographic technique which optimized extensive search and sampling (19). A fourth patient underwent a large central segmental mastectomy with node sampling. One patient died of cerebrovascular accident at 60 months of follow-up. She was clinically NED (no evidence of disease) at that time.

PATHOLOGY

The extent of the disease could be evaluated completely in 2 patients undergoing modified radical mastectomy studied by the serial subgross technique. These exhibited Paget's disease of the skin of the nipple–areolar complex and involvement of one or more lactiferous ducts to the depths of 8 and 15 mm within the nipple. There was no evidence of more diffuse or multicentric duct carcinoma in situ or occult invasion and no metastases to axillary lymph nodes sampled. One patient with Paget's disease was treated with bilateral mastectomy at another hospital. Ipsilateral duct carcinoma in situ limited to two lactiferous duct profiles to a depth of 8.5 mm was demonstrated at mastectomy. The patient undergoing segmental mastectomy demonstrated residual disease in the nipple and subareolar ducts only. Lymph nodes were negative. Six patients undergoing segmental resection of the nipple–areolar complex permitted a reasonable estimate of the extent of disease since the resection encompassed all of the histologically identified in situ carcinoma. Two of these exhibited Paget's disease confined to the epidermis and in one case a sebaceous gland, while 3 exhibited associated in situ duct carcinoma involving the most distal lactiferous ducts to depths of 4, 8 and 6 mm (Table 2).

RECURRENCES

A single patient developed an invasive event in the follow-up to date (Table 3). This patient had previously undergone a nipple–areolar resection revealing duct carcinoma in situ intermittently occurring in a single lactiferous

TABLE 2 PAGET'S DISEASE OF THE NIPPLE: PATHOLOGY OF MINIMAL INVOLVEMENT[a]

| Case no. | Extent | | Treatment |
	Epidermis	Lactiferous ducts (mm)	
1	+	0	SR and mam. BX
2	+	0	SR and AX
3	+	4	SR and mam BX
4	+	8	SR and 4 quad BX
5	+	6	SR
6	+	15	M and AX
7	+	8	M and AX
8	+	8.5	Bilateral M
9	+	ND	SR
10	+	6	SR

Treatment: M=total mastectomy; SR=segmental resection of nipple–areolar complex; underlying lactiferous ducts; AX=axillary lymph node dissection or sample; ND=not determined. BX=biopsy.
[a] Minimal involvement: no clinical mass lesion, no mammographic lesion and N1/P1 parenchymal Wolfe pattern.

TABLE 3 PAGET'S DISEASE OF THE NIPPLE: FOLLOW-UP OF SEGMENTAL RESECTION TREATMENT GROUP

Case no.	Age at diagnosis	Follow-up (months)	Status
1	67	60	DOC
2	50	89	Areolar skin, 15 months
3	74	84	NED
4	43	74	Inv. duct 15 mm T_1N_1 at 65 months
5	66	60	NED
6	61	2	NED
7	73	1	NED

DOC, died of other causes. NED, no evidence of disease.

duct profile to 8 mm depth, as well as focal lobular carcinoma in situ and atypical duct hyperplasia in the immediate vicinity. Four quadrant blind biopsies had revealed minimal duct hyperplasia only. She developed an interval invasive duct carcinoma 15 mm in maximum diameter in the upper outer quadrant at 65 months of follow-up. A segmental mastectomy including a contiguous axillary dissection was performed. One of 23 lymph nodes contained a 6 mm metastasis. She underwent radiation therapy but developed a chest wall recurrence at 74 months.

One patient developed multiple recurrences of Paget's disease in residual areolar skin following her refusal to permit a complete resection of the nipple–areolar complex or more extensive surgery. A most recent nipple skin biopsy in this patient showed residual Paget's disease but there is no clinical or mammographic lesion at 86 months of follow-up. Paone and Baker (20) note 6 patients treated by segmental resection only. All were without recurrence or evidence of axillary metastases at the time of their report.

In one patient the appearance of Paget's disease was itself a recurrence of noninvasive carcinoma. The patient had previously undergone an adequate excision biopsy for a mammographically detected focus of duct carcinoma in situ, 9 mm in maximum extent (22), and subsequently developed clinical Paget's disease at 12 months of follow-up. She was treated by nipple–areolar resection and additional biopsy at that time and is currently NED at 82 months. A number of authors have previously documented metachronous Paget's disease often after adequate treatment of the primary lesion (22, 23).

The distribution of in situ duct carcinoma in the nipple–areolar resections and the mastectomy material is similar to that previously described by Cheatle (24). In patients with histologically confirmed Paget's disease, and without a clinically or mammographically identifiable lesion, breast carcinoma would appear to be most likely limited to the most distal lactiferous ducts immediately adjoining the nipple skin and usually in continuity with the intraepidermal Paget cells, or to be limited to the epidermis itself. This would suggest that Paget's disease is a 'multicentric' manifestation of breast carcinogenesis, one limited to the epidermis. This multicentric involvement was alluded to by Paget in his initial description when he referred to the uninvolved breast

tissue separating the nipple skin and the subsequent carcinoma.

Unlike Paget's experience in which every one of the 'about fifteen' cases developed cancer 'within at the most two years, and usually within one year', only one of 6 patients treated other than by total mastectomy developed subsequent invasive cancer, at 65 months. That patient clearly had a multicentric lesion distantly located in the upper outer quadrant and which could be documented mammographically not to have been present 18 months previously.

Although Paget's disease will remain for most patients a malignant sign of underlying carcinoma, it is important to realize that some few patients can be offered breast conserving options at little risk. These fortunate patients permit a re-examination of our own perception of Paget's disease of the breast and allow a reappraisal of this unusual neoplasm.

REFERENCES

1 Paget J. On disease of the mammary areola preceding cancer of the mammary gland. St Bartholomew's Hosp Rep 1874; 10: 87.
2 Darier J. Sur une nouvelle forme de psorospermose cutanée: la maladie de Paget du mamelon. C R Soc Biol 1889; 1: 294.
3 Ashikari R, Park K, Huvos AG et al. Paget's disease of the breast. Cancer 1970; 26: 680.
4 Lagios MD, Gates EA, Westdahl PR et al. A guide to the frequency of nipple involvement in breast cancer. Am J Surg 1979; 138: 135.
5 Pierard-Franchimont C, Pierard GE. Replication of Paget cells in mammary and extramammary Paget's disease. Br J Dermatol 1984; 111: 69.
6 Vanstapel MJ, Gatter KC, De Wolf-Peeters C et al. Immunohistochemical study of mammary and extramammary Paget's disease. Histopathology 1984; 8: 1013.
7 Nagle RB, Lucas DO, McDaniel KM et al. Paget's cells. New evidence linking mammary and extramammary Paget cells to a common cell phenotype. Am J Clin Pathol 1985; 83: 431.
8 Kariniemi AL, Forsman L, Wahlstrom T et al. Expression of differentiation antigens in mammary and extramammary Paget's disease. Br J Dermatol 1984; 110: 203.
9 Kariniemi AL, Ramaekers F, Lehto VP et al.

Paget cells express cytokeratins typical of glandular epithelia. Br J Dermatol 1985; 112: 179.

10 Kirkham N, Berry N, Jones DB et al. Paget's disease of the nipple. Immunohistochemical localization of milk fat globule membrane antigens. Cancer 1985; 55: 1510.

11 Lee AK, DeLellis RA, Rosen PP et al. Alpha-lactalbumin as an immunohistochemical marker for metastatic breast carcinomas. Am J Surg Pathol 1984; 8: 93.

12 Bussolati G, Pich A. Mammary and extra-mammary Paget's disease: An immunocytochemical study. Am J Pathol 1975; 80: 117.

13 Mazoujian G, Pinkus GS, Haagensen DE Jr. Extramammary Paget's disease—evidence for an apocrine origin. An immunoperoxidase study of gross cystic disease fluid protein—15, carcinoembryonic antigen, and keratin proteins. Am J Surg Pathol 1984; 8: 43.

14 Tamaki K, Hino H, Ohara K et al. Lectin-binding sites in Paget's disease. Br J Dermatol 1985; 113: 17.

15 Nadji M, Morales AR, Girtanner RE et al. Paget's disease of the skin. A unifying concept of histogenesis. Cancer 1982; 50: 2203.

16 Lagios MD, Westdahl PR, Rose MR et al. Paget's disease of the nipple. Alternative management in cases without or with minimal extent of underlying breast carcinoma. Cancer 1984; 54: 545.

17 Sagami S. Electron microscopic studies in Paget's disease. Med J Osaka Univ 1963; 14: 173.

18 Sagebiel R. Ultrastructural observations on epidermal cells in Paget's disease of the breast. Am J Pathol 1969; 57: 49.

19 Lagios MD, Westdahl PR, Rose MR. The concepts and implications of multicentricity in breast carcinoma. Path Ann 1981; 16: 83.

20 Paone JF, Baker RR. Pathogenesis and treatment of Paget's disease of the breast. Cancer 1981; 48: 825.

21 Lagios MD, Westdahl PR, Margolin FR et al. Duct carcinoma in situ. Relationship of extent of noninvasive disease to the frequency of occult invasion, multicentricity, lymph node metastases, and short term treatment failure. Cancer 1982; 50: 1309.

22 Shearman CP, Watts GT. Paget's disease of the nipple after subcutaneous mastectomy for cancer with primary reconstruction. Ann R Coll Surg Engl 1986; 68: 17.

23 Plowman PN, Gilmore OJ, Curling M et al. Paget's disease of the nipple occurring after conservation management of early infiltrating breast cancer. Br J Surg 1986; 73: 45.

24 Cheatle GL. Benign and malignant changes in duct epithelium of the breast. Br J Surg 1920/21; 8: 21.

Textbook of Uncommon Cancer
Edited by C.J. Williams, J.G. Krikorian, M.R. Green and D. Raghavan
© 1988 John Wiley & Sons Ltd

Chapter **40**

Breast Cancer with Osteoclast-like Giant Cells

Roland Holland and
Urbain J.G.M. van Haelst
*Department of Pathology, University Hospital of Nijmegen,
Nijmegen, The Netherlands*

HISTORY

Breast cancer with multinucleated osteoclast-like giant cells represents one of the rarest types of mammary carcinomas. Since 1931 less than 40 cases have been reported. The fact, however, that some 25 of them have been published in the last 4 years may point to an increasing incidence of this neoplasm in the population.

Leroux (1) in 1931 and Duboucher et al. (2) in 1933 described a peculiar mammary tumor which could be distinguished from other breast neoplasms by the presence of both benign multinucleated giant cells and a prominent stromal angiogenesis and hemorrhage. Leroux postulated that the giant cells might arise from stromal elements as a reaction to the malignant epithelium. In an electron microscopic study, Factor et al. (3) confirmed the histiocytic nature of the giant cells and suggested that they might develop as a reaction to some antigenic stimulus associated with the tumor. The authors further noted that this peculiar tumor should be differentiated from metaplastic carcinoma and extraskeletal osteoclastoma of the breast with similar giant cells, but clearly different overall histology. In a restrospective study of 8 cases, Agnantis and Rosen (4) postulated that the same tumor-associated antigenic stimulus might elicit both the marked angiogenesis and the giant cell formation. They reported the first cases in which visceral metasteses harbored giant cells similar to those in the primary tumor. In later studies the giant cells were also observed in axillary node metastases and in tumor emboli of intra-mammary lymphatics (5–7).

We, in our own series, were able to recognize a peculiar histologic pattern of the primary tumor and called it 'adenocystic' or cribriform (7).

Recently, the (immuno)histochemical studies of Bondeson (8), Nielsen and Kiaer (9), Ichijima et al. (10) proved the nonepithelial but histiocytic nature of the giant cells. The first case of a male patient was described by Bertrand et al. (11).

PATHOLOGY AND BIOLOGY

In Table 1 relevant pathologic and clinical data of 34 recently published cases are compiled. Grossly the tumor is in general well outlined, deep brown in colour (Figure 1) and it displays a round, well-circumscribed shadow on the mammogram (Figure 2) which is radiologically often taken for a fibroadenoma or a medullary carcinoma (7, 16). In most of

TABLE 1 SUMMARY OF CLINICAL AND PATHOLOGIC DATA OF RECENTLY PUBLISHED CASES

Reference	Patient's age (years)	Tumor's size (cm)	Tumor's margin	Colour and/or hemorrhage	Histologic pattern	Nodal status	Follow-up years and status
Factor et al. (3)	45	1.5	C	H	NSR	neg.	<1
	40	10	C	H	NSR	neg.	—
Agnantis and Rosen (4)	57	1.5	C	H	IDC	pos.	11 cause unknown
	50	0.5	C	H	ILC/IDC	neg.	2 alive with metastases
	43	3.6	MC	H	ILC	neg.	7 died of the disease
	48	5	ID	H	ILC/IDC	pos.	<1 died of the disease
	53	4	MC	H	IDC	neg.	<1 died of the disease
	46	3.6	ID	H	IDC	pos.	<1
	49	2	ID	H	IDC	neg.	<1
Levin et al. (6)	53	1.5	ID	H	IDC	pos.	1
Sugano et al. (12)	45	2	C	brown	IDC with tubular structures	—	2 NED
Bondeson (8)	57	1.7	C	brown	'tubular'	—	
Volpe et al. (13)	38	1.9	ID	H	IDC with tubular structures	neg.	<1
Holland and V Haelst (7)	55	2.5	C	brown	'adenocystic'/cribriform	neg.	8 NED
	54	6	C	brown	'adenocystic'/cribriform	neg.	6 NED
	38	4	MC	yellow-white	cribriform	pos.	5 alive with metastases
	39	2	C	brown	'adenocystic'/cribriform	neg.	4 alive with metastases
	40	2.5	C	brown	'adenocystic'/cribriform	pos.	4 NED
	32	1.2	C	brown	'adenocystic'/cribriform	pos.	4 NED
Kobayashi et al. (14)	59	3	C	brown	IDC with tubular structures	neg.	1.5 NED
Nielsen and Kiaer (9)	56	2.5	C	brown	IDC	neg.	2 NED
	71	1	ID	brown	IDC with tubular structures	neg.	1.5 NED
	79	4	ID	brown	IDC/mucoid	neg.	1.5 NED
Sharma and Banerjee (15)	35	3.5	C	brown	IDC with tubular structures	—	
Pettinato et al. (16)	44	2.7	C	grayish	'adenocystic'/solid	neg.	6 NED
	47	5	MC	brown	'solid'	pos.	5 NED
	48	1 .7	C	brown	'adenocystic'	neg.	4.5 NED
	53	3	C	brown	'adenocystic'	neg.	3.5 NED
	37	2.5	C	brown	'adenocystic'	pos.	<1
	47	2.2	C	brown	'adenocystic'	pos.	<1
Bertrand et al. (11)	52 (M)	1.3	C	brown	IDC	neg.	<1
Ischijima et al. (10)	41	0.5	MC	H	'tubular'	neg.	<1
	40	4	ID	H	IDC	pos.	1
	38	1	ID	—	papillary	neg.	9 NED

C: circumscribed; MC: moderately circumscribed; ID: ill-defined; H: hemorrhage; IDC: invasive ductal carcinoma; ILC: invasive lobular carcinoma; NSR: no special remarks; NED: no evidence of disease; M, male.

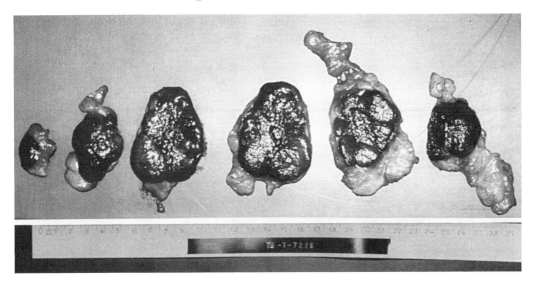

Figure 1 Characteristic gross appearance of the tumor in the tissue sections of the biopsy. A well-outlined lump with a diameter of 6 cm. The cut surface of the tumor was dark brown. *(Reproduced from reference 7 by permission of the editor of Cancer.)*

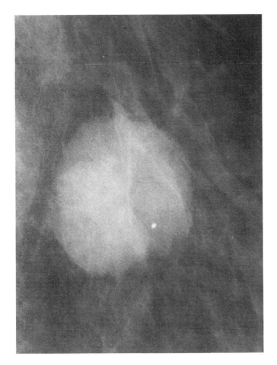

Figure 2 Magnification mammogram. This tumor displays a well-outlined round shadow reminiscent of that of a medullary carcinoma or a mucinous carcinoma. Original tumor size 1.5 cm. (Courtesy of Dr J.H.C.L. Hendriks.)

the cases the gross appearance of the tumor is characteristic enough to suggest the diagnosis.

Light Microscopic Findings

Fine Needle Aspiration Cytology

The basic cytology is characterized by three different types of cells: clusters of malignant epithelial cells, osteoclast-like multinucleated giant cells and solitary, large, mono- or binucleated cells (Figure 3). The epithelial cells are usually uniform and they have regular, oval nuclei with distinct but not especially large nucleoli and a thin rim of cytoplasm. The multinucleated giant cells, in contrast, show larger, more vesicular nuclei with more prominent nucleoli. They have abundant, often finely vacuolated cytoplasm. The mono- and binucleated cells are dispersed and they show nucleo-cytoplasmic features corresponding to those of the giant cells.

The coexistence of these three cell types is very characteristic and enables the cytologist, who is aware of this type of breast cancer, to reach the correct diagnosis (8, 11, 12, 16).

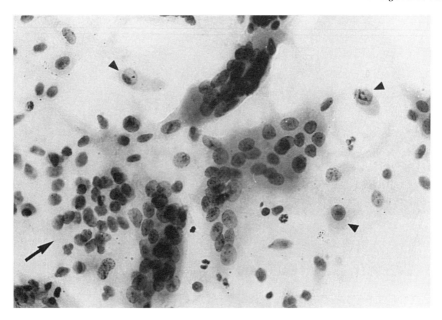

Figure 3 Fine needle aspirate showing carcinoma cell clusters (arrow), giant cells and mononucleated histiocytic cells (arrow heads) (Pap, original magnification: ×630).

Histology

In two recent papers, describing 12 cases, a distinct pattern of the invasive tumor growth has been reported (7, 16). This pattern has been called 'adenocystic' and it is characterized by tubular structures of varying sizes with round or ovoid lumina. These tubules lack myoepithelial cells on the periphery and their luminal face often shows cytoplasmic projections (apical snouts). The tubular structures are embedded in a markedly vascularized, often hemorrhagic, loose fibrous stroma (Figure 4). In other areas the tumor may display a more solid growth with branching nests and clusters of tumor cells around mucus filled lumina of different sizes (Figure 5). Earlier papers do not make a direct reference to a special growth pattern although in many of the histologic descriptions and in the illustrations the above mentioned patterns of invasive tumor can readily be recognized (3, 6, 8–15).

Obviously, the presence of the numerous multinucleated osteoclast-like giant cells is the most striking feature of the tumors (1–16). The cells histologically look benign. Their size ranges from 20 to 180 μm. The number of nuclei may vary from a few to some 40 per cent and they often show a vesicular aspect with a prominent nucleolus. The cytoplasm is well delineated, eosinophilic or amphophilic and finely granular. These cytologic features clearly differ from those of the tumor cells. On the other hand, there is a great similarity between the giant cells and the numerous mono- or binucleated polygonal cells situated intraluminally or in the stroma. They also have abundant cytoplasm with fine azurophilic granules and large, round nuclei with prominent nucleoli (Figures 5 and 6). Some of the giant cells and many of the mononuclear stromal cells contain Perls-positive iron pigment.

Bondeson (8) found nonspecific esterase activity in the giant cells in smears obtained by fine needle aspiration. However, in paraffin-embeded sections, Ichijima et al. (10) found a negative reaction in the giant cells whereas the

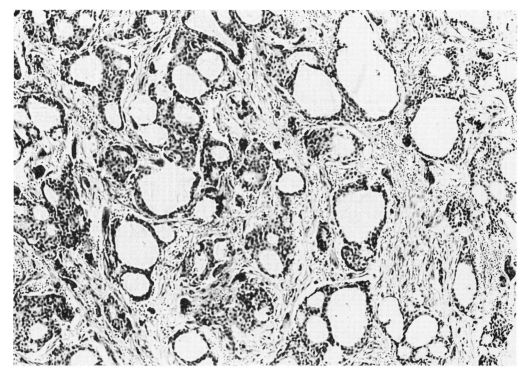

Figure 4 'Adenocystic' pattern of the invasive tumor growth with cystic tubular spaces. Scattered multinucleated giant cells in the highly vascularized stroma very close to the tubular structures (H&E. original magnification: ×100). (*Reproduced from reference 7 by permission of the editor of Cancer.*)

stromal and intraluminal mononucleated cells were positive. Acid phosphatase gave a strong reaction in both the giant cells and the mono-nucleated cells. In the same series of tumors the giant cells were negative with alkaline phosphatase and ATPase. Stains for S-100 protein, lysosyme, carcinoembryonic antigen, nonspecific cross-reacting antigen with carcinoembryonic antigen, α-1-antitrypsin, α-1-antichymotrypsin and keratin were also negative.

We had similar results in 2 recent cases, apart from a variably positive α-1-antitrypsin and α-1-antichymotrypsin reaction in both the giant and the mononuclear cells (Table 2). Nielsen and Kiaer (9) reported comparable results. Our histochemical studies demonstrated, in addition, that the positive mononuclear cells were situated not only intraluminally and in the stroma but also dispersed

among the epithelial tumor cells of the lobular structures.

The distinctive relationship between giant cells and cancer cells is noted in most recent publications. The giant cells are usually present both within the duct-like cystic spaces and in the stromal lacunae among clusters of tumor cells. A highly characteristic feature is an intimate relation between the tumor cell nests and the 'extraluminal' giant cells lying outside the tumor clusters. These giant cells are generally situated in the immediate vicinity of the marginal tumor cell row of the cluster (Figure 7) or occasionally virtually attached to it. Often pseudopodal extensions of giant cells enwrap nests of tumor cells (Figure 8). The opening of the epithelial boundary of the cystic spaces onto the stroma is another remarkable phenomenon which results in a direct contact

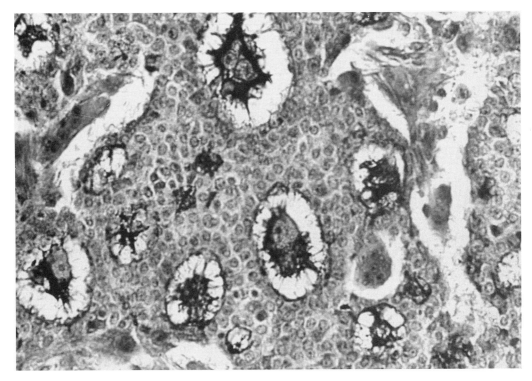

Figure 5 A more compact invasive growth of the tumor with cribriform aspect. Notice the multinucleated giant cells, the mononuclear histiocytic cells, and the mucus in the luminal spaces (PAS, original magnification: ×310). (*Reproduced from reference 7 by permission of the editor of Cancer.*)

between the lumina and the stroma on the one hand and in a continuous transition of the lining secretory cells of the duct-like spaces into the encircling cell row of the tumor cell nests on the other (Figures 9A, B).

Furthermore, the prominent vascularity and hemorrhage in the stroma is highly characteristic. Usually there is evidence of both past and recent bleeding. Nielsen and Kiaer (9) showed that some vessels were positive for factor VIII-related antigen whereas others, located in areas containing numerous giant cells, were negative. So far no explanation for this phenomenon has been given.

In the series of Agnantis and Rosen (4) the multinucleated giant cells were present in visceral metastases. We, in our series (7), observed both the giant cells and the mononuclear stromal cells in tumor emboli of intra-mammary lymphatic vessels (Figure 10) and in axillary node metastasis. Other authors as well reported on the presence of the giant cells in metastatic nodes (6, 10).

In most of the publications the carcinomatous component has been defined as ductal in origin. In only 4 cases a lobular carcinoma has been reported (4, 7), in 3 of which a combination with a ductal carcinoma was found. As alluded to above, in recent publications, a characteristic pattern of the invasive tumor has been outlined and called 'adenocystic' (7, 16). This type of tumor growth in fact does not fit comfortably in one of the two main groups of breast cancers, the ductal or the lobular. Admittedly, some tumors with more compact areas showing a cribriform-like pattern (Figure 5) suggest a ductal origin. On the other hand, even in these tumors, the neoplastic cells are characteristically small, uniform with

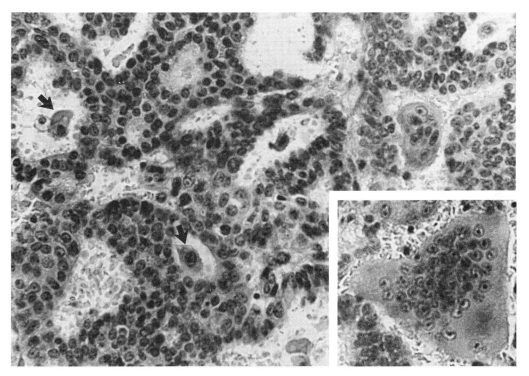

Figure 6 Mononuclear histiocytes (arrows) and multinucleated giant cell in invasive tumor growth. Inset: Another giant cell. Notice the cytologic similarity between the multinucleated giant cells and the mononuclear phagocytes. Both cells have vesicular nuclei with prominent nucleoli, and their cytoplasm shows similar density. The tumor cells lack these cytologic features (H&E, original magnification: ×310). (*Reproduced from reference 7 by permission of the editor of Cancer.*)

TABLE 2 RESULTS OF HISTOCHEMICAL AND IMMUNOHISTOCHEMICAL REACTIONS

	Giant cells	Mononuclear stromal cells	Tumor cells
Acid phosphatase	++	++	−
Anti-S-100 protein	−	−	−
α-1-antitrypsin	±	±	−
α-1-antichymotrypsin	±	±	−
Anti-keratin	−	−	+
Anti-vimentin	+	+	−

round nuclei and with few mitoses. Both intraductal (3, 4, 7, 16) and in situ lobular carcinoma (4, 7) have been found adjacent to the invasive tumor. Nevertheless, it seems most appropriate to consider these tumors as a special variant of a well- or moderately differentiated invasive ductal carcinoma.

Electron Microscopic Findings

The most striking ultrastructural feature of the multinucleated giant cells, observed by various authors (3, 7–10, 12, 14, 16), concerns the abundance of cytoplasmic organelles; that is, the large number of diffusely distributed mitochondria and free polyribosomes as well as the stacks of rough endoplasmic reticulum, often oriented towards the periphery of the cell (Figure 11). There are also numerous, membrane-bound, lysosome-like electron-dense bodies scattered throughout the cytoplasm. The nuclei are mostly irregular in shape with deep invaginations of the nuclear membrane.

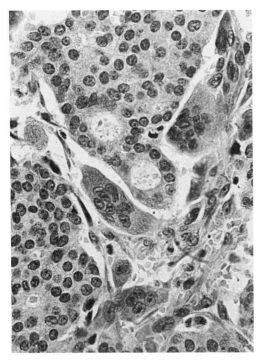

Figure 7 Multinuleated giant cells in the immediate vicinity of the tumor cell clusters (H&E,
original magnification: ×390). (*Reproduced
from reference 7 by permission of the editor of
Cancer.*)

They contain one or two prominent nucleoli. The cell surface of the giant cells is covered by microvilli or by short, irregular cytoplasmic processes. The extent of the development of these microvilli differs according to whether the giant cell is situated in the luminal spaces or in the stroma. The intraluminal giant cells have mostly a highly developed microvillous surface (Figure 12), while the giant cells situated in the stroma around the tumor cell nests have less developed and shorter micro-villi. There is often an interdigitation between the microvilli of these 'extraluminal' giant cells and the microvilli of the neighboring tumor cells indicating the close contact between the two types of cells (Figure 11).

There is an obvious similarity in the ultra-structure of the multinucleated giant cells and certain mononuclear cells situated either intra-luminally or in the stroma. These mononuclear cells also show abundant cytoplasmic orga-nelles, lysosomes, and irregular cytoplasmic borders with microvilli, reminiscent of the mononuclear histiocytes (Figure 13). In con-trast there is a significant difference between

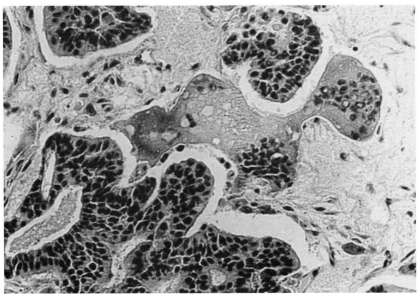

Figure 8 A bizarre giant cell with pseudopodal process. Notice the close contact
between the giant cell and the tumor cell clusters. The giant cell forms an imprint
around the tumor cell nests (H&E, original magnification: ×310). (*Reproduced
from reference 7 by permission of the editor of Cancer.*)

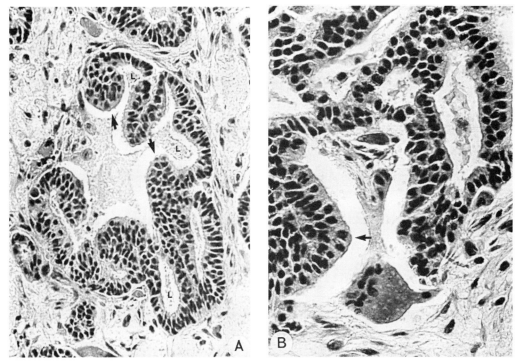

Figure 9A and 9B The opening of ductal lumina (L) of the tumor onto the stroma. Notice the continuous transition of the lining secretory cells of the previous duct into the external cell row of the tumor cell nest (arrows) (H&E, original magnification ×240). B, The same phenomenon on higher magnification. Penetration of loose stromal fibrous tissue into the original lumen. A giant cell is situated just in the opening (H&E, original magnification: ×500). (Compare this figure with the ultrastructural observations of Figure 15.) (*Reproduced from reference 7 by permission of the editor of Cancer.*)

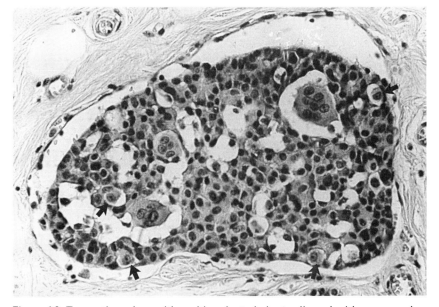

Figure 10 Tumor thrombus with multinucleated giant cells and with mononuclear phagocytes (arrows) in an intramammary lymphatic vessel (H&E, original magnification: ×310).

796 R. Holland and U.J.G.M. van Haelst

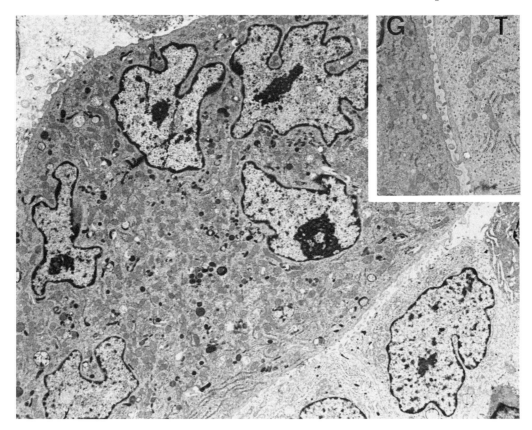

Figure 11 Electron micrograph of an 'extraluminal' multinucleated giant cell in close apposition to tumor cells in the lower right corner. The giant cell shows abundant cytoplasmic organelles (mitochondria, polyribosomes, lysosome-like electron-dense bodies, and rough endoplasmic reticulum), and nuclei with invaginations and prominent nucleoli. In contrast, the tumor cell shows a relative paucity of cytoplasmic organelles and unremarkable nucleolus (uranyl acetate and lead citrate, original magnification: ×5700). Inset: Interdigitating microvilli on the boundary of the giant cell (G) and the tumor cells (T). Notice the absence of a basal membrane (uranyl acetate and lead citrate, original magnification: ×10 000).

the ultrastructural features of the giant cells and the tumor cells, which was noted by all of the authors mentioned above, except one (14). The tumor cells have fewer cytoplasmic organelles, more regular nuclei, and unremarkable nucleoli. They are joined by desmosomal attachment (Figure 14). Some observers (3, 10) report the basement membrane around the tumor cell nests to be partially present, others (7, 9, 12, 16) as completely absent. The duct-like spaces are lined by the microvilli of tumor cells and contain mostly amorphous material, erythrocytes and often the mononuclear histio-

cytic cells or multinucleated giant cells described above. The opening of the ductal spaces onto the stroma has also been observed electron microscopically (Figure 15).

Steroid Receptors

The steroid hormone receptor protein levels of the tumors in our own series (7) provided a further discriminating feature since all but one tumor showed very low estrogen receptor (ER) levels (less than 14 fmol/mg protein), all of them had high progesterone receptor (PgR)

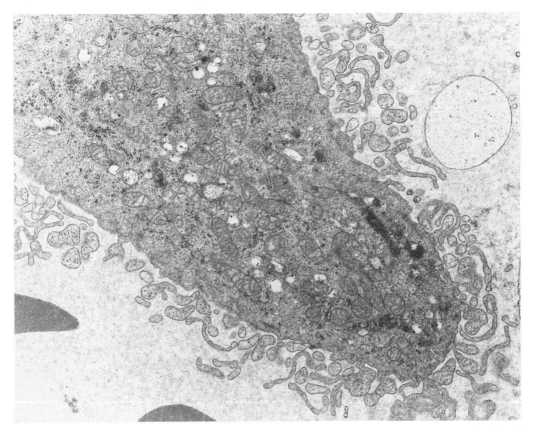

Figure 12 Electron micrograph of an 'intraluminal' giant cell marked by highly developed microvillous cytoplasmic surface (uranyl acetate and lead citrate, original magnification: ×15 600).

levels (average 270 fmol/mg protein) and, thus, very high ratios between the ER and PgR assays. Bertrand et al. (11) reported similar results in one female and one male patient. So far, this remarkable hormone receptor pattern of the tumors has not been explained.

The Origin of the Multinucleated Giant Cells

In his original description of 1931, Leroux (1) suggested that the giant cells are histiocytic in origin. Factor et al. (3) and later observers (7–10, 16) demonstrated the light and electron microscopic similarity of the mononuclear stromal cells and giant cells and proved the histiocytic origin of both. Only Kobayashi et al. (14) claimed that the giant cells might originate from the malignant epithelium. Recent studies reporting on the strong acid phosphatase (10) and nonspecific esterase reaction (8) in both cell types, provide further support to the histiocytic nature of these elements. The negative S-100 protein reaction indicates that these histiocytic cells do not belong to the T-zone lineage. There is ample evidence for the development of benign multinucleated giant cells by fusion of mononuclear histiocytes in different tumorous and granulomatous processes (17–21). Also in the present tumor, the giant cells most likely originate by fusion of the histiocytic mononuclear stromal cells.

The presence of the giant cells in different

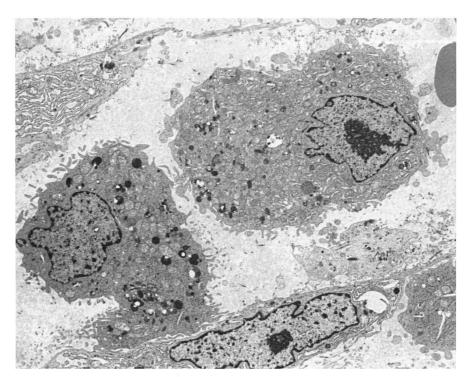

Figure 13 Two large mononuclear cells of histiocytic nature lying outside the lumina in the stroma of the tumor between myofibroblasts. Notice the ultrastructural similarity between these histiocytic cells and the giant cell of Figure 11 (uranyl acetate and lead citrate, original magnification: ×6200).

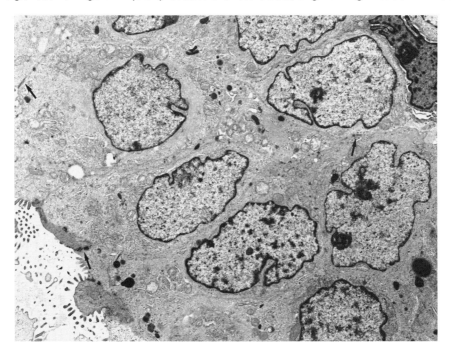

Figure 14 Electron micrograph of tumor cells lining a ductal space. The nuclei of these cells are uniform with unremarkable nucleoli. There is a relative scarcity of cytoplasmic organelles. Compare these cells with the giant cell in Figure 11. Desmosomes and tight junctions are present (arrows) between the neoplastic cells (uranyl acetate and lead citrate, original magnification: ×7800). (*Reproduced from reference 7 by permission of the editor of Cancer.*)

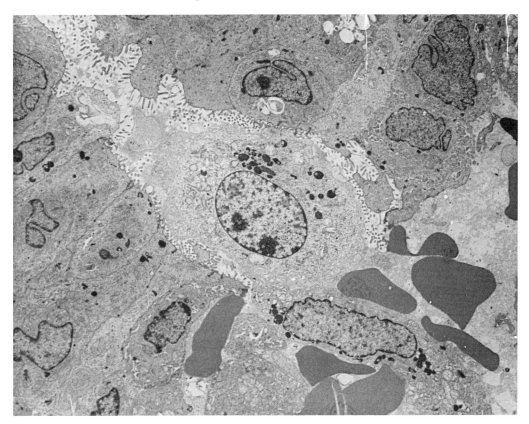

Figure 15 Opening of the lumen of a duct-like space lined by tumor cells, and containing erythrocytes as well as histiocytic cells (uranyl acetate and lead citrate, original magnification: ×5200). (*Reproduced from reference 7 by permission of the editor of Cancer.*)

sites of the metastic tumors (4, 6, 7, 10) indicates that they constitute an integral part of the neoplasm.

The intimate association of the giant cells with the tumor cell groups has been another puzzling feature of these tumors. It has been proposed that the tumor cells might produce some substances capable of eliciting giant cell formation and marked stromal angiogenesis (4). Some of our own observations provide further support to this concept (7). Firstly, the majority of the giant cells and the most pronounced stromal angiogenesis were concentrated in those areas where the tumor showed the most extensive secretion, that is, in the 'adenocystic' structures. Secondly, many of the giant cells and their probably precursors, the mononuclear histiocytes, were situated in

the luminal spaces in direct contact with the secretion produced by the tumor cells. Thirdly, the opening of the cystic spaces onto the stroma enabled a direct contact between the secretory cells and the stroma, in which tumor cells often maintained their villous surface without a delimiting basal membrane. It was on these boundaries between cell nests and stroma where the giant cells regularly appeared.

CLINICAL FINDINGS

The data of 34 recently published cases (Table 1) show that the patients are relatively young. Sixty-four percent were less than 50 years old. Data on the stage of the tumor at diagnosis fail to indicate a favourable prognosis if compared with those of the usual types of invasive breast cancer. Thirteen out of 32 women (41%) had axillary node metastasis. Out of 31 patients with an average follow-up of 3 years (range 1 to 11 years), 3 patients died of the disease, 2 patients had distant metastasis and one had a local recurrence. Obviously much longer follow-up is needed in this series of relatively young patients for a proper evaluation of the ultimate prognosis of this special type of mammary carcinoma.

REFERENCES

1 Leroux R. Réaction giganto cellulaire du stroma dans un épithélioma mammaire. Bull Cancer (Paris) 1931; 20: 692–7.
2 Duboucher H, Montpellier J, Laffargue F. Épithélioma mammaire avec réaction de type myéloplaxique. Ann Anat Pathol 1933; 70: 787-91.
3 Factor SM, Biempica L, Ratner I, Ahuja KK, Biempica S. Carcinoma of the breast with multinucleated reactive stromal giant cells: A light and electron microscopic study of two cases. Virchows Arch (Pathol Anat) 1977; 374: 1–12.
4 Agnantis NT, Rosen PP. Mammary carcinoma with osteoclast-like giant cells: A study of eight cases with follow-up data. Am J Clin Pathol 1979; 72: 383–9.
5 Bertrand G, Bidabe MCl, Bertrand AF. Le carcinome mammaire à stroma-réaction giganto-cellulaire. Etude cytologique, histologique, ultrastructurale et immunocytochimique de deux observations. Arch Anat Cytol Path 1982; 30: 5–9.
6 Levin A, Rywlin AM, Tachmes P. Carcinoma of the breast with stromal epulis-like giant cells. South Med J 1981; 74: 889–91.
7 Holland R, van Haelst UJGM. Mammary carcinoma with osteoclast-like giant cells. Additional observations on six cases. Cancer 1984; 53: 1963–73.
8 Bondeson L. Aspiration cytology of breast carcinoma with multinucleated reactive stromal giant cells. Acta Cytol 1984; 28: 313–16.

9 Nielsen BB, Kiaer HW. Carcinoma of the breast with stromal multinucleated giant cells. Histopathology 1985; 9: 183–93.
10 Ichijima K, Kobashi Y, Ueda Y, Matsuo S. Breast cancer with reactive multinucleated giant cells: report of three cases. Acta Pathol Jpn 1986; 36: 449–7.
11 Bertrand G, George P, Bertrand AF. Carcinome mammaire a stroma-réaction giganto-cellulaire. Premier cas masculin. Ann Pathol 1986; 6: 144–7.
12 Sugano I, Nagao K, Kondo Y, Nabeshima S, Murakami S. Cytologic and ultrastructural studies of a rare breast carcinoma with osteoclast-like giant cells. Cancer 1983; 52: 74–8.
13 Volpe R, Carbone A, Nicolo G, Santi L. Cytology of a breast carcinoma with osteoclast-like giant cells. Acta Cytol 1983; 27: 184–7.
14 Kobayashi S, Tobioka N, Samoto T, Kobayashi M, Iwase H, Masaoka A, Nakamura T, Shibata H, Amoh H, Matsuyama M. Breast cancer with osteoclast-like multinucleated giant cells. Acta Pathol Jpn 1984; 34: 1475–84.
15 Sharma SC, Banerjee AK. Osteoclast-like giant cells in breast carcinoma. Indian J Pathol Microbiol 1985; 28: 281–3.
16 Pettinato G, Petrella G, Manco A, di Prisco B, Salvatore G, Angrisani P. Carcinoma of the breast with osteoclast-like giant cells. Fine-needle aspiration cytology, histology and electron microscopy of 5 cases. Appl Pathol 1984; 2: 168–78.
17 Schajowicz F. Giant-cell tumors of bone (osteoclastoma): A pathological and histochemical study. J Bone Joint Surg (Am) 1961; 43: 1–29.
18 Silverman L, Shorter RG. Histogenesis of the multinucleated giant cell. Lab Invest 1963; 12: 985–90.
19 Hanaoka H, Friedman B, Mack RP. Ultrastructure and histogenesis of giant-cell tumor of bone. Cancer 1970; 25: 1408–23.
20 Mariano M, Spector WG. The formation and properties of macrophage polykaryons (inflammatory giant cells). J Pathol 1974; 113: 1–19.
21 Chambers TJ. Multinucleate giant cells. J Pathol 1978; 126: 125–48.

Textbook of Uncommon Cancer
Edited by C.J. Williams, J.G. Krikorian, M.R. Green and D. Raghavan
© 1988 John Wiley & Sons Ltd

Chapter **41**

Adenoid Cystic Carcinoma of the Breast

George N. Peters
*Department of Surgery, Baylor University Medical Center
and Sammons Cancer Center, Dallas, Texas, USA*

INTRODUCTION

Adenoid cystic carcinoma of the breast is rare and has a biological course of slow progression, local recurrence if inadequately resected, and near absence of lymph node metastases. Less than 1% of all mammary cancers are adenoid cystic (1). Billroth named this tumor 'cylindroma' in 1856 because of the well-defined cylinders of connective tissue that encased the epithelial tumor elements (2). Other synonyms include adenocystic basal cell carcinoma, adenomyoepithelioma, adenocystic carcinoma, and pseudoadenomatous basal cell carcinoma (3). Spies is credited with the term adenoid cystic carcinoma (4).

Adenoid cystic carcinoma is most frequently seen in the major and minor salivary glands. Other sites where similar tumors have been reported include the lacrimal glands, external ear, upper respiratory passage, esophagus, Bartholin gland, cervix uteri, and prostate gland. Extramammary adenoid cystic carcinoma is exemplified by a prolonged clinical course, late local recurrence, and ultimately, distant metastases and death (5). The 5-year survival in extramammary adenoid cystic carcinoma is approximately 30% and nearly one-third of the patients have regional or distant metastases at the time of initial treatment (1).

The prognosis of adenoid cystic carcinoma of the breast, in contrast, is excellent.

CLINICAL FEATURES

Up until 1977, only 95 well-documented cases had been reported in the literature (5). Since then at least another 50 cases have been documented (6–20). At the time of diagnosis, the patients ranged from 31 to 80 years of age. The presenting symptom usually is a well-demarcated, movable mass that may be tender if there is growth in the perineural spaces.

Although adenoid cystic carcinoma of the breast has a predilection for perineural infiltration, Anthony and James postulate that the tenderness is due to contractility of the myoepithelial component (21). The tumor is small with a mean diameter of 2 to 3 cm; however, a tumor up to 22 cm in size has been reported (11). These tumors occur preferentially in the area of the nipple areola with at least 26% of the reported tumors being situated beneath or adjacent to the areola. The incidence may be higher, as only a few of the reports address the location of the tumor (5–7, 10–13, 15). Although there is frequent occurrence of these tumors in the area of the areola, only two cases of bloody nipple discharge have been reported

801

(5). Fixation to the skin, nipple retraction, or invasion of the pectoral muscle are uncommon. Of the 145 cases reported in the literature, only 5 have been reported in males (5, 6). No bilateral adenoid cystic carcinomas have been reported and there is no predilection for either the left or right breast.

PATHOLOGIC FEATURES

Grossly, the tumors are roughly circumscribed, although none are encapsulated. The color of the tumor has been variably described as grey, tan, reddish grey, yellowish white with fibrous streaks, or yellowish tan with grey mucoid areas. Usually there is a yellowish hue to the tumor mass. The consistency is less hard than the usual breast cancer. On sectioning the tumor, cystic areas may be noted or the tumor may be grossly lobulated (14).

The overall microscopic pattern of adenoid cystic carcinoma of the breast is identical to that seen in the salivary gland, upper respiratory tract, and other sites. It consists of multi- ple rounded nodules of small uniform cells within which there are many small, empty spaces in a sieve-like pattern (Figure 1) (22–23).

The microscopic appearance may be quite variable in the same lesion, with examination of many fields before a classical cylindromatous and/or cribriform pattern is identified. In the histologic pattern there is a classic relationship between cells that are small, have sparse cytoplasm and uniformly hyperchromatic nuclei, and lack prominent nucleoli and stroma which is acidophilic, myxoid, or hyaline (Figure 2). The growth pattern of tumor cells within the stroma may appear cribriform, gland-forming, ductular, trabecular, or as solid masses. The stroma surrounding nests of tumor tends to be continuous with the hyalinized cores of cribriform areas occupied by either hyaline or mucoid material (Figure 3). These cores are the cylinders that are responsible for the synonym 'cylindroma'. Usually one sees the characteristic double row of epithelial cells lining ductular structures that

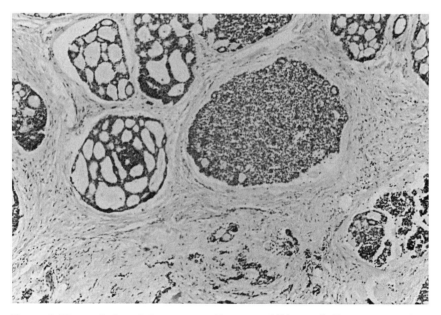

Figure 1 The majority of the tumor cell nests exhibit a cribriform pattern, but occasional solid units and tubular structures may be seen (HP&S, original magnification: ×150).

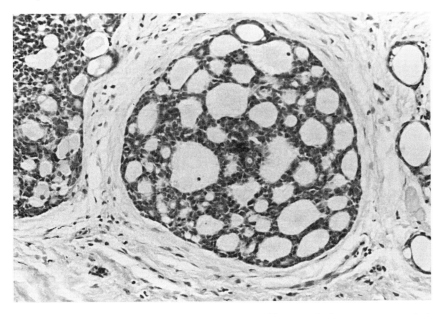

Figure 2 Typical cylindromatous pattern produced by rounded spaces surrounded by small basaloid cells with hyperchromatic nuclei (HP&S, original magnification: ×150).

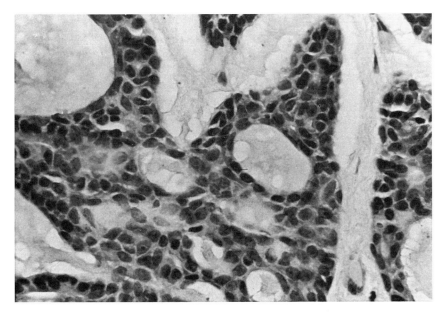

Figure 3 The majority of cystic spaces are pseudocysts continuous with the stroma surrounding the epithelial units and containing extracellular matrix varying from mucinous to hyaline (HP&S, original magnification: ×150).

are filled with myxoid material (14). These tumors are composed of two morphologic cell types: (1) cuboidal epithelial cells that line tubular duct-like structures containing neutral polysaccharides (PAS positive); (2) myoepithelial cells that elaborate acid mucopolysaccharides (alcian blue positive), giving rise to a cylindromatous appearance, focally or throughout the tumor (Figure 4) (20). Ultrastructural studies have shown that the cysts which give the tumor its name are extracellular compartments lined by a basement membrane and filled with material derived from the lamina densa (Figure 5). True ducts and intercellular spaces containing cilia are seen infrequently and there is no evidence of secreting activity in tumor cells (24).

SIMILARITY TO OTHER BREAST CANCERS

Despite its characteristic histology, adenoid cystic carcinoma can be confused with other more common breast cancers such as infiltrat-

ing duct carcinoma with a cribriform pattern, papillary carcinoma, and mucinous carcinoma. Harris described a case of cribriform intraductal carcinoma that closely resembled adenoid cystic carcinoma. Electron microscopy was used in making the differentiation. The 'pseudocysts' that are characteristic of adenoid cystic carcinomas were absent. Therefore, he determined that this was an intraductal carcinoma which he termed pseudoadenoid cystic carcinoma of the breast (25). Histologically some adenoid cystic carcinomas of the breast may bear a vague resemblance to carcinoid tumors, but Grimelius stain can help rule out any confusing cases (14, 20).

BIOLOGICAL BEHAVIOR

Adenoid cystic carcinoma of the breast (145 reported cases to date) has an excellent prognosis. As previously stated, the incidence of this rare mammary carcinoma is quoted to be less than 1%, yet a recent review of the Connecti-

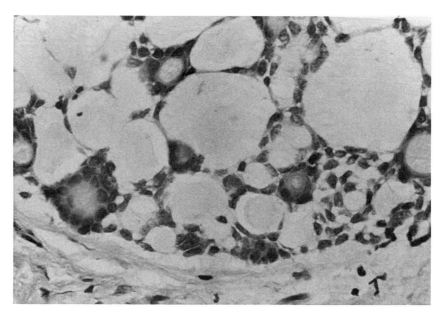

Figure 4 The biphasic cell differentiation into basaloid myoepithelial cells surrounding cylinders and cuboidal tubular cells around true glandular lumina, characterize adenoid cystic carcinoma, differentiating it from cribriform, ductal carcinoma (HP & S, original magnification: ×150).

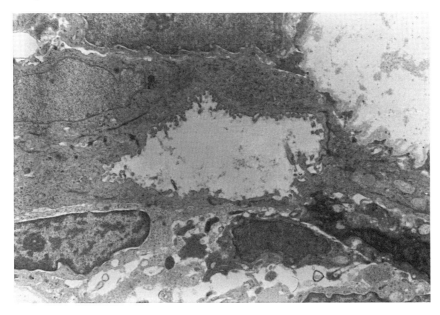

Figure 5 Electron photomicrograph showing a true lumen (in the center) and the more common pseudocyst containing basement membrane-like material (upper right corner) (original magnification: ×11 000).

cut Tumor Registry showed that the incidence was much lower (< 0.1%) (20). It is important to distinguish this cancer from other forms of breast cancer because of its excellent prognosis.

Axillary metastases at initial treatment have been reported in only 2 cases (19, 26). Several authors have cautioned against confusing adenoid cystic carcinoma with intraductal carcinoma with a cribriform pattern (21, 25, 27). Steinman et al. (7) questioned whether a second primary neoplasm might have been responsible for the metastases in the first case reported by Verani and Bel-Kahn (26). Peters and Wolff (14) suggested that this was not an adenoid cystic carcinoma, but a variant of papillary and cribriform carcinoma. The tumor contained areas of necrosis and psammoma bodies, both of which are features not considered typical of adenoid cystic carcinoma. In the second reported adenoid cystic carcinoma with axillary metastases, diagnosis was conclusive using immunocytochemistry and electron microscopy. All twelve nodes recovered contained metastatic disease,

including one node with a classic pattern of adenoid cystic carcinoma. It should be pointed out that the tumor had been present for 10–20 years and at diagnosis it was a 10 cm fungating tumor in the upper outer quadrant of the breast. Pulmonary metastases were also present. Except in a few rare cases, most of the literature has documented tumors less than 3 cm.

Only 10 cases of local recurrence in 8 patients have been documented (1, 5, 14, 18, 28–29). Two patients who initially had simple mastectomies each recurred twice. Six patients who initially had local excisions also had recurrences. Intervals from initial treatment to recurrence ranged from 6 months to 22 years. Subsequent treatment included wide excision, simple mastectomy, resection of the pectoralis muscles and axillary contents en bloc, and modified radical mastectomy. All patients were alive and well after treatment of the local recurrence.

In the literature there are now 9 cases of reported distant metastases (8, 14, 18, 19, 26,

30–32). Metastases to the lung were noted in all 9 patients; other sites of involvement included the liver, vertebrae, hilar nodes, inferior vena cava, and brain. In the only reported case of brain metastases, the patient lived 5 years after craniotomy and total excision of the tumor and was then lost to follow-up (18). Only 5 patients have died of metastatic disease. Smith (33) noted that late complications (local recurrences and/or distant metastases) occurred only in patients where primary excision was incomplete. Although 6 of the 8 initial recurrences had local excision in the breast, all 9 with distant metastases originally had either radical or modified radical mastectomies. The low incidence of local recurrence, distant metastases, and death in mammary adenoid cystic carcinoma is believed to be due to the slow growth and lack of aggressiveness of this tumor in the breast (Table 1).

Zaloudek et al. (15) did not detect either estrogen or progesterone receptors in three neoplasms that were tested. Kern (9) reported the only estrogen receptor positive tumor in the literature. When occurring in conjunction with other histologic types of breast carcinoma, the prognosis is that of the histologic type.

PROGNOSIS

Although histologically almost indistinguishable from extramammary adenocystic carcinoma, it has a much better prognosis in the

TABLE 1 SUMMARY OF 145 REPORTED CASES OF ADENOID CYSTIC CARCINOMA OF THE BREAST[a]

	No. of patients	Per cent
Axillary metastases	1[b]	<1.0
Local recurrence	8[c]	5.0
Distant metastases	9	6.0
Mortality	5	3.0

[a] Incidence 0.1–1.0%
[b] Although 2 patients have been reported with axillary metastases, there is debate whether one was from adenoid cystic carcinoma.
[c] 2 patients recurred locally twice.

breast. Whereas 5-year survival is 30% in extramammary carcinoma, in the breast only 5 patients (3%) have died from their breast cancer. Two patients died within 5 years of initial diagnosis and 3 died 11, 12 and 14 years respectively after initial diagnosis. Of the 8 patients who developed local recurrence, all were alive and disease free 10 years from initial diagnosis, except for one patient who was alive with pulmonary metastases. This patient subsequently developed brain metastases but was alive 5 years after craniotomy. A second patient developed a second local recurrence 10 years after the first recurrence.

Why adenoid cystic carcinoma of the breast is less malignant than in extramammary sites is obscure. Favorable prognosis has been attributed to the small size of breast tumors, ease of total excision of tumors in the breast compared to other sites, and a slower growth of the tumor in the breast than in similar tumors in other sites (1). Since the tumor has a chronic, slow and benign course, treatment of distant metastases from adenoid cystic carcinoma of the breast should be different from treatment in other breast cancers.

TREATMENT

Sumpio et al. (20) have suggested that wide, local excision could be curative because of the prolonged clinical course, good prognosis, and almost nonexistent lymph node involvement. However, due to the documented, albeit low, recurrence of the tumor after local excision, and because of evidence of microscopic tumor infiltration in the surrounding tissue, most authors would recommend simple mastectomy. Axillary dissection should be done only if clinically indicated. Annual physical examination and annual chest x-ray should be essential follow-up because of the possibility of local recurrence and because all patients with distant metastases had pulmonary involvement. Although one patient with pulmonary metastases had no response to radiation or chemotherapy, no conclusion can be drawn as to the effectiveness of these modalities in metastatic disease because of the inherent slow progress of the disease and because of the paucity of patients having these treatments (18).

ACKNOWLEDGEMENTS

The author wants to thank Dr Daniel Savino, Department of Surgical Pathology, Baylor University Medical Center, for his assistance in compiling and photographing the micrographs of adenoid cystic carcinoma of the breast. Also a special thanks to Ms Rose Kraft and Ms Vicki Jackson-High, Scientific Publications Office, Baylor Research Foundation, for their assistance on the manuscript.

REFERENCES

1 Cavanzo FS, Taylor HB. Adenoid cystic carcinoma of the breast. Cancer 1969; 24: 740-5.
2 Billroth T. Die Cylindergeschwalst Untersuchungen ueber die Entwicklung der Blutgefasse. Berlin: G. Reimer, 1856.
3 Groshong LE. Adenocystic carcinoma of the breast. Arch Surg 1966; 92: 424-7.
4 Spies J. Adenoid cystic carcinoma. Arch Surg 1930; 21: 365-404.
5 Qizilbash AH, Patterson MC, Oliveira KF. Adenoid cystic carcinoma of the breast. Arch Pathol Lab Med 1977; 101: 302-6.
6 Hjorth S, Magnuson PH, Blomquist P. Adenoid cystic carcinoma of the breast. Report of a case in a male and review of the literature. Acta Chir Scand 1977; 143: 155-8.
7 Steinman A, Martin P, McSwain G. Adenoid carcinoma of the breast. Southern Med J 1978; 71: 851-3.
8 Lim SK, Kevi J, Warner OG. Adenoid cystic carcinoma of the breast with metastasis: A case report and review of the literature. J Natl Med Assoc 1979; 71: 329-30.
9 Kern WH. Morphologic and clinical aspects of estrogen receptors in carcinoma of the breast. Surg Gynecol Obstet 1979; 148: 240-2.
10 Prioleau PG, Santa Cruz DJ, Buettner JB et al. Sweat gland differentiation in mammary adenoid cystic carcinoma. Cancer 1979; 43: 1752-60.
11 O'Connor T, Cornell D, Lohman H et al. Adenoid cystic carcinoma of the breast. A case report. Alabama J Med Sci 1982; 19: 17-18.
12 Lawrence JB, Mazur MT. Adenoid cystic carcinoma. A comparative pathologic study of tumors in salivary gland, breast, lung, and cervix. Hum Pathol 1982; 13: 916-23.
13 Jaworski R, Kneale KL, Ross CS. Adenoid cystic carcinoma of the breast. Postgrad Med J 1983; 59: 48-51.
14 Peters GN, Wolff M. Adenoid cystic carcinoma of the breast. Report of 11 new cases: Review of the literature and discussion of biological behavior. Cancer 1983; 52: 680-6.
15 Zaloudek C, Oertel YC, Orenstein JM. Adenoid cystic carcinoma of the breast. Am J Clin Pathol 1984; 81: 297-307.
16 Gibbs NM. Comparative study of the histopathology of breast cancer in a screened and unscreened population investigated by mammography. Histopathology 1985; 9: 1307-18.
17 Tavassoli FA, Norris HJ. Mammary adenoid cystic carcinoma with sebaceous differentiation. A morphologic study of the cell types. Arch Pathol Lab Med 1986; 110: 1045-53.
18 Koller M, Ram Z, Findler G et al. Brain metastasis. A rare manisfestation of adenoid cystic carcinoma of the breast. Surg Neurol 1986; 26: 470-2.
19 Wells CA, Nicoll S, Ferguson DJP. Adenoid cystic carcinoma of the breast: a case with axillary lymph node metastasis. Histopathology 1986; 10: 415-24.
20 Sumpio BE, Jennings TA, Sullivan PD et al. Adenoid cystic carcinoma of the breast. Data from the Connecticut Tumor Registry and a review of the literature. Ann Surg 1987; 205: 295-301.
21 Anthony PP, James PD. Adenoid cystic carcinoma of the breast. Prevalance, diagnostic criteria, and histogenesis. J Clin Pathol 1975; 28: 647-55.
22 Haagensen CD. Adenoid cystic carcinoma of the breast. In: Haagensen CD ed Diseases of the Breast, 3rd edition. Philadelphia: WB Saunders, 1986: 833-42.
23 Gallager HS. Pathologic types of breast cancer: Their prognosis. Cancer 1984; 53: 623-9.
24 Kess LG, Brannan CD, Ashikari R. Histologic and ultrastructural features of adenoid cystic carcinoma of the breast. Cancer 1970; 26: 1271-9.
25 Harris M. Pseudoadenoid cystic carcinoma of the breast. Arch Pathol Lab Med 1977; 101: 307-9.
26 Verani RR, Bel-Kahn J. Mammary adenoid cystic carcinoma with unusual features. Am J Clin Pathol 1973; 59: 653-8.
27 Galloway JR, Woolner LB, Clagett OT. Adenoid cystic carcinoma of the breast. Surg Gynecol Obstet 1966; 122: 1289-94.
28 Wilson WB, Spell JP. Adenoid cyst carcinoma of

breast: A case with recurrence and regional metastasis. Ann Surg 1967; 166: 861–4.

29 Lusted D. Structure and growth patterns of adenoid cystic carcinoma of the breast. Am J Clin Pathol 1970; 54: 419–25.

30 Nayer HR. Cylindroma of the breast with pulmonary metastases. Dis Chest 1957; 31: 324–7.

31 O'Kell RT. Adenoid cystic carcinoma of the breast. Mod Med 1964, 61: 855–8.

32 Elsner B. Adenoid cystic carcinoma of the breast. Review of the literature and clinicopathologic study of seven patients. Pathol Eur 1970; 5: 357–64.

33 Smith LC, Lane N, Rankow RM. Cylindroma (adenoid cystic carcinoma). A report of 58 cases. Am J Surg 1965; 110: 519–26.

Textbook of Uncommon Cancer
Edited by C.J. Williams, J.G. Krikorian, M.R. Green and D. Raghavan
© 1988 John Wiley & Sons Ltd

Chapter **42**

Neuroendocrine Carcinomas of the Breast

Henry F. Frierson, Jr* and
Stacey E. Mills†

*Assistant Professor of Pathology, University of Virginia
Medical Center, Charlottesville, Virginia, USA and
†Associate Professor of Pathology, University of Virginia
Medical Center, Charlottesville, Virginia, USA

OVERVIEW

A clinically and histologically diverse group of primary mammary carcinomas has features that suggest neuroendocrine differentiation. These neoplasms contain argyrophilic granules as observed histochemically (using Grimelius, Pascual, Churukian–Schenk, or Sevier–Munger stains), have membrane-bound, dense-core 'neurosecretory' granules by electron microscopy, or produce one or more hormones inappropriate to mammary tissue. This chapter will review four subgroups of mammary carcinoma with neuroendocrine features. The first section deals with carcinomas having a carcinoid-like light microscopic appearance. The second section reviews mammary carcinomas associated with aberrant hormone production. The third section discusses the rare primary small cell undifferentiated (oat cell) carcinoma of the breast. In the final section, neuroendocrine tumors metastatic to the breast, including true carcinoid tumor and oat cell carcinoma, are summarized.

MAMMARY CARCINOMAS WITH A CARCINOID-LIKE HISTOLOGIC APPEARANCE

History

In 1963, Feyrter and Hartmann documented 2 argyrophilic mucinous memmary neoplasms that they regarded as primary carcinoid tumors, based on light microscopic features (1). This report was largely ignored until 1977, when Cubilla and Woodruff described 8 neoplasms that were considered to be primary carcinoids of the breast, based on an organoid pattern of growth histologically, argyrophilia, and ultrastructural evidence of membrane-bound, dense-core granules (2).

Other reports of mammary carcinoma with carcinoid-like features followed (3–5). Kaneko et al. described bilateral carcinoid-like tumors in an elderly man (4). In a review of 3300 invasive mammary carcinomas, Fisher et al. found 3 breast neoplasms with histologic features reminiscent of carcinoid tumor (5). Using argyrophil stains and ultrastructural examination, the authors suggested that there were two variants of so-called mammary carcinoid, solid and mucinous (5).

The existence of primary carcinoid tumors of the breast as a completely distinct entity was questioned in subsequent publications (6–9). Taxy et al. recognized carcinoid-like patterns in conventional breast cancer, observing such foci in 5 of 21 otherwise ordinary infiltrating ductal and lobular carcinomas (6). These authors pointed out that so-called primary mammary carcinoids had more in common with conventional breast carcinomas than with the usual non-mammary carcinoid tumor. In a study of 20 unselected breast cancers, Clayton et al. found argyrophilia in 10 cases, dense-core granules ultrastructurally in 13 cases, and lactalbumin immunohistochemically in 7 cases (8). This study provided indirect evidence that argyrophilia and dense-core secretory granules represented lactational differentiation. Bussolati et al. subsequently reported that the apparent positivity for alpha-lactalbumin was due to a contaminant which, however, was itself a marker for endocrine differentiation (10). Other studies documented the presence of argyrophilia (6, 11–22) and membrane-bound, dense-core granules (10, 12–14, 16, 19, 21–28) in a histologically diverse assortment of breast carcinomas.

Clinical

There is no evidence that mammary carcinomas with a carcinoid-like histologic appearance differ in their biologic behavior from clinically equivalent neoplasms lacking such features. Each of the 8 patients in the Cubilla and Woodruff study presented with a painless breast mass and none had symptoms of the carcinoid syndrome (2). The prognosis for the 8 patients was related to the size and stage of the neoplasm, and was in keeping with that of conventional mammary carcinomas. Other investigators have found no differences in estrogen receptor status and prognosis for patients with conventional breast carcinomas and for those with 'endocrine' differentiation (10).

Light Microscopic

There is general agreement that, histologically, these breast neoplasms bear some resemblance to carcinoid tumors arising in the gastrointestinal tract or lung. The tumors in the Cubilla and Woodruff study were composed of nests and cords of uniform cells located in a vascularized stroma (2) (Figure 1). Occasional ribbon, papillary, glandular, and acinar patterns were also noted. The cells had round to oval nuclei with finely dispersed chromatin and one or two small nucleoli (Figure 2). Unlike most true carcinoid tumors arising in other locations, mammary carcinoid-like tumors are frequently associated with zones of typical adenocarcinoma. Three neoplasms in the Cubilla and Woodruff study had associated intraductal carcinoma and 2 had areas of infiltrating lobular carcinoma (2). The 5

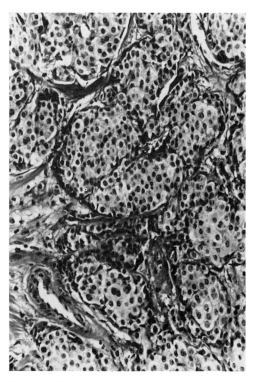

Figure 1 Mammary carcinoma with carcinoid-like features contains discrete nests of uniform cells set in a vascularized stroma.

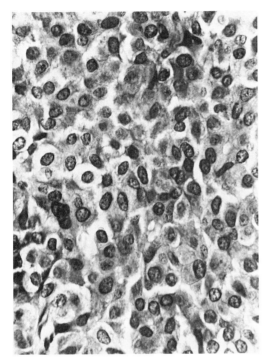

Figure 2 Carcinoid-like breast carcinomas are composed of cells with regular nuclei, stippled nuclear chromatin, and, occasionally, small nucleoli.

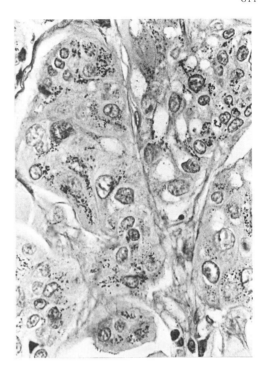

Figure 3 This carcinoma has prominent argyrophilia as seen in this Churukian–Schenk stain.

cases containing carcinoid-like foci reported by Taxy et al. were invariably associated with areas of typical ductal or lobular carcinoma (6).

Argyrophilia

The presence of argyrophilic cells in these neoplasms was initially assumed to be strong evidence for carcinoidal differentiation (Figure 3). Each carcinoid-like tumor in the Cubilla and Woodruff study had argyrophilic granules as observed in modified Grimelius stains (2). However, it soon became apparent that argyrophilia was not specific for carcinoid-like neoplasms. Fisher et al. found argyrophilia in only 1 of 3 neoplasms with light microscopic features of carcinoid tumor (5). In contrast, they noted argyrophilia in 8 of 19 mucinous carcinomas. Focal argyrophilia was

observed in 11 of the breast carcinomas (6 of 12 infiltrating lobular carcinomas and 5 of 7 infiltrating ductal carcinomas) described by Taxy and co-workers (6). Clayton et al. found focal or diffuse argyrophilia in 10 of 20 unselected breast cancers (8).

Argyrophilia in ordinary breast cancers (intraductal, infiltrating ductal, in-situ and invasive lobular, mucinous) occurs in 0% to 64% of reported series of cases (2, 5–8, 12–14, 17, 18). Overall, argyrophilic granules were identified in 20% of conventional breast cancers (175 of 889 cases). The granules may be observed in normal lactating breast (8), and, rarely, in breasts with fibrocystic changes (5). Chromogranin immunoreactivity, presently thought to be specific for neuroendocrine differentiation, was reported in 45% of argyrophilic carcinomas (10, 20) and, rarely, in histologically normal breast epithelium (20). Chromogranin-positive cells were absent in 12 infiltrating ductal carcinomas and examples of fibroadenoma, epithelial hyperplasia, and ductal papillomas (20). The finding of immunoreactivity for neuron-specific enolase in breast carcinomas does not signify neuroendocrine differentiation (10, 19, 28). Moreover, carcinoid-like tumors are immunoreactive with antibodies against human milk fat globule membrane (epithelial membrane antigen) (10), an antigen that is generally absent in true carcinoid tumors (29).

Ultrastructural

As with the light microscopic features, there is agreement that these tumors show electron microscopic findings *compatible with* carcinoid-like differentiation. Ultrastructural study of 3 tumors by Cubilla and Woodruff revealed small, uniform, membrane-bound 'neurosecretory' granules measuring 250 nm in average diameter (2). However, it must be borne in mind that dense-core granules are not diagnostic of neuroendocrine differentiation. Clayton et al. found 95 to 450 nm dense core granules in 13 of 20 unselected breast carcinomas studied by electron microscopy (8). Small membrane-bound dense-core granules have been observed in intraductal and infiltrating ductal carcinomas, lobular carcinomas, mucinous carcinomas, tubular carcinomas, and apocrine cancers (10, 12–14, 16, 19, 21–28). Membrane-bound secretory granules also have been found quite frequently in low numbers and in a few cells of the normal resting and pregnant breast and in benign breast lesions such as fibroadenoma, fibrocystic disease, and sclerosing lesions (5, 27).

Serotonin, Norepinephrine, and Ectopic Hormone Production

One of the 2 tumors in the original study by Feyrter and Hartmann (1) was found to contain small amounts of 5-hydroxytryptamine, and the urine of the second patient had elevated amounts of hydroxyindoleacetic acid. The male patient with bilateral carcinoid-like tumors reported by Kaneko et al. had a

moderate amount of urinary norepinephrine (4). Breast carcinomas with a carcinoid-like light microscopic appearance may or may not demonstrate evidence of ectopic hormone production. Sariola et al. found alpha-human chorionic gonadotropin (alpha-hCG) in 2 breast neoplasms with carcinoid-like features (30). Raju and Fine found that 2 carcinoid-like mammary tumors contained both human chorionic gonadotropin and prolactin, immunohistochemically (16). Six carcinoid-like tumors in the same study lacked immunoreactivity for serotonin, gastrin, somatostatin, cholecystokinin, or ACTH, but each was positive for carcinoembryonic antigen. A carcinoid-like neoplasm reported by Nesland et al. was immunoreactive for gastrin (19).

Summary

Mammary neoplasms with a carcinoid-like histologic appearance have been regarded as a distinct entity (2), as an endocrine subset of breast cancers that have heterogeneous histologic appearances and variable clinical outcomes (7, 10), and as a common variant of ordinary breast carcinoma (6). It is clear that both carcinoid-like tumors and conventional mammary neoplasms have overlapping clinical, light microscopic, ultrastructural, histochemical, and immunocytochemical features. As breast carcinomas with carcinoid-like features comprise a heterogeneous group without unique clinical behaviors, it seems imprudent to regard them as a distinct nosologic entity.

MAMMARY CARCINOMAS ASSOCIATED WITH ABERRANT HORMONE PRODUCTION

History

Mammary carcinomas with conventional light microscopic appearances will occasionally demonstrate ectopic hormone production, suggesting at least partial neuroendocrine differentiation at the functional level. Evidence of hormone production may be based on radioimmunoassay of tissue extracts, staining of tissue sections by immunofluorescent or immunoperoxidase techniques, or increased serum levels of specific hormones, with or without associated clinical manifestations.

ACTH Production

A few reports in the literature document patients with breast cancer who also had hypercorticism (25, 26, 31–33). Cohle et al. described such a patient with an infiltrating lobular carcinoma that contained ACTH by immunocytochemistry (26). Woodward et al. reported a patient with hypercorticism who had an infiltrating ductal carcinoma that contained ACTH as determined both by chemical extraction and immunocyto-chemistry (25). Another example of infiltrating ductal carcinoma was found to react immunocytochemically with antisera against both ACTH and hCG (15). ACTH immuno-reactivity has also been noted in apocrine carcinoma as well as in other examples of infiltrating lobular carcinoma and infiltrating ductal carcinoma (19, 28). A few cases of ductal carcinoma in situ having 'endocrine' features microscopically, were immunoreac-tive for ACTH, corticotropin-like interme-diate lobe peptide, and pro-opiomelanocortin (21).

Calcitonin and Parathyroid Hormone Production

Patients with breast cancer may have increased levels of calcitonin in their blood (34, 35). In addition, increased levels of calcitonin in cell cultures of breast cancer have been described (26). Parathyroid hormone has been demonstrated in extracts from 2 breast cancers by radioimmunoassay (36, 37).

Human Placental Lactogen and hCG Production

Human placental lactogen (HPL) and hCG were observed initially in the blood of patients with breast cancer (38–42). Using the peroxi-dase anti-peroxidase technique on formalin-fixed paraffin-embedded sections, Barry et al. found very little positive staining for HPL in a study of 46 breast carcinomas (43). Horne et al., however, employing an enzyme-bridge immunoperoxidase procedure, found that 82% of 50 breast cancers contained HPL (44). It was noted that patients whose tumors lacked HPL had longer survival times.

Using a variety of techniques, alpha-hCG has been found in 19% to 44% of mammary carcinomas (42, 45–47). Most of the breast cancers positive for hCG have been ordinary ductal cancers. Walker, in a study of 53 breast cancers, failed to find a correlation between grade of the tumor and the presence of alpha-hCG (45). She did note that the production of alpha-hCG was related to the presence of lymph node metastases.

In the largest study to date, Lee et al. stained, immunocytochemically, 233 invasive breast cancers for alpha-hCG, beta-hCG, and HPL and compared their immunoreactivity with a variety of clinical features (47). Nine-teen percent of the tumors were positive for alpha-hCG, 18% contained beta-hCG, and 30% were positive for HPL. In most instances, immunoreactivity was focal. Non-neoplastic breast tissues lacked each of the three hor-mones. It was shown that these markers had no relationship to prognostic variables including likelihood of recurrence, interval before recur-rence, and presence of metastases.

Bombesin, Vasoactive Intestinal Peptide, Pancreatic Polypeptide, Substance P, Gastrin, Somatostatin, Leu-enkephalin, Beta-endorphin, and Neurotensin Production

Immunoreactivity for each of these peptide-hormones, except leu-enkephalin and beta-endorphin, has been observed in a few exam-ples of infiltrating lobular carcinoma (19, 28). Gastrin, bombesin, leu-enkephalin, pancreatic polypeptide, and beta-endorphin have been present immunohistochemically in examples of infiltrating ductal carcinoma (19, 28). Hormone positive cells were typically few and dispersed in these neoplasms. A few cases contained more than one peptide-hormone. One case of ductal carcinoma in situ was immunoreactive for neurotensin (21).

SMALL CELL UNDIFFERENTIATED (OAT CELL) CARCINOMA

Overview

Only 3 cases of primary small cell undifferentiated carcinoma of the breast have been described. As these neoplasms are histologically identical to small cell undifferentiated carcinoma arising at other sites, it is important, before entertaining a diagnosis of primary oat cell carcinoma, to rule out a metastasis from an extramammary location.

Clinical

In the initial report of mammary oat cell carcinoma, Wade et al. described a 52-year-old woman with an 8 × 10 cm breast mass who was found to have axillary and hepatic metastases at the time of diagnosis (48). The patient was treated initially with a modified radical mastectomy. Despite postoperative chemotherapy, she died 9 months after diagnosis with widely disseminated metastases.

Toyoshima briefly described a 62-year-old woman with primary oat cell carcinoma of the breast who died almost 3 years after diagnosis (14). Jundt et al. reported an example of small cell undifferentiated carcinoma of the breast in a 52-year-old male (49). Despite radiation therapy and chemotherapy, the patient developed widespread metastases and died 14 months after the appearance of his symptoms.

It thus appears that small cell undifferentiated carcinoma of the breast follows an extremely aggressive clinical course analogous to that of pulmonary oat cell carcinoma. Distant metastases are typically present at the time of diagnosis and survival is correspond-

ingly short. Because of the poor prognosis associated with these neoplasms, they should be clearly distinguished from other forms of breast carcinoma. The words *small cell* in the diagnosis must not be confused with the family of well-differentiated small cell mammary carcinomas, including lobular and small cell ductal carcinoma. There is no evidence that these are related to small cell *undifferentiated* carcinoma. Utilizing the term oat cell carcinoma may avoid this potential pitfall.

Gross and Light Microscopic

Gross examination of the neoplasm reported by Wade et al. demonstrated a large, soft, necrotic, and hemorrhagic mass (48). Microscopically, the tumor contained sheets of polygonal to spindle-shaped cells with a high nuclear-to-cytoplasmic ratio, nuclear molding, and a high mitotic rate (Figure 4). The

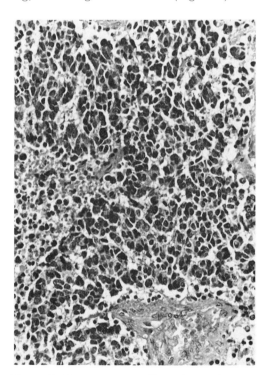

Figure 4 Mammary oat cell carcinoma is composed of sheets of small cells with hyperchromatic nuclei and scant cytoplasm. A large focus of necrosis is present (left).

tumor also formed ribbons, cords, and rosettes. necrosis and vascular invasion were prominent. The neoplasm reported by Jundt et al. had a similar light microscopic appearance (49).

Ultrastructural Features

Eighty to 120 nm membrane-bound, dense-core granules, cytoplasmic processes, and poorly formed cell junctions were observed ultrastructurally in the case reported by Wade et al. (48) (Figure 5). Coarse nuclear chromatin was often present as irregular clumps adjacent to the nuclear membrane. Ninety to 350 nm membrane-bound, dense-core granules were found in the case described by Dundt et al. (49).

NEUROENDOCRINE TUMORS METASTATIC TO THE BREAST

Carcinoid Tumor

Eleven cases of carcinoid tumor metastatic to the breast have appeared in the literature (50–60).

Clinical

The 11 patients ranged in age from 43 to 73 years (median: 58 years). Metastatic tumor in one patient was found at autopsy. Of the 8 patients who underwent mastectomy, 4 had a previous history of carcinoid tumor and 6 had symptoms of the carcinoid syndrome preoperatively. Seven tumors arose in the ileum. The

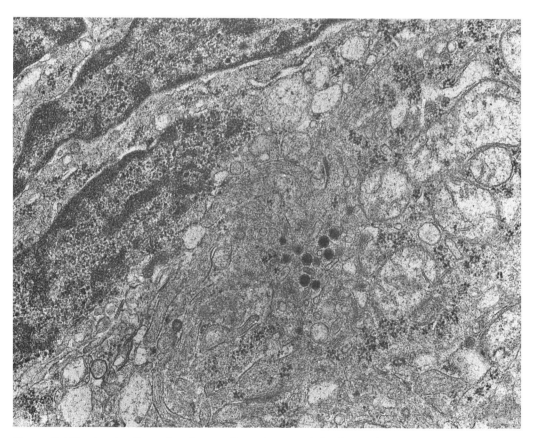

Figure 5 Ultrastructurally, cells of oat cell carcinoma of the breast have nuclei with prominent heterochromatin and cytoplasm with membrane-bound, dense-core granules.

duodenum, appendix, pancreas, and bronchus were the primary sites of one case each. Breast masses were multiple in 4 instances.

Pathologic

Seven patients had frozen section examinations of their breast neoplasms. After each was interpreted as a primary carcinoma of the breast, mastectomy was performed. Lymph nodes obtained from axillary dissections in 7 patients failed to reveal carcinoid tumor. One patient had a fine-needle aspiration of the breast that was diagnosed as a poorly differentiated carcinoma (60). It is obvious that carcinoid tumor metastatic to the breast cannot be diagnosed on tissues submitted for frozen section examination or on fine-needle aspiration cytology specimens unless a specific history of carcinoid tumor is obtained.

Small Cell Undifferentiated (Oat Cell) Carcinoma

Clinical

Four publications documenting metastatic tumors to the breast have included 10 cases of primary oat cell carcinoma of the lung (59, 61–63). In a study of cancers metastatic to the mammary gland, Hajdu and Urban reported that 5 of 51 tumors were pulmonary oat cell carcinomas (63). Oat cell carcinoma of the lung was the most frequent epithelial neoplasm to metastasize to the breast in their series. It is of interest that, in this study, the primary location of the oat cell carcinomas had not been established before breast biopsy.

Pathologic

Histologically, oat cell carcinoma metastatic to the breast is identical to the rare mammary oat cell carcinomas described above. Unlike the primary tumors, those that are metastatic sometimes manifest as multiple nodules in the superficial breast tissues (63).

REFERENCES

1 Feyrter F, Hartmann G. Uber die carcinoide Wuchsform des Carcinoma mammae, insbesondere das Carcinoma solidum (gelatinosum) mammae. Frankf Z Pathol 1963; 73: 24.

2 Cubilla AL, Woodruff JM. Primary carcinoid tumor of the breast. A report of eight patients. Am J Surg Pathol 1977; 1: 283.

3 Devitt PG. Carcinoid tumour of the breast. Br Med J (Clin Res) 1978; 2: 327.

4 Kaneko H, Hojo H, Ishikawa S, Yamanouchi H, Sumidat, Saito R. Norepinephrine-producing tumors of bilateral breasts. A case report. Cancer 1978; 41: 2002.

5 Fisher ER, Palekar AS, NSABP Collaborators. Solid and mucinous varieties of so-called mammary carcinoid tumors. Am J Clin Pathol 1979; 72: 909.

6 Taxy JB, Tischler AS, Insalaco SJ, Battifora H. 'Carcinoid' tumor of the breast. A variant of conventional breast cancer? Hum Pathol 1981; 12: 170.

7 Azzopardi JG, Muretto P, Goddeeris P, Eusebi V, Lauweryns JM. 'Carcinoid' tumours of the breast: The morphological spectrum of argyrophil carcinomas. Histopathology 1982; 6: 549.

8 Clayton F, Sibley RK, Ordonez NG, Hanssen G. Argyrophilic breast carcinomas. Evidence of lactational differentiation. Am J Surg Pathol 1982; 6: 323.

9 Anderson TJ. Carcinoid tumour of the breast (letter). Histopathology 1983; 7: 143.

10 Bussolati G, Papotti M, Sapino A, Gugliotta P, Ghiringhello B, Azzopardi JG. Endocrine markers in argyrophilic carcinomas of the breast. Am J Surg Pathol 1987; 11: 248.

11 Chabon AB, Costales F. Estrogen receptor activity in primary argyrophil carcinoma of the breast. Diagn Gynecol Obstet 1980; 2: 93.

12 Partanen S, Syrjanen K. Argyrophilic cells in carcinoma of the female breast. Virchows Arch (Pathol Anat) 1981; 391: 45.

13 Min KW. Argyrophilia in breast carcinomas: histochemical, ultrastructural, and immunocytochemical study. Lab Invest 1983; 48: 58A.

14 Toyoshima S. Mammary carcinoma with argyrophil cells. Cancer 1983; 52: 2129.

15 Juntti-Berggren L, Pitkanen P, Wilander E. Argyrophil endocrine cells with ACTH and HCG immunoreactivity in a carcinoma of the breast. Virchows Arch (Cell Pathol) 1983; 43: 37.

16 Raju U, Fine G. The controversial mammary carcinoid tumor. Lab Invest 1983; 48: 69A.

17 Fetissof F, Dubois MP, Arbeille-Brassart B, Lansac J, Jobard P. Argyrophilic cells in mammary carcinoma. Hum Pathol 1983; 14: 127.

18 Rasmussen BB, Rose C, Thorpe SM, Andersen KW, Hou-Jensen K. Argyrophilic cells in 202 human mucinous breast carcinomas. Relation to histopathologic and clinical factors. Am J Clin Pathol 1985; 84: 737.

19 Nesland JM, Memoli VA, Holm R, Gould VE, Johannessen JV. Breast carcinomas with neuroendocrine differentiation. Ultrastruct Pathol 1985; 8: 225.

20 Bussolati G, Gugliotta P, Sapino A, Eusebi V, Lloyd RV. Chromogranin-reactive endocrine cells in argyrophilic carcinomas ('carcinoids') and normal tissue of the breast. Am J Pathol 1985; 120: 186.

21 Cross AS, Azzopardi JG, Krausz T, van Noorden S, Polak JM. A morphological and immunocytochemical study of a distinctive variant of ductal carcinoma in-situ of the breast. Histopathology 1985; 9: 21.

22 Ramos CV, Boeshart C, Restrepo GL. Intracystic papillary carcinoma of the male breast. Immunohistochemical and ultrastructural study. Arch Pathol Lab Med 1985; 109: 858.

23 Goldenberg VE, Goldenberg NS, Sommers SC. Comparative ultrastructure of atypical ductal hyperplasia, intraductal carcinoma and infiltrating ductal carcinoma of the breast. Cancer 1969; 24: 1152.

24 Gould VE, Chejfec. Case 13. Ultrastruct Pathol 1980; 1: 151.

25 Woodward BH, Eisenbarth G, Wallace NR, Mossler JA, McCarty KS Jr. Adrenocorticotropin production by a mammary carcinoma. Cancer 1981; 47: 1823.

26 Cohle SD, Tschen JA, Smith FE, Lane M, McGavran MH. ACTH-secreting carcinoma of the breast. Cancer 1979; 43: 2370.

27 Ferguson DJP, Anderson TJ. Distribution of dense core granules in normal, benign and malignant breast tissue. J Pathol 1985; 147: 59.

28 Nesland JM, Holm R, Johannessen JV, Gould VE. Neurone specific enolase immunostaining in the diagnosis of breast carcinomas with neuroendocrine differentiation. Its usefulness and limitations. J Pathol 1986; 148: 35.

29 Pinkus GS, Kurtin PJ. Epithelial membrane antigen—A diagnostic discriminant in surgical pathology: Immunohistochemical profile in epithelial, mesenchymal, and hematopoietic neoplasms using paraffin sections and monoclonal antibodies. Hum Pathol 1985; 16: 929.

30 Sariola H, Lehtonen E, Saxen E. Breast tumors with a solid and uniform carcinoid pattern. Ultrastructural and immunohistochemical study of two cases. Pathol Res Pract 1985; 178: 405.

31 Lockwood CH. Studies of adrenal cortical function in three cases of carcinoma. Can Med Assoc J 1958; 79: 728.

32 Liddle GW, Givens JR, Nicholson WE, Island DP. The ectopic ACTH syndrome. Cancer Res 1965; 25: 1057.

33 Prunty FTG, Brooks RV, Dupre J, Gimlette TMD, Hutchinson JSM, McSwiney RR, Mills IH. Adrenocortical hyperfunction and potassium metabolism in patients with 'non-endocrine' tumors and Cushing's syndrome. J Clin Endocrinol Metab 1963; 23: 737.

34 Coombes RC, Easty GC, Detre SI, Hillyard CJ, Stevens U, Girgis SI, Galante LS, Heywood L, Macintyre I, Neville AM. Secretion of immunoreactive calcitonin by human breast carcinomas. Br Med J (Clin Res) 1975; 4: 197.

35 Samaan NA, Castillo S, Schultz PN, Khalil KG, Johnston DA. Serum calcitonin after pentagastrin stimulation in patients with bronchogenic and breast cancer compared to that in patients with medullary thyroid carcinoma. J Clin Endocrinol Metab 1980; 51: 237.

36 Mavligit GM, Cohen JL, Sherwood LM. Ectopic production of parathyroid hormone by carcinoma of the breast. N Engl J Med 1971; 285: 154.

37 Melick RA, Martin TJ, Hicks JD. Parathyroid hormone production and malignancy. Br Med J (Clin Res) 1972; 2: 204.

38 Braunstein GD, Vaitukaitis JL, Carbone PP, Ross GT. Ectopic production of human chorionic gonadotrophin by neoplasms. Ann Intern Med 1973; 78: 39.

39 Goldstein DP, Kosasa TS, Skarim AT. The clinical application of a specific radioimmunoassay for human chorionic gonadotropin in trophoblastic and nontrophoblastic tumors. Surg Gynecol Obstet 1974; 138: 747.

40 Sheth NA, Suraiya JN, Sheth AR, Ranadive KJ, Jussawalla DJ. Ectopic production of human placental lactogen by human breast tumors. Cancer 1977; 39: 1693.

41 Tormey DC, Waalkes TP, Simon RM. Biological markers in breast carcinoma. II. Clinical correlations with human chorionic gonadotropin. Cancer 1977; 39: 2391.

42 Cove DH, Woods KL, Smith SCH, Burnett D, Leonard J, Grieve RJ, Howell A. Tumour markers in breast cancer. Br J Cancer 1979; 40: 710.

43 Barry JD, Koch TJ, Cohen C, Brigati DJ, Sharkey FE. Correlation of immunohistochemical markers with patient prognosis in breast carcinoma: A quantitative study. Am J Clin Pathol 1984; 82: 582.

44 Horne CHW, Reid IN, Milne GD. Prognostic significance of inappropriate production of

pregnancy proteins by breast cancers. Lancet 1976; ii: 279.

45 Walker RA. Significance of alpha-subunit HCG demonstrated in breast carcinomas by the immunoperoxidase technique. J Clin Pathol 1978; 31: 245.

46 Cove DH, Smith SCH, Walker R, Howell A. The synthesis of the glycoprotein hormone alpha subunit by human breast carcinomas. Eur J Cancer Clin Oncol 1978; 15: 693.

47 Lee AK, Rosen PP, DeLellis RA, Saigo PE, Gangi MD, Groshen S, Bagin R, Wolfe HJ. Tumor marker expression in breast carcinomas and relationship to prognosis. An immunohistochemical study. Am J Clin Pathol 1985; 84: 687.

48 Wade PM Jr, Mills SE, Read M, Cloud W, Lambert MJ, Smith RE. Small cell neuroendocrine (oat cell) carcinoma of the breast. Cancer 1983; 52: 121.

49 Jundt G, Schulz A, Heitz PU, Osborn M. Small cell neuroendocrine (oat cell) carcinoma of the male breast. Immunocytochemical and ultrastructural investigations. Virchows Arch (Pathol Anat) 1984; 404: 213.

50 Zetzel L. Case records of the Massachusettes General Hospital. N Engl J Med 1957; 256: 703.

51 Chodoff RJ. Solitary breast metastasis from carcinoid of the ileum. Am J Surg 1965; 109: 814.

52 Hawley PR. A case of secondary carcinoid tumours in both breasts following excision of primary carcinoid tumour of the duodenum. Br J Surg 1966; 53: 818.

53 Turner M, Gallager DS. Occult appendiceal carcinoid. Arch Pathol 1969; 88: 188.

54 Haagensen CO. Diseases of the Breast. Philadelphia: WB Saunders, 1971. 408 9.

55 Harrist TJ, Kalisher L. Breast metastasis; an unusual manifestation of a malignant carcinoid tumor. Cancer 1977; 40: 3102.

56 Kashlan RB, Powell RW, Nolting SF. Carcinoid and other tumors metastatic to the breast. J Surg Oncol 1982; 20: 25.

57 Schurch W, Lamoureux E, Lefebvre R, Fauteux J. Solitary breast metastasis: First manifestation of an occult carcinoid of the ileum. Virchows Arch (Pathol Anat) 1980; 386: 117.

58 Ordonez NG, Manning JT Jr, Raymond AK. Argentaffin endocrine carcinoma (carcinoid) of the pancreas with concomitant breast metastasis: An immunohistochemical and electron microscopic study. Hum Pathol 1985; 16: 746.

59 Nielsen M, Andersen JA, Henriksen FW, Kristensen PB, Lorentzen M, Ravn V, Schiodt T, Thorborg JV, Ornvold K. Metastases to the breast from extramammary carcinomas. Arch Path Microbiol Scand (A) 1981; 89: 251.

60 Ahlman H, Larsson I, Gronstad K, Tisell LE, Dahlstrom A. A case of midgut carcinoid with breast metastasis and cellular localization of serotonin and substance P. J Surg Oncol 1986; 31: 170.

61 Sandison AT. Metastatic tumours in the breast. Br J Surg 1959; 47: 54.

62 Deeley TJ. Secondary deposits in the breast. Br J Cancer 1965; 19: 738.

63 Hajdu SI, Urban JA. Cancers metastatic to the breast. Cancer 1972; 29: 1691.

Textbook of Uncommon Cancer
Edited by C.J. Williams, J.G. Krikorian, M.R. Green and D. Raghavan
© 1988 John Wiley & Sons Ltd

Chapter **43**

Angiosarcoma of the Breast

Charles D. Dietzen

Assistant Professor, Department of Surgery, Louisiana State University School of Medicine, New Orleans, Louisiana, USA

HISTORY

Angiosarcoma of the breast was originally thought to have been first reported by Schmidt in 1887 (1). He documented 11 cases of breast tumors which recurred locally, failed to metastasize to regional lymph nodes, and consistently metastasized to distant organs. Steingaszner et al., on review of Schmidt's histologic description, questioned the origin of these tumors (2). Borrmann is now credited with publishing the first case of mammary angiosarcoma in 1907 (3). His patient had a tumor which appeared benign on histologic examination but recurred several times prior to the patient's death from metastatic disease.

Due to the rarity of mammary angiosarcoma most of the literature has consisted of individual case reports or series with small numbers of cases. The largest series of previously unreported cases is that of Donnell et al. with 36 patients (4). Over 185 cases of angiosarcoma of the breast have been reported since Borrmann's original case (5–13).

EPIDEMIOLOGY AND ETIOLOGY

As previously stated mammary angiosarcoma is a rare tumor and has been reported to comprise 0.05% of all breast malignancies (14). Angiosarcoma represents 8% of all sarcomas of the breast (15).

Mammary angiosarcoma is a disease of young adult females. Although it has been reported in patients from 13 (16) to 85 (17) years of age, the majority of patients develop the disease in the third and fourth decades of life (4, 5, 18). Only 3 cases have occurred in males (13, 19, 20).

The etiology of this tumor is unknown No significant genetic (with the exception of female gender) or environmental factors have been isolated. Because the majority of tumors have been in females of child bearing age a hormonal influence has been proposed (2, 7, 21). Which, if any, hormonal factors are involved have not been discovered. Cases have been diagnosed during pregnancy, and this condition offers no known protection from or predilection to development and/or progression of the disease (21–25).

PATHOLOGY AND BIOLOGY

Angiosarcoma of the breast is a malignant neoplasm of vascular origin (26). All of the following names have been applied to this tumor: benign metastasizing hemangioma (3), angiosarcoma (19), angio-endothelioma (27), hemangioblastoma (21), and hemangiosarcoma (28).

The gross appearance of the tumor is that of a soft, fleshy, hemorrhagic unencapsulated mass composed of dilated vascular spaces. The lesion usually begins deep in the breast tissue. As growth progresses foci of necrosis, penetration of the pectoralis fascia, and extension to the skin causing a purplish discoloration can occur (2, 5).

A varied histologic pattern is characteristic of this tumor. Hence, initial microscopic inspection can lead to a misdiagnosis of the lesion as a benign hemangioma. Careful search of numerous sections may be necessary to render a correct diagnosis and establish the degree of differentiation of a particular tumor.

Donnell et al. have classified mammary angiosarcoma microscopically into three groups according to degree of differentiation (4). Group I tumors are those which are most differentiated. The microscopic characteristics are those of hyperchromatic endothelial cells with interanastomosing channels in breast tissue. These characteristics are present in virtually all cases, frequently in sections at the periphery of the tumor. It is when they are the predominant microscopic features that a tumor is classified Group I (Figure 1).

Group II is an intermediate class containing, in addition to the findings of Group I, endothelial tufting, papillary formation, and mitoses (Figure 2). Group III tumors are the least differentiated and contain solid and spindle cell foci, blood lakes, and focal necrosis, in addition to the findings of Groups I and II (Figures 3 and 4).

Donnell et al. have proposed that each case be graded according to the predominant histologic characteristics. Furthermore, they feel that Group II and III features prognosticate a poorer clinical outlook (4).

Electron microscopy of mammary angiosarcoma shows a typical endothelial cells lining sinusoids with irregular growth and lacking orientation. Examination of the endothelial cells reveals occasional Weibel–Palade bodies, filaments, pinocytotic vesicles, and basal laminae (5, 29).

Cytologic analysis of angiosarcoma of the

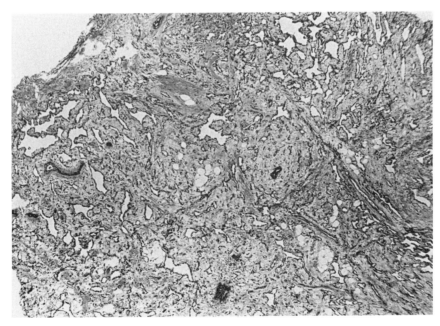

Figure 1 Note interlacing channels around breast ducts (original magnification: ×50).(*Reproduced from reference 6 by permission of the Editors of Cancer, JB Lippincott Company.*)

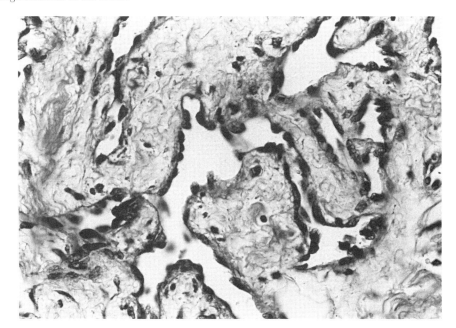

Figure 2 Note prominent, hyperchromatic endothelial cells (original magnification: ×500).(*Reproduced from reference 6 by permission of the Editors of Cancer, JB Lippincott Company.*)

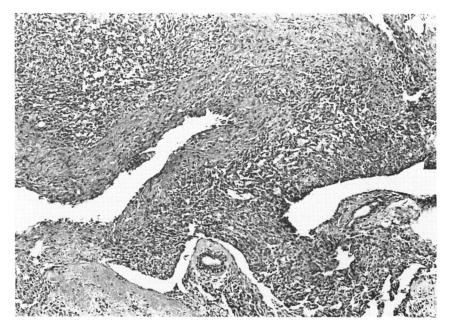

Figure 3 Note solid tumor mass around breast ducts (original magnification: ×125).(*Reproduced from reference 6 by permission of the Editors of Cancer, JB Lippincott Company.*)

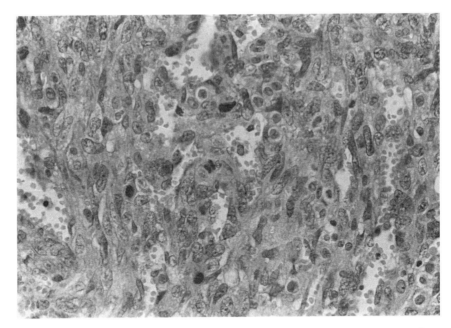

Figure 4 Note solid pattern, anaplasia, and numerous mitoses (original magnification: ×500).(*Reproduced from reference 6 by permission of the Editors of Cancer, JB Lippincott Company.*)

breast has been described (30, 31). Large sheets of ductal cells, many with papillary formation, moderate nuclear size variation, and moderate hyperchromasia are seen.

Additional studies have been performed on tumor tissue. Factor VIII-related antigen, present in endothelial cells, has been used to verify these tumors as vascular in origin. Immunoperoxidase stains with factor VIII-related antigen are described (17).

Weakly positive estrogen, progesterone, and glucocorticoid receptors have been reported in 2 patients (7). All other tests on tumor tissue have shown absence of hormone receptor sites (5, 13). The clinical significance of this is undetermined.

CLINICAL FEATURES

Angiosarcoma of the breast typically afflicts females in the third and fourth decades. Like carcinoma, the commonest presentation is that of a painless, growing breast mass; however, a painful mass may infrequently occur. A history of recent, rapid growth of the mass is often elicited. A slight right sided predominance has been noted. This is in contradistinction to the left sided predominance in carcinoma of the breast (2, 32). This is not helpful in the clinical diagnosis of mammary angiosarcoma.

As the tumor grows to the skin surface a characteristic blue, red, violaceous, or black discoloration is often seen (Figure 5). The tumor is usually mobile with respect to the chest wall. Metastasis to the regional axillary lymph nodes is rare. In cases where the regional axillary lymph nodes are palpably enlarged histologic examination shows no tumor. Only 3 cases of axillary node metastasis have been reported (16, 33, 34).

Characteristically angiosarcoma of the breast metastasizes to distant sites. Most commonly involved are the lungs, skin and subcutaneous tissue, bone, liver, brain, and ovary. Intraperitoneal bleeding from abdominal organ metastasis is known to occur (2, 22, 29, 35–39). Involvement of the contralateral breast is common, occurring in 20–25% of

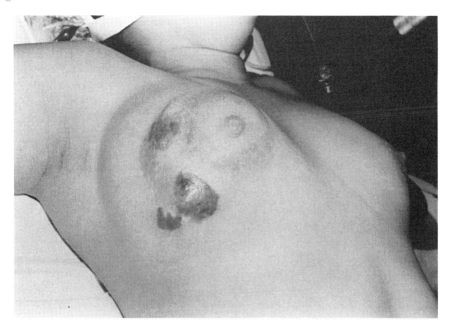

Figure 5 Note violaceous skin discoloration over a mammary angiosarcoma. (*Reproduced from reference 6 by permission of the Editors of Cancer, JB Lippincott Company.*)

cases (2, 13, 18, 21, 22, 28). It is difficult to determine whether this represents metastasis or a second primary tumor.

INVESTIGATION AND STAGING

Tissue for histologic analysis is needed to secure a diagnosis. Cytologic studies have not been helpful; there is insufficient information about the utility of core needle biopsy. Therefore, open biopsy of the breast mass is the usual confirmatory diagnostic test. Massive bleeding has been reported with this procedure (21, 28).

A thorough history and examination, chest x-ray, hematologic and chemistry studies are mandatory. As with any breast mass a mammogram should be done to evaluate the affected and contralateral breasts. A typical appearance on mammogram is that of a lobulated, solitary mass with irregular borders. However, mammographic criteria to reliably diagnose angiosarcoma have not been defined. There is literature to suggest that in a breast mass with the above mammographic appear-

ance and hyper- and hypoechoic areas on sonography angiosarcoma should be suspected (8).

The wisdom of routine additional investigation is unproven. However, if findings in the initial survey indicate possible metastatic disease, further studies, including appropriate plain x-rays, nuclear scans, and computed tomography (CT) scans are warranted.

No staging system for angiosarcoma of the breast exists. Obviously, therapeutic and prognostic implications for a case with tumor confined to the breast differ from one in which distant metastasis is present.

MANAGEMENT AND PROGNOSIS

Surgery

Management should follow the guidelines for conventional treatment of soft tissue sarcomas (40). Surgery offers the only chance of cure. Because of the tendency for microscopic extension of the tumor beyond the border of grossly palpable disease, wide excision is required. This usually necessitates total (simple) mastectomy. Axillary node dissection is seldom necessary. Extension of the tumor into the pectoral muscles is not common; however, when this occurs, the affected tissues, like the breast, should be excised with a wide margin (2, 31, 41). Surgical resection of locally recurrent lesions has been effective (36, 41–44).

Surgery for distant metastasis is indicated only for histologic confirmation. The exception would be in the case of a solitary metastatic lesion in which excision was technically feasible or when surgery for distant metastasis would provide palliation (43).

Although indeterminate, lesions in the contralateral breast should be treated as a second primary tumor. Therefore, wide excision or mastectomy should be performed unless extensive metastatic disease exists.

Radiotherapy

Radiotherapy has been used in an adjuvant and therapeutic manner for mammary angiosarcoma. To date there is insufficient data to justify the routine use of radiotherapy (5, 6, 17, 19, 29, 31, 41, 42). No reported cures exist with radiotherapy as sole treatment. Based on the efficacy of adjuvant radiotherapy, in combination with surgery, on soft tissue sarcomas this modality might provide better local control in selected cases. Additionally, palliative radiotherapy for both local recurrence and distant metastasis should be considered on an individual basis.

Chemotherapy

As with radiotherapy scattered reports exist documenting the use of chemotherapy for angiosarcoma of the breast (4, 6, 9, 17, 19, 29, 33, 41). There is evidence to suggest that actinomycin D is beneficial (4). Donnell et al. treated 11 patients with this agent on an adjuvant basis (with surgery) and found improved survival, most marked in patients whose tumors had unfavorable histologic characteristics.

Other chemotherapeutic agents which have been administered for angiosarcoma of the breast are: nitrogen mustard, mitomycin C, cyclophosphamide, vincristine, Adriamycin, methotrexate (with citrovorum rescue), 5-fluorouracil, thioTEPA, cis-platinum, and DTIC.

Metastatic Disease

Treatment of metastatic disease with any of the conventional modalities (surgery, radiotherapy, chemotherapy) has proved disappointing. However, it should be noted that long term, disease-free survival has been accomplished treating local recurrence with surgical excision and radiotherapy (41) and with surgical excision alone (44).

There is no evidence in the literature of investigational treatment of mammary angiosarcoma with other medicines or modalities. This includes steroids, antisteroidals, immunotherapy, and laser therapy.

The prognosis with angiosarcoma of the breast is generally poor. The mean survival is in the range of 1.5–2.5 years (2, 22, 33). Twenty-one patients have been reported to survive disease free greater than 5 years. All long term survivors underwent some form of wide surgical excision of the primary tumor. Some were treated with additional radiotherapy and/or chemotherapy (2, 4, 5, 12, 15, 17, 41, 42, 44, 45).

The major prognostic factors relate to tumor size and tumor grade. In long term survivors, of those with tumor size reported, the average was less than 5 cm diameter and the majority had tumors less than 4 cm diameter. Although small tumors have proven capable of distant metastasis most reviewers have acknowledged the importance of tumor size at the time of initial treatment (5, 7, 8). Not all investigators, however, have found size to be significant (13, 17).

The value of careful histologic grading as a prognostic guide has been shown. Tumor grade was especially predictive in the study of Merino et al. (17). Histologic criteria for determination of grade are described by Donnell et al. (4).

MAJOR DIFFERENCES FROM OTHER BREAST DISEASES

The major differences of mammary angiosarcoma from other breast diseases (including carcinoma) are the distinctly different rates of incidence, the relative difficulties in histologic confirmation, the recommended surgical treatments, and the prognoses.

Angiosarcoma is uncommon and this is quite different from the dominant diseases of the breast: all forms of 'fibrocystic disease'; fibroadenoma; and carcinoma. The diagnosis of these major breast diseases is usually straightforward with histologic examination. In past reports mammary angiosarcoma has frequently been mistaken for a benign lesion, commonly an angioma. Angioma of the breast is rarely a palpable lesion, and in any patient with a palpable mass this diagnosis should be viewed with suspicion (4, 5, 13, 14, 18).

Treatment of most breast lesions requires, like angiosarcoma, surgical excision; however, the extent of excision and the subsequent treatment of major breast diseases (including carcinoma) and breast sarcomas are at variance. Hence, except for the other mammary sarcomas, angiosarcoma is unique in its treatment philosophy.

The prognosis of mammary angiosarcoma has been reviewed. Only breast carcinoma in its advanced form approaches mammary angiosarcoma in mortality. All other major breast diseases have a brighter clinical outlook.

CURRENT RESEARCH

Due to its rarity there are no current ongoing studies specifically investigating angiosarcoma of the breast. However, basic and clinical research on soft tissue sarcomas is being utilized for treatment of this tumor (6).

Future clinical study will probably be in the area of determining the appropriate use of radiotherapy and chemotherapy and finding the optimum radiation modes, chemical agents, and treatment techniques.

REFERENCES

1 Schmidt GB. Ueber das Angiosarkom der Mamma. Arch Klin Chir 1887; 36: 421–7.

2 Steingaszner LC, Enzinger FM, Taylor HB. Hemangiosarcoma of the breast. Cancer 1965; 18: 352–61.

3 Borrmann R. Metastasenbildung bei histologisch gutartigen Geschwulsten (Fall von metastasierendem Angiom.) Beitr Pathol Anat 1907; 40: 372–92.

4 Donnell RM, Rosen PP, Lieberman PH et al. Angiosarcoma and other vascular tumors of the breast. Am J Surg Pathol 1981; 5: 629–42.

5 Hunter TB, Martin PC, Dietzen CD, Tyler LT. Angiosarcoma of the breast. Two case reports and a review of the literature. Cancer 1985; 56: 2099–106.

6 Antman KH, Corson J, Greenberger J, Wilson R. Multimodality therapy in the management of angiosarcoma of the breast. Cancer 1982; 50: 2000–3.

7 Brentani MM, Pacheco MM, Oshima CTF, Nagai MA, Lemos LB, Goes JCS. Steroid receptors in breast angiosarcoma. Cancer 1983; 51: 2105–11.

8 Grant EG, Holt RW, Chun B, Richardson JD, Orson LW, Cigtay OS. Angiosarcoma of the breast: sonographic, xeromammographic and pathologic appearance. A J Rl 1983; 141: 691–2.

9 Hacking EA, Tiltman AJ, Dent DM. Angiosarcoma of the breast. Clin Oncol 1984; 10: 177–80.

10 Bourlond A, Fievez C. Angiosarcome du sein. Ann Dermatol Venerol 1984; 111: 903–8.

11 Ryan JF, Kealy WF. Concomitant angiosarcoma and carcinoma of the breast: a case report. Histopathology 1985; 9: 893–9.

12 Davis JB. Angiosarcoma of the breast: a case report and review of the literature. Nebr Med J 1986; 71: 101–2.

13 Rainwater LM, Martin JK Jr, Gaffey TA, van Heerden JA. Angiosarcoma of the breast. Arch Surg 1986; 121: 669–72.

14 Stewart FW. Tumors of the breast. In: Atlas of Tumor Pathology, Section IX Fascicle 34. Washington, DC: Armed Forces Institute of Pathology 1950; 75.

15 Myerowitz RL, Pietruszka M, Barnes EL. Primary angiosarcoma of the breast. JAMA 1978; 239: 403.

16 Alvarez-Fernandez E, Salinero-Paniagua E.

Vascular tumors of the mammary gland. A histochemical and ultrastructural study. Virchows Arch (Pathol Anat) 1981; 394: 31–47.

17 Merino MJ, Carter D, Berman M. Angiosarcoma of the breast. Am J Surg Pathol 1983; 7: 53–60.

18 Chen KTK, Kirkegaard DD, Bocian JJ. Angiosarcoma of the breast. Cancer 1980; 46: 368–71.

19 Shackelford RT. Surgical disorders of the breast. In: Shackelford RT ed Diagnosis of Surgical Disease, Vol 1. Philadelphia: WB Saunders, 1968: 439–551.

20 Yadav RVS, Sahariah S, Mittal VK, Banerjee AK. Angiosarcoma of the male breast. Int Surg 1976; 61: 463–4.

21 Batchelor GB. Hemangioblastoma of the breast associated with pregnancy. Br J Surg 1958–1959; 46: 647–9.

22 McClanahan BJ, Hogg L Jr. Angiosarcoma of the breast. Cancer 1954; 7: 586–94.

23 Enticknap JB. Angioblastoma of the breast complicating pregnancy. Br Med J 1946; ii: 51.

24 Shore JH. Hemangiosarcoma of the breast. J Pathol Bacteriol 1957; 74: 289–93.

25 Tibbs D. Metastasizing hemangiomata. A case of malignant hemangio-endothelioma. Br J Surg 1952–1953; 40: 465–70.

26 Stout AP. Hemangio-endothelioma: a tumor of blood vessels featuring vascular endothelial cells. Ann Surg 1943; 118: 445–64.

27 Pulford DS Jr. Neoplasms of the blood–lymph–vascular system with special reference to endotheliomas. Ann Surg 1925; 82: 710–27.

28 Mallory TB, Castleman B, Parris EE. Case Records of the Massachusetts General Hospital. N Engl J Med 1949; 241: 241–3.

29 Hamazaki M, Tanaka T. Hemangiosarcoma of the breast: Case report with scanning electron microscopic study. Acta Pathol Jpn 1978; 28: 605–13.

30 Masin M, Masin F. Cytology of angiosarcoma of the breast: A case report. Acta Cytol 1978; 22: 162–4.

31 Savage R. The treatment of angiosarcoma of the breast. J Surg Oncol 1981; 18: 129–34.

32 Haagensen CD. The natural history of breast carcinoma. In: Haagensen CD ed Diseases of the Breast. Philadelphia: WB Saunders, 1986: 635–718.

33 Gulesserian HP, Lawton RL. Angiosarcoma of the breast. Cancer 1969; 24: 1021–6.

34 Edwards AT, Kellett HS. Hemangiosarcoma of breast. J Pathol Bacteriol 1968; 95: 457–9.

35 Davis HL Jr, Skroch EE, Ramirez G, Korbitz BC. Hemangiosarcoma of the breast. Rocky Mt Med J 1969; 66: 49–53.

36 Kessler E, Kozenitzky IL. Hemangiosarcoma of the breast. J Clin Pathol 1971; 24: 530–2.

37 Barber KW Jr, Harrison EG, Clagett OT, Pratt JH. Angiosarcoma of the breast. Surgery 1960; 48: 869–78.

38 Cauquil P, Scherrer A, Nguyen-Tan T, Belloir C, Pellier D. Métastases d'angiosarcome mammaire. A propos de deux observations. J Radiol 1985; 66: 313–16.

39 Beal JM. Surgical grand rounds. Ill Med J 1974; 146: 39–41.

40 Rosenberg SA, Suit HD, Baker LH. Sarcomas of soft tissue. In: DeVita VT Jr, Hellman S, Rosenberg SA, eds Cancer: Principles and Practice of Oncology. Philadelphia: JB Lippincott, 1985: 1243–91.

41 Morales PH, Lindberg RD, Barkley HT Jr. Soft tissue angiosarcomas. Int J Radiat Oncol Biol Phys 1981; 7: 1655–9.

42 Maddox JC, Evans HL. Angiosarcoma of skin and soft tissue. A study of forty-four cases. Cancer 1981; 48: 1907–21.

43 Saha SP, Thompson R, Still R. Angiosarcoma of the breast. South Med J 1971; 64: 1376–85.

44 Horne WI, Percival WL. Hemangiosarcoma of the breast. Can J Surg 1975; 18: 81–4.

45 Masse SR, Mongeau CJ, Rioux A. Angiosarcoma of the breast. Can J Surg 1977; 20: 341–3.

Textbook of Uncommon Cancer
Edited by C.J. Williams, J.G. Krikorian, M.R. Green and D. Raghavan
© 1988 John Wiley & Sons Ltd

Chapter **44**

Male Breast Cancer

Christopher J. Williams and
Roger B. Buchanan
Southampton University Hospitals, Southampton, UK

Male breast cancer was first described as early as in the sixteenth century (1, 2), though the first series of cases was not reported until the nineteenth century (3). The first detailed and reliable review was by Wainwright (4) and in 1972 Crichlow (5) extensively reviewed the world literature up to that time. He found 2217 documented cases and since then major reviews have added 1169 more cases, though there may have been duplication with patients reported on more than one occasion (6–14).

INCIDENCE

Cancer of the male breast is uncommon with an estimated frequency of less than 1% of the disease in women (15, 16). It accounts for only 0.2–1.5% of all cancers in Western man (5, 17). There are, each year, about 600 cases of male breast cancer in the USA and 120 cases in the UK compared with 100 000 and 29 000 cases of female breast cancer respectively. In these two countries the frequency is 0.56% of that of breast cancer in women. There is not much information on the frequency of this disease around the world but reports from Africa suggest that male breast cancer is considerably more common in the northern and central regions (18–21). In Egypt the incidence of male breast cancer has been reported to be 6% of all cases of breast cancer (18).

EPIDEMIOLOGY

In general the incidence of male breast cancer parallels that of females around the world, the only exception being in some African countries (19). Some studies have found no association between male breast cancer and race, occupation, marital status, religion and geography (20). However, the study of Schottenfeld et al. (21) described a higher death rate from breast cancer in non-white New York men and that of Crichlow has reported an excess of deaths in Jewish men (5). Despite these findings there are, overall, no clear-cut demographic features associated with the occurrence of breast cancer in men.

AETIOLOGY

A wide variety of possible factors have been proposed though they have, in general, been poorly documented (Table 1).

Altered Hormonal Metabolism

Oestrogen receptors have been found in over 80% of patients in some series (22) and it has been suggested that the disease may be associated with hyperoestrogenism. However, review of the available data does not clearly substantiate this. Crichlow (5) reviewed data on 457 men for whom information was avail-

TABLE 1 POSSIBLE AETIOLOGICAL FEATURES
ASSOCIATED WITH BREAST CANCER

Altered oestrogen metabolism
Klinefelter's syndrome
Bilharziasis (hyperoestrogenism)
Gynaecomastia
Infective orchitis
Trauma
Radiation
Familial

---

able and found only 2 with a history of prior oestrogen therapy. One of these developed breast cancer after orchidectomy and oestrogen therapy for prostate cancer. He was the only such case amongst 3000 men in a trial of oestrogen for prostatic carcinoma (23). Several studies have suggested an association with altered hormonal metabolism (6, 24–27). Though a number of studies have reported increased levels of oestrogen in small numbers of men with breast cancer (25–27), Scheike (6) failed to find any abnormalities in plasma oestradiol levels in a larger series of 19 consecutive men. More recently Ribeiro (14) has studied oestradiol, testosterone, follicle stimulating hormone and luteinizing hormone in male breast cancer and found that these were not significantly different from those of a control group.

Gynaecomastia has been cited as a predisposing factor in a number of series and in one report 20% of men have preceding gynaecomastia (23) though others have entirely failed to find the association (17). Crichlow, in his 1972 review, found only 17 cases of prior gynaecomastia among 625 patients where data were available: 7 of the cases were in one series of 40 men (23).

Testicular Abnormalities

Infectious orchitis, testicular atrophy and Klinefelter's syndrome have all been associated with male breast cancer (28). However, in a case control study only 4 of 53 men with breast cancer had preceding orchitis compared with none of 153 controls, a difference that does not

reach statistical significance (21). It has been reported (17) that men with Klinefelter's syndrome have a 66.5-fold increase in incidence of breast cancer. This observation is based on a small number of cases (6) and Crichlow (5) found only 10 men with Klinefelter's syndrome in his review of the literature. Since then several additional cases have been reported (13, 29), though only a very small minority of cases of male breast cancer are associated with Klinefelter's syndrome.

Radiation

Though several reports have linked prior exposure to radiation with male breast cancer (30, 31), Crichlow only found 5 cases in which there had been preceding irradiation. In 2 of these the radiation had been given for gynaecomastia.

Heredity

Although there have been reports of male breast cancer in families with a very high incidence of female breast cancer (21, 32) other studies have failed to support this finding (33) and certainly few men with breast cancer fall into such a high risk group.

Trauma

Trauma has been cited as an association with both female and male breast cancer (34) though only 6% of 532 evaluable patients in Crichlow's review gave a prior history of trauma.

CLINICAL FINDINGS

Male breast cancer occurs later than that in women though cases have been documented from the age of 5 years (35). The median age of diagnosis of breast cancer in men is said to be 8–10 years later than in women (36), though in the wide ranging review of Crichlow the average age was found to be 59.6 years amongst 1888 patients (5).

As in women, there is a slight predilection for the left breast compared with the right. In a literature review 552 tumours were on the right side and 590 on the left (5).

There is commonly a delay in diagnosis, though the mean time from onset of symptoms appears to have decreased from 18 months in 1927 to 9 months in 1974 (17). These data are confirmed in Crichlow's major review; data on time to diagnosis being available in 1228 patients in 22 series. The overall mean period was 18 months but in those series after 1981 it was only 10 months.

The most frequent symptom (Table 2) is a painless lump beneath the areola. Symptoms of nipple involvement and discharge are rather uncommon (less than 10%) but when present in men are associated with cancer in 75% of cases (37).

On examination, a palpable mass is almost invariably found (Table 3). There are only 2 reported cases of apparently occult carcinoma of the male breast presenting with nodal metastases (5). Axillary nodal metastases were found in about one-half of the cases in these collected series and nipple abnormalities in one-third. Single institution studies, because of their nature, include rather more detailed information and Tables 4–6 detail the clinical

TABLE 3 PHYSICAL FINDINGS IN MALE BREAST CANCER—CRICHLOW'S REVIEW 1972 (5)

Physical findings	No. of evaluable patients	Proportion involved (%)
Mass	—	Almost universal
Nipple ulceration	1034	28
Other nipple abnormality	571	37
Axillary node involvement	873	54

TABLE 4 CLINICAL ASSESSMENT OF MALE BREAST CANCER IN DENMARK 1943–72 (6)

Symptom	No of patients	%
Lump only	34	13
Lump plus		
Nipple retraction	84	33
Nipple ulceration	40	16
Nipple discharge	3	1
Skin fixation:		
Incomplete	76	30
Complete	36	14
Ulceration	67	27
Fixation to pectoralis	43	17
Chest wall fixation	13	5
Pain and tenderness	33	13
Palpable lymph nodes	106	42
Distant metastases	29	12

TABLE 2 PRESENTING SYMPTOMS OF BREAST CANCER IN 255 MEN IN DENMARK 1943–72 (6)

Symptom	No. of patients	%
Lump beneath areola	182	71
Pain and tenderness	19	8
Ulceration of skin (not nipple)	11	4
Nipple retraction	10	4
Nipple ulceration	6	
Nipple discharge	9	
Nipple iching	2	
Generalized hardness of breast	1	
Redness of skin	1	
Axillary mass	4	
Swelling of arm	1	
Symptoms of metastases	2	
No symptoms, incidental finding	5	

TABLE 5 CLINICAL STAGE (TNM) AT PRESENTATION IN DANISH MEN WITH BREAST CARCINOMA BY PERIOD OF DIAGNOSIS (6)

TNM stage	1943–72		1943–57		1958–72	
	No.	%	No.	%	No.	%
I	89	35	31	20	58	44
II	28	11	16	13	12	9
III	107	42	51	43	56	42
IV	29	12	22	18	7	5

findings in 257 men with breast cancer in Denmark between 1943 and 1972. The great majority (87%) had other abnormalities in addition to a lump. In one-third there were

TABLE 6 TUMOUR SIZE AND ULCERATION IN MALE BREAST CANCER IN DENMARK 1943–72 (6)

Tumour size (cm)	No. of patients[a]	%	Ulceration No.	%
<2	58	24	6	10
2–3	64	27	12	19
3–4	51	22	17	33
4–5	27	11	7	26
>5	39	16	23	59

[a] Total = 239 patients.

nipple changes, in nearly a half skin involvement, ulceration was seen in a quarter, and deep fixation was relatively common (1 in 5). Lymph node metastases were seen in about 40% and distant metastases in 10%. Assessment by TNM stages suggests that recently there has been an increasing number of patients who have Stage I disease though the proportion with Stage III disease remained unchanged between 1943 and 1972. The metastatic pattern of male breast cancer is very similar to that seen in women with breast cancer (38–40).

HISTOPATHOLOGY

Almost all histological types of breast cancer observed in women have been described in men (17). Most, however, are infiltrating ductal carcinomas (85%). Medullary and papillary carcinomas are both seen in about 5% of cases, papillary tumours apparently have a much better prognosis (41). Review of collected series has shown that 52% of 252 assessable patients had pathological evidence of axillary lymph node involvement.

HORMONE RECEPTOR STATUS

Oestrogen and progesterone receptor data have been reported in a number of small studies since 1980 (Table 7). Cytoplasmic receptors have been found in a majority of case studies. The overall incidence of oestrogen receptors in these collected series was 87% and for progesterone receptors the figure was 62%. These data are similar to those in a review of hormone receptor status in male breast cancer prior to 1980; the corresponding figures being 84% and 73% (46).

TREATMENT

Surgery

Because of its relative rarity there have been few series reporting a prospectively defined policy of initial surgery. Instead, most surgeons have employed an approach similar to that currently in vogue for female breast cancer at

TABLE 7 HORMONE RECEPTOR STATUS IN COLLECTED SERIES OF PATIENTS WITH MALE BREAST CANCER

Author	Receptor site	ER+ No. reported/ No. evaluated	%	PgR+ No. reported/ No. evaluated	%
Ribeiro (14)	Cytoplasmic	12/16	75	12/16	75
Pergoraro et al (42)	Cytoplasmic	12/13	92	6/9	67
	Nuclear	8/10	80	2/9	22
Ruff et al. (43)	Cytoplasmic	14/14	100	8/12	67
Nirmul et al. (44)	Cytoplasmic[a]	6/7	86	—	—
Everson et al. (45)	Cytoplasmic	29/34	85	9/14	64
Mean no. positive[b]	Cytoplasmic	76/87	87	37/60	62

[a] Some of these cases may be included in Pegoraro et al. (42)
[b] Cases in the paper by Nirmul et al. (44) have been excluded.

the time of the patient's presentation. Since many series have included patients over time periods of more than 30 years there have been major changes in approach during each individual study. This is exemplified by Ribeiro's report of 301 patients treated in one institution between 1941 and 1983 (14) (Table 8). Clearly, radical mastectomy was the standard procedure, for male and female breast cancer, in the first two decades of the study though by the final decade simple mastectomy with radiation therapy was predominent.

There are no prospective studies that suggest how extensive initial surgery should be, though several reviews have examined the role of surgery. For instance, Crichlow collected data from 14 reports; he found that of 495 men, 19% were inoperable, 13% had a simple mastectomy and 68% a radical mastectomy. However, since the pattern of surgery performed was dictated by the extent of the patient's disease and current fashion no definitive comments could be made. Despite this several authors have strongly recommended radical surgery (5, 41, 47) and others conservative surgery (23, 40). The debate about the extent of initial surgery must remain unanswered though, superficially, there is no evidence to suggest that patients having conservative procedures fare worse than those having a radical mastectomy.

Survival is generally reported to be worse than that in female breast cancer. Langlands et al. (7) compared breast cancer in 85 men and

241 women. The crude survival rates at 5 years and 10 years were 35% and 13.8% for men compared with 47.2% and 29.7% for women (p = 0.05 at 5 years and 0.01 at 10 years). However when the data are corrected for age, the differences disappeared (5- and 10-year figures for men 33.1% and 21.8% compared with 38.8% and 21.8% for the women). Similarly, in Ribeiro's study (14) there were major differences in crude survival at 5, 10 and 15 years (44%, 23%, 14%) compared with the same data corrected for intercurrent deaths (52%, 38%, 36%). Since male breast cancer occurs 8–10 years later than the female counterpart and life expectancy is shorter in males, comparison of crude survival rates in men and women is bound to be misleading.

Radiotherapy

Once again there have been no prospective studies, so that conclusions supported by sound data are difficult to come by. Despite this, there is little evidence to suggest that postoperative irradiation will improve survival, though there is likely to be a reduction in the local recurrence rate. Erlichman et al. have reported data from the Princess Margaret Hospital, Toronto (12). Twenty-eight patients underwent surgery alone and 55 surgery and radiation. Significantly more patients not receiving radiation relapsed locally, though survival was nearly identical.

TABLE 8 INITIAL SURGICAL TREATMENT BY DECADE OF PRESENTATION IN 301 PATIENTS TREATED IN MANCHESTER

		Surgical treatment		
Period	No. of patients	Radical mastectomy (%)	Simple mastectomy + radiotherapy (%)	Excision (%)
1941–51	31	77	16	7
1952–61	53	66	23	11
1962–71	49	35	47	18
1972–83	76	19	70	11

Adjuvant Chemotherapy

The National Cancer Institute (NCI) has treated 24 men with breast cancer with adjuvant chemotherapy. All patients had histological evidence of nodal involvement (Stage II) and received twelve cycles of cyclophosphamide, methotrexate and 5-fluorouracil (CMF) within 4 weeks of surgery; no postoperative radiotherapy was given. At the time of the report the actuarial 5-year survival rate was 80% (95% confidence interval, 74–100%). These results were compared with historical data and the authors concluded that such adjuvant chemotherapy may be associated with a substantial improvement in disease free and overall survival. Randomized trials of adjuvant therapy are not feasible so that decisions on therapy must be based on such studies. However, longer follow-up of more patients would strengthen the conclusions and the use of a more modern data base for the historical control would be advantageous.

Adjuvant Hormonal Therapy

Ribeiro has reported on the adjuvant use of tamoxifen in men presenting with Stage II or IIIA of breast cancer (14, 51). At the time of his report he had treated 23 patients (Stage II: 12; Stage III: 11): receptor data were only available in 8 cases, but 7 of these were positive and review data suggest that 80% of breast cancer patients have tumours which possess oestrogen receptors (Table 7). Actuarial 5-year survival in this study was 55% compared

with 28% in an historical control. Though these results appear less good than the NCI study of adjuvant chemotherapy it should be remembered that one-half of the patients in the Manchester series had more advanced disease (Stage IIIA) than in the NCI study (all Stage II). No randomized comparative trials are likely to be undertaken.

Therapy for Metastatic or Inoperable Disease

Hormonal therapy has been the mainstay of treatment and its development has paralleled that in female breast cancer. Meyskens et al. have reviewed the data on ablative therapy (Table 9) (17). They found only 70 fully evaluable patients treated by orchidectomy in eleven separate reports. Two-thirds responded for a median duration of 22 months. Only 25 patients treated by adrenalectomy were evaluable; there were 19 responders (of 11 responders to prior orchidectomy 10 responded to subsequent adrenalectomy compared with 4 of 8 non-responders to orchidectomy). Hypophysectomy was undertaken in 17 evaluable patients with 10 responses. Overall, 68% of patients undergoing an hormonal ablation of whatever type responded objectively. Such a response rate is nearly double that expected in female breast cancer (52). It is not clear why this should be though it may reflect the high incidence of positive hormone receptors found in male breast cancer (Table 7).

Surprisingly, additive hormone therapy has

TABLE 9 MALE–BREAST CANCER: REVIEW OF RESPONSE TO HORMONAL ABLATION [17]

Response	%	No. of patients	Median duration of response (months)	Median overall survival (months)
Orchidectomy				
Responder	67	47	22	56
Non-responder	33	22	—	38
Adrenalectomy				
Responder	74	14	32	74
Non-responder	26	5	—	—

been little studied. Response rates have been lower than for ablative therapy, though the data may be biased by patient selection. Indeed, in the review of Patterson et al. (Table 10) of tamoxifen there were only 31 patients in 16 collected reports (53). When these data are added to those of Ribeiro (51) only 44% of 55 patients had an objective response.

In a review Meyskens et al. (17) found few evaluable reports of therapy with oestrogens and androgens. Although there were anecdotal reports of response some patients appeared to have an exacerbation of tumour growth. They also found occasional reports of response to progestagens and corticosteroids. More recently, Ribeiro (51) reported data on 58 evaluable patients treated with diethylstilboestrol; only 21 (38%) of these patients had an objective response, though the median duration of response was particularly long (7 years). Information on response according to hormonal status is scanty. Ribeiro (51) included in his report 10 patients whose hormone receptor status was known. Seven were oestrogen receptor (ER)-positive and 3 progesterone receptor (PgR)-positive. Six of the 7 ER-positive patients responded whilst none of the receptor-negative patients responded. In the review of Patterson et al. (53), receptor data were available in only 8 cases. Of these, 5 were ER-positive and 2 PgR-positive. Four of 5 ER-positive patients responded whilst none of the receptor–negative patients responded. These data, 10 responses in 12 ER-positive patients (83%), suggest that additive hormonal therapy needs further study. Although response rates are apparently lower than for ablative therapy, this may be a result of selection of patients with more adverse factors. Until further studies are available, with hormone receptor status, orchidectomy remains standard therapy though it seems likely that additive therapy is equivalent.

Chemotherapy has been little studied. Yap et al. (49) reviewed data on 90 cases of male breast cancer at the M.D. Anderson Hospital. Only 18 patients received an adequate trial of chemotherapy. Twenty-nine trials of chemotherapy were performed in these patients with an overall response rate of 44% (Table 11).

TABLE 10 TAMOXIFEN ACTIVITY IN MALE BREAST CANCER

Source	No. of patients	No. of responders	% response rate
Patterson et al. (53)	31	15	48
Ribeiro (51)	24	9	38[a]

[a] Some patients in the Ribeiro series may have been included in the review of Patterson et al.

TABLE 11 CHEMOTHERAPY RESPONSE IN MALE BREAST CANCER: THE M.D. ANDERSON EXPERIENCE (49)

Drug	No. of patients treated	No. of patients responding
5-Fluorouracil (5Fu)	5	1
5Fu + prednisolone (Pd)	2	1
Methotrexate	3	2
Thiotepa (Ttp)	4	1
Ttp + Pd	1	1
Cyclophosphamide (cyclo)	3	2
Cyclo + Pd	2	1
Melphalan	3	2
Vinblastine (Vb)	1	0
Vb + bleomycin	1	0
Cyclo + Pd + 5Fu	1	1
Doxorubicin (Dx) + CCNU	1	0
5Fu + Dx + cyclo + BCG	2	1
Total	29	13 (44%)

Ribeiro (14) treated 10 patients with oral cyclophosphamide (150 mg/day) and had 5 complete responses; 2 of 5 patients receiving 5-fluorouracil also had complete responses. All patients in this report had soft tissue disease only.

CONCLUSIONS

Although male breast cancer is not excessively rare, it is uncommon enough to be very difficult to study. To date the literature consists mainly of single institution studies of patients collected over a long time span. Although calls for collaboration have been made (48) there are no such reports available and even international multicentre studies are unlikely to accrue enough patients for randomized studies. The following recommendations are therefore based on an historical review.

1. In general male breast cancer behaves in much the same way as female breast cancer. The incidence of hormone receptor positivity, however, appears higher in male tumours.
2. Conservative surgery is probably as effective as radical surgery.
3. Postoperative radiotherapy may reduce the rate of local recurrence but has no impact on survival.
4. Adjuvant chemotherapy may be beneficial in Stage II disease and certainly merits further study.
5. Adjuvant tamoxifen also appears to benefit in patients with Stage II and IIIA disease. Collaborative studies will need to be done to establish the role of both these adjuvant approaches.
6. Advanced male breast cancer is highly responsive to hormonal manoeuvres: although ablative procedures appear to give the highest response rates, additive therapies need further study and may prove to be equivalent to orchidectomy.
7. Cytotoxic chemotherapy has been little studied but anecdotally response rates seem to be similar to those in female breast cancer.

REFERENCES

1 Gilbert JB, Judson BC. Carcinoma of the male breast with special reference to etiology. Surg Gynecol Obstet 1933; 57: 451–66.
2 Peck ME. Malignant tumors of the male breast. Surg Clin North Am 1944; 24: 1108–25.
3 Williams WR. Cancer of the male breast, based on the records of one hundred cases; with remarks. Lancet 1889; ii: 261–3.
4 Wainright JM. Carcinoma of the male breast, clinical and pathological study. Arch Surg 1927, 14: 836–859.
5 Crichlow RW. Carcinoma of the male breast. Surg Gynecol Obstet 1972; 134: 1011–19.
6 Scheike O. Male breast cancer. 5. Clinical manifestations in 257 cases in Denmark. Br J Cancer 1973; 28: 552–61.
7 Langlands AO, Maclean N, Kerr GR. Carcinoma of the male breast: report of a series of 88 cases. Clin Radiol 1976; 27: 21–5.
8 Ramantanis G, Besbeas S, Garas JG. Breast cancer in the male: a report of 138 cases. World J Surg 1980; 4: 612–4.
9 Carlsson G, Hafstrom L, Jonsson PE. Male breast cancer. Clin Oncol 1981; 7: 149–55.
10 Appelqvist P, Salmo M. Prognosis in carcinoma of the male breast. Acta Chir Scand 1982; 148: 499–502.
11 Axelsson J., Andersson A. Cancer of the male breast. World J Surg 1983; 7: 281–7.
12 Erlichman C, Murphy KC, Elhakim T. Male breast cancer: a 13 year review of 89 patients. J Clin Oncol 1984; 2: 903–9.
13 Ouriel K, Lotze MT, Hinshaw JR. Prognostic factors in carcinoma of the male breast. Surg Gynecol Obstet 1984; 159: 373–6.
14 Ribeiro G. Male breast carcinoma—a review of 301 cases from the Christie Hospital and Holt Radium Institute, Manchester. Br J Cancer 1985; 51: 115–9.
15 Treves N, Holleb AI. Cancer of the male breast: a report of 146 cases. Cancer 1955; 8: 1239–50.
16 Haagenson CD. Diseases of the Breast, 2nd edition Philadelphia: WB Saunders, 1971: 779–92.
17 Meyskens FL, Tormey DC, Neifeld JP. Male breast cancer: a review. Cancer Treat Rev 1976; 3: 83–93.
18 El-Gazayerli MM, Abdel-Aziz AS. On bilharziasis and male breast cancer in Egypt: a preliminary report and review of the literature. Br J Cancer 1963; 17: 566–71.
19 Schottenfeld D, Lilienfeld AM. Some epidemiologic features of breast cancer among males. J Chron Dis 1963; 16: 71–9.
20 Keller AZ. Demographic, clinical and survivorship characteristics of males with primary cancer of the breast. Am J Epidemiol 1967; 85: 183–99.

21 Schottenfeld D, Lilienfeld AM, Diamond H. Some observations on the epidemiology of breast cancer among males. Am J Public Health 1963; 53: 890–7.

22 Gupta N, Cohen JL, Rosenbaum C et al. Estrogen receptors in male breast cancer. Cancer 1980; 46: 1781–4.

23 Liechty RD, Davis J, Gleysteen J. Cancer of the male breast, forty cases. Cancer 1967; 20: 1617–24.

24 Zumoff B, Fishman J, Cassovto J et al. Estrodiol transformation in men with breast cancer. J Clin Endocrinol Metab 1966; 26: 960–6.

25 Dao TL, Morreal C, Nemoto T. Urinary estrogen excretion in men with breast cancer. N Engl J Med 1973; 289: 138–40.

26 Calabresi E, De Giuli G, Beciolini A et al. Plasma estrogens and androgens in male breast cancer. J Steroid Biochem 1976; 7: 605–9.

27 Nirmul D, Pegoraro RJ, Jialal I et al. The sex hormone profile of male patients with breast cancer. Br J Cancer 1983; 48: 423–7.

28 Roswit B, Edlis H. Carcinoma of the male breast: a thirty year experience and review of the literature. Int J Rad Onc Biol Phys 1978; 4: 711–15.

29 Harnden DG, Maclean N, Langlands AO. Carcinoma of the breast and Klinefelter's syndrome. J Med Genetics 1971; 8: 460–1.

30 Mackenzie I. Breast cancer following multiple fluoroscopies. Br J Cancer 1965, 19: 1–8.

31 Wanebo CK, Johnson KG, Sato K, Thorslund TW. Breast cancer after exposure to the atomic bombings of Hiroshima and Nagasaki. New Engl J Med 1968; 279: 667–71.

32 Everson RB, Li FP, Fraumeni JF et al. Familial male breast cancer. Lancet 1976; i: 9–12.

33 Anderson DE. Genetic study of breast cancer: identification of a high risk group. Cancer 1974; 34: 1090–7.

34 Sachs MD. Carcinoma of the male breast. Radiology 1941; 37: 458–67.

35 Simpson JS, Barson AJ. Breast tumours in infants and children; a 40 year review of cases at a children's hopital. Can Med Assoc J 1969; 101: 100–2.

36 Moss NH. Cancer of the male breast. Ann NY Acad Sci 1964; 114: 937–50.

37 Seltzer MH, Perloff LJ, Kelley RI, Fitts WT. The significance of age in patients with nipple discharge. Surg Gynecol Obstet 1970; 131: 519–22.

38 Sachs MD. Carcinoma of male breast. Radiology 1941; 37: 458–67.

39 Huggins C, Taylor GW. Carcinoma of the male breast. Arch Surg 1955; 70: 303–8.

40 Greening WP, Aichroth PM. Cancer of the male breast. Br J Cancer 1965; 19. 92–100.

41 Holleb AI, Freeman HP, Farrow JH. Cancer of the male breast. NY State J Med 1968; 68: 544–53.

42 Pegoraro RJ, Nirmul D, Joubert SM. Cytoplasmic and nuclear estrogen and progesterone receptor in male breast cancer. Cancer Res 1982; 42: 4812–14.

43 Ruff SJ, Bauer JE, Keenan EJ. Hormone receptors in male breast cancer. J Surg Oncol 1981; 18: 55–9.

44 Nirmul D, Pegoraro RJ, Jialal I. The sex hormone profile of male patients with breast cancer. Br J Cancer 1983; 48: 423–7.

45 Everson RB, Lippman ME, Thompson EB, et al. Clinical correlations of steroid receptors and male breast cancer. Cancer Res 1980; 40: 991–7.

46 Everson RB, Lippman ME. Male breast cancer. In: McGuire WL ed Breast Cancer: Advances in Research and Treatment, Vol 3. New York: NY Publishing Corp, 1979; 239–67.

47 Corwin JH, Ferguson EF, Moseley T, Willey EN. Carcinoma of the male breast. South Med J 1967; 60: 777–80.

48 Bagley CS, Wesley MN, Young RC, Lippman ME. Adjuvant chemotherapy in males with cancer of the breast. Am J Clin Oncol 1987; 10: 55–60.

49 Yap HY, Tashima CK, Blumenschein GR et al. Male breast cancer; a natural history study. Cancer 1979; 44: 748–54.

50 Robison R, Montague ED. Treatment results in males with breast cancer. Cancer 1982; 49: 403–6.

51 Ribeiro GG. Tamoxifen in the treatment of male breast cancer. Clin Radiol 1983; 34: 625–8.

52 Powles TJ. Present role of hormonal therapy. In: Bonadonna G. ed Breast Cancer: Diagnosis and Management. Chichester: John Wiley, 1984; 205–28.

53 Patterson JS, Battersby LA, Bach BK. Use of tamoxifen in advanced male breast cancer. Cancer Treat Rep. 1980; 64: 801–4.

Connective Tissue and Skin Tumours

Chapter **45**

Osteoblastoma, Osteoclastoma, Postradiation Sarcoma of Bone, and Sarcoma Arising in Paget's Disease

David C. Dahlin

Emeritus Consultant, Section of Surgical Pathology, Mayo Clinic and Mayo Foundation; Emeritus Professor of Pathology, Mayo Clinic, Rochester, Minnesota, USA

OSTEOBLASTOMA

Osteoblastoma is a benign osteoblastic tumor that has also been called giant osteoid osteoma and is similar to osteoid osteoma (1–3). The histologic pattern is dominated by osteoblasts that produce trabeculae of osteoid and variable mineralization. The irregularly shaped osteoid seams, containing and mantled by osteocytes and osteoblasts, are separated by benign fibrocytes and capillaries, which may be prominent enough to be suggestive of the diagnosis of hemangioma (Figure 1). Unlike osteoid osteoma, the typical benign osteoblastoma does not have a limited growth potential. Furthermore, patients with benign osteoblastoma frequently do not have the characteristic pain of the ordinary osteoid osteoma, and the lesion usually does not have a surrounding zone of sclerotic bone. Occasionally, there are lesions that have composite features which place them midway between osteoblastoma and osteoid osteoma. McLeod and co-workers (4) have resolved this problem by arbitrarily

regarding an equivocal lesion as an osteoblastoma if it is more than 1.5 cm in diameter.

In the older literature, benign osteoblastoma of the vertebral column is found under various diagnoses. These include giant cell tumor, osteoid osteoma, ossifying (or osteogenic) fibroma, and sarcoma. Osteoblastoma, of course, lacks the more aggressive quality of genuine giant cell tumor or of sarcoma.

Whether all osteoblastomas are correctly classed with the true neoplasm is questionable because they sometimes regress or become arrested after incomplete surgical removal. Areas within some osteoblastomas resemble aneurysmal bone cysts. This feature, plus the similar clinical findings in patients with either lesion, suggests that osteoblastomas may be a manifestation of a reaction to some as yet unknown agent.

Of 8542 bone tumors seen at the Mayo Clinic, 2028 of which were benign, 63 have been osteoblastomas (Figure 2). Most of the patients with osteoblastoma were in the second and third decades of life (Figure 1). Twenty-

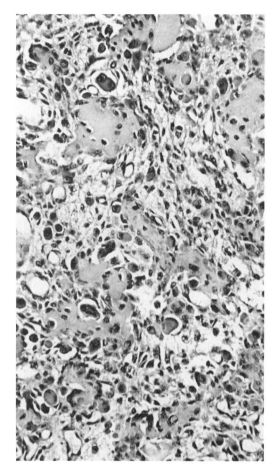

Figure 1 Osteoblastoma with prominent osteoid trabeculae. There are scattered benign giant cells. Note that between the osteoid tabeculae are completely benign fibroblasts and capillaries. (H&E, original magnification: ×250).

on adjacent structures, such as the spinal cord or the emerging nerves; and the pain usually lacks the intrinsic severity that is seen with the ordinary and smaller osteoid osteoma. With involvement of the spinal cord or nerves, weakness or paraplegia may develop. Scoliosis, muscle spasms, and various neurologic symptoms may occur. Pain may be referred to a site distant from the tumor. The lesion usually develops slowly, and the duration of symptoms has been more than 2 years before the patient sought medical advice.

Roentgenographic study may disclose only a circumscribed area of bone destruction, which is not always suggestive of a benign process. Especially when a long bone is involved, the site of the lesion is sometimes surrounded by a dense sclerotic zone (Figure 3B), like that seen with the usual small osteoid osteoma. Many osteoblastomas arise in cancellous bone, which may account for the frequent absence of perifocal sclerosis. Sometimes the lesion is surrounded by a thin layer of bone beneath expanded periosteum, making it simulate an aneurysmal bone cyst. In previously treated or older lesions, ossification of the tumor tissue may make it resemble osteoma or chronic osteomyelitis. McLeod and co-workers (4) found that 76% of long bone tumors were located in the diaphysis and that nearly 40% contained mineral densities; most of the appendicular lesions were associated with new bone formation. In their total series, some of the lesions were as large as 10 cm in diameter.

Grossly, the tumor tissue is granular, friable, and hemorrhagic because of its osteoid component and vascularity. The vascularity may be so pronounced as to make hemostasis a problem for the surgeon. Older lesions have enough mineralization of osteoid matrix that they resemble cancellous bone. Follow-up studies have indicated that the younger lesions are more lytic.

Several peculiarities of osteoblastoma must be recognized (4, 6). Pseudosarcomatous change occurs in the nucleus of 1% to 2% of lesions (7) (Figure 4). These nuclear changes are probably a consequence of degenerative

five of the tumors involved the vertebrae (Figure 3A), including the sacrum. In 1986, Bohlman and co-workers (5) found that 2 of 13 benign tumors of the cervical spine were osteoblastomas. The remainder of the osteoblastomas affected a wide variety of bones, but 7 were in the mandible; several of the mandibular lesions had features of the so-called cementoblastoma—a tumor coapted to the roots of a tooth, often a molar.

Pain related to the tumor is the cardinal symptom. Sometimes the pain is due to pressue

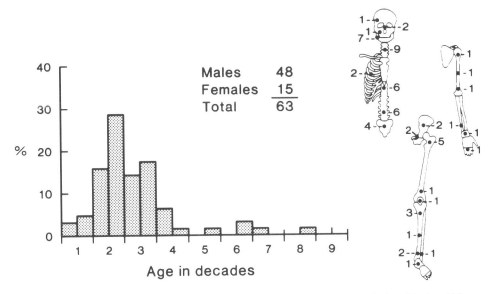

Figure 2 Distribution of osteoblastomas by age and sex of patient and site of lesion (Mayo Clinic, series to 1984). (From Dahlin DC, Unni KK. Bone Tumors: General Aspects and Data on 8,542 Cases, 4th edition. Springfield, Illinois: Charles C Thomas, 1986. *Reproduced by permission of the Mayo Foundation*.)

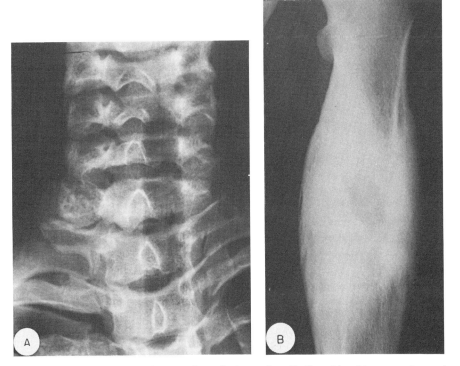

Figure 3 Osteoblastoma. A, Lateral mass of cervical vertebra. B, Considerable secondary sclerosis in femur. (From Dahlin DC. Bone Tumors: General Aspects and Data on 6,221 Cases, 3rd edition. Springfield, Illinois: Charles C Thomas, 1978. *Reproduced by permission of the publisher*.)

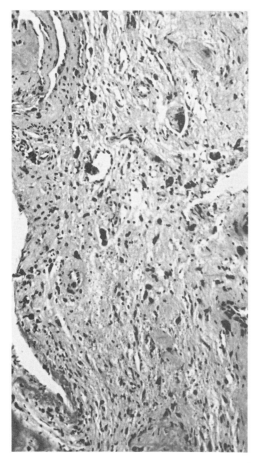

Figure 4 Pseudomalignant osteoblastoma with large hyperchromatic cells but with complete absence of mitotic figures. Although this lesion of the radius was believed to be osteosarcoma, a good result was obtained by conservative therapy. (H&E, original magnification: ×160).

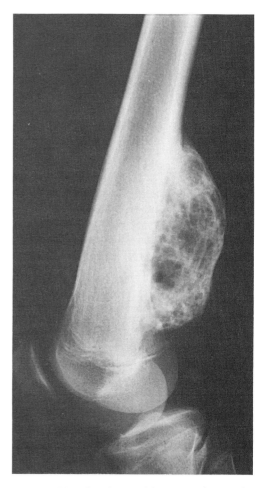

Figure 5 Multifocal osteoblastoma of posterior femur. Much nonneoplastic bone has been produced around the islands of tumor. (From McLeod et al. (4). *Reproduced by permission of the American Roentgen Ray Society*.)

changes, such as are commonly seen in neurilemomas of the eighth cranial nerve. Absence of mitotic activity and a benign quality of the roentgenogram are the evidence that such lesions are benign. Multifocality of osteoblastoma within one osseous area sometimes produces a notable bulge in the affected bone (Figure 5). Such lesions may be 8 cm or more in greatest dimension. Histopathologic appraisal discloses small islands of osteoblastoma separated by nonneoplastic trabeculae of bone and benign fibroblastic tissue. This pattern is an unusual expression of osteoblastoma, seen in only about 2% of the lesions, and it should be differentiated from a malignant tumor. The component cells are benign. As mentioned previously, some osteoblastomas are closely associated with the roots of a tooth and have been called cementoblastomas (Figure 6). An osteoblastoma that causes severe systemic toxicity and osteomalacia has been described.

Treatment requires conservative removal of the tumor. Bone grafting may be necessary after removal of the involved region. Evidence

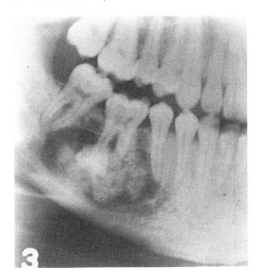

Figure 6 Osteoblastoma surrounding roots of molar. Such lesions are sometimes called cementoblastomas. (From McLeod et al. (4). *Reproduced by permission of the American Roentgen Ray Society.*)

indicates that the lesion ordinarily continues to grow until it has been removed completely. Total removal is not always necessary or desirable, especially if the lesion is in a difficult site like the sacrum or vertebra, because the residual tumor has regressed after subtotal removal. Radiation therapy may be hazardous; in one case in the Mayo Clinic series, a lethal fibrosarcoma developed in the same area 10 years after roentgen therapy had been given for an osteoblastoma of the fifth cervical vertebra.

Malignant transformation of osteoid osteoma or osteoblastoma has been reported, including one example in the Mayo Clinic files (Figure 7). Such pathologic curiosities seem bona fide and could be explained on the basis of failure to recognize that the original tumor was malignant but the malignancy was so histologically subtle that the lesion was considered benign (8–10). Aggressive and malignant osteoblastomas also have been reported. Such lesions are difficult to diagnose and to differentiate from osteosarcomas. The concept that my colleagues and I currently favor is that

osteosarcoma can resemble osteoblastoma. Bertoni and co-workers (11) found that 7 of 17 patients who had osteosarcoma with a histologic pattern similar to that of osteoblastoma died. Features suggesting that the tumors were malignant included their ability to permeate adjacent cancellous or cortical bone and their occurrence in solid sheets of tumor cells. As already indicated, benign osteoblastomas contain trabeculae separated by benign spindle cells and capillaries.

GIANT CELL TUMOR (OSTEOCLASTOMA)

Most authorities now refer to osteoclastoma as a giant cell tumor. The lesion is locally aggressive and has poorly differentiated cells of unknown origin (12–14). Histologic similarities of their nuclei indicate that the multinucleated giant cells, a constant and prominent part of these tumors, are closely related to the mononuclear cells and probably derive from them (Figure 8). A similar osteoclast-like giant cell occurs in many pathologic conditions of bone that must be distinguished from a genuine giant cell tumor. These include nonosteogenic fibroma and aneurysmal bone cyst (still frequently mistaken for giant cell tumor), as well as giant cell granuloma, giant cell epulis, benign chondroblastoma, lesions of bone in hyperparathyroidism, and osteosarcomas rich in benign giant cells. Including such 'variants' with their divergent biologic behavior has delayed the understanding of the clinical characteristics and the response to treatment of the ordinary giant cell tumor.

Of the more than 8500 bone tumors seen at the Mayo Clinic to 1984, 2028 of which were benign, 429 (425 patients) were giant cell tumors (Figure 9). Slightly more than 56% of the patients with giant cell tumor were females. In the subgroup of patients who were less than 20 years old, 72% were females. Because giant cell tumor nearly always is found in patients with mature skeletons, this sex preference in younger patients probably is related to the earlier maturation of the female. Most of these

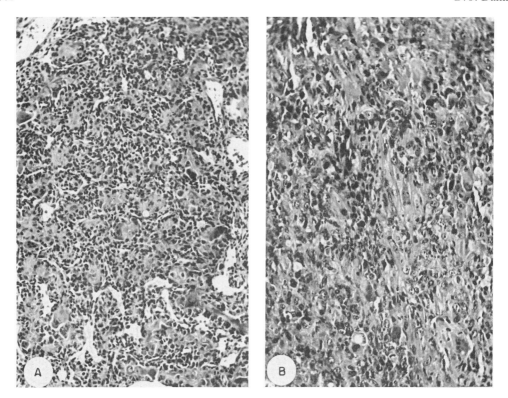

Figure 7 A, Osteoblastoma of tibia. H&E, original magnification: ×160. B, Osteosarcoma developed 4 years later from osteoblastoma shown in Figure 7A. There had been no radiation therapy. H&E, original magnification: ×160. (From McLeod et al. (4). *Reproduced by permission of the American Roentgen Ray Society.*)

younger patients were nearly 20 years old; only 3 patients were younger than 10 years. There was a gradual decrease in incidence after the third decade of life.

Most of the giant cell tumors were found in the epiphyseal region of long bones (15). More than half were found in the region of the knee (Figure 10). Lesions in the distal end of the radius and the sacrum were third and fourth, respectively, in frequency. In the Mayo Clinic series, 21 giant cell tumors were found in the pelvic bones and only 16 were in vertebrae above the sacrum. 'Variants', such as osteoblastomas and aneurysmal bone cysts, are more common in these vertebrae. The 'variants' tend to affect the posterior elements of the vertebrae, whereas the giant cell tumor usually involves the body. Only 10 of the lesions were in the small bones of the hands and feet (16).

Only 4 of the 425 patients with giant cell tumors had involvement of more than one bone. In such instances of multicentric involvement, each lesion has the characteristics of giant cell tumor, but systemic disease, such as hyperparathyroidism, must be excluded. Three giant cell tumors were in the body of the sphenoid.

Although nearly all giant cell tumors extended to the articular cartilage, a few did not. Five patients had metaphyseal tumors, and two of these had immature skeletons.

Pain and swelling are the cardinal symptoms of giant cell tumor. Some patients have weakness, limitation of motion, or signs of pathologic fracture. Sometimes the tumor is crepitant.

Roentgenographically, the features outlined by Gee and Pugh (17) were those of an

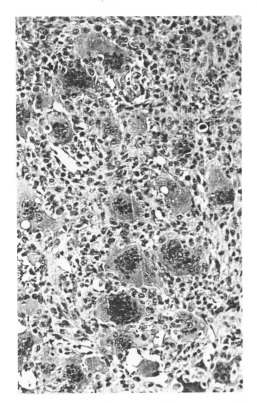

Figure 8 Giant cell tumor with monomorphic cells, producing no matrix. H&E, original magnification: ×160. (From Williams RR, Dahlin DC, Ghormley RK. Giant-cell tumor of bone. Cancer 1954; 7: 764. *Reproduced by permission of the American Cancer Society*.)

expanding zone of radiolucency, usually in the end of a long bone in an adult (see Figure 10). They stated, however, that this appearance is neither specific for giant cell tumors nor produced by all of them. Prior therapy or pathologic fracture may alter the roentgenographic appearance. The margin between the normal bone and the tumor shows a gradual alteration of density; in untreated tumors, there is no reactive sclerosis at this junction. Some radiologists have noted an aggressive capability for giant cell tumors to be more locally destructive and have employed three radiographic grades. Metaphyseal lesions are unlikely to be giant cell tumors, but 5 of the lesions in the Mayo Clinic series spared the epiphysis.

Benign giant cell tumors that implant into soft tissues often produce an ossified periphery. Cooper and colleagues (18) found visible bony shells on the roentgenograms of 10 patients with tissue implants and in 7 giant cell tumors of bone that had been sent in for consultation. Such implants, with their bony rims, are essentially diagnostic of giant cell tumor, usually recurrent (Figure 11). Occasionally, even a benign giant cell tumor that is metastatic to the lungs also shows a bony rim.

Benign giant cell lesions (19) can be a complication of Paget's disease of bone, but only one such lesion—in the ilium—was found in the Mayo Clinic experience.

Lesions other than giant cell tumor, most notably fibrosarcoma or malignant fibrous histiocytoma, may produce an osseous defect, similar to that of giant cell tumor.

Grossly, the giant cell tumor is typically soft and friable and gray to reddish brown. Previous fracture, treatment, or degeneration may result in firmer areas that show evidence of fibrosis or osteoid production. Sometimes, cystic or necrotic portions filled with blood are present. Although these are usually not a significant feature, they are sometimes so prominent as to make the lesion simulate an aneurysmal bone cyst. Variable expansion of the bone (Figure 12), with corresponding attenuation or destruction of the cortex, usually occurs. Neglected tumors usually become very large. The tumor nearly always extends to the articular cartilage, and its boundaries are not well demarcated from adjacent bone. Involvement of more than one bone in a patient with giant cell tumor is extremely unusual. As stated, only 4 patients with such involvement were found in more than 400 patients with giant cell tumor. As indicated previously, special care must be taken to exclude systemic disease when more than one giant cell tumor is suspected.

Histologically, the basic proliferating cell has a round-to-oval or even spindle-shaped nucleus. This nucleus is surrounded by an ill-defined cytoplasmic zone, and discernible intracellular substance is not being produced

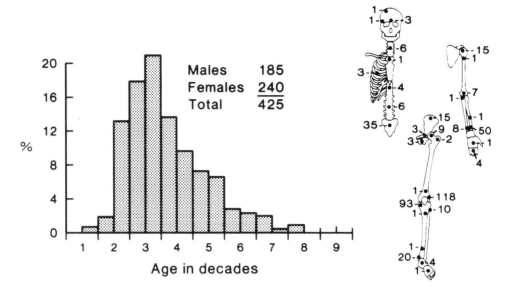

Figure 9 Distribution of 429 (425 patients) giant cell tumors by age and sex of patient and site of lesion (Mayo Clinic, series to 1984). (From Dahlin DC, Unni KK. Bone Tumors: General Aspects and Data on 8,542 Cases, 4th edition. Springfield, Illinois: Charles C Thomas, 1986. *Reproduced by permission of Mayo Foundation*.)

in the fields that are diagnostic of bona fide giant cell tumors. Every tumor contains a few mitotic figures, and sometimes they are numerous. The usual nucleus in a giant cell tumor lacks the hyperchromatism and variation in size and shape that is characteristic of the nucleus of a sarcoma. The exact interpretation may be difficult in the rare osteosarcoma that has unusually small malignant cells and an abundance of benign giant cells (20). Histochemical and ultrastructural methods for differentiating the 'variants' of giant cell tumor from true giant cell tumor have not been helpful; the pathologist must make the differentiation on the basis of correlating the sometimes subtle cytologic and histologic features with the roentgenologic findings.

The pronounced similarity of the nuclei provides the most important evidence that the multinucleated cells, that is, the giant cells, are derived from fusion of the mononuclear cells. Especially after fracture or unsuccessful treatment, some of the proliferating cells show metaplasia and are capable of producing colla-

gen or even osteoid tissue. Such osteoid or bone is commonly seen in the periphery of soft-tissue implants or in metastatic deposits of benign giant cell tumor. Chondroid differentiation is not a feature of genuine giant cell tumor, and its presence suggests that the tumor may be either a benign chondroblastoma or an osteosarcoma with cartilaginous differentiation. Zones containing iron pigment or numerous foam cells apparently result from old hemorrhage or necrosis, and such zones may not be diagnostic. Extensive necrotic foci may be present, especially after pathologic fracture. Small fragments of tissue that contain a few giant cells are inadequate for verifying the diagnosis of true giant cell tumor, so aspiration biopsy has limited usefulness.

Although benign giant cells are usually scattered throughout viable zones, some giant cell tumors contain rather large fields with slightly spindled mononuclear cells devoid of multinucleated form. Blood-filled spaces may be prominent in giant cell tumor, and sometimes even after comparison with the roentge-

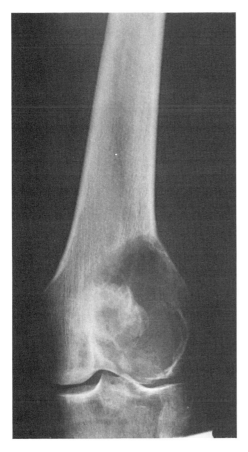

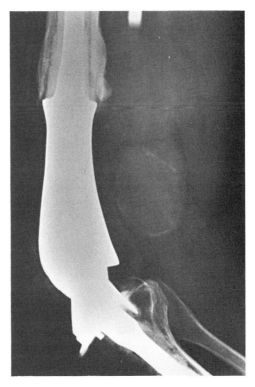

Figure 11 Ossified rim around giant cell tumor implants adjacent to femoral prosthesis. (From Cooper et al. (18). *Reproduced by permission of the Radiological Society of North America.*)

Figure 10 Giant cell tumor in commonest location, the distal femur. (From Dahlin DC. Bone Tumors: General Aspects and Data on 6,221 Cases, 3rd edition. Springfield, Illinois: Charles C Thomas, 1978. *Reproduced by permission of the publisher.*)

nographic appearance, such a lesion may be difficult to differentiate from an aneurysmal bone cyst. However, the combination of the septa having the classic appearance of a giant cell tumor and not showing fibrosis or other matrix substance is reliable evidence for the correct diagnosis of giant cell tumor. In a few tumors, extensions are found in vessels located at periphery, but this finding does not seem to correlate with increased risk. If the roentgenographic changes are those of benign giant cell tumor, mitotic activity and even worrisome cytopathologic findings may be ignored.

The grading of giant cell tumors has not been of value in predicting the lesion that is likely to become sarcomatous or even the lesion that is likely to recur. The treatment that has been used most frequently is curettage, with or without chemical cautery or thermocautery; and sometimes the defect is filled with bone chips. Wide excision or resection of the lesion is sometimes performed, especially when the tumor is located in small bones or in usual sites that show roentgenographic evidence of extensive destruction. Irradiation as a primary or adjunctive therapy is becoming less acceptable because of its sarcoma-inducing potential and the recognition that giant cell tumors are relatively radioresistant. Radiation is reserved for patients with giant cell tumors that are not amenable to surgical excision. Long-term follow-up studies have indicated that from one-

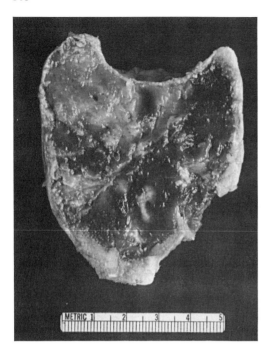

Figure 12 Giant cell tumor expanding distal end of radius. (From Dahlin DC. *Bone Tumors: General Aspects and Data on 6,221 Cases*, 3rd edition. Springfield, Illinois: Charles C Thomas, 1978. *Reproduced by permission of the publisher*).

third to one-half of giant cell tumors recur after conventional curettage, cautery, and grafting. Sarcoma complicates the course in nearly 10% of patients, especially those treated by radiation therapy. Malignant change has occurred nearly 40 years after primary therapy, although the interval is commonly 10 to 15 years. Histologic evidence of benign metastasis from giant cell tumor, especially to the lungs, has been documented in more than 30 cases (21). In the Mayo Clinic files 8 examples of such pulmonary metastases have been found; these are less than 2% of the giant cell tumors in the files. Such lesions are quasi-malignant in that sometimes they regress, and only 2 of the 8 patients have died from the consequences of such metastasis.

The literature on malignant giant cell tumor is difficult to assess (22–25) because various sarcomas with abundant benign giant cells are sometimes included. Certain dogmatic statements should be made about what constitutes malignancy in giant cell tumor. To be certain of this diagnosis, the pathologist must find zones of typical benign giant cell tumor in the malignant neoplasm under appraisal or in tissue removed previously from the same site. If an obviously malignant growth contains a few or many benign osteoclast-like giant cells, the pathologist can prove a relationship to benign giant cell tumor in no other way. Other tumors of bone, including some osteosarcomas and malignant fibrous histiocytomas, may contain many of these benign giant cells.

With this absolute definition of malignancy in giant cell tumor, 23 of 28 such tumors in the Mayo Clinic series occurred after treatment of typical giant cell tumors—tumors that contained no features to distinguish them from the remainder of the giant cell tumors (Figure 13). Of these 23 secondary malignant tumors, 21 occurred after treatment that included radiation to the original benign giant cell tumor. The interval from the treatment of the giant cell tumor to the appearance of the sarcoma averaged 13.5 years, and there was only one with residual giant cell tumor when the sarcoma was diagnosed. Two sarcomas developed without radiation therapy having been employed. One developed $1\frac{1}{2}$ years after simple curettage of the benign giant cell tumor, and the other developed 15 years after the second curettage. In spite of the increasing evidence that is being accumulated to indicate that radiation may trigger malignant transformation in various osseous lesions, and especially giant cell tumor, no such radiation had been employed in 7 cases in the Mayo Clinic series. In 5 cases, evidence of both giant cell tumor and sarcoma was present at the time of the first operation.

These 28 instances of malignancy in giant cell tumors comprised less than half of 1% of the total group of malignant tumors and only 6.6% of the giant cell tumors. The patients with malignancy in giant cell tumor were somewhat older than those with ordinary giant cell tumor. This age difference is probably

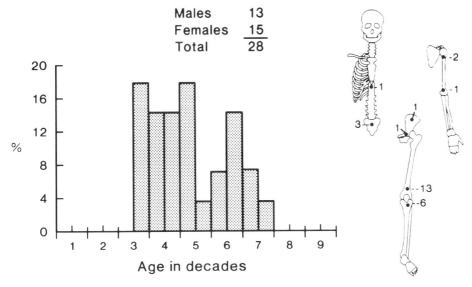

Figure 13 Sarcomas that developed after treatment of benign giant cell tumor. Distribution by age and sex of patient and site of lesion (Mayo Clinic, series to 1984). (From Dahlin DC, Unni KK. Bone Tumors: General Aspects and Data on 8,542 Cases, 4th edition. Springfield, Illinois: Charles C Thomas, 1986. *Reproduced by permission of Mayo Foundation*.)

explained by the fact that most of the tumors developed several years after treatment of the benign precursor. Most of these patients had symptoms of ordinary giant cell tumor at the outset of their disease, and the tumor later developed the more aggressive features of the sarcoma that had supervened.

The roentgenographic appearance may be similar to that of an ordinary giant cell tumor, especially when giant cell tumor and sarcoma coexist. When sarcoma, however, has developed at the site of a giant cell tumor, the roentgenographic changes usually do not differ from those seen in fibrosarcoma or osteosarcoma, except that the lesion is nearly always in the very end of the bone, when a long bone is affected.

Grossly, the tumor may simulate ordinary giant cell tumor, but more often it is firmer and more fibrous in consistency and shows local invasiveness—all features that would be expected for a genuine sarcoma of bone. To adequately assess these lesions, any portion that is grossly different must be sampled, because such areas may contain the sarcoma.

In the Mayo Clinic series, 17 of the secondary tumors were considered to be fibrosarcomas, 5 to be osteosarcomas, and 1 to be a malignant fibrous histiocytoma. As already indicated, in a few tumors, foci of benign giant cell tumor and sarcoma coexisted at the time of definitive surgery.

Primary diffusely malignant giant cell tumor (25) in which the roentgenogram is similar to that of giant cell tumor must be extremely unusual, and no such case was encountered in the Mayo Clinic series.

When malignancy is recognized in a giant cell tumor or in a zone previously occupied by one, ablative surgical treatment is the procedure of choice; and the prognosis should be that expected for the malignant tumor that has supervened.

POSTRADIATION SARCOMA

In the Mayo Clinic series, 103 sarcomas that arose in irradiated bone were seen prior to 1984 (Figure 14) (26–29). The dosage of irradiation varied from a few hundred rads to

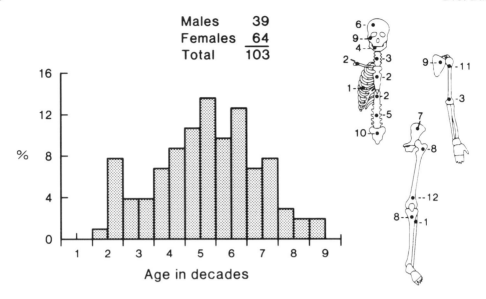

Figure 14 Sarcomas that developed in bones after radiation. Distribution by age and sex of patient and site of lesion (Mayo Clinic, series to 1984). (From Dahlin DC, Unni KK. Bone Tumors: General Aspects and Data on 8,542 Cases, 4th edition. Springfield, Illinois: Charles C Thomas, 1986. *Reproduced by permission of Mayo Foundation.*)

nearly 10 000 rads, but it generally was high. Of the 103 postradiation sarcomas, 35 were fibrosarcomas, 4 were chondrosarcomas, 8 were malignant fibrous histiocytomas, 1 was a Ewing sarcoma, 1 was a malignant lymphoma, 1 was a hemangioendothelial sarcoma, 1 was a metastasizing chondroblastoma, and 52 were osteosarcomas of various histologic types (osteoblastic, fibroblastic, and chondroblastic). All 52 osteosarcomas showed histologic evidence of osteoid production by malignant cells in at least small areas.

The primary lesion was giant cell tumor in 21 patients, including 3 who did not have histologic proof of the original diagnosis but had clinical and radiologic support for the diagnosis of giant cell tumor. In 9 additional patients, irradiation had been done for treatment of unverified osseous lesions. In 7 patients with fibrous dysplasia, sarcoma developed after radiation therapy. Sarcomatous change in fibrous dysplasia is less common in patients in whom radiation has not been done. Twelve patients had been exposed to ionizing radiation as part of the treatment for carcinoma of

the cervix, uterus, or ovaries, and 13 had ancillary radiation for carcinoma of the breast. These postradiation sarcomas had a tendency to affect the ends of the long bones (as would be expected because so many of the original lesions were giant cell tumors) or to occur in the shoulder or pelvic girdle if the primary process were malignancy of the breast or uterine region. Most of the sarcomas of the jaws developed in patients with earlier fibrous dysplasia. Twenty-three patients had primary lesions, usually tumors in the soft tissue, and 11 had miscellaneous bone lesions that were irradiated. Among the rarer primary lesions were 3 aneurysmal bone cysts, 2 chordomas, and 2 unverified brain tumors.

Data in the Mayo Clinic series do not provide information as to the risk for patients whose bones are subjected to irradiation. It seems logical, though, that radiation should not be given to patients with conditions such as fibrous dysplasia, for which radiation has no proved value, and the risk should be considered whenever such therapy is employed.

A cause-and-effect relationship was not

established unequivocally in any of the 103 cases of postradiation sarcoma seen in the Mayo Clinic experience, but there is overwhelming experimental and clinical evidence that one exists.

The interval between irradiation and the diagnosis of sarcoma may be long, thus allowing for a false sense of security. In the Mayo Clinic series, the interval ranged from $2\frac{3}{4}$ to 55 years, and the average interval was 15.1 years. It was more than 20 years in 10 patients and less than 5 years in only 8. For practical purposes, a bone subjected to radiation should be considered to be always at risk.

The sarcomas that developed were nearly as lethal as similar malignant tumors that occurred in non-irradiated bones. When fibrosarcoma or osteosarcoma develops in an older patient, the precursors, such as prior radiation or Paget's disease, should be suspected as causative. The postradiation sarcomas in the Mayo Clinic series were characteristically highly anaplastic malignant tumors and not of debatable malignancy.

SARCOMA ARISING IN PAGET'S DISEASE

This tumor is the most serious complication of Paget's disease (30). The association of sarcoma to osteitis deformans was first noted by Sir James Paget in 1877 (31–34). At the Mayo Clinic, Greditzer and co-workers (35) observed 41 cases of sarcoma of bone in Paget's disease in 1983. This entire experience at the Mayo Clinic showed that the relative frequency of sarcomatous change was 0.9%. Reports of the incidence of sarcoma in Paget's disease have ranged from 0.9% to 14%. The higher rates have been reported in the earlier literature (35), but the increased use of radiographic examinations probably accounts for the lower contemporary incidence. Although these sarcomas are a relatively uncommon complication of Paget's disease, they contribute significant mortality, because Paget's disease affects 3% of the population. Sarcomas that complicate Paget's disease are responsible

for the second peak of incidence of osteosarcomas that many studies have noted in the older age group.

Of the 41 such lesions in the Mayo Clinic experience, all but 2 were high grade (Grade 3 or 4 by Broders' method). Thirty-five of the lesions were osteosarcomas, and 6 were fibrosarcomas. In some of these sarcomas, the fibroblastic portions exhibited a storiform pattern similar to that seen in malignant fibrous histiocytoma. The distribution of these sarcomas was similar to that of uncomplicated Paget's disease except for an unusually large number of lesions of the humerus. Fifteen of the lesions were in the pelvis, 8 in the femur (Figure 15), and 7 in the humerus. Three sarcomas arose in the tibia, 3 in the skull, 2 in

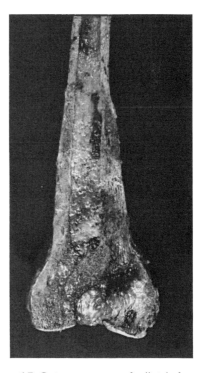

Figure 15 Osteosarcoma of distal femur in patient with Paget's disease involving distal third of femur. The 57-year-old man died 10 months after disarticulation at the hip. (From Dahlin DC. Bone Tumors: General Aspects and Data on 6,221 Cases, 3rd edition. Springfield, Illinois: Charles C Thomas, 1978. *Reproduced by permission of the publisher.*)

the scapula, 1 in the mandible, 1 in a tarsal bone, and 1 in a vertebra. In bones affected by Paget's disease, 1 giant cell tumor and 1 malignant lymphoma also were found.

Radiographically, the lesions were lytic, mixed, or sclerotic (in descending order of frequency) (Figure 16). The changes of the underlying Paget's disease sometimes obscure the developing sarcoma. Finding areas of cortical destruction is especially useful in the detection of sarcomatous development. In florid osteitis deformans, there may be osseous spicules extending into a soft-tissue mass that is contiguous with an affected bone, which at

biopsy shows only the changes of benign Paget's disease (Figure 17) (36).

The pelvis may be difficult to evaluate for malignant lesions, especially if bony detail is obscured by bowel contents. In a few cases, computed tomography will show destruction of bone and perhaps delineate a soft-tissue component of the sarcoma.

Paget's sarcomas rarely occur in patients who are less than 40 years old, as is to be expected, because Paget's disease is so uncommon in young patients. In the series of Greditzer et al. (35), only 3 patients were less than 50 years old at diagnosis. The youngest was 32

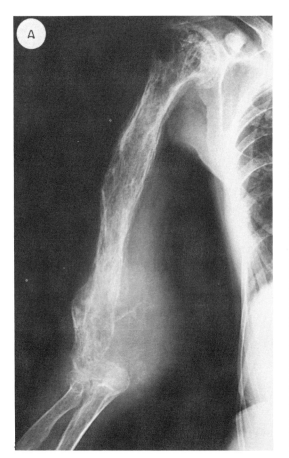
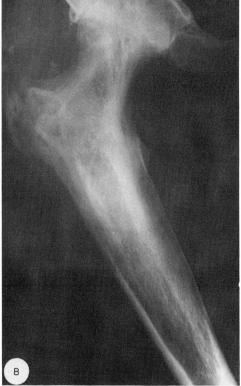

Figure 16 A, Osteosarcoma of lower humerus, showing extensive involvement by Paget's disease. Lesion is mainly lytic. B, Osteosarcoma extending above trochanter in patient with Paget's disease of femur. (From Dahlin DC. Bone Tumors: General Aspects and Data on 6,221 Cases, 3rd edition. Springfield, Illinois: Charles C Thomas, 1978. *Reproduced by permission of the publisher.*)

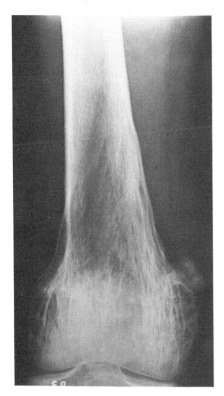

Figure 17 'Florid' Paget's diseae extending from cortex of distal part of femur of 44-year-old man. Histologically, the tumefaction was benign. (From Dahlin DC. Bone Tumors: General Aspects and Data on 6,221 Cases, 3rd edition. Springfield, Illinois: Charles C Thomas, 1978. *Reproduced by permission of the publisher*.)

years old, and the oldest was 86 years old (mean, 64 years). Sixteen of the 41 patients were women. All of their patients with sarcoma had either pain or swelling at the site of the lesion, and 37 had pain as the predominant symptom. The average duration of significant symptoms from sarcoma was 6 months.

The prognosis of patients with sarcoma complicating Paget's disease is notoriously bad, and the Mayo Clinic series provided no evidence that ancillary measures, such as radiation or chemotherapy, were helpful; but more study of the effects of chemotherapy are necessary. The overall survival rate for 5 years was only 8%, and only 3 patients survive more

than 10 years. Eighty-eight percent of the patients died within 3 years of the sarcoma being diagnosed.

REFERENCES

1 Dahlin DC, Johnson EW Jr. Giant osteoid osteoma. J Bone Joint Surg (Am) 1954; 36: 559.
2 Lichtenstein L, Sawyer WR. Benign osteoblastoma: further observations and report of twenty additional cases. J Bone Joint Surg (Am) 1964; 46: 755.
3 Schajowicz F, Lemos C. Osteoid osteoma and osteoblastoma. Closely related entities of osteoblastic derivation. Acta Orthop Scand 1970; 41: 272.
4 McLeod RA, Dahlin DC, Beabout JW. The spectrum of osteoblastoma. AJR 1976; 126: 321.
5 Bohlman HH, Sachs BL, Carter JR, Riley L, Robinson RA. Primary neoplasms of the cervical spine: diagnosis and treatment of twenty-three patients. J Bone Joint Surg (Am) 1986; 68: 483.
6 Mirra JM, Theros E, Smasson J, Cove K, Paladugu R. A case of osteoblastoma associated with severe systemic toxicity. Am J Surg Pathol 1979; 3: 463.
7 Mirra JM, Kendrick RA, Kendrick R.E. Pseudomalignant osteoblastoma versus arrested osteosarcoma: a case report. Cancer 1976; 37: 2005.
8 Schajowicz F, Lemos C. Malignant osteoblastoma. J Bone Joint Surg (Br) 1976; 58: 202.
9 Pieterse AS, Vernon-Roberts B, Paterson DC, Cornish BL, Lewis PR. Osteoid osteoma transforming to aggressive (low grade malignant) osteoblastoma: a case report and literature review. Histopathology 1983; 7: 789.
10 Dorfman HD, Weiss SW. Borderline osteoblastic tumors: problems in the differential diagnosis of aggressive osteoblastoma and low-grade osteosarcoma. Semin Diagn Pathol 1984; 1: 215.
11 Bertoni F, Unni KK, McLeod RA, Dahlin DC. Osteosarcoma resembling osteoblastoma. Cancer 1985; 55: 416.
12 Dahlin DC, Ghormley RK, Pugh DG. Giant cell tumor of bone: differential diagnosis. Proc Staff Meet Mayo Clin 1956; 31: 31.
13 D'Aubigné RM, Thomine JM, Mazabraud A, Hannouche D. Évolution spontanée et postopératoire des tumeurs à cellules géantes: indications thérapeutiques à propos de 39 cas dont 20 suivis 5 ans ou plus. Rev Chir Orthop 1968; 54: 689.
14 Goldenberg RR, Campbell CJ, Bonfiglio M. Giant-cell tumor of bone: an analysis of two

hundred and eighteen cases. J Bone Joint Surg (Am) 1970; 52: 619.

15 Campanacci M, Giunti A, Olmi R. Giant-cell tumours of bone. A study of 209 cases with long-term follow-up in 130. Ital J Orthop Traumatol 1975; 1: 249.

16 Wold LE, Swee RG. Giant cell tumor of the small bones of the hands and feet. Semin Diagn Pathol 1984; 1: 173.

17 Gee VR, Pugh DG. Giant-cell tumor of bone. Radiology 1958; 70: 33.

18 Cooper KL, Beabout JW, Dahlin DC. Giant cell tumor: ossification in soft-tissue implants. Radiology 1984; 153: 597.

19 Upchurch KS, Simon LS, Schiller AL, Rosenthal DI, Campion EW, Krane SM. Giant cell reparative granuloma of Paget's disease of bone: a unique clinical entity. Ann Intern Med 1983; 98: 35.

20 Troup JB, Dahlin DC, Coventry MB. The significance of giant cells in osteogenic sarcoma: Do they indicate a relationship between osteogenic sarcoma and giant cell tumor of bone? Proc Staff Meet Mayo Clin 1960; 35: 179.

21 Rock MG, Pritchard DJ, Unni KK. Metastases from histologically benign giant-cell tumor of bone. J Bone Joint Surg (Am) 1984; 66: 269.

22 Sanerkin NG. Malignancy, aggressiveness, and recurrence in giant cell tumor of bone. Cancer 1980; 46: 1641.

23 Murphy WR, Ackerman LV. Benign and malignant giant-cell tumors of bone: a clinical-pathological evaluation of thirty-one cases. Cancer 1956; 9: 317.

24 Hutter RVP, Worcester JN Jr, Francis KC, Foote FW Jr, Stewart FW. Benign and malignant giant cell tumors of bone: a clinicopathological analysis of the natural history of the disease. Cancer 1962; 15: 653.

25 Nascimento AG, Huvos AG, Marcove RC. Primary malignant giant cell tumor of bone: a study of eight cases and review of the literature. Cancer 1979; 44: 1393.

26 Sabanas AO, Dahlin DC, Childs DS Jr, Ivins JC. Postradiation sarcoma of bone. Cancer 1956; 9: 528.

27 Tanner HC Jr, Dahlin DC, Childs DS Jr. Sarcoma complicating fibrous dysplasia: probable role of radiation therapy. Oral Surg 1961; 14: 837.

28 Sim FH, Cupps RE, Dahlin DC, Ivins JC. Postradiation sarcoma of bone. J Bone Joint Surg (Am) 1972; 54: 1479.

29 Weatherby RP, Dahlin DC, Ivins JC. Postradiation sarcoma of bone: review of 78 Mayo Clinic cases. Mayo Clin Proc 1981; 56: 294.

30 Goldenberg RR. Neoplasia in Paget's disease of bone. Bull Hosp Joint Dis (NY) 1961; 22: 1.

31 Paget J. On a form of chronic inflammation of bones (osteitis deformans). Med Chir Trans 1877; 60: 37.

32 Porretta CA, Dahlin DC, Janes JM. Sarcoma in Paget's disease of bone. J Bone Joint Surg (Am) 1957; 39: 1314.

33 Price CHG. The incidence of osteogenic sarcoma in southwest England and its relationship to Paget's disease of bone. J Bone Joint Surg (Br) 1962; 44: 366.

34 Barry HC. Sarcoma in Paget's disease of bone in Australia. J Bone Joint Surg (Am) 1961; 43: 1122.

35 Greditzer HC III, McLeod RA, Unni KK, Beabout JW. Bone sarcomas in Paget disease. Radiology 1983; 146: 327.

36 Bowerman JW, Altman J, Hughes JL, Zadek RE. Pseudo-malignant lesions in Paget's disease of bone. Am J Roentgenol Radium Ther Nucl Med 1975; 124: 57.

Textbook of Uncommon Cancer
Edited by C.J. Williams, J.G. Krikorian, M.R. Green and D. Raghavan
© 1988 John Wiley & Sons Ltd

Chapter **46**

Adamantinoma of Bone

Gordon F. Vawter* and
Robert H. Wilkinson†

* Associate Pathologist-In-Chief, The Children's Hospi-
tal, Boston; Professor of Pathology, Harvard Medical
School, Boston, USA and † Radiologist and Associate in
Medicine, The Children's Hospital, Boston; Associate
Professor of Radiology, Harvard Medical School, Boston,
USA

HISTORY

'Adamantinoma is an uncommon malignant neoplasm of bone of uncertain origin. Its histologic pattern is reminiscent of ameloblastoma of the jaw.' Thus was adamantinoma defined in 1972 in the Atlas of Tumor Pathology published by The Armed Forces Institute of Pathology (1).

In 1913 Bernhard Fischer's classic report (2) first delineated this entity recognizing its resemblance to fetal ameloblastic tissue. This report describes a pretibial, periosteal or cortical partly cystic lens-shaped mass measuring about 11 by 3.0 cm. involving the junction of the middle and lower thirds of the tibia. The specimen was obtained by a segmental resection followed by graft from the opposite tibia by a Dr Altschuler from a 47 year old postman 11 months after a local injury followed by a hematoma and a palpable mass. Postoperative healing was satisfactory and no other site of disease was discovered during the 8-month follow-up.

The experience of the next 30 years emphasized the following points.

1. The possible pathogenetic role of remote trauma (3).

2. The gradual recognition that adamantinomas were potentially malignant as manifest by recurrence after local surgery (4) and finally by demonstration of distant metastases (5) both leading to recommendations for primary amputation. The first death attributable to adamantinoma was reported in 1943 (6). More recently the utility of segmental resection for accessible lesions has gained favor (7).

3. The predominant tibial localization was recognized in the term adamantinoma of the tibia. Later the term was expanded to adamantinoma of long bone and finally the designation adamantinoma of the appendicular skeleton was proposed (8). We prefer the term adamantinoma of bone.

By 1985 Moon had collected and reviewed 200 adamantinomas of bone including 15 personal cases and 185 from the literature (8, 9). This material includes tumors variously designated by the original authors as squamous cell carcinoma, basal cell carcinoma, eccrine carcinoma, cylindrostellate epithelioma, synovioma and angioblastoma.

While Fischer hinted that adamantinoma might be a mixed or biphasic epithelial and

855

stromal tumor, this view was clearly enunciated by Hicks in 1954 with his diagnosis of synovioma of bone (10), and this general view has gained more adherents recently (11, 12).

Beginning in 1968 the new techniques of electron microscopy and later immunoperoxidase antibody techniques demonstrated keratin to be characteristic of the epithelial component of adamantinoma, findings adding to precision of diagnosis and possibly illuminating questions of histogenesis (13, 14).

In 1978 Dahlin ventured that more than one type of tumor might be subsumed under the rubric of adamantinoma (15). Adamantinoma evolving biologically and pathologically as Ewing's sarcoma was reported beginning in 1975, a distinctive condition for which the term ewingoid adamantinoma was offered (16–18).

EPIDEMIOLOGY AND ETIOLOGY

Epidemiology

Adamantinomas have been described from all inhabited continents and subcontinents but possible racial predilection is unknown. They account for about 0.2% of all bone tumors and 0.4% of malignant bone tumors (15, 19). The male to female ratio ranges between 1 to 1 and 2 to 1. At diagnosis the youngest patient was 4 years old (19) and the oldest 74 years of age (10) with 60% of cases occurring in the second, third and fourth decades (8, 9). Moon notes that females may be somewhat younger at diagnosis than males. Bones involved have been: tibia 78%, both tibia and fibula 5.5%, femur 5%, humerus 4.5%, ulna 3.5%, fibula alone 1.5%, and other sites 2.5%. Thus 90% involve the lower extremity (8, 9).

For the tibial site Dahlin reports 18 osteosarcomas and 2 Ewing's tumors for each adamantinoma (15): Schajowicz reports 12 osteosarcomas, 3 Ewing's tumors, 4 fibrous dysplasias, and 1.5 chondromyxofibromas for each adamantinoma (19). In the latter series there were 3 fibrous dysplasias and 0.5 osteosarcomas for each adamantinoma involving the mid-shaft of the tibia.

Etiology

Cancer Diathesis

Adamantinoma preceding other cancer is known (gastric carcinoma in a 27 year old woman (20)) but remains anecdotal, since there is notable lack of extended personal or family history in the usual case report. Deaths unrelated to adamantinoma have mostly included cardiovascular diseases which do not seem unusual (8, 9).

Fibrous Dysplasia

Individuals ultimately found to have adamantinoma have been frequently considered initially to have fibrous dysplasia on the basis of protracted course, site of involvement, roentgenologic findings and characteristic histopathologic features (21). The latter were described by Fischer in the first case (2) have been reported in 0 to 100% of all adamantinomas (11, 22), and are considered as an intrinsic part of adamantinoma by an increasing number of observers who believe the tumor to be biphasic, that is to have characteristic epithelial and stromal components. Approximately 25–30% of tibial adamantinomas involve the junction of middle and distal thirds of the diaphysis. Of 2 adamantinomas associated with congenital deformity of the distal tibia, one also had pseudoarthrosis and fibrous dysplasia (19, 23). In 2 other cases symptomatic before diagnosis for 20 to 50 years, the clinical onset was around 5 years of age (20). Cohen first emphasized pathologic changes resembling fibrous dysplasia in association with adamantinoma (21). Subsequent review including Cohen's material by Unni et al. (20) indicated that inconspicuous epithelial components were usually present also. Atypical for true fibrous dysplasia are those common adamantinomas in which the lesions are purely or largely cortical (20). The incidence of polyostotic fibrous dysplasia in association with adamantinoma is unknown but if it occurs it remains anecdotal. Cutaneous melanotic pig-

mentation has not been described with adamantinoma (19, 20) but this feature is essentially only seen with polyostotic fibrous
dysplasia. Nevertheless, there remain cases
where separate foci of fibrous dysplasia coexist
with adamantinoma (24). Whether both components derive from congenital rests or
whether some adamantinomas represent a
further epithelial metaplasia and neoplastic
transformation from fibrous dysplasia cannot
yet be determined.

Remote Trauma and Aberrant Development

In 1932 Ryrie noted the high incidence of
preceding remote local trauma in tibial adamantinoma (3). As discussed by Fischer in
1913, trauma might have been incidental,
related to activation of a congenital rest or
eventuate in displacement and implantation of
epidermal tissues (2). For the 200 adamantinomas reviewed by Moon there was a history of
preceding trauma in about 30% and for those
133 with specific search for such a history the
incidence reached 60% (8, 9). Recently, possible missing links in the congenital rest/dis-
placement hypotheses have been reported:
tumors resembling adamantinoma have been
reported in deep pretibial dermis (25) and in
pretibial tissues (26), tumors which may represent way stations to the 30% or so of tibial
adamantinomas which are anterior, periosteal
or cortical (2, 27). Adamantinomas of other
'subcutaneous' bones such as ulna and fibula
might have similar pathogenesis but the 10%
of adamantinomas in deep bones such as femur
and humerus seem less easily explained (9).

Synovial Origin

On the other hand, eccentric adamantinomas
of the most proximal and distal diaphyses and
especially those rare tumors involving the
physis and metaphyseal regions could equally
well represent synovial or tendon sheath
tumors (10, 27, 28). The oft repeated statement that all bona fide soft tissue synoviomas

are such highly malignant and rapidly progressive tumors that adamantinomas of bone
cannot represent such tumors needs major
revision with the recognition that some synoviomas have a more indolent course characterized by local recurrence, and metastasis to
regional lymph nodes over a period of months
or years before hematogenous metastasis. As
will be discussed below, there is as yet no
absolute way to distinguish synovioma from
ectopic epidermal tumors.

Vascular Nature and Origin

A vascular nature and origin of adamantinoma as reflected in the term angioblastoma
has been espoused by several authorities in the
past (15, 22). Recent advances in diagnosis
suggest that this hypothesis requires further
support before it can be applied to the bulk of
adamantinomas (13, 14).

PATHOLOGY AND BIOLOGY

Pathology

Macroscopic Findings

At the time of diagnosis the maximum diameter of most lesions is 7 to 10 cm (9), ranging
from 2 cm diameter in lesions followed as long
as 4 years (7), up to involvement of virtually an
entire bone (20) especially in cases with known
osseous abnormality for several decades. The
diameter of the bone is usually increased and
bone surrounding the lesion is typically very
dense in lesions symptomatic for several years.
Perhaps lesions lacking this characteristic
should be judged more rapidly progressive.
Typically the lesion is said to be covered by a
rim of bone with little evidence of periosteal
stimulation (11). The incidence of extra-
osseous soft tissue invasion is uncertain, lacking
previous biopsy or surgery, but could
approach 40% (20). Pathologic fracture
occurs in 5 to 15%.

The abnormal tissue (Figure 1) is sharply
defined or circumscribed, may have scalloped

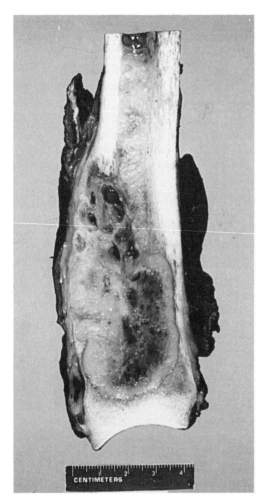

Figure 1 Adamantinoma showing characteristic macroscopic features with scalloped outline and cystic changes. Segmental resection following aspiration and secondary open biopsy. Involvement of the physis is uncommon.

outlines, is fleshy, mucoid or rarely gritty, white, grey, pale tan or faintly pink and sometimes lobulated. Cysts are frequent, small or large, round or ragged and contain clear or brown fluid or blood. Cysts may be massive with tumor reduced to a few mural placques (19, 20). The relation of these changes to trauma, pathologic fracture or previous biopsy and curettage has seldom been assessed. Arteriography and technetium-99 bone scans often indicate central hypovascularity which may

reflect cystic changes or a natural low vascular ity which may be contributory to the histopathologic patterns and to the development of cysts and propensity for hemorrhage.

Nature of Tibial Involvement

Over 97% of lesions are diaphyseal with 50% in the middle third or near the junction of the middle and distal thirds, 30% more distal and 20% more proximal (8, 9). Thirty to 40% are eccentric with major cortical involvement (Figure 1) (22), usually anteriorly and some (like Fischer's case) are periosteal. In some 11 distal lesions there has been separate or direct contiguous involvement of the fibula (8, 9, 12).

Histopathology

Characteristic stromal and epithelial patterns are present (11, 12). Since the proportion of these two elements varies between 10 and 80% (12), diagnosis often requires a generous wedge biopsy (8, 9). As the typical stromal pattern necessary for diagnosis is indistinguishable from that of fibrous dysplasia of bone, the ultimate diagnosis rests upon the epithelial pattern.

Epithelial patterns. There are four basic epithelial patterns (11, 12), often mixed together.

1. *Basaloid.* Included are two arrangements. The adamantine or cylindrostellate pattern consists of peripheral rows of cuboidal or columnar cells surrounding a central mass of stellate (epithelial reticulate) cells (Figures 2 and 8) which often are arranged loosely or in microcystic fashion (2, 15, 29, 30). The second arrangement, which resembles basal cell epithelioma (Figures 2 and 3), is comprised of compact masses of plump spindle cell epithelium with an inconstant cuboidal (basal cell) rim (1, 2, 11, 19, 20). Basaloid patterns were found in 12 of 18 adamantomas and predominated in 3 (11, 12, 22).

2. *Spindle cell.* Interrupted chains, branching cords (filigree) or solid masses of plump elongate cells with indistinct cytoplasm which lack

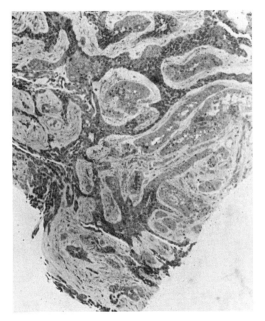

Figure 2 Basaloid pattern with basement membrane and peripheral cuboidal basal cells; 1 μm Epon embedded section, toluidine blue, original magnification: ×470.

a peripheral basal cell palisade (Figure 4), can be mistaken for sarcoma, schwannoma, or other tumors. This pattern was found in 9 of 18 adamantinomas and predominated in 5 (11, 12).

3. *Squamoid*. Nests and whorls of cells suggest squamous epithelial pearls especially when the cytoplasm becomes more plentiful and eosinophilic (Figure 5): intercellular bridges are rarely seen (11, 12, 20). The pattern was found in 5 of 18 and predominated in 1 (11, 12).

4. *Tubular*. Arrangements vary from many circular profiles suggesting glands or alveoli (adenocarcinoma) (22) or hemangioendothelioma (angioblastoma) (Figure 6) to winding double cords of cells to complexly branching irregular sinusoidal spaces lined by plump cells (Figure 7), structures which seem to arise from central degeneration of solid masses and which may contain luminal erythrocytes (1, 2, 19, 22, 29, 31). This pattern was found in 7 of 18 tumors and predominated in 4 (11, 12).

Reticulum stains are very useful since they outline groups of epithelial cells in the basaloid, squamoid and tubular patterns but may outline each individual cell in the spindle pattern (11, 12).

Stroma. For most observers the characteristic stroma of adamantinoma is an edematous, myxoid (Figure 4b) or loose whorling, cartwheel or storiform reticulogenic fibroblastic and osteogenic tissue resembling that of fibrous dysplasia of bone. Osseous (and perhaps cartilaginous) metaplasia characteristic of fibrous dysplasia is frequently present (11, 20, 21). Since these features may be predominant comprising 10 to 80% of a lesion, the clinical and radiologic setting may be crucial to ultimate diagnosis (12). Collagenization may increase in density, be sclerosing or hyalinized and assume storiform or non-specific patterns (22). Companacci et al. depict acellular hyaline stroma in previously irradiated but still recognizable adamantinoma (see Figure 5C and D in reference 12). Two other reports depict the histology of a previously irradiated adamantinomas, the irradiation dosage being unspecified (11, 31). In 2 cases we have observed stroma rich in plump spindle cells with plentiful eosinophilic cytoplasm suggesting smooth muscle cells (leiomyomatous) but it seems likely that this represents hyperplasia of fibromyoblasts (Figure 7).

Blood Supply and Vascularity

Most tibial adamantinomas arise at sites distant from major medullary vascular supply. Marginal hypervascularity seen occasionally angiographically may well be largely periosteal in origin. Microscopically, within the lesion vasculature is often inconspicuous consisting of thin sinusoidal vessels (Figure 5) or small vessels with hyperplastic endothelium. Occasional highly vascular regions seem related to degenerative change and repair. Such areas may contain hemosiderin, foam cells and multinucleate giant cells (11, 20).

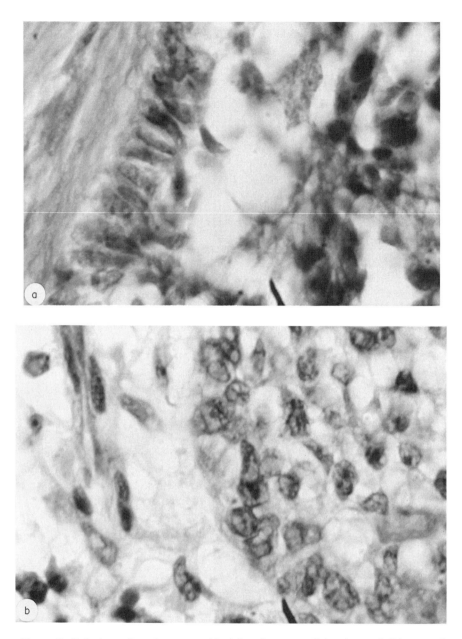

Figure 3 Cylindrostellate features with (a) columnar cell border and (b) central stellate reticular epithelial cells; 6 μm paraffin embedded sections. H&E, original magnification: ×4700.

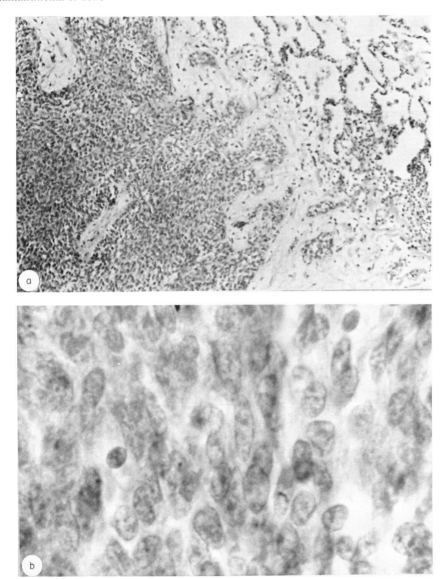

Figure 4 Spindle cell epithelial pattern: elongate nuclei with indistinct cell borders. Pulmonary metastasis: 6 μm paraffin embedded section, H&E. (a) Pulmonary metastasis. Original magnification: ×470. (b) Original magnification: ×4700.

Mitotic Activity

Mitosis is recorded in occasional adamantinomas (11, 12, 20, 31) (Figure 8). Two recent systematic studies of mitosis are difficult to interpret since different techniques were applied (11, 12). A more quantitative approach seems desirable.

Histochemistry

Mucus secretion as demonstrated by mucicarmine stains is not found in adamantinoma, a feature which may help to exclude mucus secreting adenocarcinomas. The constituents of the extracellular fluid apart from contamination with blood are poorly characterized as

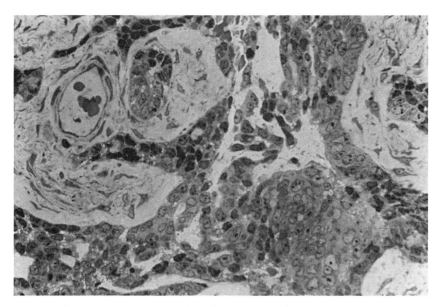

Figure 5 Squamoid pattern: on the left a cluster of plump cells with plentiful sharply defined cytoplasm suggests keratinocytes; 1 μm Epon embedded section, Toluidine blue, original magnification: ×1880.

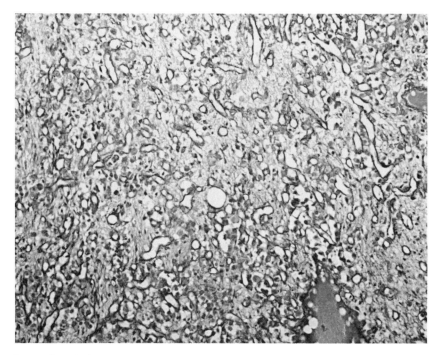

Figure 6 Tubular pattern: a rare histologic pattern of adamantinoma suggesting hemangioma or perhaps adenocarcinoma. Tumor cells contained keratin and were negative for factor VIII on immunoperoxidase staining. Tonofilaments were demonstrated by electron microscopy (see Figure 9 which is the same tumor); 6 μm section of paraffin embedded tissue. H&E, original magnification: ×250.

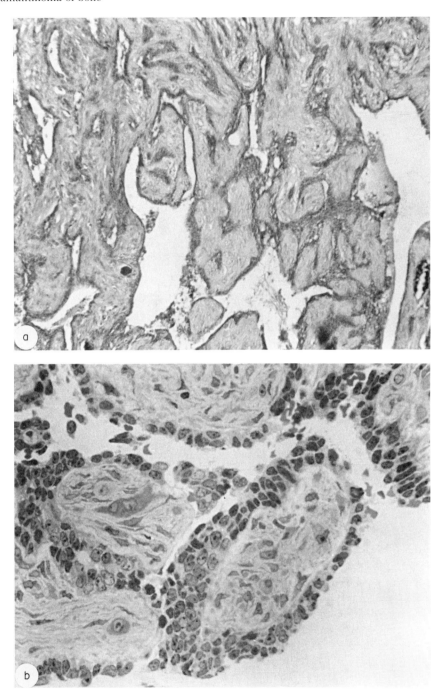

Figure 7 So-called tubular pattern. (a) A common pattern included under the term tubular. Note the pale fluid content with scattered erythrocytes and the calcospherocyte; 6 μm paraffin embedded section, H&E, original magnification: ×470. (b) 1 μm Epon embedded section, toluidine blue, original magnification: ×1880.

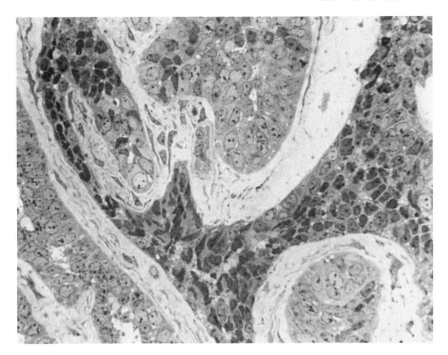

Figure 8 A basaloid adamantinoma showing mitosis and hyaline globules in the primary tumor. Pulmonary metastases were discovered following spontaneous pneumothorax 13 months after diagnosis and treatment.

having very low concentrations of protein and probably largely neutral polysaccharide (Figure 6). Hyaline globules which may be seen among epithelial cells are of unknown nature nor is it known whether these are intracellular or extracellular (Figure 8) (see Figure 11 in reference 31) (20, 31). Non-specific alkaline phosphatase, which also demonstrates but does not identify other alkaline phosphatases (such as ATPase, 5'-nucleotidase, bone specific alkaline phosphatase, glucose-6-phosphatase), is positive in the epithelium of adamantinoma of bone (31–33) and strongly positive in the stromal vasculature and in osteogenic spindle cells and this characteristic has led to an erroneous diagnosis of osteogenic sarcoma in an aspiration biopsy (31). (Adamantinoma of the jaw is negative for alkaline phosphatase (34).) One histochemical study demonstrates additional similarities between adamantinoma and eccrine sweat glands (32).

Electron Microscopy

Since the first report in 1968 of electron microscopic studies of adamantinoma by Albores Saavedra et al. (13) there have been 23 related reports referenced by Mori et al. (35) and by Moon and Mori representing study of some 28 cases (9). In 23 cases epithelial characteristics such as basal lamina, tonofilaments and desmosomes have been found with microvilli and cytoplasmic processes often noted as well (Figure 9). Actin-like microfilaments are also reported in epithelial cells of 2 of these cases (9, 35). The stroma contains fibroblasts, myofibroblasts, and collagen with spacing similar to that found in the oxytalan of teeth (36). In a report of eccrine carcinoma of the skin Albores Saavedra notes ultrastructural similarities to the findings in adamantinoma of the tibia (37).

Of the three electron microscopic studies which do not confirm the epithelial nature of

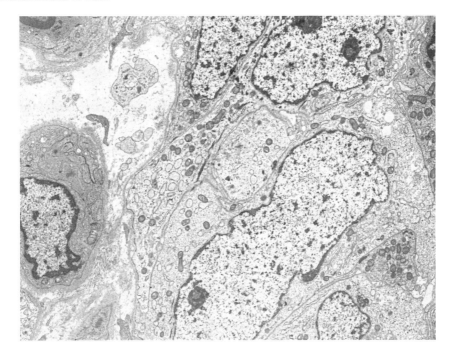

Figure 9 This electron photomicrograph of a tubular (angiomatous) adamantinoma demonstrates basal lamina, interdigitating cell contacts, tight junctions,
microvillus-like structures and keratin as tonofilaments. Keratin, which was scant
in this tumor, was confirmed by immunoperoxidase staining.

the tumor, two support endothelial–vascular origin and one is poorly differentiated with some similarities to Ewing's sarcoma (17, 38).

Immunohistochemistry

Knapp et al. (14) and Rosai and Pinkus (39) reported in 1982 that the epithelial tissues of adamantinoma contained keratin and were negative for factor VIII antigen which characterizes most vascular endothelial cells. Two subsequent studies confirm these findings (35, 36). Carcinoembryonic antigen (CEA) has been demonstrated once (32) and we have found epithelial membrane antigen (EMA) and desmin in epithelial cells by immunoperoxidase methods in the only lesion so studied. Search for a broader range of antigens by immunohistochemical techniques is a promising area of study.

Immunoperoxidase stains for polyclonal keratin molecules are positive in each of the epithelial patterns and since the technique is commercially available should be carried out in all suspected adamantinomas and especially those where the diagnosis is in doubt. Contrariwise, immunostains for factor VIII related antigens should be negative in epithelial areas and positive only in blood vessels.

Pathologic Differential Diagnoses

Erroneous diagnoses of adamantinoma have been made in tumors shown to be metastatic carcinoma, hemangiosarcoma, chordoid tumor and osteogenic sarcoma (8, 20). Other tumors with epithelioid features which might be confused with adamantinoma include malignant fibrous histiocytoma (40), epithelioid schwannoma (41) and perhaps Ewing's tumor (16–18) especially that form with a primary filigree pattern (42).

Missed histopathologic diagnoses as ada-mantinoma have most often led to erroneous diagnoses of fibrous dysplasia and benign fibro-ossesous lesion (12), but also have included aneurysmal bone cyst 19) and osteo-genic sarcoma (8, 31).

Biology

This usual disease is notoriously indolent and protracted with symptoms often preceding diagnosis for as long as 2 to 4 years and up to 50–55 years (8, 9, 20). An example of this behavior is detailed by Rock et al. (7).

Monostotic Disease

Ninety-five percent of adamantinomas (19) are monostotic at diagnosis. While many pre-sent as a solitary lytic focus, an unknown proportion show multiple lytic lesions confined to a region of bone and rarely widely separate abnormalities are demonstrated. Some of the last have been reported to be separate foci of fibrous dysplasia and of adamantinoma (19). Grouped lytic lesions may be viewed as evi-dence of origin in foci of fibrous dysplasia, multifocal origin of adamantinoma (19) or as intra-osseous metastasis. Nevertheless, the per-iosteal compartment is usually intact although within the protracted seemingly indolent course malignant behavior may already be manifest if the multiple lytic lesions represent metastasis. This hypothesis permits greater congruence in total course between those cases with distant metastasis and those with putative intra-osseous metastasis.

Monomelic, Polyostotic Disease

In 5.5% of adamantinomas there is evidence of abnormality of both tibia and fibula at diagno-sis (9). In a few instances the involvement is by direct invasion which may imply extra-osseous involvement or origin. In others some of the lesions are fibrous dysplasia and in some there are widely dispersed foci of adamantinoma which suggest metastasis (12). In some cases

the involvement appears to be asynchronous (19). The mortality of this group may be disproportionately high (12).

Polyostotic Disease

A single case reported to be polyostotic disease involving three widely separate bones is found on analysis to represent asynchronous involve-ment (43). This recalls several reports of late osseous metastasis of adamantinoma (espe-cially involving spine or ribs) developing in the absence of known pulmonary metastasis (9, 44). Such a clinical behavior has been reported both for osteosarcomas and Ewing's tumors. The question of multicentric origin cannot be resolved although techniques of molecular genetics may be helpful.

Distant Metastasis

After diagnosis the period of risk for distant metastasis may exceed 10 years if lesions reported 14 and 22 years later are metastases (8, 9, 44). At least 3% of adamantinomas have metastasized to (regional) lymph nodes either at diagnosis or up to 6 years later (9, 12), a behavior which establishes the malignant potential of the unmolested tumor and which has counterparts in basal cell carcinoma and synovial sarcoma but which would be unusual in ameloblastic fibroma or ameloblastoma. Twelve to 18% of adamantinomas metastasize to lungs (8, 9) where, as we have seen, the first manifestation (as also reported by others) may be pneumothorax (29, 45, 46) and where the course may be very indolent (up to 22 years) or rapidly progressive (11, 46). One patient was living for 6 years with known pulmonary metastasis (11). In Moon's series 2.5% had distant osseous metastasis (8, 9). Such hemato-genous spread provides no special clue as to the basic nature of the tumor.

Morbidity and Mortality

Until the present, case reports seldom assess morbidity (physical or psychologic handicap) except by inference. Several patients have had known osseous abnormality for 20 to 55 years before diagnosis, sometimes with many pathologic fractures (31) or with major deformity sufficient to assure major functional impairment (20). Local recurrence has led to recommendations for amputation but seldom is residual tumor in the specimen specifically documented. Occasionally no residual tumor is found and recorded (cases 84, 89 of reference (8)) as has been true in 2 of our own patients. Thus, 91 of the 200 patients collected by Moon had the morbidity of amputation (8, 9) but how many of these were actually necessary is impossible to judge: while most may have had persistent or recurrent tumor some of these probably were for infection, radiation osteitis, non-union of graft.

The overall known mortality of Moon's series was 18% (8, 9). About half of this mortality occurred within 3 years of original therapy.

It is tempting to propose that at least three tumors will be distinguished. First, diaphyseal tumors with the biology of basal cell carcinoma, an usually indolent and low grade malignancy whose metastatic potential may be increased by manipulation within the peculiar intra-osseous site. Second, tumors of metaphysis and physis with the biology of low to high grade synovial sarcomas. Third, highly malignant tumors representing either dedifferentiated forms of either of the two previous forms or Ewing-like tumors sui generis.

CLINICAL FEATURES

Clinical Presentation

A hard lump or osseous deformity develops insidiously over several months or years. Medical attention is sought with onset of pain, usually aching in nature, or tenderness over large lesions (20). Sharp pain might suggest micro or gross fracture (22). While the skin may be stretched or discolored over the lesion, the skin is seldom if ever fixed to the deep tissues. Siting of the lesion and history of remote trauma may lend some specificity to this complex.

Analysis of constituents of blood has been non-contributory.

Imaging

Radiography. The imaging of most lesions of bone still begins with standard radiographs. While some adamantinomas are asymptomatic and are discovered serendipitously, most cause mass or pain and are first defined by routine 'x-ray' which should be in two planes.

In the case of adamantinomas, plain films are frequently either diagnostic or show a lesion sufficiently complex to lead to biopsy of an abnormality which is clearly not a 'leave-me-alone' type of lesion.

The typical adamantinoma occurs in the tibia and has a 'bubbly' appearance with rather thick walls surrounding the small lucent areas. There is scalloping and frequently 'expansion' of the diaphysis (Figures 10–13). Involvement of outer cortex may give a characteristic saw toothed appearance (22). Active periosteal reaction is usually discordantly meager as with metastatic carcinoma (9, 20).

Tomography is useful in planning the approach for a biopsy. It rarely provides specific information which is not available on the plain films or that cannot be better displayed by other, newer modalities of imaging (Figure 12b, c).

Computed tomography. Rarely today is an orthopedic surgeon content with only plain films, and, of course, computed tomography (CT) will display the contours of the tumor with exquisite detail and definition. CT will show any soft tissue mass which may be present in an adamantinoma (47) (Figure 13d) and is useful in defining pulmonary metastasis (Figure 13f).

Arteriography. Enhancement of the vessels with an iodinated contrast material will show the overall vascularity of the lesion and its

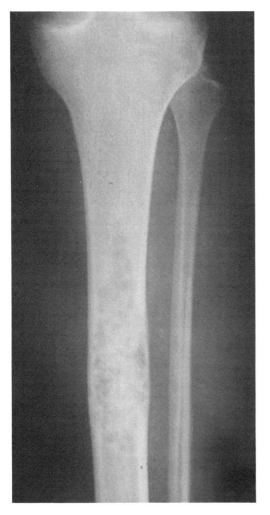

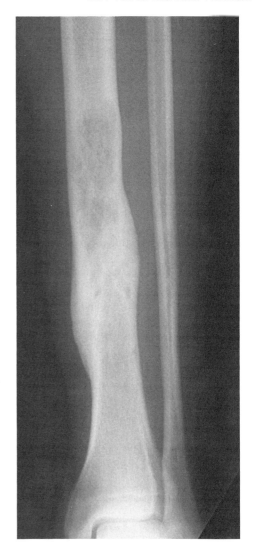

Figure 10 This 15 year old male has a lesion in the tibia at the junction of the proximal and middle thirds. There is slight expansion of the diaphysis with some endosteal scalloping but without evidence of recent periosteal new bone. There are multiple intrinsic lucencies with fairly thick margins. The tumor extends in the medullary canal both proximal and distal to the cortical extent of the disease. This is a fairly typical appearance of an adamantinoma.

This patient had pain for 4 months. An inconclusive aspiration biopsy was followed by diagnostic open biopsy and by segmental resection with autologous fibular and iliac grafts. Residual tumor at resection margin prompted a second segmental resection and bone graft at which time no residual tumor was found. No evidence of recurrence or metastasis has been found during 3 years' follow-up.

Figure 11 A man of 20 years has a lesion in the distal half of the diaphysis of the tibia. There appears to be a well healed pathologic fracture in the distal portion of the lesion. There is some endosteal scalloping proximally. The medullary lucencies are more confluent than in Figure 10 without periosteal response.

This patient sustained a pathologic fracture while skiing at 17 years of age. The fracture healed. He was admitted because of progressive deformity, with a preoperative diagnosis of fibrous dysplasia. Curettage and bone grafting was performed followed by segmental resection and bone graft. He is well 6 years later.

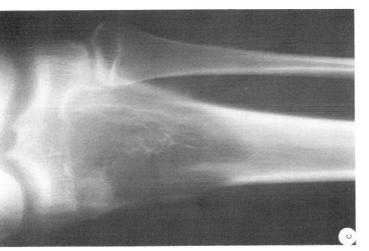

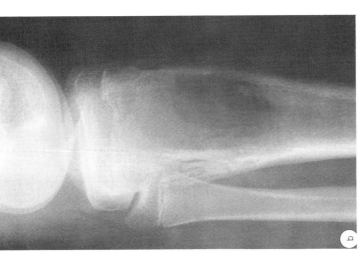

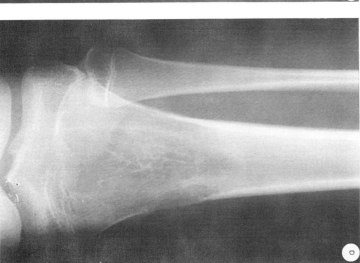

Figure 12a, b, c This girl is 14 years old. Anteroposterior and lateral radiographs of the left tibia show a primarily lytic lesion of the proximal metaphysis. There is considerable thinning of the cortex without the scalloping seen before. The physis does not appear to have been crossed, but on the anteroposterior tomogram the provisional zone of calcification is indistinct. There has been no repair bone produced. This lesion appears to be more aggressive than the earlier examples and suggest a more active, infiltrative process such as a malignant fibrous histiocytoma or lymphoma. A giant cell tumor could have this general appearance, but he open physis makes this less likely.

She presented with pain for one month; a pathologic fracture was recognized and attributed clinically to chondroblastoma. Following open biopsy, a segmental resection was done and showed involvement extending through the periosteum. She is tumor free 12 years after above the knee amputation at which time no residual tumor was demonstrated. (This tumor was reported by Perez Atayde et al (36).)

effect on adjacent vessels. This technique may have its principal usefulness in staging of adamantinoma as implied by Moon (9). The few reports known to us either show an avascular lesion, displacement of overlying vessels, or restricted patchy areas of tumor vessels (Figure 13 c, d), seemingly in contrast to a lesion which has been suspected to be of vascular origin (31, 48, 49).

Radionuclide imaging. Scintigraphic scans with ^{99m}technetium MDP will help to define the extent of the adamatinoma, especially in its medullary extent (Figure 14).

Magnetic resonance imaging (MRI). MRI was thought at first to have little utility in the diagnosis of lesions of bones. We now find it increasingly useful, especially in processes where the marrow is affected. Since most adamantinomas have a component of medullary involvement, one would expect great accuracy from MRI in defining the location and extent of the adamantinoma.

INVESTIGATION AND STAGING

Staging

A formal staging system has not been developed for adamantinoma. The system for surgical staging (SSS) of Enneking et al. (50) utilizes histologic grade of tumor (Grade I for well differentiated tumors) and extent of tumor (Stage A confined to organ or tissue of origin: Stage B touching or extending into the next adjacent organ or tissue). By inference, most adamantinomas would be Stage IA or IB preoperatively which excludes en bloc excisions in essentially all cases. A few adamantinomas may be staged IIA or IIB including those classified as ewingold adamantinoma (16–18). In keeping with Moon's conviction that incomplete surgery including biopsy and curettage potentiates malignant behavior (9), biopsy required for diagnosis must be considered to convert the lesion to Stage IB or higher, dictating removal of the biopsy site at

definitive surgery. This consideration should determine the biopsy plan.

Preoperative staging by imaging techniques is facilitated by angiography which may demonstrate displacement of major vasculature more often than tumor 'blush', by computed tomography which often serves best to demonstrate whether a rim of bone encloses the lesion and by technetium bone scans which help define intra-osseous extent of disease. The potential usefulness of MRI is unknown to us. Initial staging should include evaluation of regional lymph nodes by physical examination at least and by radiologic examination preferably computed tomography of the lungs.

Pathologic evaluation of stage and margins of excision are required for confirmation. Pathologic staging may be enhanced by standardized mitotic counts or DNA flow cytometry.

MANAGEMENT AND PROGNOSIS

Management

Surgical excision remains the treatment of choice for the primary lesion. Although curettage with bone graft has been successful in at least 7 cases with adequate long term follow-up there is no staging information in these cases, which represent between 15 and 30% of individuals treated in this manner (8, 9). Block resection has not been adequate in any reported case with adequate follow-up (8, 9). Advances in preoperative evaluation, in understanding the principles of cancer surgery, in surgical technique and in prosthetic repair support the choice of segmental resection in accessible lesions, a return to the treatment applied in Fischer's patient (2, 7). Successful surgical excision of pulmonary metastasis has been reported, although at least one patient has survived with known pulmonary metastases for many years (11).

There is a consensus that radiation therapy is not useful in adamantinoma. The basis of this consensus is anecdotal and is largely derived from experience with orthovoltage radiation,

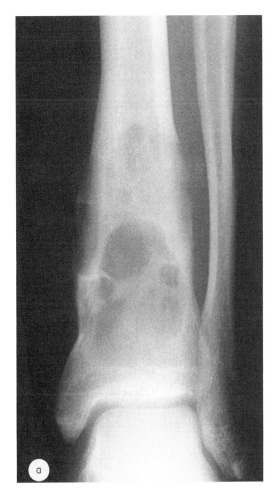
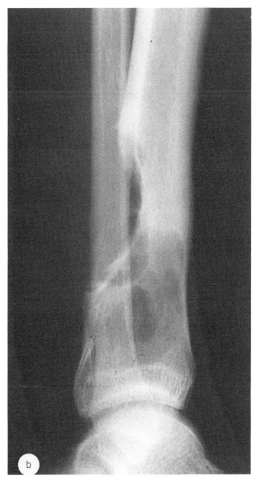

Figure 13a, b, c, d, e, f Anteroposterior and lateral radiographs of the distal portion of the left leg of an 18 year old male show a multi-loculated destructive process of the distal diaphysis and metaphysis of the tibia. There is some expansion of the bone, indicating chronicity. Many of the intrinsic margins are thin, but sharp.

The angiogram showed tumor vessels and the bowing of the posterior tibial artery testifies to the presence of a soft tissue mass.

Axial CT shows well the scalloping of the bone as well as the cortical thickening. The enlargement of the bone is evidenced on comparison with the normal leg. (Figure 1 shows the macroscopic appearance of the hemisected tumor.)

A CT of the chest shows a nodule in the right upper lobe, consistent with a metastasis.

There was a history of multiple minor athletic injuries of the shin 4 years before admission. An open biopsy was performed with preoperative diagnosis of chondromyxoid fibroma for this lesion associated with pain and deformity for 18 months. A segmental resection including distal epiphysis with reconstruction was performed. Thirteen months later he presented with pneumothorax and was found to have pulmonary metastases without disease of the bone or graft site. Seven pulmonary metastases were resected. It was thought that residual metastases were present. The chest is clear and he remains well 3 months after thoracotomy after he received multiple courses of Adriamycin, Cytoxan and vincristine.

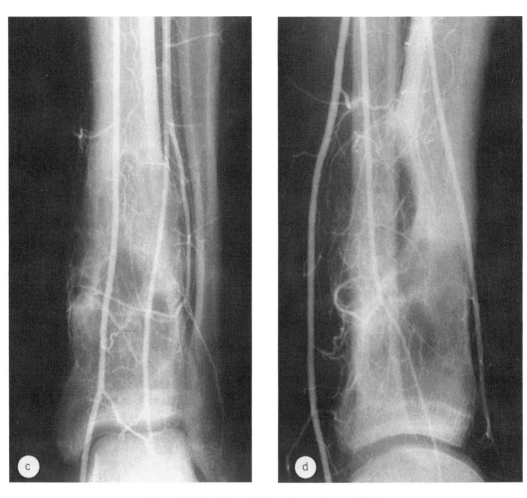

Figure 13 (*continued*) (see legend on p. 871).

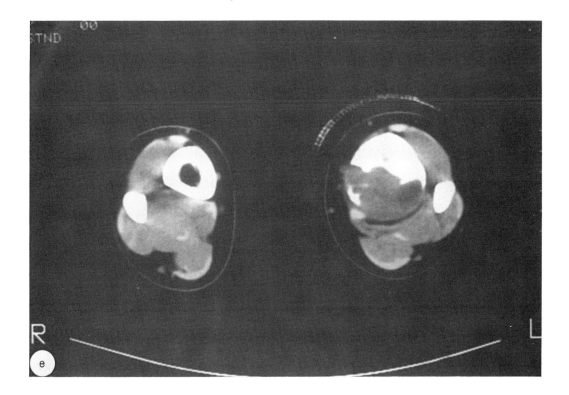

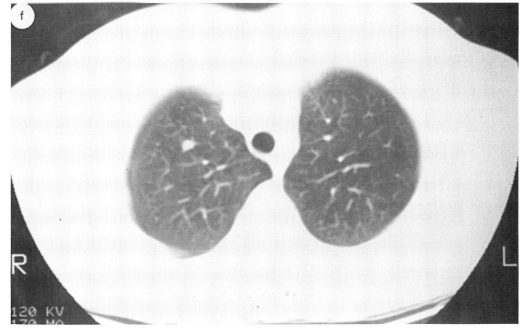

Figure 13 (*continued*) (see legend on p. 871).

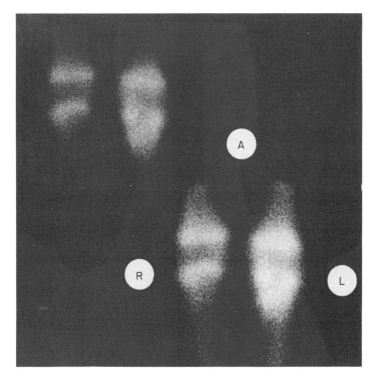

Figure 14 Technetium scan of the lesion depicted in Figure 12. Concentration of the radioactivity varies with peripheral accentuation. Although this tumor was macroscopically solid without cysts, nucleotide uptake is relatively decreased centrally.

usually with unspecified dosage. From the orthovoltage era there are reports of tumor persistent after 3500 and 5500 rad, published photomicrographs suggesting attenuated epithelium in a sclerotic acellular matrix (11) and a radiated bone with multiple pathologic fractures which showed no tumor on biopsy (31). Since there is a single report of long term local control following cobalt-60 irradiation in a primary lesion subjected only to biopsy (51), and a partial response of lung metastasis following 5500 rad radiocobalt therapy (44), the past experience deserves to be re-evaluated by radiotherapists and prospective studies should be designed and undertaken with modern protocols when surgery is precluded.

Reports of chemotherapy, usually with multiple drugs, are anecdotal, apply to patients with rapidly progressive and disseminated disease, and report little or no benefit (17–19, 46). No trials of prophylactic or adjuvant chemotherapy are reported. No trials of immunotherapy are known. Trials of perfusion therapy may have been carried out (52).

Prognosis

Moon's monumental and single handed creation of the equivalent of an International Registry of Adamantinoma suffers from the bias inherent in case reports (8, 9). This rare tumor then seems unpredictable and capricious, indolent or rapidly progressive, with substantial and probably lifelong morbidity and mortality, features which require institutional settings for meaningful analysis. Out of 77 patients collected by Moon with follow-up of more than 3 years, 71% were alive and free of disease (NED), 10% had died with disease (DWD) and 9% were alive with disease (AWD). The proportion of cases which go unreported or undiagnosed is unknown.

For those followed for 3 to 5 years 78% were NED and 8% were AWD, for those followed for 5 to 10 years 72% were NED and 6% were AWD, and for those followed over 10 years 62% were NED and 14% were AWD (8, 9).

Thus, while some 85% will recur locally after suboptimal surgery, some 20% will develop metastases and at least 10 to 15% will die because of the tumor (with perhaps half of these dying within 3 years of definitive treatment) (8, 9), it is not yet possible to clearly identify the individuals at highest risk. Standardization of methods of clinical, radiologic, pathologic, biologic analysis and therapy, if such can be accomplished, provides the greatest hope at the moment by which to unravel the mysteries of adamantinomas of bone.

Whether predominantly stromal lesions have a better prognosis than predominantly epithelial is unknown. The only recent attempt to correlate specific histologic patterns with outcome indicates that tumors with basaloid pattern metastasized more frequently (11).

CURRENT BIOLOGICAL RESEARCH—FUTURE MANAGEMENT

Tissue culture of presumed adamantinoma has only been reported in a relatively inaccessible literature. The results favor outgrowth of mesenchymal, including vascular, tissues (9, 22). Since tissues of both ectodermal and mesodermal origin may each differentiate along both epithelial and stromal lines, the question of the basic tissue of origin of adamantinoma remains unanswered, a question complicated by the possibility of intimate and interdependent interactions between ectoderm and mesoderm. For example, keratin has been identified in epithelium of ectodermal, entodermal and mesodermal origin (53). Recent studies suggest that keratin is found in Ewing's tumors raising questions about the reliability of

this finding in the diagnosis of adamantinoma (54). Other observers deny the presence of keratin in Ewing's tumor (55). Clearly further study is needed. Such questions have more than theoretical interest since chemotherapeutic agents are known to have activities that vary with the tissue of origin and the potentialities of linking chemotherapeutic agents to molecules specific to particular tumors are emerging sciences.

For the future, adamantinomas should be tested in the nude mouse system in a series large enough to demonstrate any wide variation in behavior and to permit correlation with clinical and pathologic variation. Tissue cultures should be established to permit cytogenetic analysis and molecular studies. While some molecular DNA and RNA probes are potent enough to carry out in situ hybridization on routine paraffin tissues, fresh frozen tissue stored until used is potentially worth its weight in gold for application of new techniques of molecular genetics should tissue culture fail. Studies of molecular genetics including cytogenetic analysis, the search for oncogenes or their RNA or protein differentiation products remain to be reported including characterization of collagens and keratins. Such studies should be useful in determining the etiology, pathogenesis and identity of subdivisions of adamantinoma. For example, specific tumor probes for predicting metastasis are becoming available. Whether such can be found for adamantinoma only the future will tell.

CURRENT CLINICAL RESEARCH IN PROGRESS

The usefulness of a clinical staging method such as that proposed by Enneking et al. (50) is being explored for adamantinoma (of the tibia). It seems likely that any staging method should include a descriptor of size. Methods evaluating parameters of proliferative potential such as mitotic counts should be standardized, a lack which may account for seeming discrepancies in the literature. Nuclear DNA flow cytometry, which can be adapted to formalin fixed, paraffin embedded specimens, promises another type of estimate of growth potential (56). A report of such studies suggests that this method may be very useful (57).

Moon refers to the apparent promise of wide segmental resection including normal osseous margins with allograft transplantation (9), a procedure the success of which depends upon a sound method of preoperative staging and application of modern principles of cancer surgery.

An unpublished retrospective review of the radiotherapy of adamantinoma, suggests the potential usefulness of a prospective re-evaluation of such treatment particularly in the setting of non-operable disease (58). Thus far multiagent chemotherapy has been a local option used in advanced disease. Most regimens tested have been of the sort used in sarcomas and Ewing's tumors such as VAC (vincristine, Adriamycin and Cytoxan) (16–18). Regimens incorporating agents thought useful with epithelial tumors should be considered.

REFERENCES

1 Adamantinoma. In: Spjut HJ, Dorfman HD, Fechner RE, Ackerman LV. Tumors of Bone and Cartilage: Atlas of Tumor Pathology, Second Series, Fasicle S. Washington, DC: Armed Forces Institute of Pathology, 1972: 315–23.

2 Fischer B. Uber Ein primares Adamantinom der Tibia. FrankF. Zeit. f. Pathologie. 1913; 12: 422–41.

3 Ryrie BJ. Adamantinoma of the tibia: aetiology and pathogenesis. Br Med J 1932; 2: 1000–3.

4 Dunne RE. Primary adamantinoma of the tibia. New Engl Med J 1938; 218: 634–9.

5 Baker PL, Dockerty MB, Coventry MB. Adamantinoma (so-called) of the long bones J Bone and Joint Surg (Am) 1954; 36: 704–20.

6 Shallow TA, Raker N, Fry K. Primary malignant tumors of bone with special reference to osteogenic sarcoma. J Int Coll Surg 1943; 6: 89.

7 Rock MG, Beabout JW, Unni KK, Sim FH. Mayo Clinic Tumor Rounds: Adamantinoma Orthopedics Thorofare 1983; 6: 472–7.

8 Moon NF. Adamantinoma of the appendicular skeleton. Clin Orthoped 1965, 43: 189–213.

9 Moon NF, Mori H. Adamantinoma of the

appendicular skeleton–updated. Clin Orthoped 1986; 204: 215–37.

10 Hicks JD. Synovial sarcoma of the tibia. J Pathol Bacteriol 1954; 67: 151–61.

11 Weiss SW, Dorfman HD. Adamantinoma of long bone: An analysis of nine new cases with emphasis on metastasizing lesions and fibrous-dysplasia-like changes. Hum Pathol 1977; 8: 141–52.

12 Campanacci M, Giunti A, Bertoni F, Laus M, Gitelis S. Adamantinoma of the long bones. The experiences of the Istituto Ortopedico Rizzoli. Am J Surg Pathol 1981; 5: 533–42.

13 Albores Saavedra J, Diaz Gutierrez D, Altamir-ano Dimas M. Adamantinoma de la tibia, observaciones ultrastructurales. Rev Med Hosp Gen. 1968; 31: 245.

14 Knapp RH, Wilk MR, Scheithauer BW, Unni KK. Adamantinoma of bone: An electron microscopic and immunohistochemical study. Virchows Arch (A) 1982; 398: 75–86.

15 Dahlin DC. Adamantinoma of long bone. In: Bone Tumor, General Aspects and Data on 6221 cases, 3rd edition, Chapter 23. Springfield: Charles C Thomas: 1978, 296–306.

16 Van Haelst UJ, DeHaas GM, Van Dorsser DH. A perplexing malignant bone tumor. Highly malignant so-called adamantinoma or non-typical Ewing's sarcoma. Virchows Arch (Pathol Anat) 1975: 365: 63–74.

17 Mcister P, Konrade, Hubner G. Malignant tumor of the humerus with features of adamantinoma and Ewing's sarcoma. Pathol Res Pract 1979; 1966: 112–22.

18 Lipper S, Kahn LB. Case report 235 Ewing-like adamantinoma of the left radial head. Skel Radiol 1983; 10: 61–6.

19 Schajowicz F. 'Adamantinoma' of long bones. In: Tumors and Tumor-like Lesions of Bone and Joint. New York: Springer Verlag, 1981: 383–90.

20 Unni KK, Dahlin DC, Beabout JW, Ivins JC. Adamantinoma of long bones. Cancer 1974; 34: 1796–1805.

21 Cohen DC, Dahlin DC, Pugh DG. Fibrous dysplasia associated with adamantinoma of the Long Bone. Cancer 1962: 15, 515–21.

22 Huvos AG, Marcove RA. Adamantinoma of long bones. A clinicopathologic study of fourteen cases with vascular origin suggested. J Bone Joint Surg (Am) 1975; 57: 148–54.

23 Johnson LC. Congenital Pseudarthrosis, adamantinoma of long bone and intracortical fibrous dysplasia. Lab Invest 1983; 23: 387 (Abstract).

24 Schiller A. Personal communication.

25 Bambira EA, Nogueira AMMF, Miranda D. Adamantinoma of the soft tissue of the leg

(letter). Arch Pathol Lab Med 1983: 107; 500–1.

26 Mills SE, Rosai J. Adamantinoma of pretibial soft tissues. Am J Clin Pathol 1985; 85: 108–14.

27 Lederer H, Sinclair AJ. Malignant synovioma simulating 'Adamantinoma of the Tibia''. J Pathol Bacteriol 1954; 67: 163–8.

28 Uehlinger EA. Das Skelett synoviom (Adamantinoma). In: Roentgen Diagnostik Ergebnisse. Stuttgart: Thieme, 1957: 96–103.

29 Jaffe HL. Adamantinoma of limb bones. In Tumors and Tumorous Conditions of The Bones and Joints, Chapter 14. Philadelphia: Lea and Febiger, 1958: 213–23.

30 Lichtenstein L. Dermal inclusion tumor in bone (so-called adamantinoma of limb bones). In: Bone Tumors, 4th edition, Chapter 23. St Louis: CV Mosby 1972: 343–8.

31 Changus GW, Speed JS, Stewart FW. Malignant Angioblastoma of Bone. Cancer 1957; 10: 540–59.

32 Eisenstein W, Pitcock JA. Adamantinoma of the tibia. Arch Pathol Lab Med 1984; 108: 246–50.

33 Povysil C, Matejovsky Z. Ultrastructure of adamantinoma of long bone. Virchows Arch (Pathol Anat) 1981; 393: 233–44.

34 Kabat ER, Furth J. An histochemical study of alkaline phosphatase in various normal and neoplastic tissues. Am J Pathol 1941; 17: 303–18.

35 Mori H, Yamamoto S, Hiramatsu K, Miura T, Moon NF. Adamantinoma of the tibia: Ultrastructural and immunohistochemic study with reference to histogenesis. Clin Orthop Related Res 1984; 190: 299–310.

36 Perez-Atayde AR, Kozakewich HPW, Vawter GF. Adamantinoma of the tibia: An ultrastructural and immunohistochemical study. Cancer 1985; 55: 1015–23.

37 Brandt H, Albores-Saavedra J, Mora-Tiscareno J. Eccrine sweat gland carcinoma. Its microscopic and ultrastructural similarity to adamantinoma of long bones. Pathologica (Mexico) 1977; 15: 33–43.

38 Llombart-Bosch A, Ortuno-Pacheco G. Ultrastructural findings supporting the angioblastic nature of the so-called adamantinoma of the tibia. Histopathology 1978; 2: 189.

39 Rosai J, Pinkus GS. Immunohistochemical demonstration of epithelial differentiation in adamantinoma of the tibia. Am J Surg Pathol 1982; 6: 427–34.

40 Hoffman MA, Dickersin GR. Malignant fibrous histiocytoma: an ultrastructural study of eleven cases. Hum Pathol 1983; 14: 913–22.

41 Delamonte SM, Dorfman HD, Chandra R, Malawer M. Intra-osseous schwannoma: histologic features, ultrastructure and review of the literature. Hum Pathol 1984; 15: 551–8.

42 Kissane JM, Askin FB, Foulkes M, Stratton LB, Shirley SF. Ewing's sarcoma of bone: clinicopathologic aspects of 303 cases from the Intergroup Ewing's Sarcoma Study. Hum Pathol 1983; 14: 773–9.

43 Bullough PG, Goldberg VM. Ulticentric origin of Adamantinoma of the tibia: A case report. Rev Hosp Spec Surg 1971; 1: 71.

44 Morgan AD, Mackensie DH. A metastasizing adamantinoma of the Tibia. J Bone Joint Surg (Br) 1956; 38: 892–8.

45 Winter WG Jr. Spontaneous pneumothorax heralding metastasis of adamantinoma of the tibia. J Bone Joint Surg (Am) 1976; 58: 416–7.

46 Almannsberger M, Poppe H, Schauer A. An unusual case of adamantinoma of long bone. J Cancer Res Clin Oncol 1982; 104: 315–20.

47 Sowa DT, Dorfman HD. Unusual localization of adamantinoma of long bones: report of a case of isolated fibular involvement. J Bone Joint Surg (Am) 1986; 68: 293–6.

48 Rosen RS, Schwinn CP. Adamantinoma of Long Bone: Malignant angioblastoma. AJ 1966; 97: 727–30.

49 Zidkova H, Kolar J, Matejovsky Z, Slive M. Adamantinoma koncitinovyck kosti. Cesk Radiol 1981; 35: 50–6.

50 Enneking WF, Spanier SS, Goodman MA. A system for the surgical staging of musculoskeletal sarcoma. Clin Orthop 1980; 153: 106–20.

51 Zand A, Chambers GH, Street DM. So-called 'Adamantinoma of long bone'. Clin Orthop 1972; 86: 178–82.

52 Monticelli G, Santori F-S, Folliero A, Ghera S, Cavaliere R, DiFillippo F, Cavallaro A. Antiblastic hyperthermic regional perfusion in the treatment of malignant neoplasms of the limbs. Ital J Orthop Traumatoe 1983; 9: 167–80.

53 Said JW. Immunohistochemical localization of keratin proteins in tumor diagnosis. Hum Pathol 1983; 14: 1017–19.

54 Tarbell N. Personal communication.

55 Moll R, Inchul L, Gould Ve, Berndt R, Roessner A, Frankie WW. Immunocytochemical analysis of Ewing's tumors: Patterns of expression of intermediate filaments and desmosomal proteins indicate cell type heterogeneity and pluripotential differentiation. Am J Pathol 1987; 127: 288–304.

56 Llombart—Bosch A. Personal communication.

57 Mankin HJ, Connor JF, Shiller AL et al. Grading of bone tumors by analysis nuclear DNA content using flow cytometry. J Bone Joint Surg (Am) 1985; 67: 404–13.

58 Gebhardt MA. Personal communication.

Textbook of Uncommon Cancer
Edited by C.J. Williams, J.G. Krikorian, M.R. Green and D. Raghavan
© 1988 John Wiley & Sons Ltd

Chapter **47**

Angioendotheliomatosis Proliferans Systemisata*

Jag Bhawan
Professor of Dermatology and Pathology and Head of Dermatopathology Section (Department of Dermatology), Boston University School of Medicine, Boston, Massachusetts, USA

HISTORY

Pfleger and Tappeiner in 1959 described a case characterized by cutaneous intravascular proliferation of tumor cells and believed these cells to be endothelial in origin (1). Braverman and Lerner reported the second case which in contrast to the first case had a fatal outcome (2). The original authors in 1963 termed this unusual condition angioendotheliomatosis proliferans systemisata (3). Since then many names have been given to this condition (Table 1). In the ensuing two decades the cases of angioendotheliomatosis proliferans systemisata (APS) were divided into benign and malignant types depending upon the clinical course. It was assumed that there were no histologic differences between the benign and malignant types (5). Until recently the original endothelial origin of tumor cells prevailed (6). More recently, this author has shown that there are distinct histologic differences between the benign and malignant types and that lymphoid origin is more likely in the majority of the cases (4).

EPIDEMIOLOGY AND ETIOLOGY

This neoplastic condition is quite rare. This author counted 95 cases in a recent review, 8 of which were benign (4). Recently, another case of malignant APS has been added (7). Most patients are in their fifth decade or older, while the so-called benign APS affects the younger age including infants (8). The disease has been reported in both sexes with a slight predilection for females. In most reports, where mentioned, the patients were caucasians.

The etiology of this disease is unknown and will be discussed under clinical features and histogenesis.

CLINICAL FEATURES

The disease has been divided into two main categories: benign and malignant, based upon the clinical course (Table 2). The benign form is usually associated with bacterial endocarditis (5, 9, 10) or caused by exogenous proteins such as cow's milk (11) or may have no demonstrable underlying cause. Benign APS usually responds to antibiotics and/or steroids with nonfatal outcome.

A fatal outcome with or without treatment is usual in the malignant form (2, 12) although rarely remission has been reported with chemotherapy (13). Malignant APS may be further subdivided into those associated with lymphoma (14), with carcinoma (15), with no

TABLE 1 ANGIOENDOTHELIOMATOSIS
         PROLIFERANS SYSTEMISATA:
         SYNONYMS

Angioendotheliomatosis
Cerebral angioendotheliomatosis
Diffuse malignant proliferation of vascular endothe-
  lium
Endothelioma in situ
Intravascular endothelioma
Intravascular lymphomatosis
Malignant angioendotheliomatosis
Malignant proliferating angioendotheliomatosis
Neoplastic angioendotheliosis
Neoplastic angioendotheliomatosis
Proliferating angioendotheliomatosis
Proliferating systematized angioendotheliomatosis
Reactive angioendotheliomatosis
Systemic angioendotheliomatosis
Systemic endotheliomatosis
Systemic proliferating angioendotheliomatosis
Tappeiner's angioendotheliomatosis

TABLE 2 ANGIOENDOTHELIOMATOSIS
         PROLIFERANS SYSTEMISATA:
         CLASSIFICATION

Benign
    associated with:
    (a) bacterial endocarditis
    (b) exogenous proteins
    (c) unknown etiology

Malignant
    associated with:
    (a) lymphoma
    (b) carcinoma
    (c) unknown etiology

underlying neoplasm or without any association (16).

No distinctive clinical features characterize
APS. Most of the symptomatology is caused by
clogging of vessels. Both the clinical features
and abnormal laboratory data reflect involvement of the underlying organ system. Involvement of the central nervous system and/or skin
is found in a majority of the patients. Fever
appears to be the most common sign and
symptom. The most common single laboratory
abnormality is elevated sedimentation rate.
The cutaneous manifestations are nonspecific
(17). Hemorrhagic or nonhemorrhagic nodular subcutaneous firm masses or plaques are

the most common lesions. Telangiectasia may
be prominent over the lesions. These nodules
or plaques are usually fixed to the underlying
tissue. Ulceration may be seen at times. The
usual sites of involvement are the trunk and
extremities (Figure 1), although any other site
may be involved. A wide spectrum of entities
may be entertained in the clinical differential
diagnosis of the skin lesions (Table 3). The
neurologic manifestations may be the only
presenting signs. These are confusing and
nonspecific, however, progressive dementia
being the most consistent (16). Decreased
visual acuity, homonymous hemianopia and
blindness have been reported in some cases.
Speech disturbances including aphasia may
occur. There have been reports of transient
episodes of numbness and weakness suggestive

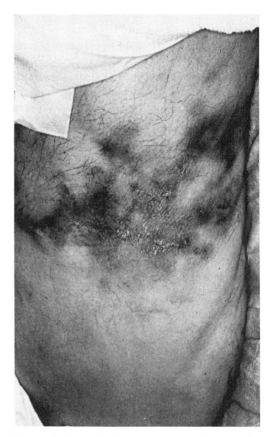

Figure 1 Clinical photograph showing irregular
hemorrhagic plaques on the thigh.

TABLE 3 ANGIOENDOTHELIOMATOSIS PROLIFERANS SYSTEMISATA: CLINICAL DIFFERENTIAL DIAGNOSIS

Leprosy
Leukemic infiltrate
Mycosis fungoides
Panniculitis
Reticulum cell sarcoma
Sarcoidosis
Syphilis
Vascular neoplasms

of transient ischemic attacks of cerebrovascular origin (18). Paraparesis, lethargy and gradual progressive paralysis have been described. Headaches have been reported (19). EEG and computerized tomography (CT) may be abnormal (16).

PATHOLOGY

The key histopathologic feature is the intravascular proliferation of tumor cells (Figure 2), with and without associated fibrin thrombi (Figure 3). The tumor cells are large with large

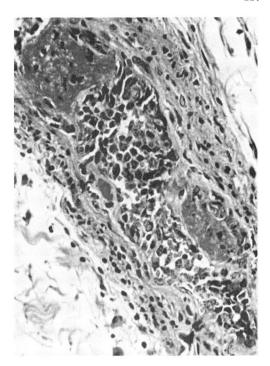

Figure 3 Intravascular tumor cells in association with fibrin thrombi. H&E, original magnification: ×330.

nuclei, show frequent pleomorphism and occlude the distended lumina to varying degree. Extravascular proliferation of tumor cells may be seen in some cases. Table 4 lists the histologic differential diagnosis. Various sized vessels of any organ system, but most commonly of skin and central nervous system, are involved, although an organ may be affected, especially in the terminal stages. Bhawan et al. have recently described new vascular changes

TABLE 4 ANGIOENDOTHELIOMATOSIS PROLIFERANS SYSTEMISATA: HISTOLOGIC DIFFERENTIAL DIAGNOSIS

Hemangioendothelioma
Lymphoma
Melanoma
Metastatic carcinoma
Metastatic sarcoma
Mycosis fungoides
Reticulum cell sarcoma
Seminoma/dysgerminoma

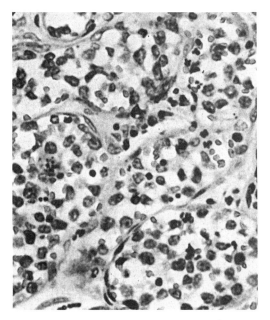

Figure 2 Intravascular proliferation of tumor cells. H&E, original magnification: ×330.

in APS (14). Both increased vascularity and tortuosity of the vessels is found. Great variation in the size of proliferating and tortuous vessels can be seen. The lumen of vessels may be folded, giving a glomerulus-like appearance (Figure 4). One micrometer thick sections (Figure 5) best demonstrate this feature, although careful examination of routine hematoxylin–eosin stained sections also reveal similar features (Figure 6). This complex luminal infolding seen in some vessels of the APS may account for some of the reports which claim to have seen the marker of endothelial cells, both on electron microscopy and immunohistochemistry (see below under histogenesis). A circulating angiogenic factor may be responsible for these vascular changes (20). Some authors have claimed that there are no histopathologic differences between clinically benign and the malignant forms (5). This concept continues to be promoted in some recent publications (8). It is apparent that the benign cases have very little cytologic atypia, if any, on review of the published photographs.

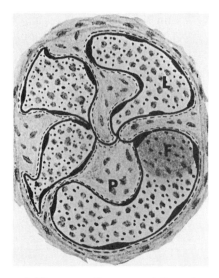

Figure 4 Diagrammatic representation of vascular change in APS. Lumen (L), pseudolumen (P) and fibrin thrombi (F). Smaller dots represent red cells and leukocytes while large ones represent the tumor cells. Thick black solid line depicts endothelial lining while dotted line is basement membrane.

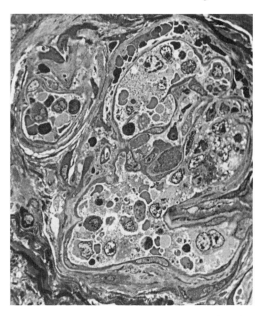

Figure 5 One micrometer thick section showing glomerulus-like intraluminal infolding of the endothelium. H&E, original magnification: ×640.

No intraluminal collection of tumor cells, as seen in the malignant type, is found and the changes are confined to the endothelium (see Figures 3 and 4 in reference 5 and Figures 1 and 2 in reference 9). The histologic features seen in the representative photomicrograph (Figure 7) taken from the actual slide of the case of Pasyk and Depowski (11) are quite different from the appearance of malignant APS (Figure 2). Fievez et al. considered their cases (21) to be of the benign type, because the patient had presumably subacute bacterial endocarditis. Review of that report, however, shows that the patient had, most likely, non-bacterial thrombotic (marantic) endocarditis rather than subacute bacterial endocarditis. Marantic endocarditis can often be seen in patients with malignancies and other debilitating conditions. Classic histologic features of malignant APS (Figure 8) were seen on review of the actual histopathologic slides. The patient died within $1\frac{1}{2}$ years of onset of illness. Thus, it is clear that their case is unjustifiably classified as benign. The histopathologic fea-

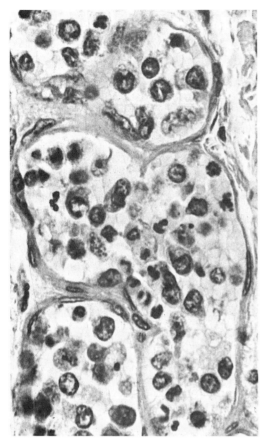

Figure 6 Intraluminal infolding of the endothe-lium. H&E, original magnification: ×640.

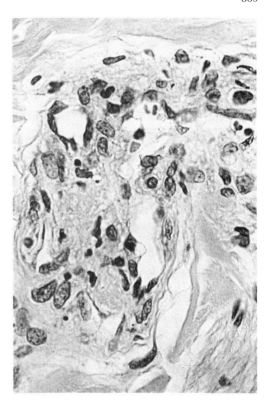

Figure 7 Photomicrograph showing the lesion in benign APS. Note endothelial swelling, partial obliteration of the lumen and absence of intra-vascular tumor cells. H&E, original magnifica-tion: ×330.

tures of benign APS are quite different from those of the malignant APS (Table 5). Reac-tive endotheliomatosis may be perhaps a more appropriate term instead of 'benign form' of APS, since both clinical and histologic features are quite distinct. The original case reported by Tappeiner and Pfleger (17) is one possible exception. The patient was alive for 7 years from the onset of illness, even though the histologic features appear to fit more that of the malignant form. However, lesions either per-sisted or recurred after 6 years. The patient was treated with steroids and has been lost to follow-up. One possible explanation for this highly unusual course for the benign APS may be that in this patient the disease was confined to skin and may represent a smoldering process such as is seen sometimes in cutaneous lympho-mas. Another explanation may be that the clinical course of this patient may be analogous to lymphomatoid papulosis where the disease clinically manifests in a benign course, but the histologic features show a malignant process (22). Follow-up has shown fatal outcome, at least in some cases of lymphomatoid papulosis (23).

HISTOGENESIS

Histogenesis of APS is the most controversial issue in this uncommon cancer. Three possibi-lities exist in the literature: (1) the endothelial original, the original hypothesis; (2) the more

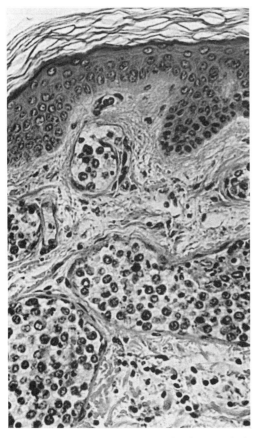

Figure 8 Intravascular tumor cells characteristic of APS. H&E, original magnification: ×400.

recent demonstration of lymphomatous origin; and (3) a nonendothelial, nonlymphomatous origin to accommodate future discoveries. There appears to be an overwhelming evidence in favor of lymphoid origin for the majority of cases of APS. These may or may not be associated with extravascular lymphomas at the time of diagnosis. Only rarely a possible endothelial origin of tumor cells is demonstrated, and there have been few reported cases of other neoplasms presenting as APS.

Endothelial Origin

The original authors described APS as the tumorous proliferation of endothelial cells (1, 2). Subsequent authors have also supported the endothelial origin of tumor cells. No concrete evidence for such a hypothesis was provided in these reports. The endothelial origin was based on the observations that the tumor cells were frequently seeen to be attached to the lining endothelial cells and were usually confined to the intravascular lumina on light microscopy. In only a few cases electron microscopy was performed (6, 14, 24–30). The best supportive evidence for endothelial origin comes from a report by Petito and his col-

TABLE 5 ANGIOENDOTHELIOMATOSIS PROLIFERANS SYSTEMISATA: HISTOLOGIC FEATURES

	'Benign'	Malignant
Intravascular occlusion by tumor cells	None	Few to complete
Lumen	Generally patent but may be partially obliterated because of endothelial swelling	Occluded to varying degree by tumor cells
Glomerulus-like intravascular infolding	Rare	Common
Endothelial swelling	Common	Common
Fibrin/hyalin thrombi	May be seen	Common
Cytologic atypia	Mild in endothelial lining cell	Moderate to severe in intra- and extravascular tumor cells
Extravascular component	None	Variable

leagues (25), subsequently cited in most publications on APS. Petito et al. reported Weibel–Palade bodies (an endothelial marker) in the tumor cells, thus confirming the endothelial nature of the cells. Critical review of their Figure 6 shows only part of a cell with a single possible Weibel–Palade body, thus likely confirming the endothelial nature of the cell. However, no evidence is presented that the cell shown is an intravascular tumor cell and not merely a part of endothelial lining cells. Figures 3A and 3B of Wick et al. (26), and Figure 6 of Kitagawa et al. (24) warrant similar citicism. It is also possible that these authors were interpreting an intraluminal endothelial cell to be a tumor cell. Even though they did not demonstrate any evidence, Scott et al. suggested an endothelial origin (28). No Weibel–Palade bodies in the luminal tumor cells which appear distinct from lining endothelial cells (Figures 9 and 10) were found by this author (14, 29). Antifactor VIII related antigen as a marker for endothelial cells has been used to attempt to confirm the endothelial nature of the tumor cells. Fulling and Gersell found positively stained tumor cells in the pancreatic vessels in one case (6). Kitagawa et al. found factor VIII related antigen positive tumor cells in 2 out of their 3 cases (24), while only 1 of the 5 cases were positive in the study reported by Schmookler et al. (31). However, factor VIII related antigen negative tumor cells were reported in the majority of publications (8, 14, 16, 26, 30, 32–34). Wick et al. proposed that the absence of factor VIII related antigen reactivity in the tumor cells may be due to their poor differentiation so that no recognizable antigens are found (26). Though this is certainly possible, the fact that some reports also have not only showed negative factor VIII related antigen, but also positive lymphoid cell markers make this explanation unlikely (14). The presence of factor VIII related antigen reactive cells in a few of the reported cases could be explained by the complex intraluminal infolding (Figure 4). This is evident in the color Figure 3 of Arnn et al. where the endothelial lining cells are strongly positive for factor VIII and one possible luminal cell which appears to be a folded endothelial cell is also positive, while hardly any tumor cells are seen in the vessel (35).

Lymphomatous Origin

Based on their electron microscopic and cell surface marker studies, Ansell et al. were the

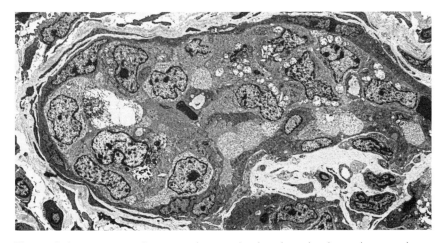

Figure 9 Low power electron micrograph showing the less electron dense intravascular tumor cells distinct from the lining endothelium. Original magnification: ×1700.

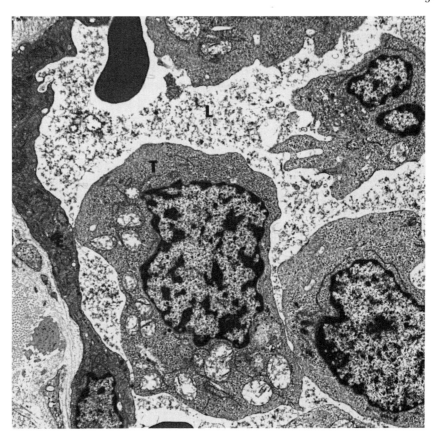

Figure 10 Higher magnification clearly shows the tumor cells (T) in the lumen (L) on the left to be distinct from the endothelial cells (E) on the right. The tumor cells lack the features of endothelial cells. Original magnification: × 7000.

first to report a patient with known histiocytic lymphoma presenting terminally as APS (29). They suggested the possibility that some published cases of APS may actually be unusual manifestations of lymphoma. Tanaka et al. reported in the Japanese literature another case of lymphoma presenting as APS in the same year (36). Another case of malignant lymphoma presenting as APS of the central nervous system was published by Yamamura et al. (32). Bhawan et al. (14) were the first to confirm the nonendothelial, lymphoid nature of the tumor cells in APS. They reported a 71 year old woman who was diagnosed as APS based on histologic features of a skin biopsy and clinical findings (14). A few days later, she underwent exploratory laparotomy for acute

abdomen and was found to have jejunal lymphoma (Figures 11 and 12). Subsequent light and electron microscopic and immuno-histochemical findings (Figures 13–15) confirmed the nonendothelial and lymphomatoid origin of APS. Others have further confirmed the lymphoid origin (30, 33, 37, 38). A case of APS in which tumor cells were positively stained for leukocyte common antigen while being negative for *Ulex europaeus* I lectin (an endothelial marker) was reported by Wrotnowski et al. (30). No associated lymphoma was found. Mori et al. (1985) found the intravascular neoplastic cells to be positively stained with anti B-lymphocyte antibody and negative with antifactor VIII related antigen (38). Another case in which the tumor cells

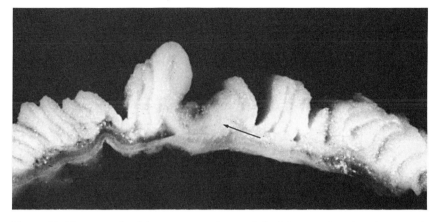

Figure 11 Photograph of the gross specimen of the jejunum showing the growth in the wall (arrow).

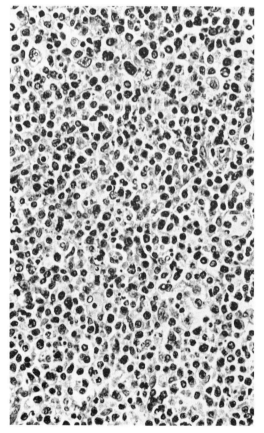

Figure 12 Diffuse cellular infiltrate of lymphoma of the jejunum. H&E, original magnification: ×315.

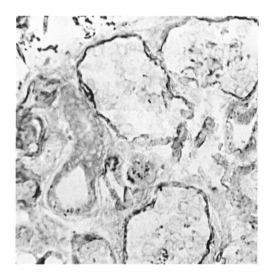

Figure 13 Immunoperoxidase staining with antifactor VIII related antigen shows positive reaction for lining endothelium and negative reaction of the intraluminal tumor cells ×340. (*Reproduced from reference 14 by permission of the editor of Cancer.*)

reacted with panleukocyte markers and IgM, but were negative for endothelial cell markers, was reported by Carroll and co-workers (37). They identified 2 other cases of lymphoma with intravascular involvement similar to that

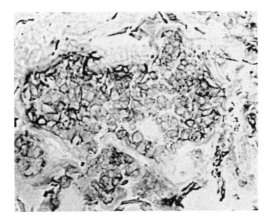

Figure 14 Intravascular tumor cells show positive immunoperoxidase staining for T200 with anti T29/33. Original magnification: ×340 (*Reproduced from reference 14 by permission of the editor of Cancer.*)

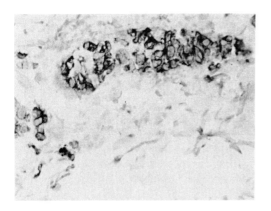

Figure 15 Intravascular tumor cells stain positively with anti-leu-4 on immunoperoxidase staining. Original magnification: ×290. (*Reproduced from reference 14 by permission of the editor of Cancer.*)

seen in APS. Wick and his colleagues reviewed 15 cases (including 5 of their earlier reported cases) and found common leukocyte antigen on malignant intravascular cells in 14 of 15 cases (34). Factor VIII related antigen was negative on tumor cells in 15 of 15 cases (34). Their electron microscopic findings were also confirmatory for nonendothelial features of the

tumor cells. Immunohistochemical markers consistent with B-lymphocyte differentiation were reported in another study (33).

It is interesting to note that review of the literature prior to the case reported by Ansell et al. (29), also shows that there is at least circumstantial evidence that APS may represent a form of lymphoma. Reticulum cell sarcoma was found on autopsy in case 1, while bone marrow examination was suggestive of lymphoma in case 2, reported by Scott et al. (28). Their case 3 had reticulum cell sarcoma involving the nasopharynx 7 years prior to the development of APS. Reticulum cell sarcoma of the ovary was suspected in another case (39). It is interesting to note that Scott et al. (28), even though they favored endothelial origin, considered the possibility that APS may be an unusual form of reticulum cell sarcoma in view of the extravascular spread. Furthermore, Braverman and Lerner (2), who were among the early authors to report APS, also felt that both clinically and histologically the lesions in the skin were similar to those seen in lymphomas, but because of the lack of involvement of the reticuloendothelial system and the predominant intravascular localization of tumor cells, concluded that it was unlikely.

Nonendothelial, Nonlymphomatous Origin

No endothelial–lymphoid origin could be demonstrated in some cases (8). One possible explanation is that even though factor VIII can be detected by immunoperoxidase techniques on paraffin embedded tissue, moist lymphoid markers are difficult to evaluate or perform in such conditions at the present state of the art. Alternatively, other tumors may present as predominantly endovascular neoplasms, just as lymphoma may be preferentially angiotropic. In fact, Dolman et al. reported 2 patients presenting as APS who were found eventually to have small carcinomas in the thyroid and pancreas, respectively (15). Similarly, another case was published in association with carcinoma of the cecum (40). Whether the intravascular tumor cells are the same as the carcinoma cells in these reported cases remains to be confirmed. Furthermore, the presence of lymphoid markers on the intravascular tumor cells had not been excluded in such cases.

INVESTIGATIONS

The diagnosis, because of the confusing symptomatology, is difficult. It should be suspected when otherwise unexplained, bizarre, neurologic manifestations are found in a patient. The patient should be investigated for underlying lymphoma, once the diagnosis of APS is established on biopsy. When cutaneous lesions are seen and a biopsy suggests APS, additional biopsies should be done and handled in a proper manner to confirm or exclude the lymphoid nature of tumor cells. At the present state of the art it can be best done by immediately freezing tissue and transporting it in the frozen state to laboratories experienced in immunohistochemistry.

MANAGEMENT

The benign APS usually responds to antibiotics and/or steroids (8, 10, 19). The treatment of the malignant APS is largely unsuccessful. Only in one case was complete remission reported with chemotherapeutic agents, on 14-month follow-up (13). However, published photomicrographs are not convincing of APS. Treatment has consisted of steroids, radiation therapy and chemotherapeutic agents. The recent findings suggesting a lymphomatous origin (4) offer hope in treatment of these patients. In patients where lymphomatous origin can be demonstrated, protocols similar to those developed for leukemia and lymphoma patients might prove to be helpful. A case of APS was reported to have been treated successfully with combination chemotherapy (41). Fibrinolytic agents may be useful when signs and symptoms pertaining to thrombosis and infarction are found.

CURRENT BIOLOGICAL RESEARCH LIKELY TO AFFECT FUTURE MANAGEMENT

Because of the rarity of this condition, there is a great need for physicians to report it. I would propose the formation of a registry of APS in order to learn more about this fatal condition. APS is largely a virgin field which needs attention, especially the therapeutic aspects. No current clinical research is in progress. The role of immunotherapy needs to be investigated. Since the disease appears to be largely confined to an intravascular compartment, particularly in the initial stages, therapeutic modalities which will selectively affect the intravascular compartment should be developed. Future prospective studies are needed in properly handled tissue for light and electron microscopic and immunohistochemical studies to further delineate this unusual and uncommon cancer. It is quite possible, in light of the histogenesis, that APS is a pathologic pattern of tumor growth common to different neoplasms or carcinoma, rather than a specific disease entity.

ACKNOWLEDGEMENT

The author wishes to express his gratitude to Drs Pasyk and Fievez for providing the original histologic material of their cases.

REFERENCES

1 Pfleger L, Tappeiner J. Zur Kenntnis der systemisierten endotheliomatose der cutanen Blutge fasse. Hautarzt 1959; 10: 359–63.
2 Braverman I, Lerner AB. Diffuse malignant proliferation of vascular endothelium. A possible new clinical and pathologic entity. Arch Dermatol 1961; 84: 72–80.
3 Tappeiner J, Pfleger L. Angioendotheliomatosis proliferans systemisata. Elin klinisch und pathohistologisch neues Krankheitsbild. Hautarzt 1963; 14: 67–70.
4 Bhawan J, Angioendotheliomatosis proliferans systemisata: An angiotrophic neoplasm of lymphoid origin. Semin Diag Pathol 1987; 4: 18–27.
5 Martin S, Pitcher D, Tschen J et al. Reactive

angioendotheliomatosis. J Am Acad Dermatol 1980; 2: 117–23.

6 Fulling KH, Gersell DJ. Neoplastic angioendotheliomatosis. Histologic, immunohistochemical and ultrastructural findings in two cases. Cancer 1983; 51: 1107–8.

7 Dominguez FE, Rosen LB, Kramer HC. Malignant angioendotheliomatosis proliferans. Report of an autopsied case studied with immunoperoxidase. Am J Dermatopathol 1986; 8: 419.

8 Gupta AK, Lipa M, Haberman HF. Proliferating angioendotheliomatosis. Case with long survival and review of literature. Arch Dermatol 1986; 122: 314–19.

9 Eisert J. Skin manifestations of subacute bacterial endocarditis. Case report of subacute bacterial endocarditis mimicking Tappeiner's angioendotheliomatosis. Cutis 1980; 25: 394–400.

10 Ruiter N, Mandema E. New cutaneous syndrome in subacute bacterial endocarditis. Arch Intern Med 1964; 113: 283–90.

11 Pasyk K, Depowski M. Proliferating systematized angioendotheliomatosis of a 5 month-old infant. Arch Dermatol 1978; 114: 1513–15.

12 Kauh YC, McFarland JP, Carnabuci GC et al. Malignant proliferating angioendotheliomatosis. Arch Dermatol 1980; 116: 803–6.

13 Keahey TM, Guerry D, Tuthill RJ et al. Malignant angioendotheliomatosis proliferans treated with Doxorubicin. Arch Dermatol 1982; 118: 512–14.

14 Bhawan J, Wolff SM, Ucci A et al. Malignant lymphoma and malignant angioendotheliomatosis: one disease. Cancer 1985; 55: 570–6.

15 Dolman CL, Sweeny VP, Magil A. Neoplastic angioendotheliosis. The case of the missed primary? Arch Neurol 1979; 36: 5–7.

16 Beal MF, Fischer MC. Neoplastic angioendotheliosis. J Neurol Sci 1982; 53: 359–75.

17 Tappeiner J, Pfleger L. Angioendotheliomatosis proliferans systemisata (diffuse malignant proliferation of vascular endothelium). In: Andrede R, Gumport SL, Popkin GL, Reeds TD eds Cancer of Skin. Philadelphia: WB Saunders, 1976: 1151–71.

18 Strouth JC, Donahue S, Ross A et al. Neoplastic angioendotheliosis. Neurology 1965; 15: 644–8.

19 Ansbacher L, Low N, Beck D et al. Neoplastic angioendotheliosis: a clinicopathological entity with multifocal presentation. J Neurosurg 1981; 54: 412–5.

20 Person J. Systemic angioendotheliomatosis: a possible disorder of circulating angiogenic factor. Br J Dermatol 1972; 96: 329.

21 Fievez M, Fievez C, Hustin J. Proliferating systematized angioendotheliomatosis. Arch Dermatol 1971; 104: 320–4.

22 McCaulay WL. Lymphomatoid papulosis: a continuing self-healing eruption, clinically benign—histologically malignant. Arch Dermatol 1968; 97: 23–30.

23 Sanchez NP, Pittelkow MR, Muller SA et al. The clinicopathologic spectrum of lymphomatoid papulosis: study of 31 cases. J Am Acad Dermatol 1983; 8: 81–94.

24 Kitagawa M, Matsubara O, Song SY et al. Neoplastic angioendotheliosis. Immunohistochemical and electron microscopic findings in three cases. Cancer 1985; 56: 1134–43.

25 Petito CK, Gottleib GJ, Dougherty JH et al. Neoplastic angioendotheliosis: ultrastructural study and review of the literature. Ann Neurol 1978; 3: 393–9.

26 Wick MR, Banks PM, McDonald TJ. Angioendotheliomatosis of the nose with fatal systemic dissemination. Cancer 1981; 48: 2510–17.

27 Madara J, Shane J, Scarlato M. Systemic endotheliomatosis: a case report. J Clin Pathol 1975; 28: 476–82.

28 Scott PWB, Silvers DN, Helwig EB. Proliferating angioendotheliomatosis. Arch Pathol 1975; 99: 323–6.

29 Ansell J, Bhawan J, Cohen S et al. Histiocytic lymphoma and malignant angioendotheliomatosis: one disease or two? Cancer 1982; 50: 1506–12.

30 Wrotnowski J, Mills SE, Cooper PH. Malignant angioendotheliomatosis. An angiotropic lymphoma? Am J Clin Pathol 1985; 83: 244–8.

31 Shmookler BM, Graham JH, Langloss JM et al. Proliferating angioendotheliomatosis. A light and electron microscopic and immunohistochemical study. Lab Invest 1983; 48: 77A.

32 Yamamura Y, Akamizu H, Hirata T et al. Malignant lymphoma presenting with neoplastic angioendotheliosis of the central nervous system. Clinical Neuropathol 1983; 2: 63–8.

33 Sheibani K, Battifora H, Winberg CD et al. Further evidence that 'Malignant Angiotheliomatosis' is an angiotropic large-cell lymphoma. N Engl J Med 1986; 314: 943–8.

34 Wick MR, Mills SE, Scheithauer BW et al. Reassessment of malignant 'Angioendotheliomatosis'. Evidence in favor of its reclassification as 'Intravascular Lymphomatosis'. Am J Surg Pathol 1986; 10: 112–23.

35 Arnn ET, Yam LT, Li C-Y. Systemic angioendotheliomatosis presenting with hemolytic anemia. Am J Clin Pathol 1983; 80: 246–51.

36 Tanaka M, Yamaguchi H, Uchiyama T et al. An autopsy case of malignant lymphoma mimicking neoplastic angioendotheliosis. Clin Neurol 1982; 22: 507–13.

37 Carroll TJ, Goeken JA, Kemp JD. Neoplastic

angioendotheliomatosis: further evidence for intravascular malignant lymphomatosis. Lab Invest 1986; 54: 10A.

38 Mori S, Itoyama S, Mohri N et al. Cellular characteristics of neoplastic angioendotheliosis. An immunohistochemical marker study of six cases. Virchows Arch (Pathol Anat) 1985; 407: 167–75.

39 Okagaki T, Richart RM. Systemic proliferating angioendotheliomatosis. A case report. Obstet Gynecol 1971; 37: 377–80.

40 Husain MM, Sun CN, White JH. Neoplastic angioendotheliosis. J Neuropathol Exp Neurol 1979; 38: 322.

41 Shiozaki H, Hoshino S, Oshimi K et al. A case report of neoplastic angioendotheliosis which responded to a combination chemotherapy (CHOP). J Jpn Soc Intern Med 1983; 73: 374.

Textbook of Uncommon Cancer
Edited by C.J. Williams, J.G. Krikorian, M.R. Green and D. Raghavan
© 1988 John Wiley & Sons Ltd

Chapter **48**

Oncogenic Osteomalacia/Rickets

Noel Weidner

Assistant Professor, Department of Pathology, Harvard Medical School, Brigham and Women's Hospital, Boston, Massachusetts, USA

HISTORY AND DEFINITION

Oncogenic or tumor-induced osteomalacia/rickets is one type of hypophosphatemic osteomalacia/rickets. The latter includes a heterogeneous group of disorders characterized by hyperphosphaturia, hypophosphatemia, normo- or hypocalcemia, elevated serum alkaline phosphatase, and osteomalacia/rickets. The clinicopathologic features of this diverse group are reviewed elsewhere (1–4). Oncogenic or tumor-induced disease will be the focus of this chapter.

Although McCance (5) probably described the first case of oncogenic osteomalacia/rickets in 1947, Prader et al. (6) first recognized the causal role of a tumor in 1959. They described an 11-year-old girl who had hypophosphatemia, inappropriate phosphaturia, and a rib tumor which they called 'giant-cell granuloma.' All of the biochemical abnormalities were corrected after resection of the tumor, and the rickets healed completely and permanently without any other form of therapy. Prader et al. (6) believed that the tumor had caused the rickets by secreting a substance that was either an antagonist to vitamin D or caused phosphaturia similar to that produced by parathyroid hormone.

Currently, 44 cases have been reported unequivocally documenting a tumor's role in causing osteomalacia/rickets (5–40). In these cases the metabolic disturbances improved or completely disappeared upon removal of the tumor. An additional 28 cases of probable oncogenic osteomalacia/rickets have been published (41–57); however, many of these patients had inoperable lesions, and the authors could not clearly establish whether removal of the tumors would have reversed the metabolic abnormalities. The clinicopathologic features of the 44 well-documented cases of oncogenic osteomalacia/rickets provide the basis of this chapter.

EPIDEMIOLOGY

The incidence of oncogenic osteomalacia/rickets is not precisely known. Although this disease is thought to be rare, it may be more common than is generally appreciated. Many cases go undiagnosed; and, indeed, some of the previously reported cases of so-called idiopathic, sporadically occurring osteomalacia/rickets may be cases of undiscovered tumor-induced disease (29, 32, 58). In addition, the syndrome often persists unrecognized for many years before tumor is discovered and removed. The mean period between onset of symptoms and excision of tumor in the reported cases was 5 years, with a range of 1 to 13 years (33).

Failure to recognize this syndrome is the consequence of two factors. First, the tumors are frequently very small and in peculiar locations. For example, my colleagues and I (33, 59) observed a maxillary sinus tumor that caused the syndrome and had a roentgenographic appearance of a mucous retention cyst. This tumor was found only in the course of an intensive search for a possible causal tumor. The patient's signs and symptoms were alleviated after initial resection, but returned 5 weeks later. Repeat surgery showed a single microscopic focus of tumor whose removal led to resolution of all symptoms and return to normal of laboratory findings. In another example, a patient was cured of osteomalacia following removal of a 1.0×1.0 cm lesion of the right big toe (14). Second, many pathologists and clinicians are not aware of this peculiar paraneoplastic syndrome. It is therefore important to emphasize that whenever a patient has acquired non-nutritional osteomalacia/rickets, the physician should consider tumor-induced disease and meticulously search for a small, inconspicuous tumor. Once these tumors are discovered and removed, the patients can have complete reversal of their often incapacitating osteomalacia/rickets (33, 59).

ETIOLOGY

Available data suggest that these tumors produce a renal phosphaturic substance or hormone that depletes total-body phosphates by reducing tubular reabsorption of phosphate (19, 60–63). When measured, tubular reabsorption of phosphate has almost always been 79% or less, usually in the 40 to 60% range, despite severe hypophosphatemia (56). Although deficiency of 1,25-dihydroxyvitamin-D3 may be contributory, after sufficient phosphate has been lost, osteomalacia or rickets develops (33, 59, 60–63).

The mediator of the phosphaturia remains obscure. Parathyroid hormone (a known phosphaturic agent) cannot be implicated because levels have been normal in most patients. In addition, the patients are usually normocalcemic, show no benefit from parathyroidectomy, and demonstrate phosphaturia greater than that encountered in hyperparathyroid states (56). There is also no evidence to implicate excessive calcitonin secretion (56).

Lau et al. (61), Popovtzer et al. (62), and Aschinberg et al. (19) have all found phosphaturic substances in saline extracts from tumors causing osteomalacia/rickets. Without increasing urinary cyclic AMP, these extracts caused phosphaturia when injected into rats or puppies, and the extracts did not contain parathyroid hormone or calcitonin (56, 62). On the other hand, Yosikawa et al. (20), using both a neutral-buffer extract and a methanol–chloroform extract, could not demonstrate phosphaturia when these extracts were injected into rats.

Because low serum levels of 1,25-dihydroxyvitamin-D3 are consistently found in oncogenic osteomalacia/rickets, some authors have suggested that deficient production of this active vitamin D metabolite is the primary metabolic defect (21, 23). These low levels occur in spite of hypophosphatemia and/or estrogen therapy, which are known to stimulate 25-dihydroxy-vitamin-D3-1-alpha-hydroxylase in the proximal nephron (the enzyme necessary for converting 25-dihydroxyvitamin-D3 to the active metabolite 1,25-dihydroxyvitamin-D3) (60). In addition, these patients have normal serum levels of 25-hydroxyvitamin-D3, indicating normal vitamin D stores and adequate vitamin-D3-25-hydroxylase activity in the liver (60).

Certainly, in some patients with oncogenic osteomalacia/rickets, the clinical and biochemical abnormalities are ameliorated by 1,25-dihydroxyvitamin-D3 therapy (56). In fact, Drezner and Feinglos (21) reported one patient who achieved complete remission of their clinical and laboratory manifestations after treatment with physiological amounts of 1,25-dihydroxyvitamin-D3. However, in many patients, symptoms and/or renal phosphate handling improve partially, or not at all, despite therapy with 1,25-dihydroxyvitamin-

D3 (or the related 1-hydroxyvitamin-D3) and normalization of serum levels (1, 23, 26, 32, 59, 61). (Drezner et al. (60) have suggested that addition of oral phosphate to 1,25-dihydroxy-vitamin-D3 therapy will increase the proportion of significant responses.) In addition, the relationship between renal phosphate wasting and decreased serum 1,25-dihydroxy-vitamin-D3 in oncogenic osteomalacia/rickets remains unclear. There is no evidence for a direct inhibitory effect of vitamin D or its metabolites on renal phosphorus excretion (32, 59). Therefore, 1,25-dihydroxyvitamin-D3 deficiency alone does not explain the hyperphosphaturia of the syndrome.

Any complete explanation of the pathogenesis of oncogenic osteomalacia/rickets must explain both the low serum levels of 1,25-dihydroxyvitamin-D3 and the aminoaciduria and glycosuria found in many patients (59). Theoretically, a tumoral substance that alters proximal nephron function could explain all the findings in oncogenic osteomalacia/rickets (59, 60). The proximal nephron is not only the site of reabsorption of glucose and amino acids (59, 60), but it is also responsible for most phosphate reabsorption (59, 60) and all 25-hydroxyvitamin-D3-1-alpha-hydroxylase activity (59, 60). Indeed, preliminary data from an animal model of osteomalacia/rickets suggest depressed 25-hydroxyvitamin-D3-alpha-hydroxylase activity in the proximal tubule in patients with this syndrome (63), a finding thus helping to explain the depressed levels of 1,25-dihydroxy-vitamin-D3 in these patients.

Chronic phosphate depletion and depressed 1,25-dihydroxy-vitamin-D3 levels may then act synergistically to produce osteomalacia/rickets in this syndrome. In fact, Drezner et al. (60) have suggested that oncogenic osteomalacia/rickets is either an abnormality of heterogeneous cause or one due to variable expression of two interlinked phenomena, abnormal vitamin D metabolism and chronic phosphaturia, both likely due to the effects of a tumor-secreted substance.

PATHOBIOLOGY

When the syndrome is well-developed, bone biopsies in these patients show the characteristic features of osteomalacia or rickets (i.e. excessive osteoid in broad seams covering a majority of the trabecular surfaces, and after tetracycline labelling, decreased mineralization rate and low mineralization-front activity) (60). In addition, in one series reported by Drezner et al. (60) bone biopsies showed no evidence of excessive bone formation or resorption, and there was no osteocytic osteolysis (perilacunar mineral deficiency) in spite of its common occurrence in other forms of hypophosphatemic osteomalacia.

Although tumor-induced osteomalacia/rickets has been reported in patients with neurofibromatosis (41, 42), fibrous dysplasia (7), oat-cell carcinoma (55), prostate carcinoma (45, 49, 53, 54), and breast carcinoma (60), this chapter will focus on the pathobiology of those tumors proven to have caused osteomalacia/rickets. In these cases the metabolic disturbances improved or completely disappeared upon removal of the tumor.

My colleagues and I (33, 59) have recently reported the pathologic features of three mesenchymal tumors causing osteomalacia, and reviewed case reports in which tumors were unequivocally documented as the cause of this fascinating syndrome. As a result of this study, we observed that pathologists often give these tumors a variety of descriptive morphologic labels. Some of these tumors are difficult to classify and, depending upon the reviewing pathologist, may be labeled with different diagnostic descriptors (Table 1) (33). This confusion persisted, because the published reports incompletely describe and illustrate many of the tumors, and because no single institution has analyzed a large number of cases. However, from our initial review it was apparent that about 87% of these tumors contained multinucleated giant cells and 80% had prominent vascularity (33). These findings, plus the histologic features of the three

TABLE 1 PHOSPHATURIC MESENCHYMAL
TUMORS: LITERATURE REVIEW.
VARIOUS DIAGNOSTIC DESCRIPTORS
USED FOR TUMORS DOCUMENTED
AS CAUSING ONCOGENIC
OSTEOMALACIA/RICKETS (*reproduced
from reference 33 by permission of the
editor of Cancer*)

[a]Ossifying mesenchymal tumor	7	(16%)
[a]Hemangiopericytoma-like tumor	7	(16%)
Osteoblastoma	5	(11%)
Nonossifying fibroma	3	(7%)
Cavernous hemangioma	2	(5%)
[a]Giant cell reparative granuloma	2	(5%)
Miscellaneous (one each)	18	(40%)
[a]Osteocartilaginous mesenchymal tumor		
[a]Soft-parts chondroma-like tumor		
[a]Benign connective tissue lesion		
[a]Chondroblastoma/chondrosarcoma		
[a]Mixed connective tissue tumor		
[a]Vascular mesenchymal neoplasm		
[a]Primitive mesenchymal tumor		
[a]Benign mesenchymal neoplasm		
[a]Giant cell tumor of bone		
[a]Sclerosing hemangioma		
[a]Fibrous histiocytoma		
Fibroangioma of skin		
[a]Benign angiofibroma		
Fibrous dysplasia		
Osteosarcoma		
Angiosarcoma		
Sarcoma, NOS		
Neurinoma		
	Total	44

[a] These tumors may represent phosphaturic mesenchymal
tumors (mixed connective tissue variant), 64% of total. NOS=
not otherwise specified.

reported cases, suggested that the so-called
'heterogeneous' group of mesenchymal tumors
causing osteomalacia/rickets could, in fact,
represent a morphologic spectrum of a unique
tumor.

To overcome these uncertainties and help
clarify this problem, a colleague and I (40)
solicited tumor material from authors who
have published cases of oncogenic osteomala-
cia/rickets. We analyzed the material
obtained, along with 5 cases already in our
possession, and reported our finding (Table 2)
(40).

It became clear that, although these mesenchymal tumors were histologically polymorphous, they were classifiable into four morphologic patterns. Within the first and largest

group (10 cases) there were mixed mesenchymal tumors that likely represented a unique
category of connective-tissue tumor. These
mixed mesenchymal tumors contained primitive-appearing stromal cells, variably prominent vessels, and/or osteoclast-like giant cells
(Figures 1 to 8). In addition, they displayed
focal microcystic changes, osseous metaplasia,
and/or poorly formed cartilage-like areas
(Figures 1B, 4A, 5C, 6, 7 and 8). The cartilage-
like areas sometimes showed considerable dystrophic calcification (Figure 7).

With one exception, tumors in this first
group occurred in soft tissue and behaved in a
benign fashion. The single malignant example
originally occurred in bone, recurred locally,
and metastasized to lung. This malignant
tumor displayed greater cytologic atypia and
increased mitotic activity when compared to
its benign counterparts. The patient remains
alive, apparently with residual tumor, 6 years
after initial diagnosis (37).

The tumors comprising the remaining three
groups (6 tumors) occurred in bone, demonstrated benign clinical behavior, and were
grouped according to their close resemblance
to tumors known to occur in bone, that is
osteoblastoma-like (3 tumors) (Figures 9 and
10), nonossifying fibroma-like (2 tumors)
(Figure 11), and ossifying fibroma-like (1
tumor) (Figure 12).

Immunohistochemical studies of the mixed
mesenchymal tumor group have revealed only
vimentin immunoreactivity, a feature of
mesenchymal cells (33, 40). All other immunohistochemical reagents (including antibodies
to desmin, factor VIII-related antigen, S-100
protein, cytokeratin, leu-M1, leukocyte common antigen, chromogranin and neuron-specific enolase) have shown no evidence of epithelial, neural, vascular, or neuroendocrine
differentiation in tumor cells. Ultrastructural
studies have shown osteoclast-like giant cells
admixed with mesenchymal cells ranging from
primitive-appearing polygonal cells with organelle-poor cytoplasm to fibrohistiocytic cells
with organelle-rich cytoplasm (Figures 3 and
8). As in numerous previous reports, no neuro-

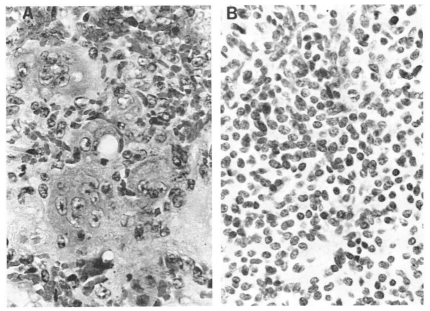

Figure 1 Case 3, mixed connective-tissue variant. A, Tumor field containing primitive-appearing stromal cells punctuated by clusters of osteoclast-like giant cells (arrows). (H&E, original magnification: ×16). B, Tumor field containing thick-walled vessels, primitive-appearing stromal cells, and numerous microcystic spaces. H&E, original magnification: ×40.

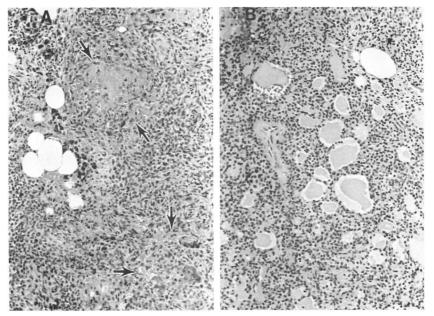

Figure 2 Case 3, mixed connective-tissue variant. A, Cluster of osteoclast-like giant cells surrounded by hemorrhagic stroma. H&E, original magnification: ×160. B, Primitive-appearing stromal cells are shown in greater detail, note the homogeneous-appearing, round to oval nuclei with scant intercellular matrix. Mitotic figures were rare. H&E, original magnification: ×160.

TABLE 2 CLINICOPATHOLOGIC FEATURES OF PHOSPHATURIC MESENCHYMAL TUMORS CAUSING OSTEOMALACIA/RICKETS

Case no. (ref.)	Age at onset/sex	Age at excision, location and initial tumor diagnosis	Giant cells	Vascularity	Microcystic spaces	Tumor bone or osteoid	Tumor cartilage	Small primitive cells	Final descriptive classification	Follow-up comments
1. (10)	34/M	38 yrs; left groin mass; 3–4 cm; 'sclerosing hemangioma with focal bone'	3+	3+	4+	1+	0	1+	Mixed mesenchymal tumor	AWED 16 yrs later
2. (10)	27/F	30 yrs; right thigh mass; 2 × 3 cm; 'sclerosing hemangioma'	3+	3+	2+	1+	0	1+	Mixed mesenchymal tumor	AWED 16 yrs later
3. (33)	35/F	39 yrs; right maxillary sinus, 'primitive mesenchymal tumor'	3+	3+	2+	0	0	4+	Mixed mesenchymal tumor	AWED 3 yrs later
4. (33)	33/M	34 yrs; left pulmonary lesion, soft tissue, 4.5 cm, 'soft parts chondroma-like with giant cells'	2+	2+	0	0	4+	1+	Mixed mesenchymal tumor	AWED 8 yrs later
5. (33)	63/F	66 yrs; left distal ulna, bone and soft tissue, 'osteocartilaginous mesenchymal tumor'	3+	2+	0	1+	2+	1+	Mixed mesenchymal tumor	AWED 2 yrs later
6. (38)	45/F	48 yrs; soft-tissue mass, right knee, 'benign angiofibroma'	0[a]	3+	2+	0	0	1+	Mixed mesenchymal tumor	AWED 9 yrs later
7. (39)	44/F	50 yrs; soft-tissue mass, left forearm, 7 cm, 'hemangiopericytoma'	1+	3+	0	2+	0	2+	Mixed mesenchymal tumor	AWED 19 mos later
8. (37)	44/M	49 yrs; cystic lesion of right femoral condyle; tumor recurred locally at 52 yrs; AKA performed; plumonary lesions resected at 53 yrs and 55 yrs; 'chondroblastoma/chondrosarcoma'	2+	3+	2+	2+	2+	2+	Mixed malignant mesenchymal tumor	Alive with disease 6 yrs later
9. (40)	61/M	61 yrs; soft-tissue mass of right deltoid region; 1.5 cm; patient also had multiple dermatofibromas; 'benign mesenchymal neoplasm'	3+	3+	2+	0	3+	2+	Mixed mesenchymal tumor	AWED 2.5 yrs later

10. (40)	57/M	57 yrs; soft-tissue mass of right ankle; 4.0 cm; 'mixed connective tissue tumor'	2+	2+	0	0	4+	2+	Mixed mesenchymal tumor	AWED 0.5 yrs later
11. (20)	13/M	18 yrs; 4th metacarpal, 'osteoblastoma'	1+	2+	0	4+	0	0	Osteoblastoma-like tumor	AWED 14 wks later
12. (20)	13/F	18 yrs; lytic lesion, upper humerus, 'osteoblastoma'	2+	2+	0	4+	0	0	Osteoblastoma-like tumor	AWED 10 wks later
13. (23)	24/F	24 yrs; lytic lesion, tibia, 4.5 cm, 'osteoid with osteoblasts'	1+	1+	0	4+	0	0	Osteoblastome-like tumor	AWED 5 mos later
14. (13)	7.5/M	12 yrs; lytic lesion, distal radius, 2.8 cm 'nonossifying fibroma'	1+	1+	0	0	0	0	Nonossifying fibroma-like tumor	AWED 1 yr later
15. (29)	13/F	14 yrs; cortical defect, left femur, 1.5 cm, 'nonossifying fibroma'	2+	1+	0	0	0	0	Nonossifying fibroma-like tumor	AWED 3 mos later
16. (30)	27/M	29 yrs; cystic mandibular lesion, 'osteosarcoma'	0	2+	0	2+	0	0	Ossifying fibroma-like	1 recurrence 1.5 mos later, treated at 2nd surgery, AWED 5 yrs later

[a] Only small segment of tumor examined.   AWED=alive without evidence of disease. AKA=above the knee amputation.

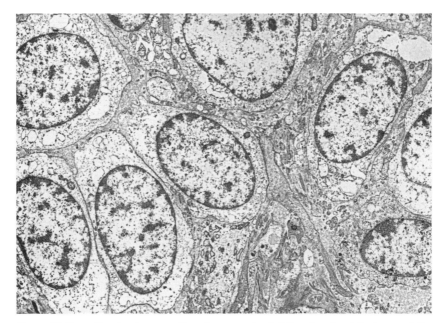

Figure 3 Case 3, mixed connective-tissue variant. Ultrastructural features of the primitive-appearing stromal cells; note organelle-poor cytoplasm, microvilli, and occasional stretches of basal lamina. No neurosecretory granules are present. Lead citrate and uranyl acetate, original magnification: ×2800.

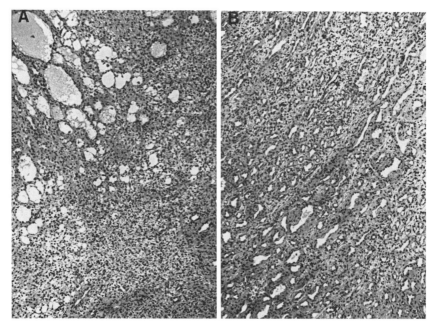

Figure 4 Case 7, mixed connective tissue variant. A, Tumor field showing primitive-appearing stroma containing numerous and variably sized icrocystic spaces, this tumor contained few osteoclast-like giant cells. (H&E, original magnification: ×10). B, Tumor field showing hemangiopericytoma-like vascularity found in some tumor fields. H&E, original magnification: ×10.

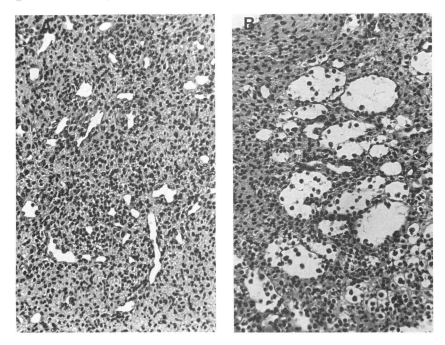

Figure 5 Case 7, mixed connective tissue variant. A, More highly magnified field of tumor showing primitive-appearing stroma containing numerous vessels forming hemangiopericytoma-like pattern. H&E, original magnification: ×100. B, More highly magnified field of tumor showing primitive-appearing stroma containing numerous microcystic spaces. H&E, original magnification: ×100.

secretory granules were observed in 6 tumors studied.

Therefore, it appears that no single mesenchymal tumor having a homogeneous morphologic pattern causes all cases of oncogenic osteomalacia/rickets. However, the first and largest group of mixed mesenchymal tumors appears to be a unique connective-tissue tumor (33, 40), a suspicion previously mentioned by both Olefsky et al. (12) and Evans et al. (11). The diagnostic terminology for these soft-tissue tumors remains controversial. Olefsky et al. (12) suggested 'ossifying mesenchymal tumor associated with osteomalacia.' However, not all tumors contain ossification. Salassa et al. (10) suggested sclerosing hemangioma, a term also favored by Mirra (64). Other authors have used diagnostic terms such as benign angiofibroma (38), hemangiopericytoma (39), chondrosarcoma (37), mixed connective tissue

tumor (40), and soft-parts chondroma-like tumor (33). The diversity of these diagnostic labels underscores the morphologic complexity of these tumors and the difficulty in developing a single, universally acceptable term.

Until the specific cell type or phosphaturic substance is characterized, we (40) favor the use of a descriptive phrase to label these tumors. For the first group of primitive mesenchymal tumors, we (40) prefer the term 'phosphaturic mesenchymal tumor (mixed connective tissue variant).' For those tumors resembling osteoblastomas, we prefer the phrase 'phosphaturic mesenchymal tumor (osteoblastoma-like variant),' and so forth.

The tumors that occurred in bone appeared to be morphologically distinct from those occurring in soft tissue. The resons for this are unclear, but possibly within bone the phosphaturic mesenchymal tumors are induced to show

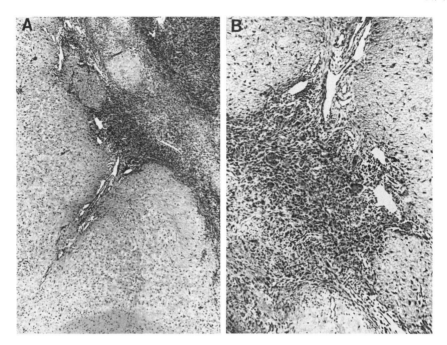

Figure 6 Case 9, mixed connective tissue variant. A, Tumor field showing lobulated, primitive-appearing stroma resembling poorly formed cartilage. This tumor was punctuated by interlobular stroma which was cellular, contained vessels, and was punctuated by clusters of osteoclast-like giant cells. In aggregate these features resembled a soft-parts chondroma. H&E, original magnification: ×10. B, Higher magnification of the interlobular stroma found in this tumor; note vessels, osteoclast-like giant cells, and primitive-appearing stromal cells. Apparent in the periphery of this photomicrograph are the stellate and spindle-shaped stromal cells forming the poorly formed cartilage-like tissue. H&E, original magnification: ×100.

bone-like differentiation. Alternatively, the bone tumors may, indeed, be separate and distinct from the unique soft-tissue tumors, but somehow they too cause secretion of a phosphaturic substance, possibly by stimulating non-neoplastic cells that are bony or inflammatory in origin.

The primitive-appearing, small stromal cells found in the unique connective-tissue tumors appear to be logical candidates for producing the putative phosphaturic substance (33). They were the predominant cells in one reported case, especially in the small microscopic recurrence that caused a relapse of osteomalacia (33, 59). However, these stromal cells tend to be organelle-poor, and they do not

have neurosecretory granules. This of course does not preclude them for secreting hormonally active substances, possibly lipid in nature.

The osteoclast-like giant cells are conspicuous in many tumors (33, 40), are likely derived from blood-borne monocytes (65, 66), and are possible candidates for secreting a phosphaturic substance. The osteoclast of bone is well-known to respond to a number of hormones and other substances, but very little is understood about biochemical messages that might be elaborated by osteoclasts (67, 68). It would not be surprising to learn that a cell specialized to mobilize phosphate, calcium, and protein from bone might also have the

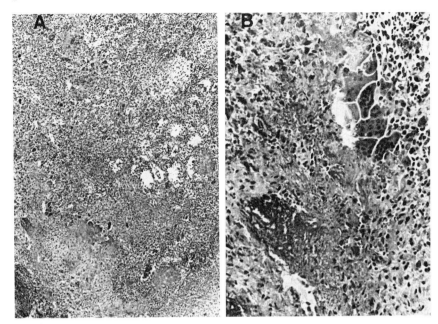

Figure 7 Case 10, mixed connective tissue variant. A, Tumor field showing primitive-appearing stroma containing numerous foci of dystrophic calcification. H&E, original magnification: ×10. B, Higher magnification showing dystrophic calcification occurring near a cluster of osteoclast-like giant cells. H&E, original magnification: ×100.

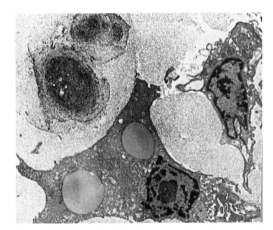

Figure 8 Case 9, mixed connective tissue variant. Ultrastructural features of primitive-appearing stromal cell from a tumor area resembling poorly formed cartilage, note the numerous profiles of rough endoplasmic reticulum, lipid vacuoles, and irregular cytoplasmic borders. No neurosecretory granules are present. These cells are surrounded by peculiar granulofibillary matrix showing early calcification (upper left-hand corner). Lead citrate and uranyl acetate, original magnification: ×3000.

ability to secrete a phosphaturic substance. Unfortunately, osteoclast-like giant cells are present in small numbers or are totally absent in some tumors causing osteomalacia/rickets. In addition, it is possible that these osteoclast-like giant cells proliferate in phosphaturic mesenchymal tumors in response to phosphate deficiency or in response to a tumor chemotactic factor. Indeed, normal osteoclasts increase in size and number in rats made deficient in calcium or phosphorus (69). Furthermore, there is good evidence that osteoclast precursors (monocytes) can be mobilized by chemotaxis (65). These same data suggest that the chemo-attractants responsible are derived from Type 1 collagen peptides and/or the bone-matrix proteins, alpha-2-HS glycoprotein and osteocalcin (65).

CLINICAL AND LABORATORY FEATURES

The mean age at which signs and symptoms of

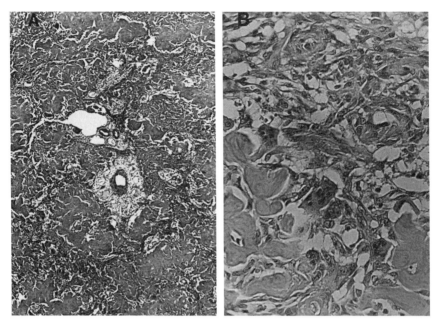

Figure 9 Case 11, osteoblastoma-like variant. A, Tumor field extensively replaced by osteoid. H&E, original magnification: ×10. B, Higher magnification showing osteoid, spindle-shaped stromal cells, and osteoclast-like giant cells. H&E, original magnification: ×100.

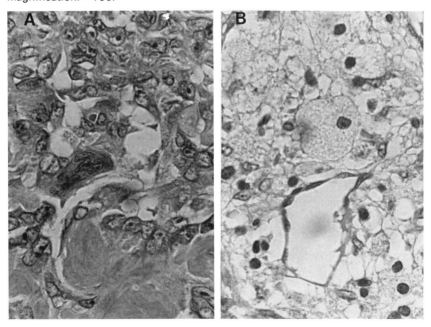

Figure 10 Case 11, osteoblastoma-like variant. A, Tumor field showing details of stromal cells and osteoid, note marked osteoblastic rimming at bottom. H&E, original magnification: ×400. B, Tumor field containing cluster of foamy histiocytes, a finding present in the three bone tumors with osteoblastoma-like features. H&E, original magnification: ×400.

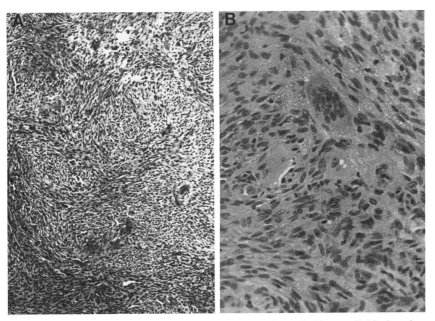

Figure 11 Case 14, nonossifying fibroma-like variant. A, Tumor field showing fascicular (sometimes storiform) growth pattern produced by the spindle-shaped tumor cells. The tumor stroma was punctated by scattered osteoclast-like giant cells. H&E, original magnification: ×16. B, Spindle-shaped tumor cells and osteoclast-like giant cells are shown in greater detail. H&E, original magnification: ×160.

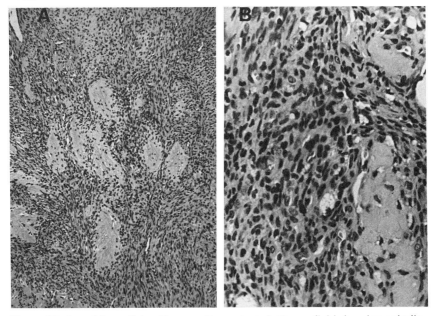

Figure 12 Case 16, ossifying fibroma-like variant. A, Tumor field showing spindle-cell stroma punctuated by islands of osteoid. H&E, original magnification: ×16. B, Higher magnification showing spindle cells forming osteoid. H&E, original magnification: ×160.

osteomalacia/rickets first develop is approximately 33 years (range 5 to 63 years). Often, however, the symptoms have persisted for a considerable time before a diagnosis of oncogenic osteomalacia/rickets is made (i.e. mean age at diagnosis is 38 years, range 1 to 13 years after symptom onset). Approximately 93% of patients have bone pain and 63% severe muscle weakness (56). Other complaints include fractures, height loss, gait disturbances, skeletal deformity, and slow growth (33, 59). In about 39% of patients the symptoms are severe enough to prevent walking (56). Men and women are equally affected.

Patients with oncogenic osteomalacia/rickets consistently show hypophosphatemia associated with inappropriate phosphaturia. In one review the mean serum phosphorus was 1.5 mg/dl (normal 2.5–4.5), which rose to a mean postoperative level of 3.5 mg/dl (60). Renal tubular resorption of phosphate is almost always less than 79%, usually in the range of 40–60% (56). These patients also show a low renal tubular maximum for the reabsorption of phosphorus per liter of glomerular filtrate (TmP/GFR), mean of 1.04 mg/dl (normal 2.45–4.55), and net gastrointestinal malabsorption of phosphorus, mean of 452 mg/day of a 1200 mg/day diet absorbed (normal 679–1059) (60). The renal phosphorus wasting and gastrointestinal malabsorption result in a negative phosphorus balance (60).

Serum calcium levels have usually been normal, but they may be slightly low at presentation (56, 60). However, if after treatment 'tertiary hyperparathyroidism' develops, serum calcium may become elevated (12, 37). Before treatment, serum parathyroid hormone levels are usually normal, even when serum calcium levels are slightly low (56, 60); however, in occasional cases parathyroid hormone has been either marginally elevated or not detectable (56). Calcitonin levels have been normal or slightly elevated (56). Like phosphorus, there is gastrointestinal malabsorption of calcium, but positive calcium balance is maintained because of renal conservation of calcium (60).

When serum vitamin D metabolites have been measured, the patients almost universally have shown low 1,25-dihydroxy-vitamin-D3 (mean 13.4 pg/ml, normal 19–50) and normal 25-hydroxyvitamin-D3 (mean 32.7 ng/ml, normal 15–18). In one patient the serum 24,25-dihydroxyvitamin-D3 was elevated (59). Serum 1,25-dihydroxyvitamin-D3 levels normalize after the tumor is removed.

Finally, serum alkaline phosphatase is consistently elevated (33) in these patients, and aminoaciduria (especially glycinuria) is present in approximately 32% (56). Glycosuria in the absence of hyperglycemia is present in about 50% of patients (56).

DIAGNOSTIC INVESTIGATION

Before any diagnostic evaluation is undertaken, it is important to consider the differential diagnostic possibilities. The common clinical causes of osteomalacia include renal failure, intestinal malabsorption, chronic acidosis, and unusual dietary habits (1–4, 56). In renal failure the serum phosphorus level is high. Although severe hypophosphatemia can occur in diabetic ketoacidosis, acute alcoholism, and severe dietary restriction of phosphorus, serum phosphorus in these conditions is usually only slightly low (1–4, 56). In all of these conditions, and in sharp contrast to oncogenic osteomalacia/rickets, the urine is virtually phosphate-free (1–4, 56).

Osteomalacia/rickets associated with both hypophosphatemia and phosphaturia can result from inherited or acquired defects of renal tubular transport of phosphate (1–4, 56). The more common conditions causing this syndrome include X-linked hypophosphatemic rickets, the Fanconi syndrome, heavy metal poisoning, idiopathic phosphate leak, and oncogenic osteomalacia/rickets (1–4, 56). X-linked hypophosphatemic rickets has a characteristic inheritance pattern and onset in early childhood (1–4, 56). The Fanconi syndrome has multiple proximal nephron dysfunctions and metabolic acidosis (1–4, 56).

Heavy metal poisoning is suggested by clinical and laboratory findings (1–4, 56).

Recently, Tieder et al. (70) reported a new hereditary syndrome of hypophosphatemic rickets and hypercalciuria in 6 affected members of a kindred. The patients have rickets associated with hypophosphatemia, phosphaturia, normocalcemia, hypercalciuria, elevated 1,25-dihydroxyvitamin-D3 levels, depressed parathyroid hormone levels, and increased gastrointestinal absorption of calcium and phosphorus. Long-term phosphate supplementation as the sole therapy resulted in reversal of all clinical and biochemical abnormalities except the renal phosphate 'leak.' Finally, it is important to separate oncogenic osteomalacia/rickets from other tumor-associated osteomalacia or hypophosphatemic syndromes, such as tumor-induced malabsorption or diarrhea (71–73), ectopic parathyroid hormone production (74–78), or phosphorus uptake by leukemia/lymphoma cells (79–82).

Oncogenic osteomalacia/rickets should be suspected in any patient who presents with hypophosphatemia and inappropriate phosphaturia (33, 59). Serum 1,25-dihydroxyvitamin-D3 is low in all cases, and serum alkaline phosphatase should be elevated. Because clinical osteomalacia or rickets may not be present when the biochemical abnormalities are first noted, a bone biopsy might be helpful in securing a diagnosis. The biopsy is best performed after tetracycline labeling.

If there is no clinical evidence to suggest one of the diseases mentioned previously, a vigorous and meticulous search for a small, inconspicuous tumor should be initiated. The mesenchymal tumors can occur in almost any location. Approximately 53% have occurred in bone, 45% in soft tissues, and 3% in skin (33). About 44% have involved the lower extremities, 27% the head-and-neck area, and 17% the upper extremities (56). The patient should be asked about the presence of a tumor and given a whole-body clinical examination. In addition, computer-assisted tomography, regional tomograms, and bone scans should be administered until a tumor is either found or ruled out. One phosphaturic mesenchymal tumor (mixed connective tissue variant) demonstrated marked uptake of 99^m-technetium methylene diphosphonate (33, 59), a property which, if present, can expedite tumor discovery.

If a phosphaturic mesenchymal tumor is not found, one should consider other tumors that have been reported to cause oncogenic osteomalacia/rickets. These tumors include prostate cancer (45, 49, 53, 54), breast cancer (60), oat-cell carcinoma (55), fibrous dysplasia (7), and soft-tissue tumors occurring in neurofibromatosis (41, 42). Unfortunately, the causal role of tumor in many of these cases cannot be proven, because of the often extensive and unresectable nature of the lesions. It is also important to consider the possibility that a small phosphaturic mesenchymal tumor may exist concomitantly with one of these 'other tumors' (e.g. carcinoma) (83). As a consequence, one should not forget to investigate these patients for an inconspicuous mesenchymal tumor as well. The dramatic cure of the osteomalacia or rickets that will result from its removal would be worth the effort and expense.

MANAGEMENT AND PROGNOSIS

Obviously, once a suspicious mass in bone, skin, or soft tissue is discovered, it needs to be surgically removed and examined by a pathologist. The morphologic features of the tumor may help confirm the diagnosis of oncogenic osteomalacia/rickets, especially if it has the unique morphologic features of a phosphaturic mesenchymal tumor (mixed connective tissue variant). Postoperatively, serum phosphate and 1,25-dihydroxyvitamin-D3 should be measured; however, it may take days to weeks for these chemistries to return to normal values (33).

If the abnormal chemistries resolve, the patient's symptoms disappear, and the tumor appears totally resected and benign, then the diagnosis is confirmed and the prognosis is excellent. However, if this does not occur and the tumor shows features not typical for phosphaturic mesenchymal tumors, then one should continue the search for the 'right' tumor or consider an alternative diagnosis. If the patient's serum chemistries and symptoms only partially improve, there may be residual tumor, especially if the tumor appears only partially resected or shows malignant cytologic features. In the latter event additional surgery, chemotherapy, and/or radiation therapy may be necessary to effect cure.

If it is not possible to find or eradicate the tumor causing the osteomalacia or rickets, then supplemental phosphorus and vitamin D therapy is indicated. The best results are achieved when both 1,25-dihydroxyvitamin-D3 (2–4 μg/day) and phosphate (2 g/day) are given orally (59, 60). Although this combined therapy has been considered to be free from harmful side effects, 2 cases have been recently reported by Firth et al. (37) that challenged this belief. In these cases long-term therapy (14 and 10 years) resulted in hypercalcemic hyperparathyroidism associated with surgically proven adenomatous hyperplasia of the parathyroids (i.e. 'tertiary hyperparathyroidism'). The ultimate prognosis of these patients with unresectable tumors will largely depend upon the nature of the underlying tumor. Most patients with high-grade malignant tumors (e.g. carcinoma) will likely succumb to their tumor. The one patient with a malignant phosphaturic mesenchymal tumor (mixed connective tissue variant) developed pulmonary metastases but remained alive with probable residual disease 6 years after diagnosis (37).

CURRENT RESEARCH AND FUTURE DIRECTIONS

As indicated, some patients with prostate carcinoma have been reported to develop osteomalacia (45, 49, 53, 54); however, the inability to completely eradicate the carcinoma has precluded direct proof that this cancer causes osteomalacia. To indirectly prove this relationship Lyles et al. (63) and Drezner et al. (60) successfully heterotransplanted tumor tissue from a patient with prostate carcinoma and osteomalacia into athymic nude mice. The tumor-bearing mice manifested many of the biochemical abnormalities found in oncogenic osteomalacia/rickets (i.e. renal phosphate wasting and hypophosphatemia). In addition, these investigators found that the mice had decreased renal 25-hydroxyvitamin-D3-1-alpha-hydroxylase activity, indicating that the defect in vitamin D metabolism found in patients with oncogenic osteomalacia/rickets is likely (at least in part) due to decreased 1,25-dihydroxyvitamin-D3 production. Of course, increased degradation of 1,25-dihydroxyvitamin-D3 may be present as well. Finally, these investigators were unable to extract the phosphaturic and hydroxylase-suppressing substance from the prostate carcinoma cells, implying that the carcinoma cells were causing non-neoplastic host cells to secrete the phosphaturic factor. Clearly, additional work will be needed with this animal model to clarify the important pathogenetic events.

The chemical nature of the putative phosphaturic substance remains unknown, but when this substance is isolated and characterized, a great deal will be learned not only about the cause of oncogenic osteomalacia/rickets but also about phosphate homeostasis in general. This discovery might also result in development of a serum assay for the phosphaturic substance, allowing patients with this syndrome to be positively identified. Certainly, a positive test would help to justify the expense and inconvenience of a vigorous and meticulous search for a small, inconspicuous tumor.

REFERENCES

1 Agus ZS. Oncogenic hypophosphatemic osteomalacia. Kidney Int 1983; 24: 113.
2 Frame B, Parfitt AM. Osteomalacia: Current concepts. Ann Intern Med 1978; 89: 966.
3 Mankin HJ. Rickets, osteomalacia, and renal osteodystrophy. J Bone Joint Surg 1974; 56-A: 101.
4 Stansbury SW. Osteomalacia. Clin Endocrinol Metab 1972; 1: 239.

5 McCance RA. Osteomalacia with Looser's nodes (Milkman's syndrome) due to a raised resistance to vitamin D acquired about the age of 15 years. Q J Med 1947; 16: 33.

6 Prader A, Illig R, Uehlinger RE, Stalder G. Rachitis infolge knochentumors. Helvet Pediatr Acta 1959; 14: 554.

7 Dent CE, Friedman M. Hypophosphatemic osteomalacia with complete recovery. Br Med J 1964; 1: 1676.

8 Yoshikawa S, Kawabata M, Hatsuyama Y, Hosokawa O, Fujita T. Atypical vitamin-D resistant osteomalacia. J Bone Joint Surg 1964; 46-A: 998.

9 Castleman B, McNeely BU. Case records of the Massachusetts General Hospital: Case #38-1965. N Engl J Med 1965; 273: 494.

10 Salassa RM, Jowsey J, Arnaud CD. Hypophosphatemic osteomalacia associated with 'nonendocrine' tumors. N Engl J Med 1970; 282: 65.

11 Evans DJ, Azzopardi JG. Distinctive tumours of bone and soft tissue causing acquired vitamin-D-resistant osteomalacia. Lancet 1972; i: 353.

12 Olefsky J, Kempson R, Jones H, Reaven G. 'Tertiary hyperparathyroidism and apparent cure' of vitamin-D-resistant rickets after removal of an ossifying mesenchymal tumor of the pharynx. N Engl J Med 1972; 286: 740–5.

13 Pollack JA, Schiller AL, Crawford JD. Rickets and myopathy cured by removal of nonossifying fibroma of bone. Pediatrics 1973; 52: 364.

14 Moser CR, Fessel WJ. Rheumatic manifestations of hypophosphatemia. Arch Intern Med 1974; 134: 674.

15 Wilhoite DR. Acquired rickets and solitary bone tumor: the question of a causal relationship. In: Proceedings of the Clinical Orthopaedic Society. Clin Orthop 1975; 109: 210.

16 Linovitz RJ, Resnick D, Keissling P, et al. Tumor-induced osteomalacia and rickets: a surgically curable syndrome. J Bone Joint Surg 1976; 58-A: 419.

17 Dent CE, Gertner JM. Hypophosphataemic osteomalacia in fibrous dysplasia. Q J Med 1976; 45: 411.

18 Wyman AL, Paradinas FJ, Daly JR. Hypophosphataemic osteomalacia associated with a malignant tumor of the tibia: report of a case. J Clin Pathol 1977; 30: 328.

19 Aschinberg LC, Solomon LM, Zeis PM, Justice P, Rosenthal IM. Vitamin-D-resistant rickets associated with epidermal nevus syndrome: demonstration of a phosphaturic substance in the dermal lesions. J Pediatr 1977; 91: 56.

20 Yosikawa S, Nakamura T, Takagi M, Imamura T, Okano K, Satoshi S. Benign osteoblastoma as a cause of osteomalacia. A report of two cases. J Bone Joint Surg 1977; 59-B: 279.

21 Drezner MK, Feinglos MN. Osteomalacia due to 1,25-dihydroxycholecalciferol deficiency. J Clin Invest 1977; 60: 1046.

22 Boriani S, Companacci M. Osteoblastoma associated with osteomalacia (presentation of a case and review of the literature). Ital J Orthop Traumatol 1978; 4: 379.

23 Fukumoto Y, Sciichiro T, Kciko T et al. Tumor-induced vitamin-D-resistant hypophosphatemic osteomalacia associated with proximal tubular dysfunction and 1,25-dihydroxyvitamin-D deficiency. J Clin Endocrinol Metab 1979; 49: 873.

24 Turner ML, Dalinka MK. Osteomalacia: uncommon causes. Am J Radiol 1979; 133: 539.

25 Sweet RA, Males JL, Hamstra AJ, DeLuca HF. Vitamin D metabolite levels in oncogenic osteomalacia. Ann Intern Med 1980; 93: 279.

26 Camus JP, Crouzet J, Prier A, Grillemant S, Ulmann A, Koeger AC. Ostéomalacies hypophophorémiques guéries par l'ablation de tumeurs bénignes du tissu conjonctif: étude de trois observations avec dosages pre- et post-opératoires des métabolites de la vitaminé D. Ann Med Intern 1980; 131: 422.

27 Parker MS, Klein I, Haussier MR, Mintz DH. Tumor-induced osteomalacia. Evidence of surgically correctable alteration in vitamin D metabolism. JAMA 1981; 245: 492.

28 Nitzan DW, Marmary Y, Azaz B. Mandibular tumor induced muscular weakness and osteomalacia. Oral Surg 1981; 52: 253.

29 Asnes RS, Berdon WE, Bassett A. Hypophosphatemic rickets in an adolescent cured by excission of a nonossifying fibroma. Clin Pediatr 1981; 20: 646.

30 Nomura G, Koshino Y, Morimoto H, Kida H. Nomura S, Tamai K. Vitamin D resistant hypophosphatemic osteomalacia associated with osteosarcoma of the manible: report of a case. Jpn J Med 1981; 21: 35.

31 Robertson A. Case of the winter season. Semin Roetgenol 1983; 18: 5.

32 Smith WS, Linsey M, Bernstein L, Yamauchi H. Nasopharyngeal angiofibroma presenting as adult osteomalacia: case report and review of the literature. Laryngoscope 1983; 93: 1328.

33 Weidner N, Bar RS, Weiss D, Strottmann P. Neoplastic pathology of oncogenic osteomalacia/rickets. Cancer 1985; 55: 1691.

34 Morita M. A case of adult onset vitamin D resistant osteomalacia associated with soft tissue tumor. Kotsudaisha (Bone Metabolism) 1976; 9: 286.

35 Lejeune E, Bouvier M, Meunier P et al. L'osteomalacie des tumeurs mesenchymateuses. Rev Rhum Mal Osteoartic 1979; 46: 187.

36 Crouzet J, Camus JP, Gatti JM, Descamps H, Beraneck L. Ostéomalacie hypophosphoremi-

que et hemangiopéricytome de la voûte du crâne. Rev Rhum Mal Ostéoartic 1980; 47: 523.

37 Firth RG, Grant CS, Riggs BL. Development of hypercalcemic hyperparathyroidism after long-term phosphate supplementation in hypophosphatemic osteomalacia. Report of two cases. Am J Med 1985; 78: 669.

38 Cotton GE, Van Puffelen P. Hypophosphatemic osteomalacia secondary to neoplasia. J Bone Joint Surg 1986; 68-A: 129.

39 Gitelis S, Ryan WG, Rosenberg AG, Templeton AC. Adult-onset hypophosphatemic osteomalacia secondary to neoplasm. J Bone Joint Surg 1986; 68-A: 134.

40 Weidner N, Santa Cruz D. Phosphaturic mesenchymal tumors. A polymorphous group causing osteomalacia or rickets. Cancer 1987; 59: 1442.

41 Hernberg CA, Edgren W. Looser-Milkman's syndrome with neurofibromatosis Recklinghausen and general decalcification of the skeleton. Acta Med Scand 1949; 136: 26.

42 Salville PD, Nassim JR, Stevenson SH, Mulligan L, Margaret C. Osteomalacia in Von Recklinghausen's neurofibromatosis: Metabolic study of a case. Br Med J 1955; i: 1311.

43 Hauge BD. Vitamin D resistant osteomalacia. Acta Med Scand 1956; 153: 271.

44 Mittal MM, Gupta MC, Sharma ML. Osteomalacia in neurofibromatosis (report of two cases). J Assoc Phys Ind 1971; 19: 823.

45 Hosking DJ, Chamberlain MJ, Shortland-Webb WR. Osteomalacia and carcinoma of the prostate with major redistribution of skeletal calcium. Br Med J Radiol 1975; 48: 451.

46 Renton P, Shaw DG. Hypophosphatemic osteomalacia secondary to vascular tumors of bone and soft tissue. Skel Radiol 1976; 1: 21.

47 Moncrieff MW, Brenton DP, Arthur LJH. Case of tumour rickets. Arch Dis Child 1978; 53: 740.

48 Daniels RA, Weisenfield I. Tumorous phosphaturic osteomalacia: report of a case associated with multiple hemangiomas of bone. Am J Med 1979; 67: 155.

49 Lyles KW, Berry WR, Haussler M, Harrelson JM, Drezner MK. Hypophosphatemic osteomalacia: association with prostate carcinoma. Ann Intern Med 1980; 93: 275.

50 Retnam VJ, Rangnekar DM, Bhandarkar SD. neurofibromatosis with hypophosphatemic osteomalacia (Von Recklinghausen-Hernberg-Edgren-Swann syndrome) (a case report). J Assoc Phys Ind 1980; 28: 319.

51 Chacko V, Joseph B. Osteomalacia associated with hemangiopericytoma. J Ind Med Assoc 1981; 76: 173.

52 Cramer CF, Aikawa M, Cebelin M. Neurosecretory granules in small cell invasive carcinoma of the bladder. Cancer 1981; 47: 724.

53 Kabadi UM. Osteomalacia associated with prostatic cancer and osteoblastic metastases. Urology 1983; 21: 65.

54 Charhon SA, Chapuy MC, Delvin EE, Valentin-Opran A, Edouard CM, Meunier PJ. Histomorphometric analysis of sclerotic bone metastases from prostate carcinoma with special reference to osteomalacia. Cancer 1983; 51: 918.

55 Taylor HC, Fallon MD, Velasco ME. Oncogenic osteomalacia and inappropriate antidiuretic hormone secretion due to oat-cell carcinoma. Ann Intern Med 1984; 101: 786.

56 Ryan EA, Reiss E. Oncogenous osteomalacia. Review of the world's literature of 42 cases and report of two new cases. Am J Med 1984; 77: 501.

57 Nortman DF, Coburn JW, Brautbar N et al. Treatment of mesenchymal tumor associated osteomalacia (MTAO) with 1,25(OH)2D3: report of a case. In: Norman AW, Schaefer K, Herrath DV et al. (eds) Vitamin D, Basic Research and its Clinical Application. Berlin: W de Greyter, 1979: 1167.

58 Dent DE, Stamp TCB. Hypophosphatemic osteomalacia presenting in adults. Q J Med 1971; 40: 303.

59 Weiss D, Bar RS, Weidner N, Werner M, Lee F. Oncogenic osteomalacia: strange tumors in strange places. Postgrad Med J 1985; 61: 349.

60 Drezner MK, Lobaugh B, Lyles KW, Carey DE, Paulson DF, Harrelson JM. The pathogenesis and treatment of tumor-induced osteomalacia. In: Norman AW, Schaefer K, Herrath DV et al. (eds) Vitamin D, Chemical, Biochemical and Clinical Endocrinology of Calcium Metabolism. Berlin/New York: de Gruyter, 1982: 949.

61 Lau K, Stom MC, Goldberg M et al. Evidence for a humoral phosphaturic factor in oncogenic hypophosphatemic osteomalacia (abstract). Clin Res 1979; 27: 421A.

62 Popovtzer MM. Tumor-induced hypophophatemic osteomalacia (TUO): evidence for a phosphaturic cyclic AMP-independent action of tumor extract (abstr). Clin Res 1981; 29: 418A.

63 Lyles KW, Lobaugh B, Paulsen DF, Drezner MK. Heteotransplantation of prostate cancer from an affected patient creates an animal model for tumor induced osteomalacia in the athymic nude mouse (abstr). Calcif Tiss Int 1982; 34: S33.

64 Mirra JM. Bone Tumors, Diagnosis and Treatment, 1st edition. Philadelphia: JB Lippincott, 1980: 500.

65 Malone JD, Teitelbaum GL, Griffin RM, Senior RM, Kahn AJ. Recruitment of osteoclast precursors by purified bone matrix constituents. J Cell Biol 1982; 92: 227.

66 Fischmann DA, Hay ED. Origin of osteoclasts

from mononuclear leukocytes in regenerating newt limbs. Anat Rec 1962; 143: 329.

67 Holtrop ME, King GJ. The ultrastructure of the osteoclast and its functional implications. In: Proceedings of the Clinical Orthopaedic Society. Clin Orthop 1977; 123: 177.

68 Bonucci E. New knowledge of the origin, function, and fate of osteoclasts. In: Proceedings of the Clinical Orthopaedic Society. Clin Orthop 1981; 158: 252.

69 Thompson ER, Baylink DJ, Wergedal JE. Increases in number and size of osteoclasts in response to calcium or phosphorus deficiency in the rat. Endocrinology 1975; 97: 283.

70 Tieder M, Modal D, Samuel R et al. Hereditary hypophosphatemic rickets with hypercalciuria. N Engl J Med 1985; 312: 611.

71 Camero DG, Warner HA, Szabo AJ. Chronic diarrhea in an adult with hypokalemic nephropathy and osteomalacia due to a function ganglioneuroblastoma. Am J Med Sci 1967; 253: 417.

72 Lewis JH. Clement S. Zollinger-Ellison syndrome presenting with osteomalacia. Va Med 1981; 108: 619.

73 Palmucci L, Bertolotto A, Doriguzzi C, Mongini T, Coda R. Osteomalacia myopathy in a case of diffuse nodular lipomatosis of the small bowel. Acta Neurol Belg 1982; 82: 65.

74 Naide W, Matz R, Spear PW. Cholangiocarcinoma causing hypercalcemia and hypophosphatemia without skeletal metastases (pseudo-hyperparathyroidism). Am J Dig Dis 1968; 13: 705.

75 Goldman JW, Becker FO. Ectopic parathyroid hormone syndrome: occurrence in a case of undifferentiated lymphoma with bone marrow involvement. Arch Intern Med 1978; 138: 1290.

76 Hirano T, Tsuchiyama H, Yanagawa M. An autopsy case of cholangiocarcinoma with hypercalcemia. Acta Pathol Jpn 1978; 28: 465.

77 Sztern M, Barkan A, Rakowsky E, Shainkin-Kestenbaum R, Raphael M, Blum I. Hypercalcemia in carcinoma of the breast without evidence of bone destruction: beneficial effect of hormonal therapy. Cancer 1981; 48: 2383.

78 Zidar BL, Shadduck RK, Winkelstein A, Zeigler Z, Hawker CD. Acute myeloblastic leukemia and hypercalcemia: a case of probable ectopic parathyroid hormone production. N Engl J Med 1976; 295: 692.

79 Akerka D, Shoenfield Y, Santo M et al. Life threatening hypophosphatemia in a patient with acute myelogenous leukemia. Acute Haematol 1980; 64: 117.

80 Zamkoff KW, Kirshner JJ. Marked hypophosphatemia associated with acute myelomonocytic leukemia: indirect evidence of phosphorus uptake by leukemic cells. Arch Intern Med 1980; 140: 1523.

81 Matzner Y, Prococimer M, Polliack A, Rubinger D, Popovtzer M. Hypophophatemia in a patient with lymphoma in leukemic phase. Arch Intern Med 1981; 141: 805.

82 Sariban E, Magrath IT. Hypophosphatemia in Burkett's Lymphoma. Arch Intern Med 1981; 142: 418.

83 Weiss D, Bar RS, Weidner N. Oncogenic osteomalacia. Ann Intern Med 1985; 102: 557.

Chapter **49**

Merkel Cell Tumours

J. Mackintosh*, E.J. Wills† and
M. Friedlander

*Departments of *Clinical Oncology* and †*Anatomical
Pathology, Royal Prince Alfred Hospital, Missenden Road,
Camperdown, New South Wales, Australia*

INTRODUCTION

Trabecular (Merkel cell) carcinoma of the skin is a rare malignant tumour that was first described in 1972 by Toker (1) and has subsequently become more commonly recognized as a distinct clinicopathological entity as evidenced by the increased frequency of case reports in the literature. These tumours are located in the dermis and immediate subcutaneous tissue and are commonly misinterpreted as being cutaneous metastases from small cell carcinoma of the lung or as being primary cutaneous neoplasms such as amelanotic melanoma or sweat gland carcinoma. Although early reports indicated that these tumours were associated with a relatively good prognosis it has become recognized more recently that they often pursue an aggressive clinical course with a considerable proportion of patients dying from widespread metastases.

Toker (1) originally proposed that these tumours arose from immature cells in the dermis or subcutis which were capable of giving rise to primitive sudoriferous structures. Subsequently, however, a primary neural crest origin appeared more probable in view of the characteristic electron microscopic findings of membrane bound neurosecretory granules within the cytoplasm (2) and the Merkel cell

was suggested as the likely cell of origin. Merkel, in 1876 (3), described a distinctive cell in the basal epidermis closely associated with nerve processes and considered to be a special sensory cell of the skin. Trabecular carcinoma was thought, therefore, on the basis of its ultrastructure, to represent malignant transformation of the Merkel cells and hence the name Merkel cell carcinoma. There is still considerable difference of opinion regarding the histogenesis of this neoplasm and the entity has been described under a variety of names including trabecular carcinoma, Merkel cell carcinoma, primary neuroendocrine carcinoma of the skin, primary small cell carcinoma of the skin, cutaneous apudoma and primary endocrine carcinoma of the skin. Objections can be raised to each of these terms but Merkel cell carcinoma appears to have found the most widespread acceptance and will be the preferred term used throughout this review.

HISTOGENESIS AND AETIOLOGY

In his original description of the entity of trabecular carcinoma of the skin, Toker (1) considered that the primary dermal location indicated likely derivation from primitive sudoriferous elements within the dermis. However, a primary endocrine derivation was also postulated because of the trabecular pattern of the tumours. The acceptance of this new entity as a distinct primary cutaneous neoplasm was delayed partly because light microscopy and histochemistry could not establish the cell of origin. With the ultrastructural identification of cytoplasmic neurosecretory granules within tumour cells in 1978 (2), the relationship to Merkel cells was postulated. The latter is one of three non-keratinocytic or branched cells in the epidermis (4) and is found in all mammals. It is the only cell in the skin known to contain neurosecretory granules and it has therefore been considered part of the APUD system (5, 6). Like Merkel cell tumours, the normal Merkel cell stains uniformly with neurone specific enolase (NSE) and as well cytoplasmic granules, spikes or filament-rich cytoplasmic processes are evident on electron microscopy. It is postulated that the Merkel cell originates in neural crest tissue and subsequently migrates to the dermal mesenchyme and epidermis in close relationship with nerve ending. More recently Merkel cells have been reported in the outer follicle of human hair (7) which may account for the location of Merkel cell tumours in the upper dermis.

Despite the close relationship with nerve processes the Merkel cell granules have never been shown to contain a specific neurotransmitter substance. Immunochemical stains for serotonin, calcitonin and adrenocorticotrophin are usually negative and biogenic amines have not yet been demonstrated within the granules of the tumour cells (8). This has led some investigators to postulate a trophic relationship between it and the neurite, rather than it being the effector cell (9). Kroll and Toker (10), on the other hand, suggest that these tumours may arise from primitive cells capable of both endocrine and exocrine differentiation rather than from Merkel cells, considering the neurosecretory granules to represent a line of differentiation rather than being indicative of the parent cell. Certainly, Merkel cell tumours appear to be no different from many others in their ability to undergo multi-

directional differentiation; instances have been reported, for example, of inappropriate peptide hormone and melanosome formation within the same tumour (11), whilst the simultaneous expression of cytokeratins with neuropeptide and other neuroendocrine markers is becoming increasingly recognized (12). Wick et al. (13) and Sidhu (14) endorse the concept of the Merkel cell tumour as a neuroendocrine neoplasm, but suggest an endodermal histogenesis to be more likely on the basis of the consistent ultrastructural finding of perinuclear filament whorls and occasional desmosomes. The coexistence of non-neuroendocrine components in some tumours (e.g. squamous differentiation) has also been considered to support the concept of an endodermal origin (15).

Merkel cell tumours occur predominantly on the head and neck or extremities whereas Merkel cells predominate in the skin of the neck and abdomen. This predilection of Merkel cell tumours for sun-exposed areas in elderly people suggests an aetiological role for ultra-violet light, similar to other primary cutaneous tumours (13). If this association is real, then fair-skinned people might be expected to be at increased risk, but as yet this association has not been reported.

PATHOLOGY

Macroscopically these dermal tumours have a fairly uniform appearance. Most usually measure less than 3.5 cm in greatest diameter at presentation, have a raised nodular shape and a firm to hard consistency. Compression of the overlying epidermis and subsequent ulceration may be evident. The cut surface is homogeneous grey-white or red-pink, with occasional small haemorrhagic foci, and may reveal infiltration into subcutaneous fat or underlying muscle fascia.

Light Microscopy

The original description by Toker (1) was of anastomosing trabeculae of cells with focal rosette-like arrangements occupying the entire thickness of the dermis and the immediate subcutis. However, a predominant trabecular growth pattern was present in only 35% of cases in a recently reported large series (16) and it is more usual to find interconnecting solid groups of cells partly demarcated by slender sheets of connective tissue or a mixed arrangement (17). There may be a prominent inflammatory cell infiltrate with lymphocytes and plasma cells at the periphery. Whilst epidermal compression is common macroscopically only a small minority of tumours (<5%) have histological evidence of epidermal invasion. Many tumours, however, show a high rate of blood vessel and lymphatic invasion at their periphery.

One of the most striking features of these tumours is their marked cellularity, with cellular crowding accentuated by the paucity of cytoplasm. Loss of cell cohesion, with formation of a lymphoma-like pattern also occurs. The tumour cells are generally round or oval and of uniform size within a particular tumour, but elongated cells, indistinguishable from oat cell carcinoma and larger pleomorphic forms may also occasionally occur. Gould et al. (18) have described three distinct morphological variants of trabecular, intermediate cell and small cell type which as discussed later were associated with differences in clinical behaviour. Others have also stressed the prognostic importance of a small cell variant (15).

The round or oval, occasionally indented, nuclei with delicate nuclear membranes are generally larger than those of normal lymphoid cells and contain finely dispersed, stippled chromatin and small, often inconspicuous nucleoli. The cytoplasm is typically scanty, acidophilic to amphophilic, and granular. Frequent mitoses and apoptotic bodies are seen. Rosette-like circular formations may also occur, as well as moulding (17); a striking 'ball in mitt' appearance (19) produced by a crescentic tumour cell closely wrapped around an oval cell and resembling a small epithelial pearl is common; this latter feature may prove very useful diagnostically.

Immunohistochemistry

NSE, which is present in normal Merkel cells (20), is the most consistent immunohistochemical marker for Merkel cell carcinoma (19, 21). Staining for the immunoreactive peptides commonly found in neuroendocrine tumours is negative in most instances (13), but occasional positivity for somatostatin, ACTH, calcitonin, insulin, met-encephalin and vasoactive intestinal peptide has been reported (11, 19).

Immunohistochemical staining for cytokeratin has also been demonstrated (12, 16, 17, 19, 21, 22) with positivity in as many as 96% (16) and 77% (21) of tumours being reported. Although keratin is also found in carcinoid and oat cell tumours as well as many undifferentiated carcinomas, a 'ball-like' immunostaining pattern resembling an inclusion body is seen only in Merkel cell tumours and some carcinoid tumours (16). This characteristic juxtanuclear globule is thought to correspond to the intermediate perinuclear filaments apparent on electron microscopy (see below).

Immunostaining with antibodies to neurofilaments may show a continuous rim around nuclei or a globular inclusion-like pattern (21–23). Recently immunostaining using a monoclonal antibody to chromogranin, the carrier protein from neurosecretory granules, has been reported (16). Six of 21 Merkel cell tumours and all of the carcinoid tumours studied stained positively.

Electron Microscopy

The characteristic ultrastructural feature of Merkel cell tumours is the presence of membrane bound (Figures 1 and 2) (2, 15, 19, 24–26), dense core neurosecretory type granules, 80–200 nm in diameter. The granules tend to be concentrated in cell processes or arranged in linear fashion at the periphery of the cell beneath the plasma membrane (13, 18, 25), but at times may be scanty and difficult to identify. Free ribosomes and polyribosomes are abundant and the Golgi zone may be prominent, but rough surfaced endoplasmic reticu-

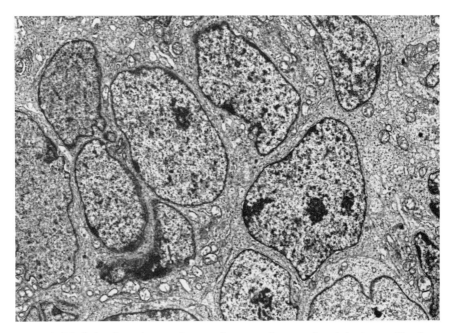

Figure 1 Merkel cell carcinoma. Survey electron micrograph, original magnification: ×6000.

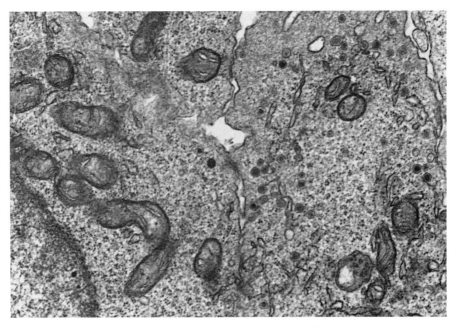

Figure 2 Electron micrograph showing cell details, including dense core granules. Original magnification: ×28 000.

lum and other cytoplasmic organelles are typically sparse. Paranuclear whorls of 10 nm intermediate filaments are often present (13, 18, 19, 25, 26), but not tonofilaments. The presence of spinous projections or microvilli containing microfilaments and secretory granules are also distinctive (17).

Nuclei vary in shape from round to oval to indented and contain evenly dispersed chromatin and one or two small nucleoli. Rodlet-type intranuclear inclusions may occur. Tumour cells often lack cohesion but may be connected by primitive intercellular junctions and a rare desmosome. An ill defined discontinuous external lamina may be present around cell clusters.

CLINICAL FEATURES AND DIFFERENTIAL DIAGNOSIS

In Toker's original description, Merkel cell tumours were misinterpreted as being cutaneous metastases from visceral malignancies in 3 of the 5 cases. The most important aspect for clinician and pathologist alike is familiarity with this unique skin tumour and its inclusion in the differential diagnosis of primary cutaneous and lymph node malignancies.

The tumour was initially described in 5 elderly patients and since then over 200 cases have been reported in the literature, mostly in patients over 60 years of age (2, 10, 13, 15, 17, 26–30). The mean age varies between 65 and 70 years with a range of 15–92 years. There is a slight predominance of females affected with a female to male ratio of 1.3 to 1. The duration of symptoms prior to presentation varies from 1 month to 2 years or longer. Most patients present with painless, non-tender, firm subcutaneous nodules. Occasionally patients have flat pigmented lesions or exuberant ulcerated lesions which may bleed. Almost half of these dermal lesions are between 1.5 and 2 cm in maximum diameter at presentation and only rarely measure greater than 4 cm. The nodules occur mainly on the head and neck (45–50%), upper (10–20%) and lower (20–30%) extre-

mities and buttocks (5–10%). Primary involvement of the trunk is very uncommon.

The location of primary lesions on predominantly sun-exposed areas of the body suggests that solar damage may be an aetiological factor and squamous cell carcinomas and other evidence of solar skin damage have been described in association with Merkel cell carcinomas (13). Silva et al. (17) found that in 21% of their 67 patients a squamous carcinoma had either been resected earlier from the skin of the same anatomical area or that the two tumours coexisted.

Initial reports (1, 2, 12) suggested that Merkel cell tumours had an indolent clinical course with a low incidence of tumour-related deaths, but with prolonged follow-up and more frequent recognition of the entity, the high propensity for local recurrence and distant metastases has become appreciated (see Table 1). Despite wide local excision, regional lymph node recurrence or occasional 'in transit' cutaneous metastases occur in 40–60% of patients, usually within 2 years of primary diagnosis and about 25% of patients die from distant metastases involving liver, lungs, bone, brain or distant lymph nodes. Involvement of regional lymph nodes may be the first clinical manifestation of the tumour, either because the small primary has been clinically unrecognized or has been previously excised and misdiagnosed.

Clinically, Merkel cell tumours may resemble primary cutaneous neoplasms such as basal and squamous cell carcinomas, amelanotic melanoma or adnexal carcinomas such as primary sweat or sebaceous gland carcinoma and primary cutaneous lymphoma. Metastatic carcinoma, although uncommon, also characteristically presents as painless nodules located within the dermis and subcutaneous tissue with an intact epidermis. These occur in less than 5% of visceral malignancies (33), most commonly with breast, gastrointestinal, lung or renal primaries. They will usually be easily distinguished from Merkel cell tumours by light microscopy, although difficulty may arise especially with metastatic small cell carci-

TABLE 1 CHARACTERISTICS OF PATIENTS WITH MERKEL CELL
CARCINOMA ACCORDING TO SITE OF PRIMARY TUMOUR

Site	% patients	Mean age (years)	% with local recurrence	% with regional disease	% with distant metastases
Head and neck	44	70	34	40	29
Leg	28	68	45	64	27
Arm	16	64	38	46	23
Buttock	9	59	14	71	43
Hand	2	75	50	100	0
Foot	1	71	0	100	0
Total	100	68	36	53	28

From Warner et al. (25).

noma. One practical clinical point which may be useful is the tendency for cutaneous metastases to occur in the region of the primary growth; hence lung cancers tend to metastasize to the skin of the anterior chest wall, back or upper extremities. Patients with cutaneous metastases from visceral malignancies generally have a poor prognosis with a mean survival of 3 months from their development (33).

Several neoplasms may appear similar by light microscopy and will need consideration in the differential diagnosis. These include primary malignant lymphoma of the skin (exclusive of mycosis fungoides), metastatic carcinoid tumours, metastatic small cell carcinoma of pulmonary or extrapulmonary origin, metastatic neuroblastoma and other metastatic neuroendocrine tumours (e.g islet cell carcinoma). A careful history for the presence of constitutional or 'B' symptoms (suggestive of lymphoma), cough, haemoptysis, dyspnoea and history of cigarette smoking (suggestive of small cell carcinoma of the lung), or features of carcinoid syndrome should be elicited. Clinical examination should be thorough especially looking for evidence of localized or generalized lymphadenopathy, other cutaneous nodules, hepatomegaly, finger clubbing or features of bronchial obstruction.

With respect to primary cutaneous lymphomas it should be realized that these are rare and most patients with cutaneous involvement

have generalized disease; hence the importance of thorough clinical examination. A point of similarity between primary cutaneous lymphomas and Merkel cell tumours is the high incidence of head and neck presentations for both. If there is regional lymph node involvement the distinction becomes even more difficult. Accurate diagnosis is essential as these malignancies require completely different treatment approaches. Histologically, a diffuse pattern of tumour cells with scanty cytoplasm and vesicular nuclei may simulate diffuse histiocytic lymphoma, the most common histological subgroup of primary cutaneous lymphomas. Ultrastructural features of neurosecretory granules and intercellular junctions together with histochemical staining for NSE in Merkel cell tumours and their absence in lymphomas are the most important differentiating features. In addition, cutaneous lymphomas will be commonly positive for leucocyte common antigen (LCA) and negative for chromagranin, neurofilaments and cytokeratin.

Metastatic carcinoid or other apudomas frequently form trabecular structures and contain numerous membrane bound secretory granules, but their morphological distinction from Merkel cell tumours should seldom cause problems. NSE may be positive in all these tumours. Careful clinical evaluation, including the search for an underlying endocrinopathy or typical carcinoid syndrome features, is essential. Although Merkel cell tumours may derive from APUD related cells, patients with coexistent clinical endocrinopathies have not been reported.

There are no reliable morphological criteria that allow distinction between Merkel cell carcinoma and metastatic small cell carcinoma of the lung (17). It remains to be seen whether immunohistochemistry (in particular for cytokeratins) will prove diagnostic. In addition, in recent years primary extrapulmonary small cell carcinomas have become well recognized and increasingly reported (34) from sites that include the oesophagus, stomach, pancreas, bowel, cervix, endometrium, breast, prostate and bladder. The biological behaviour of these tumours is not as well characterized as that of pulmonary small cell carcinoma but, with few exceptions, they do appear to share many of its features such as rapid growth, early dissemination and ectopic hormone production (34). Cutaneous metastases from any of these primary sites is possible and may make differentiation from Merkel cell tumours difficult.

Immunocytochemical staining is also of value in excluding some of the other morphologically similar tumours which may come into the differential diagnosis. For example, malignant melanoma is commonly S-100 positive and negative for neurofilaments, chromogranin and keratin, while the S-100 protein is consistently absent in Merkel cell carcinomas. NSE is not found in primary sweat gland cancer or in cutaneous metastases from anaplastic visceral malignancies. Metastatic neuroblastoma, although frequently NSE and neurofilament positive, will be cytokeratin negative.

INVESTIGATION AND STAGING

The histological features of Merkel cell tumours are often quite striking and familiarity with the entity should ensure a correct diagnosis in the majority of cases. A worthwhile policy, especially in difficult cases, may be to perform NSE histochemical staining on all suspicious skin lesions. Electron microscopy is useful for confirmation of suspected cases as well as providing an additional form of investigation of histologically undifferentiated tumours. We have also applied electron microscopy to fine needle aspirates from suspicious cases.

Once a definitive diagnosis has been made, examination for evidence of regional or distant lymph node involvement or visceral metastases should be undertaken. Careful clinical examination is also necessary to exclude cutaneous metastases from an underlying pulmonary or extrapulmonary small cell carcinoma, the most difficult pathological differential diagnosis. Staging investigations should therefore include chest X-ray, liver function tests and lymphangiography, as well as appropriate imaging of suspicious sites. Although still undergoing investigation, measurement of serum NSE levels may also be of value in staging patients. While a negative result does not necessarily indicate that the patient has no metastatic disease in our limited experience, an elevated level is highly suggestive of residual or metastatic tumour.

Recently ^{131}I-*meta*-iodobenzylguanidine (MIBG) scintigraphy has been used in the localization of a wide range of neuroendocrine tumours. MIBG is concentrated in intracellular storage vesicles by an active process and its structure confers resistance for catechol-*o*-methyltransferase (COMT) and monoamine oxidase (MAO). It was first used in the localization of phaeochromocytomas and appears to be more sensitive in demonstrating metastasis or recurrences than other imaging or biochemical tests in this tumour (35). Positive MIBG scans have also been demonstrated in carcinoid tumours, paragangliomas, medullary carcinomas of the thyroid, chemodectomas and Merkel cell tumours (36). In Merkel cell tumours MIBG scintigraphy is likely to be most useful in defining the extent and location of locoregional or metastatic disease and hence indicating therapeutic potential.

PROGNOSIS AND TREATMENT

Early descriptions of Merkel cell carcinoma highlighted the lack of specific morphological features which might predict the future clinical course. Indeed, several reports commented upon the presence (in what at that time was considered to be an indolent tumour) of malignant characteristics such as frequent mitoses, tumour cell necrosis and invasion of surrounding tissues. Gould et al. (18) have linked three distinctive morphological subsets with corresponding differences in clinical behaviour. The trabecular type was the least frequent, occurring almost exclusively on the face of elderly patients; it seemed less aggressive than the intermediate and small cell types, in which locoregional and systemic recurrences were very common. The small cell type occurred in a slightly younger patient group and often involved the extremities. The small cell variant was also found to be associated with an aggressive behaviour by Tang and co-workers (15). Others (13) addressing the same issue have failed to show a relationship between tumour differentiation and metastatic potential. Leong et al. (19) noted a high incidence of lymphatic and vascular invasion in their series and considered this an indicator of the underlying aggressive nature of this neoplasm. However, in practice it remains difficult to predict the outcome of these tumours on histological grounds. The number of dense core granules evident on electron microscopy appears to have no bearing on behaviour and it remains to be seen whether numerous desmosomes are related to a better prognosis, as has been claimed for small cell carcinoma of the lung. The anatomical site and tumour size do not influence clinical behaviour.

The early report of Tang et al. (15), suggested that Merkell cell tumours were slow growing and had a low malignant potential, as there was only one tumour related death in their 17 patients (6%). Similarly Warner et al. (25) reported 6 deaths (12%) within 3 years of diagnosis in their series of 52 patients. Two recent literature reviews (24, 27), however,

indicate a more aggressive clinical course than was previously considered, with distant metastases and death from metastatic tumour occurring in 25–35% of patients. The local recurrence rate is between 30 and 40% and regional lymph node metastases occur in over 50% of cases. These statistics indicate that the initial reports suggesting an indolent clinical course were misleading and that a reappraisal of primary therapy is warranted.

The early recommendations for treatment were surgical excision of the primary lesion with adequate resection margins, though precise details were not specified (10, 15). Given the high rates of local and regional node recurrence now recorded, with more than half the patients eventually developing regional disease, Raaf et al. (27) have recently advocated wide excision of the primary site (as for primary malignant melanoma) and prophylactic regional lymph node dissection. However, to date, in the absence of controlled clinical trials, it is not known whether such measures prolong survival. Another approach, again employed in malignant melanoma, is wide local excision and in-continuity radical regional node dissection. Obviously careful and long-term postoperative follow-up is mandatory.

It should be remembered that most patients will be over 60 years of age at the time of diagnosis and their general health and coexistent medical illnesses will determine the appropriateness and degree of aggressive primary therapy. As for malignant melanoma, the regional node drainage of the primary lesion, particularly those near the mid-line, may be uncertain. Lymphangiography or lymphoscintigraphy may be useful in this situation.

However, the roles of adjuvant postoperative radiotherapy or chemotherapy have not been tested in a controlled trial given the relative rarity of these tumours. The apparent sensitivity of metastatic deposits to these modalities, the high incidence of locoregional recurrence and the possibility that one-third of patients have occult metastases at the time of diagnosis, suggest that future studies should include both these approaches. After the primary tumour has been resected a number of investigators (17) recommend routine radiotherapy in view of the fact that Merkel cell tumours frequently occur in the head and neck area where wide excision is not always possible and because the tumours frequently have an infiltrating margin. Analysis of failures in patients treated with radiation therapy indicate that no therapy failures were observed within the treatment portals when the dose was at least 4500 rads over 5 weeks (17). All failures of radiation therapy, in one series (17), were geographic misses due to inadequate field margins and this suggests that radiation ports should be very wide to cover not only the areas of original disease, but also to include the operative bed.

Some patients will present with clinical regional lymph node involvement only. The risk of distant metastases is high in this setting and thorough clinical work up including chest x-ray, liver function tests and organ imaging of suspicious areas is mandatory. If distant metastases are not identified an aggressive therapeutic approach is recommended with wide excision of the primary lesion, radical regional node dissection and postoperative radiotherapy, if the patient's general health permits. Prolonged disease-free survival has been achieved with this approach. Once again the precise role of adjuvant chemotherapy is unknown but it may be indicated particularly in a young patient with histological features suggestive of a high malignant potential.

For metastatic disease, both radiotherapy and chemotherapy have demonstrated efficacy though complete responses and prolonged disease-free survival are rare. Irradiation, and occasionally surgical excision of localized metastatic deposits, can provide significant palliative benefit but chemotherapy is necessary for widespread metastases. In the first 30 patients reported by Kroll and Toker (10), 4 of 6 with distant metastases received chemotherapy. They described initial rapid regression with chemotherapy followed by recurrence within 6 to 12 months in all cases.

Experience with chemotherapy in Merkel cell tumours is very limited and the available data do not allow one to make conclusions about the optimum therapy. The majority of patients have been treated with combinations of drugs similar to those used in small cell carcinoma of the lung or apudomas, as there is some histological and clinical overlap between these tumours and Merkel cell tumours. There are a number of active single agents in apudomas and these include cyclophosphamide, 5-fluorouracil, streptozotocin, Adriamycin, vincristine and methotrexate. Combination chemotherapy appears to be associated with a higher response rate than that achieved with single agents. Moertel (37) reported a very high response rate with a combination of 5-fluorouracil and streptozotocin in advanced islet cell carcinomas that was superior to that achieved with streptozotocin alone. Mengel and Schaffer (38) have reported a 55% response rate with a combination of cyclophosphamide and methotrexate in 41 patients with carcinoid tumours, which is higher than the 25% response rate achieved with cyclophosphamide alone. More recently a 42% response rate has been reported using Adriamycin and cisplatin in patients with advanced apudomas (39). There is obviously a wealth of information on the chemotherapy of small cell lung cancer, but surprisingly very little reported data on the chemosensitivity of extrapulmonary small cell carcinoma. Levensen et al. (40) described 3 responders of 6 evaluable patients using a pulmonary small cell carcinoma regimen, i.e. cyclophosphamide, methotrexate, CCNU alternating with vincristine, Adriamycin and procarbazine. Other than this only isolated cases have been reported.

Merkel cell tumours have been treated with a variety of chemotherapy regimens and for the most part combinations have been used. Apart from the suggestion in one study that Adriamycin and streptozotocin in combination was more effective than 5-fluorouracil alone (27) there are little data to support the superiority of combination chemotherapy over single agents in terms of overall survival. Feun et al.

(41) reported 12 responses, including 3 complete responses, in 13 patients with metastatic disease treated with various chemotherapy regimens. Two patients with regional nodal metastases had a complete response and were alive and free of disease at 4 and 10 years respectively. The duration of response in their series ranged from 2 months to 10 years with a median of 6 months. Silva et al. (17) are currently evaluating the combination of cyclophosphamide, vincristine, doxorubicin and imidazole carboxamide, a combination that has demonstrated efficacy in small cell lung cancer, adult neuroblastoma and in the small number of patients with Merkel cell tumours treated to date. Sibley et al. (26) have obtained good, albeit transient, responses with a combination of cyclophosphamide, Adriamycin, vincristine, prednisone and bleomycin. Our group in collaboration with others is investigating the role of VP16, vincristine, cyclophosphamide and Adriamycin in extrapulmonary small cell cancers as well as Merkel cell cancers. Preliminary results, in the few patients treated to date, indicate that this is an active combination in these tumour types.

A new approach to treatment of Merkel cell tumours is the possible therapeutic role of ^{131}I-MIBG which, as described earlier, is selectively taken up by neuroendocrine tumours (36). Doses of up to 500 mCi (compared with the 0.5 mCi used for scanning purposes) are cytotoxic and have been used therapeutically in patients with metastatic phaeochromocytoma. The dose-limiting factor is bone marrow toxicity, particularly at doses greater than 500 mCi.

The available data therefore suggest that metastatic Merkel cell tumours are often chemosensitive and long-term surival may be achieved. However, as is the case with aggressive local surgery for the primary lesion, toxicity of aggressive combination chemotherapy must be carefully considered in these older patients. While the rarity of these neoplasms precludes randomized controlled trials a strong case can be made for patients to be registered in a rare tumour registry, and treated according to a common treatment plan

which may allow some conclusions to be made in the future regarding the optimum treatment of patients with these neoplasms.

REFERENCES

1 Toker C. Trabecular carcinoma of the skin. Arch Dermatol 1972; 105: 107–10.
2 Tang CK, Toker C. Trabecular carcinoma of the skin. An ultrastructural study. Cancer, 1978; 42: 2311–21.
3 Merkel, F. Tastzellen und Tastkörperchen bei den Hausthieren und beim Memschen. Arch Mikrosk Anat 1876; 11: 636–52.
4 Breathnach AS. Branched cells in the epidermis: An overview. J Invest. Dermatol 1980; 75: 6–11.
5 Winkelmann RK. The Merkel cell system and a comparison between it and the neurosecretory or APUD cell system. J Invest Dermatol 1977; 69: 41–6.
6 Winkelmann RK, Breathnach AS. The Merkel cell. J Invest Dermatol 1973; 60: 12–15.
7 Santa Cruz DJ, Bauer EA. Merkel cells in the outer follicular sheath. Ultrastruct Pathol 1982; 3: 59–63.
8 Hartschuh W, Grube D. The Merkel cell: A member of the APUD system? Arch Dermatol Res, 1979; 265: 115–22.
9 English KB. The ultrastructure of cutaneous type I mechanoreceptors in cats following denervation. J Comp Neurol 1977; 172: 137–64.
10 Kroll MH, Toker C. Trabecular carcinoma of the skin: Further clinicopathologic and morphologic study. Arch Pathol Lab Med 1982; 106: 404–8.
11 Gould VE, Memoli VA, Dardi LE, Sobel HJ, Somers SC, Johannessen JV. Neuroendocrine carcinomas with multiple immunoreactive peptides and melanin production. Ultrastruct Pathol 1981; 2: 199–217.
12 Green WR, Linnoila R, Triche TJ. Neuroendocrine carcinoma of skin with simultaneous cytokeratin expression. Ultrastruct Pathol 1984; 6: 141–52.
13 Wick MR, Goellner JR, Scheithauer BW et al. Primary neuroendocrine carcinomas of the skin (Merkel cell tumours): A clinical, histologic, and ultrastructural study of thirteen cases. Am J Clin Pathol 1983; 79: 6–13.
14 Sidhu GS. The endodermal origin of digestive and respiratory tract APUD cells: Histopathologic evidence and a review of the literature. Am J Pathol 1979; 96: 5–20.
15 Tang CK, Toker C, Nedwick A et al. Unusual cutaneous carcinoma with features of small cell (oat cell-like) and squamous cell carcinomas. Am J Dermatopathol 1982; 4: 537–48.

16 Battifora H, Silva EG. The use of antikeratin antibodies in the immunohistochemical distinction between neuroendocrine (Merkel cell) carcinoma of the skin, lymphoma and oat cell carcinoma. Cancer 1986; 58: 1040–6.

17 Silva EG, Mackay B, Goepfert H et al. Endocrine carcinoma of the skin (Merkel cell carcinoma). Pathol Annu 1984; 19 (Part 2): 1–30.

18 Gould VE, Moll R, Moll I et al. Neuroendocrine (Merkel) cells of the skin: Hyperplasias, dysplasias and neoplasms. Lab Invest 1985; 52: 334–53.

19 Leong ASY, Phillips GE, Pieterse AS, Milios J. Criteria for the diagnosis of primary endocrine carcinoma of the skin (Merkel cell carcinoma). A histological, immunohistochemical and ultrastructural study of 13 cases. Pathology 1986; 18: 393–9.

20 Gu J, Polak JM, Tapia FJ et al. Neuron-specific enolase in the Merkel cells of mammalian skin. Am J Pathol 1981; 104: 63–8.

21 Sibley RK, Dahl D. Primary neuroendocrine (Merkel cells?) carcinoma of the skin: II. An immunocytochemical study of 21 cases. Am J Surg Pathol 1985; 9: 109–16.

22 Gould VE, Lee I, Hammar SP. Neuroendocrine skin carcinoma coexpressing cytokeratin and neurofilament proteins. Ultrastruct Pathol 1985; 9: 83–90.

23 Miettinen M, Lehto VP, Virtanen I et al. Neuroendocrine carcinoma of the skin (Merkel cell carcinoma); ultrastructural and immunohistochemical demonstration of neurofilaments. Ultrastruct Pathol 1983; 4: 219–25.

24 Sibley RK, Dehner LP, Rosai J. Primary neuroendocrine (Merkel cell?) carcinoma of the skin. I. A clinical pathologic and ultrastructural study of 43 cases. Am J Surg Pathol 1985; 9: 95–108.

25 Warner TF, Uno H, Hafez GR et al. Merkel cells and Merkel cell tumours: ultrastructure, immunocytochemistry and review of the literature. Cancer 1983; 52: 238–45.

26 Sibley RK, Rosai JR, Foucar E et al. Neuroendocrine (Merkel cell) carcinoma of the skin. Am J Surg Pathol 1980; 4: 211–21.

27 Raaf JH, Urmacher C, Knapper WK et al. Trabecular (Merkel cell) carcinoma of the skin: Treatment of primary, recurrent and metastatic disease. Cancer 1986; 57: 178–82.

28 Abaci IF, Zak FG. Multicentric amyloid containing cutaneous trabecular carcinoma: Case report with ultrastructural study. J Cutan Pathol 1979; 6: 292–303.

29 De Wolf-Peeters G, Marien K, Mebis I, Desmet V. A cutaneous APUDoma or Merkel cell tumour? Cancer 1980; 46: 1810–16.

30 Sidhu GS, Feiner H, Flosse TJ et al. Merkel cell neoplasms: histology, electron microscopy, biology and histogenesis. Am J Dermatopathol 1980; 2: 101–19.

31 Pilotti S, Rilke F, Lombardi L. Neuroendocrine (Merkel cell) carcinoma of the skin. Am J Surg Pathol 1982; 6: 243–54.

32 Frigerio B, Capella C, Eusebi V et al. Merkel cell carcinoma of the skin: The structure and origin of normal Merkel cells. Histopathology 1983; 7: 229–49.

33 Reingold IM. Cutaneous metastases from internal carcinoma. Cancer 1966; 19: 162–8.

34 Ibrakim NB, Briggs JC, Corbishley CM. Extrapulmonary oat cell carcinoma. Cancer 1984; 54: 1645–61.

35 Beirwaltes WH, Sisson JC, Shapiro B et al. Malignant potential of pheochromocytoma: implications for follow-up. Abstract 131. J Nucl Med 1986; 27(6): 908.

36 Shapiro B, von Moll L, McEvan A et al. I-131-meta-iodobenzyl-guanidine (mIBG) uptake by a wide range of neuroendocrine tumours other than pheochromatocytoma and neuroblastoma. Abstract 131. J Nucl Med 1986; 27(6): 908.

37 Moertel CG. Clinical management of advanced gastrointestinal cancer. Cancer 1975; 36: 675–82.

38 Mengel CE, Schaffer RD. The carcinoid syndrome. In: Holland JF, Frei E III (eds) Cancer Medicine. Philadelphia: Lea and Febiger, 1973; 1584–94.

39 Sridhar KS, Holland JF, Brown JC et al. Doxorubicin plus cisplatin in the treatment of APUDomas. Cancer 1985; 55: 2634–7.

40 Levenson RM, Ihde DC, Matthews MJ et al. Small cell carcinoma presenting as an extrapulmonary neoplasm: sites of origin and response to chemotherapy. J Nat Cancer Inst 1981; 67(3): 607–12.

41 Feun LG, Savaraj N, Legtha S et al. Chemotherapy for metastatic Merkel cell carcinoma: Review of M.D. Anderson Hospital's experience. ASCO Proc 1986; Vol 5.

Section IX

Ophthalmic Tumours

Textbook of Uncommon Cancer
Edited by C.J. Williams, J.G. Krikorian, M.R. Green and D. Raghavan
© 1988 John Wiley & Sons Ltd

Chapter **50**

Uncommon Tumours of the Eyelids, Conjunctiva, and Orbit

John Hungerford

Consultant Ophthalmic Surgeon, St Bartholomew's Hospital, London; Consultant Surgeon, Moorfields Eye Hospital, London, UK

THE EYELID

Tumours may develop in the skin of the eyelid, in the glands it contains or in the conjunctiva with which its inner surface is lined. Frankly malignant primary tumours may appear de novo or may arise in a precancerous or in situ lesion. Less commonly a tumour may extend to the eyelid from the skin of the face or from adjacent structures including the eye, the orbit, and the paranasal sinuses. Occasionally, the eyelid may be the site of a metastatic tumour or may contain one or more deposits from a generalized malignant lymphoma or leukaemia.

Primary Cutaneous Tumours

Adenocarcinoma

Most adenocarcinomas of the eyelids are sebaceous carcinomas. The lids are a site of election for this uncommon tumour. Although second in frequency among malignant tumours of the eyelid after basal cell carcinoma (1), sebaceous carcinoma is far less common. The tumour arises in the meibomian glands of the tarsal plates, in the sebaceous-like glands of Zeis associated with eyelash follicles, or in the

sebaceous glands proper of the eyebrow hair follicles or of the caruncle (2).

The upper eyelid is more richly supplied with meibomian glands and the tumour is twice as common in this situation as in the lower eyelid (2). Mortality from sebaceous carcinoma is greater when the tumour occurs in the eyelid than when it develops elsewhere in the skin (3) and is second only to that of malignant melanoma of the eyelid (1). Metastases are frequent (3–6). Adenocarcinomas may also arise in Moll's glands. Like sebaceous carcinomas, these tumours may be highly malignant and incur a significant mortality (7).

The *clinical appearance* of a sebaceous carcinoma is of a yellowish tumour commonly arising at the lid margin (Figure 1), where it may be associated with loss of eyelashes and where it is all too often mistaken for a meibomian cyst or occasionally for a basal cell carcinoma. This tumour may also present with diffuse, pagetoid infiltration of the bulbar and palpebral conjunctiva and of the eyelid skin, simulating chronic conjunctivitis, blepharitis or keratitis (4). Sebaceous carcinoma of the eyelid may be multicentric (2, 8). Adenocarcinomas of Moll's glands tend to be firm and rubbery and such a tumour may also be

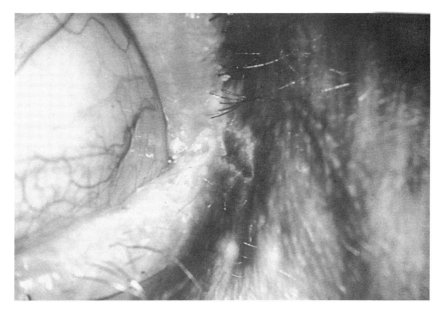

Figure 1 Sebaceous carcinoma arising in a meibomian gland at the outer canthus of the left eye.

mistaken for a meibomian cyst. A tissue *diagnosis* should be obtained as early as possible for these tumours, which tend to present late because of their tendency to masquerade as benign lesions. Sebaceous carcinoma is commonly moist and friable and the diagnosis is best achieved by a generous wedge biopsy to include all the layers of the eyelid. Tissue from a recurrent meibomian cyst should always be examined histologically. Sebaceous carcinoma is said to be more radioresistant than carcinomas of squamous cell origin. *Treatment* of all adenocarcinomas should be by wide excision where possible and should include all diffuse pagetoid spread in sebaceous carcinoma. In the presence of regional lymphadenopathy lymph node dissection should be considered. Where plastic reconstruction of the eyelid cannot be performed after adequate excision, or where the tumour invades deeper orbital structures, orbital exenteration should be considered. Radiotherapy may be offered for an unresectable tumour involving the only good eye, in the presence of metastatic disease, or when the patient refuses radical surgery.

Squamous Carcinoma

This tumour is surprisingly rare in the eyelid (9, 10). It must be distinguished from benign lesions including pseudoepitheliomatous hyperplasia, inverted follicular keratosis, seborrhoeic keratosis and keratoacanthoma, from carcinoma in situ, which is synonymous with intraepidermal carcinoma or Bowen's disease, and from the commonest of all eyelid tumours, basal cell carcinoma (11–13).

The *clinical appearance* is of an ulcer with a scaly, rolled edge and a central crater occurring most commonly on the lower lid and at the lid margin. The tumour is apt to develop from a pre-existing actinic keratosis in fair skinned individuals. A basal cell carcinoma has a much more pearly appearance and benign and premalignant simulating lesions rarely have a central ulcer crater. The *diagnosis* is preferably established by excisional biopsy but if the lesion is very large or involves more than a third of the upper eyelid incisional biopsy may be performed in the first instance. *Treatment* depends substantially on whether or not there is evidence of spread to regional lymph nodes. The preauricular and cervical glands should be examined carefully. In the absence of lymphadenopathy surgical excision of the tumour is to be preferred though radiotherapy is an alternative, particularly for very large or unfavourably situated tumours. If excision is chosen, a 4 mm margin of macroscopically healthy tissue is essential, even if a full thickness lid reconstruction is required (14). Block dissection of cervical glands can be combined with excision of the primary tumour when involved lymph nodes are mobile. More often than not an infiltrated preauricular node will be tethered in which case radiotherapy is the treatment of choice, both to the primary and the preauricular node, and to the cervical chain. Although these tumours do metastasize, death from an eyelid primary is very rare (15).

Malignant Melanoma

The occurrence of a primary malignant melanoma in the skin of the eyelid is exceedingly rare (9, 10, 16, 17). More common in this situation is an implanted deposit from a conjunctival malignant melanoma or from a distant cutaneous primary. Malignant melanoma in the eyelid may arise de novo or it may develop in a pre-existing naevus or an area of lentigo maligna and must be distinguished from these lesions. Occasionally, corresponding naevi are present at the lid margin on both the lower and the upper eyelid. These divided or 'kissing' naevi arise from one naevus by division of the eyelids during embryonic life (18). Oculodermal melanocytosis (naevus of Ota) occurs predominantly in individuals of Asian extraction. It may be distinguished from malignant melanoma by its characteristic slate grey appearance and by the extensive associated ocular involvement. Very rarely the eyelid element of this condition may undergo malignant change to melanoma (15). Another common simulating lesion is pigmented sebhorroeic keratosis, though this is much more uniformly pigmented and has a much more regular outline than an eyelid malignant melanoma. Nodular malignant melanomas of the eyelid skin have a worse prognosis than those of the superficial spreading type (17, 19) though the outlook for eyelid melanomas is generally better than for those of the skin elsewhere (17).

The *clinical appearance* is usually of a pigmented lesion, often with an irregular outline and sometimes associated with regional lymphadenopathy. As with skin melanoma elsewhere the degree of pigmentation may vary between lesions and from area to area within an individual tumour. The lesion may be raised or fairly flat. The *diagnosis* should be established by a wide excision which may also serve as the definitive *treatment* and may be followed by a plastic repair of the eyelid if necessary. Local recurrence after this approach is unlikely. Recurrent or very extensive melanomas may require orbital exenteration.

Malignant Lymphoma and Leukaemia

Although the eyelid may be the only site of involvement with these tumours they are commoner in the conjunctiva and in the orbit and will be discussed under these headings (below).

Secondary Cutaneous Tumours

The orbit and the eye are much commoner sites for metastatic tumours than the eyelids though occasional secondary deposits of tumours such as melanoma may be encountered in the lids.

THE CONJUNCTIVA

A tumour may arise at any site within the conjunctiva or in the adjacent caruncle. The outlook for any particular neoplasm may differ depending on whether the lesion is situated in the bulbar or tarsal conjunctiva, either of the two conjunctival fornices, the plica semilunaris, or the caruncle. As for eyelid tumours, conjunctival neoplasms may arise de novo or in a precancerous or in situ lesion. The conjunctiva may be invaded by an eyelid tumour.

Primary Conjunctival Tumours

Intraepithelial Squamous Carcinoma

This is a premalignant condition which may progress to invasive conjunctival carcinoma (20). Although commonly termed Bowen's disease of the conjunctiva, a parallel may be better drawn between Bowen's disease of the skin and the very earliest dysplastic changes in the conjunctiva in which the epithelial cells retain their polarity. Loss of polarity indicates a true in situ carcinoma.

The *clinical appearance* is variable. The very earliest changes may be difficult to detect in the conjunctiva but may be indicated by slight thickening, increased vascularization, and later, frank leucoplakia. The condition begins most commonly at the limbus in the conjunctiva exposed by the interpalpebral fissure. For this reason the early changes may be mistaken for a pinguecula and, as with this benign lesion, there may be a history of solar exposure. Intraepithelial carcinoma commonly spreads onto the cornea (Figure 2) where it presents a typical gelatinous appearance which facilitates

the clinical diagnosis. The *diagnosis* is usually made by excisional biopsy but may be suggested by the presence of atypical cells on exfoliative cytology. *Treatment* by wide excision may be considered but is commonly followed by recurrence. For a bulbar conjunctival lesion it is not necessary to excise the superficial fibres of the underlying sclera. It is difficult to delineate the true lateral extent of this diseases in the conjunctiva. Furthermore there may be multiple foci of dysplasia and it is likely that surgical failures result from incompletely excised and missed lesions. It is easier to determine the extent of the disease in the cornea but the friable character of the tumour makes complete excision difficult without resort to lamellar keratectomy. When the lesion involves the central cornea reduced vision from overgrowth of thickened conjunctiva will follow keratectomy if the excised tissue is not replaced by a lamellar graft. Sometimes this complication is encounted despite grafting. Recurrent lesions may be managed by further excision but previous surgical scars make it even more difficult to delineate the extent of abnormal conjunctiva. Intraepithe-

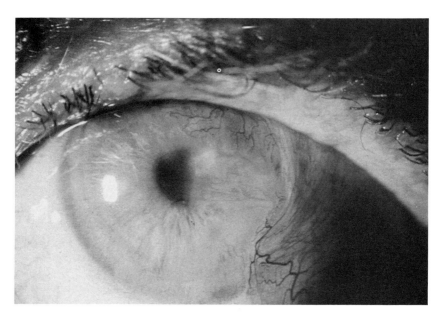

Figure 2 Intraepithelial squamous carcinoma of the conjunctiva spreading onto the cornea.

lial carcinoma is radiosensitive and its superficial distribution lends itself to the use of poorly penetrating beta rays. Eighteen to 27 Gy in two to three fractions over 7 to 10 days using a strontium-90 ophthalmic surface applicator has been found effective. The applicator should be large enough to encompass the whole lesion with a generous margin of apparently healthy tissue. Recurrences follow treatment by radiation for the same reasons as they follow treatment by surgical excision. Retinoic acid has been employed in drop form in an attempt to treat the whole conjunctiva and with encouraging results.

Invasive Squamous Carcinoma

Invasive squamous carcinoma may arise in and must be distinguished from a pre-existing in situ carcinoma of the conjunctiva (20).

The *clinical appearance* is of a pale, fleshy swelling which is seen most commonly in the interpalpebral fissure at the nasal or temporal limbus. The tumour commonly spreads across the cornea (Figure 3) and, if unchecked, may eventually protrude between the eyelids, infiltrate the sclera along blood vessels, and gain access to the orbit, eyelid, and regional lymph nodes. The tumour may be pigmented and, if so, must be distinguished from a conjunctival malignant melanoma. The *diagnosis* is best made by excision biopsy. The cornea and to a lesser extent the sclera seem resistant to invasion by conjunctival neoplasms and squamous carcinoma of the bulbar conjunctiva rarely invades the underlying scleral lamellae and very rarely the corneal lamellae (21). Tumours of the fornix or tarsal conjunctiva have easier access to deeper structures and a carcinoma may invade the orbit. If biopsy indicates complete excision, no further *treatment* will be required in the absence of regional lymphadenopathy. Incomplete excision will lead to failure of local control and may be managed by excision of residual tumour. Whilst lamellar sclerectomy or keratectomy is feasible for incompletely excised bulbar conjunctival lesions it is difficult for the surgeon to assess peroperatively the depth of penetration of the tumour. Superficial radiotherapy using surface applicators has been advocated in this situation (22) and some surgeons combine excision

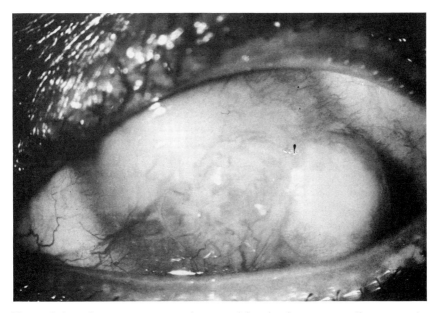

Figure 3 Invasive squamous carcinoma arising in the cornea adjacent to the corneoscleral limbus in an area of pre-existing intraepithelial carcinoma.

with cryotherapy (23). Occasionally, an aggressive tumour will be encountered which requires total excision of the conjunctiva (15). A free conjunctival graft from the patient's other eye or a mucous membrane graft will be required if a functioning eye is to be retained after this procedure. If a tumour resists all attempts at eye conservative local control, orbital radiotherapy may be considered. This will produce a dry, uncomfortable, blind eye and orbital exenteration is a practical and humane alternative in the absence of lymphadenopathy. Spread to regional lymph nodes is rare (20) but when it occurs probably results from access of tumour cells to lid lymphatics. Management is as for carcinoma of the eyelid. Death from squamous carcinoma of the conjunctiva is extremely uncommon. One death only was reported in each of two large series. One patient died from local invasion of the brain (20) and the other from metastases (21).

Precancerous Melanosis

This is a premalignant condition which may progress to intraepithelial melanoma and, in some 17% of cases (24), to invasive conjunctival malignant melanoma.

The *clinical appearance* is of flat, granular, brown pigmentation first noticed in adult life and commonly extending over many years to involve the entire conjunctiva. Precancerous melanosis is always unilateral. It must be distinguished from conjunctival involvement with ocular melanocytosis in which the pigmentation is subconjunctival and slate grey in colour, and from argyrosis resulting from exposure to silver salts. It is rare in heavily pigmented individuals and can be differentiated with relative ease from racial conjunctival pigmentation. The pigmentary changes may extend into the corneal epithelium and, not uncommonly, 'kiss lesions' are seen in which the condition involves both the bulbar conjunctiva and that area of tarsal conjunctiva in contact with it. A peculiar and notable feature of precancerous melanosis is a tendency for the degree of pigmentation to wax and

wane and for variation over time in the geographic location of the lesions within the conjunctiva.

The *diagnosis* is a clinical one and so long as there is nothing to suggest malignancy biopsy is not necessary. Progress of the disease may be documented photographically. Increased thickness, pigmentation, or vascularity of an affected area or areas is suggestive of malignant change and indicates biopsy, preferably of the excisional type, or exfoliative cytology. Malignant change commonly supervenes in several areas simultaneously and multiple biopsies are frequently necessary. Increased vascularity or pigmentation in the absence of increased thickness suggests change to an in situ or superficial spreading melanoma. *Treatment* of precancerous melanosis by excision of areas of visible pigmentary change is doomed to failure; the condition almost invariably reappears within months in some other location. The condition can even recur after an attempt at total excision of the conjunctiva. The place of selective destruction of potentially malignant pigment cells within the conjunctiva by cryotherapy or superficial beta ray therapy is not yet certain and for the time being management must be directed towards repeated observation with excision biopsy of any suspicious lesion.

Malignant Melanoma

Some 50–65% of conjunctival malignant melanomas arise in an area of precancerous melanosis or in a pre-existing naevus and the remainder arise de novo (25, 26).

The typical *clinical appearance* is of a raised, pigmented mass with prominent feeder vessels (Figure 4) situated anywhere within the conjunctiva. The tumour may be deeply pigmented, lightly pigmented or completely amelanotic and must be distinguished from a conjunctival naevus and from acquired melanosis. Rapid growth, fixation to the underlying sclera of tumours not involving the limbus, the presence of a prominent blood supply and the absence of a cystic component are strongly

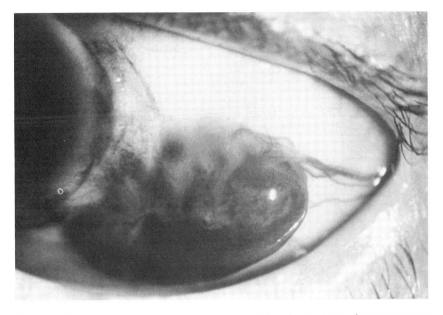

Figure 4 Conjunctival malignant melanoma arising in an area of precancerous melanosis.

suggestive of a melanoma. A lightly pigmented melanoma may simulate a squamous carcinoma and a non-pigmented tumour may be mistaken for a squamous carcinoma or lymphoma. The *diagnosis* is established by excision biopsy where possible. *Treatment* of conjunctival malignant melanoma as of melanoma elsewhere is aimed at complete and wide excision, though, if the eye is to be retained, the margin of healthy tissue cannot be nearly as generous as is considered suitable for cutaneous melanoma. The outlook depends on the location of the tumour within the conjunctiva, on the size of the lesion and in particular its thickness, and on whether or not a local cure can be obtained. These factors combine to dictate the treatment of choice. As with squamous carcinoma, the cornea and sclera appear to present a barrier to deep invasion of a melanoma of the bulbar conjunctiva; access to blood vessels and lymphatics is limited and the prognosis is correspondingly good. These tumours can be safely managed by eye conservative local excision. By contrast, melanoma in the fornix, the plica, the caruncle, and the

tarsal conjunctiva appears free to invade deeply with free access to blood vessels and lymphatics and, accordingly, a poor prognosis. It is difficult to assess depth of penetration of a tumour in one of these situations peroperatively and orbital exenteration is generally advocated. Radiotherapy has been advocated as an alternative to conservative local surgical excision (27) and is best confined to tumours involving only the bulbar conjunctiva. The survival rate is better for conjunctival melanomas as a whole than for skin melanomas and approaches 78% (26). The outlook is good for solitary tumours and for lesions involving the bulbar conjunctiva only. The prognosis is poor for tumours involving the fornix, caruncle, plica, or lid and for multiple tumours arising in precancerous melanosis.

Kaposi's Sarcoma

The cell of origin of this multifocal malignant vascular tumour is unknown. The neoplasm is most frequently encountered in skin but the conjunctiva and, very occasionally, the eyelid skin or lacrimal gland may be involved (28, 29). Kaposi's sarcoma is particularly common in Africa, where it may present in childhood. Until recently, among non-Africans, the tumour was usually seen in older adults but now affects all age groups as a concomitant of infection with HIV. Eventually, death may occur from visceral involvement or, in non-African patients, from lymphoma.

The *clinical appearance* is of redness and thickening, usually of the bulbar conjunctiva, and must be distinguished from pyogenic granuloma, angioma, lymphoma, and from a persistent subconjunctival haemorrhage (30). Except in African children, the ocular involvement is usually preceded by cutaneous lesions (30) and this may facilitate the *diagnosis* which may then be confirmed by incisional or excisional biopsy. Kaposi's sarcoma is radiosensitive and *treatment* of conjunctival tumours, of rare lesions of the eyelid skin or lacrimal gland, and of any spread to the anterior orbit, is by radiotherapy. Chemotherapy may be required for visceral involvement.

Lymphoma and Leukaemia

Conjunctival involvement in systemic lymphoma is uncommon and occurs in only 2% of cases (31). Much more frequently, the conjunctiva is an extranodal primary site for lymphoma where, like lymphoma arising in certain other extranodal sites such as oropharnx, gastrointestinal tract and bone, it carries a good prognosis (31–36), probably because these sites have their own population of lymphocytes and a tumour can develop in situ (37). Conjunctival deposits of leukaemia are much more frequent than those of systemic lymphoma.

The *clinical appearance* is of a pink conjunctival deposit and the *diagnosis* should be confirmed by incisional biopsy. A computed tomography (CT) scan should be performed to confirm that the tumour is localized and that the conjunctiva is not secondarily invaded by an orbital mass. When a lymphoma presents in the conjunctiva, systemic staging investigations should be performed to ensure that widespread disease is not present. A conjunctival deposit of leukaemia or one of lymphoma associated with a widespread tumour may respond to the systemic *treatment* indicated for the disease as a whole. Solitary deposits of lymphoma respond well to local radiotherapy.

Secondary Conjunctival Tumours

The conjunctiva is an extremely uncommon site for metastatic tumour though it may become involved by orbital metastases. Conjunctival invasion may occur from intraocular and orbital tumours and from tumours of the eyelids and paranasal sinuses.

THE ORBIT

A primary tumour may develop within the orbit or it may extend to the orbit from an origin in one of the paranasal sinuses, the postnasal space, the eyelid, or the eye. The orbit is a relatively common site for a metastatic tumour. Less commonly it may harbour a deposit from a generalized leukaemia or lymphoma and, occasionally, it appears to be the site of origin of an extranodal lymphoma. Many orbital tumours, although showing histological evidence of malignancy, have low potential for metastasis but may yet kill by aggressive and remorseless local infiltration.

Proptosis is the cardinal sign of a mass lesion within the orbit. Proptosis is said to be axial when the eye is displaced forwards but neither up or down, nor left or right. By far the commonest cause for axial proptosis is dysthyroid exophthalmos but, when a tumour is present, the neoplasm must be situated within the muscle cone. When the globe is displaced up or down, or left or right, as well as forwards, proptosis is said to be non-axial. A tumour is a common cause for non-axial proptosis and must be situated outside the muscle cone. By observing the direction in which the eye is displaced, it is generally quite easy to determine the position of the tumour within the orbit and, for a primary tumour, this in turn may indicate the structure from which the neoplasm is arising.

Orbital tumours, particularly those within the muscle cone, may be relatively inaccessible surgically. Although some may be excised via an anterior approach and with preservation of the globe with useful vision and good motility, others may require a lateral approach involving removal and replacement of the lateral wall of the orbit. Lateral orbitotomy is a much more difficult operation and there will be a significant ocular morbidity following removal of many of the posterior tumours dictating this approach. For locally invasive primary tumours, for recurrences, and for neoplasms extending to the orbit from the eye, it may be necessary to sacrifice the globe and to perform an orbital exenteration. For some tumours infiltrating bone and others extending into the orbit from surrounding structures including the paranasal sinuses, a joint approach with an ear, nose, and throat surgeon or neurosurgeon may be wise.

Primary Orbital Tumours

Malignant Vascular Tumours

Vascular malformations and benign vascular neoplasms are common causes of proptosis. They must be distinguished from malignant tumours of vascular tissue, which are much less common.

Malignant haemangioendothelioma. A tumour of vascular endothelial cells, this neoplasm, also described as angiosarcoma, is particularly uncommon (38). Malignant haemangioendothelioma may arise in the orbit de novo, may follow orbital irradiation of a benign haemangioendothelioma, or may spread to the orbit from a distant site (39). There have been reports of the tumour affecting children (40, 41). It is non-encapsulated and tends to infiltrate surrounding tissues. Local recurrence after conservative excision is frequent. Shedding of malignant endothelial cells into vascular lumina within the tumour

may explain an incidence of metastases of the order of 60% (42, 43). The cases on record are too few to describe a typical *clinical appearance.* The *diagnosis* is best made by an excisional biopsy if possible. Should local recurrence take place, *treatment* by a further local excision may be justified but the high degree of malignancy of this neoplasm suggests that orbital exenteration may be wiser.

Haemangiopericytoma. This is a relatively slow-growing malignant tumour of vascular pericytes which affects adults of all ages (44). The tumour tends to be encapsulated and may occur inside or outside the muscle cone. Local recurrence after conservative excision is uncommon unless the tumour capsule has been breached. Thereafter, the tumour can behave like a malignant haemangioendothelioma and kill by invasion of all local structures, including bone. Late recurrence is a feature of haemangiopericytoma and one tumour recurred in the orbit 18 years after primary surgery (44).

The *clinical appearance* is of slowly progressive axial, or non-axial proptosis over a period of up to 2 years. Radiological examination may assist in the *diagnosis* by revealing enlargement of the orbit without bone destruction (44). On B-scan ultrasound a haemangiopericytoma may appear partially cystic and be distinguished from fibrous histiocytoma which is acoustically solid (39). *Treatment* is by excision of the encapsulated tumour, if possible with a margin of healthy tissue, via an orbitotomy. Radiotherapy has not been shown to produce sustained local control (39) and recurrence should be managed by orbital exenteration.

Malignant Lymphoma

Abnormal accumulations of lymphocytic cells within the orbit are relatively common. Many masses of such cells are now classified as benign reactive lymphoid hyperplasia or 'pseudotumour' but there is no clear-cut dividing line between these and lymphomas. The orbit may be the presenting site of a generalized lymphoma or it may represent a primary site (45).

Any patient presenting with an orbital lymphoma should be staged to determine whether there is evidence of extraorbital tumour. These investigations may need to be repeated because half of all patients with no evidence of dissemination at the time of diagnosis of the orbital lesion develop widespread lymphoma within 5 years (45, 46). This may mean that the tumour has spread from the orbit but, more probably, it indicates that the presenting lesion was part of a systemic lymphoma which could not be demonstrated initially (47). Almost all lymphomas of the orbit are of B-cell origin; T-cell tumours are extremely rare at this site. As with lymphoma elsewhere, the prognosis is better for lower grade tumours, and a follicular pattern improves the outcome whatever the histology.

Lymphocytic lymphoma. This is the commonest orbital lymphoma in adults. Most patients with poorly differentiated lymphocytic lymphoma in the orbit have or subsequently develop systemic involvement. A few patients with well-differentiated lymphoma will develop widespread disease. It may be extremely difficult to distinguish histologically between well-differentiated lymphocytic lymphoma and benign reactive lymphoid hyperplasia, and in one series 10% of tumours classified benign ultimately became widespread (48). When widespread disease does follow a histological diagnosis of well-differentiated lymphoma or benign reactive lymphoid hyperplasia the systemic disease may be a chronic lymphatic leukaemia and run a relatively prolonged course (45).

Most orbital lymphomas present in the anterior orbit and the *clinical appearance* is of swelling of the eyelid with a rubbery, palpable lump rather than proptosis, or of a salmon-pink mass visible beneath the conjunctiva (Figure 5). On orbital CT the lesion may be shown to be more extensive than it looks. The history of the less malignant lesions may extend over months or years whereas that of the more malignant tumours tends to be measured in weeks or months. Absence of pain or of evidence of inflammation may help to distinguish lymphoma clinically from benign reactive lymphoid hyperplasia (45). A tissue *diagnosis* must be obtained by biopsy and this may be performed through the conjunctiva or orbital septum as appropriate (45). Systemic staging

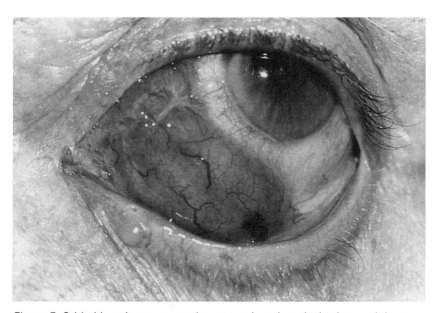

Figure 5 Orbital lymphoma presenting as a subconjunctival salmon-pink mass.

investigations are necessary in all except elderly patients in whom histology reveals a benign or well-differentiated tumour (45). *Treatment* of histologically malignant orbital lymphocytic tumours is by fractionated radiotherapy (49) to a tumour dose of 30 Gy in 3 weeks, and achieves a local control rate of virtually 100%, with little local morbidity (45) and a low recurrence rate. Patients with evidence of systemic lymphoma will require additional chemotherapy.

Histiocytic lymphoma. Ophthalmologists still call histiocytic lymphoma reticulum cell sarcoma and some ophthalmic pathologists defend the continued use of the term (37). This form of lymphoma is relatively uncommon in the orbit and is seen only in middle-aged and elderly people. It is always a manifestation of systemic 'histiocytic' lymphoma (37). Accordingly the prognosis is bad and many patients are dead within 2 years. The *clinical appearance* is notable for the relatively short history typical of more malignant lymphomas. The approach to the *diagnosis* is the same as for lymphocytic lymphoma and, histologically, it is important to distinguish 'histiocytic' lymphoma in the orbit from a deposit of acute lymphoblastic or granulocytic leukaemia. The *treatment* is as for lymphocytic lymphoma with orbital and systemic involvement.

Burkitt's lymphoma. This tumour affects predominantly young children in Africa (50). Burkitt's lymphoma commonly arises in the marrow of the maxillary bone and expands rapidly over a period of a few weeks to invade the orbit and occasionally the globe (37, 51, 52). Visceral involvement is common. The bone marrow and central nervous system may be involved and this worsens the prognosis.

The *clinical appearance* is of rapid painless proptosis and gross facial swelling. The appearances must be differentiated from those of orbit rhabdomyosarcoma, orbital extension of retinoblastoma, and from granulocytic sarcoma (chloroma) in acute myelogenous leukaemia. The *diagnosis* is made by incisional biopsy. *Treatment* of the maxillary and orbital element of the disease is by radiotherapy whilst visceral involvement will require systemic chemotherapy, and central nervous system involvement will require neuraxis radiotherapy together with intrathecal chemotherapy.

Plasmacytic Tumours

Myeloma and Waldenström's macroglobulinaemia. Soft tissue and bone deposits of myeloma have been reported in the orbit in elderly people (53, 54) and lacrimal gland and orbital deposits in Waldenström's macroglobulinaemia (55, 56).

The *clinical appearance* is of proptosis. An increase of blood viscosity in association with the typical serum protein abnormalities of these disorders results in a venous stasis retinopathy which facilitates the *diagnosis*, and may obviate the need for formal biopsy. The *treatment* is essentially that of the systemic disease but the orbital lesions may respond to radiotherapy.

Histiocytic Tumours

There are no reports of malignant histiocytosis affecting the orbit but orbital involvement occurs in the systemic differentiated histiocytoses, together referred to as histiocytosis X. Broadly, two patterns of systemic histiocytosis are recognized. The chronic form, known as Hand–Schüller–Christian disease, pursues a relatively benign course whereas the acute type, termed Letterer–Siwe disease, becomes rapidly widespread and, although not cytologically malignant, is associated with a significant mortality. Eosinophilic granuloma of bone usually remains isolated and does not share the tendency of the other histiocytoses to become multifocal. Eosinophilic granuloma cannot therefore be regarded as systemic and is no longer included under the term histiocytosis X.

Eosinophilic granuloma. The presence in

bone of a solitary or of multiple histiocytic deposits only, with no evidence of soft tissue histiocytosis, indicates a diagnosis of eosinophilic granuloma. Affected individuals are usually adults and they do not die.

The *clinical appearance* may be of a visible periorbital mass or an area of osteolysis may be a chance finding on a skull x-ray. The *diagnosis* may be confirmed by biopsy and simultaneous local curettage may effect a cure. If this fails, *treatment* by low doses of radiation may be curative. A total dose of 5 to 6 Gy should suffice and 10 Gy should not be exceeded (57). The bony deposits respond well to an intralesional injection of methylprednisolone sodium succinate (58) or methylprednisolone acetate (59), though the injection may need to be repeated (59).

Histiocytosis X. This condition usually has its onset in childhood and histiocytes accumulate throughout the body in soft tissues and in bone. The membrane bones of the skull and the sella turcica are a common site for deposition of these histiocytes. Orbital bone involvement is relatively infrequent (60) but when proptosis occurs it is usually non-axial and results from a bony deposit. Occasionally axial proptosis may be seen in association with a soft tissue deposit within the optic nerve sheath. Bony involvement is most prominent in Hand–Schüller–Christian disease and proptosis is therefore seen more often in this condition than in Letterer–Siwe disease.

The *clinical appearance* of proptosis is frequently associated with diabetes insipidus. The combination of proptosis, bone deposits, and diabetes insipidus constitutes a triad of signs which suggest a *diagnosis* of histiocytosis X. This should then be confirmed by radiological examination and by biopsy. Before beginning *treatment* the patient should be fully staged to assess the extent of the disease. Because of multifocal tumours, systemic therapy will be required. This should begin with prednisolone alone and cytotoxic drugs such as vincristine and vinblastine may be added. VP 16 may be tried for resistant disease. Since bony deposits

respond well to intralesional injection of methyl sodium succinate (58), this form of treatment is appropriate for accessible orbital lesions. The injection may need to be repeated several times before complete regression occurs (60). Lesions resistant to this approach and inaccessible deposits may be treated effectively by low dose radiotherapy as for eosinophilic granuloma.

Leukaemia

Invasion of the eye and orbit is commonest in the acute leukaemias, particularly those of the lymphoblastic type and may be bilateral (61, 62).

Chloroma. Occasionally, and particularly in children from the Middle East and Africa, deposits of blast cells may accumulate in the orbit in acute myeloid leukaemia before the disease is detected in the bone marrow or peripheral blood (63). The name derives from the green colour imparted to affected tissues by the action of the enzyme myeloperoxidase present within the tumour cells. Not all deposits are thus discoloured and chloroma has also been termed granulocytic sarcoma.

The *clinical appearance* is of proptois which may be bilateral. Chloroma must be distinguished from rhabdomyosarcoma, neuroblastoma, and malignant lymphoma, especially Burkitt's lymphoma in African patients. The *diagnosis* should be established by orbital biopsy. Tumour cells may infiltrate the eye in chloroma and *treatment* may involve both radiotherapy and chemotherapy. It has been claimed that survival is best if therapy begins before widespread tumour is detected (63).

Lacrimal Gland Tumours

Tumours of the lacrimal gland are either benign mixed neoplasms or they are carcinomas (64). It is now recognized that malignant change can occur in a benign mixed tumour and that the frequency with which this happens increases with the number of recurrences

(65). Benign mixed tumours are often encapsulated and if the diagnosis can be recognized clinically, and early and complete excision achieved by modified lateral orbitotomy, the outlook is excellent (66, 67). If, on the other hand, the diagnosis is arrived at by biopsy, the tumour capsule will be breached and local recurrence is inevitable, with an attendant risk of late malignant change. Biopsy is therefore to be avoided at all costs (45). Even if the recurrent tumour is not histologically malignant, it may follow a locally invasive course indistinguishable from that of a true carcinoma (45). Benign mixed tumours typically present in middle life usually with a greater than 12 months' history of painless, slowly progressive upper lid swelling without inflammatory symptoms or signs. A mass may be palpable in the upper outer quadrant of the orbit. Plain x-ray examination may reveal enlargement of the lacrimal fossa without invasion of bone. Even though malignant lacrimal gland tumours have a limited potential for metastasis, they are associated with a high mortality rate because they are difficult to excise and because they have a strong propensity for remorseless local spread.

Lacrimal gland carcinoma.
The commonest malignant tumour of the lacrimal gland is adenocystic carcinoma although adenocarcinoma, undifferentiated carcinoma, squamous carcinoma, and malignant mixed tumours may be encountered (68).

The *clinical appearance* is of a mass in the upper eyelid temporally, sometimes associated with lacrimation. Posterior growth of the tumour to produce proptosis is uncommon. Enlargement of the neoplasm may result in displacement of the globe and diplopia. Lacrimal gland carcinomas present quite differently from benign mixed lesions. The history is short, with rapid progression. Pain is a prominent feature, especially of adenocystic carcinoma, because this tumour tends to invade neural channels. Lacrimal gland carcinomas must be distinguished from inflammatory pseudotumours, from lymphomas, and particularly

from acute dacryoadenitis when this fails to respond to antibiotics over a period of a fortnight (45). Malignant lacrimal gland tumours are usually non-encapsulated and invasive. Nothing is to be lost by establishing the *diagnosis* by biopsy. It has been advocated that tissue should be obtained via an incision through the orbital septum and not through the periosteum to avoid extra-periosteal seeding of malignant cells (45). Radiological evidence of invasion of bone suggests a malignant tumour and the presence on x-ray of calcium within the tumour is diagnostic of malignancy (45). Prior to *treatment* the extent of any bony involvement must be assessed fully with both axial and coronal CT views: surgical excision can only be considered when there is no evidence of involvement of the orbital apex and when the tumour appears confined within the periosteum (45). When these criteria are met, orbital exenteration should be performed with the aid of a neurosurgeon, a head and neck surgeon, and a plastic surgeon to include the eyelids and portions of the lateral and superior orbital walls. Radiotherapy and chemotherapy may be considered for patients who do not fulfil the criteria for surgery or who have residual disease.

Neural Crest Tumours (see Chapter 30)

Many orbital neoplasms are derived from cells of neural crest origin. Benign and malignant tumours may arise de novo from Schwann cells, from melanocytes, and from ganglion and leptomeningeal cells (69). Also, in neurofibromatosis there is a tendency for multiple tumours to develop in any group of cells of neural crest lineage. Most of these neoplasms are benign, but the frequency with which they arise means that occasionally a malignant variant is encountered.

Malignant schwannoma.
The majority of these uncommon tumours probably arise in a pre-existing benign lesion (Figure 6). Malignant change can occur in a solitary orbital neurofibroma (70) or schwannoma (71) but

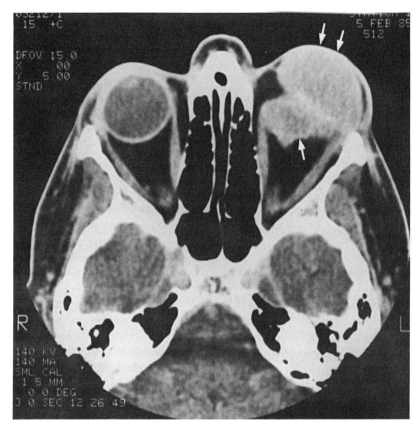

Figure 6 Orbital CT scan showing a malignant schwannoma (double arrows) which developed in a benign schwannoma which, in turn, arose in an eviscerated eye (single arrow).

probably takes place more often in patients with neurofibromatosis: up to 15% of such individuals may develop a malignancy in a pre-existing neurofibroma (72, 73).

The tumour is said to develop most commonly in the distribution of the superior orbital nerve (74) and the *clinical appearance* is usually that of a mass in the anterior orbit. Malignant schwannoma may be painful because, like adenocystic carcinoma of the lacrimal gland, it shows a marked tendency to grow along nerves. In the orbit the tumour must be distinguished from a fibrosarcoma or primary orbital melanoma. The *diagnosis* is made by orbital biopsy. The first-line *treatment* is surgical excision but the infiltrative character of malignant schwannoma makes local recurrences frequent. The tumour shows a tendency to invade the orbital apex and death may result from extension into the middle cranial fossa. Orbital exenteration offers the best chance of complete excision and post-surgical radical orbital radiotherapy may reduce the possibility of inexorable local spread.

Alveolar soft part sarcoma. This tumour is the malignant counterpart of paraganglioma (75) which in the orbit is thought to arise from non-chromaffin paraganglionic structures in the region of the ciliary ganglion (76–79).

The *clinical appearance* is of rapidly progressive proptosis which must be distinguished from rhabdomyosarcoma in a child. The *diagnosis* is made by orbital biopsy. Alveolar soft part sarcoma is unusual amongst malignant orbital tumours in having a great potential for fatal metastatic spread and *treatment* is by early orbital exenteration.

Primary orbital melanoma. Malignant change may take place in melanocytes which are present in the orbit in association with oculodermal melanocytosis (naevus of Ota), neurocutaneous melanosis, cellular blue naevus, or pigmented neurofibroma (70, 80–85). It may also occur in melanocytes which have spilled from the eye along scleral emmissary channels or along the optic nerve, and in stray melanocytes deposited in the orbit during embryonic life (36, 37).

The cases recorded are too few to define a typical *clinical appearance*. Investigations should include radiological examination to assess the extent of any bone involvement. The *diagnosis* is made by biopsy and the *treatment* is generally orbital exenteration with removal of any bone which shows signs of tumour infiltration.

Meningioma. Most orbital meningiomas arise in the sphenoid wing or basofrontal region and invade the orbit secondarily (88, 89). Much less commonly a meningioma may originate from the sheath of the intraorbital portion of the optic nerve (90). It has been suggested that meningioma may also arise within the orbit from ectopic arachnoidal cells within the muscle cone and from the periosteal lining of the orbit (91–95). As with intracranial meningioma, the tumour in the orbit is much commoner in females. The age of onset tends to be young with 40% of these tumours occurring under age 20 (70). In children, orbital meningioma behaves in a particularly aggressive fashion and survival rates are relatively poor (96). Although primary orbital meningiomas do not metastasize they are locally invasive and may penetrate the sclera (97).

The *clinical appearance* will depend on the site of origin of the tumour within the orbit. Optic nerve sheath meningiomas present first with either reduced vision or axial proptosis. These tumours are inaccessible for biopsy and the *diagnosis* is particularly dependent on ocular clinical signs and on radiological investigations. External ocular examination may reveal an afferent defect in the response of the pupil to light and papilloedema or optic atrophy may be seen on inspection of the ocular fundus. Sheath meningiomas obstruct the venous return from the eye and large shunt vessels may be seen around the optic disc. Plain x-rays may demonstrate enlargement of the optic foramen but the tumour size and location is best delineated by CT scanning. Orbital meningiomas in childhood are frequently associated with neurofibromatosis. Children with neurofibromatosis are also at risk of developing an optic nerve glioma and it may be difficult to distinguish clinically between a meningioma and a glioma in the orbital apex. The *treatment* of orbital meningioma is surgical excision, usually via a lateral orbitotomy, and complete cure rates are higher than for intracranial meningiomas. It is difficult to peel a sheath meningioma off the intraorbital portion of the optic nerve and it is generally necessary to excise a portion of the nerve when removing such a tumour. Although the eye will be blind and the pupil amaurotic the globe may be retained with normal motility.

Optic Nerve Gliomas

These rare tumours may occur anywhere along the length of the optic nerve or in the chiasm. Most optic nerve gliomas are now classified as juvenile pilocytic astrocytomas (98).

Juvenile pilocytic astrocytoma. Most examples of this uncommon tumour are histologically benign. Nevertheless, inexorable growth of some intracranial lesions leads to death. Other tumours grow episodically or cease growing without treatment (99). Ninety per cent of these benign lesions present in the first two decades of life (100) and there is evidence of neurofibromatosis in nearly 40% of affected individuals (101). By contrast, malignant optic nerve gliomas are exceptionally rare and affect adults (102). Most are of the highly malignant glioblastoma multiforme type but a Grade II astrocytoma has been reported (103).

The *clinical appearance* depends largely on whether the tumour is mainly intraorbital or intracranial (104). Most often the earliest sign of an optic nerve glioma is loss of vision. In a young child attention may be called to visual failure by the presence of a squint, of nystagmus, or of a dilated pupil. When the tumour involves the intraorbital portion of the optic nerve, axial painless proptosis is common and there may be a mechanical restriction of ocular motility. Presentation tends to be earlier with these added signs. Fundus examination usually reveals either optic disc swelling or atrophy, and pressure on the globe from an intraorbital tumour may produce retinal striae. The presence of signs of hydrocephalus, diabetes insipidus, somnolence, seizures, obesity, or hypogonadism suggest chiasmal tumour with involvement of the hypothalamus or pituitary and the possibility of raised intracranial pressure. In an older child or adult it may be possible to map a visual field defect. Chiasmal involvement is indicated by a quadrantic or hemianopic temporal field defect in the eye opposite to that with an intraorbital tumour but the absence of such a defect does not exclude chiasmal extension (99). The progress of the disease is much more rapid for the malignant variant.

The presence of evidence of neurofibromatosis on systemic examination in a patient with visual failure, optic atrophy or disc swelling, and proptosis is strongly suggestive of meningioma or optic nerve glioma and in a child the latter will be by far the most likely diagnosis. The greatest assistance in establishing the *diagnosis* will come from radiological investigations. Enlargement of the optic foramen is seen in the majority of affected individuals and a well-corticated margin is suggestive of a benign tumour. CT has largely replaced tomography and pneumoencephalography in the radiological assessment of patients with optic nerve gliomas.

The *treatment* of juvenile pilocytic astrocytoma is controversial. The propensity of the tumour for slow or episodic growth, or spontaneous arrest of progression, has made it difficult to assess the results of a policy of no treatment or one of treatment by surgical excision or radiotherapy. At one extreme is the view that these tumours are hamartomas, that their potential for growth is limited, and that the only indication for orbital surgery is severe proptosis of a blind eye and for intracranial surgery, raised intracranial pressure (102). At the other it is recommended that a tumour which appears confined to the orbit should be removed via a lateral orbitotomy, that an intracranial removal should be performed if orbital excision is incomplete or if a tumour enlarges the optic foramen, and that a combined approach should be considered for tumours which are both intraorbital and intracranial (105). The weight of evidence from very long-term follow-up studies suggests that the death rate is high if an attempt is not made to remove these tumours surgically (106), though only tumours not involving the chiasm are now regarded as resectable (99). The place of radiotherapy is uncertain (107); whilst some have claimed successes for this approach (100, 108, 109) others have suggested that any improvement is temporary (110). Such malignant optic nerve gliomas as have been reported have usually been rapidly fatal.

Tumours of Striated Muscle

Malignant tumours composed of striated muscle cells are termed rhabdomyosarcomas. The orbit is the primary site of rhabdomyosarcoma in 9% of all cases and in nearly a quarter of examples of this tumour arising in the head and neck (111).

Rhabdomyosarcoma. This malignant tumour may arise in the orbit or may invade it secondarily from the postnasal space or from the face. Seventy-five per cent of primary orbital rhabdomyosarcomas present in children under the age of 10 years and only 1% in individuals over the age of 25 (112). Males are affected more often than females in the ratio of 5:3 (112). In young and adolescent patients, most primary orbital rhabdomyosarcomas are of the embryonal type which carries a good prognosis because of a tendency to infiltrate and to metastasize relatively late. In youth these tumours probably arise from undifferentiated pluripotential mesenchymal cells in the orbital soft tissues and cannot be traced to extraocular muscles (113). Primary orbital rhabdomyosarcoma is very rare in adults but when it occurs the tumour is of the pleomorphic type. These adult tumours probably arise in striated muscle (114) and origin from an extraocular muscle has been demonstrated (115). Secondary orbital rhabdomyosarcomas are usually of the alveolar type which carries a relatively poor prognosis.

The *clinical appearance* depends on the site of origin of the tumour (45). Anterior lesions present with a palpable eyelid or subconjunctival mass, redness of the eye or lids, and oedema of the conjunctiva (Figure 7). Posterior tumours lead to rapidly progressive non-axial proptosis and occasionally to loss of vision (116) and optic disc oedema as a result of optic nerve compression. It has been claimed that the superonasal quadrant of the orbit is the most frequent presenting site for embryonal rhabdomyosarcoma (113, 116) though this has been disputed (117, 118). Not infrequently the tumour may present with ptosis (118) or strabismus. Pain (119) is relatively infrequent. An anterior tumour must be distinguished from a dermoid cyst, an orbital cellulitis, a haemangioma, or a lymphangioma. A posterior lesion must be differentiated from a deposit of neuroblastoma, agranulocytic sarcoma in association with leukaemia, haemorrhage into a haemangioma or rupture of an orbital varix, or extraocular extension of retinoblastoma.

Plain x-ray films may demonstrate bone erosion and a mass lesion may be delineated by tomography or CT. The *diagnosis* is made by biopsy and the tumour should be approached through the eyelid or orbit (119). The tumour is diffuse and friable though occasionally there is a good capsule (45). It tends to recur along the biopsy track and a transcranial route should not be employed (118). Needle biopsy is unlikely to yield sufficient tissue for special

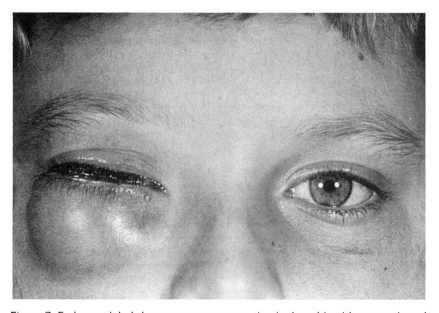

Figure 7   Embryonal rhabdomyosarcoma presenting in the orbit with proptosis and lid swelling.

histological investigations including electron microscopy.

The *treatment* of embryonal rhabdomyosarcoma in the orbit has changed radically in recent years. These tumours were formerly managed by early orbital exenteration and by radiotherapy only when this approach failed to produce local control. Radical surgery no longer has any place in the initial management of rhabdomyosarcoma in the orbit and should be reserved for disease which cannot be controlled by combined chemotherapy and radiotherapy (120, 121). Current treatment protocols employ initial chemotherapy to shrink the tumour using a combination of drugs such as cyclophosphamide, vincristine, actinomycin D or Adriamycin. This is followed by radical orbital radiotherapy employing a tumour dose of 50 to 55 Gy in 30 fractions over 42 days. Employing wedged anterior and antero-oblique megavoltage photon portals the chiasm, hypothalamus, and pituitary may receive high doses and for smaller lesions in younger patients it is permissible to choose a dose of 40 to 45 Gy in 25 fractions (120). Good local control is achieved by this approach (111) and relapse-free survival rates of the order of 90% can be achieved (122). Side effects include cataract, shortness of stature, and retarded bone growth leading to facial asymmetry (123). Radiation choroidoretinopathy when present is not severe and removal of any cataract usually results in good vision though reduced tear production may limit the wearing times of an aphakic contact lens and intraocular lens implantation may be preferable.

Tumours of Connective Tissue and Bone

The orbit may be the primary site of malignant tumours taking origin from fibroblasts, smooth muscle cells, lipocytes, chondrocytes, and osteocytes.

Fibrosarcoma. This rare tumour may be encountered in all age groups (124, 125). In youth it is seen most often as a second neoplasm in retinoblastoma survivors who have received high doses of radiation to the orbit as part of the treatment of their first tumour. Fibrosarcoma tends to recure locally but metastasis from an orbital primary does not seem to occur.

The *clinical appearance* is of proptosis with rapid onset and progression over one or two months (124, 125) and may be impossible to distinguish from that of rhabdomyosarcoma in childhood. The *diagnosis* should be established by orbital biopsy as outlined for rhabdomyosarcoma. In one reported case (125) there was a poor response to radiotherapy to a tumour dose of 38 Gy and many retinoblastoma patients will have already received high doses of radiation to the orbit which will limit further treatment by this modality. The first-line *treatment* advocated is therefore early orbital exenteration.

Fibrous histiocytoma. Orbital fibrous histiocytoma is a neoplasm of adults. Most tumours of this type occurring in the orbit are benign but a small proportion are locally aggressive. A further small group are histologically malignant (126) and, though metastasis does not occur, death may result from persistent local recurrence.

The *clinical appearance* is of proptosis with relatively slow onset over a period of months or years. In one series diplopia was a constant feature and the tumour was often situated in the upper, inner quadrant of the orbit (126). Anteriorly situated masses may feel fluctuant and be difficult to distinguish from a pseudotumour, a cyst or a haemangioma (126). The *diagnosis* must be established by orbital biopsy. Initially, most of these tumours are well circumscribed and the first-line *treatment* may be by excision of the tumour alone. Orbital exenteration is recommended for persistent local recurrence and when histology reveals the malignant variant.

Leiomyosarcoma. This tumour is extremely rare in the orbit and affects only adults. Unlike malignant orbital tumours arising from fibroblasts, leiomyosarcoma has a strong propensity to metastasize (127).

The *clinical appearance* is of proptosis with relatively gradual onset over a year or more (127). Benign leiomyomas are usually well encapsulated and this may be apparent on B scan ultrasound of the orbit (128). The slow development in an adult of an ill-defined orbital tumour should raise the possibility of leiomyosarcoma but the *diagnosis* can only be made with certainty on the basis of tissue obtained by biopsy. When a diagnosis of leiomyosarcoma has been established the patient should be staged with particular attention paid to the possibility of lung metastases. In the absence of widespread disease *treatment* by orbital exenteration may effect a cure. If metastases are present, chemotherapy should be considered but the outlook is poor and any ocular treatment may only be palliative.

Liposarcoma. Very few malignant tumours of lipocytes have been reported arising in the orbit (129). The patients have been adults and there has been a tendency towards both local recurrence and metastasis.

The *clinical appearance* in the few reported examples has been of proptosis with relatively rapid onset. The diagnosis must be established by orbital biopsy. There are insufficient data on which to base a definitive approach to *treatment* by surgery or radiotherapy. It has been suggested that local excision can be attempted initially for well-differentiated tumours (128) but recurrence and malignant variants should be managed by orbital exenteration.

Chondrosarcoma. Orbital variants of this tumour may arise in bone of cartilaginous origin at the base of the skull or in extraskeletal mesenchymal elements. Most patients have been children or young adults. Chondrosarcoma is one of the commoner second tumours seen after orbital radiotherapy for retinoblastoma. The tumour rarely metastasizes early though death may occur from pulmonary or other metastases or from local disease.

The *clinical appearance* of orbital chondrosarcoma both of extraskeletal and of bony origin has been one of rapidly progressing proptosis with diplopia, headache, and orbital pain (130–133). Following establishment of the *diagnosis* by biopsy and in the absence of evidence of widespread tumour on staging, the first-line *treatment* of extraskeletal chondrosarcoma is orbital exenteration and that of the tumour arising in the bones of the orbit is radical excision of the affected bone when accessible and radiotherapy and chemotherapy when not.

Osteogenic sarcoma. The occurrence of this tumour in the walls of the orbit is extremely uncommon (134) and most examples occur in the third decade of life. Osteogenic sarcoma is an all too frequent sequela of orbital radiotherapy. Most radiation-related osteogenic sarcomas follow treatment for retinoblastoma but not all such neoplasms occurring as second tumours arise in the irradiated orbit. Many more osteogenic sarcomas than would be expected also develop in the long bones and in individuals who have never received radiotherapy. It is now considered that survivors of retinoblastoma of the germinal type have a genetic predisposition to bone and soft tissue sarcomas (135, 136) though it is generally accepted that radiation may also contribute to the development of such of these neoplasms as occur at the edge of an irradiated field in or around the orbit. In contrast with chondrosarcoma, osteogenic sarcoma tends to metastasize early.

The *clinical appearance* is of facial swelling with pain or numbness and displacement of the eye. Radiological investigation may show increased bone density and the *diagnosis* should be confirmed by bone biopsy. *Treatment* is unsatisfactory. In one large series radiotherapy was found to be ineffective in establishing local control without extensive surgery (137). Radical orbital surgery should not be performed if systemic staging demonstrates pulmonary or other metastases. Chemotherapy is unlikely to be of avail in the presence of established metastases and in most cases will not prevent a metastatic death in patients in whom staging demonstrates no evidence of metastatic disease at the time of the diagnosis of the orbital primary.

Secondary Orbital Tumours

More than 50% of tumours arising in the orbit have spread there from a distant primary, from structures surrounding the orbit, or from within the eye (138).

Metastases

In children the commonest sources of metastases to the orbit are embryonal tumours such as neuroblastoma (139) and nephroblastoma (140), and sarcomas such as Ewing's sarcoma (141). By contrast, in adults, the source of an orbital metastasis is almost invariably a carcinoma, usually from a lung or breast primary (142) though occasionally from stomach, thyroid, kidney, or adrenal (138). Metastatic spread of a sarcoma to this site in an adult is extremely rare.

Neuroblastoma. Orbital metastases are quite common in children with neuroblastoma (141) and when they occur are bilateral in at least 50% of patients (141, 143). Theoretically, this tumour might arise from the ciliary ganglion and one case is recorded of neuroblastoma which may have originated in the orbit (144).

The *clinical appearance* is one of proptosis, often associated with a painful mass in the temple or cheek because of a tendency for neuroblastoma to deposit in the zygomatic bone. Rapid growth of the tumour within the orbit leads to early haemorrhagic necrosis and thereby to ecchymosis of the eyelids. When bilateral, this feature of orbital neuroblastoma is virtually diagnostic though, if the presence of the primary tumour is not already known, the patient should be investigated for leukaemia, aplastic anaemia, or any other cause of a bleeding tendency. Should it be considered necessary, the *diagnosis* of an orbital deposit of neuroblastoma may be confirmed by biopsy. Radiographic changes in the skull or orbit are seen in 65% of cases (143). Orbital lesions of neuroblastoma may regress following *treatment* of widespread disease by chemotherapy and are also sensitive to radiotherapy.

Ewing's sarcoma. Orbital metastases are also relatively common in children and young adults with Ewing's sarcoma (141, 145) and one of the bones of the orbit may be the primary site of this tumour.

The *clinical appearance* is similar to that of neuroblastoma with rapidly progressive proptosis, haemorrhage, and necrosis though orbital deposits of Ewing's sarcoma tend to be unilateral. If in doubt, the *diagnosis* of an orbital deposit of Ewing's sarcoma may be confirmed by biopsy. Early metastasis is a feature of the tumour and treatment of orbital deposits is largely palliative. The prognosis for Ewing's sarcoma arising in the axial skeleton is poor so that the outlook is also grave for this tumour arising at a primary site within an orbital bone. *Treatment* is by chemotherapy and radiotherapy.

Direct Extension of Extraorbital Tumours

Invasion of the orbit by intracranial meningiomas has been discussed. In addition, various malignant tumours may spread to the orbit from the eyelids and conjunctiva, the lacrimal sac, the paranasal sinuses, and the nose and pharynx.

Carcinoma. Mortality from metastatic disease is surprisingly low following invasion of the orbit by squamous carcinoma arising in the conjunctiva (146), in the eyelids, and in the lacrimal sac (147). Death from disseminated tumour is similarly rare in mucoepidermoid carcinomas but these tumours are generally much more invasive than squamous carcinomas. Orbital invasion is relatively common in sebaceous carcinoma and mortality is significant. A tendency to late presentation leads to a high mortality rate in carcinoma arising in the paranasal sinuses and the outlook is worse still for orbital invasion by carcinoma arising in the nose or nasopharynx (138).

The *clinical appearance* will depend on the extraorbital site of origin of the tumour. If proptosis is non-axial, observation of the direction in which the globe is displaced will be helpful. Ophthalmoplegia may occur late in the progress of tumours invading the orbit from the nasopharynx.

The *diagnosis* must be established by biopsy because some carcinomas are more radiosensitive than others. *Treatment* depends on surgical accessibility. Most squamous carcinomas invading the orbit from anterior structures will require orbital exenteration, particularly if local control is not established by conservative local resection. This is especially so for mucoepidermoid carcinomas (148) and sebaceous carcinomas (149). It has been estimated that 45% of all carcinomas arising in the paranasal sinuses ultimately require orbital exenteration (150) if local control is to be achieved. Carcinomas invading the orbit posteriorly from the nasopharnx are generally not amenable to surgical excision and radiotherapy should be attempted.

Sarcoma. Approximately one-fifth of tumours invading the orbit from the paranasal sinuses are sarcomas (150). To these must be added rhabdomyosarcomas invading the orbit from the nasopharynx. These latter tumours are usually of the alveolar type and have a substantially worse prognosis than embryonal rhabdomyosarcomas arising in the orbit.

The *clinical appearance* is governed by the tendency of these tumours to reach a considerable size before detection. Nasopharyngeal rhabdomyosarcomas frequently present with external ophthalmoplegia or loss of vision from invasion of the orbital apex. The *diagnosis* is usually established by biopsy via the postnatal space. *Treatment* is by radiotherapy and chemotherapy but yields a low survival rate.

Melanoma. Although spread to the orbit of malignant melanoma most commonly occurs from within the eye, direct extension may take place from the conjunctiva and, very occasionally, from a rare primary within the nasal cavity or in a paranasal sinus (138). Orbital extension of a conjunctival melanoma is commoner when the primary tumour involves the conjunctival fornix, the plica semilunaris, or the caruncle than when the tumour does not extend beyond the bulbar conjunctiva.

The *clinical appearance* depends on the site of origin of the melanoma. Brown discoloration of the conjunctiva in association with displacement of the globe suggests orbital extension of a conjunctival melanoma. On the other hand, an amelanotic conjunctival melanoma or any melanoma arising in the nose or in a paranasal sinus will be difficult to distinguish clinically from a carcinoma. The *diagnosis* may be supported by CT and should be confirmed if possible by biopsy, combined with enucleation of the eye where appropriate. *Treatment* is not associated with a good survival rate. Orbital exenteration may be considered for melanoma extending from the conjunctiva and, combined with hemimaxillectomy, for melanoma extending from a maxillary sinus provided that there is no evidence of metastatic disease. Radiotherapy may be considered for unresectable tumours and for palliative treatment dictated by the presence of metastases.

Direct Extension of Intraocular Tumours

Melanoma. Extraocular extension of uveal melanoma is usually associated with a very large intraocular tumour but occasionally a small intraocular melanoma may extend via a scleral emissary channel to produce a much larger orbital mass (Figure 8). Some 13% of eyes enucleated for malignant melanoma show histological evidence of extrascleral extension and the 5-year survival rate is 34% compared with 67% for eyes without evidence of extrascleral extension (151). Some 20% of individuals with extrascleral extension of uveal melanoma will have recurrence in the orbit.

The *clinical appearance* of proptosis of a blind eye in an adult raises the possibility of extrao-

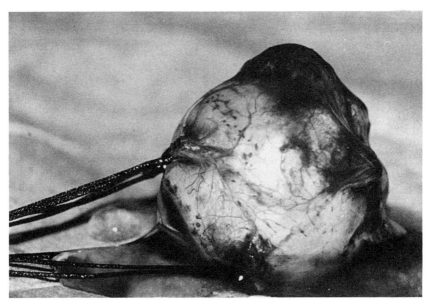

Figure 8 Enucleated eye showing encapsulated extrascleral extension of choroidal malignant melanoma.

cular extension of an intraocular melanoma. The *diagnosis* of extraocular extension can usually be confirmed by ultrasound but the extent of the orbital element is best estimated by high definition orbital CT. The place of orbital exenteration in the *treatment* of extrascleral extension of an intraocular melanoma is not yet determined (152). This procedure may be justified when a massive extrascleral extension of an intraocular melanoma is transected during enucleation but it is not known whether exenteration in these circumstances prolongs life. Orbital exenteration is not considered necessary when a nodular, encapsulated extrascleral melanoma is removed intact with the globe though there is some evidence to suggest that radical orbital radiotherapy in this situation reduces the incidence of orbital recurrence.

Retinoblastoma. If it remains undetected in the eye for a long period this tumour may rupture the globe and spread to the orbit. Though still rare, in Western countries orbital deposits of retinoblastoma are much more

commonly seen within a period of 12 to 18 months following enucleation. There is histological evidence of extrascleral spread of the tumour in the enucleated eye in half of orbital recurrences of retinoblastoma and it seems likely that this serious development can be prevented by appropriate orbital radiotherapy (153).

The *clinical appearance* will depend on whether or not the globe has been removed. When retinoblastoma recurs in the orbit following removal of an eye it usually presents with displacement or expulsion of the prosthesis. In a child who retains both eyes, and in whom the diagnosis of retinoblastoma has not yet been made, there is rapidly progressing proptosis with lid oedema and the appearances may be suggestive of orbital cellulitis or rhabdomyosarcoma. Opening the lids will reveal a disorganized eye and the *diagnosis* of retinoblastoma with orbital extension may be supported by radiological evidence of calcium within the orbit on CT or plain x-ray. *Treatment* is associated with an extremely poor survival rate and at present only individuals without evidence of widespread retinoblastoma at presentation have a chance of surviving. Children with widespread retinoblastoma at diagnosis of orbital involvement should be offered palliative therapy but with a modern approach some children with tumour apparently confined to the orbit may survive. Orbital exenteration should be reserved for children with rupture and disorganization of the globe and has been shown to play no part in the management of orbital recurrence which should be treated by a combination of lumpectomy, radical orbital radiotherapy, neuraxis radiotherapy or intrathecal methotrexate, and adjuvant systemic chemotherapy (153).

Medulloepithelioma. Although malignant examples of this tumour may metastasize late to the lungs most deaths from intraocular medulloepithelioma result from direct extension to the brain via the orbit (154). As with retinoblastoma, orbital involvement usually follows delayed enucleation and the *clinical appearance* is predominantly one of orbital recurrence. The *diagnosis* may be confirmed by biopsy and the extent of the recurrent tumour assessed by CT. *Treatment* of resectable recurrences by orbital exenteration has produced survivors but radiotherapy for extensive lesions has been much less encouraging.

REFERENCES

1 Rao NA, Hidayat AA, McLean IW, Zimmerman LE. Sebaceous carcinomas of the ocular adnexa: a clinicopathologic study of 104 cases, with five-year follow-up data. Hum Pathol 1982; 13: 113.
2 Boniuk M, Zimmerman LE. Sebaceous carcinoma of the eyelid, eyebrow, caruncle, and orbit. Trans Am Acad Ophthalmol Otolaryngol 1968; 72: 619.
3 Rulon D, Helwig E. Cutaneous sebaceous neoplasms. Cancer 1974; 33: 82.
4 Lee SC, Roth LM. Sebaceous carcinoma of the eyelid with pagetoid involvement of the bulbar and palpebral conjunctiva. J Cut Pathol 1977; 4: 134.
5 Weigent CE, Staley NA. Meibomian gland carcinoma; report of a case with electron microscopic findings. Hum Pathol 1976; 7: 231.
6 Russell WG, Page DL, Hough AJ et al. Sebaceous carcinoma of meibomian gland origin. Am J Clin Pathol 1980; 73: 504.
7 Chuo NI, Wagoner M, Kieval S, Albert DM. Tumours of the Moll's glands. Br J Ophthalmol 1984; 68: 502.
8 Cavanagh H, Green W, Goldberg H. Multicentric sebaceous adenocarcinoma of the meibomian gland. Am J Ophthalmol 1974; 77: 326.
9 Aurora A, Blodi F. Lesions of the eyelids: a clinicopathologic study. Survey Ophthalmol 1970; 15: 94.
10 Ferry A. The eyelids. In: Sorsby A ed Modern Ophthalmology, Vol 4. Philadelphia: Lippincott, 1972: 833.
11 Boniuk M. Differentiation of squamous cell carcinoma from other epithelial tumors of the eyelid. In: Boniuk M ed Ocular and Adnexal Tumors. St Louis: Mosby, 1964: 75.
12 Boniuk M, Kwitko ML, Zimmerman LE. Tumors of the eyelid with specific reference to lesions often confused with squamous cell carcinoma. I. Incidence and errors in diagnosis. Arch Ophthalmol 1963; 69: 693.
13 Jakobiec FA, Zimmerman LE. Symposium on Ophthalmic Surgical Pathology, Part I. Introduction. Human Pathology 1982; 13: 98.
14 Collin JRO. Surgery of adnexal tumours. In: Oosterhuis JA ed Ophthalmic Tumours. Dordrecht: Dr W Junk, 1985, 307.
15 Jakobiec FA, Rootman J, Jones IS. Secondary and metastatic tumors of the orbit. In: Jones IS, Jakobiec FA eds Diseases of the Orbit. Hagerstown: Harper and Row, 1979: 503.
16 Naidoff MA, Bernardino VB Jr, Clark WH Jr. Melanocytic lesions of the eyelid, skin and conjunctiva. Am J Ophthalmol 1976; 82: 371.
17 Garner A, Koornneef L, Levene A, Collin JRO. Malignant melanoma of the eyelid skin: histopathology and behaviour. Br J Ophthalmol 1985; 69: 180.
18 Hamming N. Anatomy and embryology of the eyelid: review with special reference to the development of divided nevi. J Paed Dermatol 1983; 1: 51.
19 Collin JRO, Garner A, Allen LH, Hungerford JL. Malignant melanoma of the eyelid and conjunctiva. Aust NZ J Ophthalmol 1986; 14: 29.
20 Zimmerman LE. The cancerous, precancerous, and pseudocancerous lesions of the cornea and conjunctiva. The Poklington Memorial Lecture. In: Rycroft PV ed Corneoplastic Surgery. New York: Pergamon Press, 1969: 547.
21 Illif W, Marback R, Green WR. Invasive squamous cell carcinoma of the conjunctiva. Arch Ophthalmol 1975; 93: 119.

22 Lommatzsch PK. Beta-ray treatment of malignant epithelial tumors of the conjunctiva. Am J Ophthalmol 1976; 81: 198.

23 Frauenfelder FT, Wingfield D. Management of intraepithelial conjunctival tumors and squamous cell carcinomas. Am J Ophthalmol 1983; 95: 359.

24 Reese AB. Pigmented tumors. In: Tumors of the Eye. Hagerstown: Harper and Row, 1976: 25.

25 Zimmerman L. Pigmented tumors of the conjunctiva. In: Boniuk M ed Ocular and Adnexal Tumors. St Louis: Mosby, 1964: 24.

26 Jay B. Naevi and melanomata of the conjunctiva. Br J Ophthalmol 1969; 49: 169.

27 Lederman M, Wybar K, Busby E. Malignant epibulbar melanoma: natural history and treatment by radiotherapy. Br J Ophthalmol 1984; 68: 605.

28 Ackerman LV, Murray JF. In: Ackerman LV, Murray JF eds Symposium on Kaposi's sarcoma. New York: Karger, 1962.

29 Reynolds W, Winkelmann R, Soule E. Kaposi's sarcoma: a clinicopathologic study with particular reference to its relationship to the reticuloendothelial system. Medicine 1965; 44: 419.

30 Howard G, Jakobiec F, DeVoe A. Kaposi's sarcoma: the subconjunctival hemorrhage that never clears. Am J Ophthalmol 1975; 79: 420.

31 Rosenberg SA, Diamond HD, Jaslowitz B, Craver LF. Lymphopsarcoma: a review of 1,269 cases. Medicine 1961; 40: 31.

32 McGavic JS. Lymphomatoid diseases involving the eye and its adnexa. Arch Ophthalmol 1943; 30: 179.

33 McGavic JS. Lymphomatous tumors of the eye. Arch Ophthalmol 1955; 53: 236.

34 Jones SE, Fulks Z, Bull M et al. Non-Hodgkin's lymphomas: IV. Clinicopathologic correlation in 405 cases. Cancer 1973; 31: 806.

35 Freeman C, Berg J, Cutler S. Occurrence and prognosis of extranodal lymphomas. Cancer 1972; 29: 252.

36 Boston HC, Dahlin D, Ivins J, Cupps R. Malignant lymphoma (so-called reticulum cell sarcoma) of bone. Cancer 1974; 34: 1131.

37 Jakobiec FA, Jones IS. Lymphomatous, plasmacytic, histiocytic, and hematopoietic tumors. In: Jakobiec FA, Jones IS eds Diseases of the Orbit. Hagerstown: Harper and Row, 1979: 309.

38 Carelli P, Cangelosi J. Angiosarcoma of the orbit. Am J Ophthalmol 1948; 31: 453.

39 Jakobiec FA, Jones IS. Vascular tumors, malformations, and degenerations. In: Jakobiec FA, Jones IS eds Diseases of the Orbit. Hagerstown: Harper and Row, 1979: 269.

40 Tsuda N, Takaku I. A case report of malignant vascular tumour of the orbit in a new born. Folia Ophthalmol Jap 1970; 21: 728.

41 Sekimoto T, Nakaseko H, Kondo K, et al. A case of malignant haemangioendothelioma in the orbit. Folia Ophthalmol Jap 1971; 22: 535.

42 Stout AP. Hemangio-endothelioma: a tumor of blood vessels featuring vascular endothelial cells. Ann Surg 1943; 118: 445.

43 Stout A, Lattes R. Tumors of the Soft Tissues. Armed Forces Institute of Pathology, 1968.

44 Jakobiec F, Howard G, Jones J et al. Hemangiopericytoma of the orbit. Am J Ophthalmol 1974; 78: 816.

45 Wright JE. Management of malignant orbital tumours. In: Oosterhuis JA ed Ophthalmic Tumours. Dordrecht: Dr W Junk, 1985: 229.

46 Henderson J. Orbital Tumors. Philadelphia: Saunders: 1973; 345.

47 Zimmerman LE. Lymphoid tumors. In: Boniuk M ed Ocular and Adnexal Tumors: New and Controversial Aspects. St Louis: Mosby, 1964: 429.

48 Morgan G, Harry J. Lymphocytic tumors of indeterminate nature: a 5-year follow up of 98 conjunctival and orbital lesions. Br J Ophthalmol 1978; 62: 381.

49 Foster SC, Wilson CS, Tretter PK. Radiotherapy of primary lymphomas of the orbit. Am J Roentgenol Radium Ther Nucl Med 1971; 111: 343.

50 Ziegler J. Burkitt's tumor. In: Holland J, Frei E eds Cancer Medicine. Philadelphia: Lea and Febiger, 1973: 1321.

51 Fenman SS, Niwayama G, Hapler RS, Foos RY. 'Burkitt tumor' with intraocular involvement. Survey Ophthalmol 1969; 14: 106.

52 Karp LA, Zimmerman LE, Payne T. Intraocular involvement in Burkitt's lymphoma. Arch Ophthalmol 1971; 85: 295.

53 Rodman HI, Font RL. Orbital involvement in multiple myeloma: review of the literature and report of 3 cases. Arch Ophthalmol 1972; 87: 30.

54 Benjamin I, Taylor H, Spindler J. Orbital and conjunctival involvement in multiple myeloma. Am J Clin Pathol 1975; 63: 811.

55 Little JM. Waldenström's macroglobulinaemia in the lacrimal gland. Trans Am Acad Ophthalmol Otolaryngol 1967; 71: 875.

56 Paufique L, Girard P, Schott B et al. Macroglobulino-secreting pseudolymphoma of the orbit. Ann Ocul 1969; 202: 1033.

57 Smith DG, Nesbitt ME, D'Angio GJ, Levitt SH. Histiocytosis X. Role of radiation therapy in management with special reference to dose levels employed. Radiology 1973; 106: 419.

58 Sims DG. Histiocytosis X: follow up of 43 cases. Arch Dis Child 1977; 52: 433.

59 Cohen M, Zorneza J, Cangir A, Murray JA, Wallace S. Direct injection of methyl sodium succinate in the treatment of solitary eosinophilic granuloma of bone. Radiology 1980; 136: 289.

60 Moore AT, Pritchard J, Taylor DSI. Histiocytosis X: an ophthalmological review. Br J Ophthalmol 1985; 69: 7.

61 Consul BN, Kulshrestha OP, Mehrotra AS. Bilateral proptosis in acute myeloid leukaemia. Br J Ophthalmol 1967; 51: 65.

62 Crombie AL. Proptosis in leukaemia. Br J Ophthalmol 1967; 51: 101.

63 Zimmerman LE, Font RL. Ophthalmologic manifestations of granulocytic sarcoma (myeloid sarcoma or chloroma): a clinicopathologic study of 33 cases. Am J Ophthalmol 1975; 80: 975.

64 Sanders TE. Mixed cell tumors of the lacrimal gland. Arch Ophthalmol 1939; 21: 239.

65 Font RL, Gammel JW. Epithelial tumors of the lacrimal gland. An analysis of 265 cases. In: Jakobiec FA ed Ocular and Adnexal Tumors. Birmingham, Alabama: Aesculapius, 1978: 737.

66 Wright JE, Stewart WB, Krohel GB. Clinical presentation and management of lacrimal gland tumours. Br J Opthalmol 1979; 63: 600.

67 Wright JE. Factors affecting the survival of patients with lacrimal gland tumours. Can J Ophthalmol 1982; 17: 3.

68 Forrest AW. Lacrimal gland tumors. In: Jakobiec FA, Jones IS eds Diseases of the Orbit. Hagerstown: Harper and Row, 1979: 355.

69 Jakobiec F, Ellsworth R, Tannenbaum M. Primary melanoma of the orbit. Am J Ophthalmol 1974; 787: 24.

70 Jakobiec FA, Jones IS. Neurogenic tumors. In: Jakobiec FA, Jones IS, eds Diseases of the Orbit. Hagerstown: Harper and Row, 1979: 371.

71 Schatz H. Benign orbital neurilemoma: sarcomatous transformation in von Recklinghausen's disease. Arch Ophthalmol 1971; 86: 268.

72 D'Agostino A, Soule E, Miller R. Primary malignant neoplasms of nerves (malignant neurilemomas) in patients without manifestations of multiple neurofibromatosis (von Recklinghausen's disease). Cancer 1963; 16: 1003.

73 D'Agostino A, Soule E, Miller R. Sarcomas of the peripheral nerves and soft tissues associated with neurofibromatosis (von Recklinghausen's disease). Cancer 1963; 16: 1015.

74 Grinberg M, Levy N. Malignant neurilemoma of the supraorbital nerve. Am J Ophthalmol 1974; 78: 489.

75 Welsh R, Bray D, Shipkey F, Meyer A. Histogenesis of alveolar soft part sarcoma. Cancer 1972; 29: 191.

76 Fisher E, Hazare J. Nonchromaffin paraganglioma of the orbit. Cancer 1952; 5: 521.

77 Deutsch AR, Duckworth JK. Nonchromaffin paraganglioma of the orbit. Am J Ophthalmol 1969; 68: 659.

78 Goder G. Nonchromaffin paraganglioma of the orbit. Zentralbl Allg Pathol 1970; 113: 167.

79 Wang-Huang L-F, Suzuki R, Soeno F, Ishitobi F, Watari T. A case of alveolar soft-part sarcoma of the orbit. Folia Ophthalmol Jpn 1986; 37: 552.

80 Jay B. Malignant melanoma of the orbit in a case of oculodermal melanosis (naevus of Ota). Br J Ophthalmol 1965; 49: 359.

81 Hagler W, Brown C. Malignant melanoma of the orbit arising in a nevus of Ota. Trans Am Acad Ophthalmol Otolaryngol 1966; 70: 817.

82 Reese AB. Congenital melanomas. Am J Ophthalmol 1974; 77: 798.

83 Leopold J, Richards D. Cellular blue naevi. J Pathol Bacteriol 1967; 94: 247.

84 Rodriguez H, Ackerman L. Cellular blue nevus: clinico-pathologic study of forty-five cases. Cancer 1968; 21: 393.

85 Henderson J, Farrow C. Malignant melanoma primary in the orbit: report of a case. Trans Am Acad Ophthalmol Otolaryngol 1972; 76: 1487.

86 Rottino A, Kelly A. Primary orbital melanoma: case report with review of the literature. Arch Ophthalmol 1942; 27: 934.

87 Wolter J, Bryson J, Blackhurst R. Primary orbital melanoma. Eye Ear Nose Throat Mon 1966; 45: 64.

88 Stern WE. Meningiomas in the cranio-orbital junction. J Neurosurg 1973; 38: 428.

89 Gordon E. Orbital extension of meningioma. Can J Ophthalmol 1970; 5: 381.

90 Wright JE, Call NB, Liaricos J. Primary optic nerve meningioma. Br J Ophthalmol 1980; 64: 553.

91 Craig W, Gogela L. Intraorbital meningiomas: a clinicopathologic study. Am J Ophthalmol 1949; 32: 1663.

92 D'Alena PR. Primary orbital meningioma. Arch Ophthalmol 1964; 71: 832.

93 Tan KK, Lim ASM. Primary extradural intra-orbital meningioma in a Chinese girl. Br J Ophthalmol 1965; 49: 377.

94 MacMichael IM, Cullen JF. Primary intraorbital meningioma. Br J Ophthalmol 1969; 53: 169.

95 Mandelcorn MS, Shae M. Primary orbital

perioptic meningioma. Can J Ophthalmol 1971; 6: 293.

96 Karp LA, Zimmerman LE, Borit A, Spencer W. Primary intraorbital melanomas. Arch Ophthalmol 1974; 91: 24.

97 Hannesson OB. Primary meningioma of the orbit invading the choroid: report of a case. Acta Ophthalmol 1971; 49: 627.

98 Rubinstein LJ. Tumors of the central nervous system. In: Atlas of Tumor Pathology, Second Series, Fascicle 6. Washington, DC: Armed Forces Institute of Pathology, 1972.

99 Eggers H, Jakobiec FA, Jones IS. Optic nerve gliomas. In: Jakobiec FA, Jones IS eds Diseases of the Orbit. Hagerstown: Harper and Row, 1979; 417.

100 Chutorian AM, Schwartz JF, Evans RA, et al. Optic gliomas in children. Neurology 1964; 14: 83.

101 Monschot WA. Primary tumours of the optic nerve in von Recklinghausen's disease. Br J Ophthalmol 1954; 38: 285.

102 Hoyt WF, Baghdassarian SB. Optic glioma of childhood: natural history and rationale for conservative management. Br J Ophthalmol 1969; 53: 793.

103 Gibberd FB, Miller TN, Morgan AD. Glioblastoma of the optic chiasm. Br J Ophthalmol 1973; 57: 788.

104 Crowe FW, Schull WJ. The diagnostic importance of the café-au-lait spot in neurofibromatosis. Arch Intern Med 1953; 91: 758.

105 Lloyd L. Gliomas of the optic nerve and chiasm in childhood. Trans Am Opthalmol Soc 1973; 72: 488.

106 Imes RK, Hoyt WF. Childhood chiasmal gliomas: update on the fate of patients in the 1969 San Francisco Study. Br J Ophthalmol 1986; 70: 179.

107 Editorial. Glioma of the optic nerve Lancet 1970; i: 229.

108 Taveras JM, Mount LA, Wood EH. The value of radiation therapy in the management of glioma of the optic nerves and chiasm. Radiology 1956; 66: 518.

109 Throuvalas N, Batain P, Ennuyer A. Gliomas of the chiasm and optic nerve: the place of transcutaneous radiotherapy in their treatment. Bull Cancer 1969; 56: 231.

110 Reese AB. Glioma of the optic nerve, retina and orbit. In: Tumors of the Eye. New York: Hoeber, 1963: 162.

111 Kingston JE, McElwain TJ, Malpas JS. Childhood rhabdomyosarcoma: experience of the Children's Solid Tumour Group. Br J Cancer 1983; 48: 195.

112 Knowles DM, Jakobiec FA, Jones IS. Rhabdo-

myosarcoma. In: Jakobiec FA, Jones IS eds Diseases of the Orbit. Hagerstown: Harper and Row, 1979: 435.

113 Porterfield JT, Zimmerman LE. Rhabdomyosarcoma of the orbit: a clinicopathologic study of 55 cases. Virchows Arch (Pathol Anat) 1962; 335: 329.

114 Patton RB, Horn RC. Rhabdomyosarcoma: clinical and pathological features and comparison with human fetal and embryonal skeletal muscle. Surgery 1962; 52: 572.

115 Kassel SH, Copenhaver R, Areán VM. Orbital rhabdomyosarcoma. Am J Ophthalmol 1965; 60: 811.

116 Frayer WC, Enterline HT. Embryonal rhabdomyosarcoma of the orbit in children and young adults. Arch Ophthalmol 1959; 62: 203.

117 Ashton N, Morgan G. Embryonal sarcoma and embryonal rhabdomyosarcoma of the orbit. J Clin Pathol 1965; 18: 699.

118 Jones IS, Reese AB, Krout J. Orbital rhabdomyosarcoma; an analysis of 62 cases. Trans Am Ophthalmol Soc 1965; 63: 223.

119 Knowles DM, Jakobiec FA. Rhabdomyoma of the orbit. Am J Ophthalmol 1975; 80: 1011.

120 Voûte PA, Barrett A. Rhabdomyosarcoma. In: Voute PA, Barrett A, Bloom HJG, Lemerle J, Neidhardt MK eds Cancer in Children: Clinical Management. Berlin: Springer-Verlag, 1986: 316.

121 Ghafoor SYA, Dudgeon J. Orbital rhabdomyosarcoma: improved survival with combined pulsed chemotherapy and irradiation. Br J Ophthalmol 1985; 69: 557.

122 Sutow WW, Lindberg RD, Gehan EA, Ragab AH, Roney RB, Ruymann F, Soiule EH. Three year relapse free survival rates in childhood rhabdomyosarcoma of the head and neck. Cancer 1982; 49: 2217.

123 Heyn RM, Holland R, Newton WA, Tefft M, Breslow N, Hartmann JR. The role of combined chemotherapy in the treatment of rhabdomyosarcoma in children. Cancer 1974; 34: 2128.

124 Yanoff M, Scheie HG. Fibrosarcoma of the orbit: report of two patients. Cancer 1966; 19: 1711.

125 Eifrig DE, Foos RY. Fibrosarcoma of the orbit. Am J Ophthalmol 1969; 67: 244.

126 Jakobiec FA, Howard G, Jones I, Tannenbaum M. Fibrous histiocytomas of the orbit. Am J Ophthalmol 1974; 77: 333.

127 Jakobiec F, Howard G, Rosen M, Wolff M. Leiomyoma and leiomyosarcoma of the orbit. Am J Ophthalmol 1975; 80: 1028.

128 Jakobiec FA, Jones IS. Mesenchymal and fibro-osseous tumors. In: Jakobiec FA, Jones IS

eds Diseases of the Orbit. Hagerstown: Harper and Row, 1979: 461.

129 Mortada A. Rare primary orbital sarcomas. Am J Ophthalmol 1969; 68: 919.

130 Holland M, Allen J, Ichinoise H. Chondrosarcoma of the orbit. Trans Am Acad Ophthalmol Otolaryngol 1961; 65: 898.

131 Cardenas-Ramirez L, Albores-Saavedra J, de Buen S. Mesenchymal chondrosarcoma of the orbit: report of the first case in orbital location. Arch Ophthalmol 1971; 86: 410.

132 Trzcinska-Dabrowska Z. Mesenchymal chondrosarcoma. Arch Ophthalmol 1972; 88: 85.

133 Guccion J, Font R, Enzingere F, Zimmerman L. Extraskeletal mesenchymal chondrosarcoma. Arch Pathol 1973; 95: 336.

134 Bone R, Butler H, Harris B. Osteogenic sarcoma of the frontal sinus. Ann Otolaryngol 1973; 82: 162.

135 Abramson DH, Ellsworth RM, Kitchin FD, Tung G. Second nonocular tumors in retinoblastoma survivors: are they radiation-induced? Ophthalmology 1984: 91; 1351.

136 Draper GJ, Sanders BM, Kingston JE. Second primary neoplasms in patients with retinoblastoma. Br J Cancer 1986; 53: 661.

137 Fu YS, Perzin KH. Non-epithelial tumors of the nasal cavity, paranasal sinuses and nasopharynx: a clinicopathologic study: II. Osseous and fibro-osseous lesions, including osteoma, fibrous dysplasia, ossifying fibroma, osteoblastoma, giant cell tumor and osteosarcoma. Cancer 1974; 33: 1289.

138 Henderson JW. Orbital Tumors. Philadelphia: Saunders; 1973: 444.

139 Porterfield J. Orbital tumors in children. Int Ophthalmol Clin 1962; 2: 319.

140 Apple DJ. Wilms' tumor metastatic to the orbit. Arch Ophthalmol 1968; 80: 480.

141 Albert DM, Rubenstein RA, Scheie HG. Tumor metastasis to the eye: II. Clinical study in infants and children. Am J Ophthalmol 1967; 63: 727.

142 Ferry A, Font R. Carcinoma metastatic to the eye and orbit: I. A clinicopathologic study of 227 cases. Arch Ophthalmol 1974; 92: 276.

143 Alfano JE. Ophthalmological aspects of neuroblastomatosis: a study of 53 verified cases. Trans Am Acad Ophthalmol Otolaryngol 1968; 72: 830.

144 Levy WJ. Neuroblastoma. Br J Ophthalmol 1957; 41: 48.

145 Coley B, Higinbotham N, Bowden L. Endothelioma of bone (Ewing's sarcoma). Ann Surg 1948; 128: 533.

146 Iliff W, Marback R, Green WR. Invasive squamous cell carcinoma of the conjunctiva. Arch Ophthalmol 1975; 93: 119.

147 Ryan S, Font R. Primary epithelial neoplasms of the lacrimal sac. Am J Ophthalmol 1973; 76: 73.

148 Rao N, Font R. Mucoepidermoid carcinoma of the conjunctiva: a clinicopathologic study of 5 cases. Cancer 1976; 38: 1699.

149 Boniuk M, Zimmerman LE. Sebaceous carcinoma of the eyelid, eyebrow, caruncle and orbit. Trans Am Acad Ophtholmol Otolaryngol 1968; 72: 619.

150 Conley JJ. Sinus tumors invading the orbit. Trans Am Acad Ophthalmol Otolaryngol 1966; 70: 615.

151 Starr H, Zimmerman L. Extrascleral extension and orbital recurrence of malignant melanomas of the choroid and ciliary body. Int Ophthalmol Clin 1962; 2: 369.

152 Kersten RC, Tse T, Anderson RL, Blodi FC. The role of orbital exenteration in choroidal melanoma with extrascleral extension. Ophtholmology 1985; 92: 436.

153 Hungerford J, Kingston J, Plowman N. Orbital recurrence of retinoblastoma. Ophthalmic Paediatrics and Genetics 1987; 8: 63.

154 Andersen SR. Medulloepithelioma of the retina. Int Ophthalmol Clin 1962; 2: 483.

Textbook of Uncommon Cancer
Edited by C.J. Williams, J.G. Krikorian, M.R. Green and D. Raghavan
© 1988 John Wiley & Sons Ltd

Chapter **51**

Uncommon Tumours of the Eye

John Hungerford
Consultant Ophthalmic Surgeon, St. Bartholomew's Hospi-
tal, London; Consultant Surgeon, Moorfields Eye Hospital,
London, UK

TUMOURS OF THE RETINA

Primary tumours of the retina are much less common than those of the uveal tract and most are rare. In contrast to uveal tumours, primary retinal neoplasms are substantially commoner than lesions metastatic to the retina and occur significantly more frequently in children than in adults.

Primary Tumours of the Retina

Retinoblastoma

This is an embryonal tumour of developing photoreceptors. The overwhelming majority of examples occur in very young children and the neoplasm may be congenital. Occasionally the tumour is seen in older children and adolescents but very rarely in adults. There are two distinct forms of the disease, one inherited and the other not (1). The clinical management is made complex because of the possibility of inherited susceptibility to the tumour, because multiple tumours may occur, and because there is a potential for development of new ocular tumours over a period of several years (2). Furthermore, there is a highly significant incidence of second, non-ocular tumours in survivors of the genetically determined type of retinoblastoma (3–8). Modern treatment

methods can save vision as well as life and it is essential to identify which children presenting with the neoplasm are at risk from further ocular tumours and which family members may also develop the disease. The best overall results are to be obtained by a firm policy of repeated examinations of affected individuals and repeated prospective examinations of family members at risk. The interval between each examination may be the same for already affected and for as yet unaffected children but the risk of tumour formation diminishes with increasing age and the interval between examinations may gradually be extended (9) (Table 1).

Approximately one-third of cases of retinoblastoma are genetically determined. The gene responsible behaves as an autosomal dominant with high penetrance and nearly 50% of the offspring of survivors are affected. All children of affected parents should be examined from the earliest age possible according to the plan proposed. In developing countries, nearly all genetically determined cases are sporadic and even in developed countries, where treatment has been available for several generations, only 1 in 10 new cases of retinoblastoma has a family history of the disease. Approximately 5% of patients with retinoblastoma have associated mental retardation and developmental abnormalities and in their somatic karyotype these

955

TABLE 1 PROSPECTIVE EXAMINATION OF
          CHILDREN AT RISK OF DEVELOPING
          RETINOBLASTOMA

| Examination under anaesthesia (EUA) |
| First EUA aged 2 to 4 weeks |
| Then EUAs as follows |
Year 1	every 3 months
Year 2–	every 4 months
Years 3–5	every 6 months
Examination without anaesthesia
Years 6–10 every 12 months

individuals can be shown to have a deletion of band 14 in the long arm of chromosome 13 (10). Persons with this 13q minus or 'D-deletion' syndrome also have half the normal level of a tissue enzyme of uncertain function, esterase D (11). The levels of this enzyme can be estimated in red cells (12) and reduced levels are a useful marker of the deletion (13).

There is no difference in appearance or clinical behaviour between a tumour of the genetic type and one of the non-genetic variety. Nevertheless there are clinical indicators of genetic determination in most cases where an abnormal gene is responsible. It is of the utmost importance to recognize these indicators because the clinical management of retinoblastoma of the genetic and non-genetic types is significantly different. In non-genetic retinoblastoma of the genetic and non-genetic types is significantly different. In non-genetic retinoblastoma the tumour is invariably solitary whereas in the genetic type multiple tumours are encountered in some 90% of cases and commonly affect both eyes. This is a very useful indicator; the presence of more than one tumour confirms categorically that the disease is genetically determined and indicates that more tumours may develop in the course of time. This is particularly important when two tumours are detected in one eye of a child without a family history of this disease because it means that the other eye is substantially at risk and that repeat examinations are especially necessary. The presence of only one tumour suggests that the disease is non-genetic but not categorically so because one tumour only may develop in a small proportion of genetically determined cases. Sometimes this dilemma may be resolved by another clinical feature, the age of onset. The average age of onset in genetic disease, is 8 months (9) and the majority of cases have presented by age 3 years. By contrast, the average age of onset for retinoblastoma of the non-genetic type is 17 months (9) though cases may occur well into the teens. Generally, it can be safely assumed that a child presenting with unilateral retinoblastoma over the age of 5 years has the non-genetic form of the disease but a child under that age must undergo repeat examinations because there is nearly one chance in three that he or she will develop more than one tumour.

It is now known that an allelic pair of genes exists in the normal cell, each one of which is somehow capable of preventing the development of retinoblastoma. Only loss of both alleles in a cell can lead to the development of the tumour (14). One of these alleles is missing in all somatic cells of an individual with genetically determined retinoblastoma and it is the loss of this allele which is inherited. Loss of this one allele alone is insufficient for tumour formation or the entire retina in each eye would become neoplastic; the second allele must be lost before a neoplastic transformation can take place. This does happen in nearly all genetic cases but in relatively few cells so that the total number of tumours averages only five. The time scale is variable and the tumours can occur over a period of years but is relatively short because each cell has already lost one allele. This may account for the early onset of retinoblastoma in genetic cases. It seems that the pair of genes primarily responsible for retinoblastoma may in some way suppress the development of certain non-ocular tumours (15), particularly soft tissue sarcomas and melanomas, because of an exceptionally high incidence of these neoplasms in survivors of genetic retinoblastoma. The second allele may not be lost in any retinal cell in some people with loss of the first allele in all cells. These individuals presumably also run a high risk of developing other tumours even if they do not develop retinoblastoma. More particularly, though, they are carriers and are at risk of producing more than one affected child even though there is no apparent family history. This is not a rare event; approximately one in 20 healthy parents producing a child with retinoblastoma will produce another affected child even though they have no evidence or history of the tumour themselves. For this reason all siblings under age 5 years of a child with retinoblastoma should be examined prospectively at regular intervals.

Some two-thirds of individuals with retinoblastoma have the non-genetic type and all their somatic cells are normal. For a tumour to form in the retina of such a person a single retinal cell must lose both alleles of the gene responsible for retinoblastoma. It is assumed that two separate mutational events are responsible for this loss. The chances of two such events taking place in more than one cell are remote so that the non-genetic tumours are solitary. Furthermore the extra time required for successive loss of the two alleles may explain the relatively late onset in non-genetic retinoblastoma.

The *clinical appearance* of retinoblastoma varies according to its mode of growth within the eye and the stage at which it is first detected. The most common mode of presentation in the United Kingdom is with a white pupil or 'leucocoria' (Figure 1) (9). This appearance is generally caused by a large 'endophytic' retinoblastoma growing forwards into the vitreous cavity where it may occasionally be mistaken for a granuloma caused by the nematode worm *Toxocara canis*. Leucocoria may also result from an 'exophytic' retinoblastoma growing under the retina and producing a serous retinal detachment, when it may be hard to distinguish from the retinal exudation seen in a vascular anomaly termed Coats' disease, and from retinopathy of prematurity (ROP). Coats' disease is by far the most common condition simulating retinoblastoma. A tumour may be detected at a much earlier stage if it arises at the macula. Such a lesion disturbs central vision and may result in strabismus which leads to its discovery. This is the second commonest presentation of retinoblastoma in the United Kingdom (9). A small tumour may also be found in the second eye of an individual newly discovered to have reti-

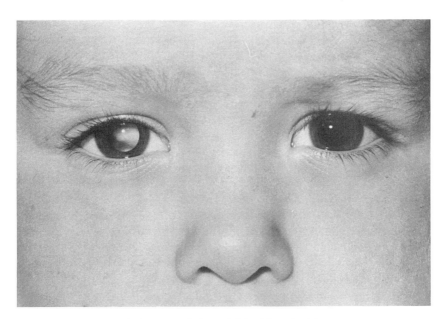

Figure 1 Leucocoria in a child with retinoblastoma.

noblastoma or it may be detected during subsequent examination of an affected child or during prospective examination of a family member at risk. The small tumour is hemispherical in contour and paler than the surrounding retina. At first it may appear translucent but later takes on a pinkish hue with fine blood vessels visible on the surface (Figure 2). Only when the tumour becomes a little larger still does it appear white. A solitary small tumour in a child without a family history of retinoblastoma may be mistaken for the astrocytic hamartoma of the retina characteristic of tuberous sclerosis in the absence of other stigmata of this disease. Clumps of tumour cells may break off a larger retinoblastoma lesion and float free in the vitreous where they may be thought to represent an inflammatory endophthalmitis (Figure 3). Very occasionally some of these cells may find their way into the anterior chamber and settle to form a psuedohypopyon which may simulate intraocular inflammation (Figure 4). When a tumour becomes very large, iris neovascularization may occur so that the irides appear of different colour. The new blood vessels may result in glaucoma which, in

a child, leads to expansion of the globe and may be mistaken for congenital glaucoma. Where medical advice is not freely available the tumour may not be detected before it has ruptured the globe (see Chapter 50) by its continued expansion and invaded the orbit where, in a child, it may simulate orbital inflammation or a primary orbital tumour (Figure 5).

The *diagnosis* of retinoblastoma is essentially a clinical one and, although certain non-invasive techniques may help to distinguish the tumour from simulating lesions, the distinction may be very difficult, even when the patient is assessed in a specialist unit. B-scan ultrasound may help to differentiate a non-neoplastic retinal detachment from one resulting from retinoblastoma and furthermore may demonstrate the presence of calcium within the lesion. Calcium is better seen on ultrasound or computed tomography (CT) (Figure 6) than on plain x-ray. Whilst not pathognomonic, calcium in certain distribution patterns is strongly suggestive of retinoblastoma. The perinatal history may suggest that ROP is possible and systemic examination may demonstrate stig-

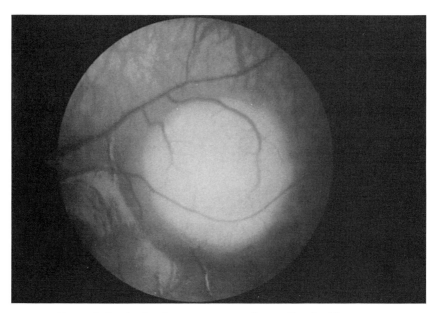

Figure 2 Ocular fundus appearance of a small retinoblastoma.

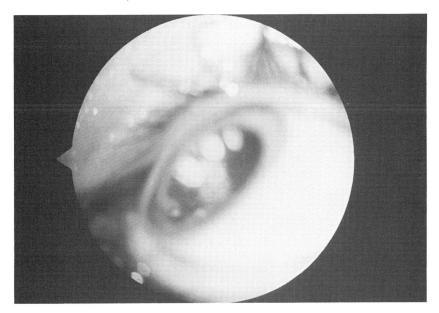

Figure 3 Vitreous seeding of retinoblastoma.

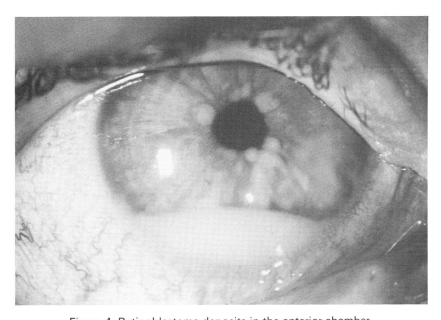

Figure 4 Retinoblastoma deposits in the anterior chamber.

mata of a generalized disorder such as tuberous sclerosis. The presence of vitreous cells may suggest a diagnosis of *Toxocara canis* infestation, though a positive enzyme-linked immunosorbent assay (ELISA) test for *Toxocara* should be regarded with caution as it is perfectly possible for a child with retinoblastoma also to have *Toxocara*. Invasive tests should be avoided if at all possible because of the very real risk of spilling retinoblastoma cells when the eye is opened and because of the very poor prognosis for a consequent orbital recurrence. Vitreous

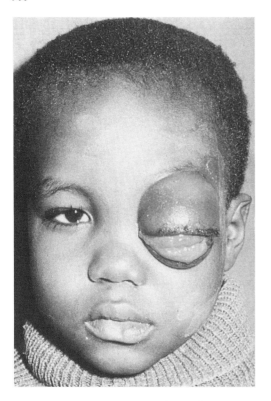

Figure 5 Orbital extension of retinoblastoma.

biopsy is extremely hazardous and should never be performed under any circumstances when a diagnosis of retinoblastoma is considered possible. Very occasionally a paracentesis and aqueous tap may be performed when cells in the anterior chamber may possibly be inflammatory. The procedure should be carried out through the clear cornea so that the needle track may subsequently be observed. The levels in aqueous of various enzymes including lactate dehydrogenase and phosphoglucose isomerase have been compared with those in serum in retinoblastoma and in other simulating conditions (16) but the results are insufficiently specific for a reliable diagnosis to be made on the basis of the test and to justify the hazard of opening the globe.

In a child presenting with leucocoria the tumour is usually sufficiently advanced that *treatment* by enucleation of the eye cannot be avoided. The decision to enucleate should be based on strict clinical criteria and the operation should not be performed simply because only one eye is affected or because one eye has more extensive tumour than the other. Clearly, when both eyes are extensively involved there may be justification for a trial of conservative therapy for the least affected eye. Enucleation should be performed whenever glaucoma is present or it is suspected that extrascleral extension of the tumour may have occurred and whenever tumour obscures the optic disc. An eye with a retinoblastoma associated with a total retinal detachment is unlikely to be retained with useful vision and should probably be removed, though a trial of conservative therapy may be justified if ultrasound indicates that the tumour is not adjacent to the optic disc. Retinoblastoma shows a pronounced tendency to grow down the optic nerve and when histological examination reveals tumour at the resected end of the nerve there is a substantial risk of incurable intracranial and meningeal spread. Surgically, therefore, every effort must be made to obtain as long a length of the orbital portion of the optic nerve as possible.

Retinoblastoma is a radiosensitive tumour and radiotherapy is the major conservative treatment modality. Most tumours treatable by this method receive external beam radiotherapy. The external beam approach is applicable to all retinoblastomas which do not fulfil the criteria for enucleation of the eye and it is considered prudent to treat the whole retina to a total dose of 40 Gy in 20 fractions over 4 weeks. When tumour extends to the ora serrata, which marks the anterior limit of the retina, and when there is evidence of extensive vitreous seeding it is necessary to irradiate the whole eye including the lens in case malignant cells have passed into the anterior chamber. When the other eye is in situ and free from disease a megavoltage anterior external beam approach is usually employed, with the beam exiting through brain. When the other eye has been removed, photons from a linear accelerator may be used and the beam directed to exit through the enucleated orbit. Should both eyes

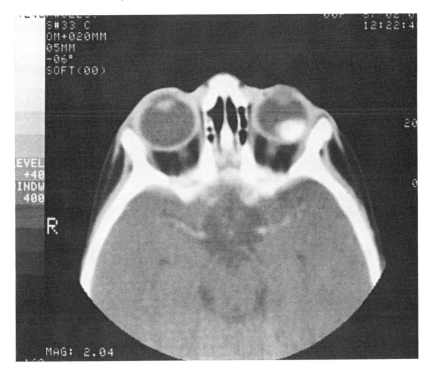

Figure 6 CT appearance of calcification in intraocular retinoblastoma.

require external beam radiotherapy, opposed lateral portals may be used, again employing a linear accelerator. Although adequate fractionation substantially reduces morbidity from radiation choroidoretinopathy a whole eye approach is inevitably followed by the development of a cataract some 2 or more years after the completion of radiotherapy. Radiation also results in lid shrinkage leading to corneal exposure. This may combine with reduced tear production, also brought about by radiotherapy, to produce a corneal opacity which limits the visual results of modern lens aspiration techniques. For tumours posterior to the ora serrata and in the absence of extensive vitreous seeding it is unnecessary to irradiate the lids, lacrimal and accessory lacrimal glands, cornea, and lens. With the aid of a contact lens acting as a fixed reference point on the eye, a collimated, penumbra trimmed beam of photons from a linear accelerator may be guided accurately behind the lens but to

deliver the full dose of 40 Gy to the whole retina (17–19).

It is unnecessary to irradiate the whole retina for certain medium-sized and small retinoblastoma situated in favourable locations and focal treatment methods may be employed, keeping whole retina irradiation in reserve for treatment failures and for new tumours in unfavourable locations. Medium-sized tumours up to 13 mm in diameter may be treated by radiation brachytherapy employing cobalt-60 (9, 20–23), ruthenium-106 (24), or iodine-125 (25) surface applicators sutured temporarily to the sclera over the base of the tumour and left in place until a dose of 40 Gy has been delivered to the apex of the neoplasm. Two surface applicators may be employed simultaneously provided the treatment fields do not overlap at the optic disc or macula to exceed a dose of 50 Gy. When more than two lesions of this size require treatment, or when such a tumour is situated adjacent to the optic disc or macula, brachytherapy is contraindicated and an external beam approach is to be preferred.

Small tumours may be treated without resort to radiotherapy. Posterior to the equator of the eye, xenon arc photocoagulation (26) through the dilated pupil is the treatment of choice for any tumour of 4 mm diameter or less which does not abut the optic disc or macula. It is essential not to treat the tumour directly for this may lead to explosive release of malignant cells into the vitreous and a subsequent, massive, diffuse recurrence which may be difficult to treat. The aim of photocoagulation is to destroy the blood supply of the retinoblastoma by surrounding it with gentle burns in healthy retina. Several treatments may be required at intervals of 2 or 3 weeks before the tumour is replaced by a flat scar which is adjudged inert. Anterior to the equator, photocoagulation is technically difficult and there may be no adequate margin of healthy retina between the tumour and the ora serrata. In this situation, triple-freeze cryotherapy (27) may be performed for tumours of 7 mm diameter or less. Treatment is applied through the sclera under indirect ophthalmosocopy control, using a probe placed in the conjunctival fornix and without the need for an incision in the conjunctiva. Triple-freeze cryotherapy is applied directly to the retinoblastoma because the lesion is destroyed by lysis of tumour cells and there is no risk that active malignant cells will be disseminated through the vitrous. The ice-ball must envelope the whole tumour mass if not during the first treatment session then, at least, during subsequent applications as the lesion shrinks. One or more treatments will be required at 2- or 3-week intervals until the tumour is replaced by a flat scar. The presence of lens opacity or vitreous opacity, sometimes as a result of previous treatment, may also preclude photocoagulation. Under these circumstances, cryotherapy may be applied behind the equator, though not to the region of the optic disc or macula. A surgical incision in the conjunctiva will be required for adequate access of the cryotherapy probe to a posterior tumour.

Once a tumour has been successfully treated by whatever form of therapy there remains the risk that a further tumour or tumours will develop. All patients should be examined prospectively as outlined in Table 1, whether they are known to have the genetically determined form of retinoblastoma or not. This risk is significantly less following external beam radiotherapy of the whole retina than after focal therapy with radioactive plaque, photocoagulation, or cryotherapy. Presumably, when the whole retina is irradiated, some tumours are destroyed when they are so small that they cannot yet be seen on ophthalmoscopy. Nevertheless, approximately 1 patient in 12 develops a further retinoblastoma after external beam radiotherapy. Further irradiation of the whole retina to a full tumour dose of 40 Gy in such a patient results in substantial loss of vision from severe radiation choroidoretinopathy (28). With adequate post-irradiation follow-up, most new tumours will be small enough for management by photocoagulation or cryotherapy and without recourse to radiation. If further radiotherapy is required, a plaque should be used if at all possible. This will limit the volume of retina and choroid receiving a double dose of radiation. Provided that the new lesion is not situated close to the optic disc or macula, a child who undergoes scleral plaque therapy after external beam irradiation will retain useful central vision. Occasionally, untreated ocular lesions of retinoblastoma may not progress or may undergo regression (29). The mechanism or mechanisms involved are not understood (30, 31).

Although excellent survival rates have been reported for retinoblastoma, some 5% of children die from deposits of the tumour in the central nervous system, bone and bone marrow, or viscera. Certain histological and clinical indicators of high risk have been identified.

Retinoblastoma may escape from the eye by invading the optic nerve, the choroid, or the sclera. Mortality from optic nerve invasion only becomes significant when the resected end of the nerve is infiltrated by tumour (32). When extension of tumour to the cut end is the only adverse histological indicator, 67% of children survive (32). The choroid must be invaded extensively by tumour before a deleterious effect on survival is seen. When extensive invasion of the choroid is the only adverse histological finding, 59% of children survive (32). A combination of optic nerve invasion by retinoblastoma to the resected end and extensive choroidal invasion reduces survival to 22% (32). Histological evidence of trans-scleral extension of retinoblastoma is accompanied by a survival rate of 36% (32).

Biopsy proven orbital recurrence of retinoblastoma is a serious adverse clinical indicator of survival. In a series of 25 patients, all children with this complication died (33) and in a more recent study of 16 cases of orbital recurrence of retinoblastoma only one child survived (6%) (34).

Histological evidence of trans-scleral extension, invasion by retinoblastoma cells of the resected end of the optic nerve, and orbital recurrence are indications for radical orbital radiotherapy. Prior to treatment, the extent of any intraorbital or intracranial mass lesion should be delineated as far as possible by a CT head scan, and meningeal involvement excluded by lumbar puncture and cerebrospinal fluid (CSF) cytology. Any orbital mass should be excised and a tissue diagnosis of retinoblastoma made before radiotherapy is commenced. Although a dose of 50 Gy in 25 fractions over 4 weeks has been found to prevent local orbital recurrence after extraocular spread of retinoblastoma, children continue to die from meningeal or distant metastatic spread. A case can be made for combining orbital radiotherapy with neuraxis irradiation when the resected end of the optic nerve is involved or when there is orbital recurrence, together with intrathecal chemotherapy when retinoblastoma cells are demonstrated on CSF cytology. If heavy choroidal invasion or trans-scleral spread of retinoblastoma is demonstrated, bone marrow aspiration and cytology

and a bone scan should be performed. Although there are very few reports of sustained remissions in established systemic retinoblastoma following the use of chemical agents, there may be a case for adjuvant chemotherapy if systemic staging investigations are negative for disseminated retinoblastoma and in addition to radiotherapy where appropriate. There is probably no case for the use of chemotherapy as a first-line treatment for intraocular retinoblastoma.

Some 2% of children with genetically determined retinoblastoma present within 6 years of the ocular diagnosis with symptoms of hydrocephalus or diabetes insipidus. On CT head scan a solitary, enhancing, midline lesion is found in the region of the pineal or the anterior end of the third ventricle. Most of these children have not had unfavourable histology and are regarded as having ectopic intracranial retinoblastomas rather than metastases (35). Despite adequate radiotherapy to the ectopic tumour all children with this condition in one large series died from widespread meningeal disease (36). If an ectopic or 'trilateral' retinoblastoma is discovered, staging investigations must include lumbar puncture and CSF cytology together with a myelogram, and current policy is to irradiate the whole neuraxis to a dose of up to 30 Gy, depending on the age of the child, with an additional 10 Gy to the main ectopic tumour and to any satellite lesions demonstrated by the myelogram. Simultaneously, adjuvant systemic chemotherapy may be given, together with appropriate intrathecal chemotherapy if CSF cytology is positive for retinoblastoma. As yet there are no long-term survivors from this approach.

Metastatic retinoblastoma remains notoriously resistant to chemotherapy. Information on the efficacy of single agents is limited but responses have been reported for cyclophosphamide (37), ifosfamide (38) and Adriamycin (39). In two drug regimens the best results have been achieved with a combination of vincristine and cyclophosphamide and, recently, the four agent combination of vincristine, cyclophosphamide, cis-platinum, and

VM26 has produced lengthy remissions in metastatic retinoblastoma.

Adenocarcinoma of the Retinal Pigment Epithelium

This very rare pigmented tumour occurs in the retinal or ciliary pigment epithelium (40–46). It is extremely difficult to distinguish clinically from a uveal melanoma, a melanocytoma, and in some instances, reactive hyperplasia of the retinal pigment epithelium. The diagnosis is almost invariably a surprise histological finding when an eye is enucleated for a presumed choroidal or ciliary body malignant melanoma (43). Histologically, it may be difficult to distinguish between a benign adenoma and an adenocarcinoma of the pigment epithelium. Even when the histology is considered malignant, the tumour rarely metastasizes.

The *clinical appearance* may help to differentiate the tumour from the much commoner alternative diagnosis of melanoma. The adenocarcinoma is jet black compared with the grey brown appearance of a melanoma. A melanocytoma is also jet black. The melanocytoma is a benign tumour and, typically, occurs adjacent to the optic disc. In this particular situation it may be especially difficult to distinguish between a carcinoma of the retinal pigment epithelium and a melanocytoma. There are no specific investigations to assist in the *diagnosis* and no data on the most appropriate *treatment*.

UVEAL TUMOURS

A tumour may develop in any of the three constituent parts of the uveal tract; the iris, the ciliary body, and the choroid. The iris is the least frequent site for tumour formation and the choroid the most frequent. Metastatic tumours are commoner than primary neoplasms of the uveal tract. By far the commonest primary tumour is malignant melanoma. Other primary malignant tumours are exceedingly rare.

Primary Tumours of the Uvea

Leiomyoma

This rare tumour of smooth muscle is much commoner in the iris and ciliary body than in the choroid. It is usually benign. In a series of 21 leiomyomas, 4 were classified as malignant but no tumour-related deaths were recorded (47).

The *clinical appearance* of a leiomyoma in the iris is of a pale, slightly elevated mass typically situated at the pupil margin, suggesting that the tumour most commonly arises from the sphincter pupillae. A ciliary body leiomyoma may expand to invade the iris root and anterior chamber. In both situations leiomyoma is extremely difficult to distinguish from an amelanotic melanoma on clinical criteria. In the iris the much rarer rhabdomyosarcoma may be mistaken for a leiomyoma. A solitary report exists of a leiomyoma arising in the choroid (48). The only certain means of establishing the *diagnosis* is by excision biopsy and this approach is indicated for a pale iris tumour which has been documented to grow. Sector iridectomy or iridocyclectomy to include the tumour mass with a small margin of healthy tissue is technically straightforward and has a low complication rate. A pale iris or ciliary body tumour is much more likely to be an amalenotic malignant melanoma and exclusion of this diagnosis by excision of the lesion more than justifies the cosmetic blemish and the minor photophobia which may follow removal of a sector of iris. Local recurrence after excision is extremely unlikely and no further *treatment* is required, even in the unlikely event of the histology indicating a malignant form of leiomyoma.

Medulloepithelioma

Medulloepitheliomas arise in the primitive medullary epithelium. This comprises the inner layer of the embryonic optic cup, derivatives of which include the non-pigmented ciliary epithelium and the iris pigment epithelium which are generally classified as uveal structures, and the neurons and neuroglia of the sensory retina which are not. Although this neoplasm has been reported outside the uveal tract in the retina (49) and in the optic nerve (50, 51), it is usually encountered in the iris or ciliary body and it will be convenient to discuss medulloepithelioma arising in all possible sites under the uveal heading. The tumour is commonly termed dictyoma by opthalmologists. It is regarded as a congenital tumour and presents most frequently in children or young adults. The neoplasm is usually benign or of low grade malignancy. In one series 6 out of 23 medulloepitheliomas (52) and in another 37 out of 56 of these tumours were classified as malignant (53). Metastasis of medulloepithelioma is rare and when death occurs it usually results from invasive local recurrence.

The *clinical appearances* are very variable. In its commoner, anterior location within uveal structures the tumour may present as a grey mass arising from the ciliary body (Figure 7) or as a pigmented mass arising from the posterior surface of the iris. It may have a predominantly cystic aspect. There may be associated glau-

coma, cataract, or persistent hyperplastic primary vitreous. In the ciliary body the tumour must be distinguished from other neoplasms, particularly retinoblastoma and amelanotic melanoma, from non-neoplastic inflammatory conditions including pars planitis, and from a granuloma due to the nematode *Toxocara canis*. Medulloepithelioma grows relatively slowly and prolonged pressure on the lens of the eye may result in a notch. In this way it should be possible to distinguish the tumour from a rapidly growing neoplasm such as retinoblastoma but less easy to make the distinction between a medulloepithelioma and a slowly growing amelanotic melanoma in a younger person. A rare medulloepithelioma in the iris may be difficult to distinguish from an even rarer, but benign, glioneuroma.

In its less common, posterior location outside the uveal tract a medulloepithelioma of the retina is reported to have presented in a child with a white pupil similar to that seen in retinoblastoma (49). A medulloepithelioma expanding the optic nerve and disc can present with loss of vision and a dilated pupil, or with proptosis. In a child or young person it may be

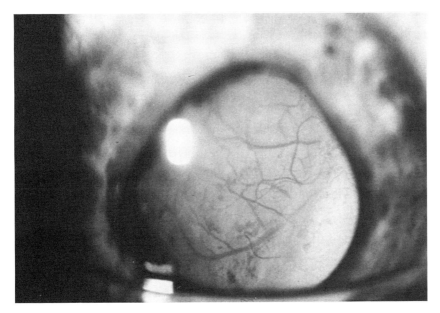

Figure 7   Medulloepithelioma arising from the ciliary body in a 7 year old boy.

difficult to distinguish from an astrocytic hamartoma unless general examination suggests that the individual has tuberous sclerosis or neurofibromatosis, which are associated with these benign astrocytic lesions. Other simulating lesions are juvenile pilocytic astrocytoma of the optic nerve or meningioma of the optic nerve sheath unless, once again, it is apparent that the patient has neurofibromatosis which predisposes to both these conditions.

Clinical *diagnosis* of medulloepithelioma depends on the appearance in a young patient of a non-pigmented tumour mass visible within the eye or, perhaps, demonstrated on orbital CT in an individual presenting with proptosis. Even with the assistance of ancillary investigations including ophthalmic ultrasound, fluorescein angiography, and the radioactive phosphorus test it may be difficult to be confident of a diagnosis of medulloepithelioma based on clinical criteria alone. A tissue diagnosis is to be preferred but in most cases histology has been obtained by enucleation of the eye. For a tumour confined to the iris an excisional biopsy is theoretically possible and may be delayed until growth of a tumour is documented (54). For a ciliary body tumour, iridocyclectomy will be required. It is difficult to achieve complete surgical clearance of this tumour by such procedures, particularly when there is a marked cystic component, and in practice few eyes are retained after attempted conservative excision. There is an inherent risk that the tumour may, after all, be a retinoblastoma and that an intraocular procedure might seriously limit a child's chances of survival (55). This possibility would seem to contraindicate retinal biopsy for a posterior lesion in the retina which statistically is very much more likely to be retinoblastoma. Medulloepithelioma involving the optic disc is not amenable to a conservative biopsy procedure although, in the unlikely event of the disc being spared, a retrobulbar optic nerve medulloepithelioma could be diagnosed by excision of the nerve via a lateral orbitotomy approach.

The *treatment* of choice for an extensive medulloepithelioma is enucleation of the eye with an adequate length of optic nerve when the latter is involved. Removal of the globe is also advised if attempted excision of a more localized tumour by iridectomy proves incomplete. Overall mortality from malignant medulloepithelioma is only 10%. Most deaths occur from direct orbital and subsequent intracranial extension rather than from metastases and the presence of extrascleral extension is the most important adverse prognostic factor (53). Orbital exenteration is indicated for extrascleral spread and radiotherapy and chemotherapy may be considered for patients relapsing locally or at a distant site.

Rhabdomyosarcoma

Within the eye, this tumour has been an unexpected histological finding on very rare occasions (56, 57) although rhabdomyosarcomatous differentiation is recognized as one of the features of malignancy in medulloepithelioma (58).

The *clinical appearance* has been of a pale iris mass indistinguishable from an amelanotic melanoma or leiomyoma. There are no specific features to aid the *diagnosis* as, to date, the tumour has been a chance finding in enucleated eyes. Accordingly there are no data on conservative *treatment*.

Malignant Lymphoma

Intraocular deposits of malignant lymphoma are uncommon. Almost all the reported examples have been of 'histiocytic' lymphoma. Lymphocytic lymphomas within the eye are exceedingly rare. Intraocular lymphoma occurs predominantly in uveal structures but the retina too may be involved and will be considered with the uveal sites.

'Histiocytic' Lymphoma 'Reticulum Cell Sarcoma'

Ophthalmologists know this tumour as 'reticulum cell sarcoma'. This term should be discarded in favour of the newer terms such as 'histiocytic' lymphoma. The tumour affects predominantly elderly people and, ultimately, is usually bilateral (59). The ocular involvement can include the iris, the choroid, the retina, the optic nerve, and the vitreous. Frequently, the ocular presentation of 'histiocytic' lymphoma is closely followed by central nervous system or systemic involvement (60). For this reason, all patients in whom this diagnosis is established should undergo periodic review for systemic and central nervous system (CNS) disease.

When iris involvement predominates, the *clinical appearance* may be indistinguishable from a granulomatous anterior uveitis or a metastasis (61). When the involvement is mainly choroidal, the differential diagnosis includes posterior uveitis (62) and, once again, metastasis (63). Copious cells within the vitreous may obscure the ocular fundus (64) and suggest a diagnosis of inflammatory vitritis. Retinal deposits are yellowish and characteristically multifocal (65). The *diagnosis* may be established by cytological examination of aqueous humour obtained by paracentesis (66) or of vitreous humour obtained by vitrectomy (67). Alternatively, where appropriate, fine needle biopsy of a visible mass may be performed. The cell yields may be poor in quantity and quality using these approaches and the best results are obtained from surgical biopsy of the iris or choroid when this is possible. Systemic staging investigations are essential and should include assessment of the CNS, and bone marrow aspiration and cytology.

The *treatment* of ocular 'histiocytic' lymphoma is fractionated radiotherapy to the whole eye to a total dose of 15 to 30 Gy. The tumour is extremely radiosensitive but the condition is notoriously difficult to diagnose and treatment is usually begun late in the course of the disease. Accordingly, the visual outlook is poor. Most patients die of systemic lymphoma within 2 years of the ocular diagnosis (61, 68) but improved survival has been reported after simultaneous irradiation of the central nervous system and the eye (69).

Lymphocytic Lymphoma

Intraocular deposits of lymphocytic lymphoma are exceedingly rare and few of the reported cases have been supported by reliable histology. Ocular involvement has been described in Hodgkin's lymphoma (70), lymphosarcoma (71), Burkitt's lymphoma (72, 73), and mycosis fungoides (74, 75). In the absence of a prior diagnosis of lymphocytic lymphoma the *clinical appearance* and indeed the histology of an intraocular deposit may be difficult to distinguish from that of 'histiocytic' lymphoma or benign reactive lymphoid hyperplasia. Even in the presence of an existing diagnosis of systemic lymphocytic lymphoma it may be difficult to distinguish clinically between an opportunistic intraocular infection with cytomegalovirus or a fungus in the immune suppressed individual and the much rarer alternative of an intraocular lymphoma deposit. The reported cases are so few that it is not possible to comment precisely on the best methods of *diagnosis* and *treatment* but a similar approach to that advised for 'histiocytic' lymphoma is advocated.

Leukaemia

The eye is a potential sanctuary site for leukaemia deposits because, developmentally, it is part of the brain. Many of the drugs used in standard chemotherapy regimens cross neither the blood–brain nor the blood–retina barrier and so do not enter the eye. The relative rarity of ocular relapse of leukaemia has to be set against the development of radiation cataract when considering radiotherapy cranioprophylaxis and the eyes are not routinely treated. All uveal structures may become involved, particularly in acute leukaemias (76). The retina and retinal pigment epithelium. the vitreous, and the optic nerve may also harbour leukaemic deposits and involvement of these structures will be considered under the uveal heading.

In iris involvement the *clinical appearance* is one of iris thickening with nodule formation and occasionally a tumour pseudohypopyon. The clinical signs may be difficult to distinguish from those of inflammation. Yellow choroidal deposits may be seen and, when the retina is involved, the picture is predominantly one of retinal infarction with intraretinal and preretinal haemorrhages and, occasionally, neovascularization (77, 78). Haemorrhage may break through into the vitreous gel. Clumping of pigment has been reported in the retinal pigment epithelium similar to the 'leopard spot' appearance seen in choroidal metastases (79, 80). Swelling of the optic nerve head may be difficult to distinguish from papilloedema due to intracranial leukaemia involvement when it is bilateral. As with lymphomas it is important to recognize that opportunistic intraocular infections may simulate leukaemia deposits. Intraocular biopsy by fine needle aspiration (81), or by surgical biopsy of choroid or retina (82) is rarely needed to establish the *diagnosis* of leukaemia for the patient as a whole because this is usually known or can be established by blood and bone marrow studies. The value of these techniques is to make the distinction between an intraocular leukaemia deposit and an opportunistic infection in order to establish the overall disease status of the patient and to determine the most appropriate ocular treatment. Ocular deposits of leukaemia respond well to fractionated radiotherapy. A dose of 24 Gy is appropriate. The visual results are good but the major indication is to establish complete clinical remission of the systemic disease.

Secondary tumours

Uveal Metastases

Metastases to the choroid are amongst the commonest of all intraocular tumours but secondary deposits in the iris, ciliary body, and retina are uncommon.

Metastatic iris tumours may be solitary or multiple. The *clinical appearance* is of one or more yellowish, vascular iris nodules (83), which, unlike most primary iris tumours, grow rapidly. Occasionally, malignant cells may settle in the anterior chamber to produce a pseudohypopyon. A similar appearance may be encountered when an intraocular tumour such as a retinoblastoma becomes dispersed throughout the eye. A ciliary body metastasis may be indistinguishable from a primary tumour such as a melanoma except in its rate of growth. Metastasis to the retina (84) has been reported and is characterized by seeding of tumour cells into the vitreous. The *diagnosis* of an intraocular metastasis can usually be made on clinical criteria. Even if a primary tumour elsewhere has not already been identified, serial observation will commonly demonstrate the rapid growth which is the hallmark of an intraocular metastasis. If a tissue diagnosis is required, this may be obtained by fine needle aspiration or by biopsy for iris and ciliary body lesions. *Treatment* is palliative and by radiotherapy.

REFERENCES

1 Hungerford JL. Recent advances in the understanding of retinoblastoma. Trans Ophthalmol Soc UK 1985; 104: 832.

2 Hungerford JL, Kingston J, Plowman N. Tumours of the eye and orbit. In: Voûte PA, Barrett A, Bloom HJG, Lemerle J, Neidhardt MK eds Cancer in Children: Clinical Management. Heidelberg: Springer-Verlag, 1986: 223.

3 Aherne G. Retinoblastoma associated with other primary malignant neoplasms. Trans Ophthalmol Soc UK 1974; 94: 938.

4 Abramson DH, Ellsworth RM, Zimmerman LE. Non-ocular cancer in retinoblastoma survivors. Trans Am Acad Ophthalmol Otolaryngol 1976; 81: 454.

5 Draper GJ, Sanders BM, Kingston JE. Second primary neoplasms in patients with retinoblastoma. Br J Cancer 1986; 53: 661.

6 François J. Retinoblastoma and osteogenic sarcoma. Ophthalmologica 1977; 175: 185.

7 Abramson DH, Ronner HJ, Ellsworth RM. Second tumors in nonirradiated bilateral retinoblastoma. Am J Ophthalmol 1979; 86: 624.

8 Abramson DH, Ellsworth RM, Kitchin FD,

Tung G. Second non-ocular tumors in retinoblastoma survivors: are they radiation induced? Ophthalmology 1984; 91: 1351.

9 Bedford MA, Bedotto C, MacFaul P. Retinoblastoma: a study of 139 cases. Br J Ophthalmol 1969; 55: 19.

10 Yunis JJ, Ramsay N. Retinoblastoma and subband deletion of chromosome 13. Am J Dis Child 1978; 132: 161.

11 Sparkes RJ, Sparkes MC, Wilson MG et al. Regional assignment of genes for human esterase D and retinoblastoma to chromosome band 123 of 14. Science 1980; 208: 1042.

12 Cowell JK, Rutland P, Jay M, Hungerford J. Effect of the esterase D phenotype on its in vitro activity. Hum Genet 1986; 74: 298.

13 Cowell JK, Thompson E, Rutland P. The need to screen all retinoblastoma patients for esterase D activity: detection of submicroscopic deletions. Arch Dis Child 1987; 62: 8.

14 Knudson AG Jr. Mutation and cancer: a statistical study of retinoblastoma. Proc Natl Acad Sci USA 1971; 68: 820.

15 Murphree AL, Benedict WF. Retinoblastoma: clues to human oncogenesis. Science 1984; 223: 1028.

16 Fellberg NT, McFall R, Shields JA. Aqueous humour enzyme patterns in retinoblastoma. Invest Ophthalmol 1977; 16: 1039.

17 Schipper J. An accurate and simple method for megavoltage radiation therapy of retinoblastoma. Radiother Oncol 1983; 1: 31.

18 Schipper J, Tan KEWP, van Peperzeel HA. Treatment of retinoblastoma by precision megavoltage radiation therapy. Radiother Oncol 1985; 3: 117.

19 Harnett AN, Hungerford J, Lambert G, Hirst A, Darlinson R, Hart B, Trodd TC, Plowman PN. Modern lateral external beam (lens sparing) radiotherapy for retinoblastoma. Ophthalmic Paediatrics and Genetics 1987; 8: 53.

20 Stallard HB. Radiotherapy of malignant ocular neoplasms. Br J Ophthalmol 1948; 32: 639.

21 Stallard HB. The irradiation of retinoblastoma. Trans Ophthalmol Soc UK 1960; 80: 589.

22 Stallard HB. The treatment of retinoblastoma. Mod Probl Ophthalmol 1968; 7: 149.

23 Buys RJ, Abramson DH, Ellsworth RM, Haik B. Radiation regression patterns after cobalt plaque insertion for retinoblastoma. Arch Ophthalmol 1983; 101: 1206.

24 Lommatzsch PK. Beta-irradiation of retinoblastoma with $^{106}Ru^{106}Rh$ applicators. Mod Probl Ophthalmol 1977; 18: 128.

25 Sealy R, LeRoux PLM, Rapley F et al. The treatment of ophthalmic tumours with low energy sources. Br J Radiol 1976; 49: 551.

26 Höpping W, Meyer-Schwickerath G. Light coagulation and cryotherapy. In: Blodi FC ed Retinoblastoma. New York: Churchill Livingstone, 1985. 95.

27 Tolentino FI, Tablante RT. Cryotherapy of retinoblastoma. Arch Ophthalmol 1972; 87: 52.

28 Abramson DH, Ellsworth RM, Rosenblatt M et al. Retreatment of retinoblastoma with external beam irradiation. Arch Ophthalmol 1982; 100: 147.

29 Smith JLS. Histology and spontaneous regression of retinoblastoma. Trans Ophthalmol Soc UK 1974; 94: 953.

30 Gallie BL, Phillips RA, Ellsworth RM, Abramson DH. Significance of retinoma and phthisis bulbi for retinoblastoma. Ophthalmology 1982; 89: 1393.

31 Margo C, Hidayat Kopelman J, Zimmerman LE. Retinocytoma; a benign variant of retinoblastoma. Arch Ophthalmol 1983; 101: 1519.

32 Hungerford J, Kingston J, Plowman N. Histological risk factors influencing survival in retinoblastoma. International Symposium on Intraocular Tumours. Czech Ophthalmological Society, Bratislava, 1986. In press.

33 Reese AB. Retinoblastoma. In: Reese AB Tumors of the Eye. London: Cassell, 1951: 67.

34 Hungerford J, Kingston J, Plowman N. Orbital recurrence of retinoblastoma. Ophthalmic Paediatrics and Genetics 1987; 8: 63.

35 Bader JL, Miller RW, Meadows AT, Zimmerman LE, Champion LAA, Voûte PA. Trilateral retinoblastoma. Lancet 1980; ii: 582.

36 Kingston JE, Plowman PN, Hungerford JL. Ectopic intracranial retinoblastoma in childhood. Br J Ophthalmol 1985; 69: 742.

37 Lonsdale D, Berry DH, Holcomb TM et al. Chemotherapeutic trials in patients with metastatic retinoblastoma. Cancer Chemother Rep 1968; 52: 631.

38 Pratt CB, Crom DB, Howarth C. The use of chemotherapy for extraocular retinoblastoma. Med Pediatr Oncol 1985; 13: 330.

39 Ragab AH, Suton WW, Komp DM, Starling A, Lyon GM, George S. Adriamycin in the treatment of childhood solid tumors. A Southwest Oncology Group Study. Cancer 1975; 36: 1572.

40 Fair JR. Tumors of the retinal pigment epithelium. Am J Ophthalmol 1958; 45: 495.

41 Garner A. Tumours of the retinal pigment epithelium. Br J Ophthalmol 1970: 54: 715.

42 Tso MOM, Albert DM. Pathological conditions of the retinal pigment epithelium: neoplasms and nodular non neoplastic conditions. Arch Ophthalmol 1972; 88: 27.

43 Shields JA, Zimmerman LE. Lesions simulating malignant melanoma of the posterior uvea. Arch Ophthalmol 1973; 89: 466.

44 Minckler D, Allen AW. Adenocarcinoma of the

retinal pigment epithelium. Arch Ophthalmol 1978; 96: 2252.

45 Vogel MH, Woltz U. Malignant epitheliomas of the retinal pigment epithelium. Klin Mbl Augenheilk 1979; 175: 592.

46 Laqua H. Tumors and tumor-like lesions of the retinal pigment epithelium. Ophthalmologica 1981; 133: 34.

47 Ashton N. Primary tumours of the iris. Br J Ophthalmol 1964; 48: 650.

48 Jakobiec FA, Witschel H, Zimmerman LE. Choroidal leiomyoma of vascular origin. Am J Ophthalmol 1976; 82: 205.

49 Mullaney J. Primary malignant medulloepithelioma of the retinal stalk. Am J Ophthalmol 1974; 77: 499.

50 Green WR, Iliff WJ, Trotter RR. Malignant teratoid medulloepithelioma of the optic nerve. Arch Ophthalmol 1974; 91: 451.

51 Reese AB. Medulloepithelioma (dictyoma) of the optic nerve. Am J Ophthalmol 1957; 44: 4.

52 Anderson SR. Medulloepithelioma of the retina. Int Ophthalmol Clin 1962; 2: 483.

53 Broughton WL, Zimmerman LE. A clinicopathologic study of 56 cases of intraocular medulloepitheliomas. Am J Ophthalmol 1978; 85: 407.

54 Morris AT, Garner A. Medulloepithelioma involving the iris. Br J Ophthalmol 1975; 59: 276.

55 Shields JA. Tumors of the nonpigmented ciliary epithelium. In: Diagnosis and Management of Intraocular Tumors. St Louis: Mosby, 1983: 322.

56 Woyke S, Chevinot R. Rhabdomyosarcoma of the iris: report of the first recorded case. Br J Ophthalmol 1972; 56: 60.

57 Naumann G, Font RL, Zimmerman LE. Electron microscopic verification of primary rhabdomyosarcoma of the iris. Am J Ophthalmol 1972; 74: 110.

58 Zimmerman LE, Font RL, Anderson SY. Rhabdomyosarcomatous differentiation in malignant intraocular medulloepitheliomas. Cancer 1972; 30: 817.

59 Barr CC, Green WR, Payne JW, Knox DL, Jensen AD, Thompson RL. Intraocular reticulum cell sarcoma: a clinicopathologic study of four cases and review of the literature. Surv Ophthalmol 1975; 19: 224.

60 Appen RE. Posterior uveitis and primary cerebral reticulum cell sarcoma. Arch Ophthalmol 1975; 93: 123.

61 Collyer R. Reticulum cell sarcoma of the eye and orbit. Can J Ophthalmol 1972; 7: 247.

62 Currey TA, Deutsch AR. Reticulum cell sarcoma of the uvea. South Med J 1965; 58: 919.

63 Stephens RF, Shields JA. Diagnosis and management of cancer metastatic to the uvea; a study of 70 cases. Ophthalmology 1979; 86: 1336.

64 Kennerdell JS, Johnson BL, Wizotskey HM. Vitreous cellular reaction; association with reticulum cell sarcoma of the brain. Arch Ophthalmol 1975; 93: 1341.

65 Gass JDM, Sever RJ, Grizzard WS, Clarkson JG, Blumenkranz M, Wind CA, Shugarman R. Multifocal pigment epithelial detachment by reticulum cell sarcoma. Retina 1984; 4: 135.

66 Shields JA. Intraocular lymphoid tumors and leukaemias. In: Diagnosis and Management of Intraocular Tumors. St Louis: Mosby: 1983; 619.

67 Michels RG, Knox DL, Erozen YS, Green WR. Intraocular reticulum cell sarcoma: diagnosis by pars plana vitrectomy. Arch Ophthalmol 1975; 93: 1331.

68 Vogel MH, Font RL, Zimmerman LE, Levine RA. Reticulum sarcoma of the retina and uvea. Am J Ophthalmol 1968; 66: 205.

69 Char DH, Margolis L, Newman AB. Ocular reticulum cell sarcoma. Am J Ophthalmol 1981; 91: 480.

70 Primbs GB. Monsees WE, Irvine AR. Intraocular Hodgkin's disease. Arch Ophthalmol 1961; 66: 477.

71 Lewis RA, Clark RB. Infiltrative retinopathy in systemic lymphoma. Am J Ophthalmol 1970; 79: 48.

72 Feman SS, Niwayama G, Hepler RS, Foos RY. "Burkitt tumor" with intraocular involvement. Surv Ophthalmol 1969; 14: 106.

73 Karp LA, Zimmerman LE. Intraocular involvement in Burkitt's lymphoma. Arch Ophthalmol 1971; 85: 295.

74 Foerster HC. Mycosis fungoides with intraocular involvement. Trans Am Acad Ophthalmol Otolaryngol 1960; 64: 308.

75 Keltner JL, Fritsch E, Cykiert RC, Albert DM. Mycosis fungoides: intraocular and central nervous system involvement. Arch Ophthalmol 1977; 95: 645.

76 Allen RA, Straatsma BR. Ocular involvement in leukaemia and allied disorders. Arch Ophthalmol 1961; 66: 490.

77 Leveille AS, Morse PH. Platelet-induced retinal neovascularization in leukaemia. Am J Ophthalmol 1981; 91: 640.

78 Morse PH, McCready JL. Peripheral retinal neovascularization in chronic myelocytic leukaemia. Am J Ophthalmol 1971; 72: 975.

79 Clayman H, Flynn J, Koch K, Israel C. Retinal pigment abnormalities leukaemic disease. Am J Ophthalmol 1972; 74: 416.

80 Jakobiec FA, Behrens M. Leukaemia retinal pigment epitheliopathy. J Pediatr Ophthalmol 1975; 12: 10.

81 Schwarz M, Schumann GB. Acute leukaemic

infiltration of the vitreous diagnosed by pars plana aspiration. Am J Ophthalmol 1980; 90: 326.

82 Taylor D, Day S, Tiedemann K, Chessels J, Marshall WC, Constable IJ. Chorioretinal biopsy in a patient with leukaemia. Br J Ophthalmol 1981; 65: 489.

83 Freeman TR, Friedman AH. Metastatic carcinoma of the iris. Am J Ophthalmol 1975; 80: 947.

84 Young SE, Cruciger M, Lukeman J. Metastatic carcinoma to the retina: a case report. Ophthalmology 1979; 86: 1350.

Section **X**

Head and Neck Tumours

Textbook of Uncommon Cancer
Edited by C.J. Williams, J.G. Krikorian, M.R. Green and D. Raghavan
© 1988 John Wiley & Sons Ltd

Chapter **52**

The Diagnosis and Management of Nasopharyngeal Carcinoma in Caucasians

Lester J. Peters*, John G. Batsakis†, Helmuth Goepfert‡ and Waun K. Hong§
*Head, Division of Radiotherapy, †Head, Division of Pathology, ‡Chairman, Department of Head and Neck Surgery and §Chief, Section of Head and Neck Medical Oncology, The University of Texas M.D. Anderson Hospital and Tumor Institute, Houston, Texas, USA

HISTORY

The first histologically confirmed case of cancer of the nasopharynx was probably that reported by Michaux (1) who in 1845 described a 45-year-old male with carcinoma of the base of the skull. There is anthropologic evidence, however, that the disease has existed for many centuries. For example, Strouhal (2) described an ancient Egyptian skull from the cemetery at Naga-ed-Der in Upper Egypt with features consistent with extensive destruction by a nasopharyngeal cancer. The first English language review of the disease is contained in Chapter 68 of the textbook 'Diseases of the Nose and Throat' by Bosworth in 1889 (3). Further details of the history of this fascinating disease may be found in the article by Muir (4).

EPIDEMIOLOGY, ETIOLOGY PATHOLOGY AND BIOLOGY

Cancer of the nasopharynx, in the generic sense, includes carcinomas, sarcomas, and lymphomas (See Chapter 53). Throughout the world, however, 'nasopharyngeal cancer' pragmatically refers to carcinoma and to a specific category of carcinoma, abbreviated as NPC. While potentially a source of confusion NPC designates non-glandular malignancies arising from the epithelium lining the surface and crypts of the nasopharynx. On the basis of ultrastructural features, all types of NPC may be regarded as variants of squamous cell carcinoma (Figure 1) and are subclassifiable into groups on the basis of their predominant pattern as viewed by the light microscope (5–9).

NPC represents a nearly unique model in human neoplasia because of its etiopathogenic relationships between viral infection, neoplastic transformation and immune response of the host (5, 10). Its clinicopathologic aspects, histology, clinical staging systems and genetic as well as environmental variables have further positioned NPC into a stalking-horse role in oncologic research (5).

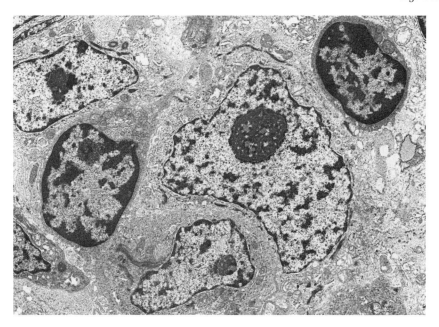

Figure 1 Electron micrograph of undifferentiated carcinoma of nasopharynx showing epidermoid characteristics, e.g. cell junctions and tonofilaments. Original magnification: ×9000.

Surgical and Microscopic Anatomy of the Nasopharynx

Anatomical Considerations

The roof of the nasopharynx begins behind the posterior nasal choanae and slopes downward where it becomes continuous with the posterior wall. The bony roof and posterior wall are formed serially by the basisphenoid, basiocciput and anterior arch of the atlas. The lateral and posterior walls are, in part, upward extensions of the boundaries of the oropharynx. In the lower part of the lateral wall, the superior constrictor muscle sends its fibers posteriorly to attach to the basisphenoid. Between the upper border of the superior constrictor and the skull's base is stretched the pharyngobasilar fascia with the eustachian tube lodged between the medial pterygoid plate and the superior constrictor. The tubal ampulla's inward bulge creates a slit-like space between it and the posterior wall; the pharyngeal recess or fossa of Rosenmüller, filled, in part, by the levator palati muscle which lies between the pharyngobasilar fascia and the mucous membrane (11).

The nasopharyngeal lymphoid tissue or adenoid is concentrated at the junction of the roof and posterior wall of the post-nasal space. There are other lymphoid aggregates about the tubal openings. The sensory nerve supply to the post-nasal space is provided by the glossopharyngeal and maxillary nerves (11).

Beneath the mucous membrane of the roof is the vestigial pharyngeal hypophysis. Lying in the midline near the vomero-sphenoidal articulation, its presence is a reminder of the embryologic origin of the anterior pituitary from Rathke's pouch. The hypophyseal vestige may be partly or completely surrounded by the basisphenoid. Also in the midline but dorsal along the roof and separated from the pharyngeal hypophysis by adenoidal tissue is an epithelial recess, sometimes called the pharyngeal bursa, an occasional locus of inflammation or cyst formation. Believed to be formed by a tethering of pharyngeal endoderm to the tip of the embryonic notochord, the recess has no relationship with Rathke's pouch (11).

Microscopic Anatomy

Batsakis et al. (5) have summarized our current knowledge of the histology of the nasopharynx's mucosa. It is composed of three basic cell types: pseudostratified columnar (respiratory) cells, squamous cells, and intermediate (pseudostratified) cuboidal cells. All three types are found during fetal development with the respiratory type being the first to evolve. There is an increase in squamous epithelium until, in the adult nasopharynx, the dominance of respiratory over squamous epithelium is reversed. A commensurate increase in the intermediate type of epithelium is not seen, but it persists at junctions between respiratory and squamous epithelia with its greatest density at the junction of the oro- and nasopharynx. In the adult, squamous epithelium covers approximately 60% of the entire nasopharyngeal surface.

The intermediate epithelium is aptly named since it is intermediate in a topographic as well as cytologic sense. Investigations in nonhuman species have indicated change of some of the intermediate cells to either ciliated respiratory or squamous cells (5). Resembling the intermediate cell layers in both respiratory and squamous epithelia, the intermediate epithelium's greatest density is in the sites of predilection for nasopharyngeal carcinomas (NPC) and it is also the closest normal histologic homologue of the nonkeratinizing or undifferentiated carcinomas of the nasopharynx (5).

Etiology and Epidemiology

The etiology of NPC is very likely multifactorial; genetic, environmental and viral (10, 12–14). There are at least three major risk factors: (1) a genetically determined predisposition allowing an Epstein–Barr virus (EBV) infection of the type that permits (2) integration of the genomes of the virus into the chromosomes of some nasopharyngeal epithelial cells, thereby priming them for (3) neoplastic transformation by some environmental cofactor. Alternatively, the environmental agent(s) may trigger the viral genome in the cells to oncogenic activity.

Although environmental factors appear to be essential, the high frequency in disparate ethnic groups points (Tables 1 and 2) to different operative agents for each group (5, 7, 10, 13–20). As judged by age-specific incidences, Scandinavians and American blacks and whites appear to have a different etiologic origin for NPC from that of Chinese Americans, or Hong Kong or Singapore Chinese. In Chinese the incidence curves rise sharply after the third decade; those for non-Chinese show a rise after the fourth or fifth decade. Native Alaskans have a curve pattern similar to that of

TABLE 1 GEOGRAPHIC INCIDENCE OF NPC PER 100 000 POPULATION PER YEAR

Geographic site: ethnic characteristic	Males	Females	Combined
Hong Kong: Chinese	35.5	15.1	—
Hong Kong: Chinese (boat people)	54.7	18.8	—
Singapore: Chinese	20.2	9.0	—
San Francisco-Oakland: Chinese	17.8	—	—
Alaska: native population	13.5	3.7	—
Tunisia: blacks	7.5	3.3	—
Japan, Korea: native population	1–2	0.4	—
North American: white (Connecticut)	0.17	0.05	0.22
Norway: native population	0.16	0.09	0.35

Adapted from Moloy et al. (19).

TABLE 2 MORTALITY OF
NASOPHARYNGEAL
CARCINOMA

Location	Annual mortality (per 100 000)
USA	0.6–0.9
Taiwan	1.5
China	
Guangdong	6.5
Zhongshan	10.4
Guangxi	4.7
Hunan	3.2
Shanxi	0.4

Adapted from Hwang (14).

Chinese, but Tunisians have a bimodal curve, with an early peak in the second decade.

Epidemiologic Features of United States

Levine and others (21) have studied demographic patterns for nasopharyngeal carcinoma in the United States. These were obtained from the Third National Cancer Survey, the Surveillance, Epidemiology, and End Results Program and the Connecticut Tumor Registry. Approximately 7 out of every 8 malignant tumors of the nasopharynx (1202 patients) were classified as NPC. While 84% of white patients with cancer of the nasopharynx had NPC, more than 90% of nonwhite patients had NPC. The preponderance of NPC in the case material held for all but the youngest patients; sarcomas were the more frequent among whites under 10 years of age. White patients had the highest frequency of squamous cell carcinomas. Undifferentiated carcinomas were more common in black and Chinese American patients and were relatively frequent in young patients of all races. Chinese Americans have a greater risk of developing NPC than any other racial/ethnic group in the United States. Whites and blacks have similar risks, except at young ages where there is a minor post-adolescent age peak in NPC risk that is more pronounced for United States blacks than for whites (22). A similar young age peak has been observed in other parts of

the world such as India, Tunisia and the Sudan but remains unexplained. The apparent excess risk in the young black United States population has been considered to be related to rural residence and low socioeconomic status (23).

The morbidity data from the United States do not show outstanding geographic or temporal variation in NPC risk for whites (21, 23). Only the relatively high mortality rate in Alaska stands out as a significant factor in mortality studies of the states and counties (18).

Epstein–Barr Virus and Biologic Implications

The Epstein–Barr virus (EBV) is ubiquitous in humans and antibodies to polypeptides of the virus are present in over 80% of human serum samples from the United States and in higher percentages from Asian and African populations (10, 13, 24). Practically no one escapes infection from this herpes-group virus. Primary infections often remain clinically inapparent or not recognized as being due to EBV, particularly in subjects under the age of 3 to 5 years.

Consequences of EBV infection vary in different populations, i.e it is associated predominantly with infectious mononucleosis in the western hemisphere, Burkitt's lymphoma in Africa, and nasopharyngeal carcinoma in Asia. Occurrence of these three EBV-associated diseases is unusual outside their normally associated populations, suggesting strongly the role of additional factors in the populations at risk. The apparent differences in geographic distribution of the three main EBV-associated diseases have also prompted suggestions that different strains of EBV are prevalent in different areas. This has not been verified and likely is not a factor (10, 13).

Clinically manifest or not, primary EBV infections establish a permanent EBV carrier state in the lymphatic system and also in the major salivary glands (25). This is reflected in the life-long persistence of EBV-specific antibodies, at almost constant titers, and an intermittent excursion of EBV into the oropharynx (10, 13, 25, 26).

Although the precise role of EBV in cellular transformation has been difficult to elucidate, it does appear to be different from that of another herpes virus (simplex) where a 'hit and run' mechanism has been proposed. EBV displays an extreme tropism for human B lymphocytes, preferentially infecting B cells in vitro and having a relationship with three B cell lymphoproliferative disorders; infectious mononucleosis, Burkitt's lymphoma and lymphomas in immunocompromised hosts. The marked affinity for the B lymphocyte relates to the existence of a B cell-specific receptor for EBV (140–145 kilodalton c3d receptor molecule CR2) on B lymphocytes, but not found on any other hematopoietic cell (10, 13, 27).

Difficult to reconcile with the lymphotropic behavior of EBV have been: (a) consistent presence of EBV genomes in malignant cells of nasopharyngeal carcinoma, (b) a similar association with so-called lymphoepithelial carcinomas of the salivary glands and thymus, and (c) replication of EBV in patients lacking antibodies to major EBV-related early antigens. It has been argued that epithelial cells are not the natural targets for EBV infection but that indirect access to such cells is obtained through their fusion with a virus-infected B cell or by formation of pseudotype particles in which EBV capsids acquire envelopes from an unrelated epitheliotropic virus.

There is, however, a growing belief that EBV can directly infect epithelial cells as evidenced by the surface expression of a functional EBV receptor on cells lining the uterine cervix and oropharynx (27). It further appears as if the expression of the receptor molecule is differentiation-linked in stratified epithelium—just as it is in B lymphocytes.

It remains for in-vitro studies to ascertain how the EBV/cell interaction may be influenced by anatomic site and/or level of differentiation of the target epithelial cells. Young and associates (27) postulate that infec-tion of receptor-positive basal epithelial cells, followed by virus replication in progeny cells could provide a self-sustaining reservoir to maintain the apparent virus carrier state of B lymphoid tumors.

Transfection studies point to an immortalizing sub-genomic fragment of EBV and these studies suggest EBV contains a gene(s) capable of immortalizing primary epithelial cells, that is stimulating them to proliferate continuously, at least in culture (28). After time in culture, epithelial cells show an unaltered chromosomal pattern and EBV DNA 'footprints' can be detected in total chromosomal DNA. Transformation of cells is not total since the epithelial cells are not able to produce tumors in immunoincompetent animals and there is limited growth in low serum and semisolid media (28).

The data from epithelial cultures are in apparent conflict with some of the studies directed towards localizing a transforming function in B lymphocytes. This may possibly be explained by the appreciation that a genome as large as EBV's (172 000 base pairs) may well have encoded within it more than one immortalizing function.

Although our knowledge of the immortalization phenomenon has increased greatly in the last few years, not much is known about the manner in which EBV imparts to its target cell the information to grow continuously. It does appear that the particular host cell in which the viral genome finds itself is a crucial determinant of the outcome of the viral infection (10, 13). In one type of cell, the virus replicates and in a different cell type, the path is towards cell transformation. For the DNA viruses involved in the causation of naturally occurring tumors, the tumorigenic action can be rapid and direct, or chronic and probably indirect, as in the case of hepatitis virus B. The papilloma viruses and EBV may merely increase a target cell population that runs the risk of undergoing malignant change. With EBV, a combination of viral immortalization and chronic infections may create a preneoplastic population of cells, partially blocked in their differentiation and at risk for a crucial chromosomal translocation that initiates the growth of an autonomous neoplastic clone.

Ubiquitous tumor viruses such as EBV have a long symbiotic history with their host and in the event this has ensured a tight surveillance system that prevents growth of transformed cells.

Pathology

Classification and Histology of Nasopharyngeal Carcinoma

Regardless of geographic distributions, the nonglandular, nonlymphomatous and nonsarcomatous malignancies are the most common neoplasms of the nasopharynx (5) (Table 3). In high risk regions these carcinomas dominate

TABLE 3 CARCINOMAS OF THE NASOPHARYNX

Nasopharyngeal carcinoma (NPC)
  Squamous cell
  Nonkeratinizing
  Undifferentiated

Adenocarcinomas
  Salivary type
  Nonsalivary type

Neuroendocrine carcinoma

Teratocarcinoma

cancer statistics for the head and neck (Table 4) (5, 7, 14, 15, 18, 19, 29).

Over the years, diversity of diagnostic nomenclature and an absence of a uniform histologic reporting system have bedeviled correlation with results of therapy and prognosis (5). Cognizant of this, the World Health Organization (WHO) has divided nasopharyngeal carcinoma into three histologic types: squamous cell, nonkeratinizing, and undifferentiated (5, 7, 9). The categories are distinct and cover the spectrum of NPC's micromorphology (Table 5).

Microscopically, *squamous cell carcinoma* of the nasopharynx is like squamous cell carcinomas in other anatomic sites of the upper aerodigestive tracts. The carcinomas manifest obvious and readily identifiable keratin products and their growth pattern is typical of that found in any squamous cell carcinoma (Figure 2). In general, the carcinoma is moderately differentiated and is accompanied by a desmoplastic host response. Since it is preponderantly a surface growth, endoscopic examination of the nasopharynx usually identifies the carcinoma. This form of NPC has little or no association with EBV and serologic titers are similar to control subjects. The average age of patients with squamous cell carcinoma of the nasopharynx is somewhat older than that for all NPC patients. It is rarely found in patients younger than 40 years of age (9).

TABLE 4 GEOGRAPHIC VARIATION OF HISTOLOGIC TYPES OF MALIGNANT NEOPLASMS OF THE NASOPHARYNX[a]

| Geographic site | NPC | Histologic types (% of all malignant neoplasms of nasopharynx) | | |
		Adenocarcinoma	Lymphoma	Others
USA	86.3	4.0	7.2	2.5
UK	70.2	2.9	21.5	5.5
Japan	79.2	2.9	15.8	2.1
Uganda	92.2	0.0	3.3	4.4
Tunisia	93.7	1.4	4.9	0.0
Taiwan	97.1	1.9	0.9	0.1
Singapore	98.7	0.3	0.7	0.3
Columbia	94.2	1.3	3.9	0.6

[a] After the compilation by Bedoya and Betancur (15).

TABLE 5 CLASSIFICATION OF NASOPHARYNGEAL CARCINOMA
(NPC)

WHO Classification	Former terminology
Type 1: Squamous cell carcinoma	Squamous cell carcinoma
Type 2: Nonkeratinizing carcinoma without lymphoid stroma With lymphoid stroma	Transitional cell carcinoma; intermediate cell carcinoma Lymphoepithelial carcinoma (Regaud)
Type 3: Undifferentiated carcinoma without lymphoid stroma With lymphoid stroma	Anaplastic carcinoma; clear cell carcinoma Lymphoepithelial carcinoma (Schmincke)

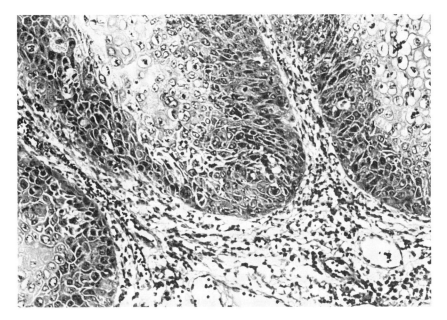

Figure 2 Keratinizing squamous cell carcinoma of nasopharynx, WHO Type 1.
H&E, original magnification: ×400.

Nonkeratinizing carcinoma of the WHO classification is distinct from both squamous cell and undifferentiated carcinomas (5, 7, 9). It is a category accommodating carcinomas that are neither keratinizing nor undifferentiated. Like the squamous carcinomas, nonkeratinizing carcinomas exhibit variable degrees of differentiation within the limits of their definition. The cells have a maturation sequence that ends without good light optic evidence of squamous differentiation (Figures 3 and 4). Growth may be papillary and/or plexiform. The cells have fairly well defined cell margins and the neoplastic islands are usually quite well delineated from the adjacent stroma. In some of the carcinomas, there is a pseudostratified arrangement of cells, not unlike that noted for the intermediate epithelium of the nasopharynx. While histologic differences between squamous cell carcinoma and nonkeratinizing carcinomas are sharp, the differences between nonkeratinizing and undifferentiated carcinomas are sometimes vague and may be arbitrary. The clinical features and the serologic association with EBV suggest that the last two carcinomas are closely related and give sup-

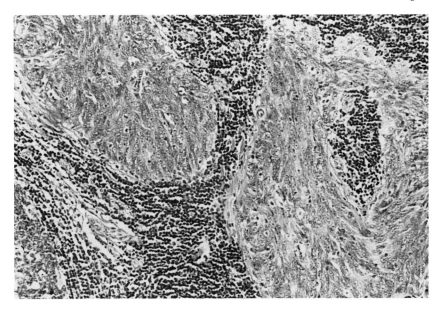

Figure 3 Nonkeratinizing carcinoma of nasopharynx, WHO Type 2. Note sharp delimitation from surrounding lymphoid tissue and in this example, a spindle character to the neoplastic cells. H&E, original magnification: ×360.

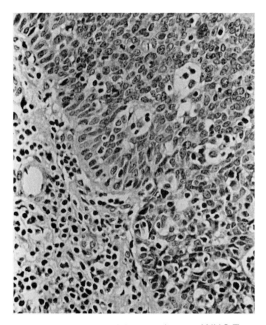

Figure 4 Nonkeratinizing carcinoma, WHO Type 2. This example manifests in addition to neoplasm–stroma demarcation, clear cells and 'intermediate-type' cells. H&E, original magnification: ×400.

port to the notion that there are really only two major subtypes of NPC; squamous cell carcinomas and the less differentiated forms (9, 19, 30).

Undifferentiated NPC carcinoma (also known as anaplastic and poorly differentiated) is composed of primitive cells whose most consistent feature is a single, prominent nucleolus and a nucleus with distinct membrane and, in many cases, nuclear vesiculation (Figure 5). In contrast to the other NPC types, the cell margins of this carcinoma are often indistinct and the tumor often has a syncytial appearance (Figure 6). The cellular arrangement, however, is variable with masses, strands, or individual cells lying in a lymphoid stroma (Figure 7).

The variety of cytoplasmic forms and growth patterns has given rise to descriptive terms such as anaplastic, clear cell, spindle cell, simplex, and lymphoepithelioma.

Undifferentiated NPC has a striking invasive and metastasizing capability and tissue reactions to the infiltrating tumor are usually

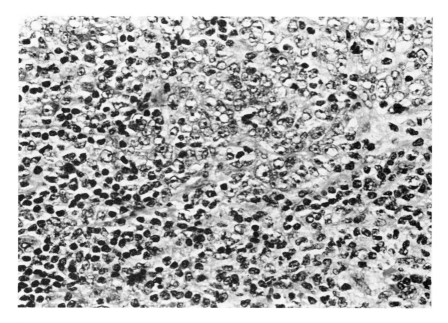

Figure 5 Type 3 WHO NPC or undifferentiated carcinoma. Vesicular nuclei, prominent nucleoli, indistinct cell membranes and a lymphoid-like character are manifested. Note intimate relationship with non-neoplastic lymphocytes. H&E, original magnification: ×420.

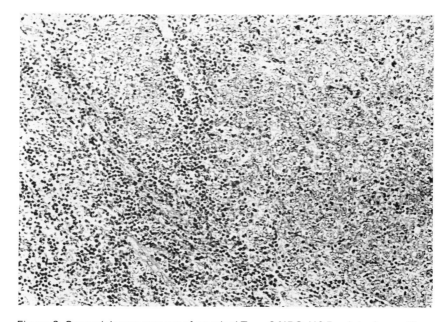

Figure 6 Syncytial arrangement of a typical Type 3 NPC. H&E, original magnification: ×100.

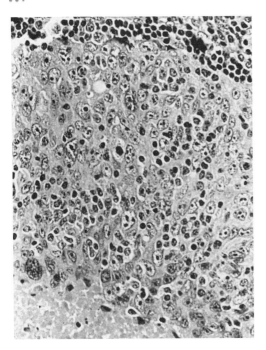

Figure 7 WHO Type 3 NPC. This example shows more nuclear irregularity than that of Figures 5 and 6, but still retains its typical cytomorphology. H&E, original magnification: ×250.

limited. Fibrosis or desmoplasia, for example, are never prominent unless there has been prior radiation therapy (9). Usually there is no discernible reaction and the carcinoma maintains an intimate relationship with lymphoid tissues.

The presence or absence of lymphocytes in NPC is not a factor in making the diagnosis. It is now firmly established that the lymphocytes are not neoplastic or integral to the carcinomas. They can be found in all three of the WHO types, but most often associated with undifferentiated carcinomas. Approximately 98% of undifferentiated, 70% of nonkeratinizing and 37% of squamous cell carcinomas of the nasopharynx are associated with lymphocytes (99). The lymphoid 'stroma' is not entirely passive. Metastases of undifferentiated NPC to nonlymphoid tissues may also have an accompaniment of lymphoid cells.

Several histologic findings of a host response

to NPC merit mention. Some may have as yet unknown prognostic value while others, in the presence of undifferentiated NPC, may mislead the surgical pathologist to a diagnosis of lymphoid neoplasm. A mixture of lymphoid cells, plasma cells, sometimes associated with polymophonuclear leukocytes, is found in nearly all forms of NPC. A mild to moderate stromal eosinophilia is evident in about a quarter of the carcinomas, most often with the undifferentiated types, where it may be a conspicuous feature. Some authors have also reported an amyloid-like material in the stroma and also sometimes in the cytoplasm of the carcinoma cells (31). The amyloid, unlikely to be of a secondary type, is found most often in association with nonkeratinizing NPC. In the lymphoid tissue immediately adjacent to undifferentiated NPC, there may be a predominance of T lymphocytes; a finding of possible significance because of the inherently B cell nature of the lymphoid tissue of the nasopharynx. T zone histiocytes (Langerhans' cells and precursors) at primary carcinoma sites may also play a role in an immune reaction (32). In lymph nodes with or without metastases from NPC and on occasion, in the nasopharynx itself, tuberculoid granulomas are found. Usually around neoplasm, the epithelioid granulomas may be accompanied by large numbers of eosinophils, fibrosis and caseous necrosis. Infective granulomas or Hodgkin's disease may be simulated.

Despite the variations in histologic appearance of the WHO types, their proposed mode of histogenesis, the lability and maturational tendencies of the nasopharyngeal epithelium, and clinicopathologic findings suggest all three types may be histologically homogeneous. The tendency for an epidermoid differentiation and the light optic findings of a mixed cell or intermediate population in otherwise prototypic histologic classes support this homogeneity, as does ultrastructure. Shanmugaratnam et al. (7) have indicated that features of more than one histologic type were present in 25% of all nasopharyngeal carcinomas studied in a Singapore population. In such instances, classification is based on the predominant type found in the primary lesion.

Carcinomas histologically similar or indistinguishable from NPC types 2 and 3 have been found elsewhere in the epithelium of Waldeyer's ring (33), in the larynx (34), the thymus (35), in major salivary glands (29), and cervix (37). The role of EBV in some of these carcinomas is strongly suggested by serologic profiles, presence of EBV-associated nuclear antigen in the carcinoma cells and by high levels of viral genomes in the DNA. A histomorphologic feature common to all is an intimacy of epithelium and lymphoid cells, not unlike that of the nasopharyngeal mucosa. This 'lymphoepithelium' is found in the base of the tongue, tonsillar and adenoidal crypts, in association with salivary ducts, laryngeal 'tonsil' and obviously in the thymus. These 'lymphoepithelial carcinomas' are infrequent, e.g. less than 5% of base of tongue and tonsil carcinomas but their biologic behavior and response to treatment qualifies them further as *carcinomas of nasopharyngeal type*.

Salivary type carcinomas, preponderantly adenoid cystic carcinomas (Figure 8), of the nasopharynx, are unusual and extremely so in Chinese. Indeed, adenoid cystic carcinomas of *any* head and neck site appear to be rare in that ethnic population; 8 of 1776 (0.45%) malignant neoplasms studied by Zhang and Deng (37). One of the adenoid cystic carcinomas arose in the nasopharynx. Yin et al. (38) indicate that 10 of 1379 patients (0.7%) had adenoid cystic carcinoma as their type of carcinoma of the nasopharynx. A higher, yet still low, incidence is expressed in studies of nonoriental populations in the United States (39).

Biology

Immunologic Aspects of NPC

Over the past several years a collaborative prospective study of North American patients with different histopathologic types of nasopharyngeal carcinoma, has identified certain

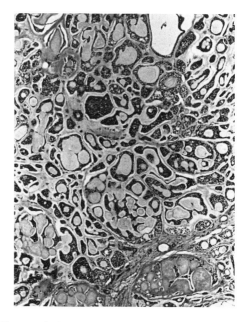

Figure 8 Adenoid cystic carcinoma of the nasopharnyx, the most common of the rarely encountered salivary type carcinomas of the nasopharynx. H&E, original magnification: ×80.

biologic characteristics of EBV that have clinical importance for diagnosis and possibly for the management of the disease (7, 9, 10, 13, 40). Immunovirologic tests having diagnostic significance include antibody titers to viral capsid antigen (VCA) and to early antigen (EA) (Table 6). The VCA (IgA) is more specific, while the EA is more sensitive. In addition, antibody dependent cellular cytotoxicity (ADCC) assays titrating EBV-induced membrane antigen complex appear to be predictive of clinical outcome and prognosis of patients with NPC Types 2 and 3. High ADCC titers at time of diagnosis are associated with a more favorable prognosis, regardless of stage of disease.

The incidence of positive titers in NPC appears to be the same regardless of size of tumor and hence can complement the diagnostic evaluation of patients. Improvement in sensitivity and specificity of the procedures will clearly enhance screening programs. Anti-EBV serologic findings distinguish WHO Type

TABLE 6 IMMUNOVIROLOGIC TESTS AND NASOPHARYNGEAL
CARCINOMAS

Test population	Viral capsid antigen (VCA-IgA)		Early antigen (IgG)	
	Percent positive	Percent negative	Percent positive	Percent negative
A. Patients with NPC				
WHO 1	16 ⎱		35 ⎱	65
WHO 2	89 ⎬ 85	11	94 ⎬ 85	6
WHO 3	84 ⎰	16	83 ⎰	17
		84		
B. Other patients				
Squamous cell carcinoma, head and neck	18	82	31	69
Nonsquamous cell carcinoma head and neck	13	87	38	62
Non-neoplastic disease, head and neck	14	86	86	37
C. Healthy controls	9	91	29	71

Modified from Neel (24).

1 from Types 2 and 3 carcinomas. Types 2 and 3 carcinomas manifest characteristic anti-EBV profiles and are more often, small, submucosal and may be clinically occult (9). They seem to be more radiation-sensitive than WHO Type 1 carcinomas. WHO Types 2 and 3 carcinomas appear to occur at an earlier age, manifest longer disease-free periods after treatment and have a better survival even though early and advanced metastases to the neck are more common (9, 24).

Electron microscopic evidence of EBV in nasopharyngeal carcinomas is tenuous (41). Some investigators claim virus-like particles with a similarity to EBV *and* coronaviruses can be found in tissue culture cells or following transplantation of neoplastic tissue to nude mice (41). The inability to define EBV by ultrastructural analysis of NPC may be related to loss of the morphological configuration of the DNA virus when the viral genome is incorporated into the DNA of the tumor cell.

Genetics

Several genetic systems have been investigated in patients with NPC. Of these, the only one

strongly associated with NPC is the HLA (5, 18, 20, 42). The HLA locus A and B antigen association in Chinese with NPC is well established. Other ethnic groups do not manifest such a relationship but it is possible that the susceptibility to NPC in Caucasians may also be codetermined by genes of the HLA region. In Chinese patients, the following rather firm conclusions can be made (42).

1. HLA-B17 and HLA-Bw46 are associated with increased risk. HLA-A11 is associated with a decreased risk.
2. There is evidence the risk is associated with haplotypes rather than with individual antigens since joint occurrences of Aw19/B17 and A2 Bw46 have a higher risk than B17 or Bw46 alone.
3. Risk with A2 Bw46 is confined only to older onset (patients over 30 years of age) but Aw19/B17 is found in both young and old onset patients and is particularly marked in patients under 30 years of age.
4. B17 is associated with poor survival.
5. There is a strong association with locus DR blank. This finding requires further immunogenetic research.

The different HLA associations with development and prognosis of NPC suggest genetic factors may influence the disease at different levels, e.g. individuals with A2B46 and Aw19/B17 profiles may be more susceptible to carcinogen(s) and once the neoplasm has developed, genetic factors may influence survival. Preliminary data do not indicate HLA correlates with EBV serology other than in a secondary correlation with survival.

CLINICAL PRESENTATION AND DIAGNOSIS OF NASOPHARYNGEAL CARCINOMA

Nasopharyngeal carcinoma, especially of the WHO Type 2 and Type 3, usually arises in the region of the fossa of Rosenmüller. The early symptoms of the disease are neither pathognomonic nor specific. The clinical presentation of NPC in the North American population has recently been documented in a collaborative prospective study (43).

Over a third of patients will notice a mass in the neck as their first symptom and about an equal number will have a sensation of unilateral ear fullness or plugging and hearing loss. A persistent serous otitis media, especially if unilateral in an otherwise healthy adult, should arouse suspicion of a carcinoma of the nasopharynx. A cancer of the nasopharynx will seldom produce choanal or nasal obstruction but initial bleeding or bloody nasal drainage is noticed by about one-fifth of the patients. The triad of a mass in the neck, a conductive hearing loss and nasal obstruction with bloody tinged drainage is frequently present by the time the diagnosis of nasopharyngeal carcinoma is made.

The proximity of foramen lacerum and thus the floor of the middle cranial fossa allows for direct tumor extension into the cranium and involvement of adjacent nerves. One-fifth of the patients will have symptoms of cranial nerve involvement at the time of diagnosis. Facial pain and paresthesias suggest tumor infiltration of the branches of the trigeminal nerve and diplopia from paralysis of the external rectus muscle is a sign of involvement of the abducens nerve. Involvement of cranial nerves III and IV indicates more advanced disease along the cavernous sinus. Tumor extension may occur laterally into the parapharyngeal space and involve cranial nerves IX, X, and XI producing a jugular foramen syndrome. The latter one is rarely seen in nasopharyngeal carcinoma. A persistent occipitotemporal headache, especially unilateral, is reported by 1 out of every 6 patients. Only very occasionally will nasopharyngeal carcinoma invade the parotid gland and cause facial nerve paralysis. Proptosis will occur when cancer invades through the posterior portion of the orbit. Trismus is an indication of pterygoid muscle invasion and cancer extension into this space.

At the time of diagnosis, 9 of every 10 patients will have palpable lymph node metastases with bilateral involvement in half of them. The lymph nodes most frequently involved are in the subdigastric area and in the chain along the spinal accessory nerve in the posterior triangle. The sentinel lymph node for NPC is located underneath the upper insertion of the sternocleidomastoid muscle. Frequently the neck mass is large and painless and it can enlarge quite rapidly due to necrosis or hemorrhage. Retropharyngeal lymph node metastasis though uncommon, produces a characteristic syndrome of pain referred to the ipsilateral neck, ear, head, forehead, and orbit. It may be associated with a stiff neck or pain when cervical dorsiflexion is attempted.

Physical examination includes inspection of the nasopharynx, either indirectly with a mirror or by direct visualization through a fiberoptic endoscope. The tumor usually appears as an asymmetric mass with telangiectasia on its friable surface and centered in the fossa of Rosenmüller. Depending upon the size of the primary tumor, distortion of the soft palate can occur. Straw-colored serous otitis media is usually unilateral. Evaluation of the cranial nerves may uncover subtle signs of tumor infiltration. The earliest signs are usually extraocular muscle dysfunction especially lateral rectus palsy, and signs of trigeminal nerve involvement such as hyperesthesia and atrophy of masticatory muscles. The relative frequency of involvement of each cranial nerve is indicated in Table 7 (44).

Biopsy of the tumor in the nasopharynx can be done under the topical anesthetic by cocaine applications through the nasal cavity. Palpation of the neck, especially in the upper third, will frequently reveal lymph node metastases that are often of large size, multiple and fixed to the surrounding structures. Differentiated squamous cell carcinomas (WHO 1) produce fewer lymph node metastases as opposed to the poorly differentiated and anaplastic lesions (WHO 2 and WHO 3).

Radiographic evaluation of the nasopharynx, the base of the skull, paranasal sinuses and the neck is mandatory for appropriate staging and treatment. Computerized tomography (CT) allows for the definition of the extent of primary tumor and the amount of invasion and infiltration of surrounding structures. Bone destruction about the floor of the sphenoid sinus, the adjacent middle cranial fossa, the clivus, and the pterygoid plates can be documented as well as the extension of tumor through the foramen lacerum into the middle cranial fossa, lateral into the parapharyngeal space, anteriorly into the nasal cavity and anterolaterally into the orbit. It is important to demonstrate invasion into the posterior ethmoid cells and adjacent portion of the maxillary antrum. Radiographic documentation of invasion through the base of skull is present in at least one-fourth of patients.

CT examination may also reveal metastatic spread to lymph nodes that is undetectable clinically. For example, Figure 9 shows a patient in whom a small but obviously involved lymph node adjacent to the transverse process of C1 was demonstrated radiographically. This node would not have been included in the high dose volume of radiotherapy using standard technique, leading inevitably to treatment failure.

The majority of patients with NPC seen in North America present with advanced disease, and at least one-fifth of the patients have occult distant metastases at the time of presentation (45, 46). Sites of predilection for metastatic spread are presented in Table 8 (47). Screening for distant metastases is usually limited to a chest x-ray and sometimes a bone scan. This is mainly to provide a baseline study for future comparison since the detection rate of bony metastases on presentation is very low.

Staging

The staging system of The American Joint Commission for Cancer (AJCC) (48) is commonly used in the United States for the clinical staging of nasopharyngeal carcinoma (Table 9). Throughout the world two other staging systems are being used. In Southeast Asia the system proposed by Ho is popular (49) (Table 10). The UICC staging (Table 11) is prevalent throughout the world and in certain aspects is similar to the AJCC system (50).

There is certainly no agreement on the single best staging system for patients with nasophar-

TABLE 7 FREQUENCY OF CRANIAL NERVE INVOLVEMENT IN CANCER OF THE NASOPHARYNX[a]

	Cranial nerves											
	I	II	III	IV	V	VI	VII	VIII	IX	X	XI	XII
No. of patients	13	114	236	207	521	600	133	49	264	233	154	358
% of frequency	0.5	4.0	8.2	7.2	18.1	20.9	4.6	1.7	9.2	8.1	5.4	12.5

[a] Based on 2871 patients of which 641 (22.3%) manifested cranial nerve involvement. Adapted from Sawaki et al. (44).

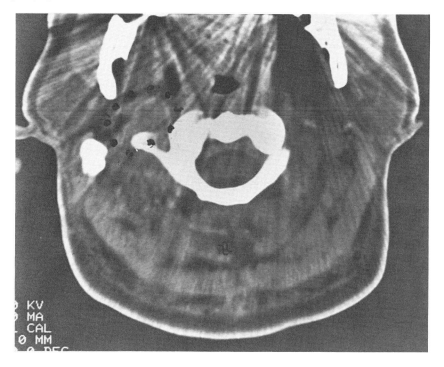

Figure 9 CT showing occult involvement of retropharyngeal nodes from NPC primary.

yngeal carcinoma. In a prospective evaluation, assessing predicted value of many variables in survival, Neel et al. (51) found none of the existing staging systems to be satisfactory, and proposed a new system of defining a prognostic score based on six individually significant variables influencing survival (see section on the prognosis score below).

MANAGEMENT AND PROGNOSIS

The main treatment modality for cancers of the nasopharynx is radiation therapy, and results of treatment with radiation alone provide the yardstick against which alternative therapeutic strategies must be measured.

The results of recent published series of nasopharyngeal cancer in Caucasian patients treated with radiotherapy are therefore reviewed, along with a consideration of patterns of relapse and prognostic variables influencing survival. This is followed by a description of modern day radiotherapy technique, and a discussion of current clinical research to investigate combined modality treatment.

TABLE 8 DISTANT METASTATIC SITES OF NASOPHARYNGEAL CARCINOMA: A STUDY OF 2637 PATIENTS

Metastatic site	No. of patients (%)
Bones	342 (41)
Lungs	256 (30)
Liver	121 (14)
Distant lymph nodes	101 (12)
Brain	18 (2)
Other	3 (1)
	841 (32)

Modified from Huang and Chu (47).

TABLE 9 AMERICAN JOINT COMMISSION STAGING SYSTEM

T	N	M	Stage
TIS= carcinoma in situ	NX= nodes cannot be assessed	MX= not assessed	I = T1 N0 M0
T1 = tumor confined to one site of nasopharynx or no tumor visible (positive biopsy only)	N0= no clinically positive node	M0= no (known) distant metastasis	II= T2 N0 M0
T2= tumor involving two sites (both postero-superior and lateral walls)	N1 = single clinically positive homolateral node less than 3 cm in diameter	M1 = distant metastasis present. Specify sites: pulmonary, osseous, hepatic, brain, lymph nodes, bone marrow, pleura, skin, eye, other	III= T3 N0 M0
T3= extension of tumor into nasal cavity or oropharynx	N2= single clinically positive homolateral node 3 to 6 cm in diameter or multiple clinically positive homolateral nodes none over 6 cm in diameter		T1 or T2 or T3, N1, M0
T4= tumor invasion of skull or cranial nerve involvement, or both	N2a= single clinically positive homolateral node 3 to 6 cm in diameter		IV=T4, N0 or N1, M0
	N2b= multiple clinically positive homolateral nodes, none over 6 cm in diameter		Any T, N2 or N3, M0
	N3= massive homolateral node(s), bilateral nodes, or contralateral node(s)		Any T, any N, M1
	N3a= clinically positive homolateral node(s), more than 6 cm in diameter		
	N3b= bilateral clinically positive nodes (each side of neck should be staged separately; ie, N3b: right=N2a, left=N1)		
	N3c= contralateral clinically positive node(s) only		

Data from American Joint Committee for Cancer Staging and End-Results Reporting (48).

TABLE 10 SOUTHEAST ASIA STAGING SYSTEM

T	N	M	Stage
T1 = T1 tumor confined to nasopharynx (space behind choanal orifices and nasal septum and above posterior margin of soft palate in resting position)	0 = N0 none palpable (nodes thought to be benign)	0 = M0 no evidence of distant metastasis	I = A tumor confined to nasopharyngeal mucosa (T1, N0, M0)
2 = T2 tumor extended to nasal fossa, oropharynx, or adjacent muscles or nerves below base of skull	1 = N1 node(s) wholly in upper cervical level bounded below by skin crease extending laterally and backward from or just below thyroid notch (laryngeal eminence)	1 = M distant metastasis present	II = B tumor extended to nasal fossa, oropharynx, or adjacent muscles or nerves below base of skull (T2) and/or N1 involvement
3 = T3 tumor extended beyond T2 limits and subclassified as follows:	2 = N2 node(s) palpable between crease and supraclavicular fossa, upper limit being line joining upper margin of sternal end of clavicle and apex of angle formed by lateral surface of neck and superior margin of trapezius		III = tumor extended beyond T2 limits or bone involvement (T3) and/or N2 involvement
4 = T3a bone involvement below base of skull (floor of sphenoid sinus is included in this category	3 = N3 node(s) palpable in supraclavicular fossa and/or skin involvement in form of carcinoma en cuirasse or satellite nodules above clavicles		IV = C N3 involvement, irrespective of primary tumor
5 = T3b involvement of base of skull			V = D hematogenous metastasis and/or involvement of skin or lymph node(s) below clavicles (M)
6 = T3c involvement of cranial nerve(s)			
7 = T3d involvement of orbits, laryngopharynx (hypopharynx), or infratemporal fossa			

Data from Ho (49).

TABLE 11 UICC STAGING SYSTEM

T	N	M	Stage
0 = no evidence of primary tumor	0 = no evidence of regional lymph node involvement	0 = no evidence of distant metastases	I = T1 N0 M0
1 = tumor confined to one site (including tumor identified from positive biopsy)	1 = evidence of involvement of movable homolateral regional lymph nodes		II = T2 N0 M0
2 = tumor involving two sites	2 = evidence of involvement of movable contralateral or bilateral regional lymph nodes	1 = evidence of distant metastases	III = T3 N0 M0
3 = tumor with extension to nasal cavity and/or oropharynx	3 = evidence of involvement of fixed regional lymph nodes	8 = minium requirements to assess presence of distant metastases cannot be met	T1 or T2 or T3, N1, M0
4 = tumor with extension to base of skull and/or involving cranial nerves	8 = minimum requirements to assess regional lymph nodes cannot be met		IV = T4, N0 or N1, M0
5 = preinvasive carcinoma (carcinoma in situ)			Any T, N2 or N3, M0
8 = minimum requirements to assess primary tumor cannot be met			Any T, any N, M1

Data from Harmer (50).

Results of Treatment with Radiotherapy Alone

Most series of nasopharyngeal cancer reported in the Western literature have been small, consistent with the incidence of this disease in the Caucasian community. The majority of patients fall into Stages III and IV of the AJCC classification. A summary of reports published since 1980 is given in Table 12 (24, 45, 52–78). Overall 5-year survival statistics range from approximately 20% to 70%, but due to differences in the patient populations in different series, one cannot necessarily attribute differences in results to radiotherapy technique. However, the fact that several series have shown an improvement in results over the last decade compared with earlier times suggests that refinement of technique and better definition of the treatment volume is indeed reflected in an improvement in therapeutic outcome.

Due to the relative rarity of this disease in Caucasians, it is important to know whether it has the same prognosis and response to therapy as nasopharyngeal cancer in Chinese. One of the most important comparative studies in this regard is that of Flores et al. (62) from the British Columbia Cancer Control Agency, Vancouver, Canada. Previous reports on this patient series have been published by Dickson (16) and Dickson and Flores (17). They had the unique opportunity to study between 1939 and 1980, 296 cases of nasopharyngeal cancer of whom 159 were Chinese and 126 Caucasian. The remaining patients were of other races. The incidence of nasopharyngeal cancer was over 100 times greater in native born Chinese than in Caucasians, and approximately six times greater in North American born Chinese than in Caucasians. In this study there were no differences in the presentation, response to treatment, or prognosis of the Chinese and Caucasian populations. However, the peak incidence of the disease in Chinese occurs at the age of 50 to 54, whereas the peak incidence (age adjusted) for Caucasians occurs approximately two decades later. Overall survival at 5 years was 39%. Patients treated after 1970 achieved a 48% 5-year survival.

This information permits one to make cautious extrapolation from the very large series of nasopharyngeal cancer emanating from China. For example, Chang et al. (79) from Shanghai reported on 511 patients treated during 1973 alone! The overall 5-year survival of these patients was 54%, ranging from 93.3% in Stage I to 31.9% in Stage IV.

Patterns of Relapse

The reported incidence of failure at the primary site is T stage dependent. Petrovich et al. (73) reported primary failure in 20% of T1 patients increasing to 88% in those with T4 disease in a series of 256 patients treated at eight VA facilities between 1956 and 1978. Corresponding figures from University of Texas M. D. Anderson Hospital reported by Mesic et al. (70) were 3% and 29% in a series of 251 patients treated between 1954 and 1977. A dose response relationship for control of nasopharyngeal cancer has been reported by Marks et al. (69).

Failure of radiotherapy to control disease in the neck is uncommon with good radiotherapy technique. For example, Mesic et al. (70) reported only 13% failure in the neck: 18.4% for squamous cell carcinoma and 7.2% for lymphoepithelioma. Moreover, failure in the neck only, without concomitant relapse at the primary site or distant metastases, occurred in only 3% of the patients.

Prognostic Variables Influencing Survival

Differences in clinical staging systems, lack of uniform histologic classifications and variable techniques, dosage and fields in radiotherapy have led to inconsistent proclamations on prognostic factors. The following represents a consensus summary.

Disease Related

T stage. Many authors cite a decrease in local

TABLE 12 SUMMARY OF RADIOTHERAPY RESULTS PUBLISHED 1980–86: CAUCASIAN SERIES[a]

Author	No. of patients	Years of study	Stage distribution (AJCC)		Survival (5-yr)	Comments
Flores et al. (62)	296	1939–80			39% overall 48% 1970–80	Same prognosis in Caucasians and Chinese
Petrovich et al. (72)	256	1956–78	82%	IV	15%	
Mesic et al. (70)	251	1954–77	80%	IV	52%	65% 5-yr surv lymphoepithelioma 42% t-yr surv SCC
Wang (78)	251	1940–71			40%	
John et al. (66)	225	1954–68			N/A	7% 10-yr survival
Robin et al. (74)	220	1957–66	28% 65%	III IV	27%	Better survival in women
Neel (24)	182		77%	IV	50%	60% 5 yr Surv WHO 2,3 20% 5 yr Surv WHO 1
Payne (45)	140	1970–76			37%	
Cellai et al. (59)	138	1959–78			39.5%	
Kajanti and Mantyla (67)	125	1958–82	80%	T3–4; N0–3	64% early 33% late	
Jenkin et al. (65)	119	1960–77	5% 91%	III IV	51% 75% T1–2	All pts <30
Marks et al. (69)	118	1950–78				20% improvement since 1974
Bedwinek et al. (55)	111	1955–76			69% T1–2; N0–1 20% late	
Vikram et al. (77) (77)	107	1970–80	87%	IV	35% 1970–76 72% 1977–80	Worse results if treatment interrupted
Ring et al. (73)	107	1950–77			29%	
Baker and Wolfe (54)	99	1951–74	67%	N+	44% age <20 14% age>60	Worse results with bilateral nodal involvement
van Andel and Hop (76)	86	1966–80	28% 63%	III IV	30%	Better survival in young
Chu et al. (60)	80	1955–80			36%	Better survival in lymphoepithelioma
Haghbin et al. (64)	79	1958–83	72%	IV	33%	
Frezza et al. (63)	78	1976–82	58%	IV	49 Disease free	Disease-free survival: significant difference between T1–2 vs T3–4; N0–1 vs N2–3; undifferentiated vs SCC
Boljesikova et al. (57)	78	1962–77	68%	N+	25%	
Schabinger et al. (75)	76	1964–79			75% Stage I 31% Stage IV	
Levendag et al. (68)	74	1966–80			35%	
Amendola et al. (52)	59	1965–77	63%	III, IV	15%	
Amornmarn et al. (53)	49	1957–76			45%	
Million and Cassisi (71)	47	1964–78	53%	T4	44%	
Cooper et al. (61)	45	1969–81	All	IV	31%	
Bey et al. (56)	42	1968–77	All	IV	39%	
Castro et al. (58)	27	1960–80	89%	N+	64%	All patients<20

[a] Where more than one report on a given patient population has been published, only the most recent has been included in the table. SCC, squamous cell carcinoma.

tumor control and worsening survival with increasing T stage. However, the important distinction appears to be whether the tumor has progressed locally beyond the nasopharynx (T3-4 versus T1-2) with intracranial extension and/or cranial nerve involvement carrying the worst prognosis.

N stage. Virtually all reports that address the issue note a decreased survival in patients with positive neck nodes compared with those who are clinically node negative. The study of Neel et al. (51) shows that the adverse influence of cervical adenopathy on survival is limited to nodes below Ho's line.

Histologic subtype. In series where an influence of histologic subtype has been demonstrated, patients with keratinizing squamous cell carcinoma have inevitably fared worse than those with tumors characterized as lymphoepithelioma.

Age. Several series document an improved survival, stage for stage, in younger patients.

Sex. When a difference has been reported, females had better survival expectation than males.

Performance status. Initial Karnovsky performance status was a highly significant prognostic factor in the large VA series of Petrovich et al. (72).

Symptomatology. Neel et al. (51) found that patients with more than seven symptoms had a poorer survival. Particularly adverse were pain syndromes and cranial nerve palsies.

EBV-induced ADCC titer. Pearson et al. (80) first reported that survival is significantly poorer in patients with low titers to EBV-induced cellular membrane antigen as measured by the antibody dependent cellular cytotoxicity (ADCC) assay.

Treatment Related

Radiation dose. No mammalian cells are totally resistant to ionizing radiation. It is therefore axiomatic that the probability of sterilizing a given tumor increases with increasing dose. However, for a variety of reasons (81) it is often difficult to establish a dose response relationship for tumor control in a heterogeneous patient series, and impossible if the technical adequacy of treatment is not assured. In spite of these difficulties, several series have demonstrated an improved disease control and survival in patients receiving the higher doses (19, 70, 72, 77).

Treatment duration. Since total dose and overall time are correlated, it is difficult in most series to assess the role of treatment duration on therapeutic response. On first principles, a shorter overall time should lead to improved tumor control (provided the total dose and dose per fraction are unchanged) by limiting the extent of tumor regeneration during treatment. This is the rationale for the concomitant boost technique (82). Evidence supporting the importance of treatment duration comes from the report of Vikram et al. (77) which shows that patients whose therapy was interrupted for any reason had a poorer survival expectation.

Radiotherapy technique. At least four series from major centers have shown improved survival in patients treated more recently (19, 62, 70, 77). This is very likely attributable to better radiotherapy techniques, both in defining disease extent and in delivery of treatment.

The Prognosis Score

Assuming treatment related variables to be standardized in their prospective study, Neel et al. (51) derived a prognosis score based on six variables having independent significance in Cox regression analysis. This scoring system, set out in Table 13, separated patients into groups with 2-year survivals ranging from 10% to 90%. However, the applicability of the scoring system to a data base other than the one from which it was derived has not yet been established.

TABLE 13 PROGNOSIS SCORE IN
          NASOPHARYNGEAL
          CARCINOMA[a]

Characteristic	Score	
Extensive tumor in nasopharynx	If yes	1
	If no	0
Nodes in lower neck	If yes	1
	If no	0
WHO Type 1 tumor	If yes	1
	If no	0
ADCC titer<1:7680 (WHO 2, 3)	If yes	1
	If no	0
Seven or more symptoms	If yes	1
	If no	0
Age>40 years	If yes	1
	If no	0

[a] Prognosis score=sum of above (range, 0 to 6; best
to worst).
Adapted from Neel et al. (61).

Radiotherapy Technique

The propensity of cancer of the nasopharynx to
metastasize and to spread locally beyond the
confines of the nasopharynx mandates large
treatment volumes for all stages of disease. The
primary tumour may extend anteriorly into
the nasal cavity, superiorly into the floor of the
sphenoid sinus or through the foramen
lacerum into the cavernous sinus, antero-
superiorly into the posterior ethmoid air cells
and orbits, laterally into the parapharyngeal
space and sphenoplatine fossa, and inferiorly
into the oropharynx (Figure 10). Lymphatic
spread involves most commonly the jugular
chain of lymphatics and the posterior cervical
chain. In addition, retropharyngeal nodes may
be involved. These lymphatic pathways are
included in the target volume for all stages of
disease. Delineation of the primary target
volume is based on the extent of disease
determined by clinical and radiologic evaluation. The latter should include both transverse and coronal CT cuts.

As in all radiotherapy, the objective of
treatment is to deliver a dose to the target
volume tailored to the amount of disease
present while respecting the tolerance of the
normal tissues irradiated. To achieve this
objective is technically difficult. Before the
advent of high energy accelerators, treatment
of the primary site through lateral fields only

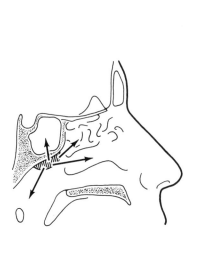
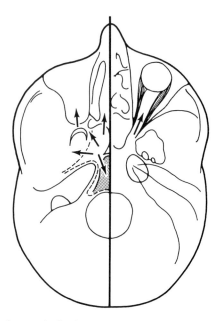

Figure 10 Potential routes of spread of primary tumor.

was limited by the high doses received by the temporal poles of the brain and the tempero-mandibular joints. Thus, boost techniques using antral fields (83) or intracavitary sources (78) were devised. The availability of high energy photons, however, permits the entire dose to be given through lateral fields. This improves the reproducibility of the set-up and permits a more uniform dose to be delivered to the primary target volume.

Standard Plan

The technique described here that is currently in use at the University of Texas M. D. Anderson Hospital for patients in whom the primary disease does not extend into the oropharynx. Treatment is delivered in two phases.

In phase I, large lateral fields, custom shaped with cerrobend blocks, are used to provide comprehensive coverage of the primary site and draining lymphatics including the retropharyngeal nodes, down to the level of the superior thyroid notch (Figure 11). These fields are angled 5° posteriorly to permit the ipsilateral external auditory canal to be excluded from the entrance beam while maintaining adequate posterior coverage of the nasopharynx. A representative port film is shown in Figure 12. The lateral fields are matched inferiorly to an anterior lower neck field with a central laryngeal shield. All phase I fields are treated with ^{60}Co gamma rays or 6 MV photons depending on the patient's thickness. If the junction line between the lateral fields and the anterior lower neck field transects an involved node, the junction line is treated in both fields. Treatment to the lateral fields proceeds at a daily tumor dose of 1.8 Gy calculated at the midline of the nasopharynx and to the lower neck at a daily given dose of 2.0 Gy. Because the separation of the lateral fields below the level of the mandible is considerably less than at the level of the nasopharynx, it is important that doses be calculated in the subdigastric plane as well as at the primary tumor reference point to avoid

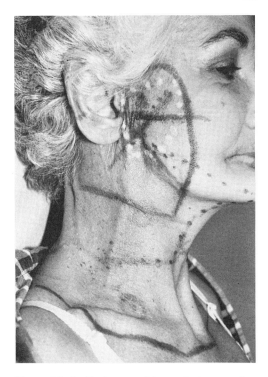

Figure 11 Radiotherapy skin marks for a patient with T4 N3b nasopharyngeal carcinoma illustrating the initial large lateral fields, anterior lower neck field, reduced lateral high energy nasopharyngeal fields, and glancing neck boost fields. Laser positioning lines and SSD points are also evident.

unnecessarily high doses to the pharyngeal axis. These portals are continued until the dose to the cervical spinal cord reaches 45 Gy.

In the second phase of the treatment, the patient is repositioned with the head in hyperextension and treatment to the primary tumor is completed using reduced 18 MV photon fields. Treatment to the neck is completed with glancing anterior and posterior fields with a midline block to protect the larynx, pharynx, and spinal cord (Figure 11). If there were no clinically palpable lymph nodes on presentation, the dose to the neck is limited to 50 Gy. If neck nodes were initially positive they are boosted either through reduced glancing fields or with appositional electron beams depending

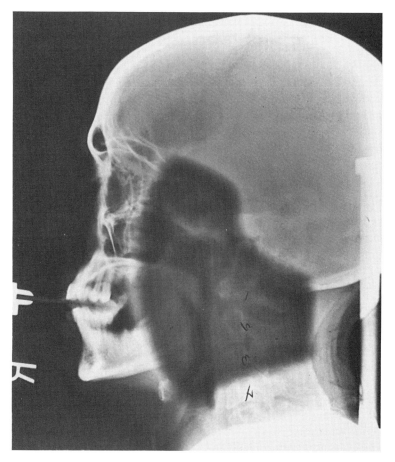

Figure 12 Port film of initial lateral fields for treatment of a patient with a T4 primary invading the base of skull. The upper margin of the field is reduced to the level of the floor of the sella for T1–2 primaries.

on their size. Because of the reduction in volume the boost dose to both the primary site and the neck is delivered at 2.0 Gy per fraction to avoid unnecessary prolongation of treatment. In certain circumstances the boost is given concomitantly with the basic treatment as a second daily fraction during the basic treatment. The total doses recommended for each stage of disease are indicated in Table 14. In general, patients with poorly differentiated NPC and lymphoepithelioma (WHO 2 and 3) receive about 4.0 Gy less, stage for stage, than those with keratinizing squamous carcinoma (WHO 1).

Modification of Plan

If the primary tumor extends into the oropharynx it is not possible to use this plan without overlap between the primary boost fields and the glancing neck fields. For this group of patients it is therefore necessary to construct compensating filters to be used from the outset so that the dose in the subdigastric plan proceeds at the same rate as that in the nasopharynx. Treatment to the compensated lateral fields proceeds until the spinal cord dose reaches 45 Gy, at which time an anterior reduction is made and treatment to the pos-

TABLE 14 RECOMMENDED DOSES[a]

Site	Keratinizing squamous cell carcinoma (WHO 1): dose (Gy)	Poorly differentiated NPC 'lymphoepithelioma' (WHO 2, 3): dose (Gy)
Primary		
T1–T2	66	62
T3	68	64
T4	70	66
Neck		
Subclinical disease	50	50
Palpable <1 cm	60	56
1–3 cm	64	60
3–6 cm	68	64
>6 cm	70+	66+

[a] Total doses delivered at 1.8 Gy per fraction for large fields and 2 Gy per fraction for boost fields.

terior strips is continued with electron beams of appropriate energy. When the midline dose reaches 50 Gy the primary fields are reduced to cover the known extensions of the primary disease and treatment is completed with 18 MV photons. Should any palpable lymph nodes lie within these high energy portals they are appropriately bolused. Other neck nodes are boosted as in the standard plan.

Preradiotherapy Evaluation

Every patient should have an audiogram and a careful dental evaluation done before treatment. Teeth that show signs of decay or periodontal disease either need to be restored or ablated. Every patient is submitted to a thorough prophylactic program (84).

Since the pituitary and hypothalamus are in either the primary beam or penumbra, patients should have baseline endocrine assessments of hypophyseal function done prior to commencement of radiotherapy. This permits early identification of hormonal deficiences to be diagnosed and appropriate replacement therapy initiated (85, 86, 83).

Immunologic screening of titers to Epstein–Barr viral antigens should also be done where facilities are available, in view of the application of such virologic data to the diagnosis and prognosis of the disease (24).

Follow-up

After completion of therapy patients are examined at regular intervals, every 2 to 3 months for the first year after, quarterly for the second and third year, and every 6 months through the fifth year after treatment. A follow-up evaluation is done every year thereafter. During follow-up the disease status is evaluated in search for recurrence at the primary site or the neck nodes and for distant metastases, especially in the lungs. Attention should be directed to possible sequelae of treatment and prevention of infectious complications in the head and neck area. The external auditory canals will be deficient in normal cerumen production and all patients should be instructed in prevention of external otitis. The auditory canal will be dry and the normal migration of the epithelium within the auditory canal is impaired. As a result, debris tends to collect and may impact. We have found that the application of 10% boric acid ointment to the external auditory meatus will prevent some of the problems secondary to this sequela of radiation therapy. Patients with carcinoma of the nasopharynx will often present with serous otitis media. After treatment, this may subside but it may persist in a chronic form. If this sequela causes bothersome symptoms, it can be managed with indwelling tympanic membrane ventilation tubes. Dental and oral cavity care should be meticulous and the application of fluoride solutions in the form of stannous fluoride or sodium fluoride by custom fitted carriers is mandatory. Dental extractions after radiation therapy should be avoided whenever possible. If extractions are unavoidable, extreme precautions are necessary to minimize the risk of osteoradionecrosis (84).

Radiation to the temporomandibular joints and masticatory muscles, especially in patients who receive systemic chemotherapy prior to radiation may cause trismus. This usually does not set in before 3 to 6 months after treatment, but is progressive. Patients need to be instructed in its prevention by encouraging active jaw exercises especially in teenagers and young adults.

The effect of irradiation on the mucosa of the sinonasal tract is a metaplastic transformation of the epithelium from ciliary-columnar respiratory epithelium to cuboidal or squamous stratified epithelium with loss of ciliary function and very often loss of the mucus secreting elements. In spite of these changes, it is rare that patients experience sinonasal infections. Nevertheless, if they do occur they should be treated promptly and aggressively to avoid undesirable necrosis of soft tissue and osteoradionecrosis of facial bones.

Irradiation of part or all of the pituitary hypothalamic axis is unavoidable, especially when there is cancerous bony invasion of the base of the skull. An annual evaluation of the pituitary function and of the thyroid and pituitary adrenal axis is therefore recommended. Proper replacement therapy should be tailored to identified deficiences (86).

Management of Recurrent or Metastatic Nasopharyngeal Carcinoma

Locally recurrent nasopharyngeal carcinoma, especially if limited to the primary site, without intracranial extension, should be considered for retreatment with radiotherapy. McNeese and Fletcher (87) reported long term disease control (1–16 years) in 10 of 30 patients retreated for local failure with high energy external beam radiotherapy. Serious complications were relatively infrequent, and resulted in the death of only 1 patient.

For recurrence in the neck and distant metastatic sites, with or without failure at the primary site, systemic chemotherapy is generally indicated (88). Because nasopharyngeal carcinoma is uncommon among the Caucasian groups, there is very little information on the role of chemotherapy in the management of metastatic nasopharyngeal cancer. Most reports on chemotherapy in head and neck cancer include only a small number of patients with nasopharyngeal cancer. Nevertheless, several chemotherapeutic agents, used primarily in combination treatment, have been tested in recurrent nasopharyngeal cancer; such as methotrexate, bleomycin, cisplatin, 5-fluorouracil, cyclophosphamide, nitrosourea, Adriamycin, and Velban. In 1978 Holoye et al. (89) reported a 40% major response rate using a combination of bleomycin, Cytoxan, methotrexate, and 5-fluorouracil (BCMF) in patients with recurrent head and neck cancer. Among these patients 4 out of 5 nasopharyngeal cancer patients achieved significant major response. In 1981 Goepfert et al. (90) reported on 18 recurrent nasopharyngeal cancer patients who were treated with either BCMF regimen or cisplatin with Adriamycin and bleomycin. The major response rate was 61% with a median duration of remission of 6 months. In 1981 Huang et al. (91) reported on 8 patients treated with bleomycin, methotrexate, vinblastine and CCNU. Dramatic tumor regression was seen in 4 of these patients. More recently, Decker et al. (92) reported the effectiveness of chemotherapy in 17 patients treated at Wayne State University in a 10-year period. Although not on a uniform protocol, 3 patients achieved complete remission on cisplatin-containing regimens, with an overall response of 53%. The median duration of partial response was 180 days with a median survival of 293 days. Multiple drug regimens achieve higher response rates than single agents. The highest response rates in head and neck cancer generally occur with platinum-containing combinations. Therefore, for palliation in patients who present with recurrent incurable tumors, it is reasonable to give one of the active platinum-containing regimens or to encourage the patient's participation in a clinical trial if available (88).

CURRENT CLINICAL RESEARCH IN PROGRESS

Adjuvant Chemotherapy Trials

As noted above, reported radiotherapeutic results for nasopharyngeal carcinoma vary considerably with reports of 5-year survival figures ranging from about 20% to 70%. Even though high survival rates can be achieved with radiotherapy alone for early stage lesions, the control of advanced nasopharyngeal tumors is poor, with most studies reporting 5-year survivals of only 20% or 30%. Advanced disease at the primary site presents a problem in local control and the risk of distant metastasis is known to be particularly high for patients with extensive nodal disease. With recent advances in chemotherapy of head and neck cancer, systemic chemotherapy has therefore been added as an adjuvant in an attempt to improve results obtained by local treatment (93). Chemotherapy given after irradiation is relatively ineffective, poorly tolerated, and produces greater toxicity. Hence, combined modality treatment of advanced squamous carcinoma of head and neck has focused on using initial induction chemotherapy followed by radiation therapy.

There is little published information about the role of adjuvant chemotherapy specifically in the management of advanced nasopharyngeal carcinoma: most reports of adjuvant chemotherapy trials involving a large series of head and neck patients include only a small number of nasopharyngeal cancer cases. Nevertheless, a number of studies of the role of adjuvant chemotherapy for advanced NPC have been reported (Table 15) (94–100).

In general, these reports indicate that nasopharyngeal carcinoma is responsive to chemotherapy when used as initial induction treatment. In general, chemotherapy was not associated with increased acute toxicity of radiation other than mucositis, but late toxicity data are lacking. Since most studies have been relatively small and uncontrolled, no firm conclusions can be made about disease-free and overall survival rates. Further trials involving a large number of patients will be required to see whether induction chemotherapy followed by radiotherapy will improve the cure rate in these tumors. Therefore, initial or simultaneous chemotherapy should not be used routinely in the management of nasopharyngeal cancer unless as part of well-designed clinical trials.

Interferon Trials

Nasopharyngeal carcinoma is almost invariably associated with evidence of Epstein–Barr virus (EBV) infection and, as discussed previously, a poor prognosis correlates with low initial antibody-dependent cytotoxicity.

Interferon has been demonstrated to have antiviral and antiproliferative activities in humans. Thus, there is rationale for using interferon in the treatment of NPC, which is a virus-associated neoplasm. Interferon is being evaluated extensively in various hematologic and other solid malignancies. However, a literature search revealed only two reports of the treatment of NPC with interferon. The first report, from Trenner et al. in 1980 (101), was the case of an 11-year-old boy with recurrent NPC after both irradiation and chemotherapy. He received gamma interferon, 4×10^6 units daily for 5 weeks followed by three applications per week at the same dose. A complete remission was documented during the subsequent 6 months.

In 1985 Connors et al. (102) reported the treatment results of recurrent NPC patients with human leukocyte interferon. Thirteen patients were treated with interferon 10×10^6 units intramuscularly daily for 3 days. Inter-

TABLE 15 ADJUVANT CHEMOTHERAPY TRIALS IN ADVANCED NPC

Investigators	No. of patients	Methods of trials	Chemotherapy regimens	Comments
Hill et al. (97)	20	Sequential CT+XRT	Vincristine Bleomycin Methotrexate 5-Fluorouracil Hydrocortisone	Initial respones to CT: 90% Final CR with XRT: 85% No acute toxicity Median survival: 40 months
Al-Kourainy et al. (94)	8	Sequential CT+XRT	Cisplatin-containing	CR after CT: 50% (4/8) CR after XRT: 75% (6/8)
	4	Simultaneous	Cisplatin	CR: 100% (4/4)
Galligioni et al. (96)	12	Sequential CT+XRT	Adriamycin Bleomycin Vinblastine Dacarbazine	Major response: 75% (9/12) CR: 33% (4/12)
Tannock et al. (100)	50	Sequential CT+XRT	Methotrexate Bleomycin Cisplatin	RR: 72% after CT 3-yr survival rate: 50% Similar to control
Kuten et al. (98)	15	Sequential CT+XRT	Methotrexate Bleomycin Cisplatin	CR after CT+XRT: 87% (13/15) Survival benefit
Al-Sarraf et al. (95)	28	Simultaneous CT+XRT	Cisplatin	CR: 82% (23/28) Survival at 1 yr: 79%
Rossi et al. (99)	113 VCA 116 No chemotherapy	Randomized after XRT Chemotherapy vs no chemotherapy	Vincristine CTX Adriamycin	Survival at 44 months: 56.5% (VCA) 56.2% (control)

feron did not affect serum anti-EBV antibody titers, either IgA or IgG antiviral capsid or early antigens. However, 4 patients did show measurable tumor regression, 3 had stable disease, and 6 patients had progression of disease. Toxicity included fever, fatigue, myalgia, and thrombocytopenia.

These two reports suggest activity of interferon in NPC patients, despite an advanced state of disease at the time of treatment and the use of relatively modest doses of interferon. This level of interferon activity justifies further investigation, perhaps as adjuvant treatment immediately after definitive irradiation for local disease. Further testing of interferon with chemotherapeutic agents in recurrent NPC should also be considered.

ACKNOWLEDGEMENTS

This investigation was supported in part by Grants CA06294 and CA16672 awarded by the National Cancer Institute, Department of Health and Human Services.

REFERENCES

1 Michaux L. Carcioma de base du crâne. In: Godfredsen E ed Ophthalmologic and Neurologic Symptoms of Malignant Nasopharyngeal Tumours. Acta Psychiat Scand 1944; 34 Suppl 1: 323.

2 Strouhal E. Ancient Egyptian case of carcinoma. Bull NY Acad Med 1978; 54: 290.

3 Bosworth FH. A Treatise on Disease of the Nose and Throat, Vol 1. New York: Wood, 1889.

4 Muir CS. Nasopharyngeal cancer—a historical vignette. CA 1983. 33: 180.

5 Batsakis JG, Solomon AR, Rice DH. The pathology of head and neck tumors: carcinoma of the nasopharynx, Part II. Head Neck Surg 1981; 3: 511.

6 Michaels L, Hyams VJ. Undifferentiated carcinoma of the nasopharynx. A light and elec-

tron microscopical study. Clin Otolaryngol 1977; 2: 105.

7 Shanmugaratnam K, Chan SH, de-The G, Goh JEH, Khor TH, Simons MJ, Tye CY. Histopathology of nasopharyngeal carcinoma. Correlations with epidemiology, survival rates and other biological characteristics. Cancer 1979; 44: 1029.

8 Taxy JB, Hidvegi DF, Battifora H. Nasopharyngeal carcinoma: Antikeratin immunohistochemistry and electron microscopy. Am J Clin Pathol 1985; 83: 320.

9 Weiland LH, Neel HB, Pearson GR. Nasopharyngeal carcinoma. Curr Hematol Oncol 1986; 4: 379.

10 Henle W, Henle G. Epidemiologic aspects of Epstein-Barr virus (EBV-associated) diseases. Ann NY Acad Sci 1980; 354: 326.

11 Watson CRR. The anatomy of the post-nasal space: its significance in local malignant invasion. Aust Radiol 1972; 16: 118.

12 Henderson BE, Louie E, Jing JS, Buell P, Gardner MB. Risk factors associated with nasopharyngeal carcinoma. N Engl J Med 1976; 295: 1101.

13 Henle W, Henle G. Epstein-Barr virus and human malignancies. Adv Viral Oncol 1985; 5: 201.

14 Hwang H-N. Nasopharyngeal carcinoma in the People's Republic of China: Incidence, treatment, and survival rates. Radiology 1983; 149: 305.

15 Bedoya V, Betancur M. Nasopharyngeal and adjacent neoplasms in Medellin, Colombia. In: Grundman E, Krueger GRF, Ablashi DV eds Nasopharyngeal Carcinomas Cancer Campaign, Vol 5. Stuttgart: Gustav Fischer Verlag, 1981; 17–30.

16 Dickson RI. Nasopharyngeal carcinoma. An evaluation of 209 patients. Laryngoscope 1981; 91: 333.

17 Dickson RI, Flores AD. Nasopharyngeal carcinoma. An evaluation of 134 patients treated between 1971–180. Laryngoscope 1985; 95: 276.

18 Lanier A, Bender T, Talbot M, Wilmeth S, Tschopp C, Henle W, Henle G, Ritter D, Terasaki P. Nasopharyngeal carcinoma in Alaskan Eskimos, Indians and Aleuts: A review of cases and study of Epstein-Barr virus, HLA, and environmental risk factors. Cancer 1980; 46: 2100.

19 Moloy PJ, Chung YT, Krivitsky PB, Kim RC. Squamous carcinoma of the nasopharynx. West J Med 1985; 143: 66.

20 Moore SB, Pearson GR, Neel HB, Weiland LH. HLA and nasopharyngeal carcinoma in North American Caucasoids. Tissue Antigens 1983; 22: 72.

21 Levine PH, Connelly RR, Easton JM. Demographic patterns for nasopharyngeal carcinoma in the United States. Int J Cancer 1980; 26: 741.

22 Greene MH, Fraumeni JF, Hoover R. Nasopharyngeal cancer among young people in the United States: Racial variations by cell type. J Natl Cancer Inst 1977; 58: 1267.

23 Easton JM, Levine PH, Hyams VJ. Nasopharyngeal carcinoma in the United States. A pathologic study of 177 US and 30 foreign cases. Arch Otolaryngol 1980; 106: 88.

24 Neel HB. A prospective evaluation of patients with nasopharyngeal carcinoma: An overview. J Otolaryngol 1986; 15: 137.

25 Wolf H, Haus M, Wilmes E. Persistence of Epstein-Barr virus in the parotid gland. J Virol 1984; 51: 795.

26 Lung ML, So SY, Chan KH, Lam WK, Lam WP, Ng MH. Evidence that respiratory tract is a major reservoir for Epstein-Barr virus. Lancet 1985; i: 889.

27 Young LS, Sixbey JW, Clark D, Rickinson AB. Epstein-Barr virus receptors on human nasopharyngeal epithelia. Lancet 1986; ii: 240.

28 Sato H, Takimoto T, Ogura H, Tanaka J, Hatano M, Glaser R. Heterogeneity of Epstein-Barr virus derived from a nasopharyngeal carcinoma that has transforming and lytic properties. J Natl Cancer Inst 1986; 76: 1019.

29 Nielsen NH, Mikkelsen F, Hansen JPH. Nasopharyngeal cancer in Greenland. Acta Pathol Microbiol Scand (Sect A) 1977; 85: 850.

30 Krueger GRF, Kottaridis SD, Wolf H, Ablashi DV, Sesterhenn K, Bertram G. Histological types of nasopharyngeal carcinoma as compared to EBV serology. Anticancer Res 1981; 1: 187.

31 Prathap K, Looi LM, Prasad U. Localized amyloidosis in nasopharyngeal carcinoma. Histopathology 1984; 8: 27.

32 Nomori H, Watanabe S, Nakajima T, Shimosato Y, Kameya T. Histiocytes in nasopharyngeal carcinoma in relation to prognosis. Cancer 1986; 57: 100.

33 Moller P, Wirbel R, Hofmann W, Schwachheimer K. Lymphoepithelial carcinoma (Schmincke type) as a derivate of the tonsillar crypt epithelium. Virchows Arch (Pathol Anat) 1984; 405: 85.

34 Micheau C, Luboinski B, Schwaab G, Richard J, Cachin Y. Lymphoepitheliomas of the larynx (undifferentiated carcinomas of nasopharyngeal type). Clin Otolaryngol 1979; 4: 43.

35 Rosai J. 'Lymphoepithelioma-like' thymic carcinoma. Another tumor related to Epstein-Barr Virus? New Engl J Med 1985; 312: 1320.

36 Mills SE. Austin MB, Randall ME. Lymphoepithelioma-like carcinoma of the uterine cervix with inflammatory stroma. Am J Surg Pathol 1985; 9: 883.

37 Zhang CX, Deng TG. Tumors in the ENT region–analysis of 1,776 cases. Chin J Oto Rhino Laryngol 1979; 14: 240.

38 Yin ZY, Wu XL, Hu YH, Gu XZ. Cylindroma of the nasopharynx. A chronic disease. Int J Radiat Oncol Biol Phys 1986; 12: 25.

39 Lee D-J, Smithe RL, Spaziani JT, Rostock R, Holliday M, Moses H. Adenoid cystic carcinoma of the nasopharynx. Case reports and literature review. Ann Otol Rhinol Laryngol 1985; 94: 269.

40 Neel HB, Pearson GR, Weiland LH, Taylor WF, Goepfert H, Philch BZ, Goodman M, Lanier AP, Huang AT, Hyams VJ, Levine PH, Henle G, Henle W. Applications of Epstein-Barr virus serology to the diagnosis and staging of North American patients with nasopharyngeal carcinoma. Otolaryngol Head Neck Surg 1983; 91: 225.

41 Arnold W. Morphological evidence of viruses in nasopharyngeal carcinoma. Acta Otolaryngol 1983; 95: 447.

42 Chan SH, Day NE, Khor TH, Kunaratnam M, Chia KB. HLA markers in the development and prognosis of NPC in Chinese. In: Grundman E, Krueger GRF, Ablashi DV eds Nasopharyngeal Carcinomas, Cancer Campaign, Vol 5. Stuttgart: Gustav Fischer Verlag, 1981: 205–11.

43 Neel HB. Nasopharyngeal carcinoma: clinical presentation, diagnosis, treatment and prognosis. Otolaryngeal Clin North Am 1985; 18: 479.

44 Sawaki S, Sugano H, Hirayama T. Analytical aspects of symptoms of nasopharyngeal malignancies. In: de-The G, Ito Y eds Nasopharyngeal Carcinoma: Etiology and Control, Publication No. 20. Lyon: IARC Scientific Publication, 1978: 147–63.

45 Payne DG. Carcinoma of the nasopharynx. J Otolaryngol 1983; 12: 197.

46 Vikram B, Mishra UB, Strong EW, Manolatos S. Patterns of failure in carcinoma of the nasopharynx. Failure at distinct sites. Head Neck Surg 1986; 8: 276.

47 Huang S-C, Chu G-L. Nasopharyngeal cancer: Study II. Int J Radiat Oncol Biol Phys 1981; 7: 713.

48 The American Joint Committee for Cancer Staging and End Results Reporting. Manual for Staging Cancer. The American Joint Committee, Chicago, 1978.

49 Ho JH. Stage classification of nasopharyngeal carcinoma: A review. IARC Sci Publ 1978; 20: 99.

50 Harmer MH (ed). TNM Classification of Malignant Tumors, 3rd edition. Geneva: International Union Against Cancer, 1978.

51 Neel HB, Taylor WF, Pearson GR. Prognostic determinants and a new view of staging for patients with nasopharyngeal carcinoma. Ann Otol Rhinol Laryngol 1985; 94: 529.

52 Amendola BE, Thrall JH, Amen dola MA, Kanellitsas C. Radiation therapy in carcinoma of the nasopharynx (Abstract). Int J Radiat Oncol Biol Phys 1981; 7: 1286.

53 Amornmarn R, Prempree T, Sewchand W, Jaiwatana J. Radiation management of advanced nasopharyngeal cancer. Cancer 1983; 52: 802.

54 Baker SR, Wolf A. Prognostic factors of nasopharyngeal malignancy. Cancer 1982; 49: 163.

55 Bedwinek JM, Perez CA, Keys DJ. Analysis of failures after definitive irradiation for epidermoid carcinoma of the nasopharynx. Cancer 1980; 45: 2725.

56 Bey P, Gueddari B, Malissard L, Pernot M. Nasopharyngeal carcinomas. A review based on 42 cases treated between 1968 and 1977. Ann Otolaryngol Chir Cervicofac 1981; 98: 43.

57 Boljesikova E, Durkovsky J, Michalikova B. Our experience with the treatment of nasopharyngeal tumors. Neoplasm 1982; 29: 351.

58 Castro VH, Mendiondo OR, Shaw DL, Jelden G, Rene JB, Someren A. Tumors of the nasopharynx in the second decade of life. Their natural history and therapeutic results. Radiodiagn Radiother 1982; 2: 25.

59 Cellai E, Chiavacci A, Olmi P, Carcangiu ML. Carcinoma of the nasopharynx. Results of radiation therapy. Acta Radiol Oncol Radiat Phys Biol 1982; 21: 87.

60 Chu AM, Flynn M, Achino E, Mendoza EF, Scott RM, Jose B. Irradiation of nasopharyngeal carcinoma: Correlations with treatment factors and stage. Int J Radiat Oncol Biol Phys 1984; 10: 2241.

61 Cooper JS, del Rowe J, Newall J. Regional stage IV carcinoma of the nasopharynx treated by aggressive radiotherapy. Int J Radiat Oncol Biol Phys 1983; 9: 1737.

62 Flores AD, Dickson RI, Riding K. Cancer of the nasopharynx in British Columbia, 1985 (in press).

63 Frezza G, Barbieri E, Emiliani E, Silvano M, Babini L. Patterns of failure in nasopharyngeal

cancer treated with megavoltage irradiation. Radiother Oncol 1986; 5: 287.

64 Haghbin M, Kramer S, Patchefsky AS, Prestipino AJ. Carcinoma of the nasopharynx. A 25 year study. Am J Clin Oncol 1985; 8: 384.

65 Jenkin RD, Anderson JR, Jereb B, Thompson JC, Pyesmany A, Wara WM, Hammond D. Nasopharyngeal carcinoma: A retrospective review of patients less than thirty years of age— a report from Children's Cancer Study Group. Cancer 1981; 47: 360.

66 John AC, Busby ER, Jones PH. Long-term survival in nasopharyngeal carcinoma. J Laryngol Otol 1980; 94: 1265.

67 Kajanti M, Mantyla M. Local control after radiotherapy of carcinoma of the nasopharynx: A retrospective analysis (Abstract). 3rd European Conference on Clinical Oncology and Cancer Nursing, June 16–20, 1985, Stockholm, Sweden, 1985, p 85.

68 Levendag PC, Huygen PL, Kazem I, van den Brock P, Slooff JL. Malignant tumours of the nasopharynx: Retrospective review of 74 cases. Clin Radiol 1983; 34: 451.

69 Marks JE, Bedwinek JM, Lee F, Purdy JA, Perez CA. Dose-response analysis for nasopharyngeal carcinoma. A historical perspective. Cancer 1982; 50: 1042.

70 Mesic JB, Fletcher GH, Goepfert H. Megavoltage irradiation of epithelial tumors of the nasopharynx. Int J Radiat Oncol Biol Phys 1981; 7: 447.

71 Million RR, Cassisi NJ. Nasopharynx In: Million RR, Cassisi NJ eds Management of Head and Neck Cancer: A Multidisciplinary Approach, Philadelphia: JB Lippincott, 1984: 445–66.

72 Petrovich Z, Cocks JD, Middleton R, Ohanian M, Paig C, Jepson J. Advanced carcinoma of the nasopharynx. Patterns of failures in 256 patients. Radiother Oncol 1985; 4: 15.

73 Ring AH, Sako K, Razack MS, Chen TY, Shedd DP. Nasopharyngeal carcinoma: results of treatment over a 27 year period, 1950 through 1977. Am J Surg 1983; 146: 429.

74 Robin PE, Powell DJ, Holme GM. Malignant tumors of the nasopharynx: 220 cases 1957–1966. Clin Otolaryngol 1980; 5: 139.

75 Schabinger PR, Reddy S, Hendrickson FR, Phillips RL, Saxena V. Carcinoma of the nasopharynx: survival and patterns of recurrence. Int J Radiat Oncol Biol Phys 1985; 11: 2081.

76 van Andel JG, Hop WC. Carcinoma of the nasopharynx. A review of 86 cases. Clin Radiol 1982; 33: 95.

77 Vikram B, Strong EW, Manolatos S, Mishra

UB. : Improved survival in carcinoma of the nasopharynx. Head Neck Surg 1984; 7: 123.

78 Wang CC. Treatment of malignant tumors of the nasopharynx. Otolaryngol. Clin North Am 1980; 13: 477.

79 Chang C, Liu T, Chang Y, Shilong C. Radiation therapy of nasopharyngeal carcinoma. Acta Radiol Oncol 1980; 19: 433.

80 Pearson GR, Neel HB et al. Antibody dependent cellular cytotoxicity and disease course in North American patients with nasopharyngeal carcinoma: a prospective study. Int J Cancer 1984; 33: 772.

81 Peters LJ. Basic principles of radiobiology in head and neck oncology. In: Larson DB, Ballantyre AJU, Guillamondegui OM eds Cancer in the Neck, New York: Macmillan 1986: 75–103.

82 Peters LJ, Ang KK. Unconventional fractionation schemes in radiotherapy. In: DeVita V, Hellman S, Rosenberg SA eds Important Advances in Oncology 1986, pp. 269–286. Philadelphia: JB Lippincott, 1986: 269–86.

83 Million RR, Fletcher GH. Nasopharynx. In: Fletcher GH ed Textbook of Radiotherapy, 3rd edition. Philadelphia: Lea & Febiger, 1980: 364–83.

84 Daly T. Dental care in the irradiated patients. In: Fletcher GH ed Textbook of Radiotherapy, 3rd edition. Philadelphia: Lea & Febiger, 1980: 229–37.

85 Perry Keene DA, Connelly JF, Young RA et al. Hypothalamic hypopituitorism following external radiotherapy for tumors distant from the adenohypophysis. 1976; 5: 373.

86 Samaan, NA, Vieto R, Schult RN et al. Hypothalamic, pituitary and thyroid dysfunction after radiotherapy of the head and neck. Int J Radiat Oncol Biol Phys 1982; 8: 1857.

87 McNeese MD, Fletcher GH. Retreatment of recurrent nasopharyngeal carcinoma. Radiology 1981; 138: 191.

88 Hong WK, Bromer R. Chemotherapy in head and neck cancer. N Engl J Med 308: 75–79, 1983.

89 Holoye PY, Byers RM, Gard DA et al. Combination chemotherapy of head and neck. Cancer 1978; 42: 1661.

90 Goepfert H, Moran MG, Lindberg R, Jesse RH et al. Chemotherapy of advanced nasopharyngeal carcinoma. Proc ASCO 1981; 22: 427.

91 Huang AT, Cole TB, Fishburns R, Baughn SG, Lucas VS. Chemotherapy for nasopharyngeal carcinoma. In: Grundman E, Krueger GRF, Ablashi DV eds Nasopharyngeal Carci-

nomas, Cancer Campaign, Vol 5. Stuttgart: Gustav Fischer Verlag, 1981.

92 Decker DA, Drelichman A, Al-Sarraf M, Crissman J, Reed ML. Chemotherapy for nasopharyngeal carcinoma: A ten year experience. Cancer 1983; 52: 605.

93 Hong WK, Dimery I. Adjuvant chemotherapy in head and neck cancer. In: Larson DL, Ballantyre AJ, Guillamondegui OM eds Cancer in the Neck. New York: Macmillan, 1986: 195–204.

94 Al-Kourainy K, Crissman J, Ensley J, Kish J, Al-Sarraf M. Excellent response to cis-platinum based combination for recurrent and previously untreated locally advanced nasopharyngeal carcinoma. Proc ASCO 1985; 4: 131.

95 Al-Sarraf M, Zundamanis M, Marcial V, Laramore G. Concurrent cis-platin and radiotherapy in patients with locally advanced nasopharyngeal carcinomas. RTOG study. Proc. ASCO 1986; 5: 142.

96 Galligioni G, Carbone A, Tirelli U, Veronesi A et al. Combined chemotherapy with doxorubicin, bleomycin, vinblastine, dacarbazine, and radiotherapy for advanced lymphoepithelioma. Cancer Treat Rep 1982; 66: 1207.

97 Hill BT, Price LA, MacRae K. The promising role of safe initial non-cisplatin containing combination chemotherapy in nasopharyngeal tumors. Proc ASCO 1985; 4: 129.

98 Kuten A, Zidan G, Cohen Y, Robinson L. Progress report on the treatment of advanced squamous cancer of the head and neck by bleomycin, methotrexate and cisplatin (BMP) followed by radiotherapy. Superior survival in complete responders and in nasopharyngeal carcinoma. Proc ASCO 1986; 5: 126.

99 Rossi A, Molinari R, Marubini E et al. Adjuvant chemotherapy after complete response to radiotherapy in nasopharyngeal cancer: Follow-up of a randomized study. Proc ASCO 1986; 5: 147.

100 Tannock I, Hewitt K, Payne D. Chemotherapy given prior to radiation for nasopharyngeal cancer produces a high rate of tumor response but does not improve survival. Proc ASCO 1986; 5: 133.

101 Trenner J, Neithammer D, Dannecker G et al. Successful treatment of nasopharyngeal carcinoma with interferon. Lancet 1980; i: 817.

102 Connors JM, Andiman WA, Howarth CB, Liu E, Mierigna TC, Jacobs C. Treatment of nasopharyngeal carcinoma with human leukocyte interferon. J Clin Oncol 1985; 3: 813.

Chapter **53**

Soft Tissue Sarcomas of the Head and Neck

R. Kim Davis* and
Milton Waner†
* Associate Professor, Division of Head and Neck Surgery,
Department of Otolaryngology, University of Utah, Salt
Lake City, Utah, USA and † Senior Lecturer, Department
of Surgery, Division of Otolaryngology, University of
Sydney, New South Wales, Australia

HISTORY

Sarcomas are malignant tumours arising from any non-epithelial mesodermal tissue. The term sarcoma is derived from the Greek 'Sarx' meaning flesh, by way of sarcoma meaning a fleshy excrescence. It was Rudolph Virchow (1892–1902) who separated sarcomas from epithelial cancers and defined them as a variety of tumour that evolved from non-epithelial and non-haematogenous tissue. Virchow distinguished six major types of sarcoma:

1. Fibrosarcoma.
2. Myxosarcoma.
3. Gliosarcoma.
4. Melanosarcoma.
5. Chondrosarcoma.
6. Osteosarcoma.

EPIDEMIOLOGY

Soft tissue sarcomas today account for approximately 4500 cases of malignancy yearly in the United States. The head and neck area accounts for approximately 15% of these cases while soft tissue sarcomas in general, compose only 0.6% of all cancers. In patients under the age of 15, 6.5% of cancers are soft tissue sarcomas. These sarcomas are the fifth most common cancer under the age of 15. The majority of childhood tumours are rhabdomyosarcomas, primarily arising in the head and neck area. In adults the incidence tends to be higher in the extremities while the head and neck is the least affected. There are no sex predilections in the occurrence of soft tissue sarcomas.

PATHOLOGY AND BIOLOGY

There are over 20 different histological diagnoses that comprise soft tissue sarcomas. The classification of these diseases by the World Health Organization, as modified by Enzinger (1), is probably the mostly widely accepted classification system. These tumours are divided into three groups:

1. Tumours of known histogenesis.
2. Tumours of specific type but uncertain histogenesis.
3. Tumours of undetermined type.

1007

As the frequency of these malignancies in the head and neck is so limited, these tumours will be divided into rhabdomyosarcomas versus all other soft tissue sarcomas. The main sarcomas in this group include malignant fibrous histiocytoma, fibrosarcoma, liposarcoma, and synovial cell sarcoma. The second sub-division of particular importance in the head and neck area is that of paediatric sarcomas (mainly rhabdomyosarcomas), versus soft tissue sarcomas in adults.

Virtually all soft tissue sarcomas of the head and neck have a common natural history, characterized by very aggressive local invasion and early distant spread of disease. These malignancies spread extensively along anatomic structures such as nerve bundles, muscle fibres and fascial planes. Microscopic extension at great distance from the primary gross tumour is common. Additionally, skip areas in soft tissue are frequently seen as a local occurrence following surgical excision of these tumours. While local recurrence following surgical excision alone has been found in approximately 50% of reported patients, this may even be higher in the head and neck. Distant metastases may also occur early in the course of this disease. The lungs are the most common site of metastases in head and neck patients. When all patients with soft tissue sarcoma are considered, 10% of patients present with pulmonary metastases at the time of initial diagnosis.

Rhabdomyosarcoma

This is the most common soft tissue sarcoma in children. The head and neck is one of the most common tumour sites for this malignancy. Rhabdomyosarcoma is a high grade tumour of striated muscle origin, which tends to infiltrate muscle bundles widely. It is a highly aggressive tumour, with a propensity to spread by local extension, by haematogenous routes, and by a lymphatic spread. These tumours often originate on or near the meninges and have a high potential to spread to the central nervous

system by direct extension as well via subarachnoid fluid.

The original histological description by Horn and Enterline divided these tumours into three categories on the basis of pathological features.

1. Embryonal tumours.
2. Alveolar rhabdomyosarcoma.
3. Pleomorphic types.

Approximately 70% are embryonal, 20% alveolar, and the remainder, undifferentiated or pleomorphic (2).

Malignant Fibrous Histiosarcoma

This is the most common soft tissue sarcoma in all patients. Approximately 3% of these lesions occur in the head and neck area. There is a male to female predominance in this malignancy of approximately 3:1 in the head and neck. A wide range of histological features are seen, and it is impossible to predict the malignant potential of these tumours solely on the basis of their histopathological features. Blitzer et al. reviewed the literature and reported that fibrous histiosarcomas of the head and neck were reported in the following locations: intraosseous, paranasal sinuses, oral cavity, major salivary glands, airway, neck and temporomandibular joint (3).

Synovial Cell Sarcoma

Synovial cell sarcoma of the soft tissues of the head and neck was first described in 1954. A review by one of the authors (R.K.D.) of 66 cases accumulated at the Armed Forces Institute of Pathology between 1948 and 1981 revealed 43 males and 23 females with an age range of 9 to 74 years. Tumour sites in order of frequency were: hypopharynx, neck, face, lateral oropharynx, larynx, retropharynx, and nasopharynx. These tumours were all well circumscribed, frequently covered by a thin fibrous capsule, and were easily dissected from surrounding structures. Histologically, two neoplastic cellular components are described;

a spindle cell component and a pseudoepithe-lioid component. This biphasic pattern is the only histological feature by which a diagnosis of synovial cell sarcoma can be made with certainty (4).

Liposarcomas

These are the most commonly encountered soft tissue sarcomas; they are extremely rare in the head and neck. Liposarcomas arise from toti-potential mesenchymal cells or lipoblasts within or adjacent to fascial and intramuscular areas. They do not arise from a pre-existing lipoma and rarely arise from subcutaneous adipose tissue (5).

Liposarcomas appear macroscopically to be encapsulated. However, this is a false capsule, caused by compression of surrounding tissue. Satelite nodules leading off from the main mass are very common and these account for the recurrence, post excision in 'shelling out' pro-cedures. The appearance of the matrix will depend on its predominant composition. The tumour is made up of fat cells, myxoid compo-nents, fibrous elements, vascular tissue and a variable amount of necrotic tissue. Batsakis divides liposarcomas into the following four sub-groups (6).

1. Myxoid.
2. Round cell type.
3. Well differentiated or adult type.
4. Pleomorphic type.

Their histological features will thus vary according to the predominant cell type. All stages in the embryological development of fatty tissue are found, from the primitive lipoblast to the mature lipocyte (6).

Fibrosarcoma

Many of the earlier studies dealing with soft tissue sarcomas designated fibrosarcoma as being the most common tumour of this variety. Unfortunately fibrosarcomas were confused with other soft tissue tumours and therefore misdiagnosis probably accounted for this pre-ponderance. Fibrosarcomas currently only account for 5.5% of soft tissue sarcomas (7).

The most common site of origin of fibrosar-coma in the head and neck appears to be the face followed by the neck. Fibrosarcomas of the paranasal sinuses are less common, and a few cases of fibrosarcoma of the nasopharynx have been reported (6).

Fibrosarcomas are slow growing, locally infiltrative, and are associated with a better prognosis than other soft tissue sarcomas of the head and neck. They metastasize rarely.

Histologically fibrosarcomas may be well differentiated, moderately well differentiated, or poorly differentiated. Well differentiated lesions are less cellular, and the fibroblasts appear uniform in size and shape, and do not exhibit much mitotic activity. The cells lie in a bed of well developed collagen, arranged in bands and bundles. Moderately differentiated fibrosarcomas are more cellular, and less well organized. Poorly differentiated tumours are highly cellular, exhibit no signs of differentia-tion and have very sparse intercellular matrix (6).

CLINICAL FEATURES

The clinical features of soft tissue sarcomas of the head and neck depend on the tumour type and the size of the lesion.

Rhabdomyosarcoma

While the orbit is the most common site lesion, the nasopharynx, ear and naso-sinus areas are also sites of predilection for this tumour. These tumours are locally invasive and will infiltrate surrounding tissues to include the sphenoid, maxillary and ethmoid sinuses. The clivus, base of skull, orbit, nasal cavity, and temporal bones are also commonly involved. Infiltration of the base of skull will result in cranial nerve deficits.

Rhabdomyosarcoma is the most common malignancy of the ear in children. In a review by Pratt and Gray (8), of 50 patients, the predominant symptoms were:

1. A mass in the region of the ear, 56%.
2. A polyp in the ear canal, 54%.
3. An aural discharge, 40%.
4. Bleeding from the ear, 30%.
5. Earache, 22%.
6. Deafness, 14%.
7. Facial nerve paralysis, 14%.

Eighty per cent of these patients were under 12 years of age and the average age was 4.4 years. These tumours were felt to originate from the palatal muscles around the eustachian tube, and spread to the middle ear and mastoid as well as the petrosal cells.

The presenting symptom of a rhabdomyosarcoma involving the nose or paranasal sinuses is often a visible mass, nasal bleeding, nasal obstruction, headache, nasal polyps, rinorrhoea, and proptosis.

Synovial Cell Sarcoma

The most common presenting symptom was that of a solitary painless mass with associated dysphagia, hoarseness, or dyspnoea depending on the site of origin. At surgery, these tumours originated mainly in the prevertebral connective tissue space, often extending from the base of skull to the hypopharynx.

Malignant Fibrous Histiosarcoma

Fibrous histiosarcomas of skin usually present as a painful, slow growing, subcutaneous mass. Duration of the tumour may vary from only a few months to many decades. Occasionally multiple subcutaneous nodules may coalesce to form a continuous plaque usually level with the skin surface, fixed to skin, but freely mobile over deeper structures. The tumour may remain in this state for many years but eventually secondary tumours appear on the surface. These vary in size from a few millimetres to several centimetres (6). The tumour may become necrotic, soft, or haemorrhagic, and eventually ulceration of the surface of the tumour may take place.

Alternatively a tumour presenting in the paranasal sinus will result in eventual obstruction of that sinus and symptoms of chronic sinusitis. Growth into surrounding structures may cause proptosis, nasal obstruction, and eventual erosion of overlying bone and the presence of a subcutaneous facial mass.

Fibrosarcoma

Fibrosarcomas appear to grow more slowly, infiltrate less extensively, and are less frequently metastatic and therefore associated with a better prognosis, when compared with other soft tissue sarcomas in the head and neck. Clinical presentation is variable and will obviously depend on the site of the tumour. Signs and symptoms therefore are not unlike those described in the foregoing paragraphs.

Liposarcomas

These present as a subcutaneous soft tissue mass of variable size. Since their origin is rarely subcutaneous, they are usually large by the time they are presented in the subcutaneous area. Their consistency will vary according to the predominant tissue component. And differentiation of these tumours from other soft tissue sarcomas is not possible on clinical examination. These tumours are both locally infiltrative and have a tendency to metastasize (6). Approximately 30% of patients with pleomorphic variants have metastases at the time of initial presentation (9, 10).

INVESTIGATIONS

The most common sites of soft tissue sarcoma in the head and neck are the neck, nasopharynx, ear, sinonasal area and parapharyngeal space. It is imperative that a tissue diagnosis be made prior to planning of treatment. The three major techniques of obtaining tissue from soft tissue sarcomas include needle biopsy, incisional biopsy, and excisional biopsy. Fine needle aspiration cytology, which has been particularly helpful in squamous cell carcinoma and salivary gland tumours, has to date been of limited value in the diagnosis of sarcomas. With the introduction of more sophisticated immunohistochemistry markers, fine needle aspiration may well become more important (11). One of the difficulties with fine needle aspiration or even needle biopsy of soft tissue masses is poor sampling of tumour tissue. Soft tissue sarcomas are often loosely adherent. Obtaining a core of tissue may thus be very difficult. As the exact histological nature of these tumours is difficult to determine, often significant amounts of tissue are required. Furthermore electron microscopy is often necessary to confirm the diagnosis of these tumours.

The preferred method of making a diagnosis of the soft tissue sarcoma is by incisional biopsy, which presents a dilemma for the head and neck surgeon. Most head and neck surgeons feel that incisional biopsy of the most frequent head and neck cancer, namely, squamous cell carcinoma, will decrease survival period. On the other hand excisional biopsy of soft tissue sarcomas is equally to be condemned. While soft tissue sarcomas often have a pseudocapsule and can in fact easily be excised, these malignancies almost always extend beyond the pseudocapsule sometimes at a great distance from the presenting mass. Excisional biopsy in this context simply spreads the tumour, leaves a greater chance of haematoma formation, which will further spread the tumour, and thus create difficulty in delineating the tumour extent with subsequent computed tomography (CT) or magenetic resonance imaging (MRI) scanning. When soft tissue sarcomas are suspected on the basis of fine needle aspiration cytology or in the case of a clinical presentation different from that commonly seen with squamous cell carcinoma, an incisional biopsy can be entertained. Such an incisional biopsy must be performed through an incision carefully placed so as not to compromise subsequent surgery. The biopsy should be obtained under direct vision with care to obtain excellent haemostasis. With soft tissue sarcomas there is no evidence that incisional biopsy leads to increased spread of these tumours. This is in contradistinction to the case of squamous cell carcinoma of the head and neck.

Since the rate of distant metastasis at the time of presentation is high, a full metastatic workup of these patients is imperative. This must include a chest CT, a bone scan and a biochemical screen (SMA-20). The use of head and abdominal CT is dictated by the patient's presenting symptoms. Imaging of the primary tumour has been done by CT, but MRI may be in fact more helpful. A recent study by Weekes et al. showed MRI to be better than CT in defining the anatomic extent of these tumours (12). Relationship of these tumours to major vascular structures was clearly defined in 80% of MRI scans as opposed to only 62% of CT scans. MRI and CT were shown to be equally effective in determining the presence or absence of bony invasion. When CT or MRI of the primary lesion is performed, it is not necessary to routinely image the neck in the absence of palpable regional disease. A study by Weingard and Rosenberg reviewing more than 2000 patients with soft tissue sarcomas showed metastases to regional lymph nodes in only 5% of patients (13).

STAGING

Several staging systems have been developed for soft tissue sarcomas. Table 1 shows the staging system proposed by the task force on soft tissue sarcomas of the American Joint Committee for Cancer Staging and the end results (14). In contrast to the staging of squamous cell carcinoma, the grade of the sarcoma is the most important single prognostic fact. Histological grades vary from well differentiated Grade I lesions to poorly differentiated or undifferentiated Grade III lesions. These grades are assigned to soft tissue sarcomas on the basis of estimates of the number of mitoses, the presence of necrosis, cellularity, pleomorphism, and cell type. In a multivariate analysis of prognostic factors related to recurrence in soft tissue sarcomas, Heise et al. demonstrated the prognostic importance of tumour location, presence or absence of direct extension to surrounding structures, symptoms related to the tumour mass, and tumour size (< 5 cm vs ⩾ 5 cm) (15). These factors were all important prognostic indications in addition to the grade of the tumour.

TREATMENT

Surgery has long been the mainstay of soft tissue sarcoma therapy. As has been suggested earlier, surgery often fails to achieve a cure due to the high local recurrence rates and the high incidence of metastases. In the various series, the local recurrence rate has ranged from 40 to 80% in adult sarcomas and as high as 90% in childhood sarcomas. This has led to the addition of radiation therapy as well as the use of adjuvant chemotherapy. As there are major differences in the response rate of childhood sarcomas vs adult sarcomas, to the different treatment regimens, and as the incidence of rhabdomyosarcoma in the head and neck in paediatric patients is notably higher than any other soft tissue sarcoma, this section on treatment will be divided accordingly. Attention will be directed to the treatment of paediatric soft tissue sarcomas divided into rhabdomyosarcomas and all other soft tissue sarcomas. The discussion of adult sarcomas will include these tumours as one group.

Historically, the treatment of rhabdomyosarcoma was primarily surgical. Surgery as a primary modality lost popularity as a result of the severe cosmetic and functional deformities seen with wide surgical excision. This was furthermore complicated by a poor overall cure rate. As megavoltage radiation units became more common, large volume irradiation was administered with curative intent and was soon accepted as a preferable alternative to massive surgical resection. With orbital rhabdomyosarcoma, high dose megavoltage irradiation has led to local control and cure in 90% of cases with the preservation of sight (16). Other head and neck sites could not be controlled as readily by radiation therapy due to the proximity of vital structures such as the brain and spinal cord, which severely limited

the total dose as well as the portals of radiation. In addition, as many patients died of systemic disease, indicating the presence of distant metastases at the time of first presentation, the need for systemic therapy was recognized.

The efficacy of a coordinated programme using surgery, radiation and triple drug combination chemotherapy was demonstrated by Pratt et al. (17). They reported 7 of 20 children who achieved tumour free survival from 3 to 39 months post-treatment. The value of adjuvant combined chemotherapy was further tested in a prospective randomized trial by the Children's Cancer Study Group (18). In this study surgical staging was accomplished followed by postoperative radiation therapy to all children. Additionally, children were treated with dactinomycin and vincristine. When complete resection was possible and postoperative radiation therapy given, followed by chemotherapy, 14 of 17 patients remained in remission for at least 2 years. This was compared to 7 of 15 patients when no adjuvant chemotherapy was used.

With these initial results, the Inter Group Rhabdomyoma Study Group, was subsequently formed, testing, in a series of protocols, the efficacy of chemotherapy and radiation therapy as a function of surgical stage. The preliminary report of this group was published in 1977 (19) with the following observations:

1. Prognosis is poor with increasing tumour burden, i.e. increased stage.
2. In localized tumours, amenable to complete resection, postoperative radiation therapy was unnecesary if the patient was given vincristine, dactinomycin, and cyclophosphamide chemotherapy.
3. Three drug regimens as above failed to show improved results over two drug regimen (vincristine and dactinomycin only) in patients with stage II disease when postoperative radiation therapy was given;
4. Any recurrence, local or metastatic, is associated with a grave prognosis.

This study did show that local control of microscopic residual disease could be obtained in 90% or more of cases when adequate radiation therapy and combination chemotherapy was used. It was shown that local control was definitely greater for tumours less than 5 cm, than for those 5 cm or greater. When chemotherapy is given, 4500–5000 rads is necessary to control microscopic disease; 5000–5500 rads is recommended for gross residual disease (19).

The value of combined chemotherapy with radiation therapy has been further confirmed by Flamant and Hill, in clinical Stage III and IV tumours of the head and neck (20). In an attempt to conserve cosmesis and function, an Amsterdam pilot study was performed in children with head and neck as well as urogenital primaries, relying on primary chemotherapy in an attempt to later use a more conservative local modality (21). Of 24 patients managed primarily with vincristine, dactinomycin and cyclophosphamide, only 7, or 29%, were alive without evidence of disease at a median survival of 37 months. Ten of the 24 children ultimately required surgical resection to achieve disease-free status with a mean survival of 50 months. Of particular concern were 7 patients who developed intracranial extension and died from locoregional uncontrolled disease. In light of this, considerable concern remains in using primary chemotherapy alone to irradiate gross disease. Chemotherapy must be combined with radiation therapy or surgery (where functionally or cosmetically acceptable).

In the case of rhabdomyosarcoma, survival in this group of patients has been compromised by meningeal spread of the tumour, seen in 20 of 57 patients in a large review by Tefft et al. (22) Eighteen of these 20 patients died. This extremely poor prognosis relates to the inability to aggressively treat these lesions.

Only 3500–4000 rads of irradiation can be delivered to the entire craniospinal meninges, owing to the poor tolerance of the nervous tissue and bone marrow. Systemic chemotherapeutic agents which are otherwise effective against rhabdomyosarcoma do not cross the blood–brain barrier well. Further intrathecal therapy must be limited to specific agents which are non-toxic and are unfortunately inadequate for the treatment of rhabdomyosarcoma.

Soft tissue sarcomas other than rhabdomyosarcoma unfortunately have a poorer prognosis. In a large series by Horowitz et al. 62 cases of other soft tissue sarcomas treated in a single institution were reviewed (23). The most common diagnosis was synovial sarcoma, occurring in 18 patients, followed by malignant schwannoma in 12 patients. The median age at diagnosis was 11 years. Ten of these 62 cases were in the head and neck. In 31 patients whose tumours could be completely resected, 26 (84%) survived free of disease. Postoperative chemotherapy, administered to one-half of this group has not produced any demonstrable gain in survival period. Only one of the 26 patients with local or gross tumour remaining after resection has survived. This is in notable contrast to rhabdomyosarcoma where irradiation and chemotherapy has resulted in cure rates in the 50–70% range. To extrapolate from the Rhabdomyosarcoma Study Group and treat these patients with only chemotherapy or radiation therapy appears inappropriate. Aggressive surgical approaches remain imperative in this group of patients.

This study should be contrasted with a recent report from the Inter Group Rhabdomyosarcoma Study in which 72 patients with sarcoma of the oral cavity, oropharynx, larynx and parotid area, cheeks, scalp and neck could be analysed. Sixty-three (88%) of these patients attained complete remission of whom 13 subsequently relapsed. The 5-year complete remission rate was 78%. Patients with primary tumours arising in sites other than neck had retained a complete response rate exceeding 90%. In contrast, 11 relapses occurred in the 26 patients with neck primaries (54% retained complete response rate). Female infants younger than age 24 months were all likely to relapse. Prognostic factors with little or no influence on relapse included tumour size, histology, regional lymph node status, clinical group, and treatment arm. Five of 6 patients with failure at the primary site either had no radiation therapy or an insufficient dose (less than 3000 rads). No patient required major organ sacrifice such as laryngectomy or pharyngectomy. Isolated failure and regional nodes did not occur. Children with non-orbital, non-parameningeal head and neck rhabdomyosarcoma treated in accordance with the Inter Group Study have an excellent rate of local control and long term survival.

Treatment of adult soft tissue sarcomas remains a very perplexing problem. There are very few series of soft tissue sarcomas in the adult head and neck. Greager et al. reported on 53 adult patients with head and neck soft tissue sarcomas treated at the University of Illinois (24). The most common anatomic location was the neck (36%), and these patients had the highest 5-year disease free interval (67%). Fibrosarcoma was the most common histological type (26%). Patients with aggressive fibromatosis had the longest mean survival (93 months). The mean overall survival was 58.7 months and the disease free, 2-year, 5-year and 10-year survival rates, were 68% and 54% and 28% respectively. Wide local excision was the treatment of choice, with adjuvant radiation therapy or chemotherapy or both, used in selected patients. In this series, all long term survivors had well differentiated (Grade I tumours) or malignancies less than 5 cm in size. This study found reasonable prognosis in patients with fibrosarcoma, synovial cell sarcoma, and haemangiopericytoma. Angiosarcoma patients had the worst prognosis of all with a mean survival of 7 months. Preliminary data from this study suggest that high grade fibrosarcomas and liposarcomas are best treated by a combination of surgery and radiation therapy. Patients with myogenic sarcoma, malignant fibrous histiocytoma, high grade synovial cell sarcoma or haemangiopericytoma, are better treated with surgery, irradiation therapy and chemotherapy.

Rhabdomyosarcomas of the head and neck are distinctly less common in adults than in children. In a series of 54 cases of embryonal rhabdomyosarcoma reported by Lloyd et al.

only 4 patients had head and neck sites of origin (25). In this series the overall 5-year survival rate was only 21%, with 79% of patients dead in an average of 17 months after the primary diagnosis was made. In the patients with tumours less than 5 cm, 80% survived 5 years. In these patients, treatment with surgery only or surgery combined with either radiation therapy or chemotherapy, showed distinctly better survival rates than patients treated with chemotherapy or radiation therapy alone. This study illustrates that the success rates seen in childhood rhabdomyosarcoma cannot be extrapolated to adults. The mainstay of therapy in this group of patients remains surgery. If disease free margins cannot be obtained, then radiation therapy must be added. As 68% of these patients developed metastatic disease, local therapy alone is certainly insufficient. The lung was the most frequent site of metastases (49%). Twenty-four per cent of metastases were to bone, 14% to liver, and 11% to the brain. Interestingly, 33% of these patients had metastases to regional lymph nodes.

Similar results were seen in a study by Newman and Rice of patients with rhabdomyosarcoma of the head and neck treated at UCLA (26). In this study, a retrospective review of all cases of rhabdomyosarcoma was undertaken. Survival prior to the advent of cyclic multi-drug chemotherapy was compared to survival with this therapy. In the group of patients with chemotherapy, survival was 150% better with gross total removal of disease than with biopsy only. This confirms the observation that radiation therapy and chemotherapy alone is not sufficient in treating this tumour in adults. Interestingly, in this study, 15% of patients developed regional node metastases. However, 75% of these patients with regional nodes developed intracranial extension and died. In addition, 19% developed late regional node metastases. Eighty per cent of the patients developing late regional disease also developed systemic metastases and died. Survival in the absence of nodal disease was 41%. This study shows that in rhabdomyosarcoma of the head and neck, regional nodal metastases at any time imply a grave prognosis and more adversely affect survival than does nodal disease in squamous cell carcinoma of adults.

Due to the paucity of reported cases of adult head and neck soft tissue sarcoma, it is not possible from the literature to definitively state the best form of therapy. Several observations, however, seem appropriate:

1. Wide local resection of these tumours to include adequate volumes of normal tissue is almost never possible.
2. Local recurrence of cancer is high and portends a grave prognosis.
3. Metastatic recurrence is very common in the presence of local recurrence.
4. Almost all survivors have either Grade I sarcomas or sarcomas less than 5 cm.
5. Irradiation therapy and chemotherapy alone is rarely curative in these tumours.

In light of these observations the following recommendations are made. Vigorous surgery should be contemplated in head and neck soft tissue sarcomas in adults. Wide margins should be obtained where possible. Postoperative radiation therapy should be given to all patients except those with Grade I tumours, to enhance local control rates. The question of whether adjuvant chemotherapy will improve survival in these patients, cannot be determined from the available literature on head and neck sarcomas alone. It should be noted, however, that studies from the National Cancer Institute, have shown a tendency towards improved disease free survival in patients treated with adjuvant chemotherapy (27). These patients underwent complete resection of gross tumour, followed by postoperative irradiation therapy to 6000–6300 rads over 7–8 weeks. Those patients who additionally received chemotherapy, had a 3-year actuarial disease free survival in the chemotherapy arm of 77% vs 49% in the non-chemotherapy arm. The 3-year overall actuarial survival in the two treatment arms, however, represented 68% vs 58%. The tendency

toward improved disease free survival was apparent amongst those treated with chemotherapy. Chemotherapy in this group consisted of doxorubicin, cyclophosphamide, and methotrexate.

When patients are not operable, it should be noted that irradiation therapy alone has some efficacy in soft tissue sarcoma. In a study by Tepper and Suit, 51 patients were treated by irradiation therapy alone (28). Eleven of 51 patients were alive at a 5-year follow-up with no evidence of disease. The overall 5-year survival and local control rates were 25.1% and 33% respectively. Of these patients treated to a dosage of greater than 6400 rads, the 5-year survival and local control rates were 28.4% and 43.5% respectively. Local control rate in tumours less than 5 cm was 87.5%, in tumours 5–10 cm, 53%, and in tumours greater than 10 cm, was 30%. In this series only 4 patients had Grade I tumours and no survival difference could be detected between Grade II and Grade III tumours. The development of distant metastatic disease portends a grave prognosis in these patients. Some patients, however, can yet be salvaged. In study by Glenn, 12 of 57 patients developed pulmonary metastases (27). Three of these 12 patients were inoperable and died shortly thereafter. Nine patients were explored using a median sternotomy incision or staged by lateral thoracotomies, and 8 patients were rendered free of gross metastatic tumour. Of these 8, 4 did not recur for follow-up periods of 3, 16 and 22 months after resection of the pulmonary lesions. Where possible pulmonary metastases should be resected, as a significant number of patients can be given prolonged survival period. In a study by Greenall et al., the efficacy of chemotherapy in distant metastatic soft tissue sarcoma was investigated (29). Adriamycin has been found to be the most active single agent for patients with metastatic sarcoma. Any combination chemotherapy regimen that omits Adriamyacin has proven ineffective in adults. The most effective regimen currently is that of cyclophosphamide, vincristine, Adriamycin, and DTIC. This regimen has produced complete response rates of 13% and partial response rates of 28% in patients. Median survival in patients with complete responses has been 20–30 months whereas those with partial responses have survived 15 months. As complete response rates are still under 15% there is definitely a need for further evaluation of new regimens. On the other hand chemotherapy should be given to these patients when surgery is not possible. Experimental therapies for soft tissue sarcomas have to date proved to be minimally helpful. In a study by Ashby and Harmer hypofractionated radiation therapy was used in an attempt to improve local control rates of soft tissue sarcomas (30). In this scheme, 7 weekly fractions of 660 rads each were administered to 64 patients. These patients were divided into two groups; group A consisted of 37 patients with measurable disease who achieved partial response rates of 22% but no complete responses. Group B consisted of 27 postoperative patients with varying degrees of completeness of surgical excision. Early radiation damage was documented in 26% but was not dose limiting or incapacitating. However, later normal tissue damage occurred in 23 out of 32 evaluable patients and was the cause of serious morbidity in 6 patients. No apparent improvement in therapeutic gain was demonstrated by this radiation therapy scheme, which had a high morbidity.

Harris et al. reported the treatment of soft tissue sarcomas using fibroblast interferon in 20 patients (31). Patients received 5×10^6 units over 10 minutes then 5×10^6 units intravenously over 3 hours daily $\times$ 10, with cycles repeated every 20 days $\times$ 3. Maintenance was given twice weekly if the disease was stable or responsive after three therapy periods. One patient had a partial response to treatment and 6 patients had stable disease over variable periods of time. It appears from this report that human fibroblast interferon in the dose and schedule used has limited value.

In an interesting study from Urano et al. of mouse fibrous sarcoma, it was demonstrated that thermochemotherapy resistant tumour cells were not identical to radioresistant cells (32); this suggested that thermochemotherapy with cyclophosphamide could be an excellent adjuvant to radiation therapy. Clearly improved chemotherapeutic agents or techniques will be necessary to allow chemotherapy with radiation therapy to be of benefit in adult soft tissue sarcomas.

SUMMARY

Therapy of paediatric and adult soft tissue sarcomas of the head and neck has been presented. Paediatric rhabdomyosarcomas clearly have the best prognosis to date and can in fact be effectively treated with regimens of radiation therapy and chemotherapy, with surgery used mostly in establishing the diagnosis. Non-rhabdomyosarcomas of paediatric patients and all adult soft tissue sarcomas currently are best treated by aggressive surgery when this is possible. Irradiation and chemotherapy alone in adult patients has minimal therapeutic efficacy. The addition of irradiation to surgery helps improve the local control rates. Adjuvant chemotherapy shows promise of further improving disease free intervals and survival. When distant metastases have developed (especially pulmonary), these should be aggressively treated where possible.

REFERENCES

1 Enzinger FM. Recent developments in the classification of soft tissue sarcomas. In: Management of Primary Bone and Soft Tissue Tumours. Chicago: Year Book, 1977.
2 Horne RC, Enterline HT. 'Rhabdomyosarcoma: A clinicopathological study and classification of 39 cases. Cancer 1958; 11: 81–99.
3 Blitzer A, Lawson W, Biller H. 'Malignant fibrous histiocytoma of the head and neck'. Laryngoscope 1977; 87: 1479–99.
4 Harrison EG Jr, Black BM, Devine KD. Synovial sarcoma primary in the neck. Arch Pathol 1961; 71: 137.
5 Sauk JJ Jr. Liposarcoma of the head and neck. J Oral Surg 1971; 29: 38.
6 Batsakis JF. Tumours of the Head and Neck, 2nd edition. Baltimore: Williams & Wilkins; 1982.

7 Thompson DE, Frost HM, Henrick JW, Horn RC Jr. Soft tissue sarcomas involving the extremities and the limb girdles. South Med Jr 1971; 64: 33.

8 Pratt J, Gray GF. Massive Neuraxial spread of aural rhabdomyosracoma. Arch Otolaryngol 1977; 103: 301–3.

9 Enterline HT, Culberson JD, Rochlin DB, Brady LW. Liposarcoma: A clinical and pathological study of 53 cases. Cancer 1960; 13: 932.

10 Kindblom LG, Angervall L, Svendsen P. Liposarcoma: A clinicopathologic, radiographic and prognostic study. Acta Pathol Microbiol Scand Suppl, 1975; 253.

11 Roholl PJM, DeJong ASH, Raemaekers FCS. Application of markers in the diagnosis of soft tissue tumors. Histopathology 1985; 9: 10–1019–1035.

12 Weekes RG, Berquist TH, McCleod RA, Zimmer WD. Magnetic resonance imaging of soft-tissue tumors: Comparison with computed tomography. Magnetic Resonance Imaging 1985; 3: 345–52.

13 Weingard DW, Rosenberg SA. Early lymphatic spread of osteogenic and soft tissue sarcomas. 1978; 84: 231.

14 Russell WO, Cohen J, Enzinger F, Hajdu SI, Heise H, Martin RG, Meissner W, Miller WT, Schmitz RL, Suit HD. A clinical and pathological staging system for soft tissue sarcomas. Cancer 1977; 40: 1562.

15 Heise HW, Myers MH, Russell WO, Suit HD, Enzinger FM, Edmonson JH, Cohen J, Martin RG, Miller WT, Hajdu SI. Recurrence-free survival time for surgically treated soft tissue sarcoma patients. Cancer 1986; 57: 172–7.

16 Cassady JR, Sagerman RH, Tretter P, Ellsworth RM. Radiation Therapy for Rhabdomyosarcoma. Radiology 1963; 91: 116–20.

17 Pratt CB, Hustu HO, Fleming ID, Pinkel D. Coordinated treatment of childhood rhabdomyosarcoma with surgery, radiotherapy, and combined chemotherapy. Cancer Res 1972; 32: 606–10.

18 Heyn RM, Holland R, Newton WA, Tefft M, Breslow N, Hartmann JR. The role of combined chemotherapy in the treatment of rhabdomyosarcoma in children. Cancer 1974; 34: 2128–42.

19 Maurer HM, Moon T, Donaldson M et al. The Intergroup Rhabdomyosarcoma Study: A preliminary report. Cancer 1977; 40: 2015–26.

20 Flamant F, Hill C. The improvement in survival associated with combined chemotherapy in childhood rhabdomyosarcoma. Cancer 1984; 53: 2417–21.

21 Voute PA, Vos A, deKraker J, Behrendt H. Rhabdomyosarcomas: Chemotherapy and limited supplementary treatment program to avoid mutilation. Natl Cancer Inst Monogram 1981; 56: 121–5.

22 Tefft M, Fernandez C, Donaldson M. Incidence of meningeal involvement by rhabdomyosarcoma of the head and neck in children: Report of the intergroup rhabdomyosarcoma study. Cancer 1978; 42: 253–8.

23 Horowitz ME, Pratt CB, Webber BL, Hustu HO, Etcubanas E, Miliauskas J, Rao BN, Fleming ID, Kumar APM, Green AA. Therapy of childhood soft-tissue sarcomas other than rhabdomyosarcoma: A review of 62 cases treated at a single institution. J Clin Oncol 1986; 4(4): 559–64.

24 Greager JA, Patel MK, Briele HA, Walker MH, Gupta TKD. Soft tissue sarcomas of the adult head and neck. Cancer 1985; 56: 820–4.

25 Lloyd RV, Hajdu SI, Knapper WH. Embryonal rhabdomyosarcoma in adults. Cancer 1983; 51: 557–565.

26 Newman AN, Rice DH. Rhabdomyosarcoma of the head and neck. Int J Pediatr Otorhinolaryngol 1983; 5(2): 115–24.

27 Glenn J, Kinsella T, Glatstein E, Tepper J, Baker A, Sugarbaker P, Sindelar W, Roth J, Brennan M, Costa J, Seipp C, Wesley R, Young RC, Rosenberg SA. A randomized, prospective trial of adjuvant chemotherapy in adults with soft tissue sarcomas of the head and neck, breast, and trunk. Cancer 1985; 55: 1206–14.

28 Tepper JE, Suit HD. Radiation therapy alone for sarcoma of soft tissue. Cancer 1985; 56: 475–9.

29 Greenall MJ, Magill GB, DeCosse JJ, Brennan MF. Chemotherapy for soft tissue sarcoma. Surg Gynecol Obstet 1986; 162: 193–8.

30 Ashby MA, Harmer CL. Hypofractionated radiotherapy for sarcomas. Int J Radiat Oncol Biol Phys 1986; 12: 13–17.

31 Harris J, Gupta TD, Vogelzang N, Badrinath K, Bonomi P, Desser R, Locker G, Blough R, Johnson C. Treatment of soft-tissue sarcoma with fibroblast interferon. Cancer Treat Rep 1986; 70: 293.

32 Urano M, Kahn J, Kenton LA. Thermochemotherapy with or without hyperglycemia as an adjuvant to radiotherapy. Int J Radiat Oncol Biol Phys 1986; 12: 45–50.

Textbook of Uncommon Cancer
Edited by C.J. Williams, J.G. Krikorian, M.R. Green and D. Raghavan
© 1988 John Wiley & Sons Ltd

Chapter **54**

Uncommon Tumours of the Cerebellopontine Angle, and the Temporal Bone

M. Waner*, W.P.R. Gibson†
and M.L. Pensak‡

* Senior Lecturer, Department of Surgery, Division of Otolaryngology, University of Sydney, New South Wales, Australia, † Professor of Surgery, Division of Otolaryngology, University of Sydney, New South Wales, Australia, and ‡ Director, Division of Neurotology; Assistant Professor, Department of Otolaryngology and Maxillofacial Surgery, University of Cincinnati Medical Center, Cincinnati, Ohio, USA

CERUMINOUS GLAND TUMOURS

Ceruminous glands are modified apocrine sweat glands. These glands are found deep in the dermis of the cartilaginous portion of the external auditory canal. The term ceruminoma has until recently been used in referring to both benign and malignant tumours arising from these glands. Although the term hybridoma had been previously used to describe these tumours, (since these were tumours of sweat glands) Batsakis et al. and Juby felt that the term ceruminoma was more appropriate since they were tumours of specialized sweat glands. Furthermore there were sufficient clinical features as well as histological appearances of these tumours to justify the term ceruminoma (1, 2). Since ceruminoma refers to a heterogeneous group of both malignant and benign tumours, with different clinical presentations and behaviour, more appropriate terminology was suggested by Althaus and Ross

in 1970 and subsequently by Wetli et al. in 1972 (3, 4). Wetli et al. classified these tumours into the following four subdivisions:

1. Ceruminous adenoma.
2. Pleomorphic adenoma (mixed tumour).
3. Ceruminous adenocarcinoma.
4. Ceruminous adenoid cystic carcinoma.

This more precise terminology is in accordance with the histological characteristics of these tumours, and is more appropriate in terms of planning treatment and prognostication.

Epidemiology and Aetiology

Ceruminous gland tumours are extremely rare. Approximately 90 documented cases have been reported. A review of the literature by Wetli et al. reveals that men and women are about equally affected, the average age of patients is 48 years, and malignant tumours

1019

are more common than benign tumours by a ratio of 2.5:1. The most common variant is the adenoid cystic carcinoma. Malignant varieties are more common in younger age groups whereas benign tumours are more common in older age groups (4).

The origin of ceruminous gland tumours is almost certainly from modified sweat glands. The possibility of some tumours originating in nests of salivary tissue has been suggested (5). An interesting observation is that whilst ceruminous glands are modified apocrine sweat glands, the tumours derived from these glands strongly suggest that they are of eccrine origin (6). It should be remembered that the external auditory canal is one of the few places devoid of eccrine sweat glands (7). It would thus appear that although the tumours arise from apocrine glands, they differentiate into an eccrine structure. It has also been suggested that the proliferation of myoepithelial cells may account for this discrepancy (4).

Pathology and Biology

Ceruminous Adenoma

These tumours represent a well differentiated, benign, localized proliferation of ceruminous gland tissue, and are histologically similar to normal ceruminous glands. Both cystic and papillary variations may be found. These tumours are well circumscribed and are non-invasive.

Pleomorphic Adenoma (Mixed Tumour)

These tumours are lobulated, localized, benign, but locally invasive tumours resembling pleomorphic adenomas of salivary gland tissue. They consist of nests of epithelial cells embedded in a myxoid and/or pseudocartilaginous or hyalinized stroma of myoepithelial origin.

Ceruminous Adenocarcinoma

The histological appearance of ceruminous adenocarcinomas is somewhat similar to that of the benign adenoma. There is, however, usually more pleomorphism and occasionally more mitotic activity. The hallmark of these tumours, however, is the fact that they infiltrate locally into soft tissue and cartilage. This infiltration is often extensive. Although all grades of adenocarcinoma have been reported, the well differentiated forms predominate (3).

Adenoid Cystic Carcinoma

This tumour bears close resemblance, both histologically and pathologically, to adenoid cystic tumours found in salivary glands. It consists of nests of small dark cells, with cystic spaces or hyaline cylinders. Perineural spread and a tendency to distant metastases to lung and kidney have been reported (8). These tumours may also infiltrate soft tissue, bone and cartilage.

Clinical Presentation and Investigations

The clinical presentation of ceruminous gland tumours varies according to the histological type of tumour.

Ceruminous Adenoma

These tumours may be present for some time before discovery. Batsakis et al. reported a case that had been present for 20 years before the patient sought medical advice (1). It may also be discovered as a coincidental finding during physical examination, or may present with an aural discharge due to obstruction of the external auditory canal and secondary otitis externa.

Pleomorphic Adenoma

The presentation of these tumours is similar to that of ceruminous adenoma, i.e. the patient may present with a skin covered aural polyp found coincidently during routine head and neck examination, or as a result of secondary otitis externa, with an aural discharge and pain.

Adenocarcinoma and Adenoid Cystic Carcinoma

These tumours usually present with signs and symptoms of bony destruction. Aural discharge, aural pain, and facial nerve palsy are the most common presenting symptoms. Clinical findings will obviously depend on the extent of the tumour. A skin covered aural polyp, pedicled on the wall of the external auditory canal, with or without a discharge and with or without local tissue invasion and destruction, is the usual presentation.

Investigation of tumors of the external auditory canal should include routine mastoid x-rays as well as a computed tomography (CT) scan of the temporal bone. Pure tone audiometry usually reveals a conductive hearing loss in the presence of extensive local infiltration. A sensorineural hearing loss may also be present. Biopsy of these lesions is mandatory. Sufficient tissue should be provided for an accurate histological diagnosis. This will enable adequate appropriate operative planning. Where adenocarcinoma has been diagnosed a search must be undertaken for a primary tumour, since metastatic deposits of adenocarcinoma have been reported in the external auditory canal (9).

Treatment

Ceruminous Adenoma and Pleomorphic Adenoma

Both these tumours are benign; the latter, however, has a tendency to recur locally if incompletely excised. Wide excision with a rim of surrounding normal tissue is advocated. These patients should be followed up so that any local recurrence can be promptly dealt with.

Adenoid Carcinoma and Adenoid Cystic Carcinoma

More aggressive therapy is indicated for these tumours. Appropriate surgical excision will obviously depend on the location and extent of the tumour. In general this will include wide excision of the external auditory canal and a radical mastoidectomy, with or without removal of cranial nerve VII. Postoperative radiation therapy has been advocated, although it is not yet clear whether this is of any added benefit (4–12). A radical or functional neck dissection in the absence of palpable lymphadenopathy is unnecessary. Close long-term follow-up is mandatory since, as with similar tumors of the salivary glands, recurrence may occur several years after initial treatment was undertaken.

CEREBELLOPONTINE ANGLE MENINGIOMAS (Chapter 29)

Although the term meningioma was first used by Cushing in 1922, reference to tumours of the dura mata date back to 1774 (13).

Meningiomas may affect both young and old. The peak incidence, however, is around 45 years (14). The tumour appears to be more common in females, with about 60% of cases reported in a number of series (15–17).

Pathology and Biology

Less than 10% of all meningiomas occur in the posterior fossa and about half of these occur on the posterior surface of the temporal bone (16–20). Meningiomas, however, account for only 3% to 12% of the cerebellopontine angle mass lesions (21, 22). It is now accepted that the cells from which meningiomas arise are the same cells that give rise to arachnoid villi and arachnoid endothelium. These cells probably originate from the neural crest and are pluripotential cells; hence the numerous variants of meningiomas (23).

Meningiomas are usually solitary supratentorial tumours. Occasional multiple meningiomas have been reported. In addition to this multiple meningiomas have been reported in association with the central form of neurofibromatosis (von Recklinghausen's disease) (24). Most meningiomas are lobulated, well circumscribed, non-invasive tumours. The surface of these tumours takes on a course granular appearance; these granules represent calcified 'psammona' bodies.

The classification of meningiomas, as proposed by Cushing and Eisenhardt, is long and complex, involving nine types with 20 subdivisions (25). The most widely accepted classification, however, is based on the predominant cell group and pattern, of which five subtypes are described (14, 26).

1. Meningotheliomitis meningioma (most common).
2. Fibroblastic meningioma.
3. Mixed or transitional meningioma.
4. Angioblastic meningioma.
5. Sarcomatous meningioma.

The vast majority or meningiomas are benign although a few cases have been reported with metastases through the cerebrospinal fluid, or to lung (14). In children and adolescents, however, meningiomas tend to be more frequently malignant.

Clinical Features

The classic description by Cushing in 1917 of the syndrome of cerebellopontine angle compression as a progression of symptoms consists of the following (27):

1. Auditory and vestibular changes.
2. Headache.
3. Ataxia.
4. Involvement of adjacent cranial nerves.
5. Hydrocephalus.
6. Dysarthria and dysphagia.
7. Cerebellar and brainstem changes.

Stages 5, 6 and 7 are very rarely seen today. However, an analysis of the charts of 32 patients by Granek et al. (28) found that the most common symptoms were hearing loss, vertigo or imbalance, and tinnitus. Additional symptoms include alteration of facial sensation, headache, visual changes, facial pain and difficulty in swallowing (28).

This variable clinical presentation has led to a high degree of initial misdiagnosis, with a delay of 3 to 7 years between presentation and diagnosis reported in one series (29). It is hoped that the increased use of CT scanning and more lately magnetic resonance imaging (MRI) will substantially shorten this interval.

Examination of these patients usually reveals a unilateral hearing loss. Other signs such as hypothesia, or loss of sensation in the distribution of cranial nerve V, as well as facial weakness or a complete seventh nerve palsy are the most frequent cranial nerve deficits. Other cranial nerves affected include IX, X and XII. Changes of these are, however, rarely found.

Special Investigation and Staging

Results of routine audiometry are similar to those found with seventh nerve schwannomas. These include unilateral sensory neural hearing loss, poor speech discrimination and acoustic reflex decay or absence. These findings merely suggest the presence of a cerebellopontine angle (CPA) lesion. They do not, however, differentiate meningiomas from any other CPA lesion. Brainstem evoked response audiometry (BERA) usually demonstrates abnormal latency or absence of the fifth wave. Vestibular testing may show a spontaneous or positional nystagmus, and caloric stimulation may show either a directional preponderance or a canal paresis.

Radiological evaluation is often more helpful in distinguishing meningiomas from acoustic neuromas. Acoustic neuromas usually widen or erode the internal auditory meatus. Meningiomas on the other hand are usually found on the posterior surface of the petrous temporal bone, are often not centred on the internal auditory meatus, and thus do not show widening or erosion of this canal. They do, however, display certain additional characteristics which are helpful in differentiating them from acoustic neuromas (30, 31). These include the following.

1. The tumour density is higher than surrounding brain tissue on a non-contrast scan. They are therefore more often demonstrated on non-contrast scanning, and with contrasting infusion, they appear as very dense, homogeneous masses.
2. They display a flat surface attachment to the temporal bone.
3. They almost invariably demonstrate some evidence of calcification.

The recent addition of MRI as a routine investigation of patients with suspected CPA tumours has resulted in some encouraging findings. Meningiomas are more vascular than schwannomas and therefore appear much darker on MRI.

Management and Prognosis

The treatment of CPA meningiomas is, in the main, surgical removal. Where possible complete surgical excision is desirable. The morbidity and mortality of posterior fossa surgery has greatly improved since the early 1960s, the major factor being the introduction of and employment of microsurgical techniques. The major surgical approaches are suboccipital, translabyrinthine, translabyrinthine/suboccipital, and middle fossa. The translabyrinthine approach provides good access to the internal auditory canal and is suitable for small tumours where there is no valuable hearing left to preserve. Tumours larger than 3 cm are best managed by the combined translabyrinthine/suboccipital approach. The middle fossa approach is good for small to medium sized tumours. Unfortunately, it allows only limited access to the posterior fossa and the surgeon may thus have difficulty in controlling haemorrhage. The major advantage of the suboccipital approach is that it affords wide access to the posterior fossa and is thus suitable for large tumours. The only disadvantage of this approach is that there is a high incidence of air embolism and extruded lumbar discs where

the sitting or semi-sitting position is used. The preferred surgical approach is therefore dependent on: the size of the lesion, the level of hearing acuity on the involved ear, and the training and philosophy of the surgeon.

Although meningiomas have been reported to be radioresistant, radiation therapy should be considered where the tumour has not been completely removed or where the patient is unfit for surgery. The coincidental finding of a small CPA meningioma on CT scan in an otherwise unfit patient can usually be treated conservatively.

CEREBELLOPONTINE ANGLE LIPOMAS (Chapter 29)

Intracranial lipomas are extremely rare. A collective series of brain tumours showed that 0.1% were of a fatty nature, and that the majority of these lesions were mid-line (32, 33). Only 13 cases of CPA lipomas have appeared in the world literature.

Pathology and Biology

Although the behaviour of lipomas is generally innocuous, Batsakis noted that if the vascularity of the lesion is much greater than that of a simple lipoma the designation 'angiolipoma' is appropriate (34). Further work by Lim and Lim describe two types of angiolipoma, an infiltrating and a non-infiltrating variety. The infiltrating angiolipoma is unencapsulated and is capable of infiltrating neural as well as bony tissue, and can simulate a malignant neoplasm. This renders surgical exenteration difficult. The non-infiltrating variety is usually encapsulated and does not recur even after enucleation (35). The work of Penzak et al. (36), Fukui et al. (37), Leibrock et al. (38) and Budka (39), suggests that CPA lipomas are of the infiltrating variety. These tumours are thus firmly adherent to both the brainstem as well as surrounding cranial nerves, rendering surgical removal extremely difficult.

Clinical Features

The clinical presentation of CPA lipomas resembles that of acoustic neuromas. The most common symptom is thus a progressive unilateral hearing loss (36). Periods of intermittent paroxysmal vertigo accompanied by nausea and vomiting, as well as tinnitus, are mentioned. Seventh nerve symptoms are surprisingly absent in the cases reported, and since the tumour is slow growing, gross manifestations of gait disturbance are unusual.

Investigation and Staging

A full audiological investigation is necessary. This includes pure-tone air and bone conduction audiometry, tympanometry, speech discrimination, acoustic reflexes and tone decay. Calorimetry as well as brainstem evoked auditory potentials (BERA) are helpful. Typical findings include a unilateral sensorineural hearing loss, poor speech discrimination and tone decay. Caloric testing may show a normal response, a canal paresis, or a directional preponderance. BERA may either be normal or show a delay or absence of the fifth wave. CT scanning with contrast is mandatory. The usual finding is that of a low density mass (commensurate with fat) occupying the cerebellopontine angle. Widening of the internal auditory canal may or may not be present depending on the precise location of the tumour. Intracranial lipomas rarely produce a mass effect and therefore an indentation of the fourth ventricle or a shift of mid-line structures, should not be evident (32).

Management and Prognosis

Due to the vascularity of these tumours, and the fact that they are usually of an infiltrating variety, complete surgical removal is extremely dangerous and very often not possible. Furthermore, since no mass effect is produced by these tumours, operative intervention is usually not necessary. Continued clinical surveillance as well as serial CT evaluation is probably the most prudent management of these patients. In the face of brainstem compression, unrelenting vertigo, or the development of hydrocephalus, debulking may be necessary, and the use of laser or ultrasonic surgical aspiration (Cavatron) techniques may be invaluable (1). Although radiation therapy has not been used in the past it should be considered in the face of early recurrence of symptoms following adequate debulking.

FACIAL NERVE SCHWANNOMAS
(Chapter 29)

History

The terminology of nerve tumours remains somewhat confusing. One reason for this is that the origin of the cells forming these tumours has been disputed. The currently held theory of Cravioto (1969), based on an extensive study of auditory nerve tumours, using electron microscopy and tissue culture, has confirmed that these tumours are composed of Schwann cells, hence the term schwannoma (40, 41). Synonyms include neurilemmoma, neurinoma and neuroma.

Epidemiology and Aetiology

At least 146 cases have been reported in the world literature. Saito and Baxter report an occult incidence of 0.8% of undiagnosed tumours (42). This evidence is based on an analysis of 600 human temporal bones. All but one of the patients had normal facial movements.

Pathology and Biology

Acoustic schwannomas are known to originate at the glial–neurilemmal junction. Seventh nerve schwannomas, however, can be found anywhere along the path of cranial nerve VII. Whether or not this same process is active, is not therefore known.

Macroscopically seventh nerve schwannomas are encapsulated, well circumscribed homogeneous masses. Histological features are similar to those of acoustic neuromas. Two patterns are recognized: the fasciculated pattern with an orderly arrangement of parallel cells and interwoven bundles of intercellular fibres producing a palisading effect, and the reticular, disordered or variable pattern.

Clinical Features

The clinical presentation of these tumours is variable. This is as a result of the variable site of origin of these tumours. The tumour can originate anywhere along the course of cranial nerve VII. The main symptom, however, is a progressive peripheral facial nerve palsy over a period of months. A tumour situated within the internal auditory meatus would thus cause a sensorineural hearing loss secondary to auditory nerve compression. Such a patient may also experience intermittent episodes of vertigo. If the point of origin is located lateral to the geniculate ganglion, i.e. in the middle ear, symptoms of conductive hearing loss secondary to ossicular involvement usually precedes the facial nerve palsy. A large tumour in this situation may be visualized through the tympanic membrane. A tumour originating in the vertical segment of the facial nerve would cause progressive facial nerve palsy, and may present as an aural polyp pedicled posteriorly in the external auditory canal wall. The patient may or may not have an accompanying aural discharge, ipsilateral loss of taste in the anterior two-thirds of the tongue, as well as decreased salivary flow from the submandibular gland on the same side. An intracranial schwannoma will present as a CPA tumour. The accompanying clinical signs will therefore be a facial nerve weakness of palsy, associated with a unilateral sensorineural hearing loss, and decreased salivation and taste to the anterior two-thirds of the tongue. An intracranial mass effect with ventricular compression and a shift of mid-line structures may also be found.

Investigation and Staging

The diagnosis is usually obvious from the history. The early, slow, progressive onset of facial nerve paralysis prior to the onset of any other symptoms, is usually suggestive of facial nerve pathology. This is quite easily differentiated from Bell's palsy, which is an acute onset of facial palsy. Investigation should include a CT scan with axial and coronal cuts. Both bone windows and soft tissue windows should be evaluated. Typical audiometry findings include a sensorineural hearing loss or a conductive hearing loss (depending on the site of the tumour). The ipsilateral acoustic reflexes may be absent because of involvement of the motor fibres of cranial nerve VII. The contralateral reflex may also be absent, resulting from involvement of cranial nerve VII. BERA may show features similar to that of an acoustic neuroma. Electroneuronography will show the degree of ipsilateral facial nerve generation. The percentage degeneration will obviously depend on the size and site of the tumour. This finding is usually late in acoustic schwannomas and therefore, this test may help in differentiating an acoustic schwannoma from a seventh nerve schwannoma.

Management and Prognosis

The tumour should be surgically excised. The surgical approach will depend on the exact site of the tumour. A tumour of the internal auditory canal is best approached via the middle fossa and a more distal tumour is best approached via a transmastoid operation. Where possible a cable nerve graft should be carried out.

SCHWANNOMAS OF THE JUGULAR FORAMEN
(Chapter 29)

Schwannomas may arise on any of the cranial nerves of the posterior fossa. The most common, however, is the acoustic schwannoma, accounting for approximately 92% of tumours in this area. Only 56 cases of schwannomas arising in the jugular foramen have been reported (43).

Pathology

Schwannomas account for between 2% and 8% of intracranial neoplasms. They are typically well circumscribed, encapsulated masses that displace surrounding neural structures, without directly invading them. This is in direct contradistinction to neurofibromas, which are non-encapsulated and are usually multiple. Neurofibromas do not displace surrounding neural structures but incorporate them into the tumour (34).

Two histological types can be recognized:

1. Fasciculated (Antoni A): in this type an orderly arrangement of parallel cells and intercellular fibres form interwoven bundles producing a palisading pattern with alternating nuclear and fibrous zones.
2. Reticular (Antoni B): in this type there is a disorderly arrangement of cells of variable shapes, with intercellular cystic spaces and reticular tissue.

Clinical Features

The most common symptoms relate to cranial nerve deficits resulting from these tumours. The patients may therefore present with voice changes, shoulder weakness, or speech changes. Alternatively, the initial presentation may not be dissimilar from that of a CPA tumour. Thus a unilateral progressive sensorineural hearing loss, or intermittent periods of vertigo, may be the sole presenting feature.

Examination of these patients usually reveals cranial nerve palsies of cranial nerves IX, X, XI, and XII. Tumours expanding up to the cerebellopontine angle may also produce cranial nerve VIII changes such as progressive unilateral sensorineural hearing loss or vestibular signs.

Special Investigations

The results of routine audiometry may include a unilateral sensorineural hearing loss, poor speech discrimination and acoustic reflex decay or absence. These findings are not dissimilar from those of any other CPA tumour. BERA may show abnormal latency or absence of the fifth wave, and caloric stimulation may show either a directional preponderance or a canal paresis.

CT scanning usually shows erosion of the margin of the jugular foramen. Extension of the tumour to the petrous apex will be accompanied by erosion of the petrous temporal bone. Carotid angiography is essential to determine both the vascularity of the tumour and the integrity of the ipsilateral carotid artery, jugular bulb and sigmoid sinus, as all these structures may be compressed by a large tumour.

Management and Prognosis

Schwannomas of the jugular foramen should be surgically excised. The combined expertise of a neurosurgeon, a head and neck surgeon, and a neurotologist is usually required. The carotid artery should firstly be identified in the neck, and followed into the skull with the help of a neurotologist. The neurotologist should reroute and thus preserve the facial nerve, and continue the dissection of the carotid artery from the base of the skull to the apex of the petrous temporal bone. These procedures will then enable the neurosurgeon to extend the dissection into the posterior cranial fossa and thus complete the removal.

This approach will usually result in successful total removal of these tumours. However, loss of function of cranial nerves IX, X, and XI is almost inevitable. The postoperative morbidity is thus considerable.

CONGENITAL CHOLESTEATOMA
(Chapter 29)
History

The first description of an intracranial epidermoid was attributed to Duverney in 1683 (44). The word cholesteatoma, however, was first used by Johannes Müller in 1838, to describe intracranial deposits of keratin (44). The first reported case of congenital cholesteatoma of the petrous temporal bone, however, was published in 1938 by Jefferson and Smalley (45). House in 1953 described a case of middle ear cholesteatoma behind an intact tympanic membrane (46) and by 1977 43 cases had been reported in the literature, 22 of them by Derlacki (47). By 1980 86 cases had been reported in the world literature. The most substantial contribution to this was by House and Sheehy who added 41 additional cases (48).

Epidemiology and Aetiology

Congenital cholesteatomas are believed to develop from embryonic cell rests of squamous epithelium during the embryological development of the temporal bone. This theory was proposed by Korner in 1830 (49), but was rejected by Ruedi in 1958, who in an analysis and histological examination of 124 temporal bones, found no evidence of embryonic cell nests (50). Friedmann and Osborne also sectioned 500 temporal bones and were unable to find any evidence of these cell nests (51). The most recent theory proposed is that of Aimi (52), who concludes that the location of congenital cholesteatomas is closely related to the junction of the first and second branchial arches in the middle ear. This junction is called the tympanic isthmus. The origin therefore of cholesteatoma is probably linked to the migration of external canal ectoderm into the middle ear at an early stage of development. The tympanic ring, which normally plays an important role in limiting the medial extent of external canal ectoderm migration, has in these cases failed to exert its inhibitory function.

Pathology and Biology

Congenital cholesteatomas have a lining of keratinizing stratified squamous epithelium (matrix). The sack is filled with flaky, dry, odourless masses of desquamated keratinized epithelium. These epidermal cysts slowly enlarge as the desquamated material filling the sack accumulates. This enlargement is accompanied by bone resorption. Valvassori (53) differentiated four types of congenital cholesteatomas. These four types correspond to the four different sites commonly involved: cerebellopontine angle, jugular foramen, petrous apex, middle ear and mastoid.

Clinical Features

The clinical presentation of these tumours is variable and will obviously depend on the site of the tumour. CPA tumours usually present with one or a combination of the following symptoms: progressive unilateral sensorineural hearing loss, intermittent attacks of vertigo, or progressive unilateral facial nerve paresis. Jugular foramen cholesteatomas on the other hand may present with compression of the cranial nerves in the jugular foramen, i.e. IX, X, XI and XII. Cholesteatomas of the petrous apex usually present with progressive sensorineural hearing loss, and a cholesteatoma of the middle ear and mastoid will present with progressive conductive hearing loss with or without progressive facial nerve paresis. If the cholesteatoma has eroded through the exterior and has become secondarily infected, it may be difficult to differentiate from a secondary acquired cholesteatoma.

Investigations

High resolution CT scanning will usually demonstrate the presence of a mass as well as that of bone erosion. The tumour does not enhance and therefore it may be difficult to make a diagnosis of congenital cholesteatoma purely on the basis of a CT scan. In this regard MRI may be more helpful. Early experience by the senior author (W.P.R. Gibson) has been promising.

Management

Congenital cholesteatoma should be surgically excised. The exact approach will obviously depend on the location of the tumour. The appropriate surgical procedure should therefore be tailored accordingly. The usual treatment, however, is that of surgical exterioration of the cholesteatoma by means of a radical mastoidectomy. If, however, there is good residual hearing and the surgeon is confident that he has removed the entire tumour, a modified radical mastoidectomy with a tympanoplasty procedure may be carried out. Complete surgical removal, however, may be extremely difficult especially if extensive spread of the cholesteatoma is already present. In these cases removal of the entire matrix is often difficult and probably not necessary since reaccumulation of epithelial debris will occur very slowly in the absence of infection (54).

REFERENCES

1 Batsakis JG, Hardy GC, Hishiiama RH. Ceruminous gland tumours. Arch Otolaryngol 1967; 86: 66–9.

2 Juby HB. Tumours of the ceruminous glands—so called ceruminoma. J Laryngol 1957; 71: 832–7.

3 Althaus SR, Ross JAT Cerumin gland neoplasia. Arch Otolaryngol 1970; 92: 40–2.

4 Wetli CV, Pardo V, Millard M, Gerston K. Tumours of ceruminous glands. Cancer 1972; 29: 1169–78.

5 Hyams VJ, Michaels L. Benign adenomatous neoplasm (adenoma) of the middle ear. Clin Otolaryngol 1976; 1: 17–26.

6 Hashimoto K, Leaver WF. Appendage tumours of skin. Springfield, Illinois: Charles C Thomas, 1968: 9–47.

7 Pinkus H, Mehregan AH. A Guide to dermatohistopathology. New York: Appleton, Century Crofts, 1969.

8 Pulec JL, Parkhill EM, Devine KD. Adenoid cystic carcinoma (cylindroma) of the external auditory canal. Trans Am Acad Ophthalmol Otolaryngol 1963; 67: 673–94.

9 Stone HE, Lipa M, Douglas Bell R. Primary adenocarcinoma of the middle ear. Arch Otolaryngol 1975; 101: 702–5.

10 Lynde CW, McLean DI, Wood WS. Tumours of ceruminous glands. J Am Acad Dermatol 1984; 11: 841–7.

11 Anagnostou GD, Papademetriou DG, Segditsas TD. Ceruminous gland tumours: report of three cases. Laryngoscope 1974; 84: 438–43.

12 Hageman MEJ, Becker AE. Intracranial inva-

sion of ceruminous gland tumour. Arch Otolaryngol 1974; 100: 395–7.

13 Louis A. Mémoire sur les tumeurs fongueuse de la dure-mère. Mém Acad Roy Chir, Paris 1774; 5: 1–59.

14 Earle KM, Richany SF. Meningiomas: A study of the histology, incidence and biologic behaviour of 243 cases from the Frazier-Grant collection of brain tumours. Med Ann DC 1969; 38: 353–6.

15 Zulch KJ. Brain Tumours: Their Biology and Pathology. The Meningiomas, 2nd edition. New York: Springer Publishing, 1965: 202.

16 Markham JW. Meningiomas of the posterior fossa. Arch Neurol Psychiatry 1955; 74: 163–70.

17 Castellano F, Ruggiero G. Meningioma of the posterior fossa. Acta Radiol Suppl 104. Stockholm: Sweden, 1953.

18 Nager GT. Meningiomas involving the temporal bone. *Clinical and Pathologist Aspects.* Springfield, Illinois: Charles C Thomas, 1964.

19 Karam FK, Salman SD. Meningioma of the middle ear. A case report. Arch Otolaryngol 1964; 80: 177–179.

20 Punt N. A meningioma of the middle ear. J Laryngol 1965; 79: 347–8.

21 Brackmann DE, Bartels LJ. Rare tumours of the cerebellopontine angle. Otolaryngol Head Neck Surg 1980; 88: 555–9.

22 Thomson J. Cerebellopontine angle tumours, other than acoustic neuromas. Acta Laryngol 1976; 82: 106–11.

23 Minckler J. Pathology of the Nervous System, Vol 2. New York: McGraw-Hill, 1971: 2: 2125–44.

24 Shuangshoti S, Netsky MG, Jane JA. Neoplasma of mixed mesenchymal and neuroepithelial type with consideration of the relationship between meningioma and neurilemmoma. J Neurol Sci 1971; 14: 277–91.

25 Cushing H, Eisenhardt L. Meningiomas. Their Classification, Regional Behaviour, Life History and Surgical End Results. Springfield, Illinois: Charles C Thomas, 1938.

26 Rubinstein LJ. Tumours of the central nervous system. In Atlas of Tumour Pathology, 2nd Series, Fascicle 6. Washington, DC: Armed Forces Institute of Pathology, 1972: 169–89.

27 Cushing H. Tumours of the Nervous Acousticus and the Syndrome of the Cerebellopontine Angle. Philadelphia: WB Saunders, 1917.

28 Granick MS, Martuza RL, Parker SW, Ogemann RG, Montgomery WW. Cerebellopontine angle meningiomas: Clinical manifestations and diagnosis. Ann Otol Rhinol Laryngol 1985; 94: 34–8.

29 Yasargil MJ, Mortara RW, Curcic M. Men-

ingiomas of the basal posterior cranial fossa. In: Krayenbuhl H ed Advances and Technical Standards in neurosurgery, New York: Springer-Verlag, 1980: 32–115.

30 Parker W, Davis KR. Limitations of computered tomography in the investigation of acoustic neuromas. Ann Otol Rhinol Laryngol 1977; 86: 436–40.

31 Davis KR, Parker SW. CT is diagnosing and evaluating cerebellopontine angle abnormalities. In: Silverstein H, Norrell H, eds Neurological Surgery of the Ear, Vol II. Birmingham, Alabama: Aesculapius, 1980: 224–31.

32 Youmans JR. Neurologic Surgery, Vol V. Philadelphia: WB Saunders, 1982: 2928.

33 Wolpert SM, Carter BL, Ferris EJ. Lipomas of the corpus callosum: An angiographic analysis. Am J Radiol 1972; 115: 92–9.

34 Batsakis JG. Tumours of the Head and Neck. Baltimore: Williams and Wilkins 1979: 361.

35 Lim JJ, Lim F. Two entities in angiolipoma. A study of 459 cases of lipoma and infiltrating angiolipoma with review of literature. Cancer 1974; 34: 720.

36 Pensak ML, Glasscock ME, Gulya AJ, Hays JW, Smith HP, Dickens JRE. Cerebellopontine angle lipomas. Arch Otolaryngol Head Neck Surg 1986; 112: 99–101.

37 Fukui M, Tanak A, Kitamura K. Lipoma of the cerebellopontine angle. J Neurosurg 1977; 46: 544–547.

38 Leibrock LG, Deans WR, Loch S. Cerebellopontine lipoma. Neurosurgery 1983; 12: 697–9.

39 Budka H. Intracranial lipomatous hamartomas (intracranial lipomas): A study of 30 cases including combinations and medulloblastoma, colloid and epidermoid cysts, angiomatosis and other malformations. Acta Neuropathol 1974; 28: 205–22.

40 Cravioto H. The ultra structure of acoustic nerve tumours. Acta Neuropath 1969; 12: 116–40.

41 Cravioto H, Lockwood R. The behaviour of acoustic neuroma in tissue cultures. Acta Neuropathol 1969; 12: 141–57.

42 Saito H, Baxter A. Undiagnosed intratemporal facial nerve neurilemomas. Arch Otolaryngol Head Neck Surg 1972; 95: 415–19.

43 Kinney SE, Dohn DF, Hahn JF, Wood BJ. Neuromas of the jugular foramen. In Brackman DE ed Neurological Surgery of the Ear and Skull Base. New York: Raven Press, 1982: 361.

44 Peron DL, Schuknecht HF. Congenital cholesteatoma with other anomalies. Arch Otolaryngol 1975; 101: 498–505.

45 Jefferson G, Smalley AA. Progressive facial palsy produced by intratemporal epidermoids. J Laryngol Otol 1938; 53: 417–43.

46 House HP. An apparent primary cholesteatoma: A case report. Laryngoscope 1953; 63: 712–13.

47 Derlacki EL. Congenital cholesteatoma of the middle ear and mastoid: A third report. Arch Otolaryngol 1973; 97: 177–82.

48 House JW, Sheehy JL. Cholesteatoma with intact tympanic membrane: A report of 41 cases. Laryngoscope 1980; 90: 70–5.

49 Korner: Cited by Portmann C, Portmann M, Claverie G. The Surgery of Deafness. Valletta, Malta: Progress Press, 1964.

50 Ruedi L. Cholesteatosis of the attic. J Laryngol 1958; 72: 593–609.

51 Friedmann I. Pathology of the Ear. Oxford: Blackwell Scientific Publications, 1974.

52 Aimi K. Role of tympanic ring in the pathogenesis of congenital cholesteatoma. Laryngoscope 1983; 93: 1140–1146.

53 Valvassori GE. Benign tumours of the temporal bone. Radiol Clin North Am 1974; 12: 533–42.

54 House W, Doyle JB Jr. Early diagnosis and removal of primary cholesteatoma causing pressure to the VIII nerve. Laryngoscope 1962; 73: 1053.

Index

A